International Textbook of Diabetes Mellitus
VOLUME 2

International Textbook of Diabetes Mellitus

Edited by

K.G.M.M. Alberti
The Medical School, Newcastle upon Tyne, UK

R.A. DeFronzo
University of Texas Health Science Center, San Antonio, USA

H. Keen
United Medical and Dental Schools, Guy's Hospital, London, UK

P. Zimmet
International Diabetes Institute, Caulfield, Australia

Associate Editors

G. Viberti, E. Ferrannini, M. Gould, P. Home

VOLUME 2

JOHN WILEY & SONS
Chichester • New York • Brisbane • Toronto • Singapore

Other Wiley Editorial Offices

John Wiley & Sons, Inc., 605 Third Avenue,
New York, NY 10158-0012, USA

Jacaranda Wiley Ltd, G.P.O. Box 859, Brisbane,
Queensland 4001, Australia

John Wiley & Sons (Canada) Ltd, 22 Worcester Road,
Rexdale, Ontario M9W 1L1, Canada

John Wiley & Sons (SEA) Pte Ltd, 37 Jalan Pemimpin #05-04,
Block B, Union Industrial Building, Singapore 2057

Library of Congress Cataloging-in-Publication Data

International textbook of diabetes mellitus / edited by K.G.M.M.
    Alberti . . . [et al.]: associate editors, G. Viberti . . . [et al.].
        p.   cm.
    Includes bibliographical references and index.
    ISBN 0 471 91497 5
    1. Diabetes.   I. Alberti, K.G.M.M. (Kurt George Matthew Mayer)
    [DNLM: 1. Diabetes Mellitus.   WK 810 I60359]
    RC660.I585   1992
    616.4′62—dc20
    DNLM/DLC
    for Library of Congress   92-161
                                                                 CIP

British Library Cataloguing in Publication Data

A catalogue record for this book is available from the British Library

ISBN 0 471 91497 5 (2 vols)

Typeset by Alden Multimedia Ltd.
Printed in Great Britain at the Alden Press, Oxford

Contents

VOLUME 2

Special Problems in Management

42 **Diabetes in Childhood and Adolescence** 1025
J.V. Santiago, N.H. White and S.L. Pontious

43 **Brittle Diabetes** 1059
J.C. Pickup

44 **Clinical Insulin Resistance** 1073
D.S. Schade and G.M. Argoud

45 **Diabetes Mellitus and Pregnancy** 1085
B. Persson, U. Hanson and N.-O. Lunell

46 **Aging and Diabetes** 1103
A.L. Peters and M.B. Davidson

Acute Disturbances of Diabetes

47 **Hypoglycemia** 1131
G.B. Bolli and E.A.M. Gale

48 **Diabetic Ketoacidosis and Hyperglycaemic Non-ketotic Coma** 1151
S.M. Marshall, M. Walker and K.G.M.M. Alberti

49 **Infection, Immunity and Diabetes** 1165
W.G. Reeves and R.M. Wilson

50 **The Care of the Diabetic Patient During Surgery** 1173
G.V. Gill and K.G.M.M. Alberti

51 **Vascular Events and Diabetes: Acute Myocardial Infarction and Stroke** 1185
J.S. Yudkin and T.J. Hendra

Chronic Complications of Diabetes

52   **Complications of Diabetes: the Changing Scene**. 1213
      K. Borch-Johnsen and T. Deckert

Specific Complications

53   **The Genesis of Diabetes Complications: Blood Glucose and Genetic Susceptibility** . . . 1225
      P. Raskin and J. Rosenstock

54   **Basement Membrane Physiology and Pathophysiology**. 1245
      J.R. Williamson and C. Kilo

55   **Diabetic Nephropathy**. 1267
      G.C. Viberti, J.D. Walker and J. Pinto

56   **Diabetic Retinopathy** 1329
      M.D. Davis and L.I. Rand

57   **Diabetic Effects on Non-retinal Ocular Structures** 1367
      L.I. Rand, J.D. Cavallerano and L.M. Aiello

58   **Visual Impairment and Diabetes** 1373
      R. Klein and S.E. Moss

59   **Diabetic Neuropathy** 1385
      J.D. Ward

60   **Connective Tissue Disorders in Diabetes**. 1415
      A.L. Rosenbloom

Macrovascular Disease

61   **Cellular Mechanisms of Diabetic Large Vessel Disease** 1435
      T. Ledet, L. Heickendorff and L.M. Rasmussen

62   **Clotting Disorders in Diabetes** 1447
      D.E. McMillan

63   **Epidemiology of Macrovascular Disease and Hypertension in Diabetes Mellitus** 1459
      R.J. Jarrett

64   **Metabolic Control and Macrovascular Disease** 1471
      M. Uusitupa, K. Pyörälä and M. Laakso

65   **Clinical Features of Ischemic Heart Disease in Diabetes Mellitus** 1487
      E.H. Wittels and A.M. Gotto

66   **Clinical Features and Treatment of Peripheral Vascular Disease in Diabetes Mellitus** . 1509
      F.W. LoGerfo and M.S. Rosenblatt

Other Complications

67 **Arterial Hypertension in Diabetes Mellitus**. 1521
H.H. Parving

68 **The Diabetic Foot** 1535
M.E. Edmonds and P.J. Watkins

69 **The Prevention and Screening of Diabetic Complications**. 1549
M. McGill and D.K. Yue

Diabetes and Public Health

70 **Screening for Diabetes and Other Categories of Glucose Intolerance**. 1565
G. Dowse, P. Zimmet and K.G.M.M. Alberti

71a **Organization of Care: The Diabetic Clinic—A Center of Knowledge**. 1589
U. Rosenqvist

71b **Organisation of Care: The Diabetes Care Centre—A Focus for More Effective Diabetes Treatment and Prevention** 1593
J.J. Bending and H. Keen

71c **Organisation of Care: Problems in Developing Countries—India** 1601
A. Ramachandran and M. Viswanathan

71d **Organization of Care: Problems in Developing Countries—Malaysia** 1607
B.A.K. Khalid

71e **Organisation of Care: Problems in Developing Countries—Tanzania**. 1611
D.G. McLarty

71f **Organization of Care: Diabetes Community Programs as Part of Primary Health Care in the Community** 1619
J. Tuomilehto

72 **Diabetic Life Problems: Insurance, Driving, Employment** 1631
L.P. Krall

73 **The Economics of Diabetes Care** 1643
T.J. Songer

74 **Primary Prevention of Diabetes Mellitus** 1655
J. Tuomilehto, E. Tuomilehto-Wolf, P. Zimmet, K.G.M.M. Alberti and H. Keen

Index 1675

VOLUME 1

Contributors xvii

Foreword (H. Nakajima) xxv

Introduction (H. Keen, G. Alberti, R. DeFronzo and P. Zimmet) xxvii

Diagnosis, Epidemiology and Aetiology of Diabetes

1   **Classification of Diabetes Mellitus and Other Categories of Glucose Intolerance** . . .   3
     M.I. Harris and P. Zimmet

2   **Diabetes Diagnosis**   19
     H. Keen

3   **Genetics of Diabetes Mellitus**   31
     C.M. Vadheim and J.I. Rotter

4   **Epidemiology of Insulin Dependent Diabetes Mellitus: Approaches to Study**   99
     E.S. Tull and R.E. LaPorte

5   **Aetiopathogenesis of Type 1 Diabetes in Western Society**   107
     F. Dotta and G.S. Eisenbarth

6a   **Epidemiology and Etiopathogenesis of IDDM in Asia**   117
     Y. Goto

6b   **Epidemiology and Etiopathogenesis of IDDM in Other Ethnic Groups**   129
     J.M. Ekoé

7   **Epidemiology and Natural History of NIDDM: Non-obese and Obese**   147
     P.H. Bennett, C. Bogardus, J. Tuomilehto and P. Zimmet

8   **Diabetes in the Tropics**   177
     V. Mohan and K.G.M.M. Alberti

9   **Diabetes Secondary to Acquired Disease of the Pancreas**   197
     S. Del Prato and A. Tiengo

Biochemistry and Pathophysiology of Diabetes

10   **Morphology of the Pancreas in Normal and Diabetic States**   223
     G. Klöppel, W. Gepts and P.A. In't Veld

11   **Insulin Biosynthesis and Secretion In Vitro**.   261
     W.J. Malaisse

12   **Insulin Secretion in the Normal and Diabetic Human**   285
     B.J. Wallum, S.E. Kahn, D.K. McCulloch and D. Porte, Jr

13   **C-Peptide and Proinsulin**   303
     S. Madsbad, S.G. Hartling and O.E. Faber

14   **Biosynthesis, Secretion and Action of Glucagon**.   333
     P.J. Lefèbvre

15   **Somatostatin and Pancreatic Polypeptide**   341
     G. Williams and S.R. Bloom

16   **Insulin Receptors in Normal and Disease States**   357
     B.J. Goldstein and C.R. Kahn

17   **Actions of Insulin on Intracellular Processes**   385
     R.M. Denton and J.M. Tavaré

18a **Insulin Actions In Vivo: Glucose Metabolism**.   409
     E. Ferrannini and R.A. DeFronzo

18b **Insulin Actions In Vivo: Insulin and Lipoprotein Metabolism**   439
     A.H. Kissebah

18c **Insulin Actions In Vivo: Its Role in the Regulation of Ketone Body Metabolism**   459
     M. Walker and K.G.M.M. Alberti

18d **Insulin Actions In Vivo: Protein Metabolism**   467
     R.A. DeFronzo and E. Ferrannini

19   **The Assessment of Insulin Action In Vivo**   513
     G.R. Fulcher, M. Walker and K.G.M.M. Alberti

20   **Clinical Disorders of Insulin Resistance**   531
     H. Beck-Nielson

21   **Biochemistry of Obesity in Relation to Diabetes**   551
     P. Björntorp

22   **Pathogenesis of NIDDM: A Precarious Balance between Insulin Action and Insulin
     Secretion**.   569
     R.A. DeFronzo, R.C. Bonadonna and E. Ferrannini

23   **Glucose Toxicity**.   635
     D.C. Simonson, L. Rossetti, A. Giaccari and R.A. DeFronzo

24   **Glycation of Macromolecules**   669
     M. Brownlee

Management of Diabetes

25a **Dietary Management of Diabetes Mellitus in Europe and North America** 685
J.I. Mann and N.J. Lewis-Barned

25b **Dietary Management of Diabetes Mellitus in India and South East Asia** 701
J.S. Bajaj

25c **Dietary Management of Diabetes Mellitus in Japan** 707
S. Baba

25d **Dietary Management of Diabetes Mellitus in Africa** 711
Z. Lukmanji

25e **Dietary Management of Diabetes Mellitus in China** 719
Chi Zhi-sheng and Du Shou-fen

26 **Exercise** 725
F.W. Kemmer and M. Berger

27 **Sulfonylureas: Basic Aspects and Clinical Uses** 745
H.E. Lebovitz and A. Melander

28 **Biguanides: Basic Aspects and Clinical Uses** 773
L.S. Hermann and A. Melander

29 **New Drugs for the Treatment of Diabetes Mellitus** 797
D.G. Johnson and R. Bressler

30 **Hypolipidemic Agents: Their Role in Diabetes Mellitus** 817
M.-R. Taskinen and P.J. Nestel

31 **Insulin Therapy** 831
P.D. Home and K.G.M.M. Alberti

32 **Alternative Routes for Insulin Delivery** 865
G. Slama

33 **The Artificial Endocrine Pancreas** 871
A.M. Albisser

34 **Complications of Insulin Therapy** 883
E.A.M. Gale

35a **Pancreas Transplantation: Islets** 895
R. Sutton, D.W.R. Gray and P.J. Morris

35b **Pancreas Transplantation: Whole Organ and Segmental** 915
G. Pozza, J. Traeger and A. Secchi

36a **Education of the Diabetic Patient** 923
J.L. Day and J.-P. Assal

36b **Computer-assisted Diabetes Education** 949
M. Cohen

37 **General Care of the Diabetic Patient by the Nurse and Doctor** 955
P.L. Hoskins and J.R. Turtle

38 **Urine Testing: Its Place in the 1990s** 967
M. Cohen

39 **Self-monitoring of Blood Glucose** 971
P.P.B. Yeo, A.C. Thai and M. Cohen

40 **Glycation of Hemoglobin and Serum Proteins** 985
L. Kennedy

41 **Computers: Applications in Diabetes Care, Education and Research** 1009
R. Mazze and K. Matsuoka

Special Problems in Management

42

Diabetes in Childhood and Adolescence

Julio V. Santiago, Neil H. White and Sharon L. Pontious

*Washington University School of Medicine, St Louis, MO, USA; Diabetes Research and Training
Center, Washington University School of Medicine, St Louis, MO, USA; Division of Pediatric
Endocrinology and Metabolism, St Louis Children's Hospital, St Louis, MO, USA*

EPIDEMIOLOGY

Approximately 1 in every 400 to 600 school-age children under age 18 years in North America is known to have insulin dependent diabetes mellitus (IDDM) [1]. Thus, IDDM is slightly more common in children than cancer of all causes, over 4 times more common than cystic fibrosis and over 12 times more common than muscular dystrophy. The yearly incidence of IDDM, defined as the number of new cases per 100 000 children at risk, is highly variable in different parts of the world. It is approximately 25 in Finland and Sweden, 14 in the USA, Denmark and Scotland, 4 in Israel and France and less than 1 in Japan [2]. The reasons for this wide range of incidence are largely unknown; however, it does not seem to be attributable to differences either in methods of ascertainment or in definitions of IDDM. Although there is likely to be a genetic component to the variable incidence of IDDM in different populations, environmental factors are also likely to have a role. The incidence of diabetes is 2–3 times greater among children of Japanese origin living in Hawaii than among children in Japan [3]. The

incidence of diabetes is also greater among French-Canadian children living in Quebec than among children in France [4]. Whether these differences are due primarily to climatic, dietary or other unidentified environmental causes is not known; they do not appear to be due to racial admixtures in the relocated populations.

LaPorte et al have noted a striking positive relationship ($r = 0.76$) between distance from the equator and the incidence of IDDM in 13 countries between 25 and 65 degrees latitude from the equator [5]. IDDM incidence has also been negatively correlated ($r = -0.55$) with average yearly temperatures between 5°C and 28°C.

The initial diagnosis of IDDM can be made at any age but is most often made during puberty. In the Pittsburgh study, the prepubertal incidence of IDDM is about 5 cases per 100 000 per year, and increases to 10 per 100 000 in girls aged 10–12 years and in boys aged 12–14 years [1, 6]. In Denmark, the annual incidence increases from approximately 10 per 100 000 before puberty to over 20 per 100 000 at puberty before declining to 12 cases per 100 000 after puberty [7]. As in the Pittsburgh study, the surge in risk

International Textbook of Diabetes Mellitus. Edited by K.G.M.M. Alberti, R.A. DeFronzo, H. Keen and P. Zimmet
© 1992 John Wiley & Sons Ltd

occurs 2 years earlier in girls than in boys. Overall, the prevalence of diabetes at age 18 years is similar in boys and girls in both countries [1, 4, 7]. The cause for the higher incidence of IDDM during puberty is not known. Sex hormone or growth hormone changes, changes in insulin sensitivity [8] or changes in susceptibility to immune-mediated pancreatic B-cell damage and immunologic tolerance, could all play a part.

The incidence of childhood IDDM is also influenced by racial factors. For example, IDDM has been reported to be substantially less common in Americans of African origin than in Americans of European origin [9]. This may be due to the apparent rarity of IDDM in West Africa, the origin of many African-Americans. This could be due to the fact that there is a high rate of mortality from disorders that could mimic ketoacidotic dehydration.

ETIOLOGIC CONSIDERATIONS

Before the 1980s, viruses were commonly implicated as possible causative or contributing factors in the development of IDDM [10]. This notion was derived from the observation that certain viruses (encephalomyocarditis, coxsackie B4, rubella) were diabetogenic in certain rodent models of IDDM. In some of these models the development of diabetes occurs only in certain strains or gender of the animals. As in human IDDM, associated immunologic phenomena such as development of islet cell autoantibodies and an increased prevalence of antibodies against thyroid, adrenal and gastric parietal cells have been reported in some of these animal models [11].

In humans, the strongest link between viruses and IDDM is the 20% or higher incidence of IDDM in children with congenital rubella [12]. In these children there is a higher incidence of diabetes among those with HLA-DR3 and/or HDL-DR4 haplotypes, and autoantibodies against islets and other endocrine tissues are common.

Outbreaks of IDDM sometimes occur within small geographic areas. Some of these clusters of new cases have been associated with antecedent coxsackie B or mumps epidemics. However, prospective studies among newly diagnosed children with IDDM have failed to link IDDM with any specific viral infection. The case for a

significant role for *recent* viral infection as a common cause of IDDM is not strong [13]. Nevertheless, a *remote* viral infection could set into motion a series of immunologic events, such as exposure of previously masked antigenic determinants on pancreatic B cells or development of crossreactive antibodies, that could lead to cell-mediated and/or antibody-mediated immune destruction of pancreatic B cells several months or years later.

In the 1980s many centers reported that immune abnormalities such as antibodies against pancreatic islets and insulin often preceded, by months or years, the development of early impairment of insulin release after the intravenous administration of a bolus of glucose, as well as the subsequent development of glucose intolerance and overt insulin dependency [14–18]. These studies have failed to identify any specific viral agent as the initiator of autoimmune destruction of pancreatic B cells in children with IDDM, but do support the idea of a long prodromal phase in many patients with IDDM. This prodromal phase may be longer in IDDM patients with onset of disease after the start of puberty than in prepubertal children [18]. These observations have been used to support the concept that there may be considerable heterogeneity in causation, susceptibility and clinical presentation of the IDDM syndrome in humans [19].

It is likely that non-specific viral infections could actually cause either insulin resistance or increased lymphokine activity that could, in concert with hyperglycemia, reduce insulin secretion acutely [20]. One could thus propose a scenario in which a pre-existent, indolent autoimmune reaction directed against pancreatic B cells is exacerbated by an intercurrent infection that results in acute hyperglycemia and the clinical diagnosis of diabetes. In children or young adults with newly diagnosed IDDM, recovery from such an acute infection could restore sufficient insulin secretory capacity to render these patients insulin independent for several months or longer. Treatment with cyclosporin or other forms of immune suppression [21–23] may help prolong this 'honeymoon phase' of IDDM in 50% or more of these individuals. Aggressive insulin therapy aimed at diminishing endogenous insulin secretion may have a similar effect. Again, there is substantial heterogeneity in the response to these interventions as well as in the quantitative and temporal aspects of recovery of insulin secretory potential.

Several chemical agents have been used to induce diabetes in animals [24]. These include streptozotocin, alloxan and Vacor. A few pharmaceutical agents (pentamidine, L-asparaginase and cyclosporin) and the rodenticide Vacor have been shown to be occasional causes of diabetes in children [25]. In certain strains of mice, streptozotocin at lower doses does not cause acute diabetes but instead initiates an autoimmune reaction against islets and other endocrine tissues that resembles that of IDDM [26]. Other toxic agents may act in a similar, indirect way [27].

In the majority of cases, IDDM is currently thought to represent a syndrome in which immune processes in susceptible children lead to the selective destruction of pancreatic B cells [28, 29]. Numerous lines of evidence (see Chapter 5) support this idea. They include (a) a round-cell infiltration around pancreatic islets (insulitis) of recently diagnosed IDDM patients [30]; (b) an increased prevalence of IDDM among kindreds with multiple autoimmune endocrinopathies [31]; (c) the presence of antibodies against islets and/or insulin in 80–90% of children with IDDM [16, 18]; (d) the existence of non-obese diabetic (NOD) mouse, Bio-Breeding (BB) rat and other animal models of diabetes, such as the previously described low-dose streptozotocin-treated mouse, which clinically and immunologically mimic many features of human IDDM [11]; (e) the strong association of IDDM with certain class II antigen genes located on the short arm of chromosome 6 that mediate immune responses and also confer either protection against, or susceptibility to, IDDM [28–29, 32]; and (f) the fact that immunosuppressive agents such as cyclosporin A often induce or extend transient 'honeymoon' periods in children and young adults with newly diagnosed IDDM [21–23].

It is not known whether complement-fixing or other antibodies directed against pancreatic islets, B cells or insulin are primary causes of IDDM. These antibodies could simply signify responses to exposure of the immune system to islet antigens, such as the 64-kDa GABA-synthesizing enzyme glutamic acid decarboxylase, which have been unmasked by a previous cellular immune response or injury by a toxic agent or virus [33]. Furthermore, it is possible that islet

or insulin antibodies may not, of themselves, be sufficient to provide the signal required for T-cell mediated pancreatic B-cell injury. Such a signal could be a still unidentified peptide smaller than 64 kDa, that regulates macrophage presentation of a processed islet B-cell antigen or T-lymphocyte mediated destruction of the B cell [34].

Initial negative and positive associations of IDDM with specific HLA haplotypes were first made with class I transplantation antigens, i.e. specific haplotypes of HLA-A and B loci found on most cells [35]. IDDM was one of many disorders with such an association. Subsequently, these class I antigen associations were shown to be secondary to linkage disequilibria of these genes with certain class II antigen genes [36, 37]. For example, individuals with HLA-DR2 were protected from IDDM, and those with HLA-DR3 or DR4 (or their surrogates in non-Caucasians) were more susceptible to IDDM, independent of any class I antigen association. More recently, by analysis of fragments of genes obtained by molecular cloning, evidence has been developed incriminating disease susceptibility to specific amino acids (the aspartic acid at position 57) in the B chain of the class II HLA-DQ locus [38–40]. Whether the previously described class II DR antigen associations with IDDM are independent of DQ associations requires further study. Nevertheless, the association between various class II antigens and IDDM and other autoimmune diseases may be related to these molecules' important role as qualitative and quantitative regulators of cell-mediated immunity. One theory, for example, postulates that macrophages or other antigen-presenting cells that express class II antigens serve to scavenge and process foreign, altered or newly exposed antigens and then 'present' them to the immune system [34, 35, 41]. The processed foreign antigen is not 'presented' alone but as a bimolecular complex with the antigen-presenting cell's class II antigen. In certain forms of thyroiditis the antigen-presenting cell may be the thyroid cell itself, rather than a macrophage or dendritic cell, and a similar role has been proposed for islet cells modified by viral or toxic agents in IDDM [42]. Whether the antigen-presenting cell is a macrophage, an islet endothelial cell or a B cell, its own class II antigen type could confer either susceptibility to, or protection from, cell-mediated autoimmune destruction and thus explain some of the heterogeneity that seems to exist in the manifestation of the IDDM syndrome. For example, the presence of an aspartic acid residue could modify the DQ molecule's structure so that it does not allow the T-cell receptor to 'lock in' to the processed antigen–class II molecule complex. Furthermore, mechanisms that regulate T-cell cytotoxic and suppressor activity at the level of the thymus may help explain why some individuals have only a transient appearance of islet antibodies without later developing IDDM and why the majority of individuals with diabetes-associated class II antigens never develop IDDM [43].

Research into the mechanisms for HLA associations and immune disturbances in IDDM may some day help to ascertain how various triggers and contributing or protective variables influence the development of this disorder so that those children most likely to develop IDDM can be identified and treated. For example, siblings with specific HLA haplotypes might merit close monitoring for early development of antibodies or T cells directed against pancreatic islets or other early markers for IDDM. The hope, so far unfulfilled, is that information from human and animal studies will allow early immune modulation to prevent or delay the progression from a prodromal phase to overt hyperglycemia in IDDM [41, 44].

Our current state of ignorance regarding causes, variability and susceptibility to diabetes presents problems in genetic counseling in IDDM. This disorder seems to result from an interplay between two or more genes or susceptibility factors as well as from a growing list of potential environmental events. For example, over half of monozygotic siblings of children with IDDM never develop diabetes even though it may be assumed that they were born with most, or all, of the genes necessary to develop this disorder [45]. Fathers with diabetes seem to be more likely than mothers with diabetes to confer to their children susceptibility to IDDM [46]. The reasons for this are not known, but may include protection of the newborn, through increased tolerance or other mechanisms by the IDDM mother in utero, or postnatally through breast milk [47]. Only about 5% of siblings of children with IDDM will develop diabetes and less than 10% of white children will have a parent with IDDM. Genetic counseling of current or prospective parents in families with IDDM is thus based on cautious estimates of probability ratios rather than firm predictions [48].

Less Common Causes of Diabetes in Children

Neonatal diabetes refers to a syndrome in which neonates develop severe hyperglycemia within days after birth. We have seen 4 of these children at our center over the last 20 years, during which time we have seen approximately 1000 children with IDDM. These babies are very small for gestational age and have pronounced absence of subcutaneous fat. They respond dramatically to relatively low doses of insulin with rapid weight gain and accelerated growth. The most intriguing feature of the syndrome is that these babies, who are severely insulinopenic and produce little or no insulin at diagnosis, often recover their ability to produce insulin after 2–4 months [49]. Mothers of these infants are usually not themselves diabetic, and islet cell antibodies are not demonstrable in either mothers or patients. This rare syndrome may be due to a maturational defect in the development of normal insulin secretion, similar to that which occurs perinatally in rats. One of the 4 children with neonatal diabetes that we have seen during the last decade failed to recover insulin secretory capacity and had major cardiac anomalies so that this disorder is not always transient or benign. The remaining 3 had transient neonatal diabetes and developed their ability to produce insulin between 2 and 4 months of age, had no congenital anomalies or exposure to rubella and have since remained normoglycemic.

Diabetes is also found in a number of other syndromes. These include Wolfram's syndrome (diabetes insipidus, diabetes mellitus, optic atrophy, and nerve deafness; DIDMOAD), Friedreich's ataxia, Refsum's syndrome, Klinefelter's syndrome, Turner's syndrome and Down's syndrome. Severe insulin resistance with diabetes is also seen in children with infantile obesity (Alstrom's, Prader–Willi and Laurence–Moon–Biedl syndromes), lipoatrophy (Seip–Lawrence syndrome) and premature aging (Werner's syndrome) [50].

School-age children can develop a relatively mild, non-ketosis-prone form of diabetes that is diagnosed during routine screening for diabetes or during investigation of kindreds, in which diabetes is passed on through two or more generations in an autosomal dominant inheritance pattern [51]. These children are not insulin dependent and most are not obese. The syndrome may account for between 1% and 3% of diabetes in childhood. Islet cell antibodies are negative and the usual HLA antigen associations seen with type 1 diabetes are not present. These patients are said to have MODY (maturity onset diabetes of youth). Treatment is as for type 2 or adult onset diabetes. As adults, these children develop the same long-term complications seen in adult onset or type 2 diabetes, although their less severe hyperglycemia may be partially protective against early development of microvascular disease. Unlike children with IDDM, genetic counseling can be more specific for these families because of the autosomal dominant nature of the disorder.

About 5–10% of children with cystic fibrosis who survive past age 18 years develop diabetes [52]. Their diabetes is thought to be caused by chronic inflammatory pancreatic disease and most often appears during puberty or after administration of high doses of corticosteroids. There are no HLA associations and islet cell antibodies are not usually present at diagnosis. These children pose difficult therapeutic problems because their cystic fibrosis management commonly includes a high-carbohydrate diet and pancreatic enzyme replacement to help them maintain adequate weight. Insulin requirements are sometimes increased during intermittent periods of infection, corticosteroid use and prolonged stress. Adolescents with diabetes secondary to cystic fibrosis rarely develop ketoacidosis. In addition, diabetes is often viewed as a less severe or immediate problem than the life-threatening pulmonary disease of cystic fibrosis. Therefore, some families and primary treatment physicians are reluctant to institute aggressive and complex treatment regimens in these patients in hopes of reducing the relatively low probability of clinically significant long-term complications in the future [52]. However, very poorly controlled diabetes can contribute to impaired growth and sexual development in these children and young adults, and therefore good control is important even in these patients.

About 2–3% of children treated with L-asparaginase, a drug used to treat childhood leukemia, develop severe hyperglycemia and symptomatic diabetes [53]. This hyperglycemia occurs more commonly among children also given high doses of corticosteroids and often resolves spontaneously when L-asparaginase is discontinued. Because over 50% of children with acute leukemia can now expect either long-term remissions or cures, we do not usually recommend stopping L-asparaginase treatment because of transient hyperglycemia. Long-term studies are lacking regarding the subsequent development of diabetes in these children.

DIAGNOSTIC TESTS FOR IDDM

Oral glucose tolerance tests are rarely indicated in the evaluation of children suspected of having diabetes [54]. Approximately 90% of children present with classic symptoms related to hyperglycemia and an osmotic diuresis: nocturia, polydipsia and polyuria. About 75% will have experienced weight loss or fatigue; most of these will have glycosuria, ketonuria and plasma glucose values well above 200 mg/dl (11.1 mmol/l). About 25–40% will present in ketoacidosis and 5–10% in coma. No further diagnostic tests are needed in these children and oral glucose challenges are contraindicated.

Sometimes children present without weight loss or symptoms of hyperglycemia but with a randomly taken plasma glucose level above 200 mg/dl (11.1 mmol/l). In these children a repeat plasma glucose value above 200 mg/dl 2 hours after a meal readily confirms the diagnosis of diabetes [54]. No further diagnostic tests are needed in these children, although the presence of islet cell antibodies may be helpful in determining whether these patients are simply early presentations of typical IDDM or whether they have other types of diabetes [55].

When fasting plasma glucose values are between 115 mg/dl and 140 mg/dl and 2-hour postprandial values below 200 mg/dl, an oral glucose tolerance test (OGTT) can be done. Adequate preparation is necessary before performing an OGTT. This preparation should include (a) no febrile illness for 2 or more weeks; (b) adequate carbohydrate intake (at least 200 g/m² per day) for several days; (c) the child should be fasted overnight, unstressed and resting comfortably; (d) 1.75 g/kg (up to 75 g) of a glucose solution should be given and blood drawn before and at 1, 2 and 3 hours after oral glucose administration. Two values above 200 mg/dl confirm the diagnosis of diabetes. If these diabetic children are islet antibody positive we routinely start them on at least one daily injection of insulin in the hope that aggressive early treatment with reduction of hyperglycemia will help to prolong endogenous insulin secretion [56, 57].

The diagnosis of diabetes should not be made on the sole basis of family history, presence of islet cell antibodies or HLA typing. Over 50% of identical twins of patients with IDDM never develop diabetes, and some children with HLA-DR3 or DR4 who are islet cell antibody positive and are relatives of subjects with IDDM, subsequently become antibody negative without developing diabetes during the subsequent 5 or more years [58, 59]. In most cases where parental anxiety is a major factor we ask families to be watchful for signs of early diabetes such as nocturia and to perform postprandial blood glucose testing when this occurs.

After careful discussion with parents, some pediatricians also perform HLA typing and monitor islet cell antibody levels yearly [55]. There are currently no interventions that have been shown to better the long-term progression to diabetes. Therefore, at present we cannot recommend this approach in all children unless the child is part of a clinical research study of epidemiology or early immune intervention.

DIABETIC KETOACIDOSIS

The pathophysiology of ketoacidosis is described in detail elsewhere in this book (see Chapter 48). Relative or absolute insulin deficiency is a prerequisite and the presence of increased levels of important counterregulatory hormones (primarily glucagon and catecholamines but also cortisol and growth hormone) are major contributing factors in its development. In children with known IDDM the two most common causes of diabetic ketoacidosis (DKA) are failure to take insulin, and failure to increase insulin doses during infection or other forms of insulin resistance. Binge eating alone does not usually produce sufficient decrements in insulin levels or increments in counterregulatory hormones to result in the marked lipolysis and ketogenesis characteristic of DKA in children.

Failure to take insulin includes circumstances in which polymerized, aggregated or denatured insulin is administered. Insulin doses required to maintain normoglycemia increase substantially

during most febrile illnesses, during the pubertal growth spurt, with some forms of chronic stress and with the administration of corticosteroids. Although development of high titers of antibodies against injected insulin were causes of insulin resistance and DKA before 1970, the increased purity of insulin preparations used since that time has made insulin antibody-induced insulin resistance a rare cause of DKA in children with IDDM. We have seen only a single case during the last 15 years in children attending our two centers.

In our centers, the most common cause of hospital admission for DKA in children is newly diagnosed IDDM. About 25–40% of newly diagnosed children with IDDM will present with DKA. This figure may be higher among children where parental observation is poor or psychosocial factors delay early medical attention.

In children, the most important early clues leading to a diagnosis of IDDM include enuresis and nocturia. Although some normal children awake once or twice to urinate during the night, they usually do not also drink large amounts of water, a characteristic of children with early IDDM. Nocturia or enuresis in a previously 'dry' child should lead to an evaluation of possible urinary tract infection or stress as well as to possible diabetes. In these patients glycosuria is readily demonstrated if the cause of the nocturia or enuresis is diabetes.

Weight loss is a common symptom or sign at the time of initial diagnosis and typically occurs in spite of an excellent, sometimes increased appetite. Evidence of increased energy intake from carbohydrate-containing fluids is common. Much of the weight loss results from proteolysis with conversion of muscle-derived amino acids and glycogen into glucose carbon skeletons via hepatic gluconeogenesis from three-carbon intermediates such as alanine, glutamine, lactate and pyruvate. Marked proteolysis is often accompanied by weakness and fatigue. Negative nitrogen balance, nocturia, polydipsia and weight loss can sometimes persist for several months and result in growth failure.

Sudden metabolic deterioration and development of DKA is seen when an intervening infection causes insulin resistance, a decrease in already waning insulin secretion, and interference with the ability to drink and retain large volumes of fluid occurs. Within a few hours lipolysis and ketoacid formation increase markedly. Hyperglycemia, which has been previously fairly stable for days or weeks at glucose concentrations of 180–360 mg/dl because of urinary elimination of 100 g or more of glucose daily, increases as severe dehydration and decreased urine production set in. Once severe DKA has occurred, the patient's medical condition will deteriorate rapidly.

Severe ketosis results in anorexia, delayed gastric emptying, gastric dilatation and ileus with resultant abdominal pain or vomiting severe enough to be confused with appendicitis or gastroenteritis. Metabolic acidosis stimulates hyperventilation which can be confused with asthma, anxiety or other primary pulmonary problems. A distinct odor of 'ketones' on the breath is common. Generally, abdominal pain, vomiting and hyperventilation indicate a serum bicarbonate level below 10 mmol/l and arterial pH levels below 7.2 in children with overt DKA. Altered mental status and coma are seen with prolonged, severe DKA and are best correlated with the hyperosmolality rather than the severity of acidosis. Children with full-blown DKA often have lost 10–15% of their previous body weight.

Almost all episodes of severe DKA can be prevented in children with known IDDM with optimal medical care by the family and health care system. The best single preventive measure is a reliable, stable family which has undergone extensive family education and training. Written instructions that include clues to early diagnosis and recommendations for appropriate actions should be reviewed regularly and kept available by the family for ready reference [60]. Whenever a child is sick for *any* reason these 'sick day' management rules should be set into motion. These include blood glucose and urine ketone measurements every 2–4 hours and having a specific number to call 24 hours a day so that a knowledgeable health professional (physician or nurse) can provide immediate assistance. We routinely ask patients to call us immediately if (a) the child vomits twice in less than 8 hours or appears sick for any reason, (b) there are moderate or large amounts of ketones for more than 4 hours, or (c) blood glucose values are over 400 mg/dl (22.2 mmol/l) for more than 6–8 hours. Repeated hospital admissions for DKA are most common among adolescents with behavioral or adjustment problems, and in disrupted or unstable families in which adult supervision is inadequate [61].

Common problems in the management of IDDM that can lead to recurrent DKA include (a) failure to resolve behavioral, psychiatric or family problems that result in a child or adolescent not being given or allowed not to take insulin, (b) omitting insulin because a child is too sick to eat, (c) waiting several hours into an illness so that the child can be seen at a time more convenient for the family or doctor, (d) failure to maintain adequate hydration with appropriate fluids, (e) failure to monitor for ketones when a child is sick or hyperglycemic, and (f) confusing the vomiting or hyperventilation due to ketosis with gastroenteritis or asthma in a previously undiagnosed child. Children with IDDM who are vomiting repeatedly or cannot drink fluids, those who are hyperventilating, and those who have severe abdominal pain or altered mental status should be seen immediately by a person experienced in managing children with IDDM.

DKA is easily diagnosed in the office or hospital when the blood glucose concentration is over 240 mg/dl (13.3 mmol/l); a moderate to large degree of ketonuria or ketonemia is present and the plasma bicarbonate level is below 15 mmol/l or arterial pH below 7.25. Ketonemia can be ascertained by placing a drop of plasma on a crushed Acetest tablet or ketone body reagent strip. Immediate measurement of electrolytes, blood glucose and arterialized blood gases and pH are ordered. We obtain routine blood, urine and throat cultures in any child with DKA presenting with fever. An electrocardiogram is obtained if the child is hypotensive, severely acidotic, or plasma potassium levels are grossly abnormal (below 3.5 mmol/l or above 6.0 mmol/l).

A rapid assessment should be made of the adequacy of the child's airway and ventilation, mental status, presence of ketones on breath, hydration status and possible sources of infection. The child's weight should be noted to help estimate recent weight loss and repeated every 6–12 hours to help estimate the effectiveness of rehydration. All children with DKA should be evaluated by an experienced diabetologist or pediatrician as soon as the decision is made to admit to hospital for further treatment or before the decision is made to send the child home after rehydration. Most hospitalized children with severe DKA require close monitoring of heart rate, blood pressure and mental status as well as review of clinical and laboratory progress at least every 2 hours. Children with DKA who cannot drink and retain ample amounts of fluids without developing abdominal pain, and those who are still drowsy or hyperventilating, should not be sent home. Referral to or telephone consultation with a center with appropriate resources and experience in handling children with severe DKA should be considered as soon as the child's condition is stabilized and appropriate treatment begun.

TREATMENT OF DKA

The mainstays of therapy for DKA include fluid therapy (to correct dehydration and electrolyte imbalance), insulin (to inhibit ketogenesis and reduce hyperglycemia), identification and correction of the underlying precipitating cause of the episode (e.g. infection or failure to follow appropriate preventive measures) and measures designed to reduce complications of treatment such as cerebral edema, aspiration pneumonia and appendicitis presenting with DKA [62–64]. (See also Chapter 48.)

Fluids

Patients with ketonuria and hyperglycemia who are able to drink and tolerate fluids and who are alert can often be rehydrated orally without intravenous fluid therapy. For those in more severe DKA (arterial blood pH below 7.2 and serum bicarbonate below 10 mmol/l) and in patients unable to tolerate oral fluids, intravenous hydration is usually required.

Volume expansion is initially given as an isotonic solution such as 0.15 mol/l (0.9%) saline or Ringer's lactate solution at 20 ml/kg (rarely more than 1 liter). This is administered over the first 60 minutes. Subsequently, fluids may be half isotonic (e.g. 0.45% saline) unless the clinical picture is complicated by hyponatremia (plasma sodium less than 130 mmol/l), hypotension or shock. Blood glucose levels may fall by 100–300 mg/dl (5.6–16.7 mmol/l) during the first 2 hours of rehydration, even before insulin is given.

Fluids and electrolytes are administered to provide requirements, correct existing deficits, and replace continuing losses over the next 24–36 hours. If severe hyperosmolality (marked hyperglycemia along with a normal or elevated serum sodium) is present at diagnosis, we recommend that total fluid deficits be replaced more slowly (over 36–48 hours). The initial fluid deficit in patients with severe DKA is usually estimated to be 10% of total body weight [62–64]. After the initial 20 ml/kg body weight administration of isotonic fluids, rehydration can usually be accomplished using 0.45% saline at a rate of 3 l/m^2 body surface area per day. We sometimes give fluids at higher rates (4–5 l/m^2 per day) if relatively large fluid losses are occurring. Such losses are primarily the result of osmotic diuresis and vomiting, and can be decreased by reducing and maintaining the blood glucose at 150–250 mg/dl. However, this higher rate of rehydration is rarely needed for more than the usual 4–8 hours it takes to lower blood glucose levels to 250–300 mg/dl. All fluids should be given intravenously until it is shown that oral fluids can be tolerated without abdominal pain or vomiting. At this time, oral fluids can substitute for intravenous hydration, but total fluid intake (oral and intravenous) needs to be considered in the calculation of fluid replacement. An accurate accounting of fluid intake and output should be kept and analyzed carefully to ensure adequate rehydration and urine output. Weighing the patient every 6–12 hours is often helpful.

While the plasma glucose level is above 250–300 mg/dl, intravenous fluids should contain no glucose. We add 5% glucose to the hydrating fluids when the hourly monitored blood glucose level falls to about 250 mg/dl. We then attempt to maintain the hourly monitored blood or plasma glucose value between 150 mg/dl and 200 mg/dl. If glucose levels fall below 150 mg/dl, solutions containing 7.5% or 10% glucose are started or the insulin infusion rate is reduced by 25–50%. The latter option is employed only after the plasma bicarbonate level has risen above 12 mmol/l or the arterial pH above 7.2.

Insulin

The only insulin appropriate in the treatment of DKA is rapidly acting regular insulin. For mild DKA, especially if intravenous hydration is not indicated, insulin can be given subcutaneously or intramuscularly in a dose of 0.25 U/kg every 2–6 hours. In more severe DKA, continuous intravenous insulin infusion is preferable. Although subcutaneous or intramuscular regular insulin can be given (0.20 U/kg every 2 hours), this should never be used when peripheral perfusion is poor, such as in severe dehydration or shock.

Continuous intravenous insulin infusion therapy of DKA is initiated with an intravenous bolus of 0.1 U/kg. This is followed within the next hour by continuous infusion at a rate of 0.1 U/kg per hour [65, 66]. Regular insulin can be mixed in normal saline at a concentration of 0.25–1.0 U/ml, so that the fluid delivery rate (0.1 U/kg per hour) is about 10–20 ml per hour. Alternatively, the weight of the patient in kilograms is used to calculate the number of units of regular insulin added per 100 ml of saline, and this separate solution is given at a fixed rate of 10 ml per hour. Thus, in a 40-kg child, 40 units of regular insulin are mixed with 100 ml of saline and given at 10 ml per hour.

We administer the insulin using an electronically controlled, reliable infusion pump or controller 'piggybacked' into the same intravenous line as the rehydration fluid. We do not recommend mixing the insulin with the rehydration fluid because the insulin infusion rate and the fluid rate or composition often require independent adjustments. Some centers recommend adding albumin or several ml of a patient's own plasma to the insulin solution to reduce adherence to plastic infusion tubing. We find this to be unnecessary, recommending instead that about 50 ml of the insulin solution be flushed through the tubing and discarded before initiating insulin delivery to the patient. This procedure saturates the infusion line with insulin and allows predictable insulin delivery to the patient.

Insulin has two primary roles in the treatment of DKA: to reduce excessive ketogenesis and the resultant metabolic acidosis, and to lower blood glucose levels by inhibiting excessive gluconeogenesis and enhancing glucose uptake by muscle and other insulin-sensitive tissues. Insulin should lower plasma glucose by 60–100 ml/dl per hour. If the glucose values are not falling at this rate after the first 2 hours of continuous insulin infusion, the insulin administration should be verified and the dose should be doubled. If glucose values are falling more rapidly than this, glucose may be given to reduce the rate of fall or the insulin infusion rate may be reduced. Regardless of the rate of fall, when the hourly monitored glucose value drops to 250 mg/dl, glucose should be added to the rehydrating solution.

The insulin infusion should be continued at the full effective rate until severe acidosis has begun to resolve (total plasma CO_2 above 10 mmol/l or arterial pH above 7.2). Urine ketones may remain strongly positive for up to 24–48 hours, and should not be used to decide when acidosis is resolving and insulin rates can be reduced. It is convenient to stop intravenous insulin at the time of a regularly scheduled subcutaneous insulin injection, such as before breakfast or supper. However, since the half-life of intravenously administered insulin may be as short as 7–15 minutes, intravenous insulin can be continued for the first 30–60 minutes after the first subcutaneous insulin is given, to provide continuous coverage and to prevent rebound hyperglycemia.

Electrolytes

Diabetic ketoacidosis in children is associated with severe, sometimes life-threatening losses of potassium, phosphate, sodium and other electrolytes. Serum potassium can be high, normal or low at the onset of therapy for DKA. Nevertheless, severe total body potassium depletion (100–200 mmol/m² body surface area) is present in nearly all cases, and potassium administration is nearly always required. Correction of metabolic acidosis and insulin infusion both lower serum potassium levels substantially during the first few hours of treatment by redistributing potassium from the extracellular to the intracellular space. Thus, even with elevated initial plasma potassium levels, prompt initiation of potassium replacement and periodic monitoring of the potassium level are usually essential during the first 2–4 hours of treatment.

At our center, potassium (30–40 mmol/l) is usually administered in the first bag of fluid after the initial volume expansion with normal saline or Ringer's lactate. Early administration of potassium is essential if the patient is 'normokalemic' or overtly hypokalemic at the onset of treatment. In these cases the concentration of potassium is adjusted upwards (40–60 mmol/l) as indicated by frequent monitoring. Hypokalemia can cause cardiac arrest, respiratory paralysis or ileus. If severe hyperkalemia (potassium values greater than 6.0 mmol/l) or acute renal failure is present, it may be necessary to withhold potassium until adequate urine flow is established or the serum potassium begins to fall. However, this is not common, and potassium is still an important part of the therapy of DKA even if significant hyperkalemia and azotemia are present initially. More frequent monitoring of electrolytes and fluid status is required in this situation, as well as bladder catheterization in the patient who is in shock or coma or unable to void regularly.

Subjects with DKA are usually phosphate-depleted as a result of urinary losses secondary to osmotic diuresis and acidosis. During treatment of DKA, serum phosphate tends to fall, often to below 2.0 mmol/l. Although this theoretically could lower ATP or 2,3-diphosphoglycerate (2,3-DPG) levels resulting in tissue hypoxia, it is unclear whether or not prevention of hypophosphatemia during treatment of DKA has any clinical value in preventing cardiac, respiratory or neurologic problems secondary to severe hypophosphatemia [62–64, 67, 68].

Three potassium salts are available: potassium phosphate, potassium acetate and potassium chloride. In our experience, the use of potassium chloride as the only source of potassium ion often compounds the hyperchloremic acidosis commonly seen after correction of DKA. Therefore, we use solutions containing 15–20 mmol/l each of potassium acetate and potassium phosphate. The phosphate helps offset some of the hypophosphatemia. The acetate, like lactate, is converted to bicarbonate by the patient and helps correct the metabolic acidosis. In hospitals where acetate solutions are not readily available, solutions containing a mixture of phosphate and chloride can be used. Potassium phosphate solution used alone can produce hypocalcemia.

During the correction of severe hyperglycemia, serum sodium levels should rise by about 1.6 mmol/l per 100 mg/dl decrement in blood glucose. Thus a fall in serum sodium to —or failure of sodium to increase from—levels approximating 130 mmol/l has been used as a criterion to switch to a hydrating fluid containing 100–150 mmol/l of sodium (i.e. 0.9% saline or Ringer's solution). As urine sodium losses from osmotic diuresis are usually about 50–70 mmol/l, this approach helps prevent hyponatremia and an excessive decline in hypertonicity during the first 24 hours of treatment.

We rarely find it necessary to use bicarbonate unless the initial blood pH is below 7.0. It has been our experience that severely ketoacidotic children usually do well without bicarbonate and that risks of bicarbonate use (hypokalemia, central nervous system acidosis and hypoxia, hypernatremia, and rebound alkalosis) generally outweigh its potential benefits [64, 69, 70]. If bicarbonate is used, bolus administration should be avoided; 44–88 mmol of bicarbonate can be added per liter of 0.2% saline and used as the hydration fluid. Bicarbonate should certainly be discontinued when arterial pH rises above 7.1 or when the venous CO_2 rises above 10 mmol/l.

Monitoring

Although the treatment of DKA in children often runs smoothly, attention must be paid to details [62–64]. If close monitoring and immediate laboratory support are not available, a well-coordinated transfer to an adequate hospital facility should be made early. Glucose should be checked hourly (bedside monitoring with glucose reagent strips is adequate) during continuous insulin infusion. Electrolytes, with special attention to potassium, sodium and CO_2, should be monitored at least every 2 hours initially and every 4–6 hours when the clinical situation has stabilized. Accurate accounting should be kept of fluid intake and output to be sure that fluid administration is adequate. Vital signs and neurologic checks should be made at least every 60 minutes during the first 8–12 hours or until the patient is alert and able to eat. Maintenance of an adequate airway and prompt intervention at the earliest signs of ventilatory failure are essential. Severe headache, urinary incontinence, cardiac arrhythmias, unstable blood pressure, blurred optic disks, fluctuating level of consciousness or apnea may be signs of impending cerebral edema. Lethargy, arreflexia or ileus may indicate hypokalemia or hypophosphatemia. Fever warrants evaluation and treatment for possible underlying infection. Appropriate studies to rule out underlying urinary or meningeal bacterial infection may be indicated. Gastric decompression and nasogastric drainage are advised in severe cases, especially if abdominal pain or repeated vomiting is present or the level of consciousness is reduced. Appendicitis should be considered and surgical consultation obtained early for severe or persistent abdominal pain. If abdominal surgical exploration is needed, it is better delayed several hours until severe acidosis is corrected.

Cerebral Edema

Children treated for DKA occasionally die soon after initiation of treatment in the setting of rapid and unexpected neurological deterioration [71–73]. These deaths commonly occur during the first 8–24 hours of treatment at a time when hyperglycemia, acidosis and dehydration are being corrected and patients appear to be improving clinically. Cerebral edema is the most common anatomical finding, although some patients may also exhibit vascular thrombosis, brain infarcts and intra or extracerebral hemorrhage.

Cerebral edema or an acute neurologic catastrophe was demonstrable or strongly suspected in 50% of 20 children who died within the first weeks after initial diagnosis of IDDM in the Pittsburgh area, but in only 9 (26%) of 35 deaths in children with longer than 1 month of known diabetes [74]. Cerebral edema thus constitutes the single leading cause of death among children with diabetes, particularly among children who die during treatment of new-onset diabetes. Delayed diagnosis seems the main factor contributing to death from cerebral edema in children with DKA [64, 74].

There is no single accepted explanation for cerebral edema or why cerebral edema seems to occur more commonly in children than in adults. Four categories of explanations have been proposed:

(1) rapid shifts in extracellular and intracellular osmolality;
(2) central nervous system acidosis;
(3) cerebral hypoxia;
(4) excessive fluid administration.

During the development of DKA, hyperglycemia increases the serum osmolality by approximately 1 mosm per 18 mg/dl increment in blood glucose. A child with an initial plasma glucose concentration of 900 mg/dl will tend to have an osmotic burden of 50 mosm secondary to hyperglycemia. This extracellular hyperosmolality is in part compensated for by movement of water out of cells with a resultant decrease in serum sodium by about 1.6 mmol/l per 100 mg/dl increment in plasma glucose [75].

Thus, in a patient with a plasma glucose concentration 800 mg/dl above normal, sodium levels would have decreased by 13 mmol/l. This water shift partially compensates for extracellular hyperosmolality, but still leaves the child in a dehydrated, hyperosmolar state.

Chronic hyperglycemia and hypertonicity result in the accumulation of osmotically active substances in the brain. Only about 50% of the accumulated osmoles are accounted for by glucose and its metabolites so that the remainder have been referred to as 'idiogenic osmoles' [76]. The formation of these osmoles may serve to protect brain cells from exhibiting marked shrinkage and the consequent vascular disaster that would occur if a shrunken brain mass were to tear away from the cranial vault and its bridging veins during development or correction of hypertonicity.

During treatment of DKA, large amounts of non-glucose-containing fluids and insulin are given. These rapidly reduce both serum osmolality and dehydration. During recovery, water is drawn into the relatively hypertonic brain cells and modest degrees of cerebral swelling and increased cerebrospinal fluid pressure are common [77, 78].

Although the mechanisms responsible for the more excessive swelling of brain cells in the 1–2% of children recovering from DKA who develop cerebral edema are unknown, it is likely that insulin has a critical role [64, 71–73, 79]. Cerebral edema does not occur in some animals whose hypertonicity is corrected rapidly, unless insulin is given [76, 80], and rarely occurs before insulin is given to children with DKA.

Van Der Meulen et al have proposed a hypothesis attempting to explain the development of cerebral edema [79]. Their model is based on the Na^+/H^+ antiport plasma membrane transporter which exchanges intracellular hydrogen ions with extracellular sodium. In ketoacidosis, excess ketoacids cross the blood–brain barrier and accumulate in brain cells. The *intracellular* hydrogen ion of the ketoacids is exchanged with *extracellular* sodium by means of activation of the Na^+/H^+ exchanger. The accumulation of excess sodium within brain cells neutralizes the anions of the ketoacids and helps restore intracellular pH. Osmotically obliged transport of water from the extracellular fluid space, due to increased intracellular osmolality and sodium ions, would cause brain cell swelling.

Several features of this model are attractive. First, the accumulation of excess ketoacids in brain cells would require relatively prolonged ketosis. Cerebral edema would not be expected with a rapid increase in glucose or correction of hyperosmolality without antecedent keto-acidosis. Second, the Na^+/H^+ transporter's activity is normally greatly *activated*, through allosteric regulation, by intracellular acidosis and *suppressed* by extracellular acidosis. Cerebral swelling would thus be expected during more rapid correction of extracellular than intracellular acidosis. Third, the Na^+/H^+ transporter's activity is enhanced by insulin. Thus, one could envisage a scenario in which development of ketoacidosis itself does not cause brain swelling because Na^+/H^+ transporter activity is held in check by low plasma insulin concentrations as well as by low extracellular pH. However, as insulin is given to treat DKA and/or extracellular acidosis is reduced rapidly, transporter activity increases suddenly, as persistent intracellular acidosis and insulin enhances transporter activity. Activation of the transporter causes expulsion of unwanted hydrogen ion but the consequent rapid intracellular shift of sodium and water causes cell swelling. In this model, too-rapid correction of systemic acidosis or the sudden exacerbation of intracellular acidosis (as with large amounts of bicarbonate administration) could help explain the paradoxical development of cerebral edema in patients who are initially improving. This model also accepts a contributing role for excessive iatrogenic decrements in serum osmolality and the movement of free water into relatively hypertonic brain cells. Clinical studies to test this hypothesis are lacking but might involve the use of pharmacologic agents such as amiloride that reduce Na^+/H^+ transporter activity [79].

It is known that bicarbonate administration in DKA can result in paradoxical intracerebral acidosis. This is due to the fact that carbon dioxide equilibrates more rapidly than bicarbonate across the blood–brain barrier. A sudden increase in serum bicarbonate with an increase in carbon dioxide (from reduction of hyperventilation) would result in accumulation of excess carbonic acid intracerebrally [81]. However, it is not likely that this paradoxical acidosis is the sole explanation for cerebral edema since this complication is seen even when large boluses of bicarbonate are not given, and more cautious bicarbonate administration has little effect on the relative acidosis of cerebrospinal fluid commonly seen during treatment of DKA [82].

Cerebral hypoxia sometimes leads to subsequent cerebral edema and has been incriminated as a cause of cerebral edema in children recovering from DKA. In DKA there is a marked depletion of 2,3-DPG which regulates the dissociation of oxygen from hemoglobin. The resultant tendency for decreased oxygen delivery to cells is partially compensated for by systemic acidosis which increases oxygen dissociation from hemoglobin. Rapid correction of systemic acidosis without restoration of decreased 2,3-DPG could thus exacerbate cerebral hypoxemia in the patient recovering from DKA. Administration of phosphate during DKA has been recommended as a measure to prevent and correct the severe hypophosphatemia that commonly accompanies recovery from DKA and may contribute to depletion of 2,3-DPG. However, restoration of 2,3-DPG levels does not occur until hours or days after full clinical recovery from DKA, and phosphate administration has never been shown to prevent the development of cerebral edema during recovery from DKA [67, 68]. Thus, although hypoxia may be a contributing factor in development of cerebral edema in children or myocardial infarction in adults, the use of phosphate to reduce these complications is not of any proven value.

Cerebral edema has been associated with initial rates of rehydration that exceed $4.0 \, l/m^2$ body surface area per day [71–72]. Patients who developed cerebral edema were more often given fluids at these higher rates than those who did not develop cerebral edema. A rapid fall in plasma sodium concentrations, absolute or values corrected for hyperglycemia (1.6 mmol per 100 mg/dl) are thought to reflect a relative excess of antidiuretic hormone that may increase the risk for cerebral edema [72, 83]. Other investigators, although not denying that excessive replacement with hypotonic fluids may be responsible for some cases of cerebral edema, point out that in many cases no evidence for excessive fluid replacement or rapid decrements in sodium are present at the time that cerebral edema is diagnosed in children with DKA [64, 73, 85]. Furthermore, higher rates of fluid replacement may have been chosen because of relatively more severe or prolonged dehydration and keto-acidosis in children who progressed to cerebral edema, in comparison to those who did not. Even the proponents of the excess hydration–hyponatremia theory of cerebral edema admit that in some cases, somewhat more than $4.0 \, l/m^2$ hydration may be required for short periods in the rare patient in whom urinary excretion rates equal or exceed hydration rates during the first 6–8 hours of treatment [72].

Fluid administration rates sometimes recommended for the treatment of DKA are largely derived from replacement rates recommended to correct (within 24 hours) childhood non-keto-acidotic dehydration due to diarrhea where cerebral edema is not a likely problem. What may be perfectly adequate treatment for dehydration associated with diarrhea may not be optimal for treating hypertonic dehydration where a more cautious approach may be more prudent. Slower rehydration during DKA may be better than the rapid approach because of some of the reasons considered above.

Because the incidence of cerebral edema may be only 1–2% or less of all children treated for DKA, clinical studies comparing the efficacy of various fluid-infusion rates will have a low power to detect a reduction in rates of cerebral edema unless very large numbers of patients are studied in a carefully controlled clinical trial.

There is evidence to suggest that some degree of cerebral edema may be common in children with DKA and that early intervention may reduce its occurrence [73, 85]. The use of computerized tomography and intracranial pressure monitors to assess cerebral edema may help in management [64]. More helpful are very close monitoring of the patient for the presence or development of early signs of cerebral edema and prompt initiation of treatment in suspect cases [85]. Treatment involves use of intravenous mannitol, reduction in the rates of fluid administration and possibly mechanical hyperventilation to help reduce brain swelling. Dexamethasone and furosemide are frequently administered but are of no proven value. Early consultation with a neurologist and/or neurosurgeon is indicated. Although relatively large doses (1 g/kg body weight) of mannitol have been used [72], we prefer relatively smaller doses (0.2 g/kg over 30 minutes) with repeated doses at hourly intervals as indicated by the clinical response. Supportive measures and intensive monitoring are essential. Patients who present with evidence of brain herniation and diabetes insipidus due to acute cerebral edema seldom recover and many die [73, 85].

LONG-TERM TREATMENT

Goals for long-term therapy of IDDM should include (a) avoidance of severe ketosis and hypoglycemia; (b) maintenance of clinical and psychological well-being, including normal growth and development; (c) reduction of symptomatic hyperglycemia or hypoglycemia; and (d) institution of preventive measures for long-term complications such as retinopathy, neuropathy, nephropathy and macrovascular disease [62–64]. The day-to-day therapeutic regimen for the management of IDDM includes six major components: insulin, meal plan, exercise, monitoring, education and family psychosocial support.

Insulin

Insulin regimens used to treat IDDM vary from a single daily injection of intermediate-acting insulin—neutral protamine Hagedorn (NPH) or Lente—to highly intensive regimens requiring three or more daily injections or continuous subcutaneous insulin infusion (CSII, or the 'insulin pump'). After the first year of IDDM, most children with type 1 diabetes cannot achieve freedom from symptoms and clinical well-being with a single daily injection of NPH or Lente insulin. On the other hand, few children and adolescents require or do best on highly intensive insulin regimens requiring insulin injections and blood glucose monitoring four or more times a day. Therefore, the most common regimen used in children is the so-called 'split-mixed' regimen. Regular and NPH insulin are mixed in the same syringe and administered twice a day, usually before breakfast and supper. We do not recommend premixing these insulins in the bottle because this makes independent adjustments of the rapid and intermediate-acting insulins impossible and could reduce the rapid absorption of the regular insulin. We usually start newly diagnosed patients on total daily doses of 0.60–0.75 U/kg. Rapidly growing adolescents, and those recently recovering from DKA or those with an infection, can be expected to be somewhat insulin resistant and may need more; patients diagnosed before the onset of ketonuria and who are unusually lean or active often need less.

About two-thirds of the total starting insulin dose is given in the morning, and one-third is given before supper. The pre-breakfast dose consists of about one-third of regular insulin and two-thirds of NPH insulin, whereas the starting pre-supper dose is usually divided into equal amounts of regular and NPH insulin. If the morning fasting glucose measurement before initiation of insulin therapy is under 150 mg/dl and there are no ketones, the NPH portion of the evening dose is often omitted.

We do not recommend spending several days calculating total insulin requirements using regular insulin every 4–6 hours and then starting twice-daily mixtures. We prefer instead to give both regular and NPH from the outset of therapy, as soon as DKA has resolved, and to make initial adjustments during the first 2–3 days. After education is complete, more realistic adjustments of insulin dose are made by telephone consultations at home.

After initiation of therapy, insulin doses can be adjusted based on blood glucose monitoring and symptoms of hypoglycemia and hyperglycemia. During the first few weeks of therapy, many children will begin to produce some insulin again and very little insulin may be needed to achieve excellent glycemic control during this time—the 'honeymoon period'. There is now evidence suggesting that endogenous insulin secretion can be sustained for longer periods with efforts that maintain lower mean blood glucose levels during this 'honeymoon period' [56–57]. As discussed earlier, this period can last months or longer in some adolescents and young adults, but tends to be of shorter duration in prepubertal children. As the honeymoon period comes to an end, insulin requirements will increase gradually over several weeks or months. Before puberty, most children will require about 0.6–0.9 U/kg per day. During puberty, however, insulin requirements can increase to as much as 1.0–1.5 U/kg per day as the growth spurt reaches its peak [86]. As the pubertal growth spurt ends, insulin needs will often drop to below 1.0 U/kg per day.

Ideally, the rapid-acting insulin given before breakfast and supper (or lunch if an intensive regimen is being used) should be given at least 30 minutes before the meal so that higher plasma

Table 1 Insulin timing and adjustment algorithm

Blood glucose (mg/dl)	Minutes before meal	Dosage change
Below 70	15	Subtract 2 U regular insulin
70–150	30	None
150–180	45	None
Above 180	60	Add 1 U regular insulin
Above 240	60	Add 2 U regular insulin

insulin levels coincide with peak insulin needs during the first 60 minutes after eating. We instruct patients to vary the timing of the insulin injection relative to the meal, depending on self-measured blood glucose levels before breakfast and supper. For blood glucose measurements in the normal or slightly elevated range, insulin is given 30 minutes before meals; for higher pre-meal blood glucose values, a longer delay is recommended; and for lower glucose values, a shorter delay [62, 87]. An example of such a timing and dose adjustment algorithm is shown in Table 1. Typical supplemental doses are 1–2 U for a 20-kg child and 2–4 U for a 60-kg adolescent.

The use of 'waiting times' is based on our experience (as well as that of others [62, 87, 88]) that allowing 30–60 minutes extra for absorption of subcutaneous regular insulin will greatly reduce postprandial glucose excursions. An alternative response to preprandial hyperglycemia is to increase the preprandial insulin dose by a few units to compensate for hyperglycemia. Although this approach may reduce hyperglycemia before the next meal, it is less effective in reducing postprandial hyperglycemia than is waiting an extra 30–60 minutes for a lower dose to work. Using a longer waiting time also minimizes the risks of subsequent hypoglycemia due to relative hyperinsulinemia seen 3–6 hours after subcutaneous injection when large increases in insulin doses are used in a 'sliding scale' pattern [89].

Normal physiologic patterns of insulinemia with more rapid increments in plasma insulin levels during the first hour and rapid decrements after the first hour are currently impossible to replicate with the insulin preparations available at present. This situation could be remedied with more rapidly absorbed forms of insulin. One approach would be to give insulin via the nasal route using a fine spray of insulin that is modified to increase absorption [90]. This approach has not gained widespread use because of problems with inefficient and erratic absorption and possible harmful effects to the nasopharyngeal mucosa. New insulin analogs of 'custom tailored' or monomeric insulins, produced by recombinant DNA technology, are under development to allow for more rapid absorption and use as optimal 'pre-meal' insulins [91].

After the initial dosage adjustments, further changes in insulin dose are made, based on glucose monitoring before meals, at bedtime and sometimes at 2 a.m. Two types of adjustments can be made [89]. The first is to adjust the dosage because of a persistent pattern of hypoglycemia or hyperglycemia at a specific time of day. Such patterns should be present over a period of 1–2 weeks before a change is made. Adjustments of the insulin dose should be made primarily when no other preventable causes for the high or low blood glucose levels are found. For example, it makes no sense to reduce a morning regular insulin dose on a Tuesday if an individual low blood glucose value before lunch on Monday resulted from an irregular period of morning exercise that day. When an adjustment is being made, the insulin dosage most likely to be responsible for the abnormal glucose should be increased or decreased by 1–3 U every 3–4 days until the desired effect is seen. We wait to see the effect of this change over several days before making further adjustments. This form of adjustment in insulin dose is possible only when families have been shown how to measure blood glucose reliably at home, and is made initially under professional supervision based on blood glucose measurements performed at home by the patient or family while the patient is following a preplanned meal plan and a normal level of physical activity. With practice, adolescents and families are often able to make these adjustments on their own with periodic assistance from a physician or nurse specialist. Indeed, a major goal of modern outpatient management is to transfer much of the responsibility for intermediate-term management to the well-instructed, well-motivated and increasingly self-sufficient patient and family.

A second type of insulin dosage adjustment occurs in response to individual blood glucose measurements or circumstances in which insulin needs are likely to be different. These changes include increasing (or decreasing) the dose and waiting time between injection and meals if a blood glucose measurement is high (or low) before a specific meal, as in Table 1, and adjustments due to anticipated changes in usual dietary intake or exercise. Alterations of this kind may also be necessary during common febrile illnesses [60] (see 'Sick Day Management' later), during prolonged stress or at certain times in the menstrual cycle in young women. Once again, these changes, referred to by some as a 'sliding scale', 'sliding time' or 'sliding dose', should be made based on blood glucose measurements by patients who have been thoroughly trained, are carefully supervised, can be relied upon to take and record accurate readings and who have been shown to be able to follow telephone and written instructions reliably. These changes cannot be made based on urine glucose measurements.

These new self-management techniques are fairly sophisticated. They are characteristic of changes in treatment approaches developed during the 1980s which have now become standard practice in larger specialty centers. They rely on individual 'consumer training', with transfer of much of the responsibility for day-to-day management from the physician to the patient and an 'empowered' patient approach. Training can be tedious and time-consuming, and requires resources of patient educators who are in short supply in some areas of North America and who are often poorly compensated by short-sighted third-party insurance coverage. Because of this, it is our opinion that all children and adolescents with newly diagnosed IDDM should obtain intensive education in modern self-management in a center with the necessary resources and experience to conduct training and assume responsibility for follow-up care. These programs, described later in this chapter, often involve 20 or more hours of individual instruction over a period of 4–5 days.

We start all newly diagnosed patients on human insulin. However, no systematic attempt is made to switch patients using beef or pork insulin to human insulin preparations unless poor metabolic control, allergy or significant lipodystrophy necessitates a change in insulin type. We instruct patients not to switch from one species of insulin to another without careful supervision because the pharmacokinetics of different insulins may vary between species and manufacturer. Generally, it is assumed that human intermediate-acting insulins have a slightly more rapid absorption and shorter duration than comparable pork insulins [92]. In some patients this can cause problems with hypoglycemia at 3–5 hours, or more often hyperglycemia at 6–12 hours after injection.

There is some concern that human insulin, because it is more lipophilic, might have a different action in nervous tissue [93–95]. The reported increase in severe hypoglycemia and hypoglycemia unawareness after the transfer from pork to human insulin has been thought to be related to the simultaneous intensification of treatment in these patients, as well as to the new understanding that some degree of hypoglycemia unawareness is a common, unavoidable problem in all patients with IDDM as one attempts to sustain lower glycemic levels [95–99].

Noctural hypoglycemia (hypoglycemia between midnight and 8 a.m.) and the 'dawn phenomenon' (rising blood glucose between 4 a.m. and 8 a.m.) are common in children with diabetes of several years' duration who attempt to achieve optimal glycemic control with a twice-daily injection regimen. This problem is partly due to the fact that nocturnal insulin requirements are lower at 1 a.m. to 3 a.m. than at 6 a.m. to 8 a.m. [100–101]. Attempting to replace overnight insulin requirements using a 5 p.m. to 6 p.m. dose of NPH or Lente insulin to normalize 6–8 a.m. blood glucose levels tends to produce hypoglycemia at 1–3 a.m. In children and young adults treated with two daily insulin injections, nocturnal hypoglycemia rarely results in hyperglycemia at 6–8 a.m. (Somogyi phenomenon) unless there has been dietary overtreatment of hypoglycemia [102, 103]. Adjustments in nocturnal insulin should be made based on 1–3 a.m. as well as pre-breakfast blood glucose measurements. Occasionally, the pre-supper NPH or Lente dose has to be moved from 5–6 p.m. to bedtime, increasing the total number of daily injections from two to three but reducing the problems associated with too much insulin at 1–3 a.m. as well as too little insulin at dawn. Long-acting insulin (Ultralente) may also be helpful in this setting.

Over the last decade, intensive insulin therapy using multiple (three or more) daily insulin injections (MDII) or CSII has increased in popularity [89]. Intensive insulin therapy is not discussed here. However, it has been our experience that CSII or MDII therapy is complex and should be reserved for exceptionally well-motivated and well-organized families. For the most part, the use of intensive insulin therapy regimens (using targets [89] that may or may not be appropriate for extraordinarily motivated adults) in children and adolescents is not nearly as successful as it is in the carefully selected and highly motivated adult subjects often reported in the literature [104–107]. Intensive insulin therapy should not be used in children who repeatedly fail to monitor their blood glucose, to take their insulin regularly and to follow detailed instructions [105]. In these children simpler, not more arduous, treatment methods and higher glucose targets are used. Insulin infusion pumps and complex treatment regimens probably create more problems than they solve in adolescents with behavioral, psychiatric or adjustment problems trying to escape from their responsibilities.

Meal Plan

The primary goals of dietary management of IDDM in children and adolescents are to provide adequate nutrition for normal growth and development and to provide predictable composition and distribution of nutrients so that the insulin dose can be calculated to give a relatively stable pre-meal blood glucose concentration. Except in obese subjects or in the rare obese teenager with type 2 diabetes, energy restriction is not a primary goal of dietary management in children with IDDM [105]. Therefore, we prefer the term 'meal plan' to the term 'diet' [62]. The meal plan should be derived as much as possible from the patient's previous eating habits and food preferences ascertained by an experienced dietitian.

In order to meet these dietary goals, we utilize an American Diabetes Association (ADA) exchange diet [105]. The ADA diet provides 15–20% of daily energy intake from protein, 30–35% from fat and the remainder (45–65%) from carbohydrate. Attempts should be made to reduce cholesterol intake to below 300 mg per day and maintain a ratio of polyunsaturated to saturated fat (P : S ratio) of at least 2 : 1. These restrictions in dietary fat are not necessary in children below school age. Carbohydrates should be varied, but attempts should be made to minimize the ingestion of highly refined simple sugars.

The overall energy needs of children and adolescents with well-controlled IDDM are similar to those of children without IDDM. These energy needs vary with age, sex, pubertal status, level of activity and other factors. We use a 'rule of thumb' to provide an initial estimate of total daily energy needs as 1000 kcal plus 100 kcal per year of age. During puberty and in vigorously active children, this calculation may underestimate the actual needs. After puberty, this calculation usually overestimates the needs, and reduction in energy intake is often needed, especially in relatively sedentary girls. The above calculation is only used as an initial guideline. The energy intake is individually adjusted for each patient based on his or her appetite and pattern of weight gain. Normal-weight children rarely have to go to extremes in calculating total daily energy intake precisely, but should not have to resort to regular 'cheating' in order to gain access to, or avoid, food.

Consistency in the distribution of energy intake, especially carbohydrate-derived energy, throughout the day is the most important factor in the meal plan. We utilize three meals and two or three snacks per day. Breakfast, lunch and supper each contain approximately 25–30% of the daily energy intake. A midafternoon snack (to correspond to the peak action of the pre-breakfast NPH or Lente insulin) provides about 5–10% of the energy. A bedtime snack (to help prevent nocturnal hypoglycemia) provides another 5–10%. We recommend some protein in the bedtime snack in the hope that it will delay carbohydrate absorption and provide more protection against nocturnal hypoglycemia. Midmorning snacks are not taken by all but are suggested in the very young child (younger than 7–8 years old) or in those prone to pre-lunch hypoglycemia as a result of long delay (more than 4–5 hours) between breakfast and lunch.

We utilize an 'exchange system' in which foods are divided into six groups: bread, fruit, milk, meat, fat and vegetable. Items in each group contain similar amounts of carbohydrate, protein and fat. Initially, families are taught to measure and weigh foods to be sure that the correct quantity is given. However, this is rarely necessary beyond the first few weeks.

Exercise

Regular exercise is an important and often underutilized component of diabetes management. Exercise lowers blood glucose concen-

tration acutely by increasing the glucose uptake of exercising muscle and by enhancing insulin absorption from subcutaneous injection sites. In addition to improving insulin sensitivity and diabetic control, exercise tends to lower blood pressure and plasma cholesterol and helps control weight.

Like the meal plan, exercise is best if done on a consistent schedule. However, as this is not always feasible, patients who exercise irregularly should either eat extra food before unscheduled vigorous or prolonged exercise or should measure blood glucose before and during exercise and consume extra carbohydrate if the glucose level is so low that a decline of 50–60 mg/dl per hour is likely to cause a problem.

Two specific precautions regarding exercise need to be considered in children with IDDM. First, in the face of ketonuria and severe hyperglycemia, exercise can result in worsening hyperglycemia and ketosis or can even precipitate ketoacidosis. In this situation, some insulin should be administered and allowed to 'start working' before a bout of exercise is initiated. Second, the risk of hypoglycemia may be increased for at least 12 hours after a period of prolonged exercise. Patients should be alerted to this possibility and encouraged to monitor the effects of vigorous exercise on their own. They should take individualized preventive measures the night following vigorous exercise; these measures could include eating a larger bedtime snack or having a parent measure their blood sugar at 2 a.m.

Monitoring

As stated previously, blood glucose determinations, using reagent strips with or without reflectance meters, have replaced urine monitoring as the preferred method of monitoring glycemic control of IDDM. Careful instruction of the patient regarding techniques and what to do with the information is essential, as are measures to ensure accurate monitoring over the long term. We request that our patients measure blood glucose before each meal and at bedtime. However, children and adolescents often prefer not to measure blood glucose before lunch. Urine glucose measurements are not necessary in patients who measure blood glucose regularly, but they should be used for those who refuse to perform daily self-monitoring of blood glucose. Although a variety of glucose meters have built-in memories, we nevertheless ask children to write down their results in a log-book which is analyzed weekly by the family and at each visit to the office (usually every 2–4 months) or as needed over the telephone between office visits.

Ketonuria is an indicator of starvation or insulin deficiency and can result from inappropriate insulin dosage, infection or prolonged stress. We recommend measurement of urinary ketones whenever blood glucose is above 240 mg/dl for more than 4 hours or during any illness regardless of blood glucose. The presence of moderate to large amounts of urinary ketones is an indicator that 'sick day rules' may need to be implemented [60].

Glycated hemoglobin or HgbA$_{1c}$ levels are used as a measure of long-term glycemic control and reflect the average blood glucose concentration over the preceding 2–3 months. Methods and normal ranges for glycated hemoglobin vary considerably between laboratories. Therefore, it is best to use one reliable laboratory for all samples. We rarely measure glycated hemoglobins more often than once a month or less often than every 4 months.

It is inappropriate to state specific goals for blood glucose or glycated hemoglobin levels that can be applied to all patients. Goals need to be determined in association with the more general goals of therapy outlined earlier. Few subjects with IDDM can achieve and maintain normal blood glucose and glycated hemoglobin levels long term. After the first year of IDDM, we most often set goals of preprandial blood glucose between 80 mg/dl and 200 mg/dl (4.4–11.1 mmol/l) and glycated hemoglobin below 9.0%, which correspond to mean glucose values below 200 mg/dl. Unrealistic goals often lead to failure, frustration and non-compliance.

Special Considerations of Criteria for Metabolic Control in Children

A major practical problem in managing families in which a child is affected by IDDM arises when the anxiety, fear and helplessness seen at diagnosis are replaced within a few weeks by the reassurance, confidence and feeling of accomplishment of the 'honeymoon period'. Hard work seems to be rewarded by good results with blood glucose values rarely rising above 200 mg/dl, even after dietary indiscretions or failures to maintain a rigid schedule. However, at the end of the honeymoon period, blood glucose control deteriorates and major unexplained fluctuations in blood glucose are common or result from trivial deviations from the treatment plan. At this time parents commonly blame themselves for becoming too lax and attempt to restore 'good control' with overzealous attention to details of diet, insulin and other forms of badgering. Children rapidly learn that their parents' concern and anxiety as well as their own welfare are not well served by reporting too high or too low blood glucose values, or admitting that they have deviated from their treatment plan. These reactions are not helped if physicians or other health professionals assume attitudes that encourage patients to conclude that wider fluctuations in blood glucose control are the consequence of poor motivation, inability to follow instructions or some other family or adolescent deficiency, rather than realize that the prescribed treatment is suboptimal or that the rigid goals of the honeymoon period are no longer practical, realistic or safe.

We try to help children and families during this transition period by predicting its occurrence as well as by helping them learn how to adjust their regimen to their evolving absolute insulin deficiency [106, 107]. One helpful strategy is to widen the level of acceptable control so that insulin dose adjustments are made on a weekly basis. For example, during the honeymoon period patients may be asked to analyze their morning and evening glucose measurements over 7 consecutive days. If a simple majority of the morning glucose results are over a given upper limit (for example) 160–180 mg/dl), a 1–2 unit increase in the evening NPH insulin is made and the impact of this and other changes assessed on successive weeks. In the meantime, adjustments are made on a daily basis (see Table 1) in response to individual glucose values, and occasional fluctuations are accepted as a natural evolution of IDDM.

As daily insulin requirements increase at the end of the honeymoon period, simply increasing insulin doses results in more frequent episodes of severe hypoglycemia. As this occurs, the target limits can be expanded so that fluctuations of preprandial glucose values below 70 mg/dl or over 200 mg/dl once or twice a week are not viewed as sufficient criteria to adjust insulin doses long term. The goal is to have patients accept occasional glucose deviations as a manifestation of the inherent weaknesses of the treatment regimen, rather than to view them as a failure to comply with a perfect regimen. The regimen is not perfect. The patient who at 3 months after diagnosis has a mean blood glucose (measured three or four times daily) of 140 mg/dl (7–8 mmol/l) will have a $HgbA_{1c}$ concentration of 7%. By the end of the first year of IDDM, mean $HgbA_{1c}$ levels commonly increase to 9%, indicating a 60 mg/dl increase in mean blood glucose to 200 mg/dl; in addition, wider fluctuations in individual glucose values are present. Efforts to intensify the treatment regimen to bring $HgbA_{1c}$ values back to 7% or below will double or triple the risk of severe hypoglycemia [108, 109].

Based on the treatment methods that evolved during the 1980s in a growing number of specialized treatment centers for patients with IDDM, new criteria have been proposed to define good and poor metabolic control [105]. These criteria are centered, in part, on previous criteria of normal growth, development and adjustment, with avoidance of severe hypoglycemia and ketoacidosis and absence of signs and symptoms related to polyuria [62–64]. They now include three additional criteria: daily blood glucose measurements, periodic assays of glycated hemoglobin, and measurements of blood lipids and of blood pressure.

In our center we no longer routinely employ urine glucose measurements in the day-to-day management of IDDM. All children, even neonates, are expected to have two to four blood glucose measurements every day. Urine glucose measurements are done in fewer than 2% of our diabetic patients; mostly those with NIDDM, mentally deficient patients and a few patients who have refused to switch to blood glucose measurements because of phobia to blood sampling. Patients treated with two or three daily injections of insulin are considered to be in poor metabolic control if mean preprandial glucose values are over 200 mg/dl, and in excellent control if mean preprandial glucose values are below 160 mg/dl ($HgbA_{1c}$ values of 9% and 7%, respectively). Children with glycated hemoglobin values below 7% who have frequent (more than three episodes per year) severe hypoglycemia requiring glucagon or hospitalization are not considered to be in good metabolic con-

trol. In infants and toddlers, the glycemic goals are slightly higher.

Glycated hemoglobin assays provide reliable estimates of mean blood glucose levels over the previous 8–12 weeks. Using high-performance liquid chromatography of red cells treated to eliminate labile (aldimine) glucose adducts, normal $HgbA_{1c}$ values are $5.0 \pm 1.0\%$ (mean $\pm 2\,SD$). Assays that measure total $HgbA_1$ by ion-exchange chromatography usually have normal values 1–2% higher. Both of these assays may produce 'falsely elevated' values in the presence of hemoglobin F which comigrates with $HgbA_1$ and 'falsely low' values with certain hemoglobin variants (e.g. hemoglobin S or C). Median $HgbA_{1c}$ values in a large population of IDDM patients attending the Steno Memorial Hospital clinics in Copenhagen are 9.0% with less than 10% of patients below 7.0% (C. Binder, personal communication). The majority of patients are treated with two or three daily insulin injections and only 2–3% are on insulin pumps. In the Diabetes Control and Complications Trial the mean $HgbA_{1c}$ values between 1984 and 1989 among patients treated with two daily injections of insulin was 9.0–9.3%, whereas more intensively treated patients (three or more injections in all, about one-third on insulin pumps) had mean values of 7.0–7.3% between 1983 and 1989 [109]. Very few (less than 5%) of patients maintained $HgbA_{1c}$ in a normal range (below 6.0%) except during pregnancy.

Results in a large population-based study of IDDM patients diagnosed before age 30 years in Wisconsin revealed mean total glycated hemoglobin values of 13.5% (comparable to a $HgbA_{1c}$ value of 11.8%); 25% of these patients' values were above 14.2% and 25% below 10.8% [110]. These patients were followed for 4 years during the 1980s, and their initial total glycated hemoglobin value was found to be a very potent predictor of both the progression of minimal background retinopathy as well as the development of proliferative retinopathy. Those with total glycated hemoglobin values on the initial examination above 13.5% were 3–6 times more likely to have retinal deterioration than those with values below 10.8% or an equivalent $HgbA_{1c}$ value of 9.1%. Similar results were observed among diabetic children followed in Denver where mean glycated hemoglobin values during the early and mid-1980s were correlated with the development of early retinopathy and microalbuminuria [111]. These data suggest that $HgbA_{1c}$ values below 9% confer some protection against the development of microvascular disease when compared with values above 11%.

In the DCCT, efforts were made during the 1980s to reduce baseline mean $HgbA_{1c}$ from 9% to below 6% and to maintain this difference for 7–10 years. This large clinical trial is still ongoing so that the extent of reduction of $HgbA_{1c}$ on initial appearance or progression of early retinopathy, the time needed to achieve any reductions and the overall cost–benefit ratio remain to be determined [109]. Already determined, however, is the fact that highly intensive therapy resulted in higher $HgbA_{1c}$ values in adolescents than adults and increased the rates of severe hypoglycemia threefold [108, 109].

The American Diabetes Association guidelines, and our own, for the treatment of IDDM are based largely on results similar to those indicated above [105, 112, 117]. Good control for young patients with IDDM is now defined as patients who are well adjusted, do not have frequent severe hypoglycemia and have $HgbA_{1c}$ values of 7–9%. Patients having $HgbA_{1c}$ values above 11% (or total hemoglobin A_1 values above 12–13% depending on the assay used) are considered to be in poor control and at higher risk for complications of the eyes and kidneys.

It should be noted that the prepubertal child with IDDM is relatively protected against the development of microvascular complications [113]. The mechanisms responsible for this protection are unknown but could involve an interplay between growth factors, sex steroids, hemodynamic factors and other undefined factors. Furthermore, it is possible that the children under school age may be at higher risk for developing unwanted neurologic sequelae following repeated bouts of severe hypoglycemia [114]. Thus, we recommend that prepubertal children be treated somewhat less aggressively than young adults in terms of target glucose levels.

Approximately 30% of children with IDDM have serum total cholesterol or triglyceride values above the 95th percentile for normal values adjusted for age, sex and race [115]. Elevations are usually modest, and are most common with $HgbA_{1c}$ values above 11%. They are only minimally affected by restriction of cholesterol intake and saturated fat intake, but are reduced by lowering $HgbA_{1c}$ values. Well-controlled IDDM patients should also have

normal blood pressure, as hypertension can have a negative impact on microvascular disease in young adults with IDDM.

Education and Psychosocial Support

During the first few days after initial diagnosis, the families of diabetic children must be taught the skills of diabetes-related care and must acquire a good understanding of the principles underlying the pathophysiology of diabetes and its symptoms. This is often best done by healthcare professionals other than physicians, such as nurse educators, social workers and dietitians, working as part of an experienced team. We use one of two excellent teaching tools for children [116, 117]. The following knowledge and skills are necessary:

(1) signs and symptoms of hyperglycemia, hypoglycemia and DKA;
(2) insulin administration;
(3) techniques for measuring blood glucose, urine glucose and urinary ketones;
(4) treating hypoglycemia, including the use of glucagon;
(5) planning a meal using an ADA exchange diet;
(6) treating the patient during sick days and exercise.

These skills are taught in modules during the first 3–4 days after admission or recovery from DKA. The content of these modules is given in Tables 2–11. (Education modules for children with diabetes mellitus, developed by St Louis Children's Hospital, Department of Nursing, and Washington University's Department of Pediatrics—Endocrinology and Metabolism.)

Methods for insulin dosage adjustments are considered only after the family has had more time to make initial adjustments to the fact that a child has diabetes. Much of this instruction occurs after discharge and perhaps not until the end of the honeymoon period. It is important to realize that the sudden onset of diabetes, and the fear of the family related to this diagnosis, may reduce the ability of the family to learn effectively about the diabetic regimen. All patient education has to be adjusted appropriately to the child's intellectual development and the individual family's ability to assimilate a massive amount of new information. Diabetes education and training only begin during the initial hos-

Table 2 Module 1: initial family assessment

Date	Initial	
_____	_____	Introduce self, unit staff, dietitian, and social worker
_____	_____	Basic explanation of treatment and length of hospitalization
_____	_____	Interview family in regards to support systems: other family members, main caretakers, babysitters, working parents, religious beliefs, other diabetic relatives, educational background, daily family routines of parents and child, when parents can be present for education
_____	_____	Assess financial status and medical insurance benefits
_____	_____	Assess signs and symptoms of hyperglycemia experienced in the last two months
		If diagnosed with diabetes prior to this hospitalization assess:
_____	_____	meals and snacks (exchanges)
_____	_____	use of waiting times
_____	_____	relationship of exercise to blood glucose levels
_____	_____	blood glucose testing times
_____	_____	knowledge of insulin times
_____	_____	knowledge of insulin dosage adjustments
_____	_____	diabetic ketoacidosis experienced in last two months
_____	_____	signs and symptoms of hypoglycemia:
		severity:
		time:
		frequency:

Table 3 Module 1: initial family assessment—basic physiology and ketoacidosis

Date reviewed	Initial	Date reinforced	Initial	
_____	_____	_____	_____	Type 1 vs type 2 diabetes
_____	_____	_____	_____	Genetics and environmental triggers in children
_____	_____	_____	_____	Basic physiology of pancreas, insulin and B cells
_____	_____	_____	_____	Why insulin cannot be given as a pill
_____	_____	_____	_____	Importance of insulin
_____	_____	_____	_____	Honeymoon—explanation and consequences: reduced need for insulin
_____	_____	_____	_____	Signs of hyperglycemia (thirsty, ↑ urinating, exhausted, headache) and common reasons for their appearance
_____	_____	_____	_____	Signs of ketoacidosis (nausea, vomiting, stomach ache, Kussmaul respirations, acidotic breath) and common reasons for their appearance
_____	_____	_____	_____	Emphasize: nothing you could have done would have prevented diabetes
_____	_____	_____	_____	Emphasize: diabetes caused by several genes. *Each* parent is a carrier for mostly silent genes
_____	_____	_____	_____	Emphasize: unless your child has diabetes as a newborn or as a result of corticosteroids or L-asparaginase, it will most likely be permanent

Table 4 Module 2: hypoglycemia and insulin reactions

Date reviewed	Initial	Date reinforced	Initial	
				Hypoglycemia
___	___	___	___	Signs and symptoms of hypoglycemia (shaky, sweaty, sleepy *very* hungry, pale, dizzy, combative) during the day and reasons
___	___	___	___	Signs, symptoms of hypoglycemia (restless, sleepwalk, sleeptalk) at night and reasons
___	___	___	___	Common causes of hypoglycemia: missed meal or snack, ↑ exercise, too much insulin, alcohol
___	___	___	___	Treatment of hypoglycemia
___	___	___	___	Role of epinephrine (adrenaline) and glucagon in ↑ blood sugar
___	___	___	___	Glucagon use and storage in cool place required; not to exceed 85° F and not to freeze
___	___	___	___	If child passes out or has seizure *give glucagon IM*
				Insulin actions
___	___	___	___	Types and species (beef, pork, human)
___	___	___	___	Time actions of regular begins 1/2 hour; peaks 2–3 hours
___	___	___	___	Time actions of NPH begins 1 hour; peaks 6–8 hours
___	___	___	___	Time actions of Ultralente
___	___	___	___	Importance of peak insulin times to hypoglycemia
___	___	___	___	Effect of circadian rhythms on night-time glucose levels especially ↓ hormones and ↓ blood sugar especially with NPH peak 2–4 a.m. and ↑ hormones and ↑ blood sugar and ↓ insulin 5–8 a.m.
___	___	___	___	Relationship of food, exercise and insulin injections to blood glucose levels (food ↑ blood sugar; exercise ↓ blood sugar; insulin ↓ blood sugar)
___	___	___	___	Times and reasons for blood glucose testing and urine ketone testing at home
___	___	___	___	Need for individualized diabetic regimen schedule for both usual school and weekend home schedule
___	___	___	___	Need for individualized diabetic regimen for summer (i.e. changes in exercise schedule and increased need to check for ↓ glucose sugars, possibility of need to ↑ snacks)
___	___	___	___	Need for individualized diabetic regimen for days with unusual, prolonged physical activity

pitalization. The process of education and training continues during the following months and years and is continuously modified and individualized to meet the goals set for the patient [105, 107].

Whenever feasible, as many family members as possible need to be involved in initial education. Both parents should be taught the basics of diabetes care, even if one parent is primarily responsible for child care. In general, children over 8 years old should be taught the skills of the regimen and encouraged to perform them with parental support and supervision. Insulin injections can often be given by children as young as 8–9 years old, and should certainly be self-administered by most children aged 11–12 years.

We think that exclusion of parents from the initial education of adolescents is a bad idea, because it eliminates the parents as a source of support and a resource for continued adherence during adolescence [106, 107]. Lack of parental support during adolescence has been associated with poorer metabolic control.

As mentioned earlier, education and long-term follow-up of children with diabetes, and their families, are best performed using a team approach. This team should include a physician, a nurse educator, a dietitian, and a psychologist, psychiatrist or social worker experienced with childhood diabetes. As much as possible, patient education should be concentrated on a hospital service or clinic where the nursing and dietary

Table 5 Module 3: diabetic skills—mixing and injecting insulin and demonstration of blood glucose monitoring machines

Date reviewed	Initial	Date reinforced	Initial	
_____	_____	_____	_____	Explanation of insulin syringe parts—plunger, barrel, unit markings, 3/10 cc syringe, 5/10 cc syringe, 1 cc syringe, needle, bevel
_____	_____	_____	_____	Differences in types of insulin syringes: BD, Terumo, Monoject
_____	_____	_____	_____	Demonstration of mixing Regular and NPH insulin by RN
_____	_____	_____	_____	Demonstration of insulin injection technique by RN including: pinch up skin and fat, insert at a 90-degree angle, aspirate to check for blood, rotate syringe before removing needle
_____	_____	_____	_____	Injection sites and importance of rotating sites (from arms to abdomen one week to legs and abdomen the next week) to avoid lipohypertrophy
_____	_____	_____	_____	Return demonstration of mixing and injecting insulin by parents
_____	_____	_____	_____	Return demonstration of mixing and injecting insulin by child
_____	_____	_____	_____	Return demonstration of mixing and injecting insulin by significant others (sitters, grandparents)
_____	_____	_____	_____	Demonstration of urine ketone testing using Ketostix
_____	_____	_____	_____	Return demonstration of urine ketone testing
_____	_____	_____	_____	Storage of insulin (environmental temperature not to exceed 85° F)
_____	_____	_____	_____	Demonstration of the usage of two to three blood glucose monitoring meters
_____	_____	_____	_____	Demonstration of two to three different types of blood glucose strips (visual and machine)
				Return demonstration on meter and blood glucose strips of choice:
_____	_____	_____	_____	by child
_____	_____	_____	_____	by parents
_____	_____	_____	_____	by significant other(s)

staff are familiar with diabetes education and the specific needs of the diabetic child and family. Recently, we have demonstrated that a seven-session, year-long education and training program based on the appropriate use of self-monitoring of blood glucose and administered by a non-physician health care professional can result in substantially improved blood glucose control during the first 2 years after diagnosis of IDDM [118].

ADDITIONAL CONSIDERATIONS

Hypoglycemia

Hypoglycemia can occur in IDDM when insulin replacement is excessive, when meals are delayed or deficient in carbohydrate, or as a result of exercise. Hypoglycemia is most common before lunch and supper, after exercise, and between 1 a.m. and 4 a.m. Mild hypoglycemia activates adrenergic and cholinergic mechanisms that can result in shakiness, nervousness, palpitations, sweating and hunger; it can be expected to occur two or three times a week in most well-controlled diabetic individuals, and is treated by giving 5–15 g carbohydrate.

Severe hypoglycemia, manifested by neurologic impairment, may occur after unrecognized or inappropriately handled mild hypoglycemia, or it may occur without any warning. This latter event is more likely to occur in those with 'hypoglycemia unawareness' or 'defective glucose counterregulation'—often a result of absent glucagon and blunted epinephrine responses to hypoglycemia [119, 120]. Every attempt should be made to prevent severe hypoglycemia. If severe hypoglycemia should occur, intramuscular glucagon (0.5–1.0 mg) will raise the blood glucose concentration within 10–15 minutes but often causes vomiting. Glucagon should be followed by ingestion of carbohydrate and by examination and discussion with the physician.

Table 6 Module 4: insulin dose adjustments

Date reviewed	Initial	Date reinforced	Initial	
_____	_____	_____	_____	Explanation of times that dose will need to be increased or decreased—illness, puberty, growth spurts, increased or decreased activity, menses, times of stress
_____	_____	_____	_____	Need to keep accurate daily records of blood glucose tests
_____	_____	_____	_____	Explanation of what and how necessary information needs to be recorded in relation to insulin dosages and blood glucose values, exercise, dose adjustments and other notes
				Discuss principles of dose adjustments
				Explanation of how much the dose will need to be increased or decreased:
_____	_____	_____	_____	change by ½ unit with preschoolers
_____	_____	_____	_____	change by 1 unit with school-age
_____	_____	_____	_____	change by 1–2 units with adolescents
				Practice making dose adjustments by role playing with blood glucose diary
_____	_____	_____	_____	mother
_____	_____	_____	_____	father
_____	_____	_____	_____	child
_____	_____	_____	_____	significant other(s)
_____	_____	_____	_____	Identification of weekly or biweekly patterns of blood glucose levels and when to call for insulin dose changes
_____	_____	_____	_____	Meaning of glycated hemoglobin

Generally, a family member of every person taking insulin should be trained to administer glucagon and instructed to give it in case of severe hypoglycemia when the patient is unable to eat. Training the patient only is ineffective. Even though all families are taught how and when to give glucagon, less than half of the patients at our center use it when needed. Similar experiences have been reported by others in children [121].

Nocturnal (1 a.m. to 4 a.m.) hypoglycemia is relatively frequent and can have several causes [102]. These include 2–3 a.m. activity from the suppertime NPH, the failure to take a bedtime snack, and unusually severe physical activity the previous day. Blood glucose measurements are often recommended at 2 to 3 a.m. especially when the suppertime or bedtime dose of intermediate insulin is being adjusted to lower morning glucose levels. Every attempt should be made to keep the 2–3 a.m. blood glucose value above 65 mg/dl. This can usually be done without marked morning hyperglycemia (above 180 mg/dl). The main purpose of bedtime glucose monitoring is safety, as bedtime insulin supplements are seldom used in children except during illness. Supplements to bedtime snacks are used, however, if bedtime glucose is low. These usually consist of extra milk, cheese, peanut butter or complex carbohydrate.

Sick Day Management

Illness presents a specific management problem for subjects with IDDM [60]. Insulin administration must be continued during sick days, even if the patient is unable to eat. As infection may cause insulin resistance, the insulin dose may need to be increased. It is best to give the supplemental insulin needed during illness in the form of regular insulin. A dose equivalent to about 10–20% of the total daily dose every 4–6 hours, or more frequently, may be needed to control severe hyperglycemia and ketosis. Blood glucose monitoring is essential and should be performed every 2–4 hours. It is also essential that urinary ketones be monitored during intercurrent illness, even if blood glucose is being measured. The presence of moderate to large ketonuria is an indication for additional insulin or a visit to a physician regardless of the level of blood glucose. Carbohydrate must be given

Table 7 Module 4: application of diabetes care knowledge

Date reviewed	Initial	Date reinforced	Initial	
				Problem solving with concrete age-appropriate situations
				Hypoglycemia
———	———	———	———	shopping mall
———	———	———	———	park
———	———	———	———	float trip
———	———	———	———	camping
———	———	———	———	skiing
———	———	———	———	sport events
———	———	———	———	movie theater
———	———	———	———	night time
				Hyperglycemia
———	———	———	———	before sport events/activities
———	———	———	———	after sport events/activities
———	———	———	———	during infections, growth
				Ketoacidosis (before and after)
———	———	———	———	sport events
———	———	———	———	infection
———	———	———	———	exercise
———	———	———	———	with 'normal' blood glucose
———	———	———	———	with high blood glucose values
				Snacks
———	———	———	———	in relation to bedtime blood glucose $\leqslant 120$ mg/dl
———	———	———	———	in relation to bedtime blood glucose of 120–250 mg/dl
———	———	———	———	in relation to bedtime blood glucose > 250 mg/dl
———	———	———	———	whether or not to include a.m. and p.m. snack
				When you need to increase or decrease a snack
———	———	———	———	morning
———	———	———	———	afternoon
———	———	———	———	bedtime
———	———	———	———	with exercise
———	———	———	———	use of waiting times to keep blood glucose levels even
———	———	———	———	Need to call before traveling overseas to arrange for insulin, meals, names of foreign insulins, how to find diabetologist

during sick day management to prevent the occurrence of hypoglycemia secondary to supplemental insulin. Fluids must be taken to prevent dehydration.

The single most important factor in determining a diabetic patient's ability to cope with any given intercurrent illness is the presence of vomiting and the ability to retain liquids taken by mouth. During illness, oral hydration should be attempted. It is best to use frequent small quantities (85–225 ml every hour) of 'clear liquids'. Solid foods and milk products should be temporarily eliminated from the diet. When blood glucose values are above 250 mg/dl, ingested clear liquids should not contain carbohydrate (diet soda, unsweetened tea). After glucose levels drop below 250 mg/dl, carbohydrate-containing liquids such as regular soda, clear juices, flavored gelatin dessert or glucose drinks should be used. If fluids cannot be retained as a result of repeated vomiting, medical intervention for intravenous fluid therapy is necessary to prevent ketoacidosis, hypoglycemia or dehydration.

The etiology of an intercurrent illness should be sought and treated as necessary. It is import-

Table 8 Module 5: sick day management

Date reviewed	Initial	Date reinforced	Initial	
				What to do:
_____	_____	_____	_____	If blood glucose value is greater than 250 mg/dl, then check for ketones in urine
_____	_____	_____	_____	If child has stomach/abdominal pain, then call endocrine doctor on call
_____	_____	_____	_____	If ketones present, drink 8–12 oz fluid × 2 hours and retest, and if ketones still present call endocrine doctor on call
_____	_____	_____	_____	If child vomits × 2 or more (vomit × 1 = free), then call endocrine doctor on call
_____	_____	_____	_____	If blood glucose value in range and has ketones, then call for insulin dose
_____	_____	_____	_____	If night-time hypoglycemia occurs, then give ½ glass orange juice
_____	_____	_____	_____	How to handle emergencies:
				when to call _____
				who to call _____
				if no one answers, call; _____ ask for diabetes doctor on call immediately
_____	_____	_____	_____	If child can't eat, then use full and/or clear liquid diet

ant to remember that diabetic children are susceptible to the same illnesses as non-diabetic children. If infection is present, it should be treated. Although DKA itself can cause abdominal pain, tenderness and vomiting, appendicitis or other acute abdominal conditions must also be considered. In general, the same indications for the therapy of infection should be used in diabetic as in non-diabetic children. It is important to realize that DKA alone can cause an elevated white blood cell count and a shift to the left, even in the absence of infection. Although many over-the-counter medications and antibiotic preparations contain sugar, this is usually not a major problem, especially since more insulin may need to be given because of the illness itself and the 10–20 kcal in sweetened cough syrups, for example, is a comparatively small amount.

Surgery also presents a specific problem for the diabetic child. Minor elective surgery should be performed in the morning before breakfast. Many insulin regimens have been recommended (see Chapter 31). We recommend that about half of the usual morning dose of intermediate-acting insulin be given; small doses of regular insulin are added if the blood glucose level is high. Blood glucose should be monitored every 1–2

Table 9 Module 5: discharge planning

Date reviewed	Initial	Date reinforced	Initial	
_____	_____	_____	_____	Diabetes quiz _____ taken and passed with 80% accuracy
_____	_____	_____	_____	Incorrect or doubtful answers discussed
_____	_____	_____	_____	Discharge Rx's given—insulin, glucagon, and blood testing supplies
_____	_____	_____	_____	Follow-up appointment made to outpatient endocrine offices
_____	_____	_____	_____	Family instructed to call the endocrine fellow or nurse daily for dose adjustment
				FAX No. _____
				Telephone No. _____
				Emergency No. _____

Table 10 Module 6: nutrition checklist

Day 1	
_____	Nutritional history taken and compared to hospital ordered meal pattern
_____	Change ordered hospital diet to reflect child's usual eating pattern
_____	Provide family, and patient, if age appropriate, rationale of meal pattern, focusing on need for balance, timing of meals and consistency required
_____	Give exchange booklet and begin explanation of content
Day 2	
_____	Explanation of ADA exchanges and guidelines
_____	Importance of CHO distribution throughout day
_____	Need for balance of 20% protein, 30% fat and 50% CHO (approximate balance)
_____	Instruction on exchanges with booklet
_____	Explain how various foods affect the blood glucose level differently
_____	Provide rationale for keeping fat less than 30% of kcals
_____	Discuss 'diet', 'lite', and 'dietetic' foods
_____	Fills out hospital menu according to exchanges allowed and writes appropriate amounts of each item; child should do this with parent, if appropriate cognitive development present
_____	Assignment to write out a typical menu for use at home
Day 3	
_____	Review explanation of diet
_____	Review menu and discuss corrections if needed
_____	Give 'Eats and Treats' booklet and discuss
_____	Sick day management and basic explanation of replacement CHO
_____	Prepare sick day menu to replace CHO at each meal
_____	Explanation of exercise guidelines
_____	Discuss holiday or special days' menus
_____	Discuss importance of label reading
_____	Discuss how to convert a product with an appropriate label to exchanges
Day 4	
_____	Discuss use of 'fast foods'
_____	Prepare one meal of 'fast foods' into allotted exchanges
_____	Provide phone number for questions, encourage family to contact if any questions should arise

Dietitian _____

Date _____

hours. Intravenous glucose is used to keep the blood glucose levels between 200 mg/dl and 250 mg/dl. For major surgery or emergency surgery, intravenous insulin with intravenous fluids and hourly glucose monitoring should be used. The dose required is usually 15 ± 5 mU/kg body weight per hour with a maintenance infusion containing 5% glucose. The insulin infusion can be adjusted hourly with operating-room measurement of blood glucose. The goal of treatment is to maintain blood glucose concentration at about 150 mg/dl before, during and after surgery. Whenever possible, the patient should not be anesthetized if ketoacidosis is present.

Long-term Complications

A detailed discussion of long-term complications, their risk factors and management is presented in Chapters 52–60. However, long-term complications of diabetes mellitus can emerge during late adolescence. Background retinopathy (microaneurysms, dot hemorrhages, exudates) requires evaluation by an ophthalmologist and yearly follow-up [105]. We gen-

Table 11 Module 7: Social service checklist

Initial	*Psychosocial/family/child assessment*
_____	Assess parents' emotional response to diagnosis, family structure and supportiveness, ability to communicate with each other, life-style including daily routine, ability to learn, problem-solving ability, financial status, cultural or religious considerations
_____	Assess parent/child relationship
_____	Assess child's reaction to diagnosis and medical procedures, child's behavior at home and school, child's grades, possible learning problems, attendance record
_____	Identify family factors or stresses that might interfere with adjustment and adherence to the regimen (i.e. single-parent family, other health problems in the family, financial problems). Did family respond appropriately to child's symptoms prior to diagnosis?
	Education/support
_____	Discuss emotional reactions to diagnosis. Explain grief process
_____	Discuss prior knowledge of diabetes/parents' fears. Correct misconceptions
_____	Reassure patient and family of competence and support of medical staff. Familiarize with diabetes program and functions of diabetes team
_____	Discuss reactions of parents and child to medical procedures (testing, injections, etc.). Suggest ways to ease trauma and reinforce child's efforts. Teach parents behavioral reinforcement technique
_____	Discuss possible effects of diabetes on child's behavior, home life, social life and school performance. Discuss importance of maintaining appropriate discipline
_____	Discuss possible effects of diabetes on parents and siblings
_____	Discuss patient's return to school. Provide teacher literature. Discuss ways to keep diabetes from interference with school experience
_____	Help child anticipate return to school, including telling friends, sticking to the diet, parties, outings, etc. Discuss child's feelings, fears and concerns
_____	Help family plan diabetes care task assignments, i.e. who will do what at home. Be sure father is included and child is assigned age-appropriate tasks
_____	Discuss problem-solving approach to diabetes care and realistic expectations of diabetes control
_____	Familiarize patient and family with community supports, support groups
_____	Give family opportunity to discuss their concerns. What problems do they anticipate? Help with beginning problem-solving efforts or refer to appropriate staff for assistance
_____	Help shape effective parenting behaviors by reinforcing parents efforts to utilize learnings from diabetes classes and counseling

erally ask patients with IDDM to have a baseline examination at diagnosis and repeat examinations at 5 years after diagnosis and then yearly. Evidence of sudden worsening of vision or proliferative retinopathy (neovascularization, preretinal hemorrhage) requires immediate referral to an experienced ophthalmologist. Renal failure secondary to diabetes is rare before the age of 20 years. However, microalbuminuria can develop as a first sign of diabetic nephropathy during adolescence. Close follow-up and aggressive treatment of hypertension are necessary. Whether 'tight' glycemic control prevents or reverses the microvascular complications of diabetes remains unknown and awaits results of the DCCT. Children with IDDM commonly have limited joint mobility and stiffness of the hands and fingers, which seem to place them at

increased risk for long-term complications of the eyes and kidneys later in life [105, 122].

Diabetic neuropathy can cause paresthesia or pain (peripheral neuropathy), or autonomic dysfunction (orthostatic hypotension, gastroparesis, bladder dysfunction, impotence). Gastroparesis can be difficult to differentiate from bulimia or other eating disorders of adolescents. Paresthesia or painful peripheral neuropathy has been reported to respond to improved glycemic control, but may remit spontaneously in some cases. Other interventions to prevent, retard or reverse diabetes complications are under study.

Lastly, it is important that all children with diabetes be evaluated at least yearly by a person experienced in the care of children with this disorder. It is a mistake to consider children merely as small adults, or to communicate exclusively with the adolescent or the parent. The child must be educated, trained and managed by personnel familiar with the developmental and psychologic issues that arise commonly in children. Referral to a center specializing in the care of the preschool child and adolescent should be performed by all primary-care physicians whenever possible. In many areas, primary-care physicians do not routinely accept primary responsibility for managing children with diabetes when specialty centers are readily available.

REFERENCES

1. LaPorte RE, Fishbein HA, Kuller LH et al. The Pittsburgh insulin dependent (IDDM) registry: the incidence of insulin-dependent diabetes mellitus in Allegheny County, Pennsylvania (1965–1976). Diabetes 1981; 30: 279–84.
2. Diabetes Epidemiology Research International Group. Geographic patterns of childhood insulin dependent diabetes mellitus. Diabetes 1988; 37: 1113–19.
3. Drash A. Diabetes mellitus in the child: classification, diagnosis, epidemiology, and etiology. In Lifshitz F (ed.) Pediatric endocrinology. New York: Marcel Dekker, 1990: pp. 663–80.
4. Siemiatycki J, Colle E, Campbell S et al. Incidence of IDDM in Montreal by ethnic group and by social class and comparisons with ethnic groups living elsewhere. Diabetes 1988; 37: 1096–12.
5. LaPorte RE, Tajima N, Akerbloom H et al. Geographic differences in the risk of insulin dependent diabetes mellitus: the importance of registries. Diabetes Care 1985; 8 (suppl.): 101–7.
6. Cruick-Shanks KJ, LaPorte RE, Dorman JS et al. The epidemiology of insulin dependent diabetes mellitus: etiology and prognosis. In Ahmad PI (ed.) Coping with juvenile diabetes. Springfield, Ill: CC Thomas, 1985: pp 332–57.
7. Christau B, Kromann H, Christy M et al. Incidence of insulin-dependent diabetes mellitus (0–29 at onset) in Denmark. Acta Med Scand 1979; 624 (suppl.): 54–60.
8. Amiel SA, Sherwin RS, Simonson DC, Lauritano AA, Tamborlane WV. Impaired insulin action in puberty: a contributory factor to poor glycemic control in adolescents with diabetes. New Engl J Med 1986; 315: 215–19.
9. MacDonald MH. Hypothesis: the frequencies of juvenile diabetes in American blacks and caucasians are consistent with dominant inheritance. Diabetes 1980; 29: 110–15.
10. Rayfield EJ, Ishimura K. Environmental factors and insulin dependent diabetes mellitus. Diabetes Metab Rev 1987; 3: 925–57.
11. Kong YC, Lewis M. Animal models of autoimmune endocrine diseases: diabetes and thyroiditis. In Volpe R (ed.) Autoimmune diseases of the endocrine system. Boca Raton, Fla: CRC Press, 1990: pp 23–50.
12. Ginsberg-Fellner F, Witt ME, Fedun B et al. Diabetes mellitus and autoimmunity in patients with the congenital rubella syndrome. Rev Inf Dis 1985; 7 (suppl.): 170–6.
13. Schatz DA, Winter WE, Maclaren NK. Immunology of insulin-dependent diabetes. In Volpe R (ed.) Autoimmune diseases of the endocrine system. Boca Raton, Fla: CRC Press, 1990: pp 241–96.
14. Bruining GJ, Molenaar JL, Grobbee DE et al. Ten-year follow-up study of islet-cell antibodies and childhood diabetes mellitus. Lancet 1989; i: 1100–3.
15. Srikanta S, Ganda OP, Eisenbarth GS, Soeldner JS. Islet-cell antibodies and beta cell function in monozygotic triplets and twins initially discordant for Type I diabetes mellitus. New Engl J Med 1983; 308: 322–5.
16. Srikanta S, Ganda OP, Rabizadeh A, Soeldner JS, Eisenbarth GS. First-degree relatives of patients with Type I diabetes mellitus: islet-cell antibodies and abnormal insulin secretion. New Engl J Med 1985; 313: 461–4.
17. Gorsuch AN, Spencer KM, Lister J et al. Evidence for a long prediabetic period in type I (insulin-dependent) diabetes mellitus. Lancet 1981; ii: 1364–5.
18. Riley WJ, Maclaren NK, Krischer J et al. A prospective study of the development of diabetes in relatives of patients with insulin-dependent diabetes. New Engl J Med 1990; 323: 1167–72.
19. Everhardt MS, Wagener DK, Orchard TJ et al. HLA heterogeneity of insulin-dependent diabetes mellitus at diagnosis: the Pittsburgh IDDM study. Diabetes 1985; 34: 1247–52.
20. Nerup J, Mandrup-Poulsen T, Molvig J et al. Mechanisms of pancreatic B-cell destruction in Type I Diabetes. Diabetes Care 1988; 11 (suppl. 1): 16–23.
21. Bougnères PF, Carel JC, Castano L et al. Factors associated with early remission of type I diabetes in children treated with cyclosporine. New Engl J Med 1988; 318: 633–70.
22. Feutren G, Papoz L, Cessa R et al. Cyclosporin increases the rate and length of remissions in insulin-dependent diabetes of recent onset. Results of a multicenter double-blind trial. Lancet 1984; ii: 119–23.
23. Silverstein J, Maclaren NK, Riley W. Immunosuppression with azathioprine and prednisone in

recent-onset insulin-dependent diabetes. New Engl J Med 1988; 319: 599–604.

24. Toniolo A, Onodera T, Yoon JW, Notkins AL. Induction of diabetes by cumulative environmental insults from viruses and chemicals. Nature 1980; 288: 383–5.

25. Karam JH, Lewitt PA, Young CW et al. Insulinopenic diabetes after rodenticide (Vacor) ingestion: a unique model of acquired diabetes in man. Diabetes 1980; 29: 971–8.

26. Like AA, Rossini AA. Streptozotocin-induced pancreatic insulitis: new model of diabetes mellitus. Science 1976; 193: 415–18.

27. Karam JH, Prosser PT, Lewitt PA. Islet cell surface antibodies in a patient with diabetes mellitus after rodenticide ingestion. New Engl J Med 1979; 299: 1191.

28. Keller RJ, Eisenbarth GS. Immunopathogenesis of Type I diabetes mellitus. In Eisenbarth GS (ed.) Immunotherapy of diabetes and selected autoimmune diseases. Boca Raton, Fla: CRC Press, 1989, pp 1–23.

29. Sinhsa AA, Lopez MT, McDevitt HO. Autoimmune diseases: the failure of self tolerance. Science 1990; 248: 1380–8.

30. Gepts W, LeCompte PM. The pancreatic islets in diabetes. Am J Med 1981; 70: 105–15.

31. Bottazo GF, Florin-Christensen A, Doniach D. Islet-cell antibodies in diabetes mellitus with autoimmune polyendocrine deficiencies. Lancet 1974; ii: 1279–83.

32. Trucco M, Dorman JS. Immunogenetics of insulin-dependent diabetes mellitus in humans. Crit Rev Immunol 1989; 9: 201–45.

33. Baekkeskov S, Aanstoot H-J, Christgau S et al. Identification of the 64K autoantigen in insulin-dependent diabetes as the GABA-synthesizing enzyme glutamic acid decarboxylase. Nature 1990; 347: 151–6.

34. Unanue ER, Beller DI, Christopher YL, Allen PM. Antigen presentation: comments on its regulation and mechanism. J Immunol 1984; 132: 1–5.

35. Singal DP, Blajchman MA. Histocompatibility (HLA) antigens, lymphocytoxic antibodies and tissue antibodies in patients with diabetes mellitus. Diabetes 1973; 22: 429–32.

36. Nepom GT. Immunogenetics of HLA-associated diseases. Concepts immunopathol 1988; 5: 80–105.

37. Rodey GE, White NH, Frazer TE, Duquesnoy RJ, Santiago JV. HLA-DR specificities among Black Americans with juvenile-onset diabetes. New Engl J Med 1979; 301: 810–12.

38. Todd JA, Bell JI, McDevitt HO. HLA-DQ beta gene contributes to susceptibility and resistance to insulin-dependent diabetes mellitus. Nature 1987; 329: 599–604.

39. Morell PA, Dorman JS, Todd JA et al. Aspartic acid at position 57 of the DQ beta chain protects against type I diabetes: a family study. Proc Natl Acad Sci USA 1988; 85: 8111–15.

40. Baisch JM, Weeks T, Giles R et al. Analysis of HLA-DQ genotypes and susceptibility in insulin-dependent diabetes mellitus. New Engl J Med 1990; 322: 1836–41.

41. Atkinson MA, Maclaren NK. What causes diabetes? Scient Am 1990; July: 62–71.

42. Bottazo GF, Foulis AK, Bosi E et al. Pancreatic B-cell damage: in search of novel pathogenic factors. Diabetes Care 1988; 11 (suppl. 1): 24–8.

43. Ramsdell S, Fowlks BJ. Clonal deletion versus clonal anergy: the role of the thymus in inducing self tolerance. Science 1990; 248: 1342–8.

44. Gottlieb PA, Rossini AA, Mordes JP. Approaches to prevention and treatment of IDDM in animal models. Diabetes Care 1988; 11 (suppl.): 29–36.

45. Barnett AH, Eff C, Leslie RDG, Pyke DA. Diabetes in identical twins. A study of 200 pairs. Diabetologia 1981; 20: 87–93.

46. Warram JH, Krolewski AS, Gottlieb MS, Kahn CR. Differences in risk of insulin dependent diabetes in offspring of diabetic mothers and diabetic fathers. New Engl J Med 1984; 311: 149–53.

47. Fort P, Lanes R, Dahlam S. Breast feeding and insulin dependent diabetes mellitus in children. J Am Coll Nutr 1986; 5: 435–41.

48. Tillit H, Kobberling J. Age-corrected empirical genetic risk estimates for first-degree relatives of IDDM. Diabetes 1987; 36: 93–9.

49. Blethen S, White NH, Santiago JV, Daughaday WH. Plasma somatomedins, endogenous insulin secretion, and growth in transient neonatal diabetes mellitus. J Clin Endocrinol Metab 1981; 32: 144–7.

50. Younger D, Brink SJ, Barnett DM et al. Diabetes in youth. In Marble AE et al (eds) Joslin's Diabetes, 12th ed. Philadelphia: Lea & Febiger, 1985: pp 485–519.

51. Fajans SS. Scope and heterogeneous nature of MODY. Diabetes Care 1990; 13: 49–64.

52. Rodman HM, Doershuk CF, Roland JM. The interaction of two diseases: diabetes mellitus and cystic fibrosis. Medicine 1986; 65: 389–97.

53. Whitecare JP, Bodey GP, Hill CS, Samaan NA. Effect of L-asparaginase on carbohydrate metabolism. Metabolism 1970; 19: 581–6.

54. National Diabetes Data Group. Classification and diagnosis of diabetes mellitus and other categories of glucose intolerance. Diabetes 1979; 28: 1039–57.

55. Riley WJ, Winter WE, Maclaren NK. Identification of insulin-dependent diabetes mellitus

before the onset of clinical symptoms. J Pediatr 1988; 112: 314–16.

56. Shah SC, Malone JI, Simpson NE. A randomized trial of intensive insulin therapy in newly diagnosed insulin-dependent diabetes mellitus. New Engl J Med 1989; 320: 550–4.

57. DCCT Research Group. Effects of age, duration and treatment of insulin-dependent diabetes mellitus on residual B-cell function: observations during eligibility testing for the Diabetes Control and Complications Trial (DCCT). J Clin Endocrinol Metab 1987; 65: 30–6.

58. Riley WJ, Maclaren NK, Krischer J et al. A prospective study of the development of diabetes in relatives of patients with insulin-dependent diabetes. New Engl J Med 1990; 323: 1167–72.

59. Betterle C, Presotto F, Pedini B et al. Islet cell and insulin autoantibodies in organ-specific autoimmune patients: their behavior and predictive value for the development of type I (insulin-dependent) diabetes mellitus. A 10-year follow-up study. Diabetologia 1987; 30: 292–7.

60. Levandoski LA, White NH, Santiago JV. How to weather the sick day season. Diabetes Forecast 1983; 36: 30–3.

61. White NH, Santiago JV. Clinical features and natural history of brittle diabetes in childhood. In Pickup JC (ed.) Brittle diabetes. Oxford: Blackwell, 1985: pp 19–28.

62. White NH, Santiago JV. Diabetes mellitus in children and adolescents. In Rakel RE (ed.). Conn's Current therapy. Philadelphia: WB Saunders, 1988, pp 473–80.

63. Sperling MA. Diabetic ketoacidosis. Pediatr Clin North Am 1984; 31: 591.

64. Krane EJ. Diabetes ketoacidosis. Biochemistry, physiology, treatment and prevention. Pediatr Clin North Am 1987; 34: 935–60.

65. Heber D, Molitch ME, Sperling MA. Low-dose continuous insulin therapy for diabetic ketoacidosis: prospective comparison with 'conventional' insulin therapy. Arch Int Med 1977; 137: 1377–82.

66. Fisher JN, Shahshahani MN, Kitabchi AE. Diabetic ketoacidosis: low-dose insulin therapy by various routes. New Engl J Med 1977; 297: 238–43.

67. Keller U, Berger W. Prevention of hypophosphatemia by phosphate infusion during treatment of diabetic ketoacidosis and hyperosmolar coma. Diabetes 1980; 29: 87–92.

68. Wilson HK, Keuer SP, Lea AS et al. Phosphate therapy in diabetic ketoacidosis. Arch Int Med 1982; 142: 417.

69. Assal JP, Aoki TT, Manzano FM et al. Metabolic effects of sodium bicarbonate in management of diabetic ketoacidosis. Diabetes 1974; 23: 405.

70. Lever E, Jaspan JB. Sodium bicarbonate therapy in severe diabetic ketoacidosis. Am J Med 1983; 75: 263.

71. Duck SC, Weldon VV, Pagliara AS, Haymond MW. Cerebral edema complicating therapy for diabetic ketoacidosis. Diabetes 1976; 25: 111–15.

72. Duck SC, Kohler E. Cerebral edema in diabetic ketoacidosis. J Pediatr 1981; 98: 674–80.

73. Garre M, Boles JM, Garo B et al. Cerebral edema in diabetic ketoacidosis: do we use too much insulin? Lancet 1986; i: 220–2.

74. Dorman JS, LaPorte RE, Kuller LH et al. The Pittsburgh insulin-dependent diabetes mellitus morbidity and mortality study. Mortality results. Diabetes 1984; 33: 271–6.

75. Katz MA. Hyperglycemia-induced hyponatremia. New Engl J Med 1973; 289: 843–4.

76. Arieff AI, Kleeman CR. Studies on mechanisms of cerebral edema in diabetic comas. Effects of hyperglycemia and rapid lowering of plasma glucose in normal rabbits. J Clin Invest 1973; 52: 571–83.

77. Clements RS, Blumenthal AS, Morrison AD, Winegrad AI. Increased cerebrospinal-fluid pressure during treatment of diabetic ketoacidosis. Lancet 1971; ii: 671–5.

78. Krane EJ, Rockoff MA, Wallman JK, Wolfsdorf JI. Subclinical brain swelling in children during treatment of diabetic ketoacidosis. New Engl J Med 1985; 312: 1147–51.

79. Van Der Meulen JA, Klip A, Grinstein S. Possible mechanism for cerebral edema in diabetic ketoacidosis. Lancet 1987; ii: 306–8.

80. Clements RS, Prockop LD, Winegrad AI. Acute cerebral edema during treatment of hyperglycemia. Lancet 1968; ii: 384–6.

81. Ohman JL, Marliss EB, Aoki TT et al. The cerebrospinal fluid in diabetic ketoacidosis. New Engl J Med 1971; 284: 283.

82. Munk P, Freedman MH, Levison H et al. Effect of bicarbonate on oxygen transport in juvenile diabetic ketoacidosis. J Pediatr 1974; 84: 510.

83. Harris GD, Fiordalisi I, Fineberg L. Safe management of diabetic ketoacidemia. J Pediatr 1988; 113: 65–8.

84. Winegrad AI, Kern EFO, Simmons DA. Cerebral edema in diabetic ketoacidosis. New Engl J Med 1985; 312: 1184–5.

85. Rosenbloom AL. Intracerebral crisis during treatment of diabetic ketosis. Diabetes Care 1990; 13: 22–33.

86. Blethen SL, Sargeant DT, Whitlow MG, Santiago JV. Effect of pubertal stage and recent blood glucose control on plasma somatomedin C in children with insulin-dependent diabetes mellitus. Diabetes 1981; 30: 868–72.

87. Witt MF, White NH, Santiago JV. Roles of site

and timing of the morning insulin injection in type I diabetes. J Pediatr 1983; 103: 528–33.

88. Dimitriadis GD, Gerich JE. Importance of timing of preprandial subcutaneous insulin administration in the management of diabetes mellitus. Diabetes Care 1983; 6: 374–8.

89. Hirsch IB, Farkas-Hirsch R, Skyler JS. Intensive insulin therapy for treatment of type I diabetes mellitus. Diabetes Care 1990; 13: 1265–83.

90. Salzman R, Manson JE, Griffin GT et al. Intranasal aerosolized insulin. New Engl J Med 1985; 312: 1078–84.

91. Work in this area is being conducted by Eli Lilly in the USA, Novo-Nordisk in Denmark and other groups. (L. Heding and J. Galloway, personal communication.)

92. Galloway JA. Treatment of NIDDM with insulin agonists or substitutes. Diabetes Care 1990; 13: 1209–39.

93. Berger WG, Althaus BU. Reduced awareness of hypoglycemia after changing from porcine to human insulin in IDDM. Diabetes Care 1987; 10: 260–1.

94. Teuscher A, Berger WG. Hypoglycemia unawareness in diabetics transferred from beef/pork insulin to human insulin. Lancet 1987; ii: 382–7.

95. Gale EAM. Hypoglycemia and human insulin. Lancet 1989; 2: 1264–6.

96. Cryer PE. Human insulin and hypoglycemia unawareness. Diabetes Care 1990; 13: 538–40.

97. Heller SR, MacDonald IA, Herbert IM, Tattersall RB. Influence of sympathetic nervous system on hypoglycemic warning symptoms. Lancet 1987; ii: 359–63.

98. Simonson DC, Tamborlane WV, DeFronzo RA, Sherwin RS. Intensive insulin therapy reduces the counterregulatory hormone responses to hypoglycemia in patients with type I diabetes. Ann Intern Med 1985; 103: 184–90.

99. DCCT Research Group. Severe hypoglycemia in the DCCT. Am J Med 1991 (in press).

100. Clarke WL, Haymond MW, Santiago JV. Overnight basal insulin requirements in fasting insulin-dependent diabetics. Diabetes 1980; 29: 78–80.

101. Bolli GB, Gerich JE. The 'dawn-phenomenon' —a common occurrence in both non-insulin-dependent and insulin-dependent diabetes mellitus. New Engl J Med 1984; 310: 746–52.

102. Shalwitz RA, Farkas-Hirsch R, White NH, Santiago JV. Prevalence and consequences of nocturnal hypoglycemia among conventionally treated children with diabetes mellitus. J Pediatr 1990; 116: 685–9.

103. Tordjman KM, Havlin CE, Levandoski LA, White NH, Santiago JV, Cryer PE. Failure of nocturnal hypoglycemia to cause fasting hyperglycemia in patients with insulin-dependent diabetes mellitus. New Engl J Med 1987; 317: 1552–9.

104. Schade D, Santiago J, Rizza R, Skyler J. Intensive insulin therapy. Amsterdam: Excerpta Medica, 1988.

105. Sperling MA, ed. Physician's guide to insulin-dependent (type I) diabetes. Alexandria, Va: American Diabetes Association, 1988.

106. Anderson BJ, Miller JP, Auslander WF, Santiago JV. Family characteristics of diabetic adolescents: relationship to metabolic control. Diabetes Care 1981; 4: 586–94.

107. Drash AL, Becker DJ. Behavioral issues in patients with diabetes with special emphasis on the child and adolescent. In Rifkin H, Porte D (eds) Ellenberg and Rifkin's Diabetes mellitus: theory and practice, 4th edn. New York: Elsevier, 1990: pp 922–34.

108. DCCT Research Group. The Diabetes Control and Complications Trial (DCCT): results of the feasibility study. Diabetes Care 1987; 10: 1–19.

109. DCCT Research Group. Diabetes Control and Complications Trial (DCCT): update. Diabetes Care 1990; 13: 427–33.

110. Klein R, Klein BE, Moss SE et al. Glycosylated hemoglobin predicts the incidence and progression of diabetic retinopathy. JAMA 1988; 260: 2864–71.

111. Chase HP, Jackson WE, Hoops SL et al. Glucose control and the renal and retinal complications of insulin-dependent diabetes. JAMA 1989; 261: 1155–60.

112. Santiago JV. Control in diabetes: the good, the bad, and the complications. Hosp Practice 1989; (suppl. 1): 5–17.

113. Rogers DG, White NH, Shalwitz RA et al. The effect of puberty on the development of early diabetic microvascular disease in insulin-dependent diabetes. Diabetes Res Clin Pract 1987; 3: 39–44.

114. Tsalikian E, Becker DJ, Crumrine K et al. Electroencephalographic changes in diabetic ketosis in children with newly and previously diagnosed diabetes mellitus. Pediatrics 1981; 99: 355.

115. Santiago JV, Wolff PB, Davis JE et al. Effect of blood glucose control and a lipid-lowering diet on blood lipids in diabetic children. Ped Adolesc Endocrinol 1979; 7: 241–8.

116. Travis LB. An instructional aid on insulin dependent diabetes. Galveston: University of Texas, 1985.

117. Chase HP. Understanding insulin dependent diabetes. Denver: Children's Diabetes Foundation, 1988.

118. Delamater AM, Bubb J, Davis SG et al.

Randomized prospective study of self-management training with newly diagnosed diabetic children. Diabetes Care 1990; 13: 492–8.

119. White NH, Skor DA, Cryer PE et al. Identifying Type I diabetic patients at increased risk for hypoglycemia during intensive therapy. New Engl J Med 1983; 308: 485–91.

120. Cryer PE, White NH, Santiago JV. The relevance of glucose counterregulation systems to patients with insulin-dependent diabetes mellitus. Endocr Rev 1986; 7: 131–9.

121. Daneman D, Frank M, Perlman K et al. Severe hypoglycemia in children with insulin-dependent diabetes mellitus: frequency and predisposing factors. J Pediatr 1989; 113: 681–5.

122. Rosenbloom AL. Skeletal and joint manifestations of childhood diabetes. Pediatr Clin North Am 1984; 31: 569–90.

43
Brittle Diabetes

J.C. Pickup
Guy's Hospital, London, UK

A few lucky patients with insulin dependent diabetes mellitus maintain near-normoglycaemia, have no symptoms and lead a virtually normal life. Many more suffer moderate swings in blood glucose concentration, coping with occasional symptomatic hypoglycaemic episodes and, if they are unlucky, the odd admission to hospital for ketoacidosis.

A few patients are classed as 'brittle' because their metabolic control is so bad, with frequent and usually unpredictable lurches into hypoglycaemia or hyperglycaemia, that regular employment or schooling, family relationships and many aspects of ordinary daily life become impossible.

Brittle diabetes can be defined as a condition where metabolic instability is sufficient to cause major disruption to the life-style or to endanger the life of a diabetic patient. One reason why there is good reason to study brittle diabetes is the enormous financial, physical and emotional burden placed upon the health services and their personnel, and upon the patient and her (for the patient is usually female) family.

Even experienced students of brittle diabetes label its evaluation and treatment as 'frustrating, tedious and difficult' [1]. It is a bone of contention among physicians. Commonly there is much delay in finding a cause and instituting reasonably effective treatment, which invites accusations of failing to recognise or suspect self-induced

disease or other psychological factors in the patient or her family as a cause, and of pressing on blindly with expensive, sophisticated and potentially hazardous techniques of investigation and treatment that rarely help the patient. On the other hand, it is pointed out that much of the evidence for psychosocial disorder is uncontrolled, with inadequately validated instruments of measurement, and that dubious and unjustified connections are drawn between isolated events of 'cheating' and the root cause of brittleness.

All this is probably true, on occasion at least, and the 'truth' lies somewhere between the two extremes of mind and metabolism.

HOW TO MEASURE BRITTLENESS

It is the association of poor metabolic control and disruption of life that is the key feature of brittleness. Quantification of both problems is necessary in order to gauge the effects of treatments, to select and study control groups, and so on.

Assessment of Glycaemia

Glycaemic measures fall into four classes: indices of (a) average blood glucose control, (b) excursions, (c) the combined effects of the mean blood glucose level and the swings, and (d) day-to-day variability in glycaemia (see Tables 1 and 2).

International Textbook of Diabetes Mellitus. Edited by K.G.M.M. Alberti, R.A. DeFronzo, H. Keen and P. Zimmet
© 1992 John Wiley & Sons Ltd

Table 1   Some indices of brittleness (see text for explanation)

Average control	Excursions	Mean + Excursions	Variability
Mean HbA$_1$	SD Range MAGE	*M* value	MODD
Fructosamine	FAGE		SD of fasting blood glucose

Glucosylated albumin	No. of hypoglycaemic
	   episodes
	No. of episodes of
	   diabetic ketoacidosis		

Many of the ways of assessing the first two classes (mean glycaemia, HbA$_1$, fructosamine, range and standard deviation of glucose values) are familiar to most clinicians and require no special comment in this context. However, the two latter classes are slightly more esoteric, and these measures have been employed in several studies of 'difficult' diabetes.

The mean amplitude of glycaemic excursions (MAGE) was introduced by Service et al [2]. It is the arithmetic mean of blood glucose excursions when both limbs of the swing are greater than one standard deviation of the mean of all values (designed to exclude minor variations in blood glucose levels). Fasting ascending glycaemic excursions (FAGE) measure the 'dawn phenomenon', i.e. the tendency for blood glucose concentrations to increase in the few hours before breakfast. As defined by Schmidt et al [3], it is the difference between the fasting, pre-breakfast plasma glucose value and the nocturnal nadir between midnight and 6:00 a.m.

The *M* value of Schlichtkrull et al [4] is an attempt to express in a single number the quality of diabetic control. Because it is a logarithmic derivation of the blood glucose concentration, it has extra weighting for hypoglycaemia. In the most common form:

$$M = \Sigma \left| 10 \log_{10} \frac{BG}{standard} \right|^3 \div n$$

where BG = blood glucose values, standard = chosen euglycaemic value (say 4.4 mmol/l

80 mg/dl) and *n* = number of samples. The vertical bars indicate that the values are treated (cubed here) without respect to sign. It is not possible to tell whether a high *M* value is the result of hypoglycaemia or hyperglycaemia, or both.

A particular feature of many brittle diabetics is unpredictability of control, and three indices have been used in this context. The mean of daily differences (MODD) was devised by Molnar et al [5] and calculated from the records of 48 hours of continuous glucose monitoring. Values at 5-minute intervals were matched with values at the same time 24 hours later, the difference calculated (without respect to sign) and the mean taken. A simplified version uses the mean of the differences in glycaemia on two consecutive days in the fasting state, at 1 and 2 hours after breakfast, and at 2 hours after lunch [6].

As an alternative measure of unpredictability, Shima et al [7] used the standard deviation of 10 fasting blood glucose values.

Urine Glucose and Ketones

With the realisation that glycosuria is an unreliable index of glycaemia, and the advent of home blood glucose monitoring, urinary glucose testing has not stood the test of time as a measure of lability, although previously several workers [8–12] had commented that alternating periods of heavy glycosuria and aglycosuria were a common indicator of brittleness due to excessive insulin

Table 2   Approximate values for some indices of brittleness

Index	Normal	Stable diabetic	Brittle diabetic	Reference
MAGE (mmol/l)	2–5	4–5	7–0	2
M value (4.4 mmol/l standard)	0–1	10–30	40–300	2, 15
MODD (mmol/l)	0.5	0.5–2.0	2–9	5
SD fasting blood glucose	–	0.7–1.6	4.4–6.4	7

treatment and posthypoglycaemic hyperglycaemia (the Somogyi effect).

Disruption

Disruption can be assessed by such means as recording the number of emergency admissions to hospital in the previous year, and the time spent off work or absent from school.

POSSIBLE CAUSES OF BRITTLE DIABETES

Overinsulinisation and the Somogyi effect

From the 1930s onwards, Michael Somogyi and others [8–12] developed the notion that in some diabetics with wildly and periodically oscillating glycosuria and glycaemia, poor control was due to excessive insulin dosage. They observed that high values consistently occurred in the wake of hypoglycaemic episodes, sometimes asymptomatic, and postulated that release of counterregulatory hormones at this time caused the subsequent insulin resistance and hyperglycaemia. Several investigators described labile diabetic patients in whom there were features such as high insulin dosage, cyclic glycosuria and ketonuria, and improved control on gradual reduction of insulin dosage [9–12].

Somogyi observed that insulinoma patients can develop fluctuations between hypoglycaemia and hyperglycaemia, and in patients who received insulin for psychosis, hyperglycaemia sometimes developed and persisted for months after the induced hypoglycaemia. Thus, the absence of biochemical evidence of low blood glucose values during a few days of random testing may not exclude overinsulinisation, and if counterregulatory hormone surges are responsible for lack of control, their effect may be very long-lasting and hamper the detection of the initial increase.

Although the evidence is conflicting, it is probably true that triggering of counterregulatory responses can occur at normal or elevated blood glucose levels in some diabetics [13], indicating that evidence of relative as well as absolute hypoglycaemia should be sought.

In children, overinsulinisation is thought to be common [12], occurring in about 70% of patients. About one-third demonstrate hepatomegaly and many have clinical features similar to the Mauriac

Table 3 Clinical clues to the diagnosis of overinsulinisation (based on reference 12)

Obvious hypoglycaemic episodes
Polyuria, nocturia, enuresis
Excessive appetite
Hepatomegaly
Headaches, relieved by food
Weight gain
Exercise intolerance
Variation in glycosuria and glycaemia
Frequent ketoacidosis
Mood swings, irritability
Increasing insulin yet worsening control
Ketonuria without glycosuria
Worsening symptoms with increased insulin

syndrome, i.e. cushingoid obesity, growth failure and maturational delay, together with hepatomegaly [14].

Rosenbloom and Giordano [12] have summarised the clinical clues to the recognition of overtreatment with insulin in children. Those symptoms occurring in more than about 10% of cases are shown in Table 3.

It is impossible not to notice that many of the features of overinsulinisation are found in the rare groups of 'idiopathic' brittle diabetics unresponsive to optimised subcutaneous insulin therapy, i.e. mild obesity, high insulin requirements, frequent ketoacidosis and, occasionally, profound hypoglycaemia [15]. At least two of our patients who fall into this category have hepatomegaly and several have abdominal bloatedness and peripheral oedema.

Insulin reduction has been attempted on many occasions in this group of brittle patients but it has not been successful in most cases. Furthermore, brittle diabetics of this type are not more hyperinsulinaemic than stable diabetics, again arguing against simple overinsulinisation (see below).

Endogenous Insulin Production

Almost all severely brittle diabetic patients have undetectable C-peptide levels after stimulation [7, 16] and this, of course, in no way distinguishes them from the majority of long-standing type 1 diabetic patients who are stable in spite of this absence of residual B-cell function [17]. However, it has been reported by Shima et al [7] that insulin-requiring diabetics with the largest change in C-peptide levels after an oral glucose load have the highest predictability of control (assessed by SD of fasting blood glucose values).

All but one of their most unstable patients had no demonstrable C-peptide increases. The stabilising effect of even very small degrees of endogenous B-cell function is also hinted at by the finding of more stable control in insulin dependent diabetic patients with minimal C-peptide responses, detectable only by highly sensitive immunoassay [18].

The mechanisms underlying these observations are not clear. Does feedback control of minimal insulin secretion have profound effects when the insulin is directed to the liver, and is stability due to an associated islet factor such as glucagon which is secreted in response to hypoglycaemia and buffers any erratic downward glycaemic excursions?

Impaired Subcutaneous Absorption of Insulin

The idea of a barrier to insulin absorption at the subcutaneous site in brittle diabetes arose because several groups reported patients who were poorly controlled on large doses given subcutaneously but who achieved markedly improved control when insulin was given intravenously [19–22] or intramuscularly [23] in much smaller amounts, presumably bypassing the hindrance. Increased insulin breakdown by protease activity was at first thought to be the likely explanation because, in normal subjects, the proteaseinhibitor aprotinin (Trasylol), was reported to accelerate insulin absorption when mixed with subcutaneous injections of short-acting insulin [24]. In subcutaneously resistant brittle diabetic patients [22], mixtures of aprotinin and insulin produced euglycaemia and elevated plasma free insulin concentrations (see below).

In a very few patients, biopsies of the subcutaneous adipose tissue have shown augmented insulinolytic activity [21, 25]. However, in the vast majority of brittle subjects, insulin breakdown is not the explanation for apparent resistance. Biopsies do not shown increased ability to degrade insulin in vitro [26, 27]. Aprotinin is a potent vasodilator, and when it does speed insulin absorption it may do so through promoting local blood flow [28]; it is of interest that, in stable diabetic patients, evidence currently points to a virtual absence of insulin breakdown in the subcutaneous tissue [29].

Blood flow at the subcutaneous site of administration is often said to be a major determinant of insulin absorption [30]. In this respect, we showed that insulin itself causes prolonged hyperaemia at its injection site in normal subjects and in stable type 1 diabetic subjects, but this vascular response was virtually absent in a group of brittle patients [31]. Whether this impairment is causally related to the subcutaneous 'barrier' is unknown, but slowed absorption of insulin with sequestration at the injection site would be consistent with the lipohypertrophy which seems more common in brittle patients than in matched, stable diabetics ([15], and see below).

Nevertheless, to make matters more confusing, two groups have shown that in diabetic patients supposed to have high subcutaneous insulin requirements, both the fall in blood glucose and the increase in plasma free insulin levels after small test doses of short-acting insulin given subcutaneously lie within the range of values for stable diabetic controls [27, 32]. Had the patients been able to fake resistance? Was the test in the resting, supine, initially well-controlled subject not representative of insulin requirements during everyday conditions of life?

Accelerated Clearance of Circulating Insulin

At least two patients have been described [33, 34] with massive resistance to insulin administered by all routes.

We described [34] a 23-year-old insulin dependent diabetic woman who had variable degrees of insulin resistance for 6 years (and continues to have after almost 9 years, at the time of writing this chapter). Continuous subcutaneous insulin infusion was ineffective, at doses up to 2000 U per day, as was intramuscular and intravenous insulin infusion from a portable pump connected to an indwelling Hickman catheter in the subclavian vein. Insulin doses of up to 20 000 U per day were eventually required, although there were short periods of normal insulin sensitivity. Immunological resistance was excluded by the low anti-insulin antibody levels, the normal receptor binding of radio-labelled insulin, the ineffectiveness of steroids and the absence of hyperinsulinaemia. The insulin-degrading activity of subcutaneous tissue and whole blood was normal and aprotinin was ineffective. However, an intravenous injection of 32 U of short-acting insulin produced a relatively trivial peak plasma free insulin level of

60 mU/l and circulating insulin levels were consistently low during day-to-day intravenous infusion of huge insulin dosages. Because urinary insulin losses were also very small, we formed the conclusion that rapid removal of insulin from the circulation was the likely cause of the resistance, with periods of re-entry into the blood accounting for the occasional episodes of extended hyperinsulinaemia and hypoglycaemia. The site of clearance remains unknown, but it is interesting to note that, in addition to the well-known activities of liver and kidney in extracting and degrading insulin, the endothelium has recently been recognised as a source of insulin uptake without degradation [35]. Perhaps the latter could account for massive sequestration and later erratic re-entry of insulin into the circulation.

Abnormalities in Counterregulatory Hormones

Impairment in the secretion of counterregulatory hormones, crucially glucagon and catecholamines, is well established as a major causative factor in the delayed recovery from hypoglycaemia in diabetes [36]. Although hypoglycaemia is a common, potentially fatal and much-feared complication of diabetes, the extent to which counterregulatory hormone deficiencies have a role in brittleness (i.e. causing serious and chronic disruption of the patient's life) has not been investigated. Most attention has focused instead on the possible influence of excesses or erratic secretions of these hormones in producing hyperglycaemia and recurrent ketosis.

A comparison of 24-hour profiles of metabolites and hormones in ketoacidosis-prone brittle diabetes and a control group of stable patients found no significant differences in levels of glucagon, cortisol, growth hormone or free insulin when the patients were managed by subcutaneous injection therapy or an artificial endocrine pancreas, although, interestingly, glycaemic control and blood 3-hydroxybutyrate levels were not disordered in the brittle patients on the study day [37]. We have also been unable to detect abnormalities of these hormones during random testing in any of our brittle subjects. The fact that intermittent measurements of blood catecholamine concentrations have also been normal, and adrenergic blockade has failed to improve control, argues against an important role for catecholamines.

Intercurrent Illness

Infection is thought to be the underlying cause in about 30% of all cases of ketoacidosis in insulin dependent diabetes [38]. The prevalence of infection in diabetic patients is correlated with the level of glycaemic control in the preceding, non-infected period [39]. Among the infectious diseases particularly associated with diabetes are tuberculosis, candidiasis, mucormycosis, urinary tract infections, and injection and infusion site abscesses.

It is easy to speculate how infection, especially with its fluctuating course, could be a factor in brittleness. Changes in stress hormones, nutritional status, alterations in subcutaneous blood flow and insulin absorption with swinging fevers, and increased metabolic rate, dehydration and augmented capillary permeability could all exacerbate the metabolic state in an unpredictable manner [40]. Many of these effects will also be apparent in other intercurrent illnesses in the diabetic patient, such as malignancy.

White and Santiago [41] thought that recurrent streptococcal pharyngitis was the cause of brittleness in 3 of 44 children with the syndrome, but underlying infection or other intercurrent organic illness in adults has not been reported as a significant aetiological factor.

Of the non-diabetic endocrine conditions occurring in diabetic patients, thyrotoxicosis, hypophysectomy and other causes of panhypopituitarism such as antepartum and postpartum pituitary necrosis, hypoadrenalism and pancreatectomy are the ones most likely to cause brittleness. Chronic pancreatitis, renal failure, malabsorption and gastroparesis due to autonomic neuropathy can produce unpredictable hypoglycaemia, but in practice all of the above are usually quickly recognised and do not contribute significantly to the hard core of long-standing, superlabile patients [42].

Factitious Disease and Malingering

Some workers draw a distinction between malingering or manipulation, where patient-induced disease has a supposedly obvious motive of gain (e.g. avoiding school, work, responsibilities), and factitious disease, where self-destructive behaviour has no identifiable ulterior motive [43]. Clearly, though, the two are related; separation may largely depend on the success of the psychiatrist in uncovering any gain, and the explanation is rather a matter of opinion and speculation.

Many cases of factitious instability (used here to include any manipulation) have been described in patients presenting with either recurrent hypoglycaemia or ketoacidosis, or both [43–46]. Among the reported acts and clues to manipulation are omission of prescribed insulin (admitted, or detected by tagging the insulin vial with radioactivity), injection of foreign material subcutaneously, dilution of insulin with water, self-injection of non-prescribed insulin (observed or detected by weighing insulin vials to check loss), discovery of insulin and syringes in patient's belongings, and the absence of lability when concealed insulin is removed.

A further classic feature of brittle diabetes is failure to reproduce the instability or insulin resistance when the patient is admitted to hospital, strictly supervised and all injections given by the nursing staff. Although this makes most physicians suspect a factitious aetiology for brittleness, it clearly is not proof.

In our own patients, we have noted removal and reversal of insulin pump batteries, food refusal, disconnection of infusion catheters at Luer lock junctions, removal of central venous catheters (previously securely stitched to the skin) with consequent severe blood loss, and dilution of insulin in an infusion pump with tap water. None of our patients has admitted deliberate interference at the time of their hospital admission, but a few have confirmed it to another party (usually a fellow patient) at a later time.

Malingering or factitious instability was thought to be the explanation for brittleness in about one-half of the patients studied in one series [43]. Most reports comment on how confrontation does little to alter the subsequent course of events, that patients often refuse psychiatric help, that psychotherapy does not improve control and patients default from follow-up [46]. Particularly remarkable is that, in many cases, no pathology is detectable on referral to a psychiatrist, although of six brittle adolescent diabetics discovered to be surreptitiously taking extra insulin, Orr et al [46] recorded psychopathology in all. Depression and severe personality problems, including schizoid personality, were common in this study, and three patients displayed suicidal behaviour.

Inadvertent non-compliance may arise because of deficient information, poor understanding

Table 4 Some commonly reported psychosocial associations in patients with brittle diabetes and their families

Single parent
Parents or patient divorced
Poor living conditions an/or limited financial resources
Overprotective parents
Inadequate or uninterested parents
Family conflict
Psychiatric pathology or alcoholism in family
Illness or death in family
Poor acceptance of diabetes by subject
Manipulation of diabetes by patient
Truancy/poor performance at school
Antisocial behaviour of patient
Depression in patient
Decreased self-esteem of patient
Anxiety in patient

and inability to execute and adjust treatment regimens. There is little or no reason to think that brittle diabetes is the result of patients being badly informed, although they may be as poorly educated as most with insulin dependent diabetes. Surprisingly, though, Schade et al [43] concluded that about one-quarter of patients with incapacitating brittle diabetes had deficits in communication skills that would account for their instability. It is not clear why the patients were not improved by intensive insulin therapy under hospital supervision if psycholinguistic difficulties were the only explanation for poor control.

It is easy to formulate plausible reasons for deliberate non-compliance, including attention-seeking, cries for help, sympathy and affection, testing of parents and doctors, punishing self and others, and denial of illness. Whether these actually operate has not been tested and would be difficult to ascertain.

Psychosocial Influences

A stream of papers over the last fifty years (for example, references 15, 47–50) have described the high frequency of family conflict and dysfunction and behavioural problems in diabetic patients suffering from 'superlabile' diabetes. A recent thorough psychological assessment of 30 diabetic children and adolescents with recurrent ketoacidosis [50] showed that a majority of the subjects lived in families with substantial problems. Table 4 shows some of the psychosocial features that have commonly been reported in brittle diabetes.

Three questions spring to mind. Are these disorders worse than in control groups of non-brittle diabetics? Is the dysfunction the cause, the effect or an epiphenomenon of brittleness? If psychological factors do have a role, what is the mechanism by which they operate?

Unfortunately, the answer to the first question is not known. Evidence that many psychological and family difficulties existed before the patients developed diabetes [50] suggests that brittleness may be caused or exacerbated by life events and situations. In the conceptual model of psychosomatic illness in children proposed by Minuchin et al [48], the patient is invariably physiologically vulnerable (in this case, having diabetes) and the family displays four characteristics: enmeshment (i.e. interdependent family relationships), overprotectiveness (undue concern for each other's welfare), rigidity (maintaining the status quo) and lack of conflict resolution.

Two obvious ways in which family stress could lead to brittleness are by deliberate malefaction by the patient (omitting insulin to gain attention, for example) and the effects of the physiological accompaniments of emotional stress (hormonal and neurological).

In support of the latter theory, two studies aften cited are those of Hinkle and Wolf [51] and Baker et al [52]. The first authors observed many occasions when major fluctuations in diabetic control coincided with important and stressful life episodes in patients, such as conflict with a parent. Moreover, ketosis and hyperglycaemia (sometimes hypoglycaemia) could be induced by subjecting the patients to stressful interviews on the suspected topic of conflict for that particular subject. Baker et al [52] found that acute β-adrenergic blockade prevented the increase in blood glucose and free fatty acids after a stressful interview in one diabetic patient, and 1 year of treatment with a β-blocking agent all but reduced or abolished hospital admissions for ketoacidosis in two labile patients.

A recent study [53] failed to show an effect on metabolic control in either well-controlled or poorly controlled type 1 diabetic patients who were subjected to the stress of mental arithmetic or public speaking. Also α-adrenergic or β-adrenergic blockade (or both) has failed to be of any therapeutic value in more recent trials with brittle diabetics [37]. In seeking an explanation for these discrepancies, one may speculate that some patients (the superlabile ones) are perhaps more sensitive to stressful stimuli than others; that it is *chronic* emotional upset that attunes the body to react by producing metabolic disorder; or that, for the individual, one stimulus is stressful whereas another is not. These possibilities need testing.

Eating Disorders

In some studies of unselected female adolescents with type 1 diabetes, about 20% had clinically important eating disorders [54], and anorexia nervosa and bulimia occurred in about 6% of patients, representing an increase over the expected frequency in non-diabetic subjects of about 6 and 2 times respectively. Not surprisingly, there was evidence that poor control was a common feature in these patients. In other reports, normal eating habits have been found in adolescents with type 1 diabetes [55].

Binge eating is associated with poor control and many such patients have said they cope with overeating by reducing or omitting insulin [56].

SOME CLINICAL FEATURES OF 'IDIOPATHIC' BRITTLE DIABETES

When well-established causes of difficult diabetes have been excluded such as inappropriate insulin regimens, infection, intercurrent endocrine disorders and other illnesses, there remains a small group of patients in whom the aetiology is more obscure and nearly always proves difficult and time-consuming to unravel. These are the patients where the diagnoses of emotionally induced instability, deliberate manipulation and abnormalities of insulin handling are to be considered. These patients display certain common clinical features [15], which leads to speculation that they may share a similar pathophysiology, or if not the same aetiology then a similar metabolic disruption.

We compared 12 brittle diabetic patients with recurrent ketoacidosis as the main metabolic problem with 12 stable diabetic patients matched for age, sex and duration of diabetes [15]. The brittle subjects were young (13–27 years old); all were female and, although mildly overweight (mean body mass index 23–25), they were no more obese than the controls. The subcutaneous insulin requirement was greater than for stable patients (7.1 U/kg versus 1.0 U/kg), and there was a significant correlation between the age of

Admit to hospital: history and clinical examination, blood count, biochemical profile, ESR, thyroid function tests, C-peptide test, chest x-ray, urinary free cortisol, urinary HMMA, MSU, insulin antibodies

↓

(If clinical features indicate) Synacthen test, pituitary function tests, intestinal absorption tests, screen for drugs of abuse, tuberculin test

↓

2-Hourly blood glucose and free insulin profile for 48 h on usual therapy (detection of hypoglycemia, dawn phenomenon), psychosocial assessment, evaluation of diabetes education

↓

Insulin challenge test −0.1 U/kg SC and IV (blood glucose and free insulin)

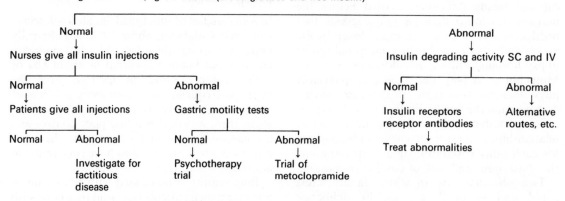

Figure 1   An algorithm for the investigation of brittle diabetes (see references 42, 57). MSU, mid-stream urine analysis; ESR, erythrocyte sedimentation rate; HMMA, 4-hydroxy-3-methoxymandelic acid

onset of brittleness and the age at menarche, hinting at a role for the hormonal and/or emotional changes at this time. Menstrual disorders were common at the time of study, and obvious lipohypertrophy at injection sites had a tendency to occur more frequently in the brittle patients. The high prevalence of psychosocial disturbances and family upsets has been mentioned above.

INVESTIGATION

Some clear instructions for the investigation of brittle diabetes have been outlined recently [42, 57], and the details in Figure 1 combine advice from several workers with experience from our own unit. Early psychological assessment is particularly recommended, because whatever other pathology is uncovered, many of the patients demonstrate abnormalities or need support to cope with chronic illness and major disruption of their lives.

The investigation of factitious disease is especially unsatisfactory. It is suggested that patients are confined to a room for 48 hours without personal possessions, insulin injections are observed, visitors banned and all food going in and out of the room checked. Regular assay

and weighing of the insulin vial should also be performed. In practice, this protocol is very difficult to accomplish. Often a room with connecting toilet and washing facilities is not available, the patient will vigorously protest and the remarkable cunning of some manipulative patients can defeat the most assiduous team.

TREATMENT APPROACHES

The general principles of management include assigning one doctor who will investigate and treat the patient and who will be available at all times by telephone for consultation by the patient or family. This is not a task for a junior. A senior decision-maker should direct and coordinate activities and adjudicate disputes, for, as Gale has said [58], the management of brittle diabetes is primarily an exercise in the organisation and delivery of medical care.

Extracorporeal Infusion Systems

In most brittle patients characterised by recurrent ketoacidosis, we have found that continuous subcutaneous insulin infusion (CSII) fails either to improve glycaemic control under closely supervised hospital conditions or to reduce further emergency admissions to hospital [23]. The technique has had most success in our hands in the group of patients with disabling attacks of hypoglycaemia. In a randomised and controlled study, 5 patients who complained of frequent, symptomatic hypoglycaemic episodes on conventional insulin injection therapy achieved a mean reduction of 57% in the number of hypoglycaemic attacks on CSII compared with injection treatment [59]. It is possible that this improved control is simply impairment of the sensation of hypoglycaemia; however, neither a change in the level of blood glucose at which the patients recognised induced hypoglycaemia nor any alteration in counter-regulatory hormone responses afterwards was detected.

Some patients who have been erratically controlled on all modern intensified injection regimens have enjoyed a dramatic reduction in biochemical and symptomatic hypoglycaemia, and a return to normal home and working life. It is also worth noting that Nathan [60], while confirming the ineffectiveness of CSII in severe brittle diabetes, was able to reduce emergency admissions and hypoglycaemic reactions, and to improve (but not to normalise) indices of labile control by employing variable basal rate subcutaneous infusion regimens using a pump, but without the preprandial supplements.

Continuous intramuscular insulin infusion (into the deltoid) using a portable pump was shown to produce a marked improvement in hospital control and in up to 1 year of outpatient control in a small group of brittle patients who were unresponsive to CSII [23]. However, the technique of inserting and securing the cannula is difficult and fibrosis occurs after a while at the infusion site. It cannot, therefore, be recommended as a long-term therapeutic option.

Continuous intravenous insulin infusion (CIVII) has received more attention [22, 61]. Patients who have proved to be resistant or unmanageable on subcutaneous insulin therapy have often been well controlled by IV infusion of insulin at rates of about 1–5 U per hour. Outpatient CIVII can be maintained for months and occasionally years, via a Silastic Hickman catheter passed into the right atrium through the subclavian vein. We have found [61] that periods of satisfactory control could be achieved in 3 of 5 brittle diabetic patients treated by CIVII, but generally control was as erratic and unpredictable as on CSII, and hospital admissions continued. In 2 patients, evidence of deliberate interference with the infusion was detected. Complications of therapy are frequent and include infection at catheter insertion sites, septicaemia, catheter blockage, and thrombosis of the subclavian vein in one subject.

Intraperitoneal insulin delivery [62] achieved a slightly improved level of control, comparable to that of CIVII but at lower insulin dosages. As with CIVII, the benefit is not maintained and overall glycaemic control is no better than on subcutaneous insulin therapy. Blockage and dislodgement of catheters and peritonitis have been reported as complications.

Implantable Pumps

At least 8 patients with incapacitating brittle diabetes and subcutaneous insulin resistance have been treated by single-rate insulin infusion from an implanted Infusaid pump delivering into the peritoneal cavity or a central vein [63–65]. This type of device consists of a titanium disc divided into two compartments by a flexible metal bellows. The upper compartment is an insulin reservoir and the lower is filled with a fluorocarbon fluid in equilibrium with its vapour. This vapour exerts pressure on the insulin chamber and forces insulin out through a bacterial filter and a pressure-drop tube to control delivery rate.

Many of the subjects had a prior history of interference with their treatment, so successful pump therapy may have had (cynics might say) a contribution from the fact that the device is so difficult to tamper with when implanted. Nevertheless, Buchwald et al [65], for example, report an impressive 99% reduction in episodes of ketoacidosis, an 89% reduction in days spent in hospital and a cost saving of an estimated $10 000 per patient month during implantable pump therapy in 5 brittle diabetic patients.

Augmented Subcutaneous Insulin Absorption

In one of the few patients in whom increased subcutaneous degradation of insulin has actually been demonstrated by measurement of this activity in biopsies, the addition of the protease inhibitor, aprotinin, to the subcutaneous insulin injections was ineffective [15]; intravenous aprotinin in this case reduced subcutaneous insulin requirements. In the many patients with subcutaneous insulin resistance and/or hyper-lability and presumed but unproved insulin degradation, aprotinin and insulin mixtures sometimes reduce insulin requirements and improve control [22, 66]; sometimes such mixtures have no benefit [66, 67]. Life-threatening anaphylaxis has been reported with aprotinin therapy [67].

White and Santiago [66] suggest that aprotinin non-responders are perhaps distinguished by requiring high intravenous insulin dosages (over 1.5 U/kg daily) as well as high subcutaneous insulin dosages. They also note that response to aprotinin may be short-lived, lasting only weeks.

In one patient with massive insulin resistance by both the subcutaneous and intravenous routes, and demonstratable accelerated insulin breakdown in subcutaneous fat tissue, Blazar et al [68] showed that oral chloroquine phosphate (500 mg thrice daily), but not aprotinin, was successful in reducing the resistance. Chloroquine is a lysosomotropic agent that inhibits insulin breakdown in liver, fat and muscle; presumably it operates through this mechanism in brittle diabetes.

Psychotherapy

Counselling and psychotherapy can take the form of individual, family or group treatment, tailored towards the needs of the particular patient. A team approach is usually recommended, with involvement of a specialist nurse, social worker, physician, psychologist and psychiatrist.

Of those patients who accept psychotherapy, most show reduced emergency hospital admissions, improved school attendances and, subjectively, are thought to be less withdrawn and depressed [48–50]. Almost always, objective measures of control such as HbA_1 are unaltered [49]. A major problem is that many patients, particularly those with factitious disease (in its broadest sense), refuse psychological help or remain poorly controlled after such treatment.

NATURAL HISTORY

Thirteen patients with disabling, CSII-unresponsive brittle diabetes were followed up for 3–6 years to assess the natural history of the condition [69]. All were young females.

One patient died of hypoglycaemia. The overall disruption of life-style was less at follow-up: 4 had no admissions to hospital in the previous year and the mean frequency of admissions had dropped from 12.5 per year to 3.5 per year. The percentage of time at work had increased from 28% to 78%. However, all of the patients (bar one) continued to suffer erratic control and episodes of unpredictable ketoacidosis or hypoglycaemia, or both. New diabetic complications appeared in 5 subjects (background and proliferative retinopathy, painful peripheral neuropathy and intermittent proteinuria). Only 3 patients consented to psychotherapy, with a short period of benefit for only one. In general, psychosocial difficulties remained unresolved.

Thus, although the effect of brittleness on life-style seems to improve, metabolic control continues to be unpredictable and the patients are at considerable risk of complications.

CONCLUSION

The pendulum is swinging more towards the emotions and self-induced decompensation as the major causes of brittle diabetes, and further away from impairment of insulin absorption and action. However, many questions are left unanswered, for example:

(1) Does the detection of one act of 'cheating' with therapy necessarily confirm that brittleness is caused by either malefaction or any psychological mechanism? Remember that psychotherapy does not usually alter glycaemic control in these patients.
(2) If CSII is ineffective because it is easily tampered with by the patients, why does switching to, say, intramuscular insulin infusion produce immediate and sustained improvement, when the system is just as open to abuse, if not more so?
(3) Why cannot early, encouraging experience with adrenergic blockade be repeated?

Perhaps more than one cause is operative in many cases. In this respect, Gill et al [42] have formulated the interesting notion that initial therapeutic manipulation leads to disruption of metabolic control; the physician intervenes with higher insulin doses; insulin resistance is induced and eventually a self-perpetuating, uncorrectable state of instability is created from which the patients cannot escape, even if they wish to.

Unfortunately the aetiology, the mechanisms and the treatment of brittle diabetes are not clear as yet.

REFERENCES

1. Santiago JV. Another facet of brittle diabetes. JAMA 1986; 256: 3263–4.
2. Service FJ, Molnar GD, Rosevear JW, Ackerman E, Gatewood LC, Taylor WT. Mean amplitude of glycemic excursions, a measure of diabetic instability. Diabetes 1970; 19: 644–55.
3. Schmidt MI, Hadjii-Georgopoulos A, Rendell M, Margolis S, Kowarski A. The dawn phenomenon, an early morning glucose rise: implications for diabetic intraday blood glucose variation. Diabetes Care 1981; 4: 579–85.
4. Schlichtkrull J, Munck O, Jersild M. The M value: an index of blood sugar control in diabetics. Acta Med Scand 1965; 177: 95–102.
5. Molnar G, Taylor WF, Ho MM. Day-to-day variation of continuously monitored glycaemia: a further measure of diabetic instability. Diabetologia 1972; 8: 342–8.
6. Lev-Ran A. Clinical observation on brittle diabetes. Arch Int Med 1977; 138: 372–6.
7. Shima K, Tanaka R, Morishita S, Tarui S, Kumahara Y, Nishikawa M. Studies on the etiology of 'brittle diabetes'. Relationships between diabetic instability and insulinogenic reserve. Diabetes 1977; 26: 717–25.
8. Somogyi M. Exacerbation of diabetes by excess insulin action. Am J Med 1959; 26: 169–91.
9. Perkoff GT, Tyler FH. Paradoxical hyperglycemia in diabetic patients treated with insulin. Metabolism 1954; 3: 110–17.
10. Bloom ME, Mintz DH, Field JB. Insulin-induced posthypoglycemic hyperglycemia as a cause of 'brittle' diabetes. Am J Med 1969; 47: 891–903.
11. Bruck E, MacGillivray MH. Posthypoglycemic hyperglycemia in diabetic children. J Pediatr 1974; 84: 672–80.
12. Rosenbloom AL, Giordano BP. Chronic overtreatment with insulin in children and adolescents. Am J Dis Child 1977; 131: 881–5.
13. Bollinger R, Stephens R, Lukert B, Diederich D. Galvanic skin reflex and plasma free fatty acids during insulin reactions. Diabetes 1964; 13: 600–5.
14. Rosenbloom AL, Clarke DW. Excessive insulin treatment and the Somogyi effect. In Pickup JC (ed.) Brittle diabetes. Oxford: Blackwell, 1985: pp 103–31.
15. Pickup JC, Williams G, Johns P, Keen H. Clinical features of brittle diabetic patients unresponsive to optimised subcutaneous insulin therapy (continuous subcutaneous insulin infusion). Diabetes Care 1983; 6: 279–84.
16. Gill GV, Home PD, Massi-Benedetti M et al. Clinical and metabolic characteristics of patients with 'brittle' diabetes. Diabetologia 1981; 21: 507 (abstr.).
17. Yue DK, Baxter RC, Turtle JR. C-peptide secretion and insulin antibodies as determinants of stability in diabetes mellitus. Metabolism 1978; 27: 35–44.
18. Fukuda M, Tanaka A, Tahara Y, Yamamoto Y, Kumahara Y, Shima K. Relationship between residual B-cell function and A-cell response to hyperglycemia. Diabetes 1987; 36 (suppl. 1): 97A.
19. Schneider AJ, Bennett RH. Impaired absorption of insulin as a cause of insulin resistance. Diabetes 1975; 24: 443 (abstr.).
20. Henry DA, Lowe JM, Citrin D, Manderson WG. Defective absorption of injected insulin (letter). Lancet 1978; ii: 741.
21. Paulsen EP, Courtney JW, Duckworth WC. Insulin resistance caused by massive degradation of subcutaneous insulin. Diabetes 1979; 28: 640–5.
22. Freidenberg GR, White NH, Cataland S, O'Dorisio TM, Sotos JF, Santiago WV. Diabetes responsive to intravenous but not subcutaneous insulin: effectiveness of aprotinin. New Engl J Med 1981; 305: 363–8.
23. Pickup JC, Home PD, Bilous RW, Keen H, Alberti KGMM. Management of severely brittle diabetes by continuous subcutaneous and intramuscular insulin infusions: evidence for a defect in subcutaneous insulin absorption. Br Med J 1981; 282: 347–50.
24. Berger M, Cuppers HJ, Halban PA, Offord RE. The effect of aprotinin on the absorption of subcutaneously injected regular insulin in normal subjects. Diabetes 1980; 29: 81–3.
25. Maberly GF, Wait GA, Kilpatrick JA, Loten EG, Gain KR, Stewart RDH, Eastman CJ, Evidence for insulin degradation by muscle and fat tissue in an insulin resistant patient. Diabetologia 1982; 23: 333–6.
26. Williams G, Pickup JC. Subcutaneous insulin degradation. In Pickup JC (ed.) Brittle diabetes. Oxford: Blackwell, 1985: pp 154–66.
27. Schade DS, Duckworth WC. In search of the subcutaneous insulin resistance syndrome. New Engl J Med 1986; 315: 147–53.
28. Williams G, Pickup JC, Bowcock S, Cooke E, Keen H. Subcutaneous aprotinin improves control in some diabetic patients. Diabetologia 1983; 24: 91–4.
29. Chisholm DJ, Kraegen EW, Hewett MJ, Furler S. Low subcutaneous degradation and slow absorption of insulin in insulin-dependent diabetic patients during continuous subcutaneous insulin infusion at basal rate. Diabetologia 1984; 27: 238–41.

30. Binder C, Lauritzen T, Faber OK, Pramming S. Insulin pharmacokinetics. Diabetes Care 1984; 7: 188–99.

31. Williams G, Pickup J, Clark A, Bowcock S, Cooke E, Keen H. Changes in blood flow close to subcutaneous insulin injection sites in stable and brittle diabetics. Diabetes 1983; 32: 466–73.

32. Williams G, Pickup JC, Collins ACG, Keen H. Subcutaneous insulin absorption and glycaemic responses in brittle diabetes. Diabet Med 1986; 3: 365–6A.

33. McElduff A, Eastman CJ, Haynes SP, Bowen KM. Apparent insulin resistance due to abnormal enzymatic insulin degradation: a new mechanism for insulin resistance. Aust NZ J Med 1980; 10: 56–61.

34. Williams G, Pickup JC, Keen H. Massive insulin resistance apparently due to rapid clearance of circulating insulin. Am J Med 1987; 82: 1247–52.

35. Jialal I, King GL, Buchwald S et al. Processing of insulin by bovine endothelial cells in culture. Internalisation without degradation. Diabetes 1984; 33: 794–800.

36. Cryer PE, Gerich JE. Relevance of glucose counterregulatory systems to patients with diabetes: critical roles of glucagon and epinephrine. Diabetes 1983; 6: 95–9.

37. Home PD, Gill GV, Husband DJ, Massi-Benedetti M, Marshall SM, Alberti KGMM. Hormonal and metabolic abnormalities. In Pickup JC (ed.) Brittle diabetes. Oxford: Blackwell, 1985: pp 167–80.

38. Nattrass M, Hale PJ. Clinical aspects of diabetic ketoacidosis. Rec Adv Diab 1984; 1: 231–8.

39. Rayfield EJ, Ault MJ, Keusch GT et al. Infection and diabetes: the case for glucose control. Am J Med 1982; 72: 439–50.

40. Hockaday TDR. Infective illness. In Pickup JC (ed.) Brittle diabetes. Oxford: Blackwell, 1985: pp 68–75.

41. White NH, Santiago JV. Clinical features and natural history of brittle diabetes in children. In Pickup JC (ed.) Brittle diabetes. Oxford: Blackwell, 1985: pp 19–28.

42. Gill GV, Walford S, Alberti KGMM. Brittle diabetes—present concepts. Diabetologia 1985; 28: 579–89.

43. Schade DS, Drumm DA, Duckworth WC, Eaton RP. The etiology of incapacitating, brittle diabetes. Diabetes Care 1985; 8: 12–20.

44. Schade DS, Drumm DA, Eaton RP, Sterling WA. Factitious brittle diabetes mellitus. Am J Med 1985; 78: 777–84.

45. O'Brien IAD, Lewin IG, Frier BM, Rodman H, Genuth S, Corrall RJM. Factitious diabetic instability. Diabet Med 1985; 2: 392–4.

46. Orr DP, Eccles T, Lawlor R, Golden M. Surreptitious insulin administration in adolescents with insulin-dependent diabetes mellitus. JAMA 1986; 256: 3227–30.

47. Rosen H, Lidz T. Emotional factors in the precipitation of recurrent diabetic acidosis. Psychosom Med 1949; 11: 211–15.

48. Minuchin S, Baker L, Rosman BL, Liebman R, Milman L, Todd TC. A conceptual model of psychosomatic illness in children. Psychosom Med 1975; 32: 1031–8.

49. Orr DP, Golden MP, Myers G, Marrero DG. Characteristics of adolescents with poorly controlled diabetes referred to a tertiary care center. Diabetes Care 1983; 6: 170–5.

50. White K, Kolman ML, Wexler P, Polin G, Winter RJ. Unstable diabetes and unstable families: a psychosocial evaluation of diabetic children with recurrent ketoacidosis. Pediatrics 1984; 73: 749–55.

51. Hinkle LE, Wolf S. Importance of life stress in course and management of diabetes mellitus. JAMA 1952; 148: 513–20.

52. Baker L, Barkai A, Kaye R, Haque N. Beta adrenergic blockade and juvenile diabetes: acute studies and long-term therapeutic trial. J Pediatr 1969; 75: 19–29.

53. Kemmer FW, Bisping R, Steingruber HJ, Baar H, Hardtmann F, Schlaghecke R, Berger M. Psychological stress and metabolic control in patients with type 1 diabetes mellitus. New Engl J Med 1986; 314: 1078–84.

54. Rodin GM, Daneman D, Johnson LE, Kenshole A, Garfinkle P. Anorexia nervosa and bulimia in female adolescents with insulin dependent diabetes mellitus: a systematic study. J Psychiat Res 1985; 19: 381–4.

55. Wing RR, Nowalk MP, Marus MD, Koeske R, Finegold D. Subclinical eating disorders and glycemic control in adolescents with type 1 diabetes. Diabetes Care 1986; 9: 162–7.

56. La Greca AM, Schwarz LT, Satin W. Eating patterns in young women with IDDM: another look. Diabetes Care 1987; 10: 659–60.

57. Schade DS, Eaton RP, Drumm DA, Duckworth W. A clinical algorithm to determine the etiology of brittle diabetes. Diabetes Care 1985; 8: 5–11.

58. Gale EAM. Basic principles in the management of unstable diabetic control. In Pickup JC (ed.) Brittle diabetes. Oxford: Blackwell, 1985: pp 183–99.

59. Ng Tang Fui S, Pickup JC, Bending JJ, Collins ACG, Keen H, Daeton N. Hypoglycemia and counterregulation in insulin dependent diabetic patients: a comparison of continuous subcutaneous insulin infusion and conventional injection therapy. Diabetes Care 1986; 9: 221–7.

60. Nathan DM. Successful treatment of extremely brittle, insulin-dependent diabetes with a novel

subcutaneous insulin pump regimen. Diabetes Care 1982; 5: 105–10.

61. Williams G, Pickup JC, Keen H. Continuous intravenous insulin infusion in the management of brittle diabetes: etiological and therapeutic implication. Diabetes Care 1985; 8: 21–7.

62. Husband DJ, Marshall SM, Walford S, Hanning I, Wright PD, Alberti KGMM. Continuous intraperitoneal insulin infusion in the management of severely brittle diabetes—a metabolic and clinical comparison with intravenous infusion. Diabet Med 1984; 1: 99–104.

63. Campbell IW, Kritz H, Najemnik G, Hagmueller G, Irsigler K. Treatment of type 1 diabetic with subcutaneous insulin resistance by a totally implantable insulin infusion device ('Infusaid'). Diabetes Res 1984; 1: 83–8.

64. Gill GV, Husband DJ, Wright PD et al. The management of severe brittle diabetes with 'Infusaid' implantable pumps. Diabetes Res 1986; 3: 135–7.

65. Buchwald H, Chute EP, Goldenburg FJ et al. Implantable infusion pump management of insulin diabetes mellitus. Ann Surg 1985; 202: 278–82.

66. White NH, Santiago JV. Enhancing subcutaneous insulin absorption. In Pickup JC (ed.) Brittle diabetes. Oxford: Blackwell, 1985: pp 241–53.

67. Pickup JC, Bilous RW, Keen H. Aprotinin and insulin resistance. Lancet 1980; ii: 93–4.

68. Blazar BR, Whitely CB, Kitabchi AE et al. In vivo chloroquine-induced inhibition of insulin degradation in a diabetic patient with severe insulin resistance. Diabetes 1984; 33: 1133–7.

69. Williams G, Pickup JC. The natural history of brittle diabetes Diabetes Res 1988; 7: 13–18.

44

Clinical Insulin Resistance

David S. Schade and Georges M. Argoud

Department of Medicine, University of New Mexico, Albuquerque, New Mexico, USA

This chapter focuses on clinical insulin resistance, in contrast to cellular insulin resistance. Although it is true that abnormalities in cellular glucose metabolism may be expressed as clinical insulin resistance, they do not always become clinically manifest. For example, a cellular defect in glucose metabolism may be unimportant in a clinical context if the defect is not rate limiting or if alternative glucose metabolic pathways exist. Furthermore, clinical insulin resistance can be caused by non-cellular abnormalities such as high-affinity insulin antibodies or anti-insulin receptor antibodies. From the viewpoint of the physician who must treat an insulin resistant patient to maintain glucose homeostasis, it is the clinical expression of insulin resistance that is of paramount importance.

This chapter is divided into two major sections. The first part describes the experimental techniques that are in current use to diagnose human clinical insulin resistance. These techniques are undergoing significant changes, and the reader should realize that new approaches are rapidly evolving. The second part of this chapter describes the presentation of patients with various etiologies of insulin resistance including diagnosis and therapy. This area is also evolving rapidly, in parallel with major advances in our understanding of the pathophysiology of insulin resistance.

EXPERIMENTAL TECHNIQUES FOR ASSESSMENT OF INSULIN SENSITIVITY

Historical Perspective

Investigations of insulin sensitivity in terms of assessing the degree of the metabolic response caused by insulin in diabetes mellitus and obesity have been undertaken since the 1930s [1]. However, in the last two decades more emphasis has been devoted to quantitation of the appropriateness of insulin's glycoregulatory actions in diabetes because of the recognition that insulin resistance is a major contributor to the pathogenesis of non-insulin dependent diabetes mellitus (NIDDM) [2–5] and insulin dependent diabetes mellitus (IDDM) [6] as well.

Various approaches have been utilized to quantitate normal and aberrant insulin sensitivity in humans. First, the glucose tolerance test has been utilized in the past to assess the degree of hyperinsulinemia with respect to the level of plasma glucose as an indication of the presence of insulin resistance. However, because of the immediate temporal interdependence of insulin and glucose during this test, it is difficult to distinguish insulin secretory defects from inadequacies of insulin action at the tissue levels [7]. Second, the insulin suppression test was developed in an effort to avoid the confounding effects of feedback between insulin and glucose

International Textbook of Diabetes Mellitus. Edited by K.G.M.M. Alberti, R.A. DeFronzo, H. Keen and P. Zimmet
© 1992 John Wiley & Sons Ltd

and, more importantly, to permit isolated evaluation of insulin action [8]. The goal of the insulin suppression test was to prevent endogenous insulin secretion with epinephrine plus propranolol (or somatostatin) infusions. Simultaneously with these infusions, standard quantities of insulin and glucose were administered so that the resulting steady state plasma glucose concentration could serve as an index of insulin sensitivity. However, there are several shortcomings of the insulin suppression test, such as occurrence of arrhythmias [9], the potential interfering effects of epinephrine, propranolol and/or somatostatin with insulin dependent metabolic processes, and the inconsistent suppression of hepatic glucose production. Because of these limitations, another technique—the glucose clamp—has been adopted by most current investigators of insulin sensitivity.

The Glucose Clamp

The glucose clamp technique involves maintaining the plasma glucose concentration at the basal level (for the euglycemic clamp) during an insulin infusion by means of a variable exogenous glucose infusion [10]. The quantity of glucose infused to maintain a stable basal glucose level during specific insulin infusion rates provides an assessment of insulin action. The changes in the plasma insulin level and the glucose infusion rate during a typical euglycemic clamp are illustrated in Figure 1. As a stable basal glycemia will prevent endogenous insulin secretion, the clamp technique permits a focused evaluation of peripheral tissue effects of insulin, i.e. insulin sensitivity, without the interfering variable of changing endogenous insulin secretion associated with fluctuating blood glucose levels. Another advantage of the euglycemic glucose clamp is avoidance of the problem of non-linear, insulin independent glucose utilization, which must be taken into account at variable plasma glucose concentrations [11].

A euglycemic clamp is usually performed under postabsorptive conditions when the rate of appearance of glucose is principally determined by hepatic glucose production, which in normal subjects in a steady state is equivalent to glucose utilization. In order to measure peripheral utilization and hepatic production of glucose, the tracer dilution technique and the equations of Steele with their later modifications [12]

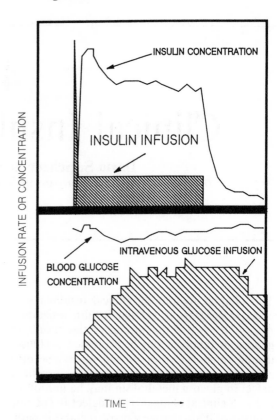

Figure 1 A representative euglycemic glucose clamp. Following a bolus intravenous injection, insulin is infused at a constant rate, resulting in a constant blood insulin concentration (top panel). Exogenous glucose is infused at a variable rate to maintain a constant (euglycemic) blood glucose concentration (bottom panel). The rate of glucose infusion is one measure of insulin sensitivity

are usually applied in combination with the glucose clamp. Thus, when hepatic glucose production is completely suppressed by exogenous insulin, the steady state glucose infusion rate is equivalent to total glucose production or glucose utilization.

The glucose clamp is an important research tool for determination of insulin sensitivity; however, its validity is dependent on careful attention to appropriate clamp procedure. For example, a crucial determinant of a successful clamp is the capacity to maintain the plasma glucose within a narrow range. Three of the more widely used methods of clamping the plasma glucose are feedback algorithms [13], the Biostator (glucose-controlled insulin infusion system) [13] and computer programs such as

PACBERG [14]. The principal function of all of these methods is to calculate the exogenous glucose infusion required to stabilize the plasma glucose during insulin administration. The drawback of feedback algorithms is that they often require manual override which introduces observer bias, while the Biostator causes a glucose profile with a sine wave configuration.

An important consideration in applying steady state turnover analysis during a glucose clamp is the principal assumption that a steady state is, indeed, achievable. A true steady state can be elusive, especially during high physiologic and supraphysiologic insulin infusions. Demonstration of changing glucose infusion rates after even 5 hours of a constant insulin infusion support the conclusion that only a quasi-steady state can be achieved [15]. Metabolic effects of the insulin plus glucose infusion, such as induction of glucose transporters, changes in rates of glycogen storage and possibly other intracellular processes involving glucose, may partially explain the instability of the 'steady state'.

Insulin Dose–Response Curves

The capacity to measure glucose turnover during the glucose clamp as a parameter of insulin action has been applied to constructing insulin dose–response curves (Figure 2). Thereafter, receptor and postreceptor processes were incorporated into the evaluation of insulin sensitivity during the insulin dose–response curve [16]. There is an analogy between the insulin receptor (in its relationship to insulin versus insulin's biologic effect) and an enzyme (in its relationship between a substrate and an enzyme-catalyzed reaction). In the pair of graphs shown in Figure 3, the terms 'V_{max}' and 'K_m' as they are applied to enzyme-catalyzed reactions and insulin dose–response curves are illustrated.

The current thesis is that, as plasma insulin concentration increases, a corresponding increase in insulin receptor recruitment leads to an incremental insulin response until a critical level of receptor activation is attained at which the maximum metabolic response (V_{max}) to insulin occurs. The plasma insulin concentrations at which half-maximal tissue response to insulin occurs is denoted K_m. Deviations of V_{max} and K_m derived from insulin dose–response curves from a population with insulin resistance, compared with V_{max} and K_m values determined in a normal

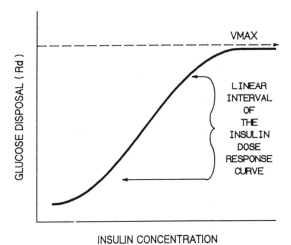

Figure 2 A representative insulin dose–response curve. The rate of glucose disposal is plotted versus the plasma insulin concentration. Different techniques may be utilized to obtain the points necessary to construct this curve. The slope and position of the linear interval of the insulin dose–response curve permits comparison of one curve to another without the necessity of having to determine V_{max}

population, have been used to draw conclusions regarding receptor and postreceptor mechanisms for insulin resistance. In Figure 4, the three types of shifts in insulin dose–response curves are shown, with the usual interpretations given to these specific shifts. An insulin receptor deficiency is suggested by an increased K_m, i.e. a rightward shift in the curve, whereas a postreceptor defect is indicated by a diminished V_{max}.

Most investigators of insulin sensitivity have combined measurement of insulin receptor binding with analysis of insulin dose–response curves. The reason for this combined approach is that numerous examples of a rightward-shifted curve being associated with normal insulin receptor binding have been reported [17, 18]. The interpretation of these findings is that a postreceptor defect is actually present which is not rate limiting in terms of the effects of in vivo, and thus V_{max} would not be decreased.

Determination of the insulin dose–response curve plus insulin receptor binding to assess the contribution of receptor versus postreceptor alterations in obesity has yielded varied results. A rightward curve shift, both normal and decreased V_{max}, and both normal and decreased insulin binding have been reported by different investigators [19]. There has also been

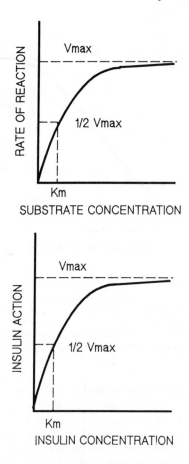

Figure 3   Similarity between an enzyme-catalyzed reaction
(top) and receptor-mediated insulin action (bottom)

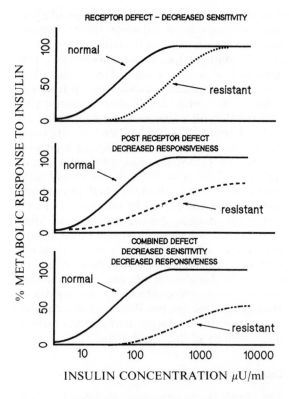

Figure 4   Theoretical changes in the insulin dose–response
curve depending upon whether there is an insulin receptor
defect, i.e. increased K_m (top); an insulin postreceptor defect,
i.e. decreased V_{max} (middle); or both an insulin receptor and
a postreceptor defect (bottom) (adapted from reference 16)

controversy regarding the contribution of receptor and/or postreceptor abnormalities to the
insulin resistance of NIDDM [20]. Methodologic
difficulties, as well as the assumptions inherent
in performance of insulin dose–response curves
and the imprecision involved in the measurement of insulin receptor binding, may contribute
to the varied results reported for these procedures in the literature.

With regard to insulin dose–response curves,
several aspects could potentially complicate
their interpretation. First, as discussed above, a
true steady state interval may be impossible to
achieve in vivo; therefore, dose–response curves
that are obtained by utilizing the steady state
glucose infusion rate as a measures of the tissue
effects of insulin are subject to variability due to
the different degrees of steady state achieved
among subjects. Second, the circulating plasma

insulin levels at which glucose utilization is
measured to delineate the dose–response curve
should be similar in the subjects with normal
and altered insulin sensitivity that are being
compared. However, substantial variation in
plasma insulin levels resulting from the same
insulin infusion rate administered to a group of
subjects is not uncommon [7]. In addition, possibly in part as a result of variation in circulating
insulin levels, a wide range of glucose utilization
rates has been reported, even in normal subjects
receiving the same insulin infusion rate [7].
Third, in some investigations 4 or more separate
days are required for determination of a dose–
response curve in a single subject, thus introducing the additional variable of day-to-day
variation in insulin-mediated glucose utilization.
Even though a mean insulin dose–response
curve determined in a group of patients with
insulin resistance is usually compared with the

mean curve obtained from a normal population, the significant variation in the two parameters that determine the dose–response curve may interfere with documentation of a curve shift. Fourth, diverse values for V_{max} and K_m in normal subjects have been reported [21, 22]. The varied values for K_m may be due to the fact that K_m is derived from the diverse V_{max}, and that determination of K_m requires estimating non-insulin dependent glucose utilization by extrapolation, which involves imprecision [21]. Thus, the discrepancies in V_{max} and K_m in normal subjects and the estimation involved in determination of K_m complicate comparison of insulin-sensitive with insulin-resistant dose–response curves. Finally, the relevance of applying dose–response curves that are based on supraphysiologic insulin concentrations and glucose disposal rates (V_{max} at plasma insulin levels of 700–10 000 μU/ml) to the clinical setting of diabetes (plasma insulin most often below 200 μU/ml) may be questioned.

Measurement of insulin receptor binding is often performed in studies of insulin sensitivity with dose–response curves to provide additional information about receptor/postreceptor mechanisms. However, determination of insulin receptor number and affinity is subject to considerable imprecision [23]. In addition, monocyte, hepatocyte, erythrocyte and adipocyte cell receptor assays have yielded disparate results [19]. It is currently not clear even whether adipose cell receptor assays in vitro correlate with human receptor activity in vivo, as less than 10% of total glucose disposal occurs in fat [19]. In spite of potential errors stemming from application of insulin dose–response curves and measurement of insulin receptor binding in the assessment of insulin sensitivity, these are still the most accepted and widely utilized methods available. However, two approaches to the evaluation of insulin sensitivity in vivo have been recently published, which do not require evaluation of V_{max} or K_m: these two approaches are termed (a) the minimal model and (b) the slope of the linear interval. A brief description of each of these approaches follows.

Pacini et al have published an alternative approach to assessing insulin sensitivity [14]. Although not yet completely validated, their approach utilizes a computerized minimal glucose model to calculate a 'sensitivity index'. The insulin sensitivity index is defined as the ratio between a change in insulin action (e.g. glucose disposal) and the change in plasma insulin that produced it. This index can be derived from data obtained during an insulin clamp study or a tolbutamide glucose tolerance test [24]. The advantage of their approach is that it can be completed within one day. The disadvantage is that the computer expertise necessary to calculate the sensitivity index is not yet widely available.

Prior to the validation by Argoud et al of the linear interval as a measure of insulin sensitivity [25], the concept of the 'inital slope' was suggested by Bergman as an approach to assess insulin sensitivity [7]. The initial slope was defined as the linear section of the insulin dose–response curve, which can be determined by evaluating steady state glucose disposal at three separate plasma insulin concentrations below 100 μM/ml. The theoretical advantages of the initial slope are that the supraphysiologic insulin levels associated with assessing V_{max} and the estimation of insulin independent glucose utilization for K_m are unnecessary. The disadvantage of this approach is that some patients with severe insulin resistance may not have sufficient data points on the initial slope at insulin concentrations below 100 μU/ml, thus complicating the determination of an adequate initial slope in such patients. Furthermore, even if three data points could be obtained, any error in measurement of the three points might greatly alter the initial slope. These problems may be overcome by expanding the concept of the initial slope to the plasma insulin range between basal levels and 400 μU/ml and by obtaining numerous data points over this entire interval, utilizing nonsteady state glucose kinetics (see Figure 2). This approach of determining insulin sensitivity has several unique advantages. First, the ability to determine the slope of the linear interval of the insulin dose–response curve in a single day eliminates the variable of day-to-day variation in glucose metabolism observed with some techniques utilized for constructing the insulin dose–response curve [22]. Second, the same protocol can be applied in subjects with normal and altered insulin sensitivity because of the wide range of plasma insulin concentrations utilized. Third, approximately 30 points (instead of only 4 by currently utilized methods) representing glucose turnover at plasma insulin concentrations between basal level and 400 μU/ml are determined, and at least 10 or more of these

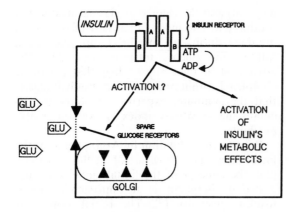

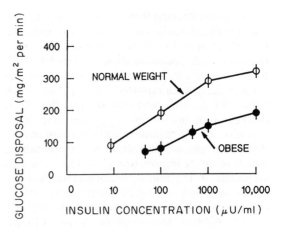

Figure 5 Interaction of insulin with its receptor on an insulin-sensitive cell. Either defects in insulin receptor binding or defects in metabolic processes of postinsulin receptor binding (or both) may lead to clinical insulin resistance (adapted from reference 19). GLU, glucose

Figure 6 Insulin dose–response curve in normal subjects and in a subpopulation of obese individuals. The curve of the obese subjects is shifted to the right and downward, suggesting the presence of both a receptor defect and a postreceptor defect respectively (adapted from reference 22)

points will lie along the linear portion of the dose–response curve. Finally, insulin sensitivity is measured at physiological instead of supraphysiological insulin concentrations.

INVESTIGATIONS OF INSULIN RESISTANCE IN DISEASE STATES

Insulin resistance is characteristic of several diseases. Because of the high prevalence of obesity and diabetes, extensive studies have been published in an attempt to understand the mechanism of these two insulin resistant states. To date, universal agreement does not exist on the pathophysiology of these disorders because of the lack of understanding of insulin mediated cellular metabolic processes. It is known that insulin interacts specifically with its receptor to initiate insulin action (Figure 5). This results in several different steps to augment insulin action, such as recruitment of spare glucose receptors from the Golgi apparatus and activation of several critical metabolic pathways. Whether the insulin does this directly, or through one or more second messengers, is not yet clear. Suffice it to say that clinical insulin resistance could result from a defect in any metabolic step that is rate-limiting within the insulin responsive cell.

The most common type of insulin resistance is that caused by obesity. In general, the degree of insulin resistance parallels the magnitude of the obesity. The resistance is secondary to the presence of excess adipose tissue, not body

weight, as muscular individuals are not insulin resistant. In a non-diabetic individual, the insulin resistance of obesity results in hyperinsulinemia. This hyperinsulinemia is observed in both the basal state and in response to insulin secretagogues, such as glucose, amino acids and sulfonylureas [19].

Much experimental work has been devoted to understanding the insulin resistance of obesity. Most studies have demonstrated that the actual number of insulin receptors per fat cell is not significantly decreased [26], although the number per cell surface area may be [19]. In contrast, the number of insulin receptors per hepatocyte in human obesity does appear to be reduced [27]. The structure of the insulin receptor in obesity does not appear to be abnormal [27]. In addition to a reduction in receptor number, some obese patients demonstrate a decreased V_{max}, suggesting a postreceptor defect in glucose metabolism [22]. Thus, obesity may be associated with both receptor and postreceptor defects in many patients (Figure 6).

The insulin resistance of NIDDM has defied a simplistic explanation. This is probably because the disease is heterogeneous and the cellular metabolic defects multiple. Several groups have reported a decrease in insulin receptor number in NIDDM [28]. Although this may be true, this reduction may not necessarily result in insulin resistance because a large number of spare receptors are present on the cell surface. In fact, only 10% of insulin receptors need to be occupied to result in maximal insulin action [7]. Furthermore, not all investigative groups have observed a decrease in insulin receptor number [7]. Thus, the specific role of insulin receptors per se in causing the insulin resistance of NIDDM is not clear.

Much effort has recently been devoted to studying defects in postinsulin receptor events as a cause of insulin resistance in NIDDM. According to this concept, normal maximal insulin action cannot be achieved because the defect is postinsulin receptor binding (Figure 6). Investigations by Olefsky and colleagues suggest that the higher the fasting blood glucose concentration, the more severe is the postreceptor defect [28]. The precise metabolic steps causing the postreceptor insulin defect are not resolved, but may involve any or all of the rate-limiting glucose metabolic pathways, such as a defect in glucose transport activity [29], altered tyrosine kinase activity at the insulin receptor [30], decreased insulin-generated mediators [31] and structural abnormalities in capillary muscle blood flow [32]. Irrespective of the defect resulting in insulin resistance in NIDDM, it is clear that the degree of resistance is altered by the degree of metabolic control. Thus, when NIDDM patients are treated with aggressive insulin therapy or sulfonylureas, an improvement in insulin resistance occurs although it is not completely reversed [33]. These observations raise the question of which abnormality is primary—the hyperglycemia or the insulin resistance. Most investigators believe that the insulin resistance, at least to some degree, antedates the hyperglycemia. Whether the insulin resistance is caused initially by a decreased capacity to secrete insulin from the B cell or is a primary cellular defect is controversial.

CLINICAL APPROACH TO THE INSULIN RESISTANT PATIENT

Although obese patients and both IDDM and NIDDM patients have measurable insulin resistance, typically the IDDM patients (and only a majority of these individuals) present with a clinical problem of insulin resistance requiring diagnosis and management. Obese patients and NIDDM patients do have metabolic abnormalities secondary to insulin resistance (e.g.

hyperlipidemia) but it is the IDDM patient presenting with frequent episodes of diabetic keto-acidosis who provides the physician with a diagnostic and therapeutic challenge.

When the physician is confronted with a patient with 'insulin resistance', what procedure should be followed? There are four important sequential steps to ensure efficient diagnosis and treatment: these steps include (1) confirmation of the insulin resistant state; (2) location and identification of the insulin resistance; (3) treatment of the pathophysiology, and (4) long-term follow-up and reassessment. Each of these steps is discussed below, on the basis of the author's experience with 50 such patients.

Confirmation of the Diagnosis

This step is the most important and most frequently omitted of the four. The reason that the physician often assumes that the patient is insulin resistant is that (1) the patient or the referring physician states that insulin resistance is present, (2) the referred patient is usually accompanied by many medical records 'proving' insulin resistance, and (3) many physicians are not certain how to confirm or refute the diagnosis. In fact, confirmation of the presence of the insulin resistant state is not difficult and does not necessarily require sophisticated testing such as a glucose clamp.

The simplest definition of 'insulin resistance' is failure of the blood glucose concentration to respond normally to insulin. Unfortunately, this definition is not clinically useful because the 'normal' response to insulin varies considerably depending on the clinical setting. For example, a reduction in blood glucose concentration is not always the normal response to subcutaneous insulin injection. In an IDDM patient who has recently ingested a large carbohydrate meal and has taken 5 U regular insulin, a normal response to this insulin dose may be a decline in the rate of rise of blood glucose concentration, not an absolute reduction in blood glucose concentration. An analogous clinical situation in which an insulin dose would not be accompanied by a hypoglycemic response is the unanticipated absorption of food from the gastrointestinal tract in a patient with delayed gastric emptying.

From the above discussion it should be apparent that to make the diagnosis of insulin resistance, all variables that might alter the blood

Table 1 Variables other than insulin that may alter glucose concentration

1. Factitious disease
2. Manipulative behavior
3. Communication disorders
4. Delayed gastric emptying
5. Excessive counterregulatory hormones
6. Surreptitious food ingestion
7. Miscellaneous—acidosis, dehydration, thyrotoxicosis, chronic hyperglycemia, medication, etc.

glucose concentration (except insulin) must be kept constant (Table 1). Factitious disease is extremely difficult to exclude in the differential diagnosis of insulin resistance (see also Chapter 20). The patient may remove the insulin from the vial and replace it with water or another substance [34]. The physician must be alert to this possibility and suspect it in all patients until it is proven otherwise by an unequivocal laboratory test result. In our experience, these patients are usually very intelligent, with no obvious psychopathology. Proof may require months of observation and retesting. Fortunately, this group constitutes the minority of patients referred with insulin resistance [35]. Manipulative behavior differs from factitious disease in that, in the former, an identifiable reason for the aberrant behavior is present. These patients are usually female diabetic teenagers who utilize their disease to obtain short-term goals such as peer acceptance and parental sympathy. However, we have also seen adult patients who utilize their diabetes to obtain narcotics and the medical benefits of having a chronic illness [35]. Communication disorders are probably the most common cause of apparent insulin resistance [36]. Surprisingly, this etiology is the most frequently overlooked by the physician. Confirmation of this etiology requires testing by a trained professional. In the simplest form of communication disorder, the diabetic patient perceives the diabetic instructions and treatment in a different manner to the physician. This difference is not apparent to either the patient or the physician; thus, the patient could be following one therapeutic regimen whereas the physician believes the patient is following another. Delayed gastric emptying should be considered in all apparently insulin resistant patients with any signs or symptoms of autonomic neuropathy or diabetes greater than 10 years' duration. A his-

tory of gastric fullness and nausea after eating are characteristic symptoms. Testing for this condition is easy, involving patient ingestion of a technetium-99 egg meal [37]. Excessive stress hormones may induce insulin resistance by their anti-insulin actions. These hormones include glucagon, catecholamines, cortisol and growth hormone. The mechanisms by which counterregulatory hormones induce insulin resistance is by increasing hepatic glucose production and/or decreasing peripheral glucose utilization. These hormones may be secreted during many types of stress, e.g. in response to fever or myocardial infarction. Chronic insulin resistance occurs in tumors that secrete these hormones (e.g. glucagonomas, pheochromocytomas and pituitary adenomas). These conditions should all be excludable with an adequate medical history, physical examination and appropriate laboratory tests. Surreptitious food ingestion often causes apparent insulin resistance because the carbohydrate absorbed negates the expected decline of blood glucose concentration following insulin injection. In our experience, this usually occurs in overweight teenagers who will not admit to not adhering to a diabetic diet. There are several miscellaneous causes of apparent insulin resistance that should be identifiable clinically, including chronic acidosis, dehydration, thyrotoxicosis, etc. Appropriate laboratory testing should alert the physician to permit identification and treatment of these conditions [38].

In concert with the exclusion of the above-mentioned factors associated with insulin resistance, the physician should directly test the patient's response to intravenously administered insulin. This can easily be done in centers familiar with the glucose clamp technique. However, in most hospitals, a simpler approach is adequate. As control data have been published for two such tests, we recommend that both tests be performed sequentially. The first test is the determination of the overnight basal insulin requirements in IDDM patients [39–41]; the second test is the glucose response to a bolus intravenous injection of 0.1 U/kg of insulin [42]. As the protocol of the second test requires the patient to be relatively euglycemic overnight, this stabilization period can also be used to provide the overnight basal insulin requirement. If the patient has overnight insulin requirements greater than 2 U insulin per hour intravenously, or responds with less than a 50 mg/dl decline in blood glucose concentration when 0.1 U/kg of insulin is injected by the physician intravenously, then insulin resistance exists. If the patient has a normal response to both these tests, then either the patient is not clinically significantly resistant to insulin or the patient has subcutaneous insulin resistance. Whether the latter condition even exists is debatable: we have been unable to confirm it in any patient, nor do we believe that any of the patients in the literature were sufficiently studied to exclude the other possibilities listed in Table 1. Exclusion of this diagnosis is relatively simple, employing a subcutaneous challenge bolus dose of insulin at 0.1 U/kg [42].

Location of the Insulin Resistance

If the patient exhibits insulin resistance by the above criteria, then the physican must identify its location. Assuming that the subcutaneous tissue is not involved, then the location for the resistance is either in the blood or at the tissue level. Two mechanisms have been reported by which blood constituents may cause insulin resistance: first, antibodies to the insulin molecule may induce insulin resistance by binding free insulin in the circulation [16, 43]; second, antibodies directed against the insulin receptor may prevent insulin from enhancing cellular glucose transport [44]. The former cause can be identified by performing a competitive insulin antibody radioimmunoassay; the second condition can be identified by performing a competitive binding assay utilizing normal erythrocyte insulin receptors and the patient's plasma. These tests are available in most diabetic research laboratories but are not routinely performed by the hospital clinical laboratories. Assuming that these two mechanisms are excluded, then the patient has insulin resistance at the tissue level. This type of insulin resistance is usually separated into receptor and postreceptor (or binding and postbinding abnormalities) (Figure 5). However, in our experience, this distinction is not clinically necessary as specific treatments for these two mechanisms are not available. Furthermore, in some patients a combined defect (or defects) may be present. This area is under intense study; specific therapy may, therefore, be available in the future.

Treatment of Insulin Resistance

Successful treatment of insulin resistance depends upon correct identification of the location and mechanism. Unfortunately, this approach is not always adhered to and the medical literature is replete with numerous empirical short-term treatment successes. However, when controlled long-term studies are performed, lack of therapeutic efficacy of empirical treatment is usually evident.

Treatment of insulin resistance located within the subcutaneous tissue would rationally be treated with delivery of insulin, either intravenously or intraperitoneally. Both approaches have been utilized with short-term success but with only minimal long-term improvement [45]. Studies in depth of patients with apparent subcutaneous resistance have failed to validate the presence of this syndrome [42]. We recommend that before the institution of treatment for subcutaneous insulin resistance, the patient should be referred to a medical center experienced in the evaluation of this syndrome. If the insulin resistance is located in the plasma, then the mechanism is either antibodies to the insulin or antibodies to the insulin receptor. If antibodies to insulin are the mechanism, then the treatment depends upon the clinical state of the patient. In rare patients with extremely high titers of anti-insulin antibodies that are inducing metabolic decompensation (diabetic ketoacidosis), high-dose steroids have been reported to be effective in disassociating the antibody-antigen complexes [43]. However, extreme care must be exercised in these patients because the sudden increase in free insulin levels may induce severe hypoglycemia and death. This entity is observed much less frequently than heretofore because of the use of purified insulins. For chronic antibody-mediated insulin resistance, treatment depends upon the specificity of the antibody. Most insulin manufacturers will provide specific titers of antibeef, antipork and antihuman insulin antibodies. Changing to a low-titer species will frequently ameliorate the insulin resistance. Low titers of anti-insulin antibodies, which may reduce the rise in plasma free insulin following insulin injection, should not induce metabolic decompensation if adequate amounts of insulin are administered to the patient.

The presence of anti-insulin receptor antibodies is of great concern to the physician as these antibodies may paradoxically induce hyperglycemia by binding with the insulin receptor. Treatment of hyperglycemia in these patients can be very difficult because very few insulin receptor sites may be available to interact with insulin. Clinically, this means that large quantities of administered insulin may have a minimal effect in these patients [46]. Our approach has been to utilize the patient's kidney to prevent severe hyperglycemia (by rapid diuresis) when the patient's blood glucose level exceeds the renal threshold. Thus, we maintain the patient in a state of volume expansion by having the patient ingest excessive quantities of salt (via popcorn, potato chips, salt tablets, etc.) and monitoring their weight as an index of hydration. Improvement may occur if the underlying disease (frequently systemic lupus erythematosus) enters a remission phase. Unfortunately, the prognosis of these patients is guarded [44].

Treatment of insulin resistance at the cellular level requires correction of the clinical condition known to induce insulin resistance at this location. Obesity, the classical cause of cellular insulin resistance, is approached with dietary weight loss therapy. Several approaches to the correction of the insulin resistance of NIDDM exist: most important is the normalization of glucose metabolism by either exogenous insulin administration or sulfonylurea therapy [47]; in some patients, the combination of insulin plus sulfonylureas may be better than either agent alone [48]. As the majority of NIDDM patients are obese, dietary therapy promoting weight loss should also be encouraged.

Long-term Follow-up and Reassessment

Although the majority of patients with insulin resistance can be correctly diagnosed and treated, a minority will have cellular resistance of obscure mechanism. These patients are extremely difficult to treat and may require continuous intravenous or intraperitoneal insulin to prevent metabolic decompensation. Until the mechanisms involved are understood, appropriate therapy will be difficult to identify.

CONCLUSION

In summary, significant advances are being made in categorizing insulin resistance based on the mechanism which may be related to blood constituents, receptor abnormalities or postreceptor defects. However, most hospitals do not have techniques such as the glucose clamp and receptor assays available for evaluating patients with insulin resistance. Nonetheless, the clinician faced with such patients can proceed with a diagnostic evaluation by recognizing factors that may be associated with insulin resistance and by utilizing overnight insulin requirements and an intravenous insulin challenge test. Such an approach will allow appropriate treatment in a majority of patients.

REFERENCES

1. Himsworth HP. Diabetes mellitus. Its differentiation into insulin-sensitive and insulin-insensitive types. Lancet 1939; i: 127–41
2. Kolterman O, Gray R, Griffin J et al. Receptor and postreceptor defects contribute to the insulin resistance in noninsulin-dependent diabetes. J. Clin Invest 1981; 68: 957–69
3. Reaven G, Berstein R, Davis B, Olefsky J. Nonketotic diabetes mellitus: insulin deficiency or insulin resistance. Am J Med 1976; 60: 809–88
4. Efendic S, Luft R, Wajngot A. Aspects of the pathogenesis of Type II diabetes. Endocr Rev 1984; 5: 395–410
5. Ginsberg H, Kemmerling G, Olefsky JM, Reaven GM. Demonstration of insulin resistance in untreated adult-onset diabetic subjects with fasting hyperglycemia. J Clin Invest 1975; 55: 454–61
6. Pedersen O, Beck-Nielsen H. Insulin resistance and insulin-dependent diabetes mellitus. Diabetes Care 1987; 10: 516–23
7. Bergman RM, Finegood DT, Ader M. Assessment of insulin sensitivity in vivo. Endocr Rev 1985; 6: 45–86
8. Greenfield MS, Doberne L, Kraemer F, Tobey T, Reaven G. Assessment of insulin resistance with the insulin suppression test and the euglycemic clamp. Diabetes 1981; 30: 387–92
9. Lampman RM, Santinga JT, Bassett BR, Savage PJ. Cardiac arrhythmias during epinephrine–propranolol infusions for measurement of in vivo insulin resistance. Diabetes 1981; 30: 618–41
10. DeFronzo RA, Tobin JD, Andres R. Glucose clamp technique: a method for quantifying insulin secretion and resistance. Am J Physiol 1979; 237: E214–23
11. Gottesman I, Mandarino L, Gerich J. Use of glucose and glucose clearance for the evaluation of insulin action in vivo. Diabetes 1984; 33: 184–90

12. Steele B, Wall JS, DeBodo RC, Altszuler N. Measurement of size and turnover rate of body glucose pool by the isotope dilution method. Am J Physiol 1956; 187: 15–24

13. Ponchner M, Heine RJ, Pernet A et al. A comparison of the artificial pancreas (glucose controlled insulin infusion system) and a manual technique for assessing insulin sensitivity during euglycemic clamping. Diabetologia 1984; 26: 420–5

14. Pacini G, Finegood DT, Bergman RN. A minimal-model-based glucose clamp yielding insulin sensitivity independent of glycemia. Diabetes 1982; 31: 432–41

15. Doberne L, Greenfield MS, Schulz B, Reaven GM. Enhanced glucose utilization during prolonged glucose clamp studies. Diabetes 1981; 30: 829–43

16. Kahn CR. Insulin resistance, insulin insensitivity, and insulin unresponsiveness: a necessary distinction. Metabolism 1978; 27: 1893–907

17. Pedersen O, Hijollunk E, Schwartz N. Insulin-receptor binding and insulin action in human fat cells: effects of obesity and fasting. Metabolism 1982; 31: 884–95

18. Lonnoth P, DiGirolamo M, Krotkiewski M, Smith U. Insulin binding and responsiveness in fat cells from patients with reduced glucose tolerance and Type II diabetes. Diabetes 1983; 32: 748–54

19. Truglia JA, Livingston JN, Lockwood DH. Insulin resistance: receptor and post-binding defects in human obesity and non-insulin-dependent diabetes mellitus. Am J Med 1985; 979 (suppl. 2B): 13–22

20. Mandarino LJ, Campbell PJ, Gottesman IS, Gerich JE. Abnormal coupling of insulin-receptor binding in non-insulin-dependent diabetes. Am J Physiol 1984; 247: E688–92

21. Rizza RA, Mandarino LJ, Gerich JE. Dose-response characteristics for effects of insulin on production and utilization of glucose in man. Am J Physiol 1981; 240: E630–9

22. Kolterman OG, Insel LJ, Saekow M, Olefsky JM. Mechanisms of insulin resistance in human obesity. Evidence for receptor and post-receptor defects. J Clin Invest 1980; 65: 1272–89

23. Gerich JE, Rizza RA, Mandarino LJ. Assessment of insulin action in humans with observations on the insulin resistance in noninsulin-dependent diabetes mellitus. In Skyler JS (ed.) Insulin update: 1982. Amsterdam: Excerpta Medica, 1982: pp 74–96

24. Beard JC, Bergman RN, Ward WK, Porte D Jr. The insulin sensitivity index in nondiabetic man. Correlation between clamp-derived and IVGTT-derived values. Diabetes 1986; 35: 362–9

25. Argoud GM, Schade DS. Validation of the dynamic nonsteady state insulin dose response curve—a new approach to insulin sensitivity. Diabetes 1987; 36 (suppl. 1): 118A–37A

26. Amatruda JM, Livingston JN, Lockwood DH. Insulin receptor interaction in human obesity. Science 1975; 188: 264–6

27. Amer P, Einarsson K, Backman L, Nilsell K, Lerea KM, Livingston JN. Studies of liver insulin receptors in non-obese and obese human subjects. J Clin Invest 1983; 72: 1729–36

28. Olefsky JM, Ciaraldi TP, Kolterman OG. Mechanisms of insulin resistance in non-insulin-dependent (Type II) diabetes. Am J Med 1985; 79 (suppl. 3B): 12–22

29. Kashwagi A, Verso MA, Andrews J, Vasquez B, Reaven G, Foley JE. In vitro insulin resistance of human adipocytes isolated from subjects with non-insulin-dependent diabetes mellitus. J Clin Invest 1983; 72: 1246–54

30. Kasuga M, Zick Y, Blithe DL, Krettaz M, Kahn CR. Insulin stimulates tyrosine phosphorylation of the insulin receptor in a cell-free system. Nature 1982; 298: 667–9

31. Larner J, Galasko J, Cheng K, DePoali-Roach AA, Huag L, Daggy P, Kellogg J. Generation by insulin of a chemical mediator that controls protein phosphorylation and dephosphorylation. Science 1979; 206: 1408–10

32. Bogardus C. Muscle histology and insulin action in vivo. Curr Concepts 1987; 40: 24–5

33. Scarlett JA, Kolterman OG, Ciaraldi TP, Kao M, Olefsky JM. Insulin treatment reverses the post-receptor defect in adipocyte 3-O-methyl glucose transport in Type II diabetes mellitus. J Clin Endocrinol Metab 1983; 56: 1195–201

34. Schade DS, Drumm DA, Eaton RP, Sterling WA. Factitious brittle diabetes mellitus. Am J Med 1985; 78: 777–91

35. Schade DS, Drumm DA, Duckworth WC, Eaton PR. The etiology of incapacitating, brittle diabetes. Diabetes Care 1985; 8: 12–22

36. Drumm DA, Schade DS. How communication disorders destabilize diabetes. Clin Diabetes 1986; 4: 16–23

37. Malmud LS, Fisher RS, Knight LC, Rock E. Scintigraphic evaluation of gastric emptying. Sem Nucl Med 1982; 12: 116–32

38. Schade DS, Eaton RP, Drumm DA, Duckworth WC. A clinical algorithm to determine the etiology of brittle diabetes. Diabetes Care 1985; 8: 5–17

39. White NH, Skor D, Santiago JV. Practical closed-loop insulin delivery. Ann Intern Med 1982; 97: 210–23

40. Lambert AE, Buysschaert M, Marchand E, Pierard M, Wojcik S, Lambotte L. Determination of insulin requirements in brittle diabetic patients by the artificial pancreas. Diabetes 1978; 27: 825–37

41. Schade DS, Argoud GM. Subclinical systemic insulin resistance—cause of apparent subcutaneous insulin resistance. Diabetes 1987; 36 (suppl 1): 118A-29A

42. Schade DS, Duckworth WC. In search of the subcutaneous-insulin-resistance syndrome. New Engl J Med 1986; 315: 147-59

43. Shipp JC, Cunningham RW, Russell RO, Marble A. Insulin resistance: clinical features, natural course and effects of adrenal steroid treatment. Medicine 1967; 44: 165-8

44. Kahn CR, Flier JS, Bar RS et al. The syndromes of insulin resistance and acanthosis nigricans: insulin-receptor disorders in man. New Engl J Med 1976; 294: 739-45

45. Husband DJ, Marshal SM, Walford S, Hanning I, Wright PD, Alberti KGMM. Continuous intraperitoneal insulin infusion in the management of severely brittle diabetes—a metabolic and clinical comparison with intravenous infusion. Diabet Med 1984; 1: 99-104

46. Eaton RP, Friedman N, Allen RC, Schade DS. Insulin removal in man: in vivo evidence for a receptor-mediated process. J Clin Endocrinol Metab 1984; 58: 555-621

47. Firth RG, Bell PM, Rizza RA. Effects of tolazamide and exogenous insulin on insulin action in patients with non-insulin-dependent diabetes mellitus. New Engl J Med 1986; 20: 1280-6

48. Schade DS, Mitchell WJ, Griego G, Addition of sulfonylurea to insulin treatment in poorly controlled Type II diabetes. JAMA 1987; 257: 2441-6

45

Diabetes Mellitus and Pregnancy

B. Persson*, U. Hanson† and N.-O. Lunell‡

**Department of Pediatrics, St Göran's Hospital; Departments of Obstetrics and Gynecology,
†Karolinska and ‡Huddinge Hospitals; Karolinska Institute, Stockholm, Sweden*

Pregnancies complicated by diabetes mellitus used to be associated with a considerably increased risk of maternal, fetal and neonatal complications. Today, the outlook for intact survival of the infant has improved markedly. The dramatic decline in perinatal mortality in diabetic pregnancy seen in most specialized units throughout the world is usually attributed to improved blood glucose control during pregnancy.

Despite major advances in clinical management we are still facing problems: perinatal morbidity is still elevated, and the incidence of malformations in the newborn has also increased—indeed, malformations have become increasingly prominent and represent today in many centers the most important single cause of perinatal mortality or severe morbidity.

DEFINITIONS

A new classification for diabetes mellitus was proposed by the World Health Organization (WHO) in 1980 and re-emphasized in 1985 [1]. The new classification is no longer based upon the age of onset (see Chapter 1), but divides the disease into three main classes as follows:

(I)   Diabetes mellitus
   (A) Insulin dependent diabetes mellitus (IDDM, type 1)
   (B) Non-insulin dependent diabetes mellitus (NIDDM, type 2)
   (C) Malnutrition dependent diabetes mellitus (MRDM)
   (D) Other types associated with certain abnormalities, for example pancreatic or Cushing's disease

(II)   Impaired glucose tolerance

(III)   Gestational diabetes mellitus (GDM)

Glucose Tolerance Test

The oral glucose tolerance test (GTT) should be performed with 75 g glucose. Impaired glucose tolerance can, by definition, be diagnosed only with an oral GTT, and the 2-hour value is diagnostic (Table 1).

Gestational Diabetes

The diagnostic criteria for GDM have been the subject of intense controversy for decades. The WHO report of 1980 suggested that GDM

International Textbook of Diabetes Mellitus. Edited by K.G.M.M. Alberti, R.A. DeFronzo, H. Keen and P. Zimmet
© 1992 John Wiley & Sons Ltd

Table 1 Diagnostic values for the 75-g oral glucose tolerance test [1]

	Glucose concentration, mmol/l			
	Whole blood		Plasma	
	Venous	Capillary	Venous	Capillary
Diabetes mellitus				
Fasting value	≥ 6.7	≥ 6.7	≥ 7.8	≥ 7.8
2 h after glucose load	≥ 10.0	≥ 11.1	≥ 11.1	≥ 12.2
Impaired glucose tolerance				
Fasting value	< 6.7	< 6.7	< 7.8	< 7.8
2 h after glucose load	6.7–10.0	7.8–11.1	7.8–11.1	8.9–12.2

Table 2 Diagnostic criteria for gestational diabetes using the 100-g oral glucose tolerance test [2, 3]

	Fasting	1 h	2 h	3 h
Venous plasma glucose, mmol/l	5.8	10.6	9.2	8.1

Table 3 Classification of diabetes according to White [5]

White's class	Age at onset yr	Duration yr	Angiopathy
A	Any		
B	≥ 20	< 10	
C	10–19	10	
D	< 10	≥ 20	Benign retinopathy
R	Any	Any	Proliferative retinopathy
F	Any	Any	Nephropathy

should be classified according to the same criteria as for impaired glucose tolerance (Table 1). The adoption of this classification is far from universal. However, many centers in Europe have replaced the 50-g glucose load with the 75-g test, which is one step towards a common standard.

At the Second International Workshop Conference on GDM [2] it was proposed that the diagnosis of GDM should be based on results of a 100-g oral GTT with venous plasma glucose determined in the fasting state and at 1, 2 and 3 hours after the glucose load [2, 3]. Two or more values equal to or exceeding those in Table 2 are diagnostic. The 75-g oral GTT, which is used for diagnosis in non-pregnant subjects, is currently being evaluated for the diagnosis of GDM [4].

White's Classification

Traditionally, diabetic women are classified according to White [5], with increasing risk of a poor outcome and increasing severity of the diabetic disease (Table 3).

PERINATAL MORTALITY

Perinatal mortality includes all losses of viable fetuses from 28 weeks' gestation, to delivery, and all deaths of liveborn babies in the first week of life. Perinatal mortality has declined markedly during the last decade. In particular, there has been a marked reduction in the rate of stillbirths and neonatal deaths due to respiratory distress syndrome. In centers with a special interest in diabetes and pregnancy, results are approaching those seen in the non-diabetic population [6–8]. Much of this improvement is probably attributable to stricter control of the maternal diabetes than was formerly possible, following the introduction of home glucose monitoring, together with a more aggressive insulin therapy. The prognostic significance of the White classification is less evident today than hitherto, when outcome of pregnancy was clearly less favorable in White's classes C, D and F than in B and A. Nephropathy (class F), especially if complicated by hypertension, is still accompanied by an increased perinatal risk, with a perinatal mortality rate almost four times higher than in classes C, D and R [9].

HORMONAL AND METABOLIC ADAPTATION IN NORMAL PREGNANCY

In normal pregnancy, both fasting and post-prandial blood glucose levels tend to decrease with gestation. At the same time there is a progressive increase in fasting levels of circulating insulin, as well as an augmented insulin response to a glucose load. This enhanced capacity to secrete insulin increases with gestational age and is most striking during the last trimester of pregnancy. Insulin secretion, measured as urinary C-peptide excretion, reaches its peak value by 28–32 weeks of gestation [10]. Rising levels of progesterone, estrogens, cortisol and human placental lactogen are held responsible for the marked increase in insulin resistance which seems to be mediated at the postreceptor level. The blood glucose level is normally regulated within a narrow interval between 3.5 mmol/l and 6.5 mmol/l [11]. Glucose is a major metabolic substrate for the fetus and traverses the placenta by facilitated diffusion. Normally there is a very close relationship between maternal and fetal glucose concentrations during both early and late gestation. During extended fasting, pregnant women develop ketonemia more rapidly and show a more pronounced fall in plasma levels of both glucose and insulin than in the non-pregnant state. This metabolic response, designated 'accelerated starvation', is suggested to be the consequence of the host–parasite relation between mother and conceptus [12].

INSULIN DEPENDENT DIABETES MELLITUS

Women with adequately controlled IDDM are no more likely to be infertile than their non-diabetic counterparts. Disturbances in the ovulation and menstrual cycle may occur when diabetes is poorly controlled.

The incidence of IDDM varies between 0.2% and 0.3% of all pregnancies [13, 14].

Embryopathy

Spontaneous Abortion

Most studies report a spontaneous abortion rate in diabetic pregnancy that is comparable to that of the non-diabetic population [15]. Early spontaneous abortion is often associated with severe fetal or placental anomalies [16]. As there is an association between high HbA$_{1c}$ in early pregnancy and increased frequency of fetal malformation [17–20], it is reasonable to expect that poor glucose control in early pregnancy could cause an increased rate of spontaneous abortion. This has also been demonstrated in recent studies [20, 21].

Congenital Malformations

Several studies show that the incidence of fetal malformation in offspring of IDDM mothers is two to three times higher than in the general population [22]. This increased incidence of fetal malformations has remained relatively constant over the years, in spite of a significant and continuous decrease in the perinatal mortality rate. More recently, however, there are reports that suggest a reduction in the incidence of fetal malformations [20, 23].

The anomalies are mainly the same as are seen in infants of non-diabetic mothers, with the exception of the caudal regression syndrome. This syndrome, with agenesis or hypoplasia of the femora, together with agenesis of the lower vertebrae appears to be strongly associated with diabetes. The susceptibility to teratogenic factors occurs mainly during the period of organogenesis which corresponds to the first 9 weeks of gestation [24]. Clinical as well as experimental data support the concept that poor metabolic control at the time of conception and organogenesis is an important teratogenic factor. Several studies have shown a strong association between elevated HbA$_{1c}$ in early pregnancy and the occurrence of congenital malformations [17–20]. Results of a nationwide prospective study in Sweden between 1982 and 1985 showed a high frequency (26%) of fetal malformation in patients with a HbA$_{1c}$ value above 11% (corresponding to the normal mean value $+7$ SD), whereas patients with a HbA$_{1c}$ below 9% had a malformation rate that was not different from that of the background population [20]. The level of HbA$_{1c}$ does not predict the severity of malformation [18–20].

The association between elevated HbA$_{1c}$ and fetal malformation has prompted the introduction of preconceptional counselling. A significantly lower incidence of fetal malformations has been demonstrated in selected groups of patients who achieved strict diabetes control during the preconceptional period, compared with mothers whose blood glucose was well regulated beyond the eighth week of pregnancy [25].

Diabetes Fetopathy

The adverse influence of maternal diabetes on the offspring during the fetal period of development, i.e. from approximately the end of the ninth week after fertilization, is referred to as diabetes fetopathy.

Clinical and experimental studies support the concept that maternal hyperglycemia leads to fetal hyperglycemia, which in turn stimulates the fetal B cell to increase insulin production and, as a consequence, increased anabolism. The maternal hyperglycemia–fetal hyperinsulinism theory has been expanded to include the stimulatory effects of free amino acids, in particular the branched chain amino acids, on fetal B-cell replication and insulin production [26–28]. The classic diabetes fetopathy is represented by the macrosomic infant, i.e. with a birthweight exceeding the 90th percentile or the normal mean by +2 SD for gestational age and sex. These infants have increased amounts of total body protein, glycogen and fat. Many of the internal organs, such as the liver, spleen, heart, adipose tissue and adrenals, as well as the islets of Langerhans, are enlarged because of cellular hyperplasia and hypertrophy. There is also evidence of extramedullary hematopoiesis. These oversized infants have a plethoric and cushingoid appearance. However, size at birth, as well as the infant's degree of functional maturity, may vary considerably. This variation can partly be attributed to differences in gestational age and degree of diabetic control during pregnancy, but also to the presence of diabetic microangiopathy. Fetal growth acceleration, or diabetes fetopathy, is usually seen in association with poor metabolic control and in particular in mothers with short duration of diabetes. The opposite, i.e. fetal growth retardation, is frequently associated with severe diabetic microangiopathy in the mother (White's classes F and R). The intrauterine-growth-retarded baby (i.e. a birthweight below the 10th percentile or 2 SD of the normal mean for gestational age and sex) has diminished stores of fat and glycogen and reduced cell size and number in many organs.

The Fetal Supply Line

The rate of fetal growth is determined by genetic, maternal, placental and fetal factors. Exactly how these factors interact is still incompletely understood. In pregnancies complicated by diabetes the normal fetal supply line may be altered in various ways: the availability of various nutrients for the fetus may be much increased; secretion and function of growth-promoting hormones of both placental and fetal origin may be exaggerated; on the other hand, uteroplacental perfusion may be reduced, resulting in diminished placental transfer of substrates.

The nutritional and hormonal growth-promoting advantages that prevail in pregnancies associated with poor metabolic control and short duration of maternal diabetes, may, however, be opposed by a reduced transfer of substrates due to placental or spiral artery lesions. Disturbances of the vasculatory support

(Figure 1) by a narrowing of the lumen of the spiral artery could result in decreased perfusion of the intervillous space and is often seen in pregnancies complicated by either essential hypertension or pre-eclampsia. The marked reduction of uteroplacental blood flow in intrauterine growth retardation can be determined using an advanced technique [29]. Patients with severe diabetic microangiopathy are more liable to develop acute hypertensive disorders during pregnancy. Maternal diabetes may also have a profound influence on the maturation and growth of the placenta (Figure 2). Fetal macrosomia is frequently accompanied by an increase of the placental mass due to prolonged proliferation of the cytotrophoblast and syncytiotrophoblast as reflected in an increased DNA content and cell number. Immature villi and also villi with syncytial knots occur more frequently in diabetes, suggesting a more active growth than normal. Whether these changes, which tend to increase the area of exchange, represent a compensatory response to tissue hypoxia or are direct effects of excess availability of nutrients and growth-promoting hormones (insulin, somatomedins) is not clear. It is difficult to assess in the individual case whether the increase in placental mass can compensate for the reduction in volume of the intervillous space caused by enhanced branching of chorionic villi. Reduced volume of the intervillous space will decrease the tolerance of the fetus to a sudden impairment of the intervillous space perfusion. It is important to underline that the structural anomalies of chorionic villi, stroma and vasculature seen in diabetic pregnancy are not unique to this condition [30].

Pathophysiology

Interest has been focused on the role of excess insulin during fetal development to explain various perinatal problems (Figure 3). Studies in vitro of human fetal pancreas obtained at legal abortions suggest that an exaggerated fetal B-cell function may be present already at around 16 weeks of gestation [31].

Experimental data suggest that fetal hyperinsulinemia per se is accompanied by excessive transfer of nutrients to the fetus and enhanced somatic growth. The tendency for offspring of mothers with diabetes to be both heavier and larger than average for their gestational age

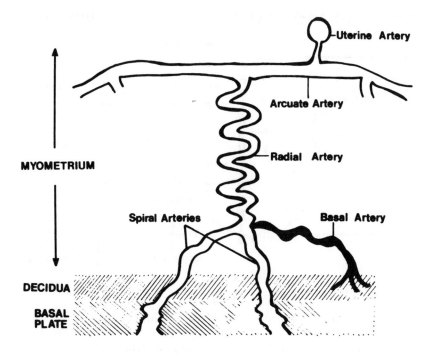

Figure 1 Maternal blood supply of the intravillous space of the placenta

and sex is clinically not manifest until after the 28th week of gestation. Severe intrauterine growth retardation seen in infants with pancreatic agenesis and who are completely devoid of insulin also seems to begin at approximately 28–30 weeks of gestation. Thus fetal insulin has a central role in fetal growth and development, at least during approximately the last 10 weeks of gestation. Both maternal and fetal somatomedins are considered as important regulators of fetal growth. Fetal macrosomia, however, has not been shown to be associated with major deviations in circulating somatomedin levels [32]. Another (though speculative) possibility

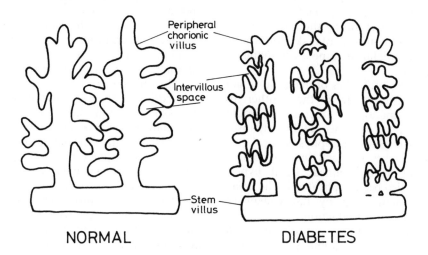

Figure 2 Term placenta with normal villous structure, contrasted with increased branching of peripheral villi in diabetic pregnancy

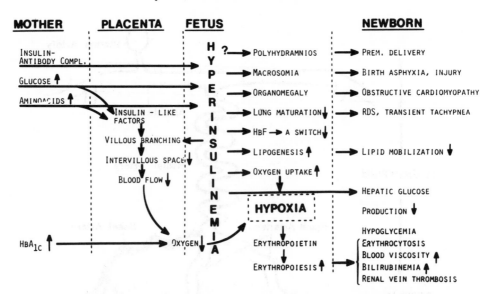

Figure 3   Proposed pathogenesis of complications in infants of diabetic mothers

that could explain enhanced fetal growth also during the second trimester of pregnancy is that excess fetal insulin and/or proinsulin bind to somatomedin receptors and thereby exert a growth-promoting effect. Meticulous control of substrate concentrations in maternal blood influences the supply line of the fetus. Indeed, increased intensity of treatment tends to normalize the infant's size, as well as appearance at birth. This reduction in size at birth can partly be attributed to a reduced amount of adipose tissue, which normally accumulates during the last 8–10 weeks of gestation. This interpretation is supported by significant correlations between maternal glucose level during the last trimester of pregnancy and both the total skinfold thickness and the mean gluteal adipose cell diameter of the newborn.

Insulin-binding antibodies of maternal origin which are transferred from the mother to the fetus represent another factor that could contribute to fetal and neonatal hyperinsulinemia [33]. The exact pathophysiological role of insulin antibodies for fetal insulin homeostasis has still to be defined. Fetal hyperinsulinism has also been implicated in the delay of fetal lung maturation by impairment of pulmonary surfactant production.

A significant delay in the onset of the switch from fetal to adult hemoglobin synthesis has also been attributed to hyperinsulinism [34]. Whether this delay in β-globin synthesis and

the resulting higher fetal oxygen affinity has any deleterious effects is unknown. Experiments in fetal lambs have demonstrated that sustained hyperglycemia–hyperinsulinemia leads to decreased fetal arterial oxygen content, due to increased peripheral oxygen consumption without a compensatory increase in placental blood flow [35]. The fetal oxygen supply may be further threatened by placental lesions and, in the case of poor diabetic control, by elevated maternal HbA_{1c} values. Increased extramedullary erythropoiesis and polycythemia could well represent the physiological responses to acute and chronic episodes of fetal hypoxia. This hypothesis is further supported by the demonstration of much-elevated concentrations of erythropoietin both in amniotic fluid and in cord blood [36]. In addition, observations in the fetal lamb suggest that the tolerance to oxygen lack is remarkably reduced in the hyperglycemic fetus. It is tempting to speculate that these derangements in fetal oxygenation could be the cause of the sudden unexpected death of the macrosomic fetus, which used to be a frequent perinatal catastrophe.

Several of the neonatal complications may be directly or indirectly associated with fetal hyperinsulinemia. Thus macrosomia predisposes to difficult deliveries, with birth injuries and asphyxia. Other possible consequences of fetal hyperinsulinemia such as cardiomegaly may be associated with impaired circulatory function, and delayed pulmonary maturation may cause respiratory distress. Metabolic deviations, such as decreased hepatic glucose production and hypoglycemia, as well as suppressed lipid mobilization, can easily be attributed to excess insulin in the newborn [37]. Enhanced extramedullary erythropoiesis and erythrocytosis will increase the viscosity of blood and may in turn predispose to cardiorespiratory distress, neurological symptoms, hyperbilirubinemia requiring treatment, and renal vein thrombosis.

Effects of Pregnancy on Microvascular Disease

Retinopathy

In non-pregnant IDDM patients, introduction of normoglycemia has been shown to be accompanied by an initial progression of retinopathy. This transient deterioration was seen after 3–6 months of tight control and was more prominent in patients who already had background retinopathy and who showed a large and rapid fall in HbA_{1c} and blood glucose values [38]. Progression of retinopathy has also been reported in diabetic pregnancy, although in most patients these changes regress to some extent following delivery [39, 40]. It is possible that rapid normalization of blood glucose could lead to hypoperfusion of the retina with impaired supply of oxygen and glucose [41]. Retinopathy may occasionally deteriorate markedly, as was recently observed in two pregnant patients who developed acute ischemic retinopathy with proliferative changes within 8–12 weeks of continuous subcutaneous insulin infusion (CSII) treatment [40]. Caution should therefore be exercised when introducing the regimen of tight blood glucose control in patients who are poorly controlled and who have background retinopathy at the beginning of pregnancy. Whenever possible, optimal regulation of the diabetic state should take place before conception. An ophthalmological examination should preferably also be done before pregnancy, but otherwise at the beginning, and thereafter in the case of background retinopathy at around monthly intervals. Patients with proliferative retinopathy and who are prone to develop systemic hypertension should be examined more frequently because they are at risk of a rapid deterioration in retinopathy. This could also include a risk of loss of vision, in which case interruption of pregnancy must be considered.

Nephropathy

Diabetic nephropathy is diagnosed in patients who before pregnancy have persistent proteinuria (greater than 0.4 g protein per 24 hours) in the absence of urinary tract infection, and who may or may not have systemic hypertension. Patients with nephropathy are at great risk of developing hypertension and/or pre-eclampsia during pregnancy. Proteinuria usually increases during pregnancy but there is no evidence that pregnancy accelerates progression of renal disease [9, 42]. Creatinine clearance usually remains stable during pregnancy, in contrast to the progressive increase that is seen in normal pregnancy. A deterioration in renal function that may occur is believed to reflect the natural history of diabetic nephropathy.

Early termination of pregnancy should be considered in White's class F patients, in particular if there is severely impaired renal function and or hypertension.

Neuropathy

Neuropathy is rarely a problem during pregnancy. Motor and sensory conduction velocities are unaffected by pregnancy in diabetic patients [43].

Medical Care

The paramount importance of achieving as normal a metabolic environment as possible for the fertilized ovum, embryo and fetus has become increasingly apparent during the past decades. The patient and her family need extensive and individualized education and support in order to create the high level of motivation that is necessary in order to attain normoglycemia.

Diabetes in pregnancy is quantitatively not a major problem. Centralized management has, therefore, obvious advantages and enables the perinatal team of obstetrician, physician and pediatrician to see a large number of patients and thus to gain the necessary experience. The introduction of self-monitoring of blood glucose has had a major impact on practical clinical management [6]. This technique, which should be applied throughout pregnancy, increases the patient's involvement in treatment, reduces the number of admissions to hospital for glucose regulation and is also cost effective.

Clinical management includes two main objectives:

(1) to attain normoglycemia, i.e. blood glucose should not exceed around 6.5 mmol/l at any time during the day and around 4 mmol/l in the fasting state;

(2) pregnancy should, when possible, be allowed to go to term (i.e. 39 weeks completed).

Diet

An individual diet tailored according to the patient's need and preferences should be prescribed, with an average energy supply from unrefined carbohydrates, fat and protein of around 50–55%, 18–20% and 30%, respectively. The energy intake of women with a normal prepregnancy weight usually amounts to 30–35 kcal/kg body weight per day, which promotes a weight gain of approximately 12 kg. In obese women (i.e. with prepregnancy weight more than 120% of ideal body weight), the energy content should be reduced to promote a weight gain of around 8 kg. Energy intake should be distributed into several small meals throughout the day, i.e. breakfast, snack, lunch, snack, dinner and a bedtime snack. The diet should contain a high content of mixed fibers, i.e. fibers from cereals, vegetables, bread and fruits, and should also be supplemented by iron and multivitamin preparations.

Insulin

Adequate metabolic control is best achieved by individualized insulin therapy and by adjusting the dose according to blood glucose values. Insulin treatment should also be given to patients who in the non-pregnant state can be adequately controlled on diet and oral hypoglycemic drugs. These drugs traverse the placenta and may cause prolonged severe hypoglycemia in the newborn.

The normal increase in insulin resistance is reflected is a marked rise in insulin requirement (approximately 30–40 U per day) as gestation proceeds. This change in insulin resistance is best compensated for by adjusting the insulin dose according to daily measurements of preprandial and 1.5 hours postprandial blood glucose values. Highly purified human insulin preparations are preferable, in order to avoid formation of insulin-binding antibodies. Various regimens of intensified conventional insulin therapy have been introduced and have become increasingly popular. A schedule with three injections per day (a mixture of short-acting and medium-acting insulin before breakfast, short-acting insulin before dinner, and medium-acting insulin at bedtime) has, in our experience, been successively replaced by multiple injections of short-acting insulin before meals and an evening dose of medium-acting insulin. Multiple preprandial injections of fast-acting insulin have physiological advantages. This regimen has gained increasing acceptance among patients following the introduction of new insulin-injection devices, i.e. the pen injectors. The experience with CSII during pregnancy is still limited. In our opinion, CSII should be considered for those very few patients who cannot be adequately controlled on daily multiple injections. The patient and her family must be thoroughly informed about how to avoid hypoglycemia. Whenever attempts are made to maintain blood glucose within the normal range, the risk of hypoglycemia increases. Hypoglycemia can easily be provoked by a missed meal, or one smaller than usual, or a sudden increase in physical activity. As gestation proceeds there also seems to be an increased susceptibility to development of nocturnal hypoglycemia; this could be prevented by a late evening snack and by appropriate adjustment of the evening dose of medium-acting insulin.

Assessment of Diabetic Control

Treatment is guided by blood glucose profiles performed at home using strip tests and, ideally, a reflectance meter. Valuable information is obtained by daily testing or urine specimens—in particular, morning urine for ketone bodies. The pregnant woman, with or without diabetes, is sensitive to starvation and prone to develop ketonemia and ketonuria. Fasting ketonuria necessitates appropriate adjustment of either diet of insulin therapy. Frequent outpatient visits (every 1 or 2 weeks) are encouraged, to meet the patient's (and her partner's) need of psychological and medical support. HbA$_{1c}$ levels, determined at monthly intervals, are a valuable index of glucose control. Optimal quality of blood glucose control is accompanied by normalization of HbA$_{1c}$ values [6, 44].

Obstetrical Care

As soon as pregnancy is verified, gestational age

is confirmed by ultrasound scanning, measuring either the crown–rump length or the biparietal diameter. Serial ultrasonic determinations of the biparietal diameter and the abdominal diameter or circumference, every 2–3 weeks from the 32nd week of gestation, will reveal the occurrence of fetal macrosomia [45]. If fetal macrosomia develops, blood glucose control should be intensified, although it is known that strict diabetic regulation does not totally exclude excessive fetal growth [46]. If the HbA_{1c} values in early pregnancy are much elevated, an extensive ultrasound examination including echocardiography is warranted around weeks 15–17 in order to detect fetal malformations. Determination of α-fetoprotein in maternal serum or amniotic fluid is also valuable for early detection of neural tube defects. Early detection of severe malformation may offer the parents the option of termination of pregnancy.

Maternal weight gain, blood pressure and urine testing for protein should be monitored at frequent intervals, especially beyond the 24th week for early detection of complication. Around 30% of all pregnant diabetics develop acute complications that necessitate hospitalization [6, 47]. This underlines the importance of well-organized and qualified obstetric supervision when the management program includes home monitoring of blood glucose during the third trimester of pregnancy. Pre-eclampsia and intrauterine growth retardation frequently occur in patients with severe diabetic angiopathy (classes F and R). Routine hospitalization of this group of patients at least from around the 32nd week of pregnancy is advisable. Patients with poor compliance to the treatment regimen are usually easily identified by psychosocial problem and 'unexplained' elevations of HbA_{1c}. Patients in this high-risk group are best cared for in hospital.

Hypertensive Disorders

A recent survey covering the period 1965–85 showed a 12% incidence of hypertension in diabetic pregnancies [48]. Pregnancy-induced hypertension has been reported to be two to three times more common in diabetic women than in non-diabetic women [49].

It is well recognized that development of hypertensive disorder parallels the severity of the diabetic disease; thus, in the 1965–85 survey, the frequency of pregnancy-induced hypertension was 16% in White's classes D, F and R, in contrast to 8% in White' classes B and C [48].

Pre-eclampsia (gestational hypertension, i.e. blood pressure above 140/90 mmHg, with proteinuria exceeding 0.3 g protein per 24 hours) in patients with nephropathy often starts early in the last trimester. If possible, pregnancy should be continued to 32–35 weeks to improve the neonatal prognosis; this will often necessitate the use of antihypertensive drugs. Studies using placental scintigraphy have demonstrated a significant reduction from normal of uteroplacental blood flow in diabetic pregnancy during the last trimester [29, 50]. Using the same technique in patients with pre-eclampsia, we have shown a significant impairment of uteroplacental blood flow by approximately 50% [51]. In severe pre-eclampsia, flow is further impaired to only 30% of normal. In view of this it is important to use an antihypertensive drug that does not further reduce the uteroplacental blood flow.

Beta-adrenergic blockers. The metabolic and hormonal responses to insulin-induced hypoglycemia in non-pregnant diabetic patients are essentially unaffected by β-blockade. Among the different β-blockers, cardioselective types seem to be preferable to the non-selective ones in patients with diabetes. The combined α,β-blocker labetalol has been given in diabetes without untoward effects.

When using β-adrenergic antagonists in pregnancy, some caution must be advised. Experiments in sheep have shown that the β-blocked fetus has a blunted hemodynamic response to moderate asphyxia, together with increased lactic acidosis and impaired cerebral function [52]. Blockade of the fetal β_1-adrenoceptors seems hazardous to the asphyctic fetus. Non-selective β-blockers without intrinsic sympathomimetic activity, such as propranolol, increase vascular peripheral resistance; this would be disadvantageous in hypertensive disease of pregnancy, which has been shown to be associated with increased vascular peripheral resistance [53].

Hydralazine, methyldopa and calcium blockers. These drugs are now rarely used outside pregnancy due to their frequent side-effects. However, during pregnancy methyldopa is still widely used in the UK and the USA, and hydralazine is used in Scandinavia. Methyldopa has been well documented to be safe but somewhat less efficient than the combined α,β-blocker labetalol [54]. Hydralazine, a vasodilator, would seem a logical choice to use in a disease characterized by increased peripheral resistance, but its effect in lowering blood pressure is weak. A combination of hydralazine and β_1-blocker (atenolol or metoprolol), or of hydralazine plus the combined α,β-blocker labetalol, has been shown to be effective. As the fetus might be compromised, a high dose of β-blocker should be avoided. In recent years calcium channel blockers, especially nifedipine, a vasodilator, has been used in pregnancy-induced hypertension [86]. Nifedipine can be an additive to labetol in severe hypertension [87]. It should be noted that angiotensin-converting enzyme (ACE) inhibitors should not be used in pregnacy because of their serious adverse effects on the offspring.

When pre-eclampsia complicates a diabetic pregnancy with angiopathy in the last trimester of gestation, the condition usually deteriorates rapidly and delivery has to be considered.

Premature Labor

Several studies have shown a high incidence (about 25%) of spontaneous premature delivery [55]. The spontaneous premature delivery rate seems to be closely related to the quality of diabetic control. Thus, patients treated with the maximal tolerated insulin dose had a prematurity rate of only 6% [56] and in our own series it was 10% [6]. The possibility of inhibition of premature uterine contractions with β_2-adrenoceptor agonists is· well established. In diabetic pregnancy these drugs induce serious metabolic side-effects due to their pronounced glycolytic, glycogenolytic and lipolytic effects [37], and extra insulin must be administered. If a premature birth with fetal lung immaturity is anticipated, corticosteroids could be used to enhance fetal lung maturation.

Fetal Monitoring

Monitoring of fetal well-being is important in view of the evidence suggesting an association between maternal hyperglycemia and fetal hypoxia. Fetal heart-rate monitoring is today the best clinical tool to detect fetal hypoxia. Registration of fetal heart rate in the non-stressed situation (non-stress test) is a valuable screening test that should be performed twice each week. If this test is normal, it has a high predictive value [47, 57]. The oxytocin challenge test (contractions stress test) is required only if the non-stressed test is abnormal or difficult to interpret. It should be recalled that maternal hypoglycemia is associated with a markedly reduced variability in fetal heart rate—'silent pattern'—that returns to normal immediately following normalization of blood glucose [58].

Evaluation of the biophysical profile based on amniotic fluid volume, fetal breathing movements, gross body movements and fetal tone is a time-consuming, subjective technique that probably cannot replace the non-stress test.

The routine determination of estriol and human placental lactogen gives limited clinical information and has been almost totally abandoned. Measurement of fetal blood flow using the Doppler technique to assess fetal condition holds promise for the future, and is currently being evaluated [59].

Timing and Mode of Delivery

The policy of delivering diabetic women prematurely because of fear of sudden intrauterine death in late pregnancy has now been abandoned. If maternal blood glucose is well regulated delivery could safely be delayed until term or after at least 39 completed weeks of pregnancy [47]. If pregnancy complications occur, or if there is coexisting severe diabetic angiopathy (White's classes F and R), the mode and time of delivery must be individualized. If there are maternal indications for delivery before completion of 36 weeks of gestation, amniocentesis should be considered for evaluation of fetal lung maturation by determination of phosphatidylglycerol.

In the case of a planned induction of labor, intracervical application of prostaglandin jelly may first be necessary to ripen the cervix and may then be followed by oxytocin and amniotomy. During vaginal delivery, fetal heart rate should be monitored continuously and pH measurements performed when indicated. Cesarean section should be performed as a result of general obstetrical indications and also where there is severe exacerbation of retinal changes.

During labor, insulin requirement decreases

markedly [60]. Therefore, on the day of elective delivery the morning insulin dose should be reduced by approximately 50%. During labor and delivery (induced labor, cesarean section or spontaneous labor) it is essential to attain normoglycemia (i.e. blood glucose around 5–6 mmol/l). Blood glucose should therefore be monitored every 30–60 minutes. Continuous intravenous infusion of glucose, together with multiple subcutaneous injections of fast-acting insulin (or as infusion) should be given according to blood glucose results.

Following delivery, and in the immediate postpartum period, insulin requirement normally decreases to about one-third of that needed during the days before delivery.

Lactation

Breastfeeding should be encouraged. The newborn should be put to the breast as early as possible after delivery. Early initiation of breastfeeding is associated with an increased prevalence of breastfeeding at 3 months after delivery [61]. The carbohydrate content of the diet should be increased during lactation by approximately 50 g per day. The insulin requirement during lactation is similar to, or slightly lower than, that recorded during the prepregnancy period.

The Newborn Infant

Routine Care

Ideally, the delivery of the baby should be planned, and a pediatrician experienced in resuscitation of the newborn should be present whether the delivery is vaginal or by cesarean section. For some practical and routine procedures, see reference [37].

Neonatal Morbidity

Despite the marked decline in perinatal mortality rate, there is still a high frequency (around 30–50%) of neonatal morbidity [6]. However, the frequency of severe morbidity such as respiratory distress (surfactant deficiency) is far lower than hitherto. This improvement has been attributed to improved maternal blood glucose control. This view is supported by excellent results with only minimal perinatal morbidity in a small

series of selected and highly motivated insulin dependent patients, who were able to attain normoglycemia throughout pregnancy [44]. It is, however, well recognized that infants of diabetic mothers constitute a heterogeneous group, not only with regard to differences in degree of blood glucose control but particularly also as regards differences in the occurrence of diabetic microangiopathy. Results of a large consecutive series of women with IDDM, who performed home monitoring of blood glucose, clearly demonstrated that gestational age at delivery had the most significant influence on the occurrence of severe neonatal morbidity such as respiratory distress, transient tachypnea, symptomatic hypoglycemia and hyperbilirubinemia [6, 62]. There was, however, no apparent association between indices of diabetic control, such as HbA_{1c} and average glucose concentrations during the last trimester of pregnancy, and infant morbidity. Others have reported a close association between maternal HbA_{1c} and neonatal morbidity [63]. These seemingly contradictory findings could be explained by differences in quality of diabetic control.

NON-INSULIN DEPENDENT DIABETES MELLITUS

NIDDM most often occurs in women above fertile age. However, in many of the developing countries NIDDM will affect women at an earlier age and will then have a bearing on pregnancy. It is realized that many of the aims set for medical treatment and obstetrical care will be impossible to reach in the developing countries.

Little is known about the rate of congenital malformations. In a study of the Pima Indians, 11% of the infants of the diabetic mothers showed malformations in comparison with 2.5% of the non-diabetic mothers [64].

Clinical Management

In general, the same guidelines that have been given for the surveillance of the mother, fetus and neonate in IDDM will be adopted in NIDDM. As NIDDM represents a less severe form of diabetes, normoglycemia can usually be attained using a less intensive management program than that in IDDM patients.

Women with NIDDM will present themselves

early in pregnancy, some being on diet therapy alone, some on diet therapy plus insulin, and a few on diet therapy plus oral antidiabetic agents. At the outset, from the first trimester, these women should be treated with insulin: usually, a combination of short-acting medium-acting insulin twice daily is enough to attain near-normoglycemia. Monitoring of blood glucose should follow the same principles as for patients with IDDM. Obesity is more often seen in NIDDM mothers and is, as such, a risk factor for the mother and her fetus. One problem is the concomitant occurrence of chronic hypertension and pre-eclampsia with obesity. Obesity also adds extra risk of the birth of a large infant.

Macrosomia should be identified by ultra-sound scanning before the mode of delivery is decided upon. Neonates of diabetic mothers show significantly greater shoulder/head and chest/head differences than neonates of non-diabetic mothers of comparable weights [65]. This might explain why, in diabetics 30% of vaginally delivered infants weighing above 4.0 kg experience shoulder dystocia [66]. Cesarean section should therefore be considered in a diabetic pregnancy with an estimated fetal weight above 4.0 kg.

In NIDDM most pregnancies may safely continue until term, which will reduce neonatal morbidity. For high-risk NIDDM women, i.e. those with hypertension and/or a poor obstetric history, delivery should be planned at 38–39 weeks of gestation. The same guidelines that have been given for delivery in IDDM patients should be followed.

GESTATIONAL DIABETES MELLITUS

A recent review of the literature showed a remarkable difference in the frequency of abnormal glucose tolerance during pregnancy, ranging between 0.15% and 12.3% [67]. This wide variation may partly be due to ethnic differences, but more importantly to methodological differences. Thus, results from some clinical series are based on screening of selected high risk populations, including women with previous GDM.

At the Second International Workshop Conference on GDM [2], some consensus was achieved. GDM was defined as 'carbohydrate intolerance of variable severity with onset or first recognition during the present pregnancy. The definition applies irrespective of whether or not

insulin is used for treatment or the condition persists after pregnancy. It does not exclude the possibility that glucose intolerance may have antedated the pregnancy.' Furthermore, 'All pregnant women should be screened for glucose intolerance since selective screening by some clinical attributes or past obstetric history has been shown to be inadequate.'

Unfortunately, we still lack uniform diagnostic criteria. Previous studies have shown that impaired glucose tolerance during pregnancy, whether determined by intravenous testing or by the oral glucose tolerance test, is accompanied by elevated maternal concentrations of free fatty acids, ketone bodies, triglycerides and amino acids [68, 69]. The extent to which such metabolic changes (which are believed to exaggerate the fetal pancreatic B-cell function), may adversely influence perinatal outcome depends on their severity and time of onset during gestation. A minimal impairment of glucose tolerance in early pregnancy may well progress to an insulin-requiring state later on. On the other hand, if the oral GTT is normal in weeks 27–31, there is no practical value in retesting to detect GDM later on [70].

GDM is a heterogeneous disorder that may be associated with an increased perinatal morbidity rate and also if left untreated an increased perinatal mortality rate [71, 72]. In addition, a large group—around 20–50% of the mothers—will develop manifest diabetes later on in life [73]. Observations of normal-weight women with previous GDM have also shown a high frequency of decreased glucose tolerance associated with an impaired early insulin response and, in some cases, with a decreased insulin sensitivity also [74].

Screening for GDM

Some of the criteria used to select pregnant women for a diagnostic GTT are given in Table 4 [2, 11, 75]. The reproducibility of the screening test using a 50-g oral glucose load administered without regard to time of the last meal or time of the day [2] is less in patients with GDM than in women with normal glucose tolerance [76]. Repeated determination of random blood glucose increases the sensitivity of this type of screening [11]. In our opinion, the conventional screening criteria, such as family history of diabetes, obesity, previous large-for-dates

Table 4 Blood glucose screening for gestational diabetes

Method	Time during pregnancy	Criteria for diagnostic GTT	Reference
50-g oral GTT	24–28 weeks	Venous plasma glucose 1 h $\geqslant 7.8$ mmol/l	[2]
Random glucose	2–3 times each trimester	Capillary blood glucose $\geqslant 6.5$ mmol/l	[11]
Random glucose	28–32 weeks	Venous blood glucose within 2 h of meal $\geqslant 6.1$ mmol/l; more than 2 h after meal $\geqslant 5.6$ mmol/l	[75]

infant, GDM in previous pregnancy and fasting glucosuria on more than one occasion, cannot be replaced by glucose screening alone [11].

HbA$_{1c}$ measurement does not seem to be sensitive enough for detection of GDM. The use of fructosamine as a screening criterion may be helpful, but this method needs to be evaluated further.

Medical Care

All women with GDM should be given dietary advice (see above). Management must include frequent measurements of blood glucose in order to detect those who deteriorate to such an extent that insulin therapy has to be started. It has been proposed that insulin therapy should be initiated if fasting plasma glucose is above 5.8 mmol/l or the 2-hour postprandial plasma glucose exceeds 6.7 mmol/l on two or more occasions within a 2-week interval [2]. Results of a randomized trial comparing two treatment regimens, i.e. diet alone and diet plus insulin, showed that routine treatment with insulin is unnecessary [77]. All patients performed self-monitoring of blood glucose six times a day, 3 days per week. Approximately 15% of the patients who were treated with diet alone needed insulin because fasting and postprandial capillary blood glucose values exceeded 7 mmol/l and 9 mmol/l, respectively, at least three times within 1 week [77]. As the rate of GDM was around 2%, this implies that about 0.3% of all pregnant women will require insulin treatment.

Obstetrical Care

Women with GDM who require insulin therapy should be followed according to the management protocol outlined above for IDDM patients. If blood glucose is carefully control-led and insulin therapy is not necessary, there is, in our experience, no need to initiate fetal surveillance. Such patients could safely be followed until they have completed 42 weeks of gestation before induction of delivery. If there is clinical suspicion of fetal macrosomia, ultrasound examination for determination of fetal size should be performed around week 38.

Follow-up

Women with previous GDM run a considerable risk of developing diabetes later in life. They should be encouraged to be physically active and to keep a normal body weight. These women should be followed postpartum and then at (yearly) intervals for early detection of diabetes.

LONG-TERM PROGNOSIS FOR THE OFFSPRING

There is limited information on the long-term prognosis of infants born to mothers with IDDM or GDM. Follow-up studies have mainly focused on two aspects: the risk of appearance of diabetes later in life, and psychosomatic development.

Future Risk of Developing Diabetes

Children of IDDM parents show, as a group, a greater genetic susceptibility to develop diabetes than children of non-diabetic parents. The frequency of diabetes in offspring of IDDM mothers has been reported to vary between 0.2% and 10% [37]. On the basis of data from 464 children of diabetic mothers the prevalence of IDDM was calculated, using a method of age correction, to be 1.5% at an age of 25 years [78]. A recent analysis of the incidence of diabetes in the offspring of IDDM parents showed a statistically significant greater risk in the offspring of fathers with IDDM (6.1%) than of mothers with IDDM (1.3%) [79]. The exact mechanism to explain this sex difference in the transmission of IDDM is still unresolved.

Neurological deficit and/or mental retardation have been recorded to have a prevalence of 2% and 18% in different reports [37]. The largest published series included 740 children who were between 1.5 years old and 26 years old at the time of follow-up: cerebral dysfunction or related conditions occurred in 36%; major cerebral handicap was seen in 18% and was associated with high or low maternal age in pregnancy, maternal White's classes D, F and R, and low gestational age and birth weight. Similar results have been recorded by others. Subsequent studies have shown a better outcome [80, 81]: one recent study of 53 infants of IDDM mothers and 20 infants of GDM mothers who were followed for 5 years disclosed no abnormalities [82]; all subjects had normal IQ scores and no relationship was found between intellectual performance and size at birth or neonatal hypoglycemia. The previous demonstration of an adverse influence of maternal acetonuria during pregnancy on the intellectual development of the children at 4–5 years of age [83, 84] could not be confirmed [82]. Follow-up studies regarding subsequent height and weight development have yielded inconsistent results. The possible influence of the prenatal metabolic environment on the subsequent development of overweight is supported by follow-up results in the Pima Indians [85]. The study disclosed that infants of mothers with overt diabetes during pregnancy were heavier at birth and also showed excessive obesity at follow-up examinations for as long as 15–19 years compared with results in offspring of prediabetic and non-diabetic controls.

REFERENCES

1. WHO Technical Report Series 727. Geneva: WHO, 1985.
2. Freinkel N, ed. Proceedings of the 2nd International Workshop Conference on Gestational Diabetes Mellitus. Diabetes 1985; 34 (suppl. 2).
3. National Diabetes Data Group. Classification and diagnosis of diabetes mellitus and other categories of glucose intolerance. Diabetes 1979; 28: 1039–57.
4. Li DFH, Wong VCW, O'Hoy KMK, Ma HK. Evaluation of the WHO criteria for 75 g oral glucose tolerance test in pregnancy. Brit J Obstet Gynaec 1987; 94: 847–50.
5. White P. Pregnancy and diabetes. Medical aspects. Med Clin North Am 1965; 49: 1015–24.
6. Hanson U, Persson B, Enochsson E et al. Self-monitoring of blood glucose by diabetic women during the third trimester of pregnancy. Am J Obstet Gynecol 1984; 150: 817–21.
7. Freinkel N, Dooley SL, Metzger BE. Care of the pregnant woman with insulin-dependent diabetes mellitus. New Engl J Med 1985; 313: 96–103.
8. Molsted-Pedersen L, Kuhl C. Obstetrical management in diabetic pregnancy: the Copenhagen experience. Diabetologia 1986; 29: 13–16.
9. Kitzmiller JL, Brown ER, Phillippe M et al. Diabetic nephropathy and perinatal outcome. Am J Obstet Gynecol 1981; 141: 741–51.
10. Nordlander E, Hanson U, Persson B, Stangenberg M. Pancreatic B-cell function during normal pregnancy. Diabetes Res 1987; 6: 133–6.
11. Stangenberg M, Persson B, Nordlander E. Random capillary blood glucose and conventional selection criteria for glucose tolerance testing during pregnancy. Diabetes Res 1985; 2: 29–33.
12. Freinkel N, Metzger BE, Nitzan M, Daniel R, Surmaczynska B, Nagel T. Facilitated anabolism in late pregnancy: some novel maternal compensations for accelerated starvation. In Malaisse WJ, Pirart J, Vallance-Owen J (eds) International Congress Series 312. Amsterdam: Excerpta Medica, 1974: pp 474–88.
13. Traub AI, Harley JMG, Cooper TK, Maguiness S, Hadden DR. Is centralized hospital care necessary for all insulin-dependent pregnant diabetics? Brit J Obstet Gynaec 1987; 94: 957–62.
14. Connell FA, Vadheim C, Emanuel I. Diabetes in pregnancy: population-based study of incidence, referral for care, and perinatal mortality. Am J Obstet Gynecol 1985; 151: 598–603.
15. Kalter H. Diabetes and spontaneous abortion: a historical review. Am J Obstet Gynecol 1987; 156: 1243–53.
16. Kline I, Stein Z. Spontaneous abortion (miscarriage). In Bracken MB (ed.) Perinatal epidemiology. New York: Oxford University Press, 1984: pp 23–51.
17. Leslie RDG, Pyke DA, John PN, White JM. Haemoglobin A_1 in diabetic pregnancy. Lancet 1978; ii: 958–9.
18. Millner E, Hare JW, Cloherty JP et al. Elevated maternal hemoglobin A_{1c} in early pregnancy and major congenital anomalies in infants of diabetic mothers. New Engl J Med 1981; 304: 1331–4.
19. Ylinen K, Raivio K, Teramo K. Hemoglobin A_{1c} predicts the perinatal outcome in insulin-dependent diabetic pregnancies. Brit J Obstet Gynaec 1981; 88: 961–7.

20. Hanson U, Persson B, Thunell S. The relation between HbA$_{1c}$ in early diabetic pregnancy and the occurrence of spontaneous abortion and malformation in Sweden. Diabetologia 1990; 33: 100–4.

21. Miodovnik M, Mimouni F, Tsang RC, Ammar E, Kaplan L, Siddiqi TA., Glycemic control and spontaneous abortion in insulin-dependent diabetic women. Obst Gynec 1986; 68: 366–9.

22. Kucera J. Rate and type of congenital anomalies among offspring of diabetic women. J Reprod Med 1971; 7: 61–70.

23. Molsted-Pedersen L. Pregnancy and diabetes. In Alberti KGMM, Krall LP (eds) Diabetes annual. Amsterdam: Elsevier, 1985: pp 238–56.

24. Mills J. Malformations in infants of diabetic mothers. Teratology 1982; 25: 385–94.

25. Fuhrmann K, Reiher H, Semmler K et al. Prevention of congenital malformation in infants of insulin-dependent diabetic mothers. Diabetes Care 1983; 6: 219–23.

26. Milner RD, Hill DJ. Fetal growth control: the role of insulin and related peptides. Clin Endocrinol 1984; 21: 415–33.

27. Freinkel N, Metzger BE. Pregnancy as a tissue culture experience: the critical implications of maternal metabolism for fetal development. In Elliot K, et al (eds) Pregnancy, metabolism, diabetes and the fetus. Ciba Foundation Symposium 63. Amsterdam: Excerpta Medica, 1979: pp 3–23.

28. Persson B, Pschera H, Lunell N-O, Barley J, Gumaa KA. Amino acid concentrations in maternal plasma and amniotic fluid in relation to fetal insulin secretion during the last trimester of pregnancy in gestational and type I diabetic women and women with small-for-gestational age infants. Am J Perinatol 1986; 3: 100–5.

29. Nylund L, Lunell NO, Lewander R, Persson B, Sarby B. Utero-placental blood flow in diabetic pregnancy. Measurements with indium-113 m and a computer-linked gamma camera. Am J Obstet Gynecol 1982; 144: 298–302.

30. Fox H. The development and structure of the placenta. In Fox H (ed.) Major problems in pathology, Vol. 7. London: WB Saunders, 1978.

31. Reiher H, Fuhrmann K, Noack S et al. Age-dependent insulin secretion of the endocrine pancreas in vitro from fetuses of diabetic and non-diabetic patients. Diabetes Care 1983; 6: 446–51.

32. Susa JB, Widness JA, Hintz R et al. Somatomedins and insulin in diabetic pregnancies: effects on fetal macrosomia in the human and rhesus monkey. J Clin Endocrinol Metab 1984; 58: 1099.

33. Heding LG, Persson B, Stangenberg M. Betacell function in newborn infants of diabetic mothers. Diabetologia 1980; 19: 427–32.

34. Perrine SP, Greene MF, Faller DV. Delay in the fetal globin switch in infants of diabetic mothers. New Engl J Med 1985; 312: 334–8.

35. Carson BS, Philipps AF, Simmons MA, Battaglia FC, Meschia G. Effects of a sustained insulin infusion upon glucose uptake and oxygenation of the ovine fetus. Pediatr Res 1980; 14: 147–52.

36. Widness JA, Susa JA, Garcia JH et al. Increased erythropoiesis and elevated erythropoietin in infants born to diabetic mothers and in hyperinsulinemic rhesus fetuses. J Clin Invest 1981; 67: 637–42.

37. Persson B, Gentz J, Lunell NO. Diabetes in pregnancy. Rev Perinat Med 1978; 2: 1–55.

38. Dahl-Jorgensen K, Brinchmann-Hansen O, Hanssen KF, Sandvik L, Aagenaes O. Rapid tightening of blood glucose control leads to transient deterioration of retinopathy in insulin dependent diabetes mellitus. The Oslo study. Br Med J 1985; 290: 811–15.

39. Moloney JBM, Frury MI. The effect of pregnancy on the natural course of diabetic retinopathy. Am J Ophthalmol 1982; 93: 745–56.

40. Laatikainen L, Teramo K, Hieta-Heikurainen H, Koivisto V, Pelkonen R. A controlled study of the influence of continuous subcutaneous insulin infusion treatment of diabetic retinopathy during pregnancy. Acta Med Scand 1987; 221: 367–76.

41. Brichmann-Hansen O, Dahl-Jorgensen K, Hanssen KF, Sandvik L. Effects of intensified insulin treatment on various lesions of diabetic retinopathy. Am J Opthalmol 1985; 100: 644–53.

42. Grenfell A, Brudenell JM, Doddridge MC, Watkins PJ. Pregnancy in diabetic women who have proteinuria. Quart J Med 1986; 228: 379–86.

43. Nylund L, Brismar T, Lunell N-O, Persson A, Persson B, Stangenberg M. Nerve conduction in diabetic pregnancy. A prospective study. Diabetes Res Clin Pract 1985; 1: 121–3.

44. Jovanovic L, Peterson CM, Saxena BB, Dawood Y, Saudek CD. Feasibility of maintaining normal glucose profiles in insulin-dependent pregnant women. Am J Med 1980; 68: 105–12.

45. Ogata ES, Sabbagha R, Metzger BE et al. Serial ultrasonography to assess evolving fetal macrosomia. JAMA 1980; 243: 2405–8.

46. Knight G, Worth RC, Ward JD. Macrosomy despite a well-controlled diabetic pregnancy. Lancet 1983; ii: 1431.

47. Gillmer MDG, Holmes SM, Moore MP et al. Diabetes in pregnancy: obstetric management 1983. In Sutherland HW, Stowers JM (eds) Carboyhdrate metalbolism in pregnancy and the newborn. Edinburgh: Churchill Livingstone, 1984: pp 102–18.

48. Cousins L. Pregnancy complications among

diabetic women: review 1965–85. Obstet Gynaecol Surv 1987; 42: 140–9.

49. Lufkin G, Nelson R, Hill L et al. An analysis of diabetic pregnancies at Mayo Clinic 1950–79. Diabetes Care 1984; 7: 539–47.

50. Semmler K, Kirsch G, Zöllner P, Fuhrmann K, Jutzi E. Die Messung der uteroplazentären Durchblutung mit 113 m-In in der diabetischen Schwangerschaft. Zentralbl Gynäkol 1985; 107: 793–802.

51. Lunell NO, Nylund L, Lewander R, Sarby B. Uteroplacental blood flow in pre-eclampsia. Measurements with indium-113 m and a computer-linked gamma camera. Clin Exp Hypertens 1982; 1: 105–17.

52. Kjellmer I, Dagbjartsson A, Hrbeck A, Karlsson K, Rosén KG. Maternal beta-adrenoceptor blockade reduces fetal tolerance to asphyxia. Acta Obstet Gynecol Scand 1984; suppl. 118: 75–80.

53. Nisell H, Hjemdahl P, Lind B, Beskow C, Lunell NO. Sympathoadrenal and cardiovascular reactivity in pregnancy-induced hypertension. III. Responses to mental stress. Am J Obstet Gynecol 1986; 68: 531–6.

54. Symonds EM, Lamming GD, Jadoul F, Broughton-Pipkin F. Clinical and biochemical aspects of the use of labetalol in the treatment of hypertension in pregnancy: Comparison with methyldopa. In Riley A, Symonds EM (eds) the Investigation of Labetalol in the management of hypertension in pregnancy. International Congress Series 591. Amsterdam: Excerpta Medica, 1982: pp 62–76.

55. Beard RW, Lowry C. The British survey of diabetic pregnancies. Brit J Obstet Gynaec 1982; 89: 783–5.

56. Roversi GD, Gargiulo M, Nicolini V et al. A new approach to the treatment of diabetic pregnant women. Report of 479 cases seen from 1963–1975. Am J Obstet Gynecol 1979; 135: 567–76.

57. Gabbe SG. Management of diabetes mellitus in pregnancy. Am J Obstet Gynecol 1985; 153: 824–8.

58. Stangenberg M, Persson B, Stånge L, Carlström K. Insulin-induced hypoglycemia in pregnant diabetics. Maternal and fetal cardiovascular reactions. Acta Obstet Gynecol Scand 1983; 62: 249–52.

59. Bracero L, Schulman H, Fleischer A et al. Umbilical artery velocimetry in diabetes and pregnancy. Obst Gynec 1986; 68: 654.

60. Golde SH, Good-Anderson B, Montoro M, Artal R. Insulin requirements during labor: a reappraisal. Am J Obstet Gynecol 1982; 144: 556–9.

61. Whichelow MJ, Doddridge MC. Lactation in diabetic women. Br Med J 1983; 287: 649–50.

62. Ylinen K, Raivio K, Teramo K. Hemoglobin A_{1c} predicts the perinatal outcome in insulin-depen-

dent diabetic pregnancies. Brit J Obstet Gynaec 1981; 88: 961–7.

63. Hanson U, Persson B, Stangenberg M. Factors influencing neonatal morbidity in diabetic pregnancy. Diabetes Res 1986; 3: 71–6.

64. Bennett PH, Webner C, Miller M. Congenital anomalies and the diabetic and prediabetic pregnancy. In Elliot K et al (eds) Pregnancy metabolism, diabetes and the fetus. Ciba Foundation Symposium 63. Amsterdam: Excerpta Medica, 1979: pp 207–18.

65. Modanlou HD, Komatsu G, Dorchester W, Freeman RK, Bosu SK. Large for gestational age neonates: anthropometric reasons for shoulder dystocia. Obst Gynec 1982; 60: 417–23.

66. Acker DB, Sachs BP, Friedman EA. Risk factors for shoulder dystocia. Obst Gynec 1985; 66: 762.

67. Hadden DR. Geographic, ethnic, and racial variations in the incidence of gestational diabetes mellitus. Diabetes 1985; 34 (suppl. 2): 8–12.

68. Persson B, Lunell NO. Metabolic control in diabetic pregnancy. Am J Obstet Gynecol 1975; 1221: 737–45.

69. Metzger BE, Phelps RL, Freinkel N, Navickas IA. Effects of gestational diabetes on diurnal profiles of plasma glucose, lipids and individual amino acids. Diabetes Care 1980; 3: 402–9.

70. Jovanovic L, Peterson CM. Screening for gestational diabetes. Optimum timing and criteria. Diabetes 1985; 34 (suppl. 2): 21–3.

71. Warner RA, Cornblath M. Infants of gestational diabetic mothers. Am J Dis Child 1969; 117: 678.

72. O'Sullivan JB, Mahan CM, Dandrow RV. Gestational diabetes and perinatal mortality rate. Am J Obstet Gynecol 1973; 116: 901–4.

73. O'Sullivan BO. Subsequent morbidity among gestational diabetic women. In Sutherland HW, Stowers JM (eds) Carbohydrate metabolism in pregnancy and the newborn. Edinburgh: Churchill Livingstone, 1984: pp 174–80.

74. Efendic S, Hanson U, Persson B, Wajngot A, Luft R. Glucose tolerance, insulin release, and insulin sensitivity in normal-weight women with previous gestational diabetes mellitus. Diabetes 1987; 36: 413–19.

75. Lind T. Antenatal screening using random blood glucose values. Diabetes 1985; 34 (suppl. 2): 17–20.

76. Fuhrman K. Reproducibility of oral glucose tolerance test in pregnancy. In Diabetes and Pregnancy Study Group. 18th Annual Meeting, Berlin, 1987 (abstr.).

77. Persson B, Stangenberg M, Hanson U, Nordlander E. Gestational diabetes mellitus (GDM). Comparative evaluation of two treatment regimens, diet versus insulin and diet. Diabetes 1985; 34 (suppl. 2): 101–5.

78. Köbberling J, Bruggeboes B. Prevalence of

diabetes among children of insulin-dependent diabetic mothers. Diabetologia 1980; 18: 459–62.

79. Warram JH, Krolewski AS, Gottlieb MS, Kahn CR. Differences in risk of insulin-dependent diabetes in offspring of diabetic mothers and diabetic fathers. New Engl J Med 1984; 311: 149–52.

80. Cummins M, Norrish M. Follow-up of children of diabetic mothers. Arch Dis Child 1980; 55: 259–64.

81. Hadden DR, Byrne E, Trotter I, Harley JMG, McClure G, McAuley RR. Physical and psychological health of children of Type 1 (insulindependent) diabetic mothers. Diabetologia 1984; 26: 250–4.

82. Persson B, Gentz J. Follow-up of children of insulin-dependent gestational diabetic mothers. Acta Paediatr Scand 1984; 73: 349–58.

83. Churchill JA, Berendes HW, Nemore J. Neuropsychological deficits in children of diabetic mothers. Am J Obstet Gynecol 1969; 105: 257–68.

84. Stehbens JA, Baker GL, Kitchell M. Outcome at ages 1, 3, and 5 years of children born to diabetic women. Am J Obstet Gynecol 1977; 127: 408–13.

85. Pettitt DJ, Baird R, Aleck KA, Bennett PH, Knowler WC. Excessive obesity in offspring of Pima Indian women with diabetes during pregnancy. New Engl J Med 1983; 308: 242–5.

86. Walters BNJ, Redman CWG: Treatment of severe pregnancy-associated hypertension with the calcium antagonist nifedipine. Br J Obstet Gynaecd 1984; 91: 230–336.

87. Greer IA, Walker JJ, Björnsson S, Calder AA. Second line therapy with nifedipine in severe pregnancy induced hypertension. Clin Exp Hypertens (B) 1989; 8(2): 277–92.

46
Aging and Diabetes

Anne L. Peters and Mayer B. Davidson

Cedars-Sinai Medical Center, Los Angeles, California, and UCLA School of Medicine, Los Angeles, California, USA

Aging is associated with the development of an increasing number of chronic illnesses, diabetes mellitus among them. Approximately 40% of individuals 65–74 years of age and 50% of individuals older than 80 years have impaired glucose tolerance (IGT) or diabetes, and in approximately half the disease is undiagnosed [1]. In this chapter, IGT is used to designate patients who fulfil specific criteria described subsequently, whereas the term 'glucose intolerance' describes raised glucose concentrations following meals or oral glucose that do not reach the levels specified for IGT. The population in Westernized societies is aging: in 1920 only 4.6% of the population of the USA was over 65 years old; by 2020, 20% of the population will be in this age group, with a particularly large increase in the number of people over 85 years old (Figure 1). The number of elderly people with diabetes will therefore increase dramatically in the next few decades. Although diabetes is treated similarly in both younger and older patients, there are some important differences that need to be addressed. First, older populations need to be screened carefully for the presence of diabetes, because older patients with diabetes are often asymptomatic, yet the prevalence of the disease in this population is increased. Second, the development of the chronic microvascular and neuropathic complications of diabetes is related to the duration of the diabetes. This implies that patients who live longer with diabetes are more likely to suffer from diabetic retinopathy, nephropathy and neuropathy. Third, the elderly often have multiple chronic diseases and as a result are receiving a variety of medications. This can alter the response to the drug and insulin therapy of diabetes, and cardiovascular disease may limit the degree of hypoglycemia tolerated as maintenance of near-euglycemia is attempted. Finally, social, functional and psychological problems often create barriers that make adequate diabetes management difficult. However, in spite of the difficulties associated with managing diabetes in the elderly, an effective diabetes management plan needs to be implemented in each individual to avoid the acute and chronic complications of diabetes that can develop in these patients.

In spite of the increasing need for diabetes care in the elderly, data on the impact of the various therapeutic modalities on morbidity and mortality in this population are lacking.

PREVALENCE OF IMPAIRED GLUCOSE TOLERANCE AND DIABETES WITH AGE

The prevalence of IGT and type 2 diabetes increases with advancing age. Spence first noted an impairment of glucose tolerance in response to an oral glucose tolerance test in people over

International Textbook of Diabetes Mellitus. Edited by K.G.M.M. Alberti, R.A. DeFronzo, H. Keen and P. Zimmet
© 1992 John Wiley & Sons Ltd

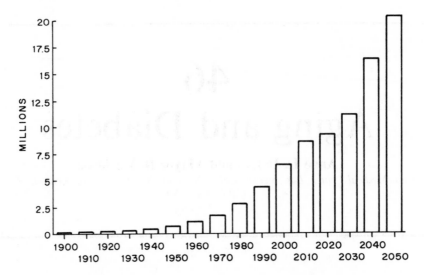

Figure 1 Actual and projected increase in population 85 years of age and older, 1900–2050 (from reference 1, reproduced with permission of the American Diabetes Association, Inc.)

60 years old in 1920 [2]. Since that time many studies have been published which confirm this observation. In 1979, a review of the literature [3] evaluated the data from 64 papers that examined the response to oral glucose tolerance tests in older subjects: in 61 of the studies, a worsening of glucose tolerance with age was seen.

More recent studies have used the National Diabetes Data Group (NDDG) [4] and the World Health Organization (WHO) [5] for the diagnosis of IGT and diabetes mellitus in various populations. A summary of the NDDG and WHO criteria for IGT and diabetes is as follows. After a 10-hour to 16-hour overnight fast, a 75-g oral glucose tolerance test (OGTT) is performed. The NDDG criteria for the diagnosis of diabetes are that the venous fasting plasma glucose concentration (FPG) is $\geqslant 7.8$ mM *or* that a mid-test (0.5, 1.0 or 1.5 hour value) *and* the 2-hour plasma glucose value are $\geqslant 11.1$ mM. The NDDG criteria for IGT require that the FPG is < 7.8 mM, a mid-test value is $\geqslant 11.1$ mM *and* the 2-hour value is between 7.8 and 11.1 mM. The WHO criteria involve only a fasting and a 2-hour value. The criteria for diabetes are a venous FPG $\geqslant 7.8$ mM *or* a 2-hour plasma glucose value $\geqslant 11.1$ mM. IGT is defined as an FPG < 7.8 mM *and* a 2-hour sample between 7.8 and 11.1 mM. As these values are so much higher than previously used

criteria, age adjustments are no longer deemed necessary. Finally, normal values are a venous FPG < 6.4 mM, a mid-test value < 11.1 mM and a 2-hour value < 7.8 mM.

The largest study using these criteria for diagnosis of IGT and diabetes was done in the USA as part of the second National Health and Nutrition Examination Survey (NHANES II). This study was conducted by the National Center for Health Statistics in order to determine the prevalence of various diseases in the United States population [6]. As the initial phase of the study, 15 357 people selected from the 1970 census report were interviewed and a medical history was obtained. Based on the reports of the presence of diabetes, estimates for the prevalence of the diagnosis of diabetes were made: 5901 of these subjects had a physical examination and 3772 people without a history of diabetes underwent an OGTT to determine the prevalence of undiagnosed IGT and diabetes mellitus.

The results from this study can be seen in Figure 2. Using NDDG criteria, the total diabetes prevalence was 6.6%, with the prevalence of undiagnosed diabetes nearly equal to that of previously diagnosed diabetes (3.2% and 3.4%, respectively). There was a marked increase in the rates of diabetes with increasing age: the rate was 2.0% in the group aged 20–44 years, increasing to 17.7% in the group aged

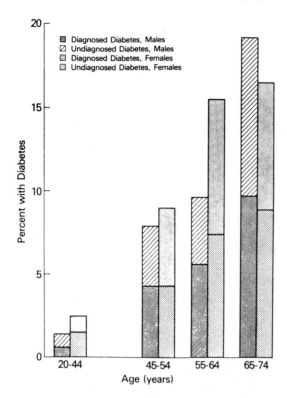

Legend:
- Diagnosed Diabetes, Males
- Undiagnosed Diabetes, Males
- Diagnosed Diabetes, Females
- Undiagnosed Diabetes, Females

Figure 2 Percentage of US population aged 20–74 years with diabetes (from reference 6, reproduced with permission of the American Diabetes Association, Inc.)

Table 1 Prevalence of impaired glucose tolerance diagnosed by WHO criteria in selected studies

Study	Age (yr)	Prevalence rate (%)	
		Men	Women
NHANES II [6],	20–44	4.7	7.8
n = 3772, 1976–80;	45–54	13.1	16.3
general US population	55–64	17.2	13.4
	65–74	22.8	22.7
Rural Italy [7], n = 1154,	18–39	2.0	3.4
1981–82	40–59	5.1	9.1
	60+	9.2	12.1
Western Australia [8],	35–44	1.8	1.3
n = 3197, 1981	45–54	2.8	0.3
	55–64	5.1	4.2
	65–74	6.5	8.6
	75+	18.9	11.8
Mauritius [9], n = 4931,	25–34	6.8	15.5
1987; Indian, Creole and	35–44	16.3	19.9
Chinese	45–54	15.7	22.1
	55–64	19.5	24.7
	65–74	24.0	26.4

Adapted from reference 10, with permission of the American Diabetes Association, Inc.

65–74 years. The prevalence of IGT also increased with age, and was higher when diagnosed according to the WHO criteria than when diagnosed by the NDDG standards (prevalence rates for diabetes were similar). Based on WHO criteria, 6.4% of the population aged 22–44 years had IGT, which increased to 22.8% in the group aged 65–74 years. In this study patients with undiagnosed IGT and diabetes were more likely to be obese or to have a family history of diabetes than those who had normal glucose tolerance.

The prevalence of IGT and diabetes in various populations [6–11] using WHO criteria are summarized in Tables 1 and 2, respectively. All of these studies confirm the increase in prevalence of IGT and diabetes mellitus with age. However, it is important to note that the 2-hour blood glucose value following an OGTT is often the value that makes the diagnosis of diabetes, not the fasting plasma glucose concentration, which tends to rise much less dramatically with age. In

the study by Wingard et al [10], 64.6% of the subjects classified as diabetic according to the WHO criteria were given the diagnosis based solely on their postglucose challenge value. In the NHANES II study [6], 75% of subjects who had no previous history of diabetes had the diagnosis made based on their 2-hour postglucose value. Thus, an increasing body of evidence supports the findings that the prevalence of both IGT and diabetes increases with age in a population, and up to 50% of the people who have diabetes are undiagnosed.

MECHANISMS FOR GLUCOSE INTOLERANCE OF AGING

The glucose intolerance of aging is manifested primarily by an increase in the postprandial blood glucose and insulin response, to both an oral glucose challenge [3, 12–17] (Figure 3) as well as to a mixed meal [13, 14, 18] (Figure 4). Fasting blood glucose values are generally not significantly elevated—it is estimated that fasting glucose levels increase by 0.055 mM (1 mg/dl) per decade, while 1-hour to 2-hour postglucose challenge values increase by 0.3–0.7 mM (6–13 mg/dl) per decade [3, 19]. The

Table 2 Prevalence of diabetes mellitus diagnosed by WHO criteria in selected studies

Study	Age (yr)	Prevalence rate (%)	
		Men	Women
NHANES II [6],	20–44	1.4	2.5
n = 3772, type	45–54	7.9	9.1
1 + 2 DM, 1976–80;	55–64	9.9	16.4
general US population	65–74	20.1	17.4
Rural Italy [7], n = 1154,	18–39	1.0	0.4
type 2 DM, 1981–82	40–59	9.3	6.2
	60+	12.6	18.1
Western Australia [8],	25–34	1.4	1.3
n = 3197, type	35–44	2.6	1.0
1 + 2 DM, 1981	45–54	2.8	0.3
	55–64	5.1	4.2
	65–74	6.5	8.6
	75+	18.9	11.8
Mauritius [9], n = 4931,	25–34	3.1	3.0
mostly type 2 DM, 1987;	35–44	10.6	8.7
Indian, Creole and	45–54	21.6	16.5
Chinese	55–64	20.7	26.0
	65–74	28.0	31.4
Rancho Bernardo,	45–54	3.6	1.9
California [10],	55–64	11.4	4.9
n = 2249, type 2 DM,	65–74	11.9	12.9
1984–87; upper middle	75–84	19.6	14.8
class, white population	85–94	19.5	20.5
Starr County, Texas [11],	25–34	2.6	0.4
n = 1931, type	35–44	3.3	5.7
1 + 2 DM, 1981–82;	45–54	12.6	10.8
Mexican-Americans	55–64	16.5	19.0
	65–74	16.7	17.0
	75+	17.6	8.0

Adapted from reference 10, with permission from the American Diabetes Association, Inc.

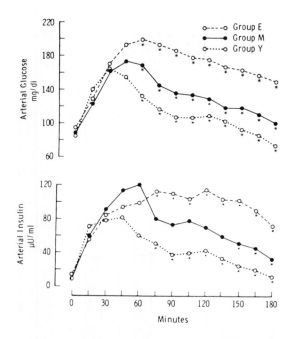

Figure 3 Mean plasma glucose and serum insulin responses to 100-g glucose tolerance test in elderly (group E, 70–83 yr), middle-aged (group M, 30–45 yr) and younger (group Y, 19–24 yr) normal men (from RA Jackson, PM Blix, JA Matthews, Influence of ageing on glucose homeostasis, J Clin Endocrinol Metab, 55: 840–8, 1982, with permission)

increase in postprandial blood glucose concentrations may be greater in women than men [19].

Poor diet, physical inactivity, decreased lean body mass, decreased relative insulin secretion and peripheral insulin antagonism have all been suggested as possible mechanisms for the development of glucose intolerance of aging [3]. It is probably attributable to a multiplicity of causes, and some or all of these factors may contribute to the development of glucose intolerance in any given individual. At least one study shows a much greater variability during euglycemic insulin clamps (see below) in the glucose metabolic clearance rate (an index of insulin sensitivity) [20] in the elderly compared with younger age groups, which probably reflects the multifactorial nature of the disorder.

Furthermore, there is a spectrum of glucose abnormalities in the elderly, ranging from the 'youthful' glucose tolerance seen in the highly trained older person, to the usual rise of postprandial glucose levels associated with aging, to true IGT as defined by NDDG criteria, to overt type 2 diabetes. Where an elderly individual fits into this definition of glucose tolerance depends on many factors (e.g. diet, level of physical activity, degree of obesity, use of drugs that impair glucose tolerance). A genetic factor is probably also important in the deterioration of IGT to diabetes.

Insulin Resistance

There is a large body of literature to suggest that the primary effect of aging is to cause a peripheral resistance to the action of insulin, probably due to a postreceptor defect. Peripheral sensitivity to insulin can be measured in a variety of ways. In a hyperglycemic clamp [21], intravenous glucose is given to raise the blood

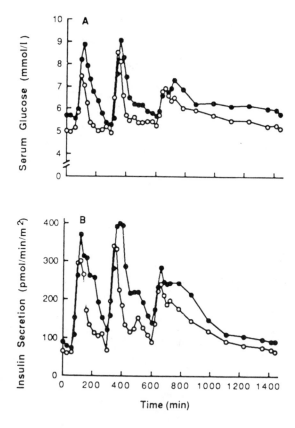

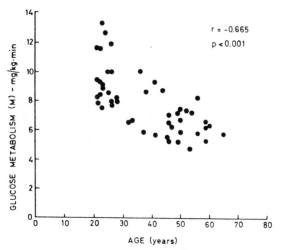

Figure 5 Correlation between age and the amount of glucose metabolized (M) during a hyperglycemic clamp study (from reference 23, reproduced with permission from the American Diabetes Association, Inc.)

Figure 4 Mean serum glucose levels (A) ($P < 0.01$ by analysis of variance [ANOVA]) and mean insulin secretion (B) ($P < 0.02$ by ANOVA) in elderly (solid circles, 60–72 yr, $n = 10$) and young (open circles, 20–35 yr) normal subjects during 24-hour meal profile (from reference 18, reproduced with permission of the American Diabetes Association, Inc.)

glucose to a chosen elevated blood glucose concentration. This is maintained for the duration of the study by a continuous, variable infusion of glucose. This technique allows for quantitation of both the early and late phase insulin response to intravenous glucose (see below), as well as an estimate of the total amount of glucose metabolized, which, when divided by the plasma insulin response, gives an index of tissue sensitivity to insulin. In a euglycemic clamp [21] a predetermined insulin infusion rate is given, and the amount of dextrose infused to maintain euglycemia is measured. The amount of dextrose given depends on the tissue sensitivity to insulin: the more dextrose needed at any given insulin infusion rate, the greater the sensitivity to insulin. Another technique to measure insulin sensitivity is to perform frequently sampled IV

glucose tolerance tests and use a computer method (called the minimal model approach) to determine insulin sensitivity, insulin independent glucose disappearance, insulin clearance and first-phase and second-phase B-cell responsiveness [22].

Insulin resistance in the older population has been documented with the hyperglycemic clamp [23] (Figure 5), the euglycemic clamp [15, 24–27] (Figure 6), a modification of the hyperglycemic clamp [28] (Figure 7) and the minimal model technique [29, 30]. Differences between young and old subjects were present even when expressed per kilogram of lean body mass [15, 24, 25, 28] (Figure 7B), ruling out decreased lean body mass as a cause of the impaired glucose tolerance associated with aging.

Insulin Secretion

The literature on insulin secretion and aging is substantial. Virtually all studies in which insulin concentrations were measured after oral glucose or meals have shown normal or increased levels, although in some instances there is a delay in the maximum response [3, 17, 23, 31]. Following intravenous glucose, these is normally a rapid release of insulin within several minutes (first phase) followed by a second phase that is lower but more substantial. A few studies have found a decreased first phase of insulin release [3, 18,

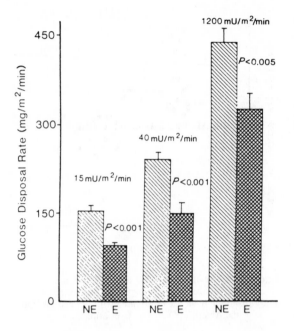

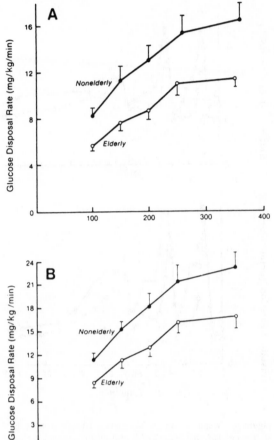

Figure 6 Mean glucose disposal rates determined by a euglycemic clamp technique at insulin infusion rates of 15, 40 and 1200 mU/m^2 per min in non-elderly (NE—23–58 yr, $n = 27$) and elderly (E—60–82 yr, $n = 17$) non-obese subjects (from reference 15; reproduced from the *Journal of Clinical Investigation*, 1983, 71, 1523–35, by copyright permission of the American Society of Clinical Investigation)

29, 31] in the elderly, whereas in others it has been normal [3, 17, 23, 31]. A possible complicating factor in interpreting insulin concentrations in the older population is the decreased metabolic clearance rate of insulin (MCR$_I$) found in a few studies [27, 32, 33]. As this would lead to higher insulin concentrations, the lowered MCR$_I$ might mask a defect in insulin secretion. This seems unlikely because not only has the decrease in the MCR$_I$ been small, but the MCR$_I$ has been normal in other studies [17, 18, 26]. Thus, decreased insulin secretion does not account for the glucose intolerance of aging.

Insulin Binding

A decrease in insulin binding could explain the decrease in insulin sensitivity with age. However, although some studies show a decrease in insulin binding to erythrocytes [12] and isolated adipocytes [26, 34, 35] with increasing age, others do not. No change in binding to monocytes [15, 16, 25, 30], erythrocytes [30],

Figure 7 (A) Glucose disposal rates at increasing plasma glucose concentrations during glucose clamp studies in elderly (60–70 yr, $n = 11$) and non-elderly (21–40 yr, $n = 10$) normal subjects. (B) Glucose disposal rates expressed as mg/kg lean body mass (LBM) (from reference 28; reproduced from the *Journal of Clinical Investigation*, 1986, 77, 2034–41, by copyright permission of the American Society of Clinical Investigation)

lymphocytes [36] or adipocytes [15] was seen with age in other studies. In one study [34] in which a decrease with adipocyte binding was seen with age, the decrement was greatest between the group aged 22–24 years and the group aged 30–46 years. The decrease in binding was much less pronounced between the group aged 30–46 years and the group aged 51–59 years, although increasing peripheral resistance to insulin occurred progressively with increasing age. Subjects older than 59 years were not studied. Few studies correlated in-vitro changes in binding with in-vivo changes in insulin sensitivity, and in one study that did [25], no correlation between a decrease in insulin binding and an increase in insulin resistance was found. Overall, the data do not suggest that changes in insulin binding play a role in the decrease of insulin sensitivity with age.

Glucose Transport

Changes in the ability of cells to transport glucose intracellularly in response to insulin is one potential cause of peripheral insulin resistance. In one study [28] in which glucose transport in isolated human adipocytes was measured, the affinity (K_m) for glucose transport was unchanged, whereas the maximal velocity for glucose transport was reduced by 34% in the elderly. In another study [37], maximal insulin-stimulated glucose transport was reduced in the elderly compared with non-elderly controls, and this measurement in vitro of glucose transport correlated significantly with measurements in vivo of glucose tolerance: those with the greatest impairment of glucose transport had more marked abnormalities on glucose tolerance testing (Figure 8). Another study found an impairment of glucose transport at submaximal levels of insulin only [26]; the maximally stimulated rate of transport was similar in the elderly and the young. These findings suggest that a decrease in glucose transport exists in the elderly and contributes to the impairment of insulin action with age.

Glucose Absorption

Alterations in the absorption of glucose do not appear to have a role in the deterioration of glucose tolerance seen with age [38, 39]. Glucose absorption is either normal [39] or slightly delayed [38], but overall delivery of glucose to the periphery does not differ between older and younger people.

Hepatic Glucose Production

Basal hepatic glucose production is not altered with age [15, 23, 27, 34, 40]. Similarly, in most studies overall suppression of hepatic glucose output by insulin is not decreased in the elderly [23, 27, 38, 40]. There may be alterations in the timing of the suppression of hepatic glucose output in the elderly, with a delay seen in the initial suppression of hepatic glucose output by insulin [38]. Overall, changes in hepatic glucose production and suppression by insulin do not explain the glucose intolerance seen with aging.

Non-insulin Mediated Glucose Uptake

Non-insulin mediated glucose uptake is probably not altered with aging. Although one study did find some impairment of non-insulin mediated glucose uptake in the basal state [41], a second study using the minimal model method [29] found no evidence for age-related changes in insulin independent glucose uptake after glucose administration.

Lean Body Mass

Lean body mass decreases with age: approximately 30% of the muscle mass is lost by the seventh decade and 40–45% by the eighth decade [42]. It has been hypothesized that a loss of lean body mass causing a decrease in available muscle for the uptake and storage of ingested glucose causes the impairment of glucose tolerance seen with aging; this has not been shown to be true, however. As already pointed out, in a number of the studies described above [15, 24, 25, 28] (Figure 7) data were corrected for differences in lean body mass and decrements in glucose tolerance with aging were still found. In one study [43] in which lean, elderly subjects were matched with younger subjects who had an equal percentage of body fat (13.4% in the older group and 13.7% in the younger), glucose tolerance was still impaired in the older, lean subjects (Figure 9). Jackson, in a recent review [19], also comments on the fact that women in their third decade with normal glucose tolerance have less overall muscle mass than healthy men aged 70–79 years. Therefore, changes in glucose tolerance with age cannot be explained by changes in lean body mass.

Effect of Diet

Some elderly patients eat a diet that is lower in carbohydrate content [44] than people in younger age groups. Decreased glucose tolerance occurs after periods of low carbohydrate intake [45] in normal subjects. Increasing the

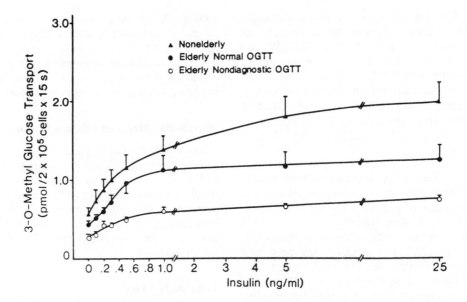

Figure 8 Dose–response curves for insulin-stimulated glucose transport (3-*O*-methyl glucose uptake) in adipocytes from non-elderly subjects (27–50 yr, $n = 11$), elderly subjects with normal oral glucose tolerance tests (60–79 yr, $n = 10$) and elderly subjects with a non-diagnostic glucose tolerance test by NDDG criteria (66–82 yr, $n = 4$) (from RI Fink, OG Kolterman, M Kao, JM Olefsky. The role of the glucose transport system in postreceptor defect in insulin action associated with human aging. J Clin Endocrinol Metab, 58, 721–5, 1984, with permission)

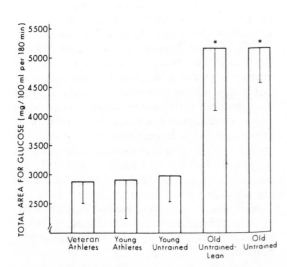

Figure 9 Mean total area under the glucose curve, following a 100-g oral glucose tolerance test in: older extremely trained athletes (60 ± 2 yr, 10.7 ± 0.5% body fat, $n = 14$), young athletes (26 ± 1 yr, 11.0 ± 0.7% body fat, $n = 15$), young untrained men (28 ± 1 yr, 13.7 ± 0.9% body fat, $n = 15$), older untrained lean men (61 ± 2 yr, 13.4 ± 0.5% body fat, $n = 9$) and older untrained men (62 ± 1 yr, 20.8 ± 0.6% body fat, $n = 12$) (from reference 43, with permission)

carbohydrate composition of the diet (to 85%) does improve insulin sensitivity in the elderly [44, 46], but age-related differences in glucose tolerance persist [44]. Therefore, decreased carbohydrate intake in older people cannot be the sole cause of the glucose intolerance of aging.

Exercise

Aerobic capacity, as measured by the maximum oxygen consumption ($\dot{V}_{O_2}$max) declines linearly with age [47]. This has led to speculation that the peripheral insulin resistance associated with advancing age is secondary to decreased physical activity and the decrease in $\dot{V}_{O_2}$max. Most of the studies on physical activity and its effects on glucose tolerance have been done in younger people. In these studies, physical exercise improves glucose tolerance and insulin sensitivity in normal [48, 49] and obese [50] non-diabetic subjects, as well as in people with IGT [51] and non-insulin dependent diabetes [51, 52]. However, the beneficial effects of exercise are lost rapidly: 7 days of bed rest [53] or 5–14 days of inactivity in previously trained individuals

[48, 54] causes a deterioration in glucose tolerance; these changes occur before any change in $\dot{V}o_2$ max or body weight. Similarly, a single bout of exercise can improve insulin-stimulated glucose disposal during a euglycemic clamp in patients with type 2 diabetes [55] and will restore glucose tolerance to previous levels in athletic individuals who have been detrained for 10 days [54]. Therefore, the effect of exercise on glucose metabolism is short-lived.

Only a few studies on exercise have been performed in older subjects. Older extremely trained athletes have the same glucose tolerance as do younger subjects, both trained and untrained. Their glucose tolerance is significantly better than that of a group of older untrained controls, both lean and of normal body weight (Figure 9) [43]. In a study of 20 active and inactive subjects, aged 60–75 years [56], there was a significant direct correlation between $\dot{V}o_2$ max and measurements of insulin action in vivo, i.e. those who were more physically active had improved glucose disposal during a hyperinsulinemic euglycemic clamp. However, this was a cross-sectional study and there was a considerable amount of overlap in the rate of insulin-stimulated glucose disposal between the sedentary and more active groups.

In another study [57], 11 older subjects with normal glucose tolerance underwent a 12-week training program. In these subjects an improvement in peripheral insulin sensitivity during a euglycemic clamp was seen with exercise. However, the improvement in insulin sensitivity did not correlate with changes in $\dot{V}o_2$ max and did not restore insulin sensitivity to the level found in younger people. Therefore, while extremely vigorous exercise can reverse the peripheral insulin resistance associated with aging, the moderate exercise that older people are more likely to be capable of performing does not normalize insulin sensitivity. This suggests that the glucose intolerance associated with aging cannot be wholly explained by physical inactivity.

Counterregulatory Hormones

Changes in levels of glucagon [58] or catecholamines [59] do not seem to be responsible for the glucose intolerance of aging, although hepatic sensitivity to physiologic increases in glucagon may be enhanced [58].

Free Fatty Acids

Abnormalities of fatty acid metabolism may contribute to the development of IGT and diabetes [60]. Elevated free fatty acid levels can cause a decrease in insulin-mediated glucose uptake and stimulate hepatic glucose output [61, 62]. In general, the data on the importance of this effect in diabetic patients are conflicting, and findings in the elderly are variable. In earlier studies, basal free fatty acid levels were found to be elevated in most of the published reports [3]. However, some recent studies have shown that basal [14, 27] and day-long [14] free fatty acid levels may be normal in the elderly, and their suppression by insulin is normal [14, 16, 27] or enhanced [17]. Therefore, the data on the role of free fatty acids in glucose intolerance in the elderly are contradictory; however, they probably do not have a major role in the glucose intolerance of aging.

Summary

The glucose intolerance of aging appears to be due to an increase in peripheral insulin resistance that occurs with aging. The exact mechanism for this defect remains unknown, but is probably associated with post receptor defect(s) in insulin action. Subtle abnormalities of insulin release, insulin binding and hepatic glucose suppression by insulin may exist, but these do not seem to play a major part in the glucose intolerance associated with aging. Changes in degree of physical fitness and carbohydrate content of the diet affect insulin sensitivity, and may underlie part of the insulin resistance noted in the elderly. The loss of lean body mass that occurs with aging is not relevant.

COMPLICATIONS OF DIABETES IN THE ELDERLY

The complications of diabetes add to the morbidity associated with aging. Microvascular (retinopathy and nephropathy) and neuropathic (peripheral and autonomic) complications all increase in frequency with increasing duration of diabetes in an individual, which make them common problems in the elderly diabetic patient. The overall goal of the treatment of diabetes is to forestall or prevent development of these problems by maintaining near-euglycemia for as many years as possible. Once diabetic patients become elderly, the risks of hypoglycemia must be balanced against the benefits of tight diabetic control. When complications do develop, an understanding of their diagnosis and treatment in the elderly is needed to help minimize their impact.

Diabetic Eye Disease

Diabetic retinopathy is the leading cause of blindness in the USA between the ages of 25 years and 74 years. In patients with type 1 diabetes, after 30 years of duration, 22% have some degree of visual impairment and the prevalence of legal blindness (visual acuity in the better eye of 20/200 or worse) increases to 12% [63]. In type 2 diabetes, legal blindness can occur early after the diagnosis of the disease, but increases less dramatically with duration of diabetes than it does in patients with type 1 diabetes [63]. Overall, in diabetic patients who become legally blind, diabetic retinopathy is the sole or a major contributing cause in 86% of patients with type 1 diabetes and 33% of patients with type 2 diabetes. Thus, older patients with diabetes often have other ocular diseases in addition to diabetic retinopathy which contribute to their visual impairment. In the Framingham study [64], nearly one-third of the subjects with diabetes had one or more of the four major ocular diseases looked for—senile cataract, senile macular degeneration, open-angle glaucoma and diabetic retinopathy. Senile macular degeneration was twice as prevalent in diabetic as in non-diabetic subjects (10.5% versus 5.2%). Senile cataract was also more prevalent in diabetic patients (19.1% versus 11.6%), with a slight increase in the prevalence of open-angle glaucoma in the diabetic patients (2.4% versus 1.8%) as well. In another study [65], cataracts were found at a higher rate in people with diabetes than in those without diabetes. In patients who had diabetes diagnosed before the age of 30 years, duration of disease was the single most important determinant of whether or not a cataract was present. Age, diabetic retinopathy, diuretic usage and a higher glycated hemoglobin value at the time of the study were also significantly associated with the presence of cataract. In subjects who developed diabetes after the age of 30 years, age at examination was the most important determinant of the presence of cataract, followed by

increasing severity of diabetic retinopathy and the use of diuretics. Therefore, as this diabetic population aged, they not only had an increased risk for developing cataracts, they also were at risk of developing diabetic retinopathy at the same time.

Prevention of the development of diabetic retinopathy through improved blood glucose control is one of the ultimate goals of current diabetic management. Should proliferative retinopathy or macular edema develop, photocoagulation therapy can delay or halt the progression to blindness [66, 67]. However, in order for treatment to be given, the retinal changes need to be detected. In a Wisconsin study [68], approximately 26% of the younger-onset and 36% of the older-onset patients with diabetes had never had an ophthalmic examination. Factors that contributed to a lack of eye care included living outside a metropolitan area, older age at diagnosis of diabetes, shorter duration of diabetes, fewer years of education, care provided by a family or general practitioner and better visual acuity. Eleven per cent of younger-onset patients and 7% of older-onset patients found to have high-risk retinal characteristics for visual loss had not been examined within 2 years of the study. Thus, older patients with recently diagnosed diabetes are both at risk for having diabetic retinopathy that may benefit from photocoagulation and are less likely to seek ophthalmologic care. Therefore, all older patients (as well as all patients with diabetes in general) should be encouraged to conform to the ADA guidelines for eye care [69], which state that all patients with type 2 diabetes should see an ophthalmologist at the time of the diagnosis of their diabetes and then at least yearly thereafter.

Elderly diabetic patients should also be encouraged to have their other ocular diseases treated to help enhance their visual acuity. Although following intraocular lens implant surgery, improvement in visual acuity is worse in patients with diabetes than in non-diabetics (65% of diabetic surgical eyes had a final visual acuity better than 20/40 compared with 90% of non-diabetic eyes) [70], However, this was not because of a decreased ability of patients with diabetes to benefit from the surgery, but rather because they had a higher prevalence of other ocular diseases, particularly non-proliferative diabetic retinopathy (proliferative diabetic retinopathy is a relative contraindication to lens implantation). When other pre-existing ophthalmic diseases were taken into account, diabetic and non-diabetic patients had an equally good chance (93% versus 96%) of achieving visual acuity better than 20/40. Therefore, elderly diabetic patients with and without non-proliferative retinopathy in need of cataract surgery may benefit from the procedure, as long as they are carefully evaluated and treated by an ophthalmologist familiar with use of lens implantation in patients with diabetes [70].

Diabetic Nephropathy

The prevalence of diabetic nephropathy increases with duration of diabetes and age [71]. Normal aging is also associated with a progressive decline in renal function: a reduction in renal mass and volume of 20–30% occurs from the third to the eighth decade [72]. A serum creatinine level of $88.4 \mu M$ (1 mg/dl) in a person in their third decade corresponds to a creatinine clearance of 2 ml/s (117 ml/min); a serum creatinine level of $88.4 \mu M$ (1 mg/dl) in a healthy individual in their eighth decade corresponds roughly to a creatinine clearance of 1.1 ml/s (64 ml/min) [73]. In addition to normal aging and diabetes, the older diabetic patient is at risk for developing the other causes of renal insufficiency that occur in the elderly—arteriosclerosis, hypertension, congestive heart failure, drugs, infection and cancer [72], as well as drug-induced renal problems.

In patients with diabetes, renal failure is a major cause of morbidity and mortality. In a series of diabetic patients followed at the Joslin Clinic from 1956 to 1964 [74], renal disease accounted for 48% of deaths in patients who developed diabetes before the age of 30 years, and was the cause of death in 5.3% of patients who were diagnosed with diabetes after the age of 39 years. In a study that examined renal mortality rates for people with and without diabetes [75], renal mortality rates were higher at all ages for people with diabetes compared with those without diabetes, particularly in older white women.

In the USA, data from the enrolment of the Medicare end-stage renal disease program revealed that diabetes was the cause of the renal failure in 28% of newly enrolled patients in 1985 —the single largest reason for patients to present

with renal failure [76]. Of all patients enrolled in 1985, 36% were 65 years or older. The number of people in this age group receiving renal transplants from 1978 to 1985 has steadily increased.

At the time of diagnosis of type 2 diabetes, approximately 8% of patients will have persistent proteinuria [77]. These patients will develop renal failure at a more rapid rate than those without proteinuria at the time of diagnosis. However, progression of renal dysfunction following the discovery of fixed proteinuria may be slower in patients with type 2 diabetes than in patients with type 1 diabetes [78]. Renal failure in elderly patients with diabetes is often not attributable to diabetic nephropathy: in one study [79], 32% of renal failure in patients with type 2 diabetes was due to non-diabetic renal disease.

Hyporeninemic hypoaldosteronism is found more frequently in older than in younger diabetic patients [80]. The mean age for diagnosis of the syndrome was 65 years, with a range of 32–82 years. In general, these patients present with asymptomatic hyperkalemia, mild renal insufficiency and a hyperchloremic acidosis. Half of them have diabetes mellitus. Those with symptoms (25%) have muscle weakness and cardiac arrhythmias. Treatment, when necessary, consists of the use of mineralocorticoid replacement (usually in the form of fludrocortisone acetate). In the elderly patient with cardiac disease and hypertension, this drug needs to be used with caution as it can lead to sodium and fluid retention, worsening hypertension and congestive heart failure. Other possibilities for treatment include the use of potassium-wasting diuretics (e.g. furosemide) and sodium bicarbonate. In general, if the serum potassium is not persistently 6.0 mM or greater, and there are no electrocardiographic changes attributable to the hyperkalemia, the risks of treatment in the elderly outweigh the benefits. Drugs that exacerbate hyperkalemia, such as potassium-sparing diuretics, prostaglandin inhibitors, heparin, β-blockers and angiotensin converting enzyme inhibitors should be avoided. Serum potassium levels and renal function should be followed frequently to detect any worsening of the hyperkalemia that would require treatment.

Prevention and treatment of diabetic nephropathy in the elderly is similar to that in the younger diabetic patient. Renal impairment may be noted early after the diagnosis of diabetes, however, and the elderly are at risk for having other conditions such as hypertension and atherosclerotic disease that could also contribute to the development of renal insufficiency. Adequate control of blood glucose levels and aggressive treatment of hypertension, once it develops, should be attempted. In the elderly, however, the side-effects of antihypertensive agents, such as orthostatic hypotension and a depression of cardiac output, may be less well tolerated. A low-protein diet may help retard progression to renal failure [81], but should be prescribed in the elderly only after a complete assessment of individual overall nutritional needs has been made. Care should be taken to avoid use of nephrotoxic drugs. Patients should undergo studies using radiocontrast dye only when absolutely necessary, as these dyes may cause acute renal failure, especially in diabetic patients with underlying renal insufficiency [82]. If a patient is to undergo a dye study, adequate hydration should be given before and after the procedure. Finally, in the USA, active, otherwise healthy elderly patients with renal failure are being treated successfully with dialysis and transplantation, which are options available if prevention fails.

Nervous System Abnormalities

As with the other complications of diabetes, the frequency of diabetic neuropathy increases with age and duration of diabetes [83]. In general, signs and symptoms of peripheral and autonomic neuropathy are manifested similarly in the elderly as in the young, causing the same morbidity and difficulties in treatment. As with the other complications of diabetes in the elderly, the presence of coexisting chronic diseases makes adaptation to yet another medical disorder all the more difficult. An elderly patient with a decrease in lower extremity sensation due to a peripheral neuropathy, coupled with arthritis that limits movement, and cataracts that decrease vision, may be unable to perform daily foot examinations. This can increase the risk for development of foot ulcers and infection, and of possible amputation. Medical treatment for neuropathy may also be more poorly tolerated in the elderly. For example, the use of tricyclic antidepressants for control of the pain associated with peripheral neuropathy may be limited due to side-effects of

the drugs such as orthostatic hypotension and a depression of mentation which are poorly tolerated in the elderly [84].

There are a few neurologic syndromes associated with diabetes that occur almost exclusively in the elderly: two such syndromes are diabetic amyotrophy and diabetic neuropathic cachexia. Diabetic amyotrophy is a poorly defined syndrome of asymmetrical motor weakness and wasting that occurs in the proximal lower extremities (particularly in the iliopsoas muscles and quadriceps) [85]. Pain is often present, with a loss of reflexes, but no sensory loss. The exact cause of the syndrome is unknown, although it is probably a form of radiculopathy. Usually the syndrome resolves spontaneously, albeit slowly. However, it has recurred on the opposite side of the body after resolving at the initial site.

Diabetic neuropathic cachexia is a striking neurologic disorder seen in elderly diabetic men. This syndrome of disabling pain, depression and profound weight loss can be so severe as to suggest the presence of malignancy [86]. Spontaneous recovery also occurs in this syndrome after 12–18 months, but supportive care with pain medication and antidepressants may be required.

Another possible effect of diabetes on the central nervous system is the finding that cognitive function is impaired in older diabetic patients when compared with age-matched controls. Diabetic patients older than 65 years have been found to have a variety of cognitive deficits on various tests of psychological performance, particularly those that involve complex mental tracking, verbal learning, memory and attention [87]. Other studies [88, 89] have suggested that older subjects with diabetes have a deficiency in recent memory retrieval when compared with non-diabetic subjects of similar age. In one study [89] an abnormal electroencephalography (EEG) pattern was seen in the patients with diabetes which was not found in the non-diabetic subjects, even when they were rendered hyperglycemic during EEG monitoring. Tests of verbal fluency, however, showed no differences between diabetic and non-diabetic subjects [90].

The cause of these cognitive deficits is not known. They have been associated with increased glycated hemoglobin levels in some studies [88] but not in others [89]. They may be associated with peripheral diabetic neuropathy. Clinically unrecognized strokes (see below) may occur in patients with diabetes and contribute to a decline in cognitive function. Recurrent episodes of hypoglycemia may contribute to these deficits in some people. Regardless of the mechanism of development of these deficits, they may make it harder for elderly diabetic patients to learn, process and retrieve new information. These patients may require more repetition of educational material before new techniques are mastered.

Depression is a common disorder in the elderly [91]: clinically significant symptoms of depression are found in at least 10% of the older population at any given time [84]. Depression also may be more common in patients with diabetes [92]. Depression can be severe, and at times virtually incapacitating for older patients who lack support systems and have other significant medical problems. It may also hamper their ability to process and learn new information. If an elderly patient is suffering from depression, referral should be made to the appropriate mental health resources for treatment. The elderly, like any age group, can recover from depression and learn how to cope with the challenges and difficulties imposed by their life situation [93].

Macrovascular Disease

The Framingham heart study identified hypertension and vascular disease [94] as being more prevalent in older subjects with diabetes than in those without diabetes (Figure 10). In elderly diabetic patients, 50–70% of deaths are due to macrovascular disease, i.e. coronary artery disease, cerebral vascular disease and peripheral vascular disease [95]. The major cause of death is coronary artery disease, causing an increased incidence of fatal myocardial infarction in diabetic patients compared with non-diabetics.

Diabetes is one of several other risks (hypertension, smoking, obesity, hyperlipidemia and genetic factors) for the development of atherosclerosis. Patients often already have coronary artery disease at the time that type 2 diabetes is diagnosed [96]. Ideally, people should be treated to decrease their cardiac risk factors long before they reach old age. However, improvement in a variety of factors—weight reduction, smoking cessation, increased exercise, improved diet, hyperlipidemic therapy, and adequate control of hypertension and diabetes—may work in concert to improve cardiovascular profiles, even in older patients [97]. Moreover, the prognosis

after a myocardial infarction, in terms of mortality, cardiogenic shock, cardiac failure and risk of reinfarction, is higher in patients with diabetes than those without diabetes [98–102]. Patients with diabetes may have an increased incidence of silent ischemia [103]. Treadmill testing or Holter monitoring may be necessary to evaluate patients for the presence of silent ischemia.

The majority of central nervous system morbidity and mortality in the elderly patient with diabetes is due to vascular events. Patients with diabetes mellitus have an increased risk of stroke [104–106]. In the Honolulu heart project [104], the incidence of thromboembolic stroke in diabetic patients was double that of a non-diabetic cohort. Furthermore, higher glucose levels in the non-diabetic subjects were associated with an increased risk of stroke—those in the 80th percentile for serum glucose level had a rate of thromboembolic stroke 1.4 times higher than subjects who had serum glucose values in the 20th percentile [104].

Patients with diabetes who suffer a stroke have a poorer prognosis than patients without diabetes [107–109]: they have an increased risk of death and recurrent stroke, and fewer have complete functional recovery. Even patients without diabetes who have hyperglycemia at the time of stroke have an increased mortality and poorer functional recovery compared with those who present with normal blood glucose values [110]. Part of the increased poststroke mortality in diabetic patients is due to an increased frequency of cardiac disease and a higher subsequent cardiac mortality; however, this does not completely account for their poorer prognosis.

Overall life expectancy is decreased in diabetic patients, with the degree of decrement related to the age of onset of diabetes (the earlier the onset, the more years lost) [95]. However, if diabetes develops after 70 years of age, life expectancy is not further decreased compared with that of non-diabetics [95]. One area in which aging particularly alters mortality is in terms of survival following an episode of diabetic ketoacidosis or hyperosmolar non-ketotic syndrome [111, 112] (Figure 11). The mortality following an episode of diabetic ketoacidosis and hyperosmolar non-ketotic syndrome rises markedly after the age of 50 years [112], with causes of death including pneumonia, sepsis, adult respiratory distress syndrome, myocardial infarction and gastrointestinal hemorrhage [112, 113].

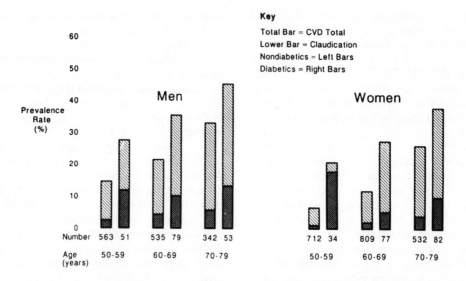

Figure 10   Prevalence of vascular disease in diabetic and non-diabetic subjects aged 50–79 years from the Framingham heart study. CVD, cardiovascular disease (from reference 94, with permission)

SCREENING FOR DIABETES

Although an OGTT is a useful tool for use in epidemiologic studies, it has less utility in clinical practice [114]. It is a time-consuming test, and is a non-physiologic stimulus designed to screen for a physiologic impairment of glucose toler-ance, before overt diabetes occurs [115]. The results of OGTTs are only poorly reproducible [116] and can be affected by a variety of factors, including diet [45], diurnal variation, drugs, exercise and acute illness [117].

Use of glycated hemoglobin values has been proposed as a screening tool for diabetes [115,

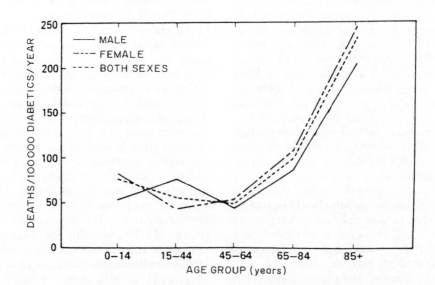

Figure 11   Age-specific average mortality rates from diabetic acidosis or hyperosmolar non-ketotic syndrome in diabetic patients in the USA from 1970–78 (from reference 111, with permission)

118–124]. Initial reports using ion chromatography methodology (HbA$_1$ and HbA$_{1c}$) found that although there was a positive correlation between progressively more abnormal OGTTs and elevations in glycated hemoglobin levels, the test varied in its sensitivity for diabetes, although it was very specific [115, 118–122]. In these studies the ability of the glycated hemoglobin value to detect diabetes ranged from 80% to 96% (i.e. 4% to 20% of patients with diabetes had normal glycated hemoglobin levels). The specificity of a markedly elevated glycated hemoglobin was even higher: in virtually all cases this was indicative of overt diabetes. In two studies an affinity chromatography method was used for measuring glycated hemoglobin levels [123, 124]. With this technique there was a clear separation between diabetic and non-diabetic subjects, i.e. there was no overlap between diabetes and normal. Regardless of the methodology employed, glycated hemoglobin values did not correlate well with IGT. Many subjects with IGT as diagnosed by an OGTT had normal glycated hemoglobin values [115, 118, 120–124]. The advantages of using glycated hemoglobin measurement to diagnose diabetes are that it requires only one venipuncture, can be drawn at any time of day, and reflects glucose homeostasis over weeks, rather than at one point in time. For a clear separation between normal patients and those with diabetes, glycated hemoglobin levels should be measured by affinity chromatography.

Given the limitations of the OGTT and the utility of glycated hemoglobin values for making the diagnosis of diabetes, we propose the clinical approach outlined in Figure 12 for diabetes screening. A fasting plasma glucose (FPG) value should be obtained as the initial laboratory test. If elevated, in an asymptomatic patient, it should be repeated for verification. On the basis of the FPG, patients can be classified as normal (no diabetes), definitely diabetic, and those who have either IGT or mild diabetes and need further evaluation. This evaluation consists of obtaining a 1-hour to 2-hour postprandial plasma glucose level, which if less than 10 mM requires no further evaluation. A postprandial plasma glucose level of 10 mM or over should be followed by a glycated hemoglobin measurement. Although this algorithm may not distinguish between IGT and mild diabetes, this distinction is not important in clinical practice

because all of these patients need to be counseled regarding diet and exercise. The carbohydrate metabolism of these patients should be monitored routinely, as some will progress to overt diabetes. This is especially important during periods of illness or other stresses.

TREATMENT

The treatment of diabetes mellitus in the elderly is similar to the treatment of diabetes in younger persons, but with several modifications. Patients with type 1 (ketosis-prone) diabetes of any age need to be treated with insulin. As described above, people who have a 1-hour to 2-hour postprandial plasma glucose concentration of over 10 mM or a glycated hemoglobin level more than 1.5% above the upper limit of normal of the assay used, may need to be treated with medication for diabetes. Elderly patients with type 2 diabetes are generally treated following the same approach as in younger patients with type 2 diabetes—a trial of dietary therapy first, followed by use of oral hypoglycemic agents and ultimately insulin if the first two fail. Treatment plans must be individualized on the basis of functional ability, the presence of coexisting diseases and life expectancy. However, as discussed below, there are basic principles that can be applied to most elderly patients with diabetes, which are modified based on individual needs.

Evaluation

In any age group, obtaining an adequate history is important. In the elderly a particular focus is necessary on variations in life-style that may hinder compliance with treatment regimens. It is important to obtain records of the patient's previous medical care and to incorporate input from relatives or friends who may be the ones responsible for providing care and insuring compliance with the diabetes treatment regimen [1]. During the physical examination an assessment both of mental and of the functional status should be performed. There are a variety of age-related changes that can alter a patient's ability to perform the skills necessary to treat diabetes [125–127]. For instance, loss of visual acuity can interfere with self-monitoring of blood glucose (SMBG) and insulin administration; arthritis of the hands or the presence of

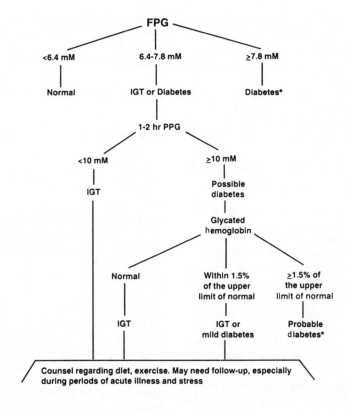

Figure 12   An algorithm for screening for diabetes. FPG, fasting plasma glucose; 1–2 hr PPG, 1–2 hour postprandial plasma glucose concentration; IGT, impaired glucose tolerance. *See Figure 13 for treatment of type 2 diabetes

tremor can impede all of the diabetes-related tasks requiring manual dexterity (food preparation, SMBG, insulin injections, etc.); anorexia can lead to hypoglycemia. The psychosocial issues that can also cause difficulty in diabetes management in the elderly are legion [126, 127]: they include poverty, a lack of access to medical care, difficulties in finding adequate housing, loneliness and grief caused by the death of a spouse and friends, inadequate social support systems and an increased risk of violent crime [126]. Table 3 summarizes a host of factors, both medical and social, that need to be considered when assessing the functional abilities of an elderly patient.

Diet

The dietary recommendations for the older patient with diabetes are not substantially different from those for younger patients with diabetes [128]. It has been shown that older,

obese patients with type 2 diabetes are capable of losing weight in a supervised weight-loss program, with a marked improvement in their glucose tolerance, even though no patient reached their ideal body weight [129]. A lifetime of dietary habits may be difficult to alter, however, and practical guidelines should be given with an emphasis on how these changes can be incorporated into an individual's pre-existing diet pattern. Meal plans should be simplified in patients with cognitive dysfunction or those with a tendency towards anorexia.

Anorexia is a serious problem in the elderly. It has been estimated that 16% of the population over 60 years of age in the USA consume less than 1000 kcal per day [130]. The anorexia of aging is a multifactorial process (Table 4) which includes many of the psychosocial issues that interfere with management of diabetes, such as social isolation, a lack of companionship at meal-times, and depression; physiologic changes such as alterations in the sense of taste and a

Table 3 Factors that can affect the control of diabetes in the elderly

Altered sense
Decreased vision
Decreased smell
Altered taste perception
Decreased proprioception
Difficulties in food preparation and consumption
Tremor
Arthritis
Poor dentition
Alterations in gastrointestinal function and nutrient absorption
Altered recognition of hunger and thirst
Altered renal and hepatic function
Effects of other diseases
Acute: infections
Chronic: systemic, neoplasia
Decreased exercise and mobility
Drugs
Other medications
Alcohol
Neuropsychiatric problems
Bereavement
Depression
Cognitive impairment and dementia
Social factors
Inadequate education
Poor dietary habits
Living alone
Poverty

From reference 127, with permission.

Table 4 Causes of the anorexia of aging

Social
Isolation
Financial
Physical
Normal physiologic changes with aging
Decreased basal metabolic rate
Decreased taste and smell
Abnormal changes
Decreased ability (cerebrovascular accident, Parkinson's disease and chewing difficulty)
Systemic disorders interfering with eating (chronic obstructive pulmonary disease, abdominal angina, constipation, cancer, and cardiomyopathy)
Nutritional deficiency (zinc)
Psychosocial
Depression
Cognitive impairment
Miscellaneous
Drugs
Decreased feeding drive
Increased satiety

Reproduced, with permission, from Morley JE, Mooradian AD, Silver AJ et al. Nutrition in the elderly. Ann Intern Med 1988; 109: 890–904.

decrease in basal metabolic rate; and chronic illness and use of a variety of medications that can depress appetite [131]. Even seemingly simple mechanical problems can contribute to the anorexia of aging: 50% of people aged 65 years or more in the USA are edentulous and many are in need of dental work [127]. Poorly fitting dentures can make eating painful and therefore an activity that is avoided. Chronic gastrointestinal problems, such as decreased gastrointestinal motility due to diabetic autonomic neuropathy, can also decrease energy intake in the elderly.

In an asymptomatic or mildly symptomatic patient with type 2 diabetes, regardless of age, a trial of diet is the first treatment employed. A dietitian should assess the patient's current dietary patterns and ability to follow dietary instructions, and formulate a meal plan based on this information. The patient should be reassessed after a 1-month trial of dietary therapy. If obese patients are losing weight and blood glucose control is improving (in obese or lean patients), dietary therapy can be continued until glycemic goals are met. If the patient's glycemic control is not improving after a trial of dietary therapy, drug therapy should be initiated.

Exercise

Exercise should be used as an adjunct to other forms of therapy for diabetes in the elderly. Older people are capable of undertaking an exercise program, regardless of whether or not they were athletic earlier in life [132, 133]. An assessment of cardiovascular status and of the presence of medical conditions that may affect the ability to exercise should be performed [134]. Limitations to exercise include cardiovascular disease, osteoarthritis, proliferative retinopathy, autonomic and peripheral neuropathy, and peripheral vascular disease. Patients treated with insulin or sulfonylurea agents may experience hypoglycemia following exercise and adjustments in food intake and insulin doses may be required. Exercise should be moderate—70–80% of the patient's maximal heart rate should be achieved at each session [135]. Exercise should be performed for 20–30 minutes, three to five times per week. Duration and frequency of training sessions, as well as the type of exercise undertaken, should be tailored to individual needs.

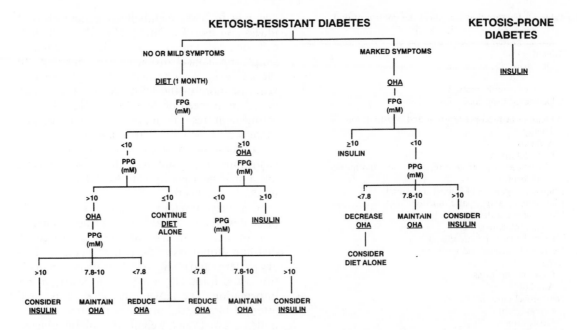

Figure 13 An algorithm for the treatment of diabetes in the older patient (adapted from reference 153). OHA, oral hypoglycemic agent; FPG, fasting plasma glucose concentration; PPG, 1–2 hour plasma glucose concentration. Adapted from Davidson MB, *Diabetes Mellitus—Diagnosis and Treatment*, Churchill Livingstone, New York, 1991, with permission

Sulfonylurea Agents

If a trial of dietary therapy is unsuccessful, treatment with an oral hypoglycemic agent should be initiated (Figure 13). Table 5 lists suggested starting doses of the sulfonylurea agents currently available in the USA. Although the pharmacology of these agents is discussed in

Table 5 Recommended initial drug doses for treatment of type 2 diabetes in older patients

Agent	Initial dose (mg)	
	Asymptomatic diet failures*	Markedly symptomatic patients†
Tolbutamide	500	—
Acetohexamide	250	—
Tolazamide	100	500
Chlorpropamide‡	100	250
Glyburide (glibenclamide)	1.25	7.5
Glipizide	2.5	15
Metformin	500	—

* Relatively asymptomatic patients should be treated with diet alone initially. See text for discussion.
† Increase drug dose quickly after one week if no response is seen.
‡ Chlorpropamide should not be a first-line agent in patients over 65 years old.
From Davidson MB, *Diabetes Mellitus—Diagnosis and Treatment*, Churchill Livingstone, New York, 1991, with permission.

Chapter 27, a few points are of particular importance when using these drugs in older patients.

First, the duration of action of these agents (Table 6) is of particular concern in the elderly, because of the possibility of anorexia and decreased food intake leading to hypoglycemia. Chlorpropamide has a half-life of 36 hours and duration of action of up to 60 hours—the longest of any of the sulfonylurea agents; tolbutamide has the shortest duration of action —6–12 hours. The other sulfonylurea agents fall in between, with durations of action of 10–24 hours. Sites of drug metabolism and elimination are also important in the elderly, because they may have hepatic or renal dysfunction. Tolbutamide and glipizide are both oxidized in the liver to inactive metabolites which are excreted by the kidneys. Acetohexamide is degraded by the liver and kidneys and one of its metabolites has hypoglycemic activity that is 2.5 times more potent than the parent compound [136]; this extends its duration of biologic activity to 12–24 hours (even though the half-life of the parent compound is only 1–2 hours). Glyburide and tolazamide are both degraded to metabolites that have some (although minimal)

Table 6 Selected properties of drugs used to treat type 2 diabetes

Generic name	US trade name	Tablet sizes (mg)	Usual daily dose range (mg)	Maximal dose (mg)	Duration of action (hr)
Tolbutamide	Orinase	250, 500	500–2000 (divided)	3000	6–12
Chlorpropamide	Diabinese	100, 250	100–500 (single)	750	60
Acetohexamide	Dymelor	250, 500	250–1500 (single or divided)	1500	12–24
Tolazamide	Tolinase	100, 250, 500	100–750 (single or divided)	1000	12–24
Glyburide	Micronase, Diabeta	1.25, 2.5, 5.0	2.5–20 (single or divided)	20	12–24
Glipizide	Glucotrol	5.0, 10.0	5–25 (single or divided)	40	10–24
Metformin	—	500, 850	1500–2000 (divided)	2500	8–12

From Davidson MB, *Diabetes Mellitus—Diagnosis and Treatment*, Churchill Livingstone, New York, 1991, with permission.

hypoglycemic activity. The metabolites of tolazamide are excreted by the kidney, whereas those of glyburide are excreted in equal quantities into the bile and urine. Chlorpropamide is partially degraded in the liver and excreted by the kidney. Therefore, in a patient with renal impairment, tolbutamide would be the drug of choice, as it is degraded by the liver and has the shortest half-life of any of the oral hypoglycemic agents. Chlorpropamide should not be used in people over the age of 65 years, both because of its long duration of action which can lead to hypoglycemia, and because of the association of hyponatremia (discussed below) which makes it an undesirable first-line agent in the elderly.

Chlorpropamide, and occasionally tolbutamide, have been associated with the development of the syndrome of inappropriate antidiuretic hormone secretion (SIADH). This is because these drugs both stimulate the non-osmolar release of ADH from the hypothalamus and enhance the effects of ADH on the renal tubule. This promotes the development of hyponatremia, which can have significant neurologic sequelae. In a retrospective study from Japan [137], the medical records of 338 patients with type 2 diabetes on oral hypoglycemic agents were reviewed for hyponatremia. Patients with other known causes for hyponatremia were not included in the study. At the time of the chart review, 25.6% of the patients receiving chlorpropamide had documented hyponatremia (serum sodium $\leqslant 134$ mM); 6.3% of the patients on chlorpropamide had a serum sodium $\leqslant 129$ mM. Those who developed hyponatremia were older (a mean of 67.9 years versus 54.5 years) and were more likely to have been taking thiazide diuretics. A review of the literature on hyponatremia associated with the use of chlorpropamide also confirmed these findings [138]: in this review, 85% of the patients who

developed hyponatremia were older than 60 years, 85% were female and most were on maximal doses of chlorpropamide.

The most serious risk of the use of sulfonylurea agents is the development of hypoglycemia. As mentioned above, a drug such as chlorpropamide with a long duration of action is more likely to cause this phenomenon. All sulfonylurea agents can cause hypoglycemia, however, which is often associated with a decrease in carbohydrate intake [139], ranging from missing only one or two meals to chronic starvation. A study from Sweden [140] reviewed 57 cases of hypoglycemia associated with glyburide (glibenclamide). Those who developed hypoglycemia were older, with a mean age of 75 years, with 21% over the age of 85 years. In those who did not develop hypoglycemia on glyburide, the mean age was 70 years, with only 5% over the age of 85 years. Ten patients had fatal outcomes from their episodes of hypoglycemia; these episodes were observed even with small doses of the drug, early in the initiation of treatment. Besides increasing age, the risk of developing hypoglycemia was also increased by a previous history of stroke or cardiovascular disease, as well as impaired renal function, decreased food intake, diarrhea, alcohol ingestion and interaction with other drugs, particularly sulfonamides.

This last point must be remembered when prescribing medication to the elderly patient with diabetes: drug interactions can occur that increase the hypoglycemic effects of sulfonylurea agents [141]. These drugs act by displacing sulfonylurea agents from their binding sites, thus potentiating their action. Table 7 lists some of these medications.

In summary, the elderly are at increased risk for the development of hypoglycemia when treated with sulfonylurea agents. They need to

Table 7 Drugs that potentiate the hypoglycemic effects of the sulfonylurea agents

Generic name	Trade names in the USA
Sulfonamides	
Sulfisoxazole	Gantrisin, Sodiozole, Sosol, Unisulf
Sulfaphenazole	Orisul, Sulfabid
Sulfadiazine*	Coco-Diazine, Microsulfon
Sulfamethizole*	Thiosulfil, Utrasul, Microsul, Azotrex
Sulfadimethoxine	Madribon
Sulfadimidine	
Sulfafurazole	
Chloramphenicol	Chloromycetin
Bishydroxycoumarin	Dicumarol
Phenylbutazone	Butazolidin
Oxyphenbutazone	Tandearil
Clofibrate	Atromid-S

* Combination of these two sulfonamides is marketed as Suladyne.
From Davidson MB, *Diabetes Mellitus—Diagnosis and Treatment*, Churchill Livingstone, New York, 1991, with permission.

be encouraged to maintain their routine oral intake, or to notify a member of their health care team if intake changes. Small doses of these drugs should be used initially, and increased gradually (every 2–3 weeks) until therapeutic goals are reached. Sulfonamide antibiotics should be used with caution in patients on sulfonylurea agents, in order to prevent precipitating hypoglycemia. Chlorpropamide should also be used with caution in the elderly because of its long duration of action and its potential to cause hyponatremia in this population.

Metformin

Metformin is a biguanide antidiabetic agent currently available throughout much of the world, but not yet approved for use in the USA (see also Chapter 28). It lowers blood glucose levels in patients with type 2 diabetes through mechanisms that differ from those of sulfonylurea agents [142], and as a result can be used alone (usually in obese patients) or in combination with a sulfonylurea agent to lower blood glucose values when single drug therapy has failed. Metformin does not cause hypoglycemia in well-nourished normal or diabetic subjects. Its plasma half-life is short (1.5–2.8 hours) and it is eliminated unchanged by the kidney [143].

The fact that metformin does not cause hypoglycemia should make it a preferred drug for use in the elderly, who tolerate hypoglycemia

poorly. Biguanides have been associated with the occurrence of lactic acidosis; however, this occurs rarely in patients taking metformin. Metformin is not tightly protein bound and is metabolized much more rapidly than phenformin. When lactic acidosis does occur in patients on metformin, patients usually have a serious medical problem in addition to diabetes, especially renal insufficiency. Other associated conditions include hepatic dysfunction, cardiorespiratory disease, acute infection or alcoholism [144]. Because of the decline in renal function associated with age it has been suggested that metformin should not be used in patients over 70 years old [144]. However, the mortality from severe hypoglycemia associated with sulfonylurea agents may exceed the mortality from severe lactic acidosis with metformin [145, 146].

If metformin is to be used in any patient, elderly or otherwise, the patient must have normal renal and hepatic function tests and be free of significant cardiovascular or pulmonary disease and alcoholism. Renal function should be checked routinely and if the serum creatinine is raised, the drug should be discontinued. The drug should also be temporarily stopped if a patient is being treated with a nephrotoxic medication, is undergoing a dye study or develops a significant acute illness.

Gastrointestinal side-effects, such as metallic taste, anorexia, abdominal pain, discomfort and distention, diarrhea, nausea and vomiting occur in 5% to 50% of patients started on the drug [147–149]. These symptoms are related to the dose of the drug, and usually resolve with its continued use. To decrease the occurrence of these gastrointestinal side-effects, metformin should be started at the lowest possible dose, increased gradually (every 2 weeks) and taken with meals.

Metformin, unlike sulfonylurea agents, does not cause weight gain, and may even cause an initial weight loss [150]. This is a desirable effect in an obese patient with type 2 diabetes. However, in an elderly patient prone to anorexia with a marginal nutritional status, the gastrointestinal side-effects and weight-reducing effects of metformin may exacerbate their poor nutritional status. Metformin has also been associated with decreased levels of vitamin B_{12} [151]. Therefore, slender, elderly patients who are on metformin should have their weight and general nutritional status monitored while on the drug, and all patients on the drug should have their serum vitamin B_{12} level measured every year.

Treatment of Symptomatic Patients

Patients who present with marked symptoms of uncontrolled diabetes (polyuria, polydipsia, weight loss) should be started on a larger dose of a hypoglycemic agent in order to control their hyperglycemic symptoms more rapidly (right panel, Figure 13 and Table 5). Sulfonylurea agents, not metformin, should be used initially, as metformin should only be started at a low dose because of its gastrointestinal side-effects. For patients who are markedly dehydrated, however, especially those with cardiovascular disease, hospitalization may be necessary.

Insulin

If a patient does not respond satisfactorily to oral hypoglycemic agent therapy (Figure 13), insulin should be started. Therapy with insulin should be used as in any other patient (keeping in mind the increased risk of hypoglycemia in elderly patients with cardiovascular disease). In patients poorly controlled on insulin, some authors advocate the use of combined insulin and oral hypoglycemic agent therapy [152]. Overall, this form of treatment lowers glycated hemoglobin levels by approximately 1%, from a mean of 11% to 10% [153]. As the goal of diabetes therapy is to achieve near-euglycemia, combination therapy is unsatisfactory and usually insulin doses should be increased in these patients. However, in an older person where life expectancy is limited and in whom oral agent therapy is failing, use of an intermediate-acting insulin at bedtime (with maintenance of maximal doses of the oral agent) may improve their symptoms and glycemic control [154]. A bedtime injection of insulin might also help 'introduce' a patient to the use of insulin. After several months of nightly injections, some patients become motivated to use twice-daily insulin in an attempt to achieve near-euglycemia. Elderly patients who have the cognitive and physical capacity to perform SMBG are capable of doing so [155] and it improves compliance with their diabetes regimen.

Treatment Goals

Throughout this treatment schema, blood glucose goals are similar to those recommended for younger patients with diabetes: a fasting plasma glucose (FPG) and 2-hour postprandial plasma glucose (PPG) value less than or equal to 10 mM, with a glycated hemoglobin value within 1.5% of the upper limit of normal of the assay used. This is because there is increasingly compelling evidence in favor of attempting to normalize the blood glucose values in patients with diabetes [156], as the microvascular complications of diabetes are related to both hyperglycemia and increasing duration of diabetes [83]. Although an 85-year-old newly diagnosed patient with diabetes may not live long enough to develop the complications of diabetes, the predicted remaining life expectancy for a woman 70–74 years old is 13.9 years [157]. As patients with type 2 diabetes may have had the disease for many years before its diagnosis [158], a 72-year-old newly diagnosed women with type 2 diabetes is not only at risk for having had the disease long enough to develop diabetic complications but also may live long enough to develop further complications that might have been prevented by near-normalization of glycemia. However, weighed against the desire to achieve near-euglycemia is the increased risk associated with hypoglycemia in the elderly patient with cardiovascular or cerebrovascular disease. Therefore, treatment goals must be individualized on the basis of the risks and potential benefits for each patient treated for diabetes.

CONCLUSION

Diabetes mellitus in the elderly is often undiagnosed and, when diagnosed, can be difficult to manage. The population is aging, and advancing age causes increasing glucose intolerance, primarily due to peripheral resistance to the action of insulin. Many of the elderly who develop diabetes already have such severe cardiovascular disease that diabetes has no significant effect on their mortality. However, as we become increasingly capable of prolonging life in patients with diabetes—either type 1 or type 2—increasing numbers of elderly people will suffer from the microvascular, neuropathic and macrovascular complications of diabetes, because their development is associated with increasing duration of the disease. Although the complications of diabetes can be disabling at any age, they can be particularly debilitating in the elderly, who often have coexisting chronic disorders and lack the resources—financial, social and emotional —to deal with the limitations the complications create. For the reasons discussed in this chapter, caring for older patients with diabetes can be a rewarding, if challenging, experience.

REFERENCES

1. Minaker KL. What diabetologists should know about elderly patients. Diabetes Care 1990; 13 (suppl. 2): 34–46.
2. Spence JC. Some observations on sugar tolerance, with special reference to variations found at different ages. Quart J Med 1920–21; 14: 314–26.
3. Davidson MB. The effect of aging on carbohydrate metabolism: a review of the English literature and a practical approach to the diagnosis of diabetes mellitus in the elderly. Metabolism 1979; 28: 688–705.
4. National Diabetes Data Group. Classification and diagnosis of diabetes mellitus and other categories of glucose intolerance. Diabetes 1979; 28: 1039–57.
5. WHO Expert Committee on Diabetes Mellitus. Second report. WHO Technical Report Series 646. Geneva: WHO, 1980: pp 8–14.
6. Harris MI, Hadden WC, Knowler WC, Bennett PH. Prevalence of diabetes and impaired glucose tolerance and plasma glucose levels in US population aged 20–74 yr. Diabetes 1987; 36: 523–34.
7. Verrillo A, de Teresa A, La Rocca S, Giarrusso PC. Prevalence of diabetes mellitus and impaired glucose tolerance in a rural area of Italy. Diabetes Res 1985; 2: 301–6.
8. Glatthaar C, Welborn TA, Stenhouse NS, Garcia-Webb P. Diabetes and impaired glucose tolerance: a prevalence estimate based on the Busselton 1981 survey. Med J Austr 1985; 143: 436–40.
9. Dowse GK, Gareeboo H, Zimmet P et al. High prevalence of NIDDM and impaired glucose tolerance in Indian, Creole and Chinese Mauritians. Diabetes 1990; 39: 390–6.
10. Wingard DL, Sinsheimer P, Barrett-Connor EL, McPhillips JB. Community-based study of prevalence of NIDDM in older adults. Diabetes Care 1990; 13 (suppl. 2): 3–8.
11. Hanis CL, Ferrell RE, Barton SA et al. Diabetes among Mexican Americans in Starr County, Texas. Am J Epidemiol 1983; 118: 659–72.
12. Fulop T, Nagy JT, Worum I, Foris G, Mudri K, Varga P, Udvardy M. Glucose intolerance and insulin resistance with aging—studies on insulin receptors and post-receptor events. Arch Geront Geriatr 1987; 6: 107–15.
13. Fink RI, Kolterman OG, Olefsky JM. The physiological significance of the glucose intolerance of aging. J Gerontol 1984; 39: 273–8.
14. Fraze E, Chiou M, Chen I, Reaven GM. Age-related changes in postprandial plasma glucose, insulin, and free fatty acid concentrations in nondiabetic individuals. J Am Ger Soc 1987; 35: 224–8.
15. Fink RI, Kolterman OG, Griffin J, Olefsky JM. Mechanisms of insulin resistance in aging. J Clin Invest 1983; 71: 1523–35.
16. Jackson RA, Blix PM, Matthews JA et al. Influence of ageing on glucose homeostasis. J Clin Endocrinol Metab 1982; 55: 840–8.
17. Ratzmann KP, Witt S, Heinke P, Schulz N. The effect of ageing on insulin sensitivity and insulin secretion in non-obese healthy subjects. Acta Endocrinol 1982; 100: 543–9.
18. Gumbiner B, Polonsky KS, Beltz WF, Wallace P, Brechtel G, Fink RI. Effects of aging on insulin secretion. Diabetes 1989; 38: 1549–56.
19. Jackson RA. Mechanisms of age-related glucose intolerance. Diabetes Care 1990; 13 (suppl. 2): 9–19.
20. Rosenthal M, Doberne L, Greenfield M, Widstrom A, Reaven GM. Effect of age on glucose tolerance, insulin secretion, and in vivo insulin action. J Am Ger Soc 1982; 30: 562–7.
21. DeFronzo RA, Tobin JD, Andres R. The glucose clamp technique. A method for quantifying insulin secretion and resistance. Am J Physiol 1979; 237: E214–23.
22. Bergman RN, Ider YZ, Bowden CR, Cobelli C. Quantitative estimation of insulin sensitivity. Am J Physiol 1979; 236: E667–77.
23. DeFronzo RA. Glucose intolerance and aging. Evidence for tissue insensitivity to insulin. Diabetes 1979; 28: 1095–101.
24. Fukagawa NK, Minaker KL, Rowe JW, Matthews DE, Bier DM, Young VR. Glucose and amino metabolism in aging man: differential effects of insulin. Metabolism 1988; 37: 371–7.
25. Rowe JW, Minaker KL, Pallotta JA. Characterization of the insulin resistance of aging. J Clin Invest 1983; 71: 1581–7.
26. Pagano G, Cassader M, Cavallo-Perin P et al. Insulin resistance in the aged: a quantitative evaluation of in vivo insulin sensitivity and in vitro glucose transport. Metabolism 1984; 33: 976–81.
27. Meneilly GS, Minaker KL, Elahi D, Rowe JW. Insulin action in aging man: evidence for tissue-specific differences at low physiologic insulin levels. J Gerontol 1987; 42: 196–201.
28. Fink RI, Wallace P, Olefsky JM. Effects of aging on glucose-mediated glucose disposal and glucose transport. J Clin Invest 1986; 77: 2034–41.
29. Chen M, Bergman RN, Pacini G, Porte D Jr. Pathogenesis of age-related glucose intolerance in man: insulin resistance and decreased beta-

cell function. J Clin Endocrinol Metab 1985; 60: 13–19.

30. Pacini G, Valerio A, Beccaro F, Nosadini R, Cobelli C, Crepaldi G. Insulin sensitivity and beta-cell responsivity are not decreased in elderly subjects with normal OGTT. J Am Ger Soc 1988; 36: 317–23.

31. DeFronzo RA. Glucose intolerance and aging. Diabetes Care 1981; 4: 493–501.

32. Fink RI, Revers RR, Kolterman OG, Olefsky JM. The metabolic clearance of insulin and the feedback inhibition of insulin secretion are altered with aging. Diabetes 1985; 34: 275–80.

33. Reaven GM, Greenfield MS, Mondon CE, Rosenthal M, Wright D, Reaven EP. Does insulin removal rate from plasma decline with age? Diabetes 1982; 31: 670–3.

34. Bolinder J, Ostman J, Arner P. Influence of aging on insulin receptor binding and metabolic effects of insulin on human adipose tissue. Diabetes 1983; 32: 959–64.

35. Pagano G, Cassader M, Diana A, Pisu E, Bozo C, Ferrero F, Lenti G. Insulin resistance in the aged: the role of the peripheral insulin receptors. Metabolism 1981; 30: 46–9.

36. Helderman JH. Constancy of pharmacokinetic properties of the lymphocyte insulin receptor during aging. J Gerontol 1980; 35: 329–34.

37. Fink RI, Kolterman OG, Kao M, Olefsky JM. The role of the glucose transport system in the postreceptor defect in insulin action associated with human aging. J Clin Endocrinol Metab 1984; 58: 721–5.

38. Jackson RA, Hawa MI, Roshania RD, Sim BM, DiSilvio L, Jaspan JB. Influence of aging on hepatic and peripheral glucose metabolism in humans. Diabetes 1988; 37: 119–29.

39. Tonino RP, Minaker KL, Rowe JW. Effect of age on systemic delivery of oral glucose in men. Diabetes Care 1989; 12: 394–8.

40. Robert J-J, Cummins JC, Wolfe RR et al. Quantitative aspects of glucose production and metabolism in healthy elderly subjects. Diabetes 1982; 31: 203–11.

41. Meneilly GS, Elahi D, Minaker KL, Sclater AL, Rowe JW. Impairment of noninsulin-mediated glucose disposal in the elderly. J Clin Endocrinol Metab 1989; 68: 566–71.

42. Cohn SH, Vartsky D, Yasumura S et al. Compartmental body composition based on total-body nitrogen, potassium and calcium. Am J Physiol 1980; 239: E524–30.

43. Seals DR, Hagberg JM, Allen WK, Hurley BF, Dalsky GP, Ehsani AA, Hollaszy JO. Glucose tolerance in young and older athletes and sedentary men. J Appl Physiol 1984; 56: 1521–5.

44. Chen M, Halter JB, Porte D. The role of dietary carbohydrate in the decreased glucose tolerance of the elderly. J Am Ger Soc 1987; 35: 417–24.

45. Wilkerson HLC, Butler FK, Franics JO. The effect of prior carbohydrate intake on the oral glucose tolerance test. Diabetes 1960; 9: 386–91.

46. Chen M, Bergman RN, Porte D Jr. Insulin resistance and beta-cell dysfunction in aging: the importance of dietary carbohydrate. J Clin Endocrinol Metab 1988; 67: 951–7.

47. Dehn MM, Bruce RA. Longitudinal variations in maximal oxygen intake with age and activity. J Appl Physiol 1972; 33: 805–7.

48. Mikines KJ, Sonne B, Tronier B, Galbo H. Effects of training and detraining on dose-response relationship between glucose and insulin secretion. Am J Physiol 1989; 256: E588–96.

49. Rodnick KJ, Haskell WL, Swislocki ALM et al. Improved insulin action in muscle, liver, and adipose tissue in physically trained human subjects. Am J Physiol 1987; 253: E489–95.

50. DeFronzo RA, Sherwin RS, Kraemer N. Effect of physical training on insulin action in obesity. Diabetes 1987; 36: 1379–85.

51. Holloszy JO, Schultz J, Kusnierkiewicz J et al. Effects of exercise on glucose tolerance and insulin resistance. Acta Med Scand 1986; suppl. 711: 55–65.

52. Ruderman NB, Ganda OP, Johansen K. The effect of physical training on glucose tolerance and plasma lipids in maturity onset diabetes. Diabetes 1979; 28 (suppl. 1): 89–92.

53. Mikines KJ, Dela F, Tronier B, Galbo H. Effect of 7 days of bed rest on dose–response relation between plasma glucose and insulin secretion. Am J Physiol 1989; 257: E43–8.

54. Heath GW, Gavin JR, Hinderliter JM et al. Effects of exercise and lack of exercise on glucose tolerance and insulin sensitivity. J Appl Physiol 1983; 55: 512–17.

55. Devlin JT, Hirshman M, Horton ED, Horton ES. Enhanced peripheral and splanchnic insulin sensitivity in NIDDM men after a single bout of exercise. Diabetes 1987; 36: 434–9.

56. Hollenbeck CB, Haskell W, Rosenthal M, Reaven GM. Effect of habitual physical activity on regulation of insulin-stimulated glucose disposal in older males. J Am Ger Soc 1984; 33: 273–7.

57. Tonino RP. Effect of physical training on the insulin resistance of aging. Am J Physiol 1989; 256: E352–6.

58. Simonson DC, DeFronzo RA. Glucagon physiology and aging: evidence for enhanced hepatic sensitivity. Diabetologia 1983; 25: 1–7.

59. Chen M, Halter JB, Porte D. Plasma catecholamines, dietary carbohydrate, and glucose tolerance: a comparison between young and old men. J Clin Endocrinol Metab 1986; 62: 1193–8.

60. Randle PJ, Garland PB, Hales CN, Newsholme

EA. The glucose fatty-acid cycle: its role in insulin sensitivity and the metabolic disturbances of diabetes mellitus. Lancet 1963; i: 785–9.

61. Ferrannini E, Barrett EJ, Bevilacqua S, DeFronzo RA. Effect of fatty acids on glucose production and utilization in man. J Clin Invest 1983; 72: 1737–47.

62. Reaven GM, Chen Y-DI. Role of abnormal free fatty acid metabolism in the development of non-insulin-dependent diabetes mellitus. Am J Med 1988; 85 (suppl. 5A): 106–12.

63. Klein R, Klein BEK, Moss SE. Visual impairment in diabetes. Ophthalmology 1984; 91: 1–9.

64. Framingham Eye Study. The four major diseases and blindness. Surv Ophthalmol 1980; 24 (suppl.): 458–62.

65. Klein BEK, Klein R, Moss SE. Prevalence of cataracts in a population-based study of persons with diabetes mellitus. Ophthalmology 1985; 92: 1191–6.

66. Diabetic Retinopathy Study Group. Photocoagulation treatment of proliferative diabetic retinopathy: clinical application of diabetic retinopathy study (DRS) findings. DRS Report 8. Ophthalmology 1981; 88: 583–600.

67. Early Treatment Diabetic Retinopathy Study Research Group. Photocoagulation for diabetic macular edema. ETDRS Report 1. Arch Ophthalmol 1985; 103: 1796–806.

68. Witkin SR, Klein R. Ophthalmologic care for persons with diabetes. JAMA 1984; 251: 2534–7.

69. Eye care guidelines for patients with diabetes mellitus. Diabetes Care 1988; 11: 745–6.

70. Straatsma BR, Pettit TH, Wheeler N, Miyamasu W. Diabetes mellitus and intraocular lens implantation. Ophthalmology 1983; 90: 336–43.

71. Herman WH. Eye disease and nephropathy in NIDDM. Diabetes Care 1990; 13 (suppl. 2): 24–9.

72. Roy AT, Johnson LE, Lee DBN, Brautbar N, Morley JE. Renal failure in older people. J Am Ger Soc 1990; 38: 239–53.

73. Lamy PP, Michocki RJ. Medication management. Clin Geriatr Med 1988; 4: 623–38.

74. Marks HH, Krall LP. Onset, course, prognosis, and mortality in diabetes mellitus. In Marble A, White P, Bradley RF, Krall LP (eds) Joslin's Diabetes mellitus, 11th ed, Philadelphia: Lea & Febiger, 1971: pp 209–54.

75. Geiss LS, Herman WH, Teutsch SM. Diabetes and renal mortality in the United States. Am J Publ Health 1985; 75: 1325–6.

76. Eggers PW. Effect of transplantation on the Medicare end-stage renal disease program. New Engl J Med 1988; 318: 223–9.

77. Humphrey LL, Ballard DJ, Frohnert PP et al. Chronic renal failure in non-insulin-dependent diabetes mellitus. Ann Intern Med 1989; 111: 788–96.

78. Fabre J, Balant LP, Dayer PG, Fox HM, Vernet AT. The kidney in maturity onset diabetes mellitus: a clinical study of 510 patients. Kidney Int 1982; 21: 730–8.

79. Grenfell A, Bewick M, Parsons V et al. Non-insulin-dependent diabetes and renal replacement therapy. Diabet Med 1988; 5: 172–6.

80. DeFronzo RA. Hyperkalemia and hyporeninemic hypoaldosteronism. Kidney Int 1980; 17: 118–34.

81. Cohen D, Dodds R, Viberti G. Effect of protein restriction in insulin dependent diabetics at risk of nephropathy. Br Med J 1987; 294: 795–8.

82. Parfrey PS, Griffiths SM, Barrett BJ et al. Contrast material-induced renal failure in patients with diabetes mellitus, renal insufficiency, or both: a prospective controlled study. New Engl J Med 1989; 320: 143–9.

83. Pirart J. Diabetes mellitus and its degenerative complications: a prospective study of 4400 patients observed between 1947 and 1973. Diabetes Care 1978; 1: 168–88.

84. Thompson TL, Moran MG, Nies AS. Psychotropic drug use in the elderly. New Engl J Med 1983; 308: 194–9.

85. Thomas PK, Ward JD, Watkins PJ. Diabetic neuropathy. In Keen H, Jarrett J (eds) Complications of diabetes, 2nd ed. London: Edward Arnold, 1982: pp 117–18.

86. Ellenberg M. Diabetic neuropathic cachexia. Diabetes 1974; 23: 418–23.

87. U'Ren RC, Riddle MC, Lezak MD, Bennington-Davis M. The mental efficiency of the elderly person with type 2 diabetes. J Am Ger Soc 1990; 38: 505–10.

88. Perlmuter LC, Hakami MK, Hodgson-Harrington C, Ginsberg J, Katz J, Singer DE, Nathan DM. Decreased cognitive function in aging noninsulin-dependent diabetic patients. Am J Med 1984; 77: 1043–8.

89. Mooradian AD, Perryman K, Fitten J, Kavonian GD, Morley JE. Cortical function in elderly non-insulin dependent diabetic patients. Arch Intern Med 1988; 148: 2369–72.

90. Perlmuter LC, Tun P, Sizer N, McGlinchey RE, Nathan DM. Age and diabetes related changes in verbal fluency. Exper Aging Res 1987; 13: 9–14.

91. Blazer D, Williams CD. Epidemiology of dysphoria and depression in an elderly population. Am J Psychiatr 1980; 137: 439–44.

92. Wing RR, Marcus MD, Blair EH, Epstein LH, Burton LR. Depressive symptomatology in obese patients with type II diabetes. Diabetes Care 1990; 13: 170–2.

93. Lakshmanan M, Mion LC, Frengley JD. Effective low dose tricyclic antidepressant treatment for depressed geriatric rehabilitation patients. J Am Ger Soc 1986; 34: 421–6.

94. Wilson PWF, Anderson KM, Kannel WB. Epidemiology of diabetes mellitus in the elderly.

The Framingham study. Am J Med 1986; 80 (suppl. 5A): 3–9.

95. Panzram G. Mortality and survival in type 2 (non-insulin-dependent) diabetes mellitus. Diabetologia 1987; 30: 123–31.

96. Uusitupa M, Siitonen O, Aro A, Pyorala K. Prevalence of coronary heart disease, left ventricular failure and hypertension in middle-aged, newly diagnosed type 2 (non-insulin-dependent) diabetic subjects. Diabetologia 1985; 28: 22–7.

97. American Diabetes Association. Role of cardiovascular risk factors in prevention and treatment of macrovascular disease in diabetes. Diabetes Care 1989; 12: 573–9.

98. Molstad P, Nustad M. Acute myocardial infarction in diabetic patients. Acta Med Scand 1987; 222: 433–7.

99. Rytter L, Troelsen S, Beck-Nielsen H. Prevalence and mortality of acute myocardial infarction in patients with diabetes. Diabetes Care 1985; 8: 230–4.

100. Yudkin JS, Oswald GA. Determinants of hospital admission and case fatality in diabetic patients with myocardial infarction. Diabetes Care 1988; 11: 351–8.

101. Ulvenstam G, Aberg A, Bergstrand R et al. Long-term prognosis after myocardial infarction in men with diabetes. Diabetes 1985; 34: 787–92.

102. Abbott RD, Donahue RP, Kannel WB, Wilson PWF. The impact of diabetes on survival following myocardial infarction in men vs women. The Framingham study. JAMA 1988; 260: 3456–60.

103. Nesto RW, Phillips RT, Kett KG et al. Angina and exertional myocardial ischemia in diabetic and nondiabetic patients: assessment by exercise thallium scintigraphy. Ann Intern Med 1988; 108: 170–5.

104. Abbott RD, Donahue RP, MacMahon SW, Reed DM, Yano K. Diabetes and the risk of stroke. The Honolulu Heart Program. JAMA 1987; 257: 949–52.

105. Gordon T, Kannel WB. Predisposition to atherosclerosis in the head, heart, and legs. The Framingham study. JAMA 1972; 221: 661–6.

106. Laakso M, Ronnemaa T, Pyorala K, Kallio V, Puukka P, Penttila I. Atherosclerotic vascular disease and its risk factors in noninsulin dependent diabetic and nondiabetic subjects in Finland. Diabetes Care 1988; 11: 449–63.

107. Pulsinelli WA, Levy DE, Sigsbee B, Scherer P, Plum F. Increased damage after ischaemic stroke in patients with hyperglycemia with or without diabetes. Am J Med 1983; 74: 540–4.

108. Olsson T, Viitanen M, Asplund K, Eriksson S, Hagg E. Prognosis after stroke in diabetic elderly patients. A controlled prospective study. Diabetologia 1990; 33: 244–9.

109. Topic E, Pavlicek I, Brinar V, Korsic M. Gly-

cosylated haemoglobin in clarification of the origin of hyperglycaemia in acute cerebrovascular accident. Diabet Med 1989; 6: 12–15.

110. Gray CS, Taylor R, French JM et al. The prognostic value of stress hyperglycaemia and previously unrecognized diabetes in acute stroke. Diabet Med 1987; 4: 237–40.

111. Holman RC, Herron CA, Sinnock P. Epidemiologic characteristics of mortality from diabetes with acidosis or coma, United States, 1970–1978. Am J Publ Health 1983; 73: 1169–73.

112. Carroll P, Matz R. Uncontrolled diabetes mellitus in adults: experience in treating diabetic ketoacidosis and hyperosmolar nonketotic coma with low-dose insulin and a uniform treatment regimen. Diabetes Care 1983; 6: 579–85.

113. Khardori R, Soler NG. Hyperosmolar hyperglycemic nonketotic syndrome. Report of 22 cases and brief review. Am J Med 1984; 77: 899–904.

114. Home P. The OGTT: gold that does not shine. Diabet Med 1988; 5: 313–14.

115. Verrillo A, de Teresa A, Golia R, Nunziata V. The relationship between glycosylated haemoglobin levels and various degrees of glucose intolerance. Diabetologia 1983; 24: 391–3.

116. Ganda OP, Day JL, Soeldner JS et al. Reproducibility and comparative analysis of repeated intravenous and oral glucose tolerance tests. Diabetes 1978; 27: 715–25.

117. Siperstein MD. The glucose tolerance test: a pitfall in the diagnosis of diabetes mellitus. Adv Int Med 1975; 20: 297–323.

118. Little RR, England JD, Wiedmeyer HM et al. Relationship of glycosylated hemoglobin to oral glucose tolerance. Diabetes 1988; 37: 60–4.

119. Kesson CM, Young RE, Talwar D et al. Glycosylated hemoglobin in the diagnosis of non-insulin-dependent diabetes mellitus. Diabetes Care 1982; 5: 395–8.

120. Dods RF, Bolmey C. Glycosylated hemoglobin assay and oral glucose tolerance test compared for detection of diabetes mellitus. Clin Chem 1979; 25: 764–8.

121. Lev-Ran A, VanderLaan WP. Glycohemoglobins and glucose tolerance. JAMA 1979; 241: 912–14.

122. Flock EV, Bennett PH, Savage PJ et al. Bimodality of glycosylated hemoglobin distribution in Pima Indians. Diabetes 1979; 28: 984–9.

123. Hall PM, Cook JGH, Sheldon J et al. Glycosylated hemoglobins and glycosylated plasma proteins in the diagnosis of diabetes mellitus and impaired glucose tolerance. Diabetes Care 1984; 7: 147–50.

124. John WG, Richardson RW. Glycosylated haemoglobin levels in patients referred for oral glucose tolerance tests. Diabet Med 1986; 3: 46–8.

125. Riesenberg D. Diabetes mellitus. In Cassel CK,

Riesenberg DE, Sorensen LB, Walsh JR (eds) Geriatric medicine, 2nd ed. New York: Springer 1990: pp 228–38.

126. Holvey SM. Psychosocial aspects in the care of elderly diabetic patients. Am J Med 1986; 80 (suppl. 5A): 61–3.

127. Lipson LG. Diabetes in the elderly: diagnosis, pathogenesis and therapy. Am J Med 1986; 80 (suppl. 5A): 10–21.

128. Mezitis NHE, Pi-Sunyer FX. Dietary management of geriatric diabetes mellitus. Geriatrics 1989; 44: 70–8.

129. Reaven GM. Beneficial effect of moderate weight loss in older patients with non-insulin-dependent diabetes mellitus poorly controlled with insulin. J Am Ger Soc 1985; 33: 93–5.

130. Abraham S, Carroll MD, Dresser CM et al. Dietary intake of persons 1–74 years of age in the United States. In Advance data from vital and health statistics of the National Center for Health Statistics 6. DHEW Publication No. (HRA) 77-1647. Rockville, MD: US Dep of Health, Education and Welfare, 1977.

131. Morley JE, Mooradian AD, Silver AJ et al. Nutrition in the elderly. Ann Intern Med 1988; 109: 890–904.

132. Benestad AM. Trainability of old men. Acta Med Scand 1965; 178: 321–7.

133. DeVries HA. Physiological effects of an exercise training regimen upon men aged 52 to 88. J Gerontol 1970; 25: 325–36.

134. Wheat ME. Exercise in the elderly. West J Med 1987; 147: 477–80.

135. Bruce RA. Exercise, functional aerobic capacity, and aging—another viewpoint. Med Sci Sports Exer 1984; 16: 8–13.

136. Galloway JA, McMahon RE, Culp HW et al. Metabolism, blood levels and rate of excretion of acetohexamide in human subjects. Diabetes 1967; 16: 118–27.

137. Kadowaki T, Hagura R, Kajinuma H et al. Chlorpropamide-induced hyponatremia: incidence and risk factors. Diabetes Care 1983; 6: 468–71.

138. Tanay A, Firemann Z, Yust I, Abramov AL. Chlorpropamide-induced syndrome of inappropriate antidiuretic hormone secretion. J Am Ger Soc 1981; 29: 334–6.

139. Seltzer HS. Drug-induced hyponatremia—a review of 1418 cases. Endocr Metab Clin N Amer 1989; 18: 163–83.

140. Asplund K, Wiholm BE, Lithner F. Glibenclamide-associated hypoglycemia: a report on 57 cases. Diabetologia 1983; 24: 412–17.

141. Hansen JM, Christensen LK. Drug interactions with oral sulphonylurea hypoglycemic agents. Drugs 1977; 13: 24–34.

142. Bailey CJ. Metformin revisited: its actions and indications for use. Diabet Med 1988; 5: 315–20.

143. Sirtori CR, Franceschini G, Galli-Kienle M et al. Disposition of metformin (N, N-dimethylbiguanide) in man. Clin Pharmacol Ther 1978; 24: 683–93.

144. Herman LS. Metformin: a review of its pharmacological properties and therapeutic use. Diabète Métab 1979; 5: 233–45.

145. Campbell IW. Metformin and sulphonylurea derivatives: the comparative risks. In Krans HMJ (ed.) Diabetes and metformin: a research and clinical update. London: Royal Society of Medicine, 1985; 79: 43–50.

146. Berger W. Incidence of severe side effects during therapy with sulfonylureas and biguanides. Horm Metab Res 1985; 15 (suppl. 1): 111–15.

147. Dandona P, Fonseca V, Mier A, Beckett AG. Diarrhea and metformin in a diabetic clinic. Diabetes Care 1983; 6: 472–4.

148. Campbell IW, Duncan C, Patton NW et al. The effect of metformin on glycaemic control, intermediary metabolism and blood pressure in non-insulin-dependent diabetes mellitus. Diabet Med 1987; 4: 337–41.

149. Cairns SA, Shalet S, Marshall AJ, Hartog M. A comparison of phenformin and metformin in the treatment of maturity-onset diabetes. Diabète Métab 1977; 3: 183–8.

150. Rains SGH, Wilson GA, Richmond W, Elkeles RS. The effect of glibenclamide and metformin on serum lipoproteins in type 2 diabetes. Diabet Med 1988; 5: 653–8.

151. Adams JF, Clark JS, Ireland JT et al. Malabsorption of vitamin B_{12} and intrinsic factor secretion during biguanide therapy. Diabetologia 1983; 24: 16–18.

152. Lebovitz HE, Pasmantier RM. Combination insulin-sulfonylurea therapy. Diabetes Care 1990; 13: 667–75.

153. Davidson MB. Diabetes mellitus—diagnosis and treatment, 3rd edn. New York: Churchill Livingstone, 1991.

154. Riddle MC. Evening insulin strategy. Diabetes Care 1990; 13: 676–86.

155. Gilden JL, Casia C, Hendryx M, Singh SP. Effects of self-monitoring of blood glucose on quality of life in elderly diabetic patients. J Am Ger Soc 1990; 38: 511–15.

156. Hanssen KF, Dahl-Jorgenson K, Lauritzen T et al. Diabetic control and microvascular complications: the near-normoglycemia experience. Diabetologia 1986; 29: 677–84.

157. Katz S, Branch LG, Branson MH et al. Active life expectancy. New Engl J Med 1983; 309: 1218–24.

158. West KM. Epidemiology of diabetes and its vascular lesions. New York: Elsevier, 1978: p 162.

Acute Disturbances of Diabetes

47

Hypoglycemia

Geremia B. Bolli* and Edwin A.M. Gale†

*Istituto di Patologia Medica, University of Perugia, Italy, and †Department of Diabetes and Metabolism, St Bartholomew's Hospital, London, UK

Clinical experience with insulin induced hypoglycemia can be divided into three main periods of about 20 years each. The first, from 1922 to 1939, was the 'age of anecdote'. Many of our clinical beliefs were acquired at this time and research was active but unsystematic. Hypoglycemia seemed a small price to set against the life-giving benefits of insulin. The second period, from 1940 to 1960, can be thought of as the 'age of neuroglycopenia'. Interest was centred on the central nervous system (CNS) because of experience with insulin shock therapy, studies of pathological changes in brain tissue following severe hypoglycemia, and the introduction of electro-encephalography. Hypoglycemic unawareness was described for the first time in patients receiving repeated insulin shock therapy or long-term insulin treatment for diabetes. Further, depot insulin preparations came into general use in the 1940s, and were blamed by some observers for an apparent increase in the morbidity and mortality of insulin treatment. The third period, heralded by the introduction of radioimmunoassay and other methods of metabolic investigation, can be termed the 'age of counterregulation'. It is still perhaps too early to predict the trend of the current 20-year period, but a renewed emphasis upon hypoglycemia as a disorder of the CNS seems likely, aided by the introduction of non-invasive means of imaging human brain structure and function.

Hypoglycemia is the most common and most serious complication of insulin therapy. It is the major obstacle to improved glycemic control by means of intensified insulin therapy. Nor should it be forgotten that for many patients (and their families) it is the most terrifying and disabling aspect of the diabetic condition.

DEFINITIONS AND TERMINOLOGY

Strictly speaking, hypoglycemia is a biochemical term and can be expressed as a statistical deviation below the normal blood glucose range. The mechanism by which the CNS perceives and responds to low blood glucose levels is little understood, but a complex set of neuroendocrine changes is generated, and clinicians and physiologists naturally seek to incorporate these responses into their description of the state. Endocrine responses include major increases in a wide range of hormones, detectable at fasting glucose levels of 60–70 mg/dl. Neurophysiological and psychomotor changes can already be identified at this level, and EEG abnormalities appear at around 50 mg/dl. These physiological changes are reasonably reproducible in healthy subjects under experimental conditions, although allowance has to be made for the

International Textbook of Diabetes Mellitus. Edited by K.G.M.M. Alberti, R.A. DeFronzo, H. Keen and P. Zimmet
© 1992 John Wiley & Sons Ltd

method of insulin administration. In diabetes, these responses may be modified in important respects by factors such as the state of metabolic control, autonomic neuropathy and the integrity of the counterregulatory system.

Terminology

There is still some confusion surrounding the terminology for the clinical manifestations that develop at low blood glucose levels. 'Hypoglycemia' should ideally be reserved for the biochemical condition rather than the clinical state, and is conventionally said to exist at plasma levels below 3.3 mmol/l (60 mg/dl) [1]. This level may actually be too low, as neurophysiological and counterregulatory changes can be detected at levels as high as 4 mmol/l. Marks has proposed the term 'neuroglycopenia' to cover *all* clinical manifestations of hypoglycemia [2]. This seems justified by the recent finding that the threshold for early signs of neuroglycopenia *and* release of counterregulatory hormones (approx 4 mmol/l) is greater than that for symptoms (about 3 mmol/l) [3]. In common usage, however, the peripheral manifestations (tremor, tachycardia, sweating) are lumped under the term *adrenergic* (ignoring the fact that sweating is cholinergic), as contrasted with the central or *neuroglycopenic* changes which develop in patients who have lost or fail to perceive these symptoms. 'Neurogenic' and 'autonomic' have been proposed as terms preferable to 'adrenergic' [4]. For the sake of simplicity we prefer to talk of 'peripheral' and 'central' manifestations of hypoglycemia.

The term 'loss of warning' is used to describe the transition from predominantly peripheral symptoms to central symptoms that many patients experience. 'Hypoglycemic (or hypoglycemia) unawareness' is a loosely used and self-explanatory expression covering both failure to develop and failure to perceive peripheral changes. There is some disagreement about the use of the terms 'low' and 'high threshold'; purists will argue that a patient who secretes epinephrine at unusually low glucose levels has a 'high threshold' for response. Despite this, we prefer to stick with the majority and consider 'low threshold' as equivalent to 'low blood glucose'.

Table 1 Classification of hypoglycemia

1. Asymptomatic (biochemical)
   a) Awake
   b) Asleep
2. Mild symptomatic (patients can treat themselves)
3. Severe symptomatic (help needed)
4. Coma

CLASSIFICATION

The straightforward classification of hypoglycemia in Table 1 is sometimes hard to translate into clinical practice. The frequency of 'biochemical' hypoglycemia under everyday conditions is impossible to know because by definition episodes are not perceived, while the ability to self-test blood glucose may be impaired. Inpatient profiles overcome these problems but may be unrepresentative of real life. Mild episodes are hard to assess because the symptoms are non-specific and their relationship to blood glucose levels variable. Another problem is that some patients underreport severe hypoglycemia, whether because of retrograde amnesia or (more often) emotional denial. In cases of doubt there is no substitute for a careful enquiry in the presence of someone who knows the patient well.

FREQUENCY

How Common is Hypoglycemia?

Intermittent asymptomatic (biochemical) hypoglycemia is an almost inevitable consequence of adequate treatment with insulin. Mild symptomatic episodes are common and are most likely to develop before meals and during or after exercise. It has been suggested that the frequency is around one episode per week in those on conventional therapy and twice that on intensified treatment—equivalent to 2000–4000 episodes in a lifetime on insulin [4]. For obvious reasons sleeping patients are less likely to be aware of symptoms, but between one-quarter and one-third of all patients on standard therapy experience nocturnal hypoglycemia, with a peak incidence around 3 a.m. [5]; patients on continuous subcutaneous insulin therapy (CSII) may reach trough values later in the night. Unperceived hypoglycemia may persist for hours and give rise to non-specific symptoms such as a headache on waking or lassitude and malaise during the day [6]. A typical patient

Table 2 Frequency of severe hypoglycemia in prospective studies

	No. of patients	Percentage experiencing severe hypoglycemia per year
Conventional therapy		
Goldstein, 1981 [8]	147 (children)	4
Potter, 1982 [9]	1200	9
Casparie, 1985 [10]	400	9
Muhlhauser, 1985 [11]	384	10
DCCT, 1987 [12]	132	9.8
DCCT, 1989 [13]	not stated	6.1
Bergada, 1989 [14]	350 (children)	6.8
CSII/Intensified therapy		
Mecklenburg, 1989 [15]	248	7
Steno, 1983 [16]	16	40
DCCT, 1987 [12]	146	26.0
DCCT, 1989 [13]	not stated	23.3

probably has two to four symptomatic episodes of nocturnal hypoglycemia yearly, but the frequency is hard to assess because these often present in clusters with long intervals in between.

Estimates of the frequency of severe hypoglycemia vary but the rate reported in prospective studies is often surprisingly—and unacceptably—high. As a rough guide, it has been suggested that a 'rule of thirds' applies to adult patients on conventional therapy [7]. According to this:

(1) one in three will experience hypoglycemic coma at some point in his or her treatment;
(2) one in three of these (i.e. 10% of the total) will have experienced coma in the previous year;
(3) one in three of these (2–3% of the total) have very real disruption of their lives because of recurrent hypoglycemia.

More formal estimates of the yearly rate are given in Table 2.

It will be seen from Table 2 that (at least from published evidence) children experience severe hypoglycemia rather less often than adults. The implication of the rule of thirds is that susceptibility to severe hypoglycemia is very unevenly distributed within the patient population—after all, 60–70% never experience hypoglycemic coma—but is remarkably uniform from one center to another. This suggests that patterns of individual susceptibility may be the determining factor rather than different strategies of management.

Early studies with intensified therapy prod-

uced conflicting results, but the Diabetes Control and Complications Trial (DCCT) has now made it clear that the incidence of severe hypoglycemia is markedly increased, with an annual rate around 25% [12]. In the course of the study the rate of severe hypoglycemia has fallen in each group [13] but the ratio between the two has not decreased (Table 2). Differences in rates between studies may relate primarily to the mean level of glucose control achieved [17], and the high rate of severe hypoglycemia reported in the course of diabetic pregnancy is probably due to attempts to achieve near-normoglycemia.

HYPOGLYCEMIA AND THE CENTRAL NERVOUS SYSTEM

Physiology

The brain has high energy requirements, estimated as 1 mg/kg of glucose per minute, or about 100 g per 24 hours in an adult, but low energy reserves. The energy is needed to maintain the ionic gradient across nerve membranes. In theory the brain is able to oxidise substrates other than glucose under normal conditions, but in practice these are either excluded by the blood–brain barrier or circulate at concentrations too low to be taken up in useful quantities [18]. Glucose oxidation thus normally provides more than 90% of the energy needed for brain function. As the brain cannot synthesize glucose, and has reserves sufficient for only a few minutes, its function is almost totally dependent upon an uninterrupted supply by the circulation. Under normal circumstances the rate-limiting step for glucose uptake is phosphorylation within the cell by the enzyme hexokinase. The glucose carrier transport system through the blood–brain barrier does however become the rate-limiting step as the plasma glucose concentration falls, even though the brain can augment the fractional extraction of glucose during hypoglycemia [19].

Neuropsychological Consequences of Hypoglycemia

Small acute decrements of less than 20% of the postabsorptive plasma glucose concentration are sufficient to impair brain oxidative metabolism and to produce evidence of cortical brain dysfunction in the absence of symptoms [3]. Neuropsychological performance deteriorates at plasma glucose levels of 55–65 mg/dl in a substantial proportion of patients, usually well in advance of the first warning symptoms [20, 21]. General psychomotor dysfunction, as assessed for example by simple arithmetic and ability to concentrate on tasks, is quite prominent. More specific abnormalities such as sense of time elapsed [20] and colour sense [22] have also been described. In practical terms this implies that driving or work ability may deteriorate appreciably without individual insight into the situation, clearly a matter of considerable concern to all diabetic patients and their doctors.

Hypoglycemia and the EEG

During symptomatic hypoglycemia, symmetrical electroencephalographic abnormalities appear in a relatively narrow blood glucose range of 2–2.5 mol/l (36–45 mg/dl). Early changes include slowing of the EEG. At lower levels still, bursts of low-frequency activity occur with bifrontal delta waves. These changes are not specific for hypoglycemia, but resemble those seen in hypoxia and other metabolic encephalopathies [23].

Neuropathology of Hypoglycemia

There is an old belief that hypoglycemia spares the deeper (and phylogenetically older) regions of the brain, since these have lower energy requirements than the neocortex [24]. This is consistent with pathological reports regarding patients who have died in severe hypoglycemia:

these show widespread degeneration and laminar necrosis of nerve cells and corresponding glial proliferation in the cerebral cortex (especially the temporal lobes), hippocampus and basal ganglia, with lesser changes, in the cerebellum and little visible damage to the brain stem [25, 26].

Symptom Complexes

Three main categories are recognized: acute, subacute and chronic neuroglycopenia [2].

Acute Neuroglycopenia

Obvious symptoms may be preceded by lassitude, unease or mild exhilaration, progressing to light-headedness. A prickling sensation in the skin heralds the onset of a cold sweat, although some patients feel hot. Tremor develops together with a moderate tachycardia and awareness of a forceful heart beat. Many patients feel peaceful and detached at this stage but others are restless and apprehensive. Passivity is marked; a patient may be intellectually aware of the situation but not bother to fetch glucose. Sounds are heard as from a distance and the eyes become unfocused. Time seems to pass more quickly and sleep often supervenes. Prolonged hypoglycemia becomes progressively more unpleasant, leading to irritability and a drained feeling. Reversal leads to a sensation of cold or actual shivering and may be followed by an unpleasant occipital or frontal 'pressure' headache.

Subacute Neuroglycopenia

Subacute neuroglycopenia is common in insulin treated patients and almost endlessly variable in its manifestations, although each patient tends to follow a pattern. The premonitory symptoms described above may seem abbreviated or be absent. Movement and thought are slow, and spontaneous activity is reduced to a minimum. A relative will spot the changes before the patient does, often by recognizing such signs as immobility, slow speech, an air of detachment, unusual irritability or (most commonly) some indefinable change in the eyes. In the words of Joslin, 'Diabetics in such a condition respond to questions like automata and somehow give the impression that they may become unconscious, or quite the reverse, become emotionally unstable'.

A form of automatism may develop and has important medicolegal consequences [27]. Routine tasks may be performed with subsequent amnesia. Office workers may sit immobile at their desks for hours, or drivers go miles past their turning home. Confusion may be drowsy or manic; the patient may appear passive but fly into a fury if disturbed, refuse sugar or fight off those trying to help.

Chronic Neuroglycopenia

This rare form is seen in occasional obsessional diabetics and in some patients with insulinomas. Obvious symptoms are absent but blood glucose may be subnormal for hours on end; patients can present with features of a personality disorder or apparent dementia.

Symptom Generation

How Are the Symptoms Produced?

As blood glucose falls below the normal range, a complex and progressive neuroendocrine response is generated. The typical 'adrenergic' symptoms reflect sympathomedullary activation but are not due simply to epinephrine secretion; adrenalectomized [28] or sympathectomized [29] patients break into a sweat and have many of the other symptoms apart from tachycardia. In contrast, paraplegic patients with high cervical transection of the cord lose epinephrine secretion *and* the autonomic response to hypoglycemia, and simply fall into a deep sleep [30].

The brain lacks a blood glucose 'alarm' and can only perceive its danger by recognizing the peripheral changes generated by neuroglycopenia. In this paradoxical situation the CNS has to depend on recognizing its own malfunction—and not surprisingly often fails to do so. In a classic experiment, Sussman induced hypoglycemia in 44 diabetic patients. The patients were asked to report the onset of symptoms, while the observer noted the onset of physical signs. Free fatty acid (FFA) levels were used as an index of metabolic (adrenergic) response. Sussman recognized three groups as listed in Table 3. The majority of those who failed to recognize hypoglycemia showed physical changes such as sweating which were easily identified by an informed observer [31].

Table 3

Group (no.)	Symptoms	Signs	Rise in FFA
I (23)	Yes	Yes	Yes
II (16)	No	Yes	Yes
III (5)	No	No	No

From reference 31, with permission.

Factors Modifying Symptoms

Glycemic Thresholds

Cortical brain function, as assessed by potentials related to auditory events, becomes impaired at plasma glucose decrements of about 15 mg/dl below fasting levels [3]. Impairments of both cognitive function [20] and counterregulatory hormone release appear at around 60 mg/dl, preceding the onset of symptomatic awareness [3, 32]. Thus brain function is exquisitely sensitive even to minor reductions in the circulating glucose level. It has long been noticed that some diabetic patients report hypoglycemic symptoms at relatively high plasma glucose levels, whereas others deny any symptoms at all even when the glucose level is subnormal. Amiel and colleagues [33] demonstrated that patients on intensified insulin therapy showed lower plasma glucose levels during insulin infusion, released epinephrine later, and experienced symptoms at lower plasma glucose levels than poorly controlled patients and non-diabetics (Figure 1). This was associated with a failure of overall counterregulatory ability. Conversely, it has been shown that poorly controlled patients experience symptoms at a higher level than non-diabetics, although thresholds for counterregulatory hormone release did not differ [34].

One possible explanation for these observations is that the CNS adapts to prevailing glucose concentrations, for example by increasing or decreasing the fractional extraction of glucose. On this basis the neuroendocrine response would reflect the rate of glucose entry and hence the cerebral energy balance rather than the level of circulating glucose. As against this, it has been shown that the threshold for EEG changes is not lowered in patients on intensified therapy with a delayed epinephrine response [35]. If adaptation has in fact not occurred, the increased vulnerability of patients on intensified therapy to severe hypoglycemia is easy to comprehend.

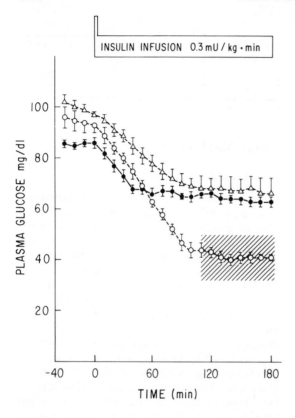

Figure 1 Demonstration that counterregulatory ability is impaired in well-controlled patients with IDDM. In this figure the non-diabetics are represented by solid circles, the poorly controlled diabetics by triangles and the well-controlled patients by open circles. The fall in plasma glucose was markedly greater in the well-controlled patients, and 4 of 11 required glucose infusion to maintain glucose levels greater than 40 mg/dl (shaded area). (From reference 34, with permission)

Duration of Diabetes

As has been seen, glycemic control has a direct effect upon the ability to recognize and respond to hypoglycemia. Duration of diabetes is another variable. About 30% of patients report a change in their warning symptoms, usually with a waning of peripheral features and increasing reliance on central symptoms, after 10 years or more of diabetes. A proportion—the overlap has yet to be established—develop impaired epinephrine secretion over a similar time-scale. This is taken to be an indication of diabetic autonomic neuropathy [36–39]. It is often said that 'loss

of warning' is due to autonomic neuropathy but in fact there is no simple association between the two except that both occur in longstanding diabetes. Many patients with autonomic neuropathy have perfectly good warning symptoms, while those with frequent unheralded comas often have little evidence of autonomic neuropathy. It is important to remember that in the clinical situation patients often drift into hypoglycemia and that symptoms may first develop long after the plasma glucose level has become subnormal.

Alcohol

Alcohol infusion will induce hypoglycemia in healthy, fasted individuals, and represents an additional hazard for insulin dependent patients. Moderate alcohol consumption seriously impairs awareness of hypoglycemia, and heavy intoxication inhibits gluconeogenesis and thereby reduces hepatic glucose output. This becomes particularly important if food is omitted, since gluconeogenesis is the mainstay of glucose production during fasting. Counterregulatory responses may also be impaired [40]. Finally, onlookers are likely to assume that coma is alcohol-induced, so that prolonged hypoglycemia may pass untreated. Fatal hypoglycemia may easily result [41].

Insulin Type

There has been considerable controversy as to whether patients transferred from animal to human insulin show altered symptomatic perception of hypoglycemia. At an anecdotal level, occasionally patients do report a marked reduction in symptoms. Attempts have been made to investigate the phenomenon, either by crossover studies in which hypoglycemia has been induced with pork or human insulin, or in clinical surveys, mostly retrospective. Published evidence supporting a systematic impairment of warning symptoms on human insulin is weak or unconvincing [42]. Human and pork insulin are however not identical, and altered pharmacokinetics due to more rapid absorption of human insulin might have some influence upon symptom recognition. More recently, a number of unexplained deaths at night have been reported in patients on human insulin, and this is discussed below.

Age

Although enormous numbers of elderly people are treated with insulin or sulfonylureas, almost no research has been undertaken concerning responses to hypoglycemia in this age group. There is a clinical impression that the elderly are vulnerable to hypoglycemia and more prone to develop mental confusion in its early stages.

PHYSIOLOGY OF GLUCOSE COUNTERREGULATION

Normal Glucose Balance

The plasma glucose concentration in the post-absorptive state is the net result of the rate of glucose production, almost exclusively by the liver, and glucose utilization by peripheral tissues. The minute-to-minute glucose balance depends on the interactions between insulin and the counterregulatory system.

Insulin suppresses glucose production by the liver and stimulates glucose utilization by insulin-sensitive peripheral tissues. The liver is more sensitive to insulin than peripheral tissues (Chapter 18a) as an increase in portal venous plasma insulin concentration of only 5–7 μU/ml results in half-maximal suppression of hepatic glucose production [43], whereas peripheral plasma insulin concentrations have to rise three to four times to produce half-maximal stimulation of glucose utilization by peripheral insulin sensitive tissues [44]. Thus, both in experimental hypoglycemia and in clinical situations such as insulinoma [45] or insulin dependent diabetes mellitus (IDDM) [36], insulin causes hypoglycemia primarily by suppressing hepatic glucose output, and only secondarily—and at much higher plasma levels—by increasing peripheral glucose utilization.

The most important counterregulatory hormones have direct hyperglycemic effects at low glucose concentrations. These are glucagon, epinephrine, cortisol and growth hormone, and possibly the neurotransmitters norepinephrine and acetylcholine. In addition, there are factors that increase plasma glucose concentration indirectly. These include suppression of insulin secretion [50] and metabolic changes secondary to a low plasma glucose; increased concentrations of gluconeogenic precursors, and high levels of FFA [76] and ketones. Increased insulin resistance or hyperresponsiveness to counterregulatory

hormones may also protect against hypoglycemia, and the latter may be important in insulin treated diabetic patients.

Glucagon and epinephrine are 'rapid' counterregulatory hormones and raise plasma glucose within a few minutes, primarily by increasing hepatic glucose output, through powerful yet transient stimulation of glycogenolysis. However, should hypoglycemia be prolonged, both glucagon and epinephrine [78] can cause a sustained increase in hepatic glucose production by activation of gluconeogenesis. Epinephrine has sustained effects in limiting glucose utilization by muscle and adipose tissue. Its hyperglycemic effects are therefore prolonged, whereas those of glucagon are more transient. The direct hyperglycemic actions of epinephrine are mediated by β_2-adrenergic receptors; it also has indirect hyperglycemic effects mediated by β_2-adrenergic receptors. The most important of these is suppression of endogenous insulin secretion. Although it has been claimed that the effect of these hormones upon hepatic glucose output is transient, this applies mainly to glycogenolysis; the effect on gluconeogenesis is more prolonged.

Norepinephrine has a lower affinity for β_2-adrenergic receptors, and similar but less marked hyperglycemic effects. Because it is a neurotransmitter, most turnover occurs at the synaptic cleft and it is difficult to judge this hormone's counterregulatory role on the basis of plasma levels.

Growth hormone and cortisol are 'slow' counterregulatory factors and it takes at least 3 hours for their anti-insulin effect to become evident. Their effects only become evident in the late phase of prolonged hypoglycemia [46, 47], and they act both by increasing hepatic glucose production (probably via gluconeogenesis) and suppressing peripheral glucose utilization.

Experimental Models of Glucose Counterregulation

Our understanding of glucose counterregulatory mechanisms in normal humans has been based on studies of short-term hypoglycemia induced by boluses of intravenous insulin [48]. It has been concluded that glucagon has a primary role in restoration of euglycemia; that epinephrine is normally not important, but plays a critical part only when secretion of glucagon is absent; and that waning of injected insulin, suppression of

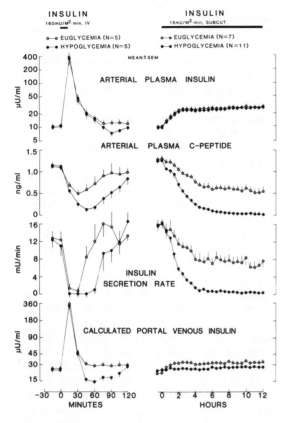

Figure 2 Arterial plasma insulin and C-peptide concentrations, calculated rates of endogenous insulin secretion and estimated portal plasma insulin concentration in a model of acute hypoglycemia induced by an IV insulin bolus (left panel) or prolonged hypoglycemia induced by continuous subcutaneous infusion of insulin (right panel). Compared to a euglycemic control experiment, the suppression of endogenous insulin secretion during prolonged hypoglycemia limits the increase in portal plasma insulin concentration (bottom panel). (Reprinted with permission from P. De Feo et al, *Diabetes*, Vol 35, May 1986. Copyright © 1986 by the American Diabetes Association)

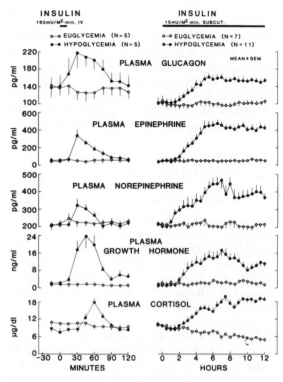

Figure 3 Responses of plasma counterregulatory hormones to acute (left panel) and to prolonged hypoglycemia (right panel). (Reprinted with permission from P. De Feo et al, *Diabetes*, Vol 35, May 1986. Copyright © 1986 by the American Diabetes Association)

endogenous insulin secretion and other potentially important factors have no role in acute glucose counterregulation. In the clinical situation, however, whether induced by an insulinoma or insulin dependent diabetes [36], hypoglycemia may be prolonged over several hours, and counterregulatory mechanisms [49, 50] may differ substantially from those derived from models of acute hypoglycemia [18].

During prolonged hypoglycemia, normal subjects suppress endogenous insulin secretion virtually completely (Figure 2). This appears to be a major factor in glucose recovery, because low

portal insulin concentrations facilitate the effects of other hormones in increasing hepatic glucose production. Counterregulatory hormones rise rapidly during both acute and prolonged hypoglycemia (Figure 3), but restoration of euglycemia only occurs when insulin levels fall, as after an IV bolus injection of insulin (Figure 4, left panel). It does not occur when hyperinsulinemia is maintained by a continuous infusion (Figure 4, right panel). Thus, waning of insulin and not activation of glucose counterregulation is the crucial factor for restoration of euglycemia after hypoglycemia. Even so, the increase in counterregulatory hormones is critical in limiting the fall in plasma glucose, and if the hormonal response is prevented or blocked, more severe hypoglycemia develops [50]. Thus, activation of hormonal counterregulation is crucial to prevent severe insulin induced hypoglycemia, but counterregulatory mechanisms

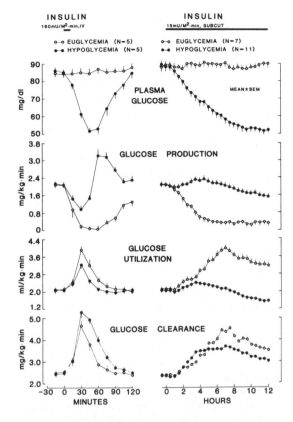

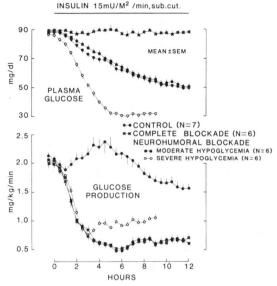

Figure 5 Demonstration of hepatic autoregulation: hepatic glucose production increases in response to severe (open circles), but not moderate hypoglycemia (solid squares) during pharmacological blockade of neurohumoral counterregulation as compared to euglycemia (complete blockade, asterisks). In the control experiment (counterregulation allowed to occur, solid circles), the increased rate of hepatic glucose production in response to moderate hypoglycemia is shown. (Reproduced from the *Journal of Clinical Investigation*, 1985, 75, 1623, by copyright permission of the American Society of Clinical Investigation)

Figure 4 Plasma glucose concentration, and rates of glucose production, utilization and clearance during acute (left panel) and prolonged hypoglycemia (right panel). (Reprinted with permission from P. De Feo et al, *Diabetes*, Vol 35, May 1986. Copyright © 1986 by the American Diabetes Association)

can only restore euglycemia when insulin levels have fallen.

In this model of prolonged hypoglycemia, two defensive mechanisms are involved—increased glucose production, and suppression of peripheral glucose utilization (Figure 4). Glucose production is increased in response to very small (10 mg/dl) decreases in plasma glucose, and this increase persists while hypoglycemia lasts, primarily because of increased gluconeogenesis [40]. Suppression of peripheral glucose utilization occurs 2–2.5 hours later and persists throughout hypoglycemia. Thus, increased hepatic glucose output is the first line of defense against hypoglycemia. Should hypoglycemia be prolonged for any reason, then suppression of peripheral glucose utilization—the second line of defense against hypoglycemia—supervenes.

Increased hepatic glucose production in this situation involves glucose autoregulation (i.e. the ability of the liver to increase glucose output autonomously in response to hypoglycemia) as well as hormonal changes. Autoregulation [51] becomes important only during severe hypoglycemia (below 40 mg/dl] and therefore represents a late defense against neuroglycopenia (Figure 5). Above these levels counterregulatory hormones account for nearly 100% of the increase in glucose production in response to hypoglycemia. The mechanisms of glucose counterregulation during prolonged hypoglycemia are summarized in Table 4.

A diminished response of one counterregulatory hormone during prolonged hypoglycemia is not fully compensated for by greater increases in the others. For example, failure of either glucagon or epinephrine results in more severe hypoglycemia despite larger increases in the unaffected 'rapid' hormone, and in the 'slow' hormones growth hormone and cortisol. Failure

Table 4 Mechanisms of glucose counterregulation to moderate (plasma glucose < 3 mM) and prolonged insulin-induced hypoglycemia in normal humans

	Glucose production	Glucose utilization	Endogenous insulin secretion	Counterregulatory hormones			
				Glucagon	Catecholamines	Growth hormone	Cortisol
Early phase of hypoglycemia (0–2 hours)	After transient suppression (~ $\frac{3}{4}$ hours) it rebounds early primarily because of glycogenolysis	Not involved	Suppressed	Limits initial suppression of glucose production and contributes to ↑glucose production	Contributes to ↑glucose production	Not involved	Not involved
Late phase of hypoglycemia (after 2 hours)	Sustained increase primarily because of ↑gluconeogenesis	Sustained ↓	Suppressed virtually to zero	Contributes to ↑glucose production	Contributes to ↑glucose production	Contributes to ↑glucose production and glucose production	Contributes to ↑glucose production and ↓glucose production

of *both* rapid hormones causes more severe hypoglycemia, whereas absence of growth hormone or cortisol results in a decrease in blood glucose 3–4 hours after the onset of hypoglycemia. Since each hormone is critical for prevention of severe hypoglycemia in this situation, counterregulatory mechanisms are not redundant, nor indeed synergistic. Nor is there a true hierarchy or synergy among counterregulatory hormones. Glucagon is not more or less 'important' than epinephrine; rather, each hormone has a unique and crucial role depending on the phase of hypoglycemia (early or late) and on its site of action (liver and/or periphery) [79].

Pathophysiology of Glucose Counterregulation in IDDM

Almost all patients with IDDM have some abnormalities in glucose counterregulatory mechanisms, except at or soon after clinical onset of the disease [37]. Partial or total deficiency of the glucagon response to hypoglycemia is seen in almost all patients, and many have multiple defects in secretion of glucagon, epinephrine, growth hormone and cortisol.

A deficient glucagon response develops early in the course of insulin dependent diabetes [37]; the mechanism is unknown [18]. It is a selective defect, as responses to other stimuli such as epinephrine or arginine infusion have been found to be normal. It does not appear to be the result of diabetic autonomic neuropathy, because the glucagon response to hypoglycemia is independent of neural signalling by the CNS to the islets [18], and because the deficient glucagon response does not correlate with the response of pancreatic polypeptide (a marker of parasympathetic autonomic neuropathy) in patients with IDDM [38]. This aggravates the severity of hypoglycemia despite larger increases in the other counterregulatory hormones, primarily because of lack of increase in hepatic glucose production [36]. In this situation the early phase of counterregulation is mediated predominantly by epinephrine.

This compensatory contribution of epinephrine is inversely proportional to the glucagon deficit, and is mediated by β_2-adrenergic receptors [52]. Thus propranolol delays glucose recovery in diabetic patients, whereas metoprolol has no effect at low doses. At larger doses of meto-

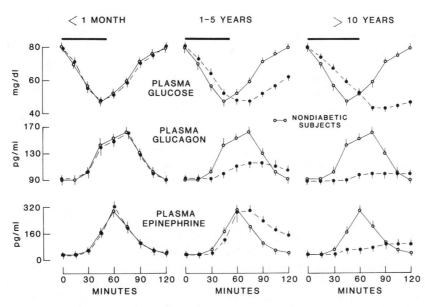

Figure 6 Plasma glucagon and epinephrine responses to insulin-induced hypoglycemia in three groups of patients with type 1 diabetes mellitus of different duration (solid circles): new-onset diabetes (left panel); 1–5 year diabetes duration (middle panel); and diabetes duration greater than 10 years (right panel). Normal subjects are shown as open circles. In new onset diabetes glucose counterregulation is normal. In patients with 1–5 year diabetes duration, the responses of plasma glucagon to hypoglycemia become impaired, but plasma glucose recovery is normal because of larger, compensatory responses of epinephrine. In long-term diabetes, since the responses of glucagon to hypoglycemia are virtually absent, and those of epinephrine become blunted, glucose counterregulation is impaired. (From reference 37, with permission)

prolol there is loss of selectivity for β_1-adrenergic blockers, and its effects are similar to those of propranolol.

Many patients, especially those with long-standing diabetes, also have deficient epinephrine responses to hypoglycemia. It is likely that in some at least, these deficient responses of epinephrine are part of the more general syndrome of diabetic autonomic neuropathy. Some, but not all, studies suggest that deficient epinephrine responses are invariably present in patients with diabetic autonomic neuropathy [37], and cosegregate with deficient pancreatic polypeptide responses, a marker of parasympathetic neuropathy in patients with IDDM [38]. From the principles of counterregulation discussed previously, it is clear that patients with IDDM who lack both 'rapid' counterregulatory hormones have severe counterregulatory failure to hypoglycemia (Figure 6, right panel).

In general, growth hormone and cortisol responses to hypoglycemia are not deficient in patients with IDDM, although defects may occur, increasing the risk of prolonged hypoglycemia.

COMPLICATIONS OF HYPOGLYCEMIA

Somogyi Effect

There are possibly as many ways of interpreting this effect as there are ways of pronouncing the name Somogyi. In his classic paper, published 30 years ago, Somogyi reported that overtreatment with insulin could be a direct cause of hyperglycemia [53]. He reached this conclusion after meticulous studies in five 'brittle' patients with IDDM in whom he noted a 'general pattern', in which the urine became sugar-free between 10 p.m. and 2 a.m. followed by a 'glycosuric tide' from 4 a.m. until 2 hours after the morning injection of insulin. He concluded that the absence of glucose in the urine between 10 p.m. and 2 a.m. indicated asymptomatic hypoglycemia and that this, in accordance with the flight/fight doctrine of Cannon, stimulated secretion of anti-insulin hormones. In the normal subject, their effect would be neutralized by pancreatic insulin secretion, whereas in the patient with IDDM they would act unopposed to cause 'rebound hyperglycemia'. Thus, the solution to high blood sugar levels before breakfast was to avoid nocturnal hypoglycemia by decreasing the insulin dose, and one of his patients showed 'spectacular clinical improvement' when this was done.

Although these were wide-ranging observations, the concept of the Somogyi effect or 'rebound hyperglycemia' became attached to one particular concept: that insulin overtreatment could result in unperceived nocturnal hypoglycemia, which in turn would generate a counterregulatory response leading to fasting hyperglycemia. The Somogyi effect is therefore based upon an apparent paradox—that hyperglycemia can be abolished by *reducing* the dose of insulin. Beguiling and intellectually attractive though this concept may be, it receives little support from the literature, which contains few if any well-documented examples. Even in Somogyi's index case, the main improvement in control was achieved on a fixed dose of 55 units of insulin, before insulin reduction was attempted. The improvement can be attributed to a multiple injection regimen and strikingly modern ideas about diet [54].

On the other hand, both nocturnal hypoglycemia and fasting hyperglycemia are common problems of insulin therapy. What, if any, is the link between the two? Declining insulin levels have been shown to be the major determinant of posthypoglycemic hyperglycemia [55], and development of an experimental model confirmed this effect, while going on to demonstrate an important contributory role for counterregulatory hormone secretion [36]. A series of studies examined the link between nocturnal hypoglycemia and fasting hyperglycemia in patients admitted for overnight observation while on their normal diet and insulin [5, 56, 57]. In no case was the link established, and indeed the trend was for lower rather than higher fasting glucose levels. Two further studies looked at the effect of induced hypoglycemia at night. Tordjman et al [58], using insulin infusions superimposed upon conventional therapy to produce hypoglycemia, also found that this resulted in lower fasting glucose levels. In this study hypoglycemia was induced relatively late (after 3:30 a.m.) by relatively high levels of insulin. Perriello et al [59] induced hypoglycemia between 1 and 2 a.m. by superimposing intravenous insulin infusions upon basal subcutaneous infusion therapy in a group of tightly controlled patients, achieving rather lower post-

hypoglycemic insulin levels. In this study, fasting glucoses were modestly (1.1 mmol/l) elevated by previous hypoglycemia, with more marked postprandial hyperglycemia, suggesting that effects are more prominent in the fed rather than the fasted state. Taken together, these observations would not support a major role for rebound hyperglycemia, although a minor effect could still be postulated.

The Somogyi effect, which began in one paradox, appears to end in another: why should the well-documented and potent posthypoglycemic changes induced by counterregulatory hormone secretion have so little apparent effect upon the clinical situation? It will be recalled that the 'slow hypoglycemia' model developed by Bolli and colleagues demonstrated a major permissive effect of declining insulin levels upon glucose recovery (see above, and Chapter 18a), although counterregulatory hormone secretion had a crucial role in preventing the development of even more severe hypoglycemia. In patients on conventional insulin therapy, nocturnal hypoglycemia results from excessive levels of circulating insulin, and these in turn depend upon the absorption of intermediate or long-acting insulin from subcutaneous injection sites—a notoriously erratic process. Furthermore, as injected insulin inevitably peaks during the night and declines steadily thereafter, it is not surprising that nocturnal hypoglycemia is common but that subsequent changes in glucose levels are highly variable. Nor is it surprising that the effects of insulin generally outweigh those of counterregulatory hormone secretion in this situation. Since nocturnal hypoglycemia may produce prolonged insulin resistance, hypoglycemia would be expected to give way rapidly to hyperglycemia if overtreated with carbohydrate. Many patients undoubtedly eat too much in response to symptoms of hypoglycemia, and this is a common cause of unstable control.

The 'dawn phenomenon' is another potential cause of fasting hyperglycemia. This results from a transient decrease in hepatic as well as extrahepatic sensitivity to insulin, occurring between 5 a.m. and 8 a.m., not preceded by hypoglycemia, and caused by nocturnal surges in growth hormone [60]. Because diabetic patients cannot respond with endogenous insulin secretion, their blood glucose increases at this time of day, especially if plasma insulin concentrations fall because of waning of the intermediate-acting insulin given the evening before.

Convulsions

Marks comments that convulsions are common in children but not in adults [2]. The frequency of true grand mal seizures is probably exaggerated, often resting on the testimony of a witness who has seen twitching movements or extreme restlessness. There is no evidence that the prevalence of idiopathic epilepsy is increased in diabetic patients, and fits in a patient on insulin should be assumed to be due to hypoglycemia until proved otherwise. Non-specific EEG abnormalities have often been described in diabetic patients, and may lead to a misdiagnosis of epilepsy.

Hemiplegic Hypoglycemia

Hemiplegic hypoglycemia is the most striking of the many focal neurological events that may occur during hypoglycemia. It was first reported in 1928 [61]. Typically noticed on waking, the hemiplegia may correct itself within minutes of glucose injection. Alternatively several hours may be needed for resolution, and the patient may reach hospital fully conscious and with a normal blood glucose. This easily gives rise to diagnostic uncertainty or to confusion with transient ischaemic attacks. Recurrent episodes usually favour the same side, but alternating episodes have been reported [62]. The pathogenesis remains uncertain, but is probably a combination of local cerebral hypoperfusion and generalized neuroglycopenia. Animal experiments have shown that carotid stenosis leads to reversible focal paralysis during hypoglycemia, and there is one clinical report of carotid stenosis in association with recurrent hemiplegic hypoglycemia [63]. There are no published clinical series, but experience suggests that most patients have normal arteriograms and that routine arteriography is not called for unless indicated on other grounds.

Hypothermia

Hypoglycemia has been reported in association with hypothermia in a wide variety of clinical conditions and in several animal species as well as in humans. In experimental hypoglycemia,

core temperature falls by an average of 1°C. During hypoglycemia oxygen consumption rises, probably due to the thermogenic actions of epinephrine. This, however, is more than compensated for by rapid surface cooling due mainly to sweating. Normal individuals shiver when exposed to a cold environment, but this can be suppressed by moderate hypoglycemia. As a result severe hypothermia (below 35°C) develops rapidly. Glucose infusion restores shivering within a matter of seconds, producing a rapid rise in temperature [64].

Hypokalemia

Potassium levels fall during hypoglycemia in a dose dependent manner. It has been shown that hypokalemia in the induction stage of experimental hypoglycemia is due to insulin-induced influx of potassium into the cells. Once hypoglycemia has developed, further falls in potassium levels can be blocked with propranolol, suggesting that this phase of the response is mediated by β-adrenoceptor stimulation by epinephrine [65]. The clinical relevance of this phenomenon has not been addressed, but there is a potential for dangerous hypokalemia in, for example, insulin-treated patients on diuretic therapy.

Ischemic Heart Disease

There is no doubt that hypoglycemia induces changes in heart rate, cardiac output and electrocardiographic configuration, but evidence that it may provoke episodes of angina in those who suffer with this condition, or may occasionally precipitate dysrhythmic episodes, is largely anecdotal. In one study patients with angina were subjected to experimental hypoglycemia without developing symptoms [66].

Prognosis

Is Hypoglycemia Dangerous?

This is really two questions: what is the risk of a single severe episode, and what are the risks of recurrent minor episodes? Death or recognized brain injury are complications of hypoglycemia, and it has been estimated to cause 1–5% of deaths in groups of patients with IDDM followed for many years [67]. Even this may be an overestimate, since hypoglycemia is difficult to diagnose at autopsy because of metabolic changes post mortem. Patients with serious sequelae often prove to have taken deliberate overdoses of insulin. Patients with brain damage usually end in institutional care, and are readily recognizable by their air of detachment and 'thousand mile stare'. In general, the longer an episode of coma, the more likely that brain damage will ensue, but late recovery may sometimes occur.

The relatively benign prognosis traditionally extended to insulin induced hypoglycemia has, however, been challenged in a recent investigation in the UK. Following media reports of sudden unexplained death at night in young patients with IDDM, a national survey was conducted for the year 1989. Twenty-two unexplained deaths were identified in patients aged 12–43 years; 20 of these were found lying in an undisturbed bed [68]. Because of difficulties in the postmortem diagnosis of hypoglycemia, it is not clear that this was the cause of death, although it remains the most likely explanation. Since death was apparently sudden, a cardiac dysrhythmia may have been responsible, possibly precipitated by changes in potassium levels associated with hypoglycemia [42]. All these deaths occurred in patients on human insulin. Since almost all young patients in the UK are taking this type of insulin, and accurate figures are almost impossible to obtain for unexplained deaths in previous years, there are at present no grounds for attributing the deaths to human insulin.

The second question, as to the frequency of brain damage after recurrent but less severe hypoglycemia, is also difficult to answer. There have been no follow-up studies of defined cohorts of patients with appropriate controls, and cross-sectional studies have been inadequate and unconvincing. Some pediatricians believe that the immature brain is more susceptible to hypoglycemic damage; it is certainly true that convulsions with their attendant risks are more common in children, and that abnormal EEGs are more frequent in diabetic children than in controls. It is difficult to prove that hypoglycemia has impaired intellectual development in a child, because there is no accurate way of comparing achieved with potential development.

ORAL HYPOGLYCEMIC AGENTS AND HYPOGLYCEMIA

Hypoglycemia is the most serious potential complication of therapy with sulfonylurea agents. The risk is best documented with chlorpropamide and glibenclamide, while tolbutamide has the best safety record in this respect, probably related to its shorter duration of action. There is no doubt that sulfonylurea hypoglycemia is both underdiagnosed and underreported, and newer sulfonylurea drugs cannot as yet be assumed to be safe in this respect. There are few data as to the frequency of the condition, but in a 2-year prospective trial 2% of patients experienced symptomatic hypoglycemia and 0.4% required hospitalization for this reason [69]. The risk of severe hypoglycemia rises with age, intercurrent illness and poor nutrition, and the case fatality appears to be much higher than that for insulin-induced hypoglycemia [70].

When prescribing sulfonylureas for elderly patients, certain precautions are essential. Chief among these is the need to avoid unnecessarily stringent targets for glucose control, and to withhold drug therapy wherever possible. The patient (or relatives) should be warned of the possible risk and asked to report symptoms. Tablets should be stopped and medical advice sought if for any reason the patient is unable to eat. Hepatic and renal function should be assessed, since drugs excreted by the kidney will accumulate in the presence of renal impairment, as will those metabolized by the liver in the presence of liver disease. Potential drug interactions, especially with aspirin, β-blockers and other sulfonamide-based preparations, also need to be considered. The authors believe that tolbutamide is the drug of choice in patients over 70 years old.

Patients with sulfonylurea-induced hypoglycemia often present with mental confusion, coma or an apparent stroke. Hospital admission is mandatory: this is because sulfonylureas 'prime' the B cells to respond to glucose, so that glucose infusion may easily result in a rebound into hypoglycemia. For this reason the initial glucose injection must be followed by intravenous glucose infusion, and both glucose and potassium levels should be monitored until the patient has made a full recovery.

CAUSES OF HYPOGLYCEMIA IN IDDM

Excessive insulin doses, omission of a meal after an insulin injection, or sudden increases in peripheral glucose uptake and insulin sensitivity such as occur during or after exercise, are common precipitating causes of hypoglycemia. The role of two underlying factors that predispose to severe hypoglycemia in insulin dependent patients, namely inappropriate peripheral (and portal) hyperinsulinemia and impaired secretion of counterregulatory hormones in response to developing hypoglycemia, also need to be considered.

Hyperinsulinemia. Insulin therapy inevitably produces hyperinsulinemia in the peripheral (systemic) circulation, and it has been shown that the rate of peripheral insulin delivery required to normalize hepatic glucose production and plasma glucose levels in patients with IDDM produces plasma insulin levels at least twice as high as those of non-diabetic subjects. Under the less ideal conditions of everyday life even greater plasma insulin concentrations may be observed. Therapeutic hyperinsulinemia thus predisposes to hypoglycemia, although the risk may be balanced by insulin resistance in patients with insulin dependent diabetes [71].

It should also be emphasized that the mean blood glucose achieved with a given therapeutic regimen is the major determinant of the frequency of hypoglycemia [17]. When the target mean blood glucose concentration is several mmol/l above the upper limit of the normal range, hypoglycemia is less likely, but when near-normoglycemia is the goal, its frequency increases [12]. Long-term near-normoglycemia also reduces warning symptoms and counterregulatory responses to hypoglycemia in patients with IDDM [72], further increasing the risk of hypoglycemia.

Impaired glucose counterregulation. When identical doses of insulin are injected into normal, non-diabetic subjects and patients with IDDM, hypoglycemia develops in both groups, but is more severe in the diabetic patients despite similar plasma insulin concentrations [36]. Impaired glucose counterregulation is therefore an important risk factor for severe hypoglycemia, especially when treatment aims for normoglycemia. Thus, any attempt to normalize blood glucose in patients with IDDM results in an increased frequency of hypoglycemia because it necessarily involves inappropriate and fluctuating levels of hyperinsulinemia. The clinical consequences in terms of severe cerebral dysfunction will, however, depend predominantly on the residual efficiency of the counterregulatory mechanisms.

TREATMENT

Minor Episodes

The standard advice is to rest and take 10–20 g of carbohydrate, which is usually adequate (10 g of glucose given intravenously would raise blood levels by about 10 mmol/l). In practice patients often overtreat hypoglycemia, and this is a common cause of unstable control. They should be advised to rest quietly for 5–10 minutes after the first snack, and to repeat the dose if necessary. It is best to specify the type and amount of food in discussion with the patient, and to stress the need for both short-acting and longer-acting carbohydrate, e.g. the regimen might be half a glass of orange juice and two biscuits. When circumstances permit, symptoms should be checked by measuring a blood glucose level. This helps patients to interpret their subjective feelings correctly and avoids unnecessary treatment.

Hypoglycemic Coma

Most episodes of coma recover spontaneously (if the patient is alone or asleep) or with the help of glucose forced into the mouth by friends or relatives. As the teeth are often clenched this may not be easy, and glucose tablets are little use because the mouth is too dry to dissolve them. Glucose solutions or gels delivered into the cheek space are effective. Failing this, helpers can give an injection of glucagon. Glucagon is supplied as a powder which must be dissolved before injection, and it is essential to demonstrate the mixing technique carefully.

Medical treatment is either by injection of glucagon 1 mg IM or glucose 25 IV. Glucose is conventionally given as a bolus dose of 50% glucose (50 ml), but lower-strength glucose infusions are preferable and less likely to produce thrombophlebitis. Glucagon is claimed to be of comparable speed and efficacy to glucose, and is simpler and less traumatic to administer.

For this reason it is the treatment of choice in restless or aggressive patients. If glucagon is used, oral carbohydrate should be given following recovery to replenish liver glycogen. It is important to note that many patients with hypoglycemia arrive in the emergency room with normal or even elevated plasma glucose levels as a result of spontaneous recovery or earlier attempts at treatment. This often causes diagnostic confusion, especially when persistent neurological deficit (e.g. coma or hemiplegia) is present. Patients in prolonged coma may be postictal, or may be suffering from neurological problems associated with prolonged or severe hypoglycemia such as cerebral edema. The possibility of a deliberate, massive overdose of insulin needs to be considered. So also should other reasons for loss of consciousness such as head injury, drug overdose, subarachnoid hemorrhage, etc.

There is no generally agreed scheme of management in cases of refractory coma. Blood glucose should be monitored regularly and a glucose infusion given with the aim of maintaining moderate hyperglycemia. Core temperature and plasma potassium levels should be checked. Routine investigations will include an ECG and skull radiograph. Dexamethasone 2 mg 6-hourly is sometimes given in addition. In prolonged coma further investigations will include a CT scan of the head, a lumbar puncture and EEG recordings. The prognosis for recovery is related to the length of coma, as is the risk of intellectual impairment.

PREVENTION

Avoidance of hypoglycemia begins with education. Many patients still believe that they are likely to die during hypoglycemic coma, and this fear needs to be confronted. The fears of parents or spouses also need to be considered. A patient who lives in fear of hypoglycemia will never achieve adequate glycemic control. Appropriate education includes an emphasis on regular snacks at the right times, warnings to take special care at periods of greatest risk (before lunch and around tea), advice about driving (with special care if driving home from work) and advice on the amount of carbohydrate needed to control symptoms since, as emphasized, overtreating is a common cause of swinging control. Patients should also be warned

specifically of the dangers of excessive alcohol consumption, particularly if food is omitted. They should also know that there is a danger of delayed hypoglycemia after heavy alcohol intake or prolonged exercise.

Exercise can induce hypoglycemia by a variety of mechanisms. Peripheral glucose uptake is enhanced during exertion, and insulin absorption is accelerated if the injected limb is exercised within an hour or two of the injection. Insulin sensitivity may be increased for several hours following sustained exercise, producing a risk of delayed hypoglycemia [73]. Other modifying factors include time of day and degree of glycemic control. Plasma glucose drops rapidly during exercise in the well-insulinized diabetic patient, but relatively little in the hyperglycemic individual with low circulating insulin levels. Advice must therefore be tailored to the needs of each patient. Anticipatory downward adjustment of insulin dose is sometimes helpful, but in general it is easier to avoid hypoglycemia by taking extra carbohydrate.

Prediction of Hypoglycemia

Management of patients with a history of severe hypoglycemia will include re-education, reassurance and a determined attempt to eradicate the problem. Diet needs to be assessed carefully and, since subjective warning symptoms cannot be trusted, regular home blood glucose testing is essential. Blood glucose targets should be relaxed, but not abandoned. Multiple small injections of insulin will often reduce the amplitude of blood glucose changes produced by standard injections once or twice daily. This is particularly important in southern Europe, where dietary habits differ greatly from those of the north. Breakfast is often omitted, and lunch is taken after 1–2 p.m. If conventional insulin therapy is given in this situation, use of a depot preparation in the morning carries a high risk of severe hypoglycemia between 10 a.m. and 1 p.m.

The simplest and most compelling clinical guide to risk of severe hypoglycemia is a history of the problem. Techniques have also been developed to identify patients with impaired counterregulation with a view to exclusion from programs of intensified therapy. Plasma glucose nadir and rates of postnadir plasma glucose recovery from hypoglycemia in response to a standard insulin infusion test are reliable indices of the state of the glucose counterregulatory system [74]. Diabetic patients with impaired counterregulation in such a test exhibit high prevalence of hypoglycemic episodes during a subsequent program of intensive insulin therapy [75]. However, the test is not needed in patients with a short duration of diabetes, since the counterregulatory system is likely to be intact [37].

Nocturnal hypoglycemia presents a particular challenge, and two studies have examined its frequency in relation to blood glucose testing at bedtime and on rising [5, 76]. Pramming found that the risk of hypoglycemia (blood glucose below 3 mmol/l) was 80% if the bedtime test was below 6 mmol/l, and that if values were above this level the probability that hypoglycemia would not develop was 88%. Other studies have largely confirmed this observation, both in children [76] and patients on CSII [77], although both these studies placed the cut-off at 7 mmol/l (125 mg/dl). Whincup and Milner went on to show that augmenting the carbohydrate snack at bedtime was a useful preventive measure [76].

Enormous advances have been made in our knowledge of the physiology and pathophysiology of hypoglycemia, yet these have yet to result in any really major clinical benefit. One can sympathize with the patient who remarked that 'you doctors know everything about hypoglycemia except how to stop people from getting it!' Even so, and as this chapter has tried to show, much can be done to reduce the frequency and severity of hypoglycemia without compromising glycemic control.

REFERENCES

1. Marks V. The measurement of blood glucose and the definition of hypoglycaemia. Horm Metab Res 1986; (suppl.) 6: 1–6.
2. Marks V, Rose FC. Hypoglycaemia, 2nd edn. Oxford: Blackwell, 1980.
3. De Feo P, Gallai V, Mazzotta G et al. Modest decrements in plasma glucose concentration cause early impairment in cognitive function and later activation of glucose counterregulation in the absence of hypoglycemic symptoms in normal man. J Clin Invest 1988; 82: 436–44.
4. Cryer PE, Binder C, Bolli GB, Cherrington AD, Gale EAM, Gerich JE, Sherwin RS. Hypoglycemia in insulin dependent diabetes. Diabetes 1989; 38: 1193–9.
5. Pramming S, Thorsteinsson B, Bendtson I, Ram B, Binder C. Nocturnal hypoglycaemia in patients receiving conventional treatment with insulin. Br Med J 1985; 291: 376–9.
6. Gale EAM, Tattersall RB. Unrecognised nocturnal hypoglycemia in insulin-treated diabetics. Lancet 1979; i: 1049–52.
7. Gale EAM. The frequency of hypoglycemia in insulin-treated diabetic patients. In Serrano-Rios M, Lefèbvre PJ (eds) Diabetes 1985. Amsterdam: Elsevier, 1986: pp 934–7.
8. Goldstein DE, England JD, Hess R, Rawlings SS, Walker B. A prospective study of symptomatic hypoglycemia in young diabetic patients. Diabetes Care 1981; 4: 601–5.
9. Potter J, Clarke P, Gale EAM, Dave SH, Tattersall RB. Insulin-induced hypoglycaemia in an accident and emergency department: the tip of an iceberg? Br Med J 1982; 285: 1180–2.
10. Casparie AF, Elving LD. Severe hypoglycemia in diabetic patients; frequency, causes, prevention. Diabetes Care 1985; 8: 141–5.
11. Muhlhauser I, Berger M, Sonnenberg G, Koch J, Jorgens V, Schernthaner G, Scholz V. Incidence and management of severe hypoglycemia in 434 adults with insulin-dependent diabetes mellitus. Diabetes Care 1985; 8: 268–73.
12. Diabetes Control and Complications Trial (DCCT) Research Group. Results of Feasibility Study. Diabetes Care 1987; 10: 1–19.
13. Zinman B, Cleary P, DCCT Research Group. Long term metabolic outcome and complications with intensive therapy in the DCCT. Diabetes 1989; (suppl. 2): 81A (abstr.).
14. Bergada I, Suissa S, Dufresne J, Schiffrin A. Severe hypoglycemia in IDDM children. Diabetes Care 1989; 12: 239–44.
15. Mecklenburg RS, Benson EA, Benson JW et al. Acute complications associated with insulin infusion pump therapy. Report of experience with 161 patients. JAMA 1984; 252: 3265–9.
16. Lauritzen T, Frost-Larsen K, Larsen H-W, Deckert T, Steno Study Group. Effect of 1 year of near normal blood glucose levels on retinopathy in insulin-dependent diabetics. Lancet 1983; i: 200–4.
17. Thorsteinsson B, Pramming S, Lauritzen T et al. Frequency of daytime biochemical hypoglycemia in insulin-treated diabetic patients: relation to daily median blood glucose concentrations. Diabet Med 1986; 3: 147–51.
18. Cryer PE, Gerich JE. Glucose counterregulation, hypoglycemia and intensive insulin therapy in diabetes mellitus. New Engl J Med 1985; 313: 232–41.
19. Shapiro ET, Cooper M, Chen C-T, Given BD, Polansky KS. Change in hexose distribution volume and fractional utilization of [^{18}F]-2-deoxy-2-fluoro-O-glucose in brain during acute hypoglycaemia in humans. Diabetes 1990; 39: 175–80.

20. Pramming S, Thorsteinnson B, Thielgaard A, Pinner EM, Binder C. Cognitive function during hypoglycaemia in Type I diabetes. Br Med J 1986; 292: 647–50.

21. Heller SR, Herbert M, Macdonald IA, Tattersall RB. Influence of sympathetic nervous system on hypoglycaemic warning symptoms. Lancet 1987; ii: 359–63.

22. Harrad RA, Cockram CS, Plumb AP, Stone S, Fenwick P, Sonksen PH. The effect of hypoglycemia on visual function: a clinical and electrophysiological study. Clin Sci 1985; 69: 673–9.

23. Pramming S, Thorsteinsson B, Stigsby B, Binder C. Glycaemic threshold for changes in electroencephalograms during hypoglycaemia in patients with insulin-dependent diabetes. Br Med J 1988; 296: 665–7.

24. Himwich HE. Brain metabolism and cerebral disorders. New York: Spectrum, 1976.

25. Lawrence RD, Meyer A, Nevin S. The pathological changes in the brain in fatal hypoglycaemia. Quart J Med 1942; 44: 181–201.

26. Kalimo H, Olsson Y. Effects of severe hypoglycemia on the human brain: neuropathological case reports. Acta Neurol Scand 1980; 62: 345–56.

27. Tattersall RB. Hypoglycemia and criminal responsibility: a guide to a lawyer's view of diabetes. Diabet Med 1986; 3: 470–4.

28. Ginsburg J, Paton C. Effects of insulin after adrenalectomy. Lancet 1956; ii: 491–4.

29. French EB, Kilpatrick R. The role of adrenaline in hypoglycaemic reactions in man. Clin Sci 1955; 14: 639–51.

30. Mathias CJ, Frankel HL, Turner RC, Christensen NJ. Physiological responses to insulin hypoglycaemia in spinal man. Paraplegia 1980; 17: 319–26.

31. Sussman KE, Crout JR, Marble A. Failure of warning in insulin-induced hypoglycemic reactions. Diabetes 1963; 12: 38–45.

32. Schwartz NS, Clutter WE, Shah SD, Cryer PE. Glycemic thresholds for activation of glucose counterregulatory systems are higher than the threshold for symptoms. J Clin Invest 1987; 79: 777–81.

33. Amiel SA, Tamborlane WV, Simonson DC, Sherwin RS. Defective glucose counterregulation after strict glycemic control of insulin-dependent diabetes mellitus. New Engl J Med 1987; 316: 1376–83.

34. Boyle PJ, Schwartz NS, Shah SD, Clutter WE, Cryer PE. Plasma glucose concentrations at the onset of hypoglycemic symptoms in patients with poorly controlled diabetes and in non-diabetics. New Engl J Med 1988; 318: 1487–92.

35. Amiel SA, Pottinger R, Archibald HR, Chusney G, Cunnah D, Prior PF, Gale EAM. Effect of antecedent glucose control on cerebral function during hypoglycemia. Diabetes Care 1991; 14: 109–18.

36. Bolli G, Dimitriadis G, Pehling G, Baker BA, Haymond M, Cryer PE, Gerich JE. Abnormal glucose counterregulation after subcutaneous insulin in insulin-dependent diabetes mellitus. New Engl J Med 1984; 310: 1706–11.

37. Bolli G, De Feo P, Compagnucci P et al. Abnormal glucose counterregulation in insulin-dependent diabetes mellitus: interaction of anti-insulin antibodies and impaired glucagon and epinephrine secretion. Diabetes 1983; 32: 134–41.

38. Kennedy FP, Bolli GB, Go VL et al. The significance of impaired pancreatic polypeptide and epinephrine responses to insulin-induced hypoglycemia in patients with insulin-dependent diabetes mellitus. J Clin Endocrinol Metab 1987; 64: 602–8.

39. Kennedy F, Go W, Cryer P, Bolli G, Gerich J. Subnormal pancreatic polypeptide and epinephrine responses to insulin-induced hypoglycemia predict the development of overt autonomic neuropathy in patients with insulin-dependent diabetes mellitus. Ann Intern Med 1988; 108: 54–8.

40. Lecavalier L, Bolli G, Cryer P et al. Contribution of gluconeogenesis and glycogenolysis during counterregulation in normal humans. Am J Physiol 1989; 256: E844–51.

41. Arky RA, Veverbrants E, Abramson EA. Irreversible hypoglycemia: a complication of alcohol and insulin. JAMA 1968; 206: 575–8.

42. Gale EAM. Hypoglycaemia and human insulin. Lancet 1989; ii: 1264–6.

43. Nurjhan N, Campbell PJ, Kennedy FP et al. Insulin dose–response curve characteristics for suppression of glycerol release and conversion to glucose in humans. Diabetes 1986; 35: 1326–31.

44. Rizza R, Mandarino L, Gerich J. Dose–response characteristics for the effects of insulin on production and utilization of glucose in man. Am J Physiol 1981; 246: E630–9.

45. Rizza R, Haymond M, Verdonk C et al. Pathogenesis of hypoglycemia in insulinoma patients: suppression of hepatic glucose production by insulin. Diabetes 1981; 30: 377–81.

46. De Feo P, Perriello G, Torlone E et al. Demonstration of a role for growth hormone in glucose counterregulation. Am J Physiol 1989; 256: E835–43.

47. De Feo P, Perriello G, Torlone E et al. Contribution of cortisol to glucose counterregulation in humans. Am J Physiol 1989; 257: E35–42.

48. Rizza R, Cryer P, Gerich J. Role of glucagon, catecholamines, and growth hormone in human glucose counterregulation. Effects of somato-

statin and combined alpha and beta-adrenergic blockade in plasma glucose recovery and glucose flux rates after insulin-induced hypoglycemia. J Clin Invest 1979; 64: 62–71.

49. Bolli G, Gottesman I, Cryer P, Gerich J. Glucose counterregulation during prolonged hypoglycemia in normal man. Am J Physiol 1984; 247: E206–14.

50. De Feo P, Perriello G, De Cosmo S et al. Comparison of glucose counterregulation during short-term and prolonged hypoglycemia in normal man. Diabetes 1986; 35: 563–9.

51. Bolli G, De Feo P, Perriello G et al. Role of hepatic autoregulation in defense against hypoglycemia in humans. J Clin Invest 1985; 75: 1623–31.

52. De Feo P, Bolli G, Perriello G et al. The adrenergic contribution to glucose counterregulation in type 1 diabetes mellitus: dependency on A-cell function and mediation through beta-2-adrenergic receptors. Diabetes 1983; 32: 887–93.

53. Somogyi M. Exacerbation of diabetes by excess insulin action. Am J Med 1959; 26: 169–91.

54. Gale EAM. The Somogyi effect. In Nattrass M (ed.) Recent advances in diabetes 2. Edinburgh: Churchill Livingstone, 1986.

55. Gale EAM, Kurtz AB, Tattersall RB. In search of the Somogyi effect. Lancet 1980; ii: 279–82.

56. Lerman IG, Wolfsdorf JI. Relationship of nocturnal hypoglycemia to daytime glycemia in IDDM. Diabetes Care 1988; 11: 636–42.

57. Stephenson JM, Schernthaner G. Dawn phenomenon and the Somogyi effect in IDDM. Diabetes Care 1989; 12: 245–51.

58. Tordjman KM, Havlin CE, Levandoski LA, White NH, Santiago JV, Cryer PE. Failure of nocturnal hypoglycemia to cause fasting hyperglycemia in patients with insulin-dependent diabetes mellitus. New Engl J Med 1987; 317: 1552–9.

59. Perriello G, De Feo P, Torlone E et al. The effect of asymptomatic nocturnal hypoglycemia on glycemic control in diabetes mellitus. New Engl J Med 1988; 319: 1233–9.

60. Bolli GB. The dawn phenomenon: its origin and contribution to early morning hyperglycaemia in diabetes mellitus. Diabète Métab 1988; 14: 675–86.

61. Ravid JM. Transient insulin hypoglycemic hemiplegias. Am J Med Sci 1928; 175: 756–69.

62. Montgomery BM, Pinnir CA. Transient hypoglycemic hemiplegia. Arch Int Med 1964; 114: 680–4.

63. Portnoy HD. Transient 'ischemic' attacks produced by carotid stenosis and hypoglycemia. Neurology 1965; 15: 830–2.

64. Gale EAM, Bennett T, Green JH, Macdonald IA. Hypoglycaemia, hypothermia and shivering in man. Clin Sci 1981; 61: 463–9.

65. Petersen K-G, Schluter KJ, Karp L. Regulation of serum potassium during insulin-induced hypoglycemia. Diabetes 1982; 31: 615–17.

66. Egeli ES, Berkman R. Action of hypoglycemia on coronary insufficiency and mechanism of ECG alterations. Am Heart J 1960; 59: 527–40.

67. Deckert T, Poulsen JE, Larsen M. Prognosis of diabetics with diabetes onset before the age of thirty-one. Diabetologia 1978; 14: 363–70.

68. Tattersall RB, Gill GV. Unexplained deaths of Type I diabetic patients. Diabet Med 1991; 8: 49–58.

69. Clarke BF, Campbell IW. Long term comparative trial of glibenclamide and chlorpropamide in diet-failed maturity onset diabetes. Lancet 1975; i: 246–8.

70. Ferner RE, Neil HAW. Sulphonylureas and hypoglycaemia. Br Med J 1988; 296: 949–50.

71. DeFronzo R, Hendler R, Simonson D. Insulin resistance is a prominent feature of insulin-dependent diabetes. Diabetes 1982; 31: 795–801.

72. Simonson DC, Tamborlane WV, DeFronzo RA et al. Intensive insulin therapy reduces counterregulatory hormone responses to hypoglycemia in patients with Type I diabetes. Ann Intern Med 1985; 103: 184–90.

73. MacDonald MJ. Postexercise late-onset hypoglycemia in insulin-dependent diabetic patients. Diabetes Care 1987; 10: 584–8.

74. Bolli G, De Feo P, De Cosmo S et al. A reliable and reproducible test for adequate glucose counterregulation in Type 1 diabetes mellitus. Diabetes 1984; 33: 732–7.

75. White NH, Skor DA, Cryer PE, Levandoski L, Bier DM, Santiago JV. Identification of Type I diabetic patients at increased risk for hypoglycemia during intensified therapy. New Engl J Med 1983; 308: 485–91.

76. Whincup G, Milner RDG. Prediction and management of nocturnal hypoglycaemia in diabetes. Arch Dis Child 1987; 62: 333–7.

77. Schiffrin A, Suissa S. Predicting nocturnal hypoglycemia in patients with Type I diabetes treated with continuous subcutaneous insulin. Am J Med 1987; 82: 1127–32.

78. De Feo P, Perriello G, Torlone E et al. Evidence against important catecholamine compensation for absent glucagon counterregulation. Am J Physiol 1991; 260: E203–E212.

79. Bolli, GB. From physiology of glucose counterregulation to prevention of hypoglycaemia in Type 1 diabetes mellitus. Diab Nutr Metab 1990; 4: 333–49.

48

Diabetic Ketoacidosis and Hyperglycaemic Non-ketotic Coma

S.M. Marshall, M. Walker and K.G.M.M. Alberti

The Medical School, Newcastle upon Tyne, UK

Despite major advances in our understanding of the pathophysiology and treatment of diabetic ketoacidosis (DKA) and hyperosmolar non-ketotic coma (HONK) over the last two decades, the morbidity and mortality of these conditions remain considerable. Many cases are potentially avoidable by education of patients, health care professionals and the general public. In this chapter the epidemiology, pathophysiology and treatment of the two conditions are discussed, with particular reference to new information and to controversial areas. The reader is also referred to several recent reviews [1–6].

DIABETIC KETOACIDOSIS

Diabetic ketoacidosis may be defined as the triad of hyperglycaemia, acidosis and ketosis, the primary cause of which is insulin deficiency, either relative or absolute. The distinction between DKA and HONK is somewhat arbitrary, but in HONK hyperglycaemia tends to be more extreme and acidosis and ketosis absent or much less marked.

Epidemiology

The incidence of DKA has not declined despite advances in our understanding, and mortality remains significant, even in specialist units. Accurate figures are difficult to obtain. In the Rhode Island study, DKA accounted for 1.6% of all diabetic admissions, with 20% of the cases being in previously undiagnosed patients [7]. The annual incidence rate was 14 per 100 000 total population or 46 per 10 000 diabetic subjects. In a Danish study, the incidence was 8.5 per 100 000 total population in the years 1975–79, rising from 2.5 per 100 000 in 1960–64 [8]. Figures collected by the National Diabetes Data Group of the USA give an annual incidence of DKA of 3–8 episodes per 1000 diabetic patients, with 20–30% of new cases presenting in keto-acidosis [9].

Estimates of mortality from DKA remain at around 5–10% [7, 9, 10]. The risk increases with increasing age, hypotension, initial high blood glucose and urea and low pH [9–12]. In the older age groups, many deaths may be due to the severity of the underlying precipitating factor

International Textbook of Diabetes Mellitus. Edited by K.G.M.M. Alberti, R.A. DeFronzo, H. Keen and P. Zimmet

[9], but in the younger person, mortality is more likely to be due to the metabolic disarray and to be preventable. In a UK review of deaths in diabetic patients aged less than 50 years, the majority of deaths from DKA were deemed to be due to errors by patients, primary health care personnel or hospital staff [13].

Precipitating Factors

The importance of the most common precipitating factors of DKA, namely infection, other intercurrent illness and failure of insulin delivery, varies with the population studied. Worldwide, infection remains the most common underlying cause [8, 9]. Tuberculosis and malaria are important precipitants in developing countries [14]. The acute rise in secretion of the catecholamines, cortisol and glucagon in response to other intercurrent illnesses, such as cerebrovascular accident, acute myocardial infarction and trauma, produces predictable metabolic consequences which may result in DKA.

Malfunction of the more sophisticated insulin delivery systems such as infusers and pens may lead to DKA, particularly if the problem is not identified early [15–17]. The overall incidence of DKA on continuous subcutaneous insulin infusion (CSII) is probably higher than on injection therapy under conditions of standard clinical care [18–20], although care that is particularly intensive may reduce the risk [21]. Episodes of DKA are particularly likely to occur during the first few months of therapy with CSII and are probably reduced by increased physician and patient awareness [22, 23].

A significant proportion of cases of DKA is accounted for by a small number of patients with repeated episodes [24, 25]. These patients are likely to fall into one of two groups: the first are a group of young patients, generally female, with severe underlying psychological and social problems and in whom the underlying cause is undoubtedly omission of insulin [26–28]; the second group are elderly patients with severe, chronic underlying physical illness such as cerebrovascular disease, where repeated episodes can probably be prevented by appropriate home supervision and back-up [24].

Pathophysiology

The deranged metabolism characteristic of DKA results from absolute or relative insulin deficiency. Insulin secretion is insufficient to balance the catabolic actions of the counterregulatory hormones, present in increased amounts, and normal metabolic homeostasis is lost. The resultant hyperglycaemia, ketosis and acidosis represent a life-threatening situation.

Glucose Metabolism

In normal humans in the fasted state, blood glucose concentrations are maintained constant at 3–5 mmol/l by finely regulated hepatic output of glucose. Glycogenolysis and gluconeogenesis proceed under the stimulus of growth hormone, glucagon and catecholamines, but are held in partial restraint by low levels of circulating insulin. There is an increase in the flux of gluconeogenic precursors to the liver, with increased hepatic extraction. The key hepatic regulatory step for glycogenolysis and gluconeogenesis is the conversion of fructose 6-phosphate to fructose 1,6-bisphosphate. The forward reaction is catalysed by phosphofructokinase (PFK) and the reverse by fructose 1,6-bisphosphatase. The key regulatory substance is fructose 2,6-bisphosphate (F2,6BP) which stimulates PFK and inhibits fructose 1,6-bisphosphatase, thus increasing flux down the glycolytic pathway. Glucagon and adrenalin inhibit F2,6BP formation, and thus in the fasted state there is a switch from hepatic glycolysis to gluconeogenesis.

In peripheral tissues, the relatively low concentrations of insulin are insufficient to promote glucose uptake. The counterregulatory hormones also inhibit glucose uptake, and fatty acids and ketone bodies become the major oxidative fuels.

In diabetic ketoacidosis, insulin deficiency results in an extension of the normal fasting state. Hepatic glucose production rises rapidly for the first 2–4 hours of insulin withdrawal, before falling towards normal. Peripheral utilization of glucose also rises, but to a smaller although more sustained extent. Thus plasma glucose concentrations initially rise quickly, but reach a plateau within 4 hours of around 16 mmol/l [29]. These changes correlate most closely with the initial acute rise in blood glucagon concentrations, other counterregulatory hormones being little affected initially [30–32]. The effect of glucagon on hepatic glucose output is mediated by a decrease in the levels of F2, 6BP, thus increasing gluconeogenesis, and by stimulation of glycogenolysis. Basal hepatic glucose production in DKA is approximately twice that in stable diabetic patients, with a much smaller decrease in peripheral glucose utilisation, confirming the primacy of the liver in the pathogenesis of severe hyperglycaemia [33].

Hyperglycaemia per se decreases peripheral glucose utilisation [34, 35] and any residual insulin secretion [36], thus creating a self-fuelling vicious cycle of increasing plasma glucose concentration.

Ketone Body Metabolism

In the fasting state, ketone body production is controlled by restraint of lipolysis by low circulating concentrations of insulin in the presence of physiological concentrations of the counterregulatory hormones, and by a direct inhibitory effect of insulin on hepatic ketogenesis, independent of the supply of non-esterified fatty acids (NEFA) [37–39]. This direct effect may be mediated via the inhibition of carnitine acyl-CoA transferase 1, both directly and by an increase in the inhibitor malonyl-CoA [40]. Such changes would favour re-esterification of NEFA rather than oxidation. Insulin may also increase the peripheral clearance of ketone bodies [41].

In the absolute or relative insulin deficiency of ketoacidosis, the uninhibited actions of the counterregulatory hormones are paramount. Lipolysis is unrestrained, with a large increase in the supply of NEFA to the liver. Lack of insulin causes direct stimulation of carnitine acyl-CoA transferase 1, and high glucagon levels inhibit the formation of malonyl-CoA, further stimulating the transferase [42]. There is thus a switch away from NEFA re-esterification to oxidation, with a subsequent rise in circulating ketone bodies. Glucagon also increase levels of carnitine, further enhancing fatty acid flux into oxidation [43]. Cortisol probably enhances hepatic ketogenesis directly, while growth hormone and the catecholamines stimulate lipolysis directly.

Insulin withdrawal studies have demonstrated a continuous rise in plasma ketone body levels for 10 hours [44]. Glucagon may be of particular importance, as plasma levels rise early in DKA and correlate with ketone body and NEFA concentrations [30, 31, 44].

Acetone

Acetone is formed by spontaneous, non-enzymatic decarboxylation of acetoacetate, the production rate being linearly related to the concentration of acetoacetate, and widely variable in DKA. The urinary excretion rate of acetone remains constant at around 7% of the production rate, while the proportion expired increases with increasing formation [45]. A small proportion of acetone is converted into glucose [46, 47].

Acid–Base Balance

The two major ketone bodies, 3-hydroxybutyrate and acetoacetate, are weak acids and dissociate completely at physiological pH. In DKA, the large hydrogen ion load rapidly exceeds normal buffering capacity. Some of the excess acid is lost by hyperventilation and hydrogen ions are excreted in the urine along with phosphate and ammonium, but classically in DKA a metabolic acidosis with an increased anion gap develops. Some patients who are able to maintain salt and water intake continue to excrete ketone bodies and sodium, and thus may present with a hyperchloraemic acidosis [48, 49]. During treatment of DKA, infusion of saline may also promote the excretion of ketone salts, producing a similar disturbance. Lactic acidosis may further complicate the picture, particularly if the patient is severely hypotensive.

The hydrogen ion concentration bears no relationship to the degree of hyperglycaemia [50], and many cases of normoglycaemic ketoacidosis have been reported.

Electrolyte Changes

The total body deficit of water in DKA is of the order of 5–8 litres, with a deficit of 300–1000 mmol K^+ and 400–700 mmol Na^+. Several factors probably account for the deficit of K^+. Insulin deficiency results in a reduction of the activity of the Na^+-K^+-ATPase, with reduced exchange of Na^+ and K^+ across the cell membrane. The metabolic acidosis is thought also to cause loss of intracellular K^+, although the mechanism is debated. The acidaemia may simply promote exchange of potassium for hydrogen ions entering the cell. Both hyperglycaemia per se and hyperglucagonaemia promote intracellular loss of K^+. The final serum concentration of K^+ probably depends on the rate of loss of K^+ in the urine. Patients with prerenal azotaemia will have a high serum potassium level whereas in those in whom renal perfusion is well maintained, the concentration will be low.

Hyperkalaemia may develop more rapidly and be more severe in patients on CSII [51, 52].

Hypomagnesaemia and hypophosphataemia are common in DKA, although their clinical importance is not clear. It has been suggested that hypophosphataemia may delay the recovery of red cell 2,3-diphosphoglycerate levels and impair oxygen delivery to the tissues [53].

Haematological Changes

Thromboembolic complications are not infrequent occurrences in DKA. Several of the clotting factors are elevated [54, 55]. Platelet secretory activity may be increased, but aggregation decreased [56]. The neutrophil count is commonly raised in DKA and correlates with plasma ketone body levels, so does not necessarily imply an underlying infection [57]. Neutrophil function appears to be impaired even at modestly elevated blood glucose concentrations [58]. Dehydration will elevate the haematocrit whereas osmotic changes may falsely increase the mean corpuscular volume when estimated by Coulter counter [59, 60].

Diagnosis

Symptoms and Signs

The classic symptoms and signs of DKA can be predicted from the pathophysiology. Patients complain of polyuria, thirst and polydipsia as a result of the osmotic diuresis. In those patients with previously unknown disease and slow onset of DKA, weight loss is marked, with loss of adipose tissue and muscle. Tiredness and general malaise are frequent, with steadily increasing drowsiness lapsing into coma as the condition becomes more serious. The degree of coma correlates only with the plasma osmolality, suggesting that intracellular fluid loss from cerebral cells is a causal factor [61]. Nausea and vomiting may aggravate the fluid and electrolyte loss, and abdominal pain, thought to be secondary to ketosis, is a common complaint. Patients may notice the smell and taste of ketones.

The patient typically is drowsy, dehydrated, hypotensive with a tachycardia, peripherally vasodilated secondary to the acidosis, hypothermic and hyperventilating, with classic Kussmaul respiration. The smell of ketones on the breath is a useful sign to those able to detect the 'pear drop' odour. There may be signs of intestinal stasis or even an 'acute abdomen'.

Biochemical Diagnosis

The above features should prompt the measurement of capillary blood glucose concentration by enzymatic test strip at the bedside, with measurement of glycosuria and ketonuria if urine is obtainable. Initial therapy can then begin while laboratory confirmation is awaited. Initial tests should include blood glucose, urea and electrolytes and blood pH, pO_2 and pCO_2. If arterial puncture is impossible, an adequate reflection of arterial pH can be obtained from capillary blood gas measurement [62]. The anion gap can be calculated from the concentrations of the four major electrolytes. Plasma ketone bodies are estimated by test strips or tablets. Despite the total body deficit of hypotonic saline, plasma sodium levels are generally artificially low, because the hyperglycaemia has drawn water from the intracellular compartment, diluting plasma. It can be calculated that for every 3 mmol/l increase in blood glucose the plasma sodium falls by 1 mmol/l [63]. As discussed above, plasma potassium levels may be low, normal or elevated. The anion gap is generally increased, but in cases of hyperchloraemic acidosis may be normal. Blood pH is invariably low, with a normal or high pO_2 and low or normal pCO_2, depending on the degree of hyperventilation.

Further investigation should include full blood count, chest x-ray, electrocardiogram and cultures from blood, urine and throat. Cardiac monitoring, in addition to aiding the diagnosis of acute myocardial infarction as the precipitating factor, is also useful in assessing the plasma potassium.

Blood glucose should be checked hourly at the bedside, and laboratory measurements of glucose, electrolytes, urea and creatinine performed at presentation and after 2, 5, 8 and 24 hours of therapy. More frequent estimations may be necessary if management is complicated. Flow sheets to record the results allow easy detection of changes.

Treatment

The treatment of DKA is very rewarding but fraught with hazards for the unwary. Simple management protocols are helpful as guidelines but should be adapted to suit each individual case. The major elements of treatment are fluids, insulin, potassium and alkali.

Fluid Replacement

Fluid replacement is the cornerstone of therapy and may on its own reduce blood glucose by up to 23% simply by reopening renal perfusion and allowing loss of glucose in the urine [64]. Rehydration also reduces the levels of counterregulatory hormones [65] and tissue perfusion increases, allowing effective insulin therapy. As described above, the total body deficit is 5–8 litres of hypotonic saline. As such, the logical replacement fluid at first sight appears to be hypotonic fluid. However, infusion of large quantities of hypotonic saline has been associated with circulatory collapse and cerebral oedema [66, 67]. For these reasons, most authorities would recommend initial rehydration with 0.154 mol/l saline, switching to hypotonic (0.074 mol/l) saline or dextrose in water only if the plasma sodium rises above 155 mmol/l. Because of problems with fluid balance (see below) we have recently begun to infuse fluid more cautiously than previously. Generally 2 litres of fluid are infused over 4 hours, 2 litres over 8 hours and subsequently 1 litre every 8 hours. Obviously, this regimen should be modified according to the fluid state of the patient and guided by central venous pressure readings if performed.

Some rise in plasma sodium is inevitable with appropriate therapy, and may even be helpful, by preventing too rapid a fall in plasma osmolality as the blood glucose falls, and thus reducing the risk of cerebral oedema.

Once the blood glucose has fallen to around 14 mmol/l, infusion of 10% glucose should be substituted for saline. This will allow continued infusion of insulin to correct the metabolic acidosis and ketosis. Saline can be given simultaneously if the patient is still dehydrated.

Generally, patients who are hypotensive at presentation show some recovery after the infusion of 2 litres of saline. If the systolic blood pressure remains less than 90 mmHg, infusion of 1 or 2 litres of colloid will often produce a rapid improvement.

Insulin

The use of low-dose insulin regimens, either intravenous or intramuscular, is now generally accepted [68, 69]. Advantages over the previously used high-dose regimens include less frequent hypokalaemia and hypoglycaemia, and a more predictable response to treatment. The aims of insulin therapy are to halt the overwhelming catabolic process and return the metabolic milieu to normality as smoothly as possible. Insulin therapy, together with adequate fluid replacement, suppresses lipolysis and ketogenesis, and reduces the grossly elevated hepatic glucose output and increases peripheral uptake of glucose, although not to normal values [33].

Continuous intravenous infusion of short-acting insulin given by infusion pump at 6 U per hour will produce plasma insulin levels of around 100 mU/l, more than adequate to restrain the catabolic process. When the blood glucose has fallen to around 14 mmol/l, infusion of 10% dextrose should be substituted for saline, the insulin infusion rate reduced to 4 U per hour and adjusted thereafter according to hourly bedside blood glucose estimations. If a significant drop in blood glucose has not been observed after 2 hours of insulin therapy, then the fluid replacement schedule, blood pressure, infusion pump and lines should be checked. If these are all satisfactory, the infusion rate of insulin should be doubled.

Hourly intramuscular injection of insulin is a satisfactory alternative to continuous intravenous insulin infusion, and is especially useful if reliable infusion pumps are not available. A loading dose of 20 U insulin is given, followed by 6–10 U each hour. Adequate hydration, with good tissue perfusion, is essential for the success of the intramuscular regimen. If after the first 2 hours the blood glucose has not fallen significantly and the patient is well hydrated and not hypotensive, the doses of intramuscular insulin can be doubled or the regimen substituted by intravenous infusion.

Little difference has been found in the past between intravenous and intramuscular regimens, although a recent study in children showed that despite the administration of smaller amounts of insulin, fluids and bicarbonate, the use of intravenous insulin was associated with a faster fall in blood glucose with no increase in hypoglycaemia, a faster rise in serum sodium and an unchanged incidence of complications [70].

The acidosis and ketosis resolve more slowly than the hyperglycaemia. It is thus essential that insulin administration continues after the blood glucose has been controlled. For this reason, infusion of dextrose should be started when the blood glucose falls to around 14 mmol/l, allowing insulin administration to continue. There is some evidence to suggest that the clearance of ketones is faster when 10% rather than 5% dextrose is infused [71]. Infusion of dextrose with intravenous or intramuscular insulin should be continued until the patient is able to eat, when subcutaneous insulin therapy can be substituted.

Potassium

As discussed above, potassium levels may be low, normal or high at presentation of DKA, despite a total body deficit of 300–1000 mmol [72]. Plasma concentrations invariably fall with treatment, and hypokalaemia is a potentially preventable cause of death in DKA [73]. The fall is secondary to rehydration of both extracellular and intracellular fluid compartments, a direct effect of insulin on intracellular potassium transport, correction of acidosis and loss of potassium in the urine with restoration of urine flow.

Opinion varies as to when potassium replacement should be started: immediately [74, 75], when plasma potassium concentrations are known [2, 76] or when urine flow is established [8, 77]. As hypokalaemia is potentially more threatening to the great majority of patients, it seems prudent to begin cautious potassium replacement (20–30 mmol per hour) when insulin therapy is started. Thereafter the rate of potassium replacement should be adjusted in the light of plasma levels, urine output and electrocardiographic monitoring. It has been suggested that potassium should be infused as the phosphate salt, as there is often a concomitant deficit in phosphate [78], but as the extent of the phosphate deficit is much less than that of potassium, it seems wiser to replace the electrolytes separately.

Bicarbonate Therapy

Acidosis has profound pathophysiological effects, including negative inotropism, peripheral vasodilation, central nervous system depression and insulin resistance. However, fortunately in many cases, the classic picture of metabolic acidosis with increased anion gap will correct spontaneously simply with fluid and insulin treatment. Administration of bicarbonate is not without risk—local irritation, hypokalaemia, paradoxical worsening of cerebrospinal fluid acidosis, rebound alkalosis and impaired oxyhaemoglobin dissociation are potential complications. For these reasons, standard teaching has limited bicarbonate infusion to patients with severe DKA and arterial pH less than 7.0 [1, 3]. However, even at this level, the benefits are not clear. Several studies have not demonstrated convincing benefit from administering bicarbonate [79–81]. However, no study has been large enough to exclude with confidence any beneficial effect on cardiac function or in preventing arrhythmias. It is the authors' current practice to administer bicarbonate only if the pH is below 6.9. A dose of 100 mmol is given in 45 min, together with 20 mmol KCl. This can be repeated until the pH exceeds 7.0. In addition, small doses (50 mmol) may be useful to relieve distressing hyperventilation.

Other Electrolytes

There is also a deficit of magnesium, calcium and phosphate in DKA, although the clinical relevance and the need for replacement are not clear. Severe hypophosphataemia may develop during treatment of DKA, plasma phosphate concentrations falling to undetectable levels. It has been suggested that hypophosphataemia may prevent the recovery of the red cell 2,3-diphosphoglycerate levels [53]. However, several small trials have shown that phosphate replacement does not hasten biochemical or clinical recovery from DKA [82, 83]. It is not the authors' current practice to replace phosphate, magnesium or calcium during treatment of DKA without a specific clinical indication.

Clinical Management

The most important aspects of clinical management are careful monitoring of the patient and assiduous attention to detail. These factors are probably more important than the use of an intensive care unit for all but the most serious cases. In a personal series of 250 episodes of DKA, Moss described a low-cost, low-intervention, low-technology approach whereby only 30 patients were admitted to an intensive care unit [84]; the others were managed in a general medical ward where the nursing staff were familiar with treating DKA. There were no deaths and the average length of stay was 4.2 days. The feasibility of such an approach has also been demonstrated in the developing countries [85]. Both studies illustrate the necessity for detailed clinical care above all other considerations.

The patient's vital signs should be monitored every half-hour initially, hourly after 4 hours and then every 2–4 hours. An accurate record of hourly urine output must be made. Measurement of central venous pressure is a useful aid to fluid replacement, especially if the patient is elderly or has heart disease. If the patient is unconscious, a nasogastric tube should be passed to prevent aspiration. Urinary catheterisation may also be needed. A careful search for the underlying cause should be conducted and broad-spectrum antibiotic therapy begun, after appropriate samples for culture have been obtained, if there is any hint of infection.

DKA is a hypercoagulable state and thromboembolism is an important complication. The elderly, those in coma or with severe hyperosmolar states are particularly at risk and consideration should be given to prophylactic subcutaneous heparin treatment.

Complications of Treatment

Fluid Overload

Unless particular care is taken, fluid overload with pulmonary oedema is a potential hazard, particularly in the elderly or those with heart disease. As discussed above, monitoring of the central venous pressure may be helpful in these patients.

Cerebral Oedema

Cerebral oedema is a well-recognized complication of DKA, particularly in children. Subclinical brain swelling is evident at presentation of DKA and may worsen with treatment [66, 67]. Occasionally, catastrophic oedema occurs, with sudden deterioration in the patient's clinical condition, often as the hyperglycaemia and acidosis are improving [86]. When clinical manifestations occur, the outcome is very poor. In a review of cases in the literature, Duck found a high frequency of hyponatraemia (74% below 134 mmol/l) and high rates of fluid administration (more than 4 l/m^2 per day) [86]. It is worth noting that cerebral oedema rarely occurs if the blood glucose is maintained around 14 mmol/l. It thus seems prudent to infuse isotonic saline at least for the first few hours, to aim for slow, gradual biochemical improvement and to begin the infusion of dextrose when the blood glucose approaches 14 mmol/l.

The cause of cerebral oedema is debated. One theory expounds the role of 'idiogenic osmoles'. As DKA develops and the plasma osmolality rises, water is drawn from the intracellular space. In an effort to prevent intracellular dehydration, 'idiogenic osmoles' are generated inside cerebral cells over several days. When rehydration is begun, the plasma osmolality rapidly falls to less than that of the intracellular space. As it takes some time for the 'idiogenic osmoles' to dissipate, the osmotic gradient across the cell membrane now draws water into the cell, causing cerebral oedema.

Recently, an alternative theory has been advanced, invoking a role for the Na$^+$/H$^+$ plasma membrane transport system which is involved in regulation of cytoplasmic pH [87]. Activation of the exchanger by acidification of the cytoplasm results in transport of Na$^+$ into the cell, with subsequent cell swelling. In some tissues, insulin can also activate the transporter. Thus in developing DKA, accumulation of ketone bodies, lactate and non-esterified fatty acids occurs in both the intracellular and extracellular compartments. Because of this balance, little activation of the exchange occurs and Na$^+$ transport into the cell is limited. Therefore, at presentation of DKA, only minor brain swelling would be expected. However, as treatment is begun, the extracellular proton concentration is reduced much more rapidly than the intracellular concentration. Correction of hyperglycaemia and osmolality relieve the extracellular inhibition of the countertransporter, while the intracellular environment still favours activation. Thus, with treatment, the exchanger is activated, sodium is transported into the cell and cell swelling occurs. This hypothesis would account for the clinical observation that cerebral oedema often becomes manifest when biochemical improvement is occurring.

Adult Respiratory Distress Syndrome

This is a fortunately rare but well-documented complication of DKA, characterised by the sudden onset of dyspnoea, hypoxaemia, decreasing lung compliance and diffuse pulmonary infiltrates on chest x-ray. Mortality is high and there is no specific treatment, ventilatory support reducing the death rate from respiratory failure but not affecting overall mortality [88]. Hypotension, hypothermia and coma appear to carry an increased risk [89]. As with cerebral oedema, rapidly decreasing oncotic pressure following resuscitation with large volumes of hypotonic fluids may precipitate the problem [66]. An alternative mechanism of a specific alveolo-capillary permeability defect induced by acidosis and hyperventilation has been suggested [90].

Other Complications

Thromboembolism has been discussed above. Other rare complications include acute rhabdomyolysis, mucormycosis and spontaneous pneumomediastinum.

Pitfalls in Diagnosis and Management

Ketoacidosis without Hyperglycaemia

With the advent of selfmonitoring of blood glucose many patients manage intercurrent illnesses by increasing their insulin dose according to the capillary blood glucose concentration. This increased dose is often sufficient to prevent severe hyperglycaemia developing, but not to restrain lipolysis and ketosis; thus these patients may present with modest hyperglycaemia but marked ketoacidosis [91]. This may be especially important for patients using CSII therapy, where after disruption of insulin delivery, blood glucose values reach a plateau at around 15 mmol/l after 4 hours but ketone body levels continue to rise [92]. The importance of urine testing for ketones when ill should be stressed to all diabetic patients on insulin.

Gastrointestinal Symptoms

Classically, DKA presents with abdominal pain, nausea and vomiting which may simulate an intra-abdominal emergency. Conversely, an abdominal emergency may precipitate DKA. A non-specific rise in serum amylase commonly occurs in DKA, further complicating the diagnostic problem. It is sensible to institute treatment of the DKA promptly and to review the abdominal findings frequently. If there is no improvement within 3–4 hours, other diagnoses should be considered.

Electrocardiography

The electrolyte disturbance seen in DKA may produce ST segment changes mimicking acute myocardial infarction but which resolve on treatment of the DKA and which are not associated with any other evidence of cardiac disease [93].

Serum Creatinine

Acetoacetate interferes with the alkaline picrate methods of determining serum creatinine. Thus in DKA, serum creatinine concentrations may be falsely elevated and should not be interpreted as evidence of renal impairment [94]. The discrepancy is of the order of 120 μmol/l and is proportional to the level of acetoacetate [95].

Other Problems

Organophosphorus poisoning and alcoholic ketoacidosis are both rare conditions that may mimic diabetic ketoacidosis [96, 97].

Prevention

Most cases of DKA are avoidable. Delays in seeking and providing medical attention were thought to be major contributory factors to the deaths of 27 previously diagnosed diabetic patients in a UK survey [13]. Of the total deaths in DKA reported in the same paper, neglect of the diabetes by the patient was judged to be contributory to the fatal outcome in 40%, and delay by the family doctor in diagnosis or in taking appropriate action was implicated in 36%. The management of 46% of those who died in hospital was criticised. More effective education of the general public, diabetic patients and all health care professionals is thus vital to prevent DKA and to promote effective management when it does occur. There is evidence that an intensive education program would reduce the incidence of DKA and be cost-effective [98]. Clear guidelines for patients on how to manage intercurrent illness should be given. Of paramount importance are instructions never to stop insulin, to monitor blood glucose and urine ketones regularly, to take the usual carbohydrate intake as fluids and to seek help if hyperglycaemia greater than 20 mmol/l persists for more than 24 hours or if significant ketonuria (2+ or more) develops. Measures such as these should decrease the incidence of DKA.

HYPEROSMOLAR NON-KETOTIC COMA

There is no clear-cut division between DKA and hyperosmolar non-ketotic diabetic coma, and the two may be regarded as being at opposite ends of a spectrum. In HONK, insulin deficiency is relative rather than absolute, and hyperglycaemia is more severe and ketosis less marked than in DKA. Patients tend to be older and to have non-insulin dependent diabetes, and often the acute presentation is the first indication that the patient has diabetes.

Epidemiology

The annual incidence of HONK is approximately one-sixth to one-tenth that of DKA [9]. Patients are older than those presenting in DKA, the mean age at presentation ranging from 57 years to 70 years in four reports [99–102]. The percentage of previously undiagnosed patients is also higher [102]. It should, however, be remembered that HONK can develop in the very young [103] and in ketosis-prone insulin dependent patients [104]. Mortality is very high, approaching 60% in some series, and has changed little over the last 20 years [99, 101].

Precipitating Factors

As with DKA, infection and other acute illnesses —particularly cardiovascular disease—are the major precipitants [99, 101]. In an analysis of risk factors predisposing to HONK, female sex, newly diagnosed diabetes and the presence of infection were independent risk factors [102]. Poor social background and social isolation are also important [105]. Many drugs, particularly corticosteroids [106] and thiazide diuretics [107], may precipitate HONK.

Pathophysiology

The classic biochemical changes seen in HONK are marked hyperglycaemia and hyperosmolality with only a minor degree of ketosis and acidosis [1, 77]. There is relative insulin deficiency, and glucagon concentrations are grossly elevated [108]. The degree of hyperglycaemia is dependent on the circulating glucagon concentration [32]. Glucagon produces a massive increase in hepatic glucose output by stimulating gluconeogenesis and glycogenolysis [109, 110]. Because of the relative insulin deficiency, peripheral utilisation of glucose is reduced and lipolysis relatively unrestrained. The increased concentrations of NEFA and increased lipid oxidation rates further stimulate gluconeogenesis and hepatic glucose output [111]. It has been suggested that continued stimulation of the B cell by the hyperglycaemia results in B-cell exhaustion and a further decline in serum insulin concentrations, aggravating the situation further [112].

Many patients have pre-existing renal disease and it may be that dehydration subsequent to the osmotic diuresis results in a further fall in glomerular filtration rate in an already compromised kidney [99, 101]. Failure of the kidney to excrete the large glucose load would further exacerbate the hyperglycaemia.

There are various putative explanations for the absence of significant ketosis in HONK. The differential effect of insulin on fat and glucose metabolism is well recognised [113], hence the explanation that there is sufficient insulin peripherally to inhibit lipolysis but not to stimulate peripheral glucose uptake. However, it is difficult to reconcile this with the fact that serum insulin levels are identical in DKA and HONK [114]. Alternatively, the hypothesis of an 'insulinised' liver but diabetic periphery has been put forward [115]: here, lipolysis proceeds unrestrained and there is a large flux of NEFA to the liver; however, because the liver is adequately insulinised, NEFA enter the gluconeogenic pathway rather than being oxidised to ketone bodies. In this model, plasma NEFA levels should be as high as in DKA: this does not appear to be the case [99, 100]. Perhaps the most convincing explanation is that dehydration and hyperosmolality per se inhibit lipolysis and ketogenesis [116].

Various factors, including renal impairment

as discussed above, reduced appreciation of thirst and physical or mental inability to drink, probably contribute to the striking hyperosmolality. The hyperosmolality is closely related to the degree of mental impairment [117].

Diagnosis

Symptoms and Signs

A high index of suspicion is necessary to make an early diagnosis as patients are often drowsy with non-specific signs and symptoms. Focal neurological signs, which resolve as the metabolic state is returned to normal, may be present [118]. There may be evidence of an acute precipitating event such as myocardial infarction or infection. Dehydration is very marked and hypotension common.

Biochemical Diagnosis

Bedside measurement of capillary blood glucose suggests the diagnosis, which can be confirmed by laboratory measurement. Plasma sodium and urea are often markedly elevated, in keeping with the degree of dehydration. Plasma potassium is low or normal, and ketosis and acidosis are minimal or absent. Calculated osmolality is greater than 350 mosm/l.

Treatment

The general principles of treatment are similar to that of DKA, with rehydration being of prime importance.

Fluids

The average fluid deficit is around 9 litres of isotonic fluid. As many patients will be hypotensive, it seems logical to begin resuscitation with isotonic saline, at least until hypotension has been corrected and a good urine flow achieved. In many cases, hypernatraemia ($>$ 155 mmol/l) may necessitate a switch to hypotonic saline or 5% dextrose in water. If hypotension is marked or persistent, infusion of 1–2 litres of colloid may be necessary. Most authors aim to replace the 9-litre deficit over 24–48 hours, although some would proceed more cautiously, apparently without harm [101]. It is the authors' current practice to infuse 2 litres within the first 4 hours,

2 litres in the next 8 hours and 1 litre every 8 hours thereafter. In these elderly, frail patients, monitoring of central venous pressure is vital.

Insulin

Patients with HONK are generally said to be sensitive to low doses of insulin. However, one recent study suggested that they were markedly insulin resistant [119]. The same insulin schedule, either intravenous or intramuscular, can be followed as in DKA, with the aim of reducing blood glucose by no more than 10 mmol/l per hour. Precipitous falls in blood glucose may lead to profound extracellular dehydration, cerebral oedema and circulatory collapse [118]. When the blood glucose falls to around 14 mmol/l, infusion of 10% dextrose should be started and the insulin continued at half the previous rate.

Potassium

There is a large total body deficit of potassium, due to the long prodromal phase, intracellular fluid depletion and marked urinary losses. Extreme hyperkalaemia at presentation is rare and plasma levels often fall precipitously with treatment. Thus potassium replacement should begin early, with 20 mmol per hour until the plasma concentration is known.

Other Measures

The hyperosmolality, hyperglycaemia, age and coma all contribute to the high risk of thromboembolism in HONK [118, 120]. Prophylactic anticoagulation with low-dose subcutaneous heparin at the least should be considered.

CONCLUSION

Given the high mortality of HONK, prevention is paramount. However, many patients succumb to the precipitating event rather than to the metabolic disturbance. A large proportion of those who survive will not require long-term insulin therapy.

REFERENCES

1. Schade DS, Eaton RP, Alberti KGMM et al. Diabetic coma: ketoacidotic and hyperosmolar. Albuquerque: University of New Mexico Press, 1981.

2. Foster DW, McGarry JD. The metabolic derangements and treatment of diabetic keto-acidosis. New Engl J Med 1983; 309: 159–69.

3. Keller U. Diabetic ketoacidosis: current views on pathogenesis and treatment. Diabetologia 1986: 29: 71–7.

4. Marshall SM, Alberti KGMM. Diabetic keto-acidosis. In Alberti KGMM, Krall LP (eds) Diabetes Annual 3. Amsterdam: Elsevier, 1987: pp 498–526.

5. Walker M, Marshall SM, Alberti KGMM. Clinical aspects of diabetic ketoacidosis. Diabetes Metab Rev 1989; 5: 651–63.

6. Alberti KGMM. Diabetic emergencies. Br Med Bull 1989; 45: 242–63.

7. Faich GA, Fishbein HA, Ellis SE. The epidemiology of diabetic acidosis: a population-based study. Am J Epidemiol 1983; 117: 551–8.

8. Ellemann K, Soerensen JN, Pedersen L et al. Epidemiology and treatment of diabetic keto-acidosis in a community population. Diabetes Care 1984; 7: 528–32.

9. Fishbein HA. Diabetic ketoacidosis, hyper-osmolar nonketotic coma, lactic acidosis and hypoglycemia. In Harris MI, Hammar RF (eds) Diabetes in America (National Diabetes Group). Washington: US Department of Health and Human Sciences, 1985, pp XII-1–16.

10. Holman RC, Herron CA, Sinnock P. Epidemiologic characteristics of mortality from diabetes with acidosis or coma, United States, 1970–78. Am J Publ Health 1983; 73: 1169–74.

11. Gale EAM, Dornan TL, Tattersall RB. Severely uncontrolled diabetes in the over fifties. Diabetologia 1982; 21: 25–8.

12. Sheppard MC, Wright AD. The effect on mortality of low-dose insulin therapy for diabetic ketoacidosis. Diabetes Care 1982; 5: 111–13.

13. Tunbridge WMG. Deaths due to diabetic keto-acidosis. Q J Med 1981; 50: 502–3.

14. Rwiza HJ, Swai ABM, McLarty D. Failure to diagnose diabetic ketoacidosis in Tanzania. Diabet Med 1986; 3: 181–3.

15. Peden NR, Braaten JT, McKendry JBR. Diabetic ketoacidosis during long-term treatment with continuous subcutaneous insulin infusion. Diabetes Care 1984; 7: 1–5.

16. Mecklenburg RS, Guinn TS, Sannar CA et al. Malfunction of continuous subcutaneous insulin infusion systems: a one-year prospective study of 127 patients. Diabetes Care 1986; 9: 351–5.

17. MacRury SM, Small M, Boal A et al. Diabetic ketoacidosis during NovoPen therapy. Diabet Med 1988; 5: 87–8.

18. Helve E, Koivisto VA, Lehtonen A et al. A crossover comparison of continuous insulin infusion and conventional injection treatment of type I diabetes. Acta Med Scand 1987; 221: 385–93.

19. Ronn B, Mathiesen ER, Vang L et al. Evaluation of insulin pump treatment under routine conditions. Diabetes Res Clin Pract 1987; 3: 191–6.

20. Nosadini R, Velussi M, Fioretto P et al. Frequency of hypoglycaemic and hyperglycaemic-ketotic episodes during conventional and subcutaneous continuous insulin infusion therapy in IDDM. Diabet Nutr Metab 1988; 1: 289–94.

21. DCCT Research Group. Results of feasibility of the Diabetes Control and Complications Trial (DCCT): glycemic control, follow-up and complications of therapy. Diabetes 1986; 35 (suppl. 1): 3A.

22. Teutsch SM, Herman WH, Dwyer DM et al. Mortality among diabetic patients using continuous subcutaneous insulin-infusion pumps. New Engl J Med 1984; 310: 361–8.

23. Bending JJ, Pickup JC, Keen H. Frequency of diabetic ketoacidosis and hypoglycemic coma during routine treatment with continuous sub-cutaneous insulin infusion. Am J Med 1985; 79: 685–91.

24. Chapman J, Wright AD, Nattrass M et al. Recurrent diabetic ketoacidosis. Diabet Med 1988; 5: 659–61

25. Fulop M. Recurrent diabetic ketoacidosis. Am J Med 1985; 78: 54–60.

26. Tattersall R. Brittle diabetes. Br Med J 1985; 291: 555–6.

27. Orr DP, Golden MP, Myers G et al. Characteristics of adolescents with poorly controlled diabetes referred to a tertiary care center. Diabetes Care 1983; 6: 170–5.

28. Flexner CW, Weiner JP, Saudek CD et al. Repeated hospitalization for diabetic ketoaci-dosis: the game of 'sartoris'. Am J Med 1984; 76: 691–7.

29. Miles JM, Rizza RA, Haymond MW et al. Effects of acute insulin deficiency in glucose and ketone body turnover in man: evidence for the primary overproduction of glucose and ketone bodies in the genesis of diabetic ketoacidosis. Diabetes 1980; 29: 926–30.

30. Alberti KGMM, Christensen NJ, Iverson J et al. Role of glucagon and other hormones in development of diabetic ketoacidosis. Lancet 1975; i: 1307–11.

31. Gerich JE, Lorenzi M, Bier DM et al. Prevention of human diabetic ketoacidosis by somatostatin. Evidence for an essential role of glucagon. New Engl J Med 1975; 292: 985–9.

32. Malchoff CD, Pohl SL, Kaiser DL et al. Determinants of glucose and ketoacid concentrations in acutely hyperglycemic diabetic patients. Am J Med 1984; 77: 275–85.

33. Luzi L, Barrett EJ, Groop LC et al. Metabolic effects of low-dose insulin therapy on glucose metabolism in diabetic ketoacidosis. Diabetes 1988; 37: 1470–7.

34. Yki-Jarvinen H, Helve E, Koivisto VA. Hyperglycemia decreases glucose uptake in type I diabetes. Diabetes 1987; 36: 892–6.

35. Arnfred J, Schmitz O, Hother-Nielsen O et al. Marked impairment of the effect of hyperglycaemia on glucose uptake and glucose production in insulin-dependent diabetes. Diabet Med 1988; 5: 755–60.

36. Imamura T, Koffler M, Helderman JH et al. Severe diabetes induced in subtotally depancreatized dogs by sustained hyperglycemia. Diabetes 1988; 37: 600–9.

37. Johnston DG, Alberti KGMM. Hormone control of ketone body metabolism in the normal and diabetic state. Clin Endocrinol Metab 1982; 11: 329–61.

38. Nosadini R, Avogaro A, Doria A et al. Ketone body metabolism: a physiological and clinical overview. Diabetes Metab Rev 1989; 5: 299–319.

39. Swislocki ALM, Chen YDI, Golay A et al. Insulin suppression of free fatty acid concentration in normal individuals and patients with Type 2 (non-insulin-dependent) diabetes. Diabetologia 1987; 30: 622–6.

40. McGarry JD, Woelrje KF, Kuwajima M et al. Regulations of ketogenesis and the renaissance of carnitine palmitoyltransferase. Diabetes Metab Rev 1989; 5: 271–84.

41. Keller U, Lustenberger M, Stauffacher W. Effect of insulin on ketone body clearance studied by a ketone body 'clamp' technique in normal man. Diabetologia 1988; 31: 24–9.

42. McGarry JD, Takabayashi Y, Foster DW. The role of malonyl CoA in the coordination of fatty acid synthesis and oxidation in isolated rat hepatocytes. J Biol Chem 1978; 253: 8294–9.

43. McGarry JD, Robles-Valdes C, Foster DW. Role of carnitine in hepatic ketogenesis. Proc Natl Acad Sci USA 1975; 72: 4385–8.

44. Miles JM, Gerich JE. Glucose and ketone body kinetics in diabetic ketoacidosis. Clin Endocrinol Metab 1983; 12: 303–8.

45. Owen OE, Trapp VE, Skutches CL et al. Acetone metabolism during diabetic ketoacidosis. Diabetes 1982; 31: 224–8.

46. Hetenyi G Jr, Ferrarotto C. Gluconeogenesis from acetone in starved rats. Biochem J 1985; 231: 151–5.

47. Reichard GA Jr, Skutches CL, Hoeldtke RD et al. Acetone metabolism in humans during diabetic ketoacidosis. Diabetes 1986; 35: 668–74.

48. Adrogue HJ, Wilson H, Boyd AE et al. Plasma acid-base patterns in diabetic ketoacidosis. New Engl J Med 1982; 307: 1603–10.

49. Adrogue HJ, Eknoyan G, Suki WK. Diabetic ketoacidosis: role of the kidney in the acid-base homeostasis re-evaluated. Kidney Int 1984; 25: 591–7.

50. Brandt KR, Miles JM. Relationship between severity of hyperglycemia and metabolic acidosis in diabetic ketoacidosis. Mayo Clin Proc 1988; 63: 1071–4.

51. Knight G, Jennings AM, Boulton AJM et al. Severe hyperkalaemia and ketoacidosis during routine treatment with an insulin pump. Br Med J 1985; 291: 371–2.

52. Pickup JC. Hyperkalaemia after interruption of CSII. Diabetologia 1986; 29: 823–4.

53. Alberti KGMM, Emerson PM, Darley JH et al. 2,3-Diphosphoglycerate and tissue oxygenation in uncontrolled diabetes mellitus. Lancet 1972; ii: 2391–5.

54. Paton RC. Haemostatic changes in diabetic coma. Diabetologia 1981; 21: 172–7.

55. Greaves M, Pickering C, Knight G et al. Changes in the factor VIII complex in diabetic ketoacidosis: evidence of endothelial cell damage? Diabetologia 1987; 30: 160–5.

56. Campbell RR, Foster KJ, Stirling C et al. Paradoxical platelet behaviour in diabetic ketoacidosis. Diabet Med 1986; 3: 161–4.

57. Alberti KGMM, Hockaday TDR. Diabetic coma—a reappraisal. Clin Endocrinol Metab 1977; 6: 421–56.

58. Kjersem H, Hilsted J, Madsbad S et al. Polymorphonuclear leucocyte dysfunction during short term metabolic changes from normo- to hyperglycaemia in type I (insulin-dependent) diabetic patients. Infection 1988; 16: 215–17.

59. Evan-Wong L, Davidson RJ. Raised Coulter mean corpuscular volume in diabetic ketoacidosis, and its underlying association with marked plasma hyperosmolarity. J Clin Pathol 1982; 36: 334–6.

60. Bock HA, Fluckiger R, Berger W et al. Real and artefactual erythrocyte swelling in hyperglycaemia. Diabetologia 1985; 28: 335–8.

61. Fulop M, Tawnewbaum H, Dreyer N. Ketotic hyperosmolar coma. Lancet 1973; ii: 635–9.

62. Hale PJ, Nattrass M. A comparison of arterial and non-arterialized capillary blood gases in diabetic ketoacidosis. Diabet Med 1988; 5: 76–8.

63. Katz MA. Hyperglycemia-induced hyponatremia. Calculation of expected sodium depression. New Engl J Med 1973; 289: 843–4.

64. West ML, Marsden PA, Singer GG et al. Quantitative analysis of glucose loss during acute therapy for hyperglycaemic, hyperosmolar syndrome. Diabetes Care 1986; 9: 465–71.

65. Owen OE, Licht JH, Sapir DG. Renal function and effects of partial rehydration during diabetic ketoacidosis. Diabetes 1981; 30: 510–18.

66. Fein IA, Rackow EC, Spring CL et al. Relation of colloid osmotic pressure to arterial hypoxemia and cerebral edema during crystalloid volume loading of patients with diabetic ketoacidosis. Ann Intern Med 1982; 96: 570–5.

67. Krane EJ, Rockoff MA, Wallman JK et al. Subclinical brain swelling in children during treatment of diabetic ketoacidosis. New Engl J Med 1985; 312: 1147–51.

68. Alberti KGMM, Hockaday TDR, Turner RC. Small doses of intramuscular insulin in the treatment of diabetic coma. Lancet 1973; ii: 515–22.

69. Page MM, Alberti KGMM, Greenwood R et al. Treatment of diabetic coma with continuous low-dose infusion of insulin. Br Med J 1974; 1: 687–90.

70. Jos J, Oberkampf B, Couprie C et al. Comparison de deux modes de traitement de l'acidocétose diabétique de l'enfant. Arch Fr Pediatr 1988; 45: 15–19.

71. Mincou I, Ionescu-Tirgoviste C, Cheta D et al. Le role de l'apport de glucose dans le traitement de la céto-acidose diabétique severe. Gazette Med France 1979; 86: 1665–70.

72. Van Gaal L, De Leeuw I, Bekaert J. Serum potassium levels in untreated diabetic ketoacidosis. Diabetologia 1981; 21: 338A.

73. Soler NG, Bennett MA, Dixon K et al. Potassium balance during treatment of diabetic ketoacidosis with special reference to the use of bicarbonate. Lancet 1972; ii: 665–7.

74. Schade DS, Eaton RP. Diabetic ketoacidosis —pathogenesis, prevention and therapy. Clin Endocrinol Metab 1983; 12: 321–8.

75. Johnston DG, Alberti KGMM. Diabetic emergencies: practical aspects of the management of diabetic ketoacidosis and diabetes during surgery. Clin Endocrinol Metab 1980; 9: 437–56.

76. Watkins PJ. Diabetic emergencies. Br Med J 1982; 285: 360–3.

77. Halperin ML, Goldstein MB, Bear RA et al. Diabetic comas. In Arieff AI, DeFronzo RA (eds) Fluid, electrolyte and acid-base disorders. Edinburgh: Churchill Livingstone, 1985: pp 933–67.

78. Felts PW. Ketoacidosis. Med Clin North Am 1983; 67: 831–6.

79. Lever E, Jaspan JB. Sodium bicarbonate therapy in severe diabetic ketoacidosis. Am J Med 1983; 75: 263–8.

80. Hale PJ, Crase J, Nattrass M. Metabolic effects of bicarbonate in the treatment of diabetic ketoacidosis. Br Med J 1984; 289: 1035–8.

81. Marr TJ, Traisman HS, Traisman ES et al. Juvenile ketoacidosis: the use of sodium bicarbonate in the treatment of diabetic children. J Kansas Med Soc 1981; 892: 282–6.

82. Wilson HK, Keuer SP, Lea AS et al. Phosphate therapy in diabetic ketoacidosis. Arch Intern Med 1982; 142: 517–21.

83. Fisher JN, Kitabchi AE. A randomized study of phosphate therapy in the treatment of diabetic ketoacidosis. J Clin Endocrinol Metab 1983; 57: 177–80.

84. Moss JM. Diabetic ketoacidosis: effective low-cost treatment in a community hospital. Southern Med J 1987; 80: 875–81.

85. Lester F. Ketoacidosis in Ethiopian diabetics. Diabetologia 1980; 18: 375–7.

86. Duck SC, Wyatt DT. Factors associated with brain herniation in the treatment of diabetic ketoacidosis. J Pediatr 1988; 113: 10–14.

87. Van der Meulin JA, Klip A, Grinstein S. Possible mechanisms for cerebral oedema in diabetic ketoacidosis. Lancet 1987; ii: 306–8.

88. Shale DJ. The adult respiratory distress syndrome – 20 years on. Thorax 1987; 42: 641–5.

89. Carroll P, Matz R. Adult respiratory distress syndrome complicating severe uncontrolled diabetes mellitus: report of 9 cases and a review of the literature. Diabetes Care 1982; 5: 574–80.

90. Brun-Buisson CJL, Bonnet F, Bergeret S et al. Recurrent high-permeability pulmonary edema associated with diabetic ketoacidosis. Crit Care Med 1985; 13: 55–6.

91. Bell PM, Hadden DR. Ketoacidosis without hyperglycaemia during self-monitoring of diabetes. Diabetes Care 1983; 6: 622–3.

92. Pickup JC, Viberti GC, Bilous RW et al. Safety of continuous subcutaneous insulin infusion: metabolic deterioration and glycaemic auto-regulation after deliberate cessation of infusion. Diabetologia 1982; 22: 175–9.

93. Khardori R, Cohen B, Taylor D et al. Electrocardiographic finding simulating acute myocardial infarction in a compound metabolic aberration. Am J Med 1985; 78: 529–30.

94. Assadi FK, John EG, Fornell L et al. Falsely elevated serum creatinine concentration in ketoacidosis. J Pediatr 1985; 107: 562–4.

95. Gerard SK, Khayam-Bashi H. Characterization of creatinine error in ketotic patients: a prospective comparison of alkaline picrate methods with an enzymatic method. Am J Clin Pathol 1985; 84: 659–61.

96. Williams GE. Alcoholic hypoglycaemia and ketoacidosis. Med Clin North Am 1984; 68: 33–8.

97. Zadik Z, Blachar Y, Barak Y et al. Organophosphate poisoning presenting as diabetic ketoacidosis. Toxicology 1983; 20: 381–5.

98. Davidson JK. The Grady Memorial Hospital Diabetes Programme. In Mann JI, Pyörälä K, Teuscher A (eds) Diabetes in epidemiological perspectives. Edinburgh: Churchill Livingstone, 1983: pp 332–41.

99. Gerich JE, Martin MM, Recant L. Clinical and metabolic characteristics of hyperosmolar non-ketotic coma. Diabetes 1971; 20: 228–38.

100. Arieff AI, Carroll HJ. Nonketotic hyperosmolar coma with hyperglycaemia: clinical features, pathophysiology, renal function, acid-base balance, plasma-cerebrospinal fluid equilibria and the effects of therapy in 37 cases. Medicine (Baltimore) 1972; 51: 73–94.

101. Khardori R, Soler NG. Hyperosmolar hyperglycemic nonketotic syndrome. Am J Med 1984; 77: 899–904.

102. Wachtel TJ, Silliman RA, Lamberton P. Predisposing factors for the diabetic hyperosmolar state. Arch Intern Med 1987; 147: 499–501.

103. Ehrlich RM, Bain HW. Hyperglycemia and hyperosmolarity in an eighteen-month-old child. New Engl J Med 1967; 276: 683–4.

104. Lotz M, Geraghty M. Hyperglycemic, hyperosmolar, nonketotic coma in a ketosis-prone juvenile diabetic. Ann Intern Med 1968; 69: 1245–6.

105. Knight G, Leatherdale BA. The role of race and environment in the development of hyperosmolar hyperglycaemic non-ketotic coma. Postgrad Med J 1982; 58: 351–5.

106. Boyer MH. Hyperosmolar anacidotic coma in association with glucocorticoid therapy. JAMA 1967; 202: 1007–9.

107. Fonseca V, Phear DN. Hyperosmolar nonketotic diabetic syndrome precipitated by treatment with diuretics. Br Med J 1982; 284: 36–7.

108. Lindsey CA, Faloona GR, Unger RH. Plasma glucagon in nonketotic hyperosmolar coma. JAMA 1974; 229: 1171–3.

109. Neely P, El Maghrabi MR, Pilkis SJ et al. Effect of diabetes, insulin, starvation and refeeding on the level of rat hepatic fructose 2,6-biphosphatase. Diabetes 1981; 30: 1062–4.

110. Exton JH. The effects of glucagon on hepatic glycogen metabolism and glycogenolysis. In Unger RH, Orci L (eds) Glucagon physiology, pathophysiology and morphology of pancreatic A cells. Amsterdam: Elsevier/North-Holland, 1981: pp 195–212.

111. Bogardus C, Lillioja S, Howard BV et al. Relationships between insulin secretion, insulin action, and fasting plasma glucose concentration in nondiabetic and noninsulin-dependent diabetic subjects. J Clin Invest 1984; 74: 1238–46.

112. Seltzer HS, Harris VI. Exhaustion of insulinogenic reserve in maturity-onset diabetic patients during prolonged and continuous hyperglycemic stress. Diabetes 1964; 13: 6–13.

113. Schade DS, Eaton RP. Dose response to insulin in man: differential effects on glucose and ketone body regulation. J Clin Endocrinol Metab 1977; 44: 1038–53.

114. Vinik A, Seftel H, Joffe BI. Metabolic findings in hyperosmolar, non-ketotic diabetic stupor. Lancet 1970; ii: 797–9.

115. Joffe BI, Goldberg RB, Krut LH et al. Pathogenesis of nonketotic hyperosmolar diabetic coma. Lancet 1975; i: 1069–71.

116. Gerich J, Panhaus JC, Gutman RA et al. Effect of dehydration and hyperosmolarity on glucose, free fatty acid and ketone body metabolism in the rat. Diabetes 1973; 22: 264–71.

117. Fulop M, Rosenblatt A, Kreitzer SM et al. Hyperosmolar nature of diabetic coma. Diabetes 1975; 24: 594–9.

118. McCurdy DK. Hyperosmolar hyperglycemic nonketotic diabetic coma. Med Clin North Am 1970; 54: 683–99.

119. Rosenthal NR, Barrett EJ. An assessment of insulin action in hyperosmolar hyperglycemic nonketotic diabetic patients. J Clin Endocrinol Metab 1985; 60: 607–12.

120. Whelton MJ, Walde D, Havard CWH. Hyperosmolar non-ketotic diabetic coma: with particular reference to vascular complications. Br Med J. 1971; 1: 85–6.

49

Infection, Immunity and Diabetes

W.G. Reeves* and R.M. Wilson†

*University Hospital, Nottingham, UK, and †Royal Hallamshire Hospital, Sheffield, UK

The experience of most practitioners regarding diabetes is coloured by a minority of patients who develop severe and persistent infections and whose diabetes is poorly controlled and often associated with complications such as vascular insufficiency, neuropathy and ulceration. However, in modern practice the prevalence of infection in the well-controlled diabetic population is much less of a problem than in the past. Relatively few studies have examined the relationship between the level of hyperglycaemia and the frequency of infection and obtained comparable data in appropriately matched control subjects. It is important to distinguish between the carriage of micro-organisms and the development of infectious disease, and the incidence of the latter has to be distinguished from the outcome of infection.

It is clear that the carriage of organisms, e.g. staphylococci on the skin, fungi on mucosal surfaces and bacteria in the urine, is generally more common in the diabetic population, although in many cases this does not give rise to infective problems when adequate control is maintained. Thus, it is not too surprising that skin and mucous membrane infection, on the one hand, and pyelonephritis, papillary necrosis and bacteraemia on the other, can readily develop when other factors such as poor control, vascular insufficiency or a physical breach in normal defences, e.g. ulceration or operative intervention, coexist.

A well-matched study investigating staphylococcal colonization showed an inverse relationship with glycaemic control [1], and a review of 241 diabetic outpatients over a 1-year period showed a fairly close correlation between blood glucose levels and the overall prevalence of infection [2]. Diabetic individuals are probably at greater risk of pneumonia caused by staphylococci or gram-negative bacilli, particularly when ketoacidosis is present, although diabetes does not seem to predispose to pneumococcal pneumonia [3]. Tuberculosis used to be ten times more prevalent in the diabetic population in the 1930s, but seems to cause few problems today except in developing countries, although diabetes may predispose to the reactivation of old foci. When infection of the skin does take hold it often takes the form of a mixed aerobic and anaerobic population of micro-organisms and can lead to necrosis. This particular combination is likely to be favoured by tissue hypoxia consequent upon the vascular insufficiency and stasis associated with the macro and microangiopathic complications of diabetes.

International Textbook of Diabetes Mellitus. Edited by K.G.M.M. Alberti, R.A. DeFronzo, H. Keen and P. Zimmet
© 1992 John Wiley & Sons Ltd

Some infections occur almost exclusively in diabetes mellitus, for example malignant external otitis, rhinoculocerebral mucormycosis and emphysematous pyelonephritis and cholecystitis. These conditions usually arise in patients with poorly controlled diabetes and are often associated with a mixed anaerobic and aerobic flora. High glucose levels in the affected tissues promote gas production due to bacterial fermentation.

The fact that the abnormal milieu within the poorly controlled diabetic can promote the colonization and pathogenicity of various microbes is in little doubt, but the nature and degree of impairment of the immune system in the diabetic patient is less well understood and is most appropriately divided into (a) abnormalities induced by hyperglycaemia or ketosis, and (b) primary abnormalities which may predispose to infection.

IMMUNOLOGICAL EFFECTS CONSEQUENT UPON HYPERGLYCAEMIA OR KETOSIS

A number of investigations have examined the competence of various components of the immune system in the diabetic patient. Most have examined lymphocytes or phagocytes, although some thought has been given to possible effects on circulating molecules, e.g. immunoglobulins and complement components.

Lymphocytes

Some have observed a diminution of total T-cell numbers [4] or individual T-cell subpopulations [5], although there is conflict as to whether the deficiency predominantly affects the helper (CD4) or cytotoxic/suppressor (CD8) T-cell population. Some studies suggest that the alteration in T-cell numbers relates to the adequacy of glucose control [5]. However, examination of lymphocyte subpopulations in whole blood by flow cytometry has failed to show significant differences either in total lymphocyte numbers or the proportion of CD3, CD4 and CD8-positive cells for 42 relatively young patients with type 1 diabetes compared with controls matched for age and sex [6]. There is general agreement that the number of activated T cells in the circulation is increased in the newly diagnosed patient with type 1 diabetes (see below) and that this pro-

gressively declines along with some of the other primary immunological phenomena, e.g. islet cell antibodies.

Lymphocyte function has also been examined using responses to non-specific mitogens, recall antigens and in the mixed lymphocyte reaction, with variable and conflicting results [5]. Few investigators have endeavoured to standardize for varying degrees of metabolic control or the variable interval from the clinical onset of diabetes. A recent study in which patients presenting with type 1 diabetes were matched for age and sex with control subjects did not reveal a significant difference between the responsiveness in vitro of peripheral blood lymphocytes to recall antigens [7].

Thus is it difficult to identify any consistent change in peripheral blood lymphocyte numbers or function in the reasonably well-controlled diabetic patient, and the case that many of the immunological abnormalities present in type 1 diabetes may be due to insulin deficiency [5] is very speculative.

Phagocytes

Disturbances in various aspects of phagocyte function, e.g. adherence, cell movement, phagocytosis and intracellular killing, have been described in diabetic subjects. Depressed neutrophil movement has been documented in patients with diabetes, and even in their non-diabetic, first-degree relatives [8, 9]. In some instances, the abnormality could be reversed by insulin and may relate to ion fluxes across the neutrophil cell membrane, but more recent studies using computer-assisted image analysis have not confirmed these findings [10].

Many of the methods used to examine the processes of phagocytosis or introcellular killing are relatively imprecise and involve microscopic evaluation of particle engulfment or counting of viable colonies of bacteria following incubation with phagocytic cells. The introduction of radiometric assays, involving the incorporation of isotopic labels into target organisms that have not been ingested or killed by phagocytic cells, offers greater precision, but their use is based on the assumption that the entire population of phagocytic cells is capable of phagocytosis. Assays involving flow cytometry allow the actual number of phagocytosing cells to be counted at any time point [11].

These variations in methodology may explain why some investigators appear to have detected perturbations of phagocytosis in the diabetic patient and have observed restoration with improvement in diabetic control [12]. However, in many instances these changes have been confined to the relatively wide range of values found in normal individuals.

Many of the documented abnormalities can be attributed to factors contained within the patient's serum used in conjunction with neutrophils during the assay procedure in vitro. We have examined neutrophil phagocytosis of *Candida albicans* in the presence of normal human serum and were unable to demonstrate any defect in phagocytosis despite the addition of 50 mmol/l glucose in vitro [13]. Phagocytosis is a robust procedure and it is very rare to observe a significant abnormality when appropriate methodology is used [14].

Intracellular killing is achieved by oxygen dependent and independent mechanisms [15]. Oxidative killing occurs early in the intracellular sequence of events and most of the respiratory activity takes place within the hexose monophosphate shunt, which provides NADPH as a fuel for the reduction of molecular oxygen. It is triggered by a membrane oxidase and culminates in the production of lytic oxygen compounds, e.g. superoxide, hydrogen peroxide, singlet oxygen, the hydroxyl radical and hypohalite. The neutrophil processes a relatively high flux of glucose through the hexose monophosphate shunt (HMPS). When insulin deficiency is present the glycolytic pathway is inhibited and this, in conjuction with the stress of hyperglycaemia, creates an excess of intracellular glucose (Figure 1), with profound effects on cell function.

Several studies point to significant changes in the bactericidal activity of neutrophils from diabetic subjects, and the stress of 50 mmol/l glucose and 20 mmol/l β-hydroxybutyrate used either independently or in combination in vitro can significantly inhibit the killing of *Candida albicans* by neutrophils taken from diabetic subjects [13]. The fact that these abnormalities were not seen when control neutrophils were incubated in a similar fashion suggests that the diabetic neutrophils possess a latent abnormality which can be demonstrated following the stress in vitro of conditions resembling diabetic ketoacidosis. Data obtained from chemilumi-

nescence studies have also shown that the same conditions in vitro suppress the generation of superoxide [16].

The importance of the polyol pathway in the development of various complications to the diabetic state is now well substantiated, and it seemed likely that this pathway is active in the neutrophil phagocyte. The excess glucose would then be converted to sorbitol following interaction with the NADPH-requiring enzyme aldose reductase (Figure 1). We have been able to identify the presence of sorbitol in biochemically stressed neutrophils, and have shown that intracellular killing can be inhibited by galactose which is unable to enter the HMPS but is readily metabolized via the polyol pathway to form another sugar alcohol—dulcitol [14]. Thus the impairment in oxidative killing seen in the diabetic neutrophil is likely to be due to competition for NADPH following induction of this pathway.

Thus, the most convincing and reproducible abnormalities of phagocyte function found in the diabetic subject are concerned with intracellular killing rather than with phagocytosis per se and are aggravated by worsening metabolic control [17]. However, many diabetic neutrophils possess a latent abnormality which can be revealed by reproducing the metabolic stress of hyperglycaemia and ketoacidosis in vitro. This is associated with induction of the polyol pathway and recent work shows that it develops comparatively slowly during the first few months of diabetes [18].

PRIMARY ABNORMALITIES PREDISPOSING TO INFECTION

Accumulating evidence points to the existence of an immunological crescendo prior to the clinical presentation of type 1 diabetes [19, 20]. Some of the pre-existing immunological abnormalities are likely to enhance susceptibility to infection. These considerations do not apply to type 2 or non-insulin dependent diabetes mellitus, in which immunological factors are largely absent [21].

Increased levels of activated T cells in the circulation of patients with type 1 diabetes is one of the most consistent findings [5]. The conflicting reports concerning alteration in individual lymphocyte subpopulations may well relate to the variable presence of lymphocyte-reactive

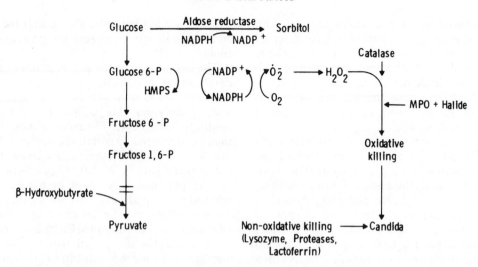

Figure 1 Glucose and β-hydroxybutyrate metabolism by polymorphonucleocytes in relation to oxidative killing. HMPS, hexose monophosphate shunt; MPO, myeloperoxidase

antibodies which in some instances shows specificity for individual T-cell subpopulations [22]. The predilection for certain viruses (e.g. coxsackie and rubella) to cause damage to islet cells, the presence of islet cell autoantibodies, as well as the close association with the possession of the HLA phenotypes DR3 and DR4, point to the likelihood that infective agents such as viruses have a triggering role in the pathogenetic sequence that culminates in the clinical expression of type 1 diabetes. With our present state of knowledge it is difficult to distinguish the primary abnormalities of the immune system which may be linked to the HLA-associated susceptibility from other changes that follow B-cell destruction. However, various studies have given indications that other component parts of the immune system may be defective ab initio, e.g. immunoglobulins and complement components, and recent work has demonstrated important abnormalities of the genes coding for these proteins. These findings will have a major impact on the way we think about the pathogenetic sequence.

Immunoglobulins

Examination of serum immunoglobulin levels in diabetic subjects has shown a significant reduction in the levels of IgG and IgA and the latter

abnormality is much more common in patients bearing the HLA-B8-DR3 haplotype [23, 24]. The levels of various kinds of specific antibody have been measured in diabetic populations and have usually been found to show no significant difference from controls, as, for example, with levels of antibody to pneumococcal polysaccharide [25]. Much attention has been focused on antibodies to the coxsackie group of viruses and a number of reports have suggested that coxsackie antibody levels are elevated in patients with type 1 diabetes of recent onset—a finding compatible with the proposal that the disease is triggered by recent infection with these viruses [26–29]. However, many of these studies are plagued by the absence of contemporary controls. Matching was possible in one study in which a large number of non-diabetic individuals had been examined as part of a viral surveillance project and this enabled matched pairs to be obtained at a time when an outbreak of coxsackie infection (of types B3, B4 and B5) occurred [30]. These data showed that antibody titres to coxsackie B3 and B4 were *lower* in the diabetic subjects and that a low antibody titre was associated with a significantly increased risk of diabetes. The other studies cited above do contain data indicating that younger subjects presenting with type 1 diabetes have lower coxsackie antibody titres than non-diabetic controls, and this association merits examination.

Complement

In addition to bearing the class I and class II HLA loci, the short arm of human chromosome 6 also carries several genes that code for components of the complement pathways, e.g. C2, C4 and factor B. Each of these gene loci show polymorphism, and patients with type 1 diabetes possess a high incidence of uncommon alleles of these components. However, it is only recently that much attention has been paid to the possibility that the serum of such patients may show a significant reduction in the quantity and functional activity of these components. Low C4 levels—often associated with the possession of the C4a null gene—are present in about 25% of patients with type 1 diabetes [31] and abnormalities of other components, e.g. C1q and C3, have also been documented [32]. The genes that code for some of these allelic variants are known to exist in linkage disequilibrium with certain HLA haplotypes, e.g. the C4a null gene is much more commonly found within the HLA-B8-DR3 haplotype [33]. It is therefore possible that the initial susceptibility to the development of type 1 diabetes is linked to deficient complement function as much as to the HLA loci themselves, and recent work indicates that genes coding for other immunologically important molecules, e.g. the lymphokine tumour necrosis factor (TNF), are also found between the class I and class II HLA loci. Studies in mice indicate that absence of these genes may be implicated in the aetiology of autoimmune disease and that disease severity can be ameliorated by administration of the deficient material [34].

It is therefore of considerable interest that more detailed analysis of this entire stretch of chromosome 6, using Southern blotting and pulsed-field gel electrophoresis, has recently revealed considerable heterogeneity for the size of some of these complement genes and the presence of large deletions in some individual haplotypes associated with susceptibility to type 1 diabetes as well as other HLA-related disorders [35, 36].

Thus, susceptibility to type 1 diabetes may be due to deficiency of component molecules of the immune system (e.g. IgA, C3, TNF) which renders the subject more prone to infection with viruses, some of which have a predilection for B cells.

CONCLUSION

The prevalence of infection in the well-controlled diabetic patient is little different from that of normal subjects. Nevertheless, the ideal of metabolic control is not achievable in all patients and the greater the tendency to hyperglycaemia and ketosis, the greater the likelihood that serious infection will develop.

High glucose concentrations and tissue hypoxia encourage the growth of mixed aerobic and anaerobic populations and some of the rare diabetes-specific problems are associated with bacterial fermentation and gas production.

The phagocyte bears the brunt of the abnormalities associated with poor metabolic control of diabetes. The biochemical events necessary for generating the oxidative burst that mediates intracellular killing are most susceptible to this abnormal milieu, and the abnormalities that ensue are associated with induction of the polyol pathway which competes for supplies of NADPH.

Several primary abnormalities pre-exist in the type 1 diabetic patient and these are also likely to predispose to infections, particularly with viruses which may have an aetiological role in its causation. Recent evidence indicates that patients bearing the HLA susceptibility genes show abnormalities of other loci which code for complement and other immunologically important components. It is therefore possible that the susceptibility to type 1 diabetes takes the form of partial immunodeficiency, which then renders the patient less able to mount an effective immune response against the triggering viruses, e.g. coxsackie and rubella.

These underlying abnormalities should make physicians think twice before proceeding with immunosuppressive regimens for the treatment or prevention of type 1 diabetes, and raise the possibility that correction of these deficiencies —possibly in conjunction with active immunization—may be a more profitable avenue to explore in the future.

REFERENCES

1. Lipsky BA, Pecoraro RE, Chen MS, Koepsell TD. Factors affecting staphylococcal colonization among NIDDM outpatients. Diabetes Care 1987; 10: 483–6.
2. Rayfield EJ, Ault MJ, Keusch GT, Brothers MJ, Nechemias C, Smith H. Infection and diabetes:

the case for glucose control. Am J Med 1982; 72: 439–50.

3. Wheat LJ. Infection and diabetes mellitus. Diabetes Care 1980; 3: 187–97.

4. Selam JL, Clot J, Andary M, Mirouze J. Circulating lymphocyte subpopulations in juvenile insulin-dependent diabetes: correction of abnormalities by adequate blood glucose control. Diabetologia 1979; 16: 35–40.

5. Drell DW, Notkins AL. Multiple immunological abnormalities in patients with type I (insulin dependent) diabetes mellitus. Diabetologia 1987; 30: 132–43.

6. Pontesilli O, Chase HP, Carotenuto P, Herberger MJ, Hayward AR. T-lymphocyte subpopulations in insulin-dependent (type I) diabetes mellitus. Clin Exp Immunol 1986; 63: 68–72.

7. Gregory R, Reeves WG. T cell reactivity in newly diagnosed diabetic patients and the effect of treatment with isophane insulins. Diabetologia 1987; 30: 525A.

8. Mowat AG, Baum J. Chemotaxis of polymorphonuclear leukocytes from patients with diabetes mellitus. New Engl J Med 1971; 284: 621–7.

9. Molenaar DM, Palumbo PJ, Wilson WR, Ritts RE. Leukocyte chemotaxis in diabetic patients and their non-diabetic first-degree relatives. Diabetes 1970; 25 (suppl. 2): 880–3.

10. Donovan RM, Goldstein TE, Kim Y et al. A computer-assisted image-analysis system for analysing polymorphonuclear leukocyte chemotaxis in patients with diabetes mellitus. J Infect Dis 1987; 155: 737–41.

11. Wilson RM, Galvin AM, Robins RA, Reeves WG. A flow cytometric method for the measurement of phagocytosis of candida by polymorphonuclear leucocytes. J Immunol Meth 1985; 76: 247–53.

12. Gin H, Brother E, Aubertin J. Influence of glycaemic normalisation by an artificial pancreas on phagocytic and bactericidal functions of granulocytes in insulin-dependent diabetic patients. J Chem Path 1984; 37: 1029–31.

13. Wilson RM, Reeves WG. Neutrophil phagocytosis and killing in insulin-dependent diabetes. Clin Exp Immunol 1986; 63: 478–84.

14. Wilson RM, Reeves WG. Neutrophil function in diabetes. In Nattrass M (ed.) Recent advances in diabetes 2. Edinburgh: Churchill Livingstone, 1986: pp 127–39.

15. Reeves WG. Lecture notes on immunology. Oxford; Blackwell, 1987.

16. Wilson RM, Tomlinson DR, Reeves WG. Neutrophil sorbitol production impairs oxidative killing in diabetes. Diabet Med 1987; 4: 37–40.

17. Miller ME. In Gupta S (ed.) Immunology

18. Wilson RM, Tebbs SE, Munro DS, Hardisty CA. Induction of neutrophil polyol pathway 1 year following diagnosis of diabetes. Diabet Med 1988; 5 (suppl): 19.

19. Eisenbarth GS. Type I diabetes mellitus—a chronic autoimmune disease. New Engl J Med 1986; 21: 1360–8.

20. Tarn AC, Al-Sakkaf L, Gale EAM. Autoimmunity in prediabetes. Clin Immun Allergy, 1987; 1: 165–86.

21. Rossini AA, Mordes JP, Handler ES. Perspectives in diabetes. Speculations on etiology of diabetes mellitus. Tumbler hypothesis. Diabetes 1988; 7: 257–61.

22. Herold KC, Huen A, Gould L, Traisman H, Rubenstein AH. Alterations in lymphocyte subpopulations in type I (insulin-dependent) diabetes mellitus: exploration of possible mechanisms and relationships to autoimmune phenomena. Diabetologia 1984; 27: 102–5.

23. Smith WI, Rabin BS, Huellmantel A, van Thiel DH, Drash A. Immunopathology of juvenile-onset diabetes mellitus. I. IgA deficiency and juvenile diabetes. Diabetes 1978; 27: 1092–7.

24. Hoddinott S, Dornan J, Bear JC, Farid NR. Immunoglobulin levels, immunodeficiency and HLA in type I (insulin-dependent) diabetes mellitus. Diabetologia 1982; 23: 326–9.

25. Lederman MM, Rodman HM, Schacter BZ, Jones PK, Schiffman G. Antibody response to pneumococcal polysaccharides in insulin-dependent diabetes mellitus. Diabetes Care 1982; 5: 36–9.

26. Gamble DR, Taylor KW, Cumming H. Coxsackie viruses and diabetes mellitus. Br Med J 1973; 4: 260–2.

27. Yoon JW, Austin M, Onodera T, Notkins AL. Virus-induced diabetes mellitus. New Engl J Med 1979; 300: 1173–9.

28. Sakurami T, Nabeya N, Nagaoka K, Matsumori A, Kuno S, Honda A. Antibodies to Coxsackie B viruses and HLA in Japanese with juvenile-onset type I (insulin-dependent) diabetes mellitus. Diabetologia 1982; 22: 375–7.

29. Banatvala JE, Bryant J, Schernthaner G. Coxsackie B, mumps, rubella and cytomegalovirus specific IgM responses in patients with juvenile onset insulin-dependent diabetes mellitus in Britain, Austria and Australia. Lancet 1985; i: 1409.

30. Palmer JP et al. Reduced Coxsackie antibody titres in type I (insulin-dependent) diabetic patients presenting during an outbreak of Coxsackie B3 and B4 infection. Diabetologia 1982; 22: 426–9.

of clinical and experimental diabetes. 1984; pp 369–83.

31. Vergani D, Johnston C, B-Abdullah N, Barnett AH. Low serum C4 concentrations: an inherited predisposition to insulin dependent diabetes? Br Med J 1983; 286: 943–8.

32. Charlesworth JA et al. The complement system in type I insulin-dependent diabetes. Diabetologia 1987; 30: 372–9.

33. Rich S, O'Neill A, Dalmasso P, Nerl C, Barbosa J. Complement and HLA. Further definition of high-risk haplotypes in insulin-dependent diabetes. Diabetes 1985; 34: 504–9.

34. Jacob CO, McDevitt HO. Tumour necrosis factor-a in murine autoimmune 'lupus' nephritis. Nature 1988; 331: 356–8.

35. Palsdottir A, Fossdal R, Arnason A. Heterogeneity of human C4 gene size: large intron (6.5 kb) is present in all C4A genes and some C4B genes. Immunogenetics 1987; 25: 299–304.

36. Kay PH, Martin E, Dawkins RL, Charoenwong P. Class III gene rearrangements in Thai/Chinese supratypes containing null or defective C4 alleles. Immunogenetics 1988; 27: 46–50.

50

The Care of the Diabetic Patient During Surgery

G.V. Gill* and K.G.M.M. Alberti†
** Walton Hospital, Liverpool, UK, and † Department of Medicine,
University of Newcastle upon Tyne, UK*

Most diabetic patients will require some sort of surgical procedure at some time in their lives. Surgery seriously interferes with normal diabetic control, and a careful and logical method of planned management is therefore required.

There are many ways in which surgery interferes with carbohydrate metabolism and glucose homeostasis. These mechanisms are outlined in Table 1. They occur in normal patients, but are greatly exaggerated in states of partial or complete relative insulin deficiency, i.e. in non-insulin dependent diabetes mellitus (NIDDM, type 2) and insulin dependent diabetes mellitus (IDDM, type 1) respectively.

The disease requiring surgical intervention may itself cause metabolic decompensation (e.g. abscesses, peritonitis, malignancy). Patient anxiety does not help, and anaesthesia can also adversely affect carbohydrate metabolism [1]. Additionally, surgery is always associated with a period of starvation, and some degree of infective risk. Finally, and perhaps most importantly, the trauma of surgical operation evokes a characteristic hormonal and metabolic response leading to catabolism, hyperglycaemia and ketogenic risks [2].

METABOLIC RESPONSES TO SURGERY

In normal subjects, the basic metabolic processes of anabolism and catabolism are finely and exactly balanced. The controlling influences on this system are essentially hormonal. Insulin is the only significant anabolic hormone, but several are associated with catabolism, notably cortisol, glucagon and catecholamines. Thus, in very basic terms, insulin will promote tissue glucose uptake, and glycogen formation in liver and muscle, as well as promoting protein synthesis and lipogenesis. Conversely, the catabolic hormones (also known as 'stress' or 'counterregulatory' hormones) will oppose the actions of insulin by stimulating glycogen breakdown, gluconeogenesis, lipolysis and inhibition of protein synthesis.

In the fed state, when insulin levels in the blood are high, anabolism predominates; on fasting, as insulin levels decline, metabolism swings towards catabolism. It should be noted, however, that even during fasting a small amount of 'basal' insulin is secreted to prevent excessive and deleterious catabolism.

The key role of insulin can thus be readily seen, in containing the catabolic drive promoted by the 'massed bands' of the counterregulatory

International Textbook of Diabetes Mellitus. Edited by K.G.M.M. Alberti, R.A. DeFronzo, H. Keen and P. Zimmet
© 1992 John Wiley & Sons Ltd

Table 1 Surgery and diabetes: factors adversely affecting diabetic control

1. Anxiety
2. Starvation
3. Anaesthetic drugs
4. Infection
5. Metabolic response to trauma
6. Diseases underlying need for surgery
7. Other drugs, e.g. steroids

ensemble. In the insulin deficient state associated with, for example, untreated IDDM, restraints to excessive catabolism are limited or non-existent. Even when a fixed amount of basal insulin is present, prolonged fasting, trauma or infection may lead to dangerously excessive glucose production and lipid breakdown.

The hormonal and metabolic changes associated with surgical trauma are well described [3], and are outlined in Table 2. Generally, the degree of metabolic change is related to the severity of trauma, and responses are exaggerated and prolonged if complications, such as sepsis, occur [1]. The prime changes are hormonal, and secretory patterns seem to be altered mainly by neural mechanisms, although the release of stimulatory 'wound hormones' is still postulated [2]. Almost immediately after the onset of trauma, the concentration of serum ACTH (and thereby of cortisol) rises, to be followed by catecholamines, glucagon and growth hormone. More variable (and less important) are rises in levels of serum aldosterone, prolactin, vasopressin and thyroid hormones. Insulin secretion is relatively reduced during trauma, and insulin resistance is commonly found [1]. This insulin insensitivity occurs even after moderate uncomplicated surgery and is a postreceptor effect [4].

The metabolic results of these hormonal changes (Table 2) are glucose release into the

Table 2 Summary of metabolic and hormonal responses to surgical trauma

Hormonal changes	Metabolic changes
'Stress hormone' secretion:	Increased gluconeogenesis
cortisol	and glycogenolysis
catecholamines	Hyperglycaemia
glucagon	Lipolysis
growth hormone	Protein breakdown
cytokines	
Relative decrease in insulin secretion	
Peripheral insulin resistance	

circulation via glycogenolysis and gluconeogenesis, as well as fat and protein breakdown. Despite the insulin resistance there is sufficient insulin to suppress lipolysis and there is thus less non-esterified fatty acid available for ketogenesis [5]. The lack of ketone bodies is associated with increased proteolysis [6], the amino acids being used for gluconeogenesis. The overall scenario is one of intense catabolism, particularly in more traumatic surgical operations. Risks of metabolic decompensation are enhanced by the preoperative and postoperative starvation that accompanies operations. The key for the diabetic patient is the inability to increase insulin secretion to counteract the increases in the catabolic hormones.

For more details of the metabolic and hormonal response to trauma in normal and diabetic humans, the reader is directed to other reviews on the subject [2, 7–10].

PRINCIPLES OF MANAGING DIABETES DURING SURGERY

Principles of management depend mainly on the ability of the patient to secrete adequate amounts of insulin [11]. Thus, patients on insulin treatment should be considered to be insulin dependent, and assumed to have no effective insulin reserves. For these patients, a management protocol must include continuous provision of insulin and glucose if the intense catabolic drives of trauma and starvation are to be survived; this is true for all grades of surgery.

Patients *not* on insulin treatment (i.e. on dietary and/or drug treatment) may be considered to be non-insulin dependent, and can be assumed to have some endogenous insulin reserves, albeit limited. Insulin therapy is less essential here for mild degrees of surgical trauma, although insulin supplementation will be needed for more severe operations. The patient's own insulin will inhibit lipolysis and ketosis, and usually prevent excessive hyperglycaemia with minor stress, but will be inadequate for more severe grades of surgery. These principles are summarized in Table 3.

RISKS OF SURGERY ASSOCIATED WITH DIABETES

In the past, diabetes was considered to be a major cause of increased mortality during sur-

Table 3 Principles of managing diabetes during surgery

Diabetics on insulin treatment	Assume to have no insulin reserves. Provide continuous insulin and glucose for all grades of surgery
Diabetics not on insulin treatment	Assume to have limited insulin reserves. Observe only (if reasonably controlled), unless surgery is major, when continuous insulin and glucose should be used as above

Table 4 Management aims for diabetic patients undergoing surgery

1. No excess mortality
2. No increase in postoperative complications (especially infective)
3. Normal wound healing
4. No increase in the duration of hospitalization
5. No hypoglycaemia
6. No ketoacidosis or severe hyperglycaemia

gery [9]. Precise and useful data from earlier years are hard to find, although one study from the USA in 1963 reported an immediate postoperative mortality rate of 24 out of 487 (4.9%) [12]. In their discussion, the authors of that report referred to considerably higher rates for other centres. The main causes of mortality were myocardial infarction, ketoacidosis and infection. Important factors underlying these unacceptable risks probably included suboptimal glycaemic control amongst the diabetic population in general at the time, and imperfect methods of operative and postoperative diabetic care.

Recent evidence, however, suggests that surgery is now safe for diabetic patients in terms of both mortality and morbidity. Thus, using treatment regimens based on the principles outlined above, Hjortrup and colleagues [13] reported a mortality of 5 out of 224 (2.2%) diabetic patients undergoing surgery, compared with 6 out of 224 (2.7%) non-diabetic controls. Postoperative complications occurred in 46 (20.5%) of each group, and in particular infections (wound, chest and urinary) were not significantly different in either group. One curious feature of this study was that diabetic subjects who developed postoperative complications had slightly but significantly *lower* blood glucose values before, during and after surgery compared with those who had uncomplicated recoveries. This lack of an increase in morbidity and mortality was confirmed in another study by the same workers [14], as well as during biliary surgery [15] and coronary artery bypass grafting [16], although there was a tendency for there to be more postoperative sepsis in the biliary surgery patients.

AIMS OF TREATMENT

When preparing detailed protocols of care for diabetic patients during surgery, it is important to be clear about the exact aims of treatment. Ideal aims are outlined in Table 4, and it will be apparent from the discussion in the previous section that the first four aims, i.e. no excess in mortality and morbidity, should be achievable provided that a logical system of diabetic care is employed. The setting of metabolic targets is more difficult, however. Excessive hyperglycaemia is to be avoided as it increases the risk of decompensation into ketoacidosis, and also promotes dehydration and electrolyte imbalance. Infection is also more likely because of impaired phagocytic function [17], and wound healing is impaired, at least experimentally [18]. On the other hand, overdiligent attempts to induce normoglycaemia may lead to hypoglycaemia—a particular hazard for anaesthetized or postoperative patients, who will have to rely on others for its detection. There is, indeed, no clear evidence that excellent glycaemic control improves outcome; indeed, as mentioned previously, the study of Hjortrup et al [13] suggested that particularly 'good' control was associated with greater risks of postoperative morbidity. A reasonable practical compromise is to aim for operative and postoperative blood glucose levels in the region of 6–12 mmol/l [11].

PREOPERATIVE ASSESSMENT OF DIABETES

All diabetic patients requiring surgery will need assessment of their diabetes, and possibly some changes in management. Table 5 outlines the requirements of preoperative assessment. Admission a little earlier than usual may be needed, and blood glucose levels must be measured regularly. This is usually done by 'bedside' monitoring with reagent test strips at least four times daily. Treatment may need to be rationalized, and in particular, excessively long-acting preparations such as the sulphonylureas, chlorpropamide and glibenclamide, and ultralente

Table 5 Preoperative assessment and management of the diabetic patient undergoing surgery

1. Admit 2–3 days prior to surgery (ideally)*
2. Make general medical assessment (cardiac, renal, etc.)
3. Avoid long-acting blood glucose lowering agents (e.g. chlorpropamide, glibenclamide, ultralente insulins)
4. Avoid metformin
5. Closely monitor blood glucose levels
6. Optimize glycaemic control—if necessary, use insulin
7. Arrange surgery in the morning
8. Cooperate closely with the anaesthetist

* It is often not possible to admit patients more than 24 hours preoperatively, and many may be dealt with as day cases. Improvement of glycaemic control, adjustment of therapy and full preoperative assessment should then be done on an outpatient basis.

Table 6 Surgical management in NIDDM

1. Ensure reasonable preoperative glycaemic control
2. Operate in the morning if possible
3. If the patient is taking oral hypoglycaemic agents, omit these on the morning of surgery
4. Avoid glucose-containing IV fluids
5. Restart oral hypoglycaemic agents with the first postoperative meal
6. Monitor glucose levels with test strips every 2 hours initially, reducing frequency later as necessary

If preoperative control is poor, or if the surgery is major, treat the patient as insulin dependent.

insulin, are best discontinued; their effect may last well into the operative and even post-operative period, and will complicate optimal management. The biguanide drug metformin is also best avoided, in case there is postoperative renal insufficiency, which is associated with lactic acidosis in metformin-treated patients.

If diabetic control needs to be improved, the treatments may include the addition of a short-acting sulphonylurea drug for those previously on diet alone, increase in drug doses for those already on sulphonylureas, or substitution with insulin if patients are on maximum doses of drugs or very poorly controlled. The insulin system used in such patients should be as flexible as possible to allow rapid adjustments. Commonly, soluble (regular) insulin is used three times daily before food, with a small amount of isophane or lente insulin at night if morning hyperglycaemia is a problem. These patients should be regarded as insulin dependent, and should be treated as such during and after surgery.

Patients with IDDM may need dose alterations to optimize control. Most patients will already be on twice-daily or multiple dose insulin injection regimens, so the basic form of treatment should not need changing. Once-daily regimens will usually require to be changed to two or three injections daily, except in insulin-treated NIDDM patients who are not using ultralente insulins and who have adequate fasting blood glucose levels. This latter is an important requirement of any preoperative diabetic treatment. If the patient is hyperglycaemic immediately preoperatively, blood glucose levels tend to remain high or may even escalate—despite reasonable protocols of operative management.

As well as attending to diabetic control, general medical assessment is essential. Particular attention should be paid to those systems affected by diabetes: heart, peripheral circulation, peripheral and autonomic nerve systems, renal function and blood pressure. Chest radiography and electrocardiography may well be needed, while renal function should be tested by measurement of serum creatinine and electrolyte levels. Urine culture should be routinely performed in older patients. Autonomic neuropathy is a particular risk because of its association with sudden death perioperatively [19]. Finally, it is vital that full and complete liaison is made with the anaesthetic staff involved, so that they are aware of the diabetic patient and any problems, as well as the operative management system planned.

Some years ago Podolsky [20] suggested that much of this preoperative assessment could be done on an outpatient basis. This is undoubtedly true, and it is regrettable that this system rarely operates. Excessive hospitalization of surgical diabetic patients almost always occurs in the preoperative phase. It is usually due to poor planning, and is very costly.

SURGICAL MANAGEMENT IN NIDDM

Management of non-insulin dependent patients for minor surgery is outlined in Table 6. There is general agreement that a conservative approach is reasonable, provided that (a) blood glucose control is reasonable, and (b) the planned surgery is not major. In the latter case, management should be as for insulin-treated patients (see next section). Otherwise, insulin is not required and only observation of blood glucose control is needed, together with omission of oral hypoglycaemic agents (OHA) immediately before surgery, if the patient is on such treatment. Glucose and insulin delivery systems are unnecessarily complex, do not give any better glycaemic control, and, indeed, may induce a rather distorted profile of blood metabolite levels [21, 22].

Morning surgery is not essential but it is helpful. If postoperative problems arise these are more easily dealt with in the afternoon or evening rather than the middle of the night! In fact, intervention is very rarely required for excessively high perioperative or postoperative blood glucose levels in response to regular monitoring. One important point is to ensure that the patient receives no glucose-containing intravenous fluids. Anaesthetists are particularly fond of 5% dextrose or dextrose–saline solutions. Similarly, lactate-containing infusion fluids (e.g. Hartmann's or Ringer-lactate solutions) should not be used as they can have hyperglycaemic effects [23]. Once again, this demonstrates the importance of liaison with anaesthetic and surgical staff.

SURGICAL MANAGEMENT IN IDDM

Historical Aspects

Twenty-five years ago, recommendations for the management of IDDM patients undergoing surgery included the complete omission of insulin until after operation [24], a system not surprisingly associated with hyperglycaemia and very significant ketotic risk (see reference 7 for review). Following this, there developed systems of continuing subcutaneous (SC) insulin and 'covering' the period of fasting with intravenous (IV) glucose infusions. These systems were generally successful, but tended to be rather complex. They remained popular up to 5–10 years ago, and a great many were described. Some recommended the usual morning SC insulin prior to operation [25], some isophane insulin only [26], some a variety of fractions of morning doses [27, 28]. Regimens of IV glucose infusion usually involved fairly arbitrary amounts of 5% or 10% dextrose (glucose). Postoperative insulin delivery with all these methods was difficult and often haphazard until the patient was able to eat. Generally, intermittent boluses of soluble insulin were suggested, often by a post hoc 'sliding scale' method. Review of the literature shows the rather poor glycaemic control obtained with the SC regimens; postoperative mean glucose levels ranged from 11.3 mmol/l [29]

to 30.2 mmol/l [30] with only one below 10 mmol/l [31]; the latter was during minor surgery.

Dissatisfaction with these complicated and inflexible regimens led to the increased popularity of intravenous insulin systems over the last decade. The first major report [26] suggested the use of a low-dose insulin infusion with separate IV glucose delivery. This has evolved to a separate-line system still frequently used. A constant glucose infusion (e.g. 100 ml 10% glucose per hour) is given preferably by electronic drip counter, while 'piggy-backed' to this (by Y-connector) is an IV insulin infusion given by syringe pump (usually 50 units short-acting insulin in 50 ml 0.9% saline, i.e. 1 unit/ml). The insulin infusion rate is altered according to regular bedside blood glucose monitoring, with the initial insulin dose usually 3 units per hour. The system is flexible and physiological, but requires special apparatus and is labour intensive. It is best reserved for situations where close attention can be paid to the patient and the infusions—for example during labour in IDDM patients, and during serious intercurrent illness requiring care on intensive therapy or coronary care units.

A variety of complex algorithms have been developed using separate IV insulin and glucose infusions. The most complex is that of Meyers et al [32]—the 'two-step' protocol, which involves complex calculations and periodic IV insulin boluses. Such a system is ripe for catastrophe in the average surgical unit. Others are more simple, such as those of Woodruff et al [33] and Watts et al [34], although the latter, perhaps inadvisably, only starts postoperatively. There has even recently been an unwelcome return to insulin-free treatment. A group of patients were given IV saline and insulin added only if blood glucose levels exceeded 11.1 mmol/l [35]. It was reported that only 40% of those previously on insulin needed this adjunctive insulin. However, no mention is made of other aspects of metabolism such as ketonaemia and protein breakdown.

A particular worry of the separate-line glucose and insulin method is that if one line should block, fail or dislodge, then danagerous hypoglycaemia or hyperglycaemia will result, depending on which infusion stops. This problem, together with the need for a simpler system, has led to the widespread introduction of combined glucose and insulin infusions.

Glucose, Potassium and Insulin Infusion

Although there are many variations in use, the
basic system of glucose, potassium and insulin
infusion remains essentially that described by
Alberti and Thomas in 1979 [7]. Infusion of
500 ml 10% dextrose containing 10 U short-acting
insulin and 10 mmol potassium chloride (KCl)
was recommended to prevent hypokalaemia.
The infusion was given at a rate of 100 ml per
hour (i.e. 500 ml in 5 hours), thus delivering 2 U
insulin, 2 mmol KCl and 10 g glucose each hour.
The system has become known as GKI (glucose–
KCl–insulin) or GIK.

It is interesting that the present GKI system
was initially described in almost its exact present
form by Galloway and Shuman in 1963 [12].
They recorded a method of management involving 'regular insulin in intravenous glucose
infusions, usually in doses ranging from 0.16 to
0.20 units per gram of glucose', which equates
with 10 U insulin in 500 ml 10% glucose.

As a result of the initial results [7] the amount
of insulin in GKI solutions was increased.
Husband and colleagues in 1985 [36] increased
the insulin to 16 U per 500 ml 10% glucose
(0.32 U/g glucose). With this mixture, over 80%
of their series of 128 patients achieved target
blood glucose levels of 5–12 mmol/l on the
operative day, and most of the apparent failures
were due to the system not being operated properly. Since the introduction of U100 insulin, the
amount added to the glucose infusion has been
adapted to the more metric 15 U of insulin
(0.3 U/g). An alternative is to use 5% dextrose
with 5–10 units per 500 ml, again given at 100 ml
per hour [37]. We prefer the 10% glucose-based
mixture as this gives more energy (5000 kJ)
rather than (2500 kJ per 24 hours).

GKI is started on the morning of surgery—
the patient receiving no food or subcutaneous
insulin—and is continued during and after surgery until diet and subcutaneous insulin can be
safely restarted. Bedside blood glucose levels are
measured regularly, and if too high, then a fresh
GKI bag contining 20 U insulin is set up. Similarly, low levels will require a reduction of GKI
to 10 U per bag. A suggested algorithm for GKI
adjustment is shown in Table 7, although in fact
such infusion changes are not often needed.

Continuous glucose and insulin infusions
are simple and flexible, and give good glycaemic results (Table 8). These results compare

Table 7 Algorithm for adjusting insulin content of GKI
infusion

1. Measure blood glucose levels with test strips every
   2 hours*
2. Adjust infusion as follows:
     blood glucose 6.5–11 mmol/l → usual GKI
     (15 U per 500 ml)
     blood glucose over 11 mmol/l → increase to 20 units
     blood glucose under 6.5 mmol/l → decrease to 10
     units
3. Continue to adjust in 5-unit increments as necessary

* Frequency of monitoring is variable and depends on the individual
clinical situation. Levels can usually be measured less frequently as time
progresses.

well with other reports of IV insulin regimens
(reviewed in reference 9). Because of the simultaneous mixed delivery of glucose and insulin,
there is a much smaller risk of unexpected
severe hypoglycaemia or hyperglycaemia compared with the separate-line system. The ratio of
insulin to glucose remains constant whatever the
infusion rate; the use of electronic dripcounters
is, therefore, not essential.

In the elderly or those with heart failure, a
standard GKI infusion may lead to fluid overload. Here, the infusion rate may be slowed a
little (e.g. to 6–8 hours per 500 ml), or the concentration of glucose can be doubled to 20%
(the rate of infusion is extended to 10-hourly or
50 ml/hour, and the potassium and insulin content also doubled). In certain predictable conditions insulin requirement may be increased.
These include severe obesity (body mass index
greater than 30), hepatic cirrhosis, sepsis and
steroid therapy (Table 9). In these situations the
initial GKI mixture should contain an appropriately increased amount of insulin.

As with all patients on intravenous fluid
therapy, plasma urea and electrolytes need to be
measured daily. The KCl content of the infusion
in particular may need altering, and for safety
plasma potassium levels should be checked 4–6
hours postoperatively. With prolonged GKI,
serious dilutional hyponatraemia may occasionally occur. If plasma sodium levels begin to fall,
and continued GKI is needed, then 0.9% (isotonic) saline infusion should be given at the same
time. Absorption of insulin on to the plastic
surfaces of infusion bags and giving sets is a
theoretical rather than a practical problem [38].
The previously suggested practices of adding

Table 8 Results of a GKI-based system of surgical diabetes care

Time	Blood glucose in mmol/l (mean ± SD)		
	NIDDM* Observation only	NIDDM** GKI infusion	IDDM** GKI infusion
Preoperative	7.4 ± 2.0	7.9 ± 2.5	8.2 ± 3.0
Postoperative	8.5 ± 3.2	10.2 ± 3.9	9.6 ± 3.4
Mean operative day	8.2 ± 1.8	9.3 ± 2.2	8.9 ± 2.3
Mean first postoperative day	8.2 ± 1.9	8.7 ± 1.6	9.4 ± 1.9
Mean second postoperative day	8.4 ± 1.9	8.8 ± 1.8	10.2 ± 2.8

* Minor surgery.
** Major and minor surgery.
Adapted from reference 36.

blood or albumin to the infusion are unnecessary, although it is wise to discard the first 25–50 ml of GKI solution by running it through the infusion set, before connecting with the patient; this is said to saturate the 'binding sites' of the plastic for insulin. Perhaps a more important problem concerns adding insulin to the drip bag via too short an insulin syringe, allowing 'trapping' of the insulin near the entry port, and inadequate mixing [39].

ORGANIZATION OF CARE FOR THE SURGICAL DIABETIC PATIENT

Thai and colleagues [40] have advocated the formation of a 'diabetic team' to supervise the care of diabetic patients undergoing surgery. The team consists of doctors belonging to the diabetic unit, who on a rotational basis act as the point of referral for diabetic surgical patients. The doctor visits appropriate surgical wards on a daily basis, making preoperative assessments, ordering operative protocols, consulting with ward and anaesthetic staff, and adjusting postoperative treatment as necessary. Compared with care by surgical or anaesthetic staff alone, better glycaemic control and more consistent management systems amongst the team-cared patients were reported by Thai and co-workers

Table 9 Conditions associated with increased insulin requirement during surgery in diabetic patients

	Insulin requirement (U/g glucose)
Uncomplicated	0.30
Liver disease	0.4–0.6
Severe obesity	0.4–0.6
Major infection/sepsis	0.6–0.8
Steroid therapy	0.5–0.8

[40]. Mortality and morbidity in both groups of patients were, however, similar.

Although attractive, the team approach is expensive in terms of physician time, and it is likely that only major teaching centres will have sufficient staff resources to mount such a scheme; most district hospitals will have to rely on surgical and anaesthetic staff to operate diabetic care in surgical patients. Certain safeguards can be taken, however: there must be full agreement between medical, surgical and anaesthetic staff on the protocol to be used, and it is up to the hospital diabetes specialist to initiate and organize this dialogue. A simple, clear and concise summary of the protocol must then be prepared (Table 10), and widely-distributed among the medical and nursing staff involved. Sufficient copies should be available so that it can be carried in any doctor's coat pocket and be seen on any notice board. The diabetes unit can then be used as a 'troubleshooting' focus only, providing advice for particularly difficult problems.

A final point of organization concerns the accuracy of bedside blood glucose monitoring. Serious errors in such extralaboratory tests can occur [41], which can seriously interfere with the smooth running and efficacy of a GKI infusion-based system. It is therefore wise to perform intermittent laboratory blood glucose level assessments on surgical diabetic patients, as a check on bedside testing. We routinely send the fasting blood glucose sample for laboratory measurement, as well as using the bedside test strip method. Additionally, all hospitals should have some form of structured education programme for test-strip blood glucose monitoring, as well as a quality control scheme to ensure its accuracy [42].

Table 10   Summarized protocol of diabetic care for surgical procedures

1. Ensure reasonable preoperative control. Operate in the morning if possible
2. Cooperate closely with anaesthetist
3. Omit patient's breakfast, and insulin or oral hypoglycaemic drug, on morning of surgery
4. **Non-insulin treated diabetic patients** having non-major surgery need observation only. Chart 2-hourly test-strip glucose results on day of surgery. If patient on oral hypoglycaemic drugs, restart with next meal
5. **Glucose–potassium–insulin** (GKI) is used in all other cases, i.e. all insulin-treated diabetic patients and for major surgery in non-insulin-treated diabetic patients

    (i) At 8–9 a.m. on morning of surgery commence GKI infusion:
        500 ml 10% dextrose
        + 15 units soluble (regular) insulin
        + 10 mmol KCl
        Infuse 5-hourly (100 ml per hour)
    (ii) Check blood glucose levels 2-hourly initially with test strips: aim for 6.5–11 mmol/l. If glucose level above 11 mmol/l, change to GKI with 20 U Actrapid; if glucose level below 6.5 mmol/l, change to GKI with 10 U Actrapid. Continue to adjust in 5-unit steps as necessary. Check plasma potassium levels 4–6 hours postoperatively
    (iii) Continue GKI till patient eats, then revert to usual treatment. If GKI is prolonged (more than 24 hours), check urea and electrolytes daily (and consider further nutritional support)

SPECIAL SURGICAL SITUATIONS

Open Heart Surgery

Although cardiac surgery is nowadays confined to specialist centres, within such centres diabetic patients represent a large proportion of the patients operated upon, because of the strong association between NIDDM and coronary artery disease. It was reported in 1981 [43] that control of diabetic patients undergoing open heart surgery was difficult, and that insulin requirements during and immediately after surgery were variable and high (about three times that during 'normal' types of operation). This has been confirmed by other workers [44] and implies severe insulin resistance [45]. This has been attributed to the severe degree of trauma, induced hypothermia and inotropic cardiac drugs. The use of glucose-containing 'priming' solutions at induction of cardiac bypass is also a major factor [43]. The hyperglycaemic problems with such solutions are now well known [46, 47], and such fluids are best avoided. Lactate solutions are also inadvisable [23], and Elliott et al [48, 49] have suggested Plasmalyte as a much less metabolically hazardous priming solution.

Correction of the priming solution problem, however, is not the entire answer. Studies using the Biostator (or artificial pancreas) [48] have shown remarkable changes in insulin requirements throughout surgery to maintain acceptable degrees of glycaemia (Table 11). Based on these observations, it has become accepted that the GKI infusion system is too inflexible, and separate-line control is needed [48, 50]. Frequent

blood glucose testing must be done, and insulin infusion altered appropriately (large and frequent changes are needed). Based on their Biostator studies, Elliott and colleagues used such an open-loop system and achieved excellent control, comparable with or even better than in the Biostator-controlled patients [48]. This group also produced computer-based algorithms to aid such glycaemic control during and after surgery. It should be noted that during bypass no glucose at all is given, just insulin.

Caesarean Section

Delivery by caesarean section in diabetic patients is nowadays usually an elective procedure. The diabetic patient in labour who eventually needs an emergency section should already be on a glucose and insulin delivery system (often a separate-line type [51]), and this can simply be continued through surgery. For elective operations, however, a GKI system is simple and acceptable. The operation is brief, and food intake is usually rapidly resumed. It should be remembered, however, that diabetic

Table 11   Insulin requirements during cardiac surgery in diabetic patients controlled by Biostator

Time	Insulin required (U/h) (mean ± SEM)
Preoperatively	1.6 ± 0.2
Skin incision to onset of bypass	3.0 ± 1.0
Bypass	5.0 ± 1.2
Immediately after bypass	8.3 ± 0.9
Postoperatively	12.3 ± 2.6

Adapted from reference 48.

patients in the later stages of pregnancy are insulin resistant, and are usually on insulin doses at least 50–100% greater than in their non-pregnant state [52]. It is thus usually sensible to start GKI with a solution containing 20 U insulin (0.4 U/g glucose), rather than the usual 15 U (0.3 U/g glucose). This insulin resistance of pregnancy rapidly disappears following delivery, in particular at delivery of the placenta, i.e. at completion of the third stage of labour. At this point, requirements drop to prepregnancy levels. A practical policy is to halve insulin delivery at this stage, whether it is being given separately or as GKI. Following this, insulin is adjusted as usual according to bedside blood glucose measurements, and subcutaneous insulin (in approximately prepregnancy amounts) is recommended when normal diet is resumed.

Emergency Surgery

Fortunately, truly urgent surgery in diabetic patients is relatively rare. If the situation does arise, then immediate assessment of metabolic status must be made. As well as a clinical history and examination, urine and plasma ketones, blood glucose and plasma urea and electrolytes will need to be measured. Metabolic status should preferably be optimized before even emergency surgery, although the urgency of the surgical situation will also have to be considered. With regard to diabetic control, the GKI system is usually applicable. The time of the last sub-cutaneous injection of insulin is important. If the injection is recent (i.e. within the last 6 hours for soluble insulin, or within the last 12 hours for intermediate-acting insulins), then the system of intravenous insulin delivery may need to be altered to account for the continued absorption of the previously injected insulin. There will need to be particularly careful monitoring of blood glucose levels, especially by the anaesthetist during the operation. In particularly unstable situations, a separate-line form of management may be advisable. In patients in whom glycaemic control is severely disturbed or where ketosis or ketoacidosis are present, treatment should be initially without glucose and with GKI substituted when glucose levels reach 12–15 mmol/l. The possibility of an 'acute abdomen' being purely due to ketoacidosis, particularly in younger patients, should also be remembered.

CONCLUSIONS

The GKI system is widely accepted and used. Some authors have, however, questioned whether it is superior to traditional methods of sub-cutaneous insulin followed by intravenous glucose—particularly in terms of glycaemic and metabolic control. Goldberg and colleagues in the USA [53] reported a study comparing the two methods in a small number of patients: no significant difference was found in blood glucose and hormonal responses, between the two groups. As well as the small numbers, however, the treatment protocols were unusual: insulin was infused at only 0.5 U per hour during surgery, and 0.5 U per hour thereafter; also, both in the intravenous and subcutaneous groups, dextrose was infused at arbitrary rates, and lactate-containing solutions were sometimes used. Glycaemic control was often at levels in excess of 15 mmol/l.

In the UK, Thomas and colleagues [29] compared the GKI system (10 U insulin per 500 ml dextrose) with subcutaneous insulin and intravenous glucose (half to three-quarters of the usual insulin dose, with 25 g IV glucose). As with the previous study, it can be seen that both regimens used here were suboptimal by modern standards. Eighteen patients were studied (12 GKI and 6 subcutaneous) and, again, no major differences were found in glucose and metabolic levels between the two groups, although blood glucose levels were lower ($P < 0.05$) at 4 hours and 72 hours postoperatively in the GKI group.

On the basis of results such as these, Hall [54] has criticized the overzealous acceptance of GKI, and has described it as a 'promise unful-filled'. Review of the literature, however, shows the clear superiority of GKI regimens (see reference 9). GKI has, however, never promised or been promoted as having dramatic metabolic advantage, but it does offer simplicity and safety. Compared with subcutaneous-based regimens it is easy to use, and requires little in the way of staff or equipment resources. Insulin therapy is, moreover, only one part of the care of the diabetic patient during surgery. Management of diabetes during surgery is an exercise in logic, organization, cooperation and communication. The diligent application of an accepted and efficacious system will result in reasonably good glycaemic control, will minimize avoidable disasters, and will ensure patterns of mortality and morbidity that are equivalent to those of the non-diabetic population.

REFERENCES

1. Allison SP, Tomlin PJ, Chamberlain MJ. Some effects of anaesthesia and surgery on carbohydrate and fat metabolism. Br J Anaesth 1979; 41: 588–93.
2. Elliott MJ, Alberti KGMM. Carbohydrate metabolism—effects of preoperative starvation and trauma. Clin Anaesthiol 1983; 1: 527–50.
3. Hume DM, Egdahl RH. The importance of the brain in the endocrine response to injury. Ann Surg 1959; 150: 697–712.
4. Nordenstrom J, Sonnenfeld J, Arner P. Characterisation of insulin resistance after surgery. Surgery 1989; 105: 28–35.
5. Foster KJ, Alberti KGMM, Binder C et al. Lipid metabolites and nitrogen balance after abdominal surgery in man. Br J Surg 1979; 66: 242–5.
6. Smith R, Fuller DJ, Wedge JH et al. Initial effect of injury on ketone bodies and other blood metabolites. Lancet 1975; i: 1–7.
7. Alberti KGMM, Thomas DJB. The management of diabetes during surgery. Br J Anaesth 1979; 51: 693–710.
8. Alberti KGMM, Gill GV, Elliott MJ. Insulin delivery during surgery in the diabetic patient. Diabetes Care 1982; 5: 65–77.
9. Alberti KGMM, Marshal SM. Diabetes and surgery. In Alberti KGMM, Krall LP (eds) Diabetes annual 4. Amsterdam: Elsevier, 1988: pp 248–71.
10. Marshal SM, Alberti KGMM, Hyperglycaemic emergencies and surgery: an update. In Alberti KGMM, Krall LP (eds) Diabetes annual 5. Amsterdam: Elsevier: 1990: pp 396–433.
11. Gill GV, Alberti KGMM. Surgery and diabetes. Hosp Update 1989; 15: 327–36.
12. Galloway JA, Shuman CR. Diabetes and surgery. Am J Med 1963; 34: 177–91.
13. Hjortrup A, Sorensen C, Dyremose E et al. Influence of diabetes mellitus on operative risk. Br J Surg 1985; 72: 783–5.
14. Hjortrup A, Sorensen C, Dyrmose E, Kehlet H. Morbidity in diabetic and non-diabetic patients after abdominal surgery. Acta Chir Scand 1985; 151: 445–7.
15. Reiss R, Deutsch AA, Nudelmann J. Biliary surgery in diabetic patients: statistical analysis of 189 patients. Dig Surg 1987; 4: 37–40.
16. Clement R, Rousou JA, Engelman RM, Breyer RH. Perioperative morbidity in diabetics requiring coronary artery bypass surgery. Ann Thorac Surg 1988; 46: 321–3.
17. Wilson RM, Reeves WG. Neutrophil phagocytosis and killing in insulin-dependent diabetes. Clin Exp Immunol 1986; 63: 478–84.
18. McMurray JF. Wound healing with diabetes mellitus. Surg Clin North Am 1984; 64: 769–78.
19. Page MMcB, Watkins PJ. Cardiorespiratory arrest with diabetic autonomic neuropathy. Lancet 1978; i: 14–16.
20. Podolsky S. Management of diabetes in the surgical patient. Med Clin North Am 1982; 66: 1361–72.
21. Thompson J, Husband DJ, Thai AC, Alberti KGMM. Metabolic changes in the non-insulin dependent diabetic undergoing minor surgery: effect of glucose–insulin–potassium infusion. Br J Surg 1986; 73: 301–4.
22. Malling B, Knudsen L, Christiansen CL et al. Insulin treatment in non-insulin dependent diabetic patients undergoing minor surgery. Diabet Nutr Metab 1989; 2: 125–31.
23. Thomas DJB, Alberti KGMM. The hyperglycaemic effects of Hartmann's solution in maturity-onset diabetics during surgery. Br J Anaesth 1978; 50: 185–8.
24. Fletcher J, Langman MJS, Kellock TD. Effects of surgery on blood glucose levels in diabetes mellitus. Lancet 1965; ii: 52–4.
25. Goldberg NJ, Wingert TD, Levin SR, Wilson SE, Viljoen JF. Insulin therapy in the diabetic surgical patient: metabolic and hormonal response to low dose insulin infusion. Diabetes Care 1981; 4: 279–84.
26. Taitelman U, Reece EA, Bessman AN. Insulin in the management of the diabetic surgical patient. Continuous intravenous administration versus subcutaneous administration. JAMA 1977; 237: 658–60.
27. Rossini AA, Hare JW. How to control the blood glucose level in the surgical diabetic patient. Arch Surg 1976; 3: 945–9.
28. Beaser SB. Surgical management. In Ellenberg M, Rifkin H (eds) Diabetes mellitus: Therapy and practice. New York: McGraw-Hill, 1970: pp 746–59.
29. Thomas DJB, Platt HS, Alberti KGMM. Insulin-dependent diabetes during the perio-operative period. An assessment of continuous glucose–insulin–potassium infusion, and traditional treatment. Anaesthesia 1984; 39: 629–37.
30. Meyer EJ, Lorenzi M, Bohannon NV et al. Diabetic management by insulin infusion during major surgery. Am J Surg 1979; 137: 323–7.
31. Christiansen CL, Schurizek BA, Malling B et al. Insulin treatment of the insulin-dependent diabetic patient undergoing minor surgery. Continuous intravenous infusion versus subcutaneous administration. Anaesthesia 1988; 43: 533–7.
32. Meyers EF, Alberts D, Gordon MO. Perioperative control of blood glucose in diabetic patients: a two-step protocol. Diabetes Care 1986; 9: 40–5.

33. Woodruff RE, Lewis SB, McLeskey CH, Graney WF. Avoidance of surgical hyperglycemia in diabetic patients. JAMA 1980; 244: 166.

34. Watts NB, Gebhart SSP, Clark RV, Phillips LS. Post-operative management of diabetes mellitus: steady-state glucose control with bedside algorithm for insulin adjustment. Diabetes Care 1987; 10: 722–8.

35. Sato T, Hoshi H, Kumon T et al. Managing diabetic surgical patients with glucose-free saline and insulin. Diabetes Res Clin Pract 1988; 5: 191–5.

36. Husband DJ, Thai AC, Alberti KGMM. Management of diabetes during surgery with glucose–insulin–potassium infusion. Diabet Med 1986; 3: 69–74.

37. Shuman CR. Diabetes mellitus and surgery. In Galloway JA, Potvin JH, Shuman CR (eds) Diabetes mellitus, 9th edn. Indianapolis: Eli Lilly, 1988: pp 242–51.

38. Petersen L, Caldwell J, Hoffman J. Insulin adsorption to polyvinylchloride surfaces with implications for constant infusion therapy. Diabetes 1976; 25: 72–4.

39. Talbot EM. Dangers of adding insulin to intravenous infusion bags with fixed needle syringes. Br Med J 1984; 289: 678–80.

40. Thai AC, Husband DJ, Gill GV, Alberti KGMM. Management of diabetes during surgery. A retrospective study of 112 cases. Diabète Métab 1984; 10: 65–70.

41. Hutchinson AS, Shenkin A. BM strips: how accurate are they in general wards? Diabet Med 1984; 1: 225–6.

42. Price CP, Burrin JM, Nattrass M. Extralaboratory blood glucose measurement: a policy statement. Diabet Med 1988; 5: 705–9.

43. Gill GV, Sherif IH, Alberti KGMM. Management of diabetes during open heart surgery. Br J Surg 1981; 68: 171–2.

44. Thomas DJB, Hinds CJ, Rees GM. The management of insulin dependent diabetes during cardiopulmonary bypass and general surgery. Anaesthesia 1983; 38: 1047–52.

45. Ekroth R, Nilsson F, Berggren H et al. Insulin sensitivity and glucose uptake in the course of surgical treatment for valvular aortic stenosis. Scand J Thorac Cardiovasc Surg 1982; 16: 137–40.

46. Stephens JW, Krause AH, Peterson CA, Bass JJ, Hartman JE, Solomon NW, Ward WK. The effect of glucose priming solutions in diabetic patients udergoing coronary artery bypass grafting. Ann Thorac Surg 1988; 45: 544–7.

47. Crock PA, Ley CJ, Martin IK, Alford FP, Best JD. Hormonal and metabolic changes during hypothermic coronary artery bypass surgery in diabetic and non-diabetic subjects. Diabet Med 1988; 5: 47–52.

48. Elliott MJ, Gill GV, Home PD, Noy GA, Holden MP, Alberti KGMM. A comparison of two regimens for the management of diabetes during open-heart surgery. Anaesthesia 1984; 60: 364–8.

49. McKnight CK, Elliott MJ, Pearson DT et al. The effects of four different crystalloid bypass pump-priming fluids upon the metabolic response to cardiac operation. J Thorac Cardiovasc Surg 1985; 90: 97–111.

50. Watson BG, Elliott MJ, Pay DA, Williamson M. Diabetes mellitus and open heart surgery. A simple practical closed-loop infusion system for blood glucose control. Anaesthesia 1986; 41: 250–7.

51. Lean MEJ, Pearson DWM, Sutherland HW. Insulin management during labour and delivery in mothers with diabetes. Diabet Med 1990; 7: 162–4.

52. Leiper JM, Paterson KR, Lunan CB, MacCuish AC. A comparison of biosynthetic human insulin with porcine insulin in the blood glucose control of diabetic pregnancy. Diabet Med 1986; 3: 49–51.

53. Goldberg NJ, Wingert TD, Levin SR, Wilson SE, Viljoen JF. Insulin therapy in the diabetic surgical patient: metabolic and hormone response to low dose insulin infusion. Diabetes Care 1981; 4: 279–84.

54. Hall GM. Diabetes and anaesthesia—a promise unfulfilled? Anaesth 1984; 39: 627–8.

51

Vascular Events and Diabetes: Acute Myocardial Infarction and Stroke

John S. Yudkin and Timothy J. Hendra

University College and Middlesex School of Medicine, Whittington Hospital, London, UK

Diabetes mellitus brings with it a substantially increased risk of large vessel disease [1–4]. In diabetic men, mortality from cardiovascular disease is approximately doubled and in women the relative risk is even higher [5–6]. Cerebrovascular disease mortality is some 2–3 times greater in both diabetic men and women than in the general population [7, 8]. In non-insulin dependent diabetes mellitus (NIDDM) the excess risk of large vessel disease seems to be unrelated to the duration of diabetes, implying that cumulative glycaemic exposure is not the major determinant [9]. In insulin dependent diabetes mellitus (IDDM), this excess risk is found mainly in patients who develop renal involvement [10], and the same may also be the case in NIDDM [11].

Several autopsy studies have shown that diabetic subjects have more extensive atherosclerosis of both coronary and cerebral vessels than age-matched non-diabetic controls [12, 13]. This more widespread atheroma increases the *incidence* of clinical manifestations of ischaemic heart and cerebrovascular disease, and abnormalities of platelets [14], fibrinogen [15], and

blood rheology [16] may also contribute to this excess incidence. However, the acute ischaemic event itself also carries a substantially higher risk in diabetic patients, and the *excess case fatality* of acute myocardial infarction, and perhaps of thromboembolic stroke, may contribute substantially to the higher total mortality (Figure 1).

In this chapter the clinical course of acute myocardial infarction and of acute stroke in diabetic patients is described and the management of these events outlined. The diabetic patient who suffers an acute myocardial infarction or stroke is at substantially increased risk of sustaining a further vascular event, and possible approaches to reducing this excess risk are considered. Finally, acute hyperglycaemia is frequently found in subjects without known diabetes who suffer a myocardial infarction or stroke, and the relevance of this abnormality is discussed.

ACUTE MYOCARDIAL INFARCTION IN DIABETIC PATIENTS

Although clinically apparent coronary heart disease is predominantly a problem of the older

International Textbook of Diabetes Mellitus. Edited by K.G.M.M. Alberti, R.A. DeFronzo, H. Keen and P. Zimmet
© 1992 John Wiley & Sons Ltd

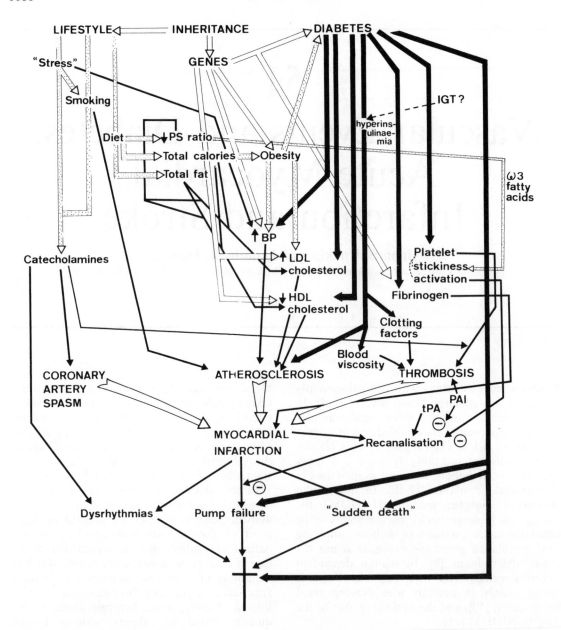

Figure 1 Factors that may contribute to the excess incidence and case fatality of myocardial infarction in diabetic patients. IGT, impaired glucose tolerance; tPA, tissue plasminogen activator; HDL, high-density lipoprotein; LDL, low-density lipoprotein; BP, blood pressure; PS, polyunsaturated/saturated; PAI, plasminogen activator inhibitor

NIDDM patient, myocardial infarction is not uncommon in diabetic patients in their third or fourth decade, and occurs as often in premenopausal women as in men of the same age [17]. Moreover, the course of myocardial infarction in a diabetic patient is likely to be a stormy one. Case series comparing diabetic and non-diabetic

subjects admitted with myocardial infarction have shown an increase in hospital mortality of between 25% and 100% among the diabetic patients [18–41]. Gwilt [42] has analysed 33 studies of hospital case fatality published over the last sixty years, and has found no evidence that this relative risk has declined since the

Table 1 Hospital mortality in diabetic and non-diabetic patients

Author	Mortality in diabetic subjects (no.)	(%)	Mortality in non-diabetic subjects (no.)	(%)	Relative risk
Partamian & Bradley, 1965 [17]	107/258	41	—	—	—
McGuire & Kroll, 1972 [18]	25/54	46	42/287	15	5.03
Soler et al, 1974 [19]	65/184[a]	35	327/1804[a,d]	18	2.47
Soler et al, 1975 [20]	113/285[a]	40	—	—	—
Henning & Lundman, 1975 [21]	86/240	36	448/1768	25	1.64
Harrower & Clarke, 1976 [22]	24/99	24	678/3568[d]	19	1.36
Lichstein et al, 1976 [23]	64/265	24	—	—	—
Kvetny, 1976 [24]	11/37[b]	30	186/560[d]	33	0.85
Tansey et al, 1977 [25]	25/89	28	110/793	14	2.43
Maempel, 1978 [26]	60/289[b]	21	94/656	14	1.57
Czyżyk et al, 1980 [27]	56/154	36	29/154	19	2.46
Weitzman et al, 1982 [28]	11/54[c]	20	28/270[c]	10	2.21
Jaffe et al, 1984 [29]	27/84	32	70/385	18	2.13
Gwilt et al, 1984 [30]	124/417	30	632/3602	18	1.99
Rytter et al, 1985 [31]	34/81[b]	42	152/751	20	2.85
Yudkin & Oswald, 1988 [32]	35/83	42	94/380[e]	25	2.22
Mølstad & Nustad, 1987 [33]	25/95	26	116/545	21	1.32
Malmberg & Rydén, 1988 [34]	20/81	25	42/260	16	1.70
Kouvaras et al, 1988 [35]	29/98	30	72/450	16	2.21
Savage et al, 1988 [36]	52/183	28	—	—	—
Day et al, 1988 [37]	42/100	42	29/100	29	1.77
Herlitz et al, 1988 [38]	9/78	12	54/709	8	1.58
Stone et al, 1989 [39]	6/85	7	8/415	2	3.86
Sewdarsen et al, 1989 [40]	62/143	43	38/277	14	4.81
Singer et al, 1989 [41]	61/228[f]	27	33/196[f]	17	1.80
Total	1063/3479	31	2955/16126	18	1.96*

[a] Patients also included in Gwilt et al, 1984 [30] so excluded from totals.
[b] Includes patients diagnosed as diabetic on basis of hyperglycaemia after infarction.
[c] 20-day mortality.
[d] Calculated from data presented in report.
[e] Excludes patients with levels of glycated haemoglobin indicating undiagnosed diabetes.
[f] 30-day mortality.
* 95% confidence interval 1.80–2.13.

introduction of modern principles of coronary care. There is also a little evidence that the absolute case fatality rate has declined in diabetic subjects over the last twenty years, despite substantial changes in treatment regimens. Table 1 summarises the more recent studies.

A number of studies have suggested that coronary heart disease mortality is increased in subjects with lesser degrees of glucose intolerance as well as in those with overt diabetes [4, 6, 43]. We have recently demonstrated that patients with levels of glycated haemoglobin exceeding the 90th centile, but without overt diabetes mellitus, have a significantly greater risk of left ventricular failure and cardiogenic shock after admission with myocardial infarction than patients with lower levels of glycated haemoglobin [44], suggesting that a higher case fatality may contribute to the excess risk of death in such people, as well as in those with known diabetes.

The Impact of Diabetes on Hospital Admission and Mortality after Myocardial Infarction

The prevalence of known diabetes among patients admitted with myocardial infarction is likely to differ substantially both in different hospitals and in different populations, as it will be determined both by the prevalence of diabetes in the at-risk population and by the referral patterns for patients developing chest pain, specifically whether they have been previously known to a particular hospital. Among 463 consecutive patients admitted to the Whittington Hospital unit over a 2-year period, 66 had previously diagnosed diabetes (14%). Because of the high case fatality of diabetic patients with myocardial infarction, these 14%

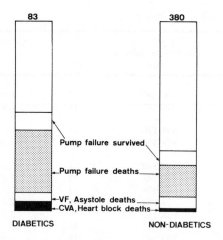

Figure 2 Causes of death and incidence of pulmonary oedema and cardiogenic shock (pump failure) in 83 diabetic patients and 380 non-diabetic subjects with levels of glycated haemoglobin excluding undiagnosed diabetes. VF, ventricular fibrillation; CVA, cerebrovascular accident [32]

of patients represented 21% of the hospital deaths [44]. Similar figures have been published from Birmingham, UK, where between 1967 and 1983, 10% of patients admitted with myocardial infarction had known diabetes, these representing 16% of hospital deaths [30]. The studies on consecutive series of patients admitted with myocardial infarction among those summarised in Table 1 give a figure of 14.6% (range 3–34%) for the prevalence of diabetes mellitus, and these patients contributed 20.3% (range 3–62%) of hospital deaths. In a major European multicentre study of intravenous atenolol for patients after acute myocardial infarction, enrolling some 16000 patients, the prevalence of known diabetes was 6%, and these patients contributed around 10% of the hospital deaths [45].

Mode of Death

There is well-documented excess risk of cardiogenic shock and congestive cardiac failure (hereafter together termed pump failure) in diabetic subjects after myocardial infarction. In our own study, the hospital mortality was 42% among 83 diabetics with confirmed myocardial infarction and 25% among 380 non-diabetics with admission levels of glycated haemoglobin excluding undiagnosed diabetes [32]. The causes of death in these subjects are shown in Figure 2, where it is seen that pump failure is the major

cause of death in both groups, but that 42% of the diabetic patients and only 24% of the non-diabetic subjects developed pump failure, defined as cardiogenic shock (with systolic pressure below 90 mmHg and oliguria or signs of hypoperfusion) or pulmonary oedema (Killip class C or D [46]). There was no difference between the two groups in the risk of dysrhythmia, conduction disorders or other causes of death [32]. Partamian and Bradley were the first to identify cardiogenic shock and congestive cardiac failure as a major risk factor for death after myocardial infarction in diabetic patients [17]. Several more recent studies have confirmed this excess risk [19, 22, 23, 25, 35, 37, 40–42]. Other reports have also noted an excess incidence of pump failure, without categorising causes of death in such a fashion [26, 29, 31, 39]. Pump failure is responsible for 80% of deaths among diabetic patients, and 75% of those in non-diabetic subjects, in studies listed in Table 1, but because the absolute case fatality is higher in diabetic patients, this represents a markedly increased incidence of pump failure (Table 2).

The risk of dysrhythmia as a cause of death in non-diabetic patients has declined since the advent of coronary care units, and this appears also to be true for diabetic patients, although non-fatal dysrhythmias were reported more frequently in some series [19, 22] (Table 2). Five recent studies have suggested that atrioventricular or intraventricular conduction disorders are more common in diabetic patients [27, 31, 34, 35, 39]. Thromboembolic disease makes a small contribution to mortality but appears to be more common in diabetic patients [17, 19, 26]. Table 2 is a summary of the clinical features of myocardial infarction taken from all the studies reviewed, and quantifies the incidence of the major complications as variously defined by individual authors.

Hospital mortality represents only some 35–40% of all deaths after myocardial infarction [47, 48] and, by their nature, studies of hospital mortality are unable to determine the risk of sudden death in diabetic patients. Two epidemiological studies have shown an increased risk of sudden death, as well as hospital fatality, in diabetic patients. The Israel Ischaemic Heart Disease Study found sudden cardiac death to be 3.6 times more frequent in diabetic patients [3]. The Framingham study suggested that the

Table 2 Characteristics and complications of diabetic and non-diabetic patients with myocardial infarction

	Diabetic	Non-diabetic	Relative risk (95% confidence interval)
Percentage women	42.3 (2941)	24.7 (7805)	2.20 (2.01–2.41)
Case fatality			
men	27.9 (906)	14.8 (2127)	2.23 (1.85–2.69)
women	37.7 (802)	20.4 (646)	2.36 (1.86–3.00)
RR*	1.57 (1.28–1.92)	1.48 (1.18–1.85)	
Case fatality			
diet	24.9 (221)		
oral	33.7 (612)		
RR oral versus diet	1.80 (1.27–2.55)		
Insulin	35.3 (399)		
RR insulin versus diet	1.65 (1.14–2.38)		
Presenting in ketoacidosis	2.5 (1130)		
Anterior	49.1 (2097)	46.3 (5249)	1.12 (1.01–1.24)
Inferior	32.5 (1501)	29.5 (3400)	1.15 (1.01–1.31)
Pump failure (cardiogenic shock, pulmonary oedema, congestive cardiac failure)	29.9 (3481)	19.0 (9873)	1.81 (1.66–1.98)
Deaths	22.1 (846)	16.9 (1059)	1.39 (1.11–1.75)
Ventricular fibrillation, tachycardia	7.3 (2454)	5.8 (9630)	1.26 (1.06–1.51)
Deaths	4.6 (898)	5.7 (1455)	0.79 (0.54–1.16)
Conduction disorders (second degree, complete heart block, left bundle branch block)	18.3 (1548)	14.0 (4644)	1.37 (1.18–1.60)
Thromboembolism (cerebrovascular accidents, pulmonary embolism, systemic embolism)	3.4 (1030)	0.9 (1661)	3.85 (2.19–6.79)
Deaths	1.6 (817)	0.5 (1455)	3.34 (1.33–8.41)

The data are collated from references 17–42 and 66. Figures given are percentages and the figures in parentheses represent the denominator number of subjects from the series in which the information is provided. As references 19, 20, 30 and 42 all represent a single consecutive case series, only one reference is employed to provide the data for any characteristic.
* Relative risks (RR) are given with 95% confidence intervals.

increased risk of sudden death was more marked in diabetic women [49].

Following hospital admission with myocardial infarction there is some difference of opinion as to the stage of inpatient stay when diabetic patients are most at risk. Tansey et al found the excess risk to apply only to the time in the coronary care unit [25], but a study from Warsaw, Poland, reported that the excess mortality of diabetic patients was found only between 2 and 7 days after admission [27]. A study from Birmingham, UK, has also suggested that late deaths are common in diabetic patients, with around 50% of the deaths occurring some 5 or more days after admission [19, 20]. The excess risk of pump failure death beyond 2–4 days after the infarct is considered in some centres as a justification for observing diabetic patients in the coronary care unit for longer than is habitual for non-diabetic patients. However, the benefits of treatment in such units for patients in cardiogenic shock or severe cardiac failure are less clear than those for the treatment of dysrhythmias, and there is no obvious excess risk of late dysrhythmias in diabetic patients.

The Relationship of Hospital Outcome to Patient Characteristics

The findings of the University Group Diabetes Program suggested that diabetic patients treated with tolbutamide and phenformin experienced a significant increase in cardiovascular mortality [50, 51]. Two earlier series suggested that oral hypoglycaemic agents were associated with an increased risk of dysrhythmias after myocardial infarction [19, 23], these patients having a relative risk of ventricular fibrillation of 2.39 (95% CI 1.05–5.44) compared with those on diet and insulin in the two studies. However, as might be expected with the diminishing contribution of dysrhythmias to total mortality, most case series have found no association between the type of hypoglycaemic therapy and hospital mortality. Amalgamating the results of all the studies suggests a better outcome in patients treated with diet alone (Table 2), but not all of these studies have documented the criteria employed in the diagnosis of diabetes in such patients. Most insulin-treated patients admitted with myocardial infarction have NIDDM, and only one study has separately presented the data on hospital mortality for IDDM and NIDDM patients [31]. There are no data available pertaining to differences in clinical course of myocardial infarction in IDDM patients [52].

In our own series of 83 diabetic patients with confirmed myocardial infarction there was no gender difference in mortality [32], but several reports have suggested that diabetic women suffer an excess case fatality compared with men after myocardial infarction [17, 20, 25, 26, 28, 31, 36, 37, 40] (Table 2). Moreover, the Framingham study described a more marked excess of cardiovascular mortality than of incidence in diabetic women compared with men [2]. No comparative data are available for case fatality in different populations or ethnic groups, despite wide geographical differences in coronary heart disease prevalence [53].

Most studies have shown no relationship between duration of known diabetes and hospital case fatality following myocardial infarction [20, 27, 31, 32, 39], but this finding is not universal [17]. It is clear, however, that most diabetic patients who sustain a myocardial infarction have NIDDM, and so the duration since diagnosis may be much shorter than the total duration of hyperglycaemia.

We have studied the relationship between prior blood glucose control, as evidenced by the admission level of glycated haemoglobin, and outcome from myocardial infarction, having demonstrated that the level of glycated haemoglobin is unaffected by a major vascular event and so can justifiably be used to reflect premorbid glycaemia [54]. In our series, there was no significant difference in levels of glycated haemoglobin between those patients developing and those not developing left ventricular failure or cardiogenic shock, or between those who died and those who survived their hospital stay [32]. Two other studies have also investigated the relationship between premorbid blood glucose control and hospital outcome, but employing clinic blood glucose levels as an index of previous control, and have found a worse outcome in patients with poor control [22, 31].

In non-diabetic patients, admission hyperglycaemia after myocardial infarction is associated with poor outcome (see below). Among the patients in our series with known diabetes, admission plasma glucose levels were higher in those who developed pump failure or died, but this difference was no longer apparent in a logistic regression analysis including infarct size [32]. Four other studies have suggested that diabetic patients admitted with hyperglycaemia after myocardial infarction do less well in hospital [20, 30, 31, 40], but in one of these studies [31] patients were defined as having newly diagnosed diabetes if they showed hyperglycaemia persisting for 3 days after admission. This may well have resulted in the misclassification of non-diabetic patients with stress hyperglycaemia.

Diabetes Mellitus and Silent Infarcts

There have been several reports suggesting that patients with longstanding diabetes are more likely to present with painless myocardial infarction than non-diabetic subjects [55, 56], the event being manifested by worsening heart failure or diabetic control, or by vomiting or collapse. It is suggested that painless myocardial infarction may result from autonomic neuropathy [56, 57].

The proportion of patients presenting with painless myocardial infarction in different series varied from 2.8% to 46.1% [18, 20, 26, 27, 36, 41], and these differences may reflect different criteria for inclusion of patients or differences in referral patterns between centres. Epidemiological observations have shown that some 25–30% of all myocardial infarcts diagnosed by sequential electrocardiograms are unrecognised as such, half of these being truly silent [58, 59]; although patients with diabetes may be more prone to unrecognised infarcts, in the Framingham population the differences were not statistically significant (39% versus 22%) [59]. The comparison of the proportion of painless infarcts in both diabetic and non-diabetic subjects could be made accurately only with a population-based study of this type.

Possible Causes of Excess Hospital Mortality in Diabetic Patients after Myocardial Infarction

The reason for the excess risk of cardiogenic shock and left ventricular failure in diabetic patients after myocardial infarction is not clear. Several possible candidates are discussed below.

Infarct Size and Site

Estimation of the size of a myocardial infarction can be performed at autopsy, or in survivors by enzymic, electrocardiographic or radioisotope techniques. A number of studies have estimated peak levels of enzyme or cumulative enzyme release after myocardial infarction in diabetic and non-diabetic patients, and have found either no greater [26, 29, 32–34, 38, 60] or, indeed, smaller [39, 41] infarct size in the diabetic group. Several of these studies [29, 32, 37, 39, 60] have demonstrated that the diabetic patient is more at risk of left ventricular failure, cardiogenic shock or death at any level of enzyme release (Figure 3). There are, however, three major problems in measuring infarct size by this method. First, survival for 48 hours is a prerequisite for this assessment, and consequently the technique may select the patients with smaller infarcts. Secondly, it has been demonstrated that more cardiac enzyme is released following spontaneous, as well as pharmacological, reperfusion of the infarcted myocardium [61, 62]. As spontaneous reperfusion is associated with an improvement in left ventricular function [63], such patients may well have spuriously high estimates of infarct size with a good outcome. Finally, studies of peak enzyme levels are even less satisfactory than those of cumulative enzyme release. One study which employed QRS scoring of the

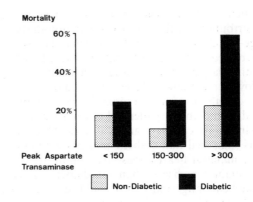

Figure 3 Hospital mortality after myocardial infarction in 50 diabetic and 136 non-diabetic patients according to peak levels of asparate transaminase (IU/l)

electrocardiogram to estimate infarct size has suggested that diabetic patients do have larger areas of infarction than matched non-diabetic subjects [64]. However, because certain criteria had to be satisfied before such analyses were possible, only 23% of the electrocardiograms of the diabetic patients admitted with myocardial infarction were analysed. Gwilt et al were unable to confirm these findings using similar techniques in a smaller number of patients [60]. Furthermore, a recent study using radionuclide techniques has shown that diabetes causes impaired left ventricular function independently of QRS-score estimates of infarct size [65]. Although a combination of radioisotopic imaging techniques and autopsy studies would be necessary to elaborate clearly the contribution of infarct size to excess mortality in diabetic subjects, the consensus of evidence is that this is not the cause of their higher risk.

Weitzman et al [28] have suggested that the excess mortality after infarction in diabetic subjects is limited to those having an anterior infarct, and that these are more common in diabetic than non-diabetic subjects below 60 years of age. We have found no significant differences in infarct site between diabetic and non-diabetic subjects [66], but the data in Table 2 suggest that anterior infarcts are marginally more common in diabetic patients.

Diffuse and Widespread Atherosclerosis in Diabetic Patients

Several autopsy studies have indicated that

patients with diabetes have more widespread distribution of atherosclerosis than non-diabetic age-matched controls [11–13]. There is also an increased prevalence of complicated atheroma, with plaque fissuring and calcification [11]. However, few studies have compared the severity or distribution of atheroma between diabetic and non-diabetic patients known to have, or dying from, coronary artery disease. One study has suggested that diabetic patients with clinically manifest heart disease have more frequent left main stem disease than non-diabetic patients matched for age and sex [67], but found no other differences between the groups.

We have found that the excess risk of pump failure and death is apparent in diabetic patients, whether or not they have a previous history of myocardial infarction [32]. We have also studied the possible effects of critical ischaemia in non-infarcted areas of the heart by the use of electrocardiographic reciprocal change. This comprises the finding of ST-segment depression in the non-infarcted areas of the heart and is said to reflect ischaemia in these areas. Although patients showing reciprocal change had a worse outcome from their myocardial infarct, whether or not they had diabetes, the risk of pump failure or hospital death was not related to an excess of reciprocal change among diabetic patients [66]. A similar finding was reported in a small number of patients in another series [60].

Spontaneous Coronary Artery Reperfusion and Haemostatic Abnormalities in Diabetes

Myocardial infarction occurs as a result of thrombosis in a coronary artery, but the fate of this thrombus has a major influence on outcome. Both spontaneous reperfusion [63] and that induced pharmacologically [68] produce improvement in myocardial function, whereas patients in cardiogenic shock are more likely to have persistent occlusive thrombus [69]. It is likely that reperfusion limits the eventual size of the infarct [63] although, as pointed out above, this is difficult to estimate from levels of enzyme release because of the limitations of that method in estimating infarct size.

Following coronary thrombosis, there is likely to be an equilibrium between further platelet aggregation and thrombus proliferation on the one hand, and thrombolysis on the other [70], but the factors that determine the fate of the thrombus in the coronary artery are not known. It is possible that the recognised abnormalities of haemostasis and fibrinolysis in diabetic patients are responsible for a failure of thrombolysis, with consequent pump failure in these patients after myocardial infarction. In patients admitted with myocardial infarction, elevated levels of fibrinogen and factor VIII are associated with radiographic evidence of left ventricular failure [71], while elevated fibrinogen and factor VII levels predict 5-year mortality from ischaemic heart disease [72]. The role of the fibrinolytic system would seem likely to be of importance in determining recanalisation, but fibrinolytic activity, as estimated by dilute clot lysis time, was not significantly lower in myocardial infarct patients dying within 6 weeks [71]. Nevertheless, an important component in the control of fibrinolysis is the circulating inhibitor of tissue plasminogen activator, PAI-1. Elevated levels of this inhibitor are found in survivors of myocardial infarction [73], and also predict recurrent infarction [74]. Diabetic patients have elevated concentrations of PAI-1 [75–78]. Insulin appears to stimulate hepatic synthesis of PAI-1 [77–79], but in subjects with NIDDM, proinsulin-like molecules, rather than insulin, may have an important role in determining the elevated levels of PAI-1 [80]. Recent work in our laboratory has shown that diabetic patients admitted with myocardial infarction have higher levels of PAI-1 than do non-diabetic infarct patients [81], perhaps reducing the likelihood of spontaneous thrombolysis, or increasing the risk of reocclusion after pharmacological thrombolysis [82, 83].

We have reported that diabetic patients, and hyperglycaemic patients with cardiogenic shock, have increased serum levels of platelet β-thromboglobulin compared with non-diabetic patients with uncomplicated myocardial infarcts [84]. These elevated levels of platelet α-granule proteins correlated with levels of both glucose and adrenaline, but were further increased in the presence of pump failure [84]. This suggests that excessive platelet activation in vivo may contribute to the failure of coronary artery recanalisation in diabetic and hyperglycaemic patients after myocardial infarction [85], and may also predispose to reinfarction [86].

Cardiomyopathy

Patients with diabetes mellitus have a substantially increased risk of developing congestive heart failure compared with non-diabetic subjects. The Framingham study showed an excess risk of 3.8 in diabetic men and 5.5 in diabetic women when those with previous coronary heart disease were excluded [49]. Whether this risk is related to diffuse coronary fibrosis [87, 88], to microangiopathy [89], or to glycation of cardiac myosin or other proteins [90, 91], is not clear. However, it is possible that cardiac reserve following myocardial infarction is decreased in diabetic patients.

Metabolic Abnormalities

One possible reason for the excess risk of pump failure in diabetic subjects after myocardial infarction is the metabolic effect of the relative or absolute deficiency of insulin [92, 93]. In the presence of elevated levels of cortisol and catecholamines, hyperglycaemia is further increased, with inhibition of cell membrane glucose transport and of glycolysis. These hormonal abnormalities also stimulate lipolysis, producing a marked rise in levels of non-esterified fatty acids (NEFA). Elevated NEFA levels may impair myocardial metabolism directly and have been shown to reduce contractility, increase oxygen consumption [94] and increase ischaemic injury [95]. It has also been proposed that these elevated levels act synergistically with elevation of catecholamine levels in inducing ventricular dysrhythmias [92], although this, as already noted, has not been recorded as a particular problem in diabetic patients.

One further possible effect of elevated NEFA levels relates to the theory of free radical damage following ischaemia. It has been proposed that spontaneous or pharmacological reperfusion of an ischaemic tissue may produce further cell damage as a result of free radical production [96]. McCord has proposed that xanthine dehydrogenase is converted to xanthine oxidase during myocardial ischaemia, and when molecular oxygen is reintroduced, free radicals are produced [96]. Moreover, a recent study has shown that successful thrombolytic therapy is associated with an increase in markers of lipid peroxidation [97], and that left ventricular ejection fraction is inversely correlated with the rise in concentrations of these markers [98]. Diabetic subjects may be more susceptible to free radical damage [99] and, in particular, elevated levels of free fatty acids in lipolytic states may include a high concentration of free-radical-damaged, diene-conjugated species with abnormal physical and chemical characteristics [100]. However, we have compared levels of free-radical products in circulating phospholipids between diabetic and non-diabetic subjects after myocardial infarction, and have found lower, and not higher, levels in diabetic subjects 48 hours after admission [101].

Evidence against the importance of insulin deficiency per se in determining the poor outcome from myocardial infarction is the lack of a clear independent relationship of outcome with blood glucose concentrations, as noted above. There have also been a number of studies of insulin infusion in diabetic patients after myocardial infarction and these are considered further below.

Autonomic Neuropathy

Patients with longstanding diabetes who have symptoms of autonomic neuropathy are unlikely to increase heart rate or stroke volume to compensate for damage from a myocardial infarction [102]. However, several studies have found no relationship between duration of diabetes and mortality following myocardial infarction, which would make this explanation appear unlikely [20, 27, 31, 32]. Similarly, the well-recognised reduction in peak catecholamine levels found in longstanding diabetic subjects is unlikely to represent the explanation for poor outcome in these subjects [102, 103]. We have found no significant difference ($P > 0.1$) in admission levels of adrenaline or noradrenaline between 9 diabetic and 14 non-diabetic subjects admitted after myocardial infarction [84].

Differences in Referral Patterns

Although most studies comparing diabetic and non-diabetic patients admitted to hospital after myocardial infarction have not discussed possible confounding variables (such as time of admission following onset of symptoms, duration of hospital stay and referral patterns for diabetic and non-diabetic patients), it appears improbable that the consistent differences in outcome between the groups could be explained on these bases [42].

In summary, it is not clear why the prognosis of myocardial infarction in diabetic patients is so poor. Myocardial function may be severely impaired even after small infarcts, and this might result from diffuse vascular or heart muscle disease. However, the possibility that metabolic abnormalities or haemostatic function are responsible for this excess risk indicates the need for good therapeutic trials, despite the problems in their implementation outlined below.

Long-term Prognosis of Patients with Diabetes after Acute Myocardial Infarction

Several studies have reported an approximately threefold increase in long-term mortality of diabetic patients surviving the acute stage of myocardial infarction [29, 34, 38, 39, 41, 104–106]. As in non-diabetic patients, manifestations of poor left ventricular function are important indicators of poor prognosis [29, 39, 104]. A Swedish study [105] followed 73 diabetic and 1229 non-diabetic subjects for up to 8 years after myocardial infarction and found a 2.3-fold increase in mortality and 1.7-fold increase in reinfarction rate. The excess risk remained after allowing for age and other cardiac risk factors [105]. Data from the Framingham study [106] suggest that this excess risk of recurrent myocardial infarction and death may be limited to women with diabetes, an observation also made in another study from the USA [39].

Studies of Intervention in Diabetic Patients after Acute Myocardial Infarction

Patients with diabetes mellitus represent between 6% and 10% of all patients admitted with myocardial infarction. The probable benefit from most interventions employed after infarction is a reduction in mortality of around 20%, and this implies that most intervention studies in patients with myocardial infarction that employ mortality as an end-point are performed as multicentre studies. In order to recruit sufficient numbers of diabetic patients, such studies would have to be conducted in 10 times the number of centres, or over 10 times the duration, which is the reason why conclusions on efficacy of therapy for diabetic patients after

myocardial infarction are usually based on small numbers of patients with historical controls, or on subgroup analyses of large therapeutic trials in patients admitted with myocardial infarction. In order to demonstrate a 20% reduction in mortality among diabetic subjects admitted with myocardial infarction, and assuming a hospital mortality in the control group of 40%, it would be necessary to randomise 1120 subjects between two groups to show a significant difference at the 5% level with a power of 80%.

Management of Diabetic Patients after Myocardial Infarction

Blood Glucose Control

Admission hyperglycaemia is very common in diabetic patients admitted after myocardial infarction. In our own series, 33% of such patients had a plasma glucose level on admission of over 20 mmol/l and 8% had levels over 30 mmol/l. In the Birmingham series of 453 diabetic patients admitted with myocardial infarction, 3% were in ketoacidosis on admission [42], while in all studies summarised in Table 2, ketoacidosis was present in 2.2%.

The theoretical benefits of tight blood glucose control, or of correcting the metabolic abnormalities of insulin deficiency, have been touched on above. There are, however, also some theoretical risks associated with inducing normoglycaemia by insulin infusion following acute myocardial infarction. Hypoglycaemia is associated with a marked increase in the production of counterregulatory hormones, and among these both adrenaline and vasopressin are capable of inducing platelet activation [107–109]. Hypoglycaemia can therefore increase the risk of thrombotic episodes. If, then, there exists an equilibrium between thrombosis and thrombolysis after myocardial infarction, it is important that any insulin regimen designed for use in patients after myocardial infarction must avoid the risk of hypoglycaemia as well as being designed to correct hyperglycaemia.

Three groups have described insulin infusion regimens for patients after myocardial infarction [30, 110–112]. All of these studies have also reported outcome in the insulin-infused group and a matched control group, but in no case was a randomised study performed. Gwilt et al [30] compared outcome in 64 patients admitted between 1981 and 1983 and given intravenous insulin infusion with that in 353 controls admitted between 1967 and 1981, of whom 224 (63.5%) were given subcutaneous insulin and the remainder continued on previous therapy. They reported no difference in mortality between the infusion and control group, or between those given insulin and those continued on previous treatment among the historical controls. The regimen of insulin employed was reported to reduce mean blood glucose levels to less than 10 mmol/l by 6–8 hours after starting the infusion [110], and the levels on the day after admission were 9.9 (SD 3.6) mmol/l in the treated group and 12.4 (SD 5.9) mmol/l in the control group [30]. Husband et al [111] described subcutaneous and intravenous insulin regimens of benefit in controlling blood glucose levels following myocardial infarction, and these also achieved a mean blood glucose concentration of less than 10 mmol/l over the first 48 hours. Interestingly, blood glucose control was better in those patients given intravenous insulin, glucose and potassium than those given thrice-daily subcutaneous insulin, despite the fact that the former regimen was reserved for the more seriously ill patients. They noted a mortality in patients in whom the regimens were used (18.6%) that was no different from that in historical controls (24.4%). The mean blood glucose level was 9.6 (SD 2.7) mmol/l and 12.9 (SD 4.0) mmol/l on the first day after infarction in the two groups [111].

The third report on the effects of insulin infusion after acute myocardial infarction came from Dundee, UK [112]. This reported the results of insulin infusion over a 12-month period during which 29 patients with diabetes were admitted with acute myocardial infarction, and compared outcome with that in the preceding year when 33 such patients were admitted. In the control year, 15 of the 33 patients were treated with subcutaneous insulin, the remainder continuing on their previous therapy of diet alone or oral hypoglycaemic drugs. In the subsequent year, all patients whose previous therapy comprised either insulin or oral hypoglycaemic agents were converted to an intravenous insulin regimen, the dose of porcine highly purified soluble insulin being varied between 0 U and 4 U per hour according to blood glucose concentrations. Although admission blood glucose levels were similar, follow-up levels in the two

groups were not reported. The mortality was reduced from 42% to 17%, which, when expressed as a relative risk compared with non-diabetics, represented a reduction from 5.5 in the control year to 1.3 in the active treatment year. There are many problems in accepting the findings of this study without reservation, the main ones being the employment of a historical control group, and the fact that, as 10 patients during the active treatment year continued on diet alone, the significant reduction in mortality during that year was demonstrated in only 19 patients. The mortality from dysrhythmias during the control year was unexpectedly high, and it is possible that the outcome in this small number of historical controls could represent a chance finding during a single year. Nevertheless, the findings of this study warrant a randomised trial of intravenous insulin in diabetic patients after myocardial infarction, and such a study is being conducted in a number of centres at present.

In this unit, we have developed an algorithm for the management of known diabetic patients admitted with acute myocardial infarction. The aim is to reduce the blood glucose concentration to between 4 mmol/l and 8 mmol/l during the first 4 hours following admission and to maintain this degree of glycaemic control for 72 hours. The regimen employs an intravenous infusion of human soluble insulin, diluted to 1 U/ml in sodium chloride solution 154 mmol/l, which is given via an intravenous infusion pump. The infusion rate is shown in Table 3, and is adjusted hourly on the basis of bedside reflectance meter blood glucose estimations. These are correlated with a laboratory blood glucose estimation every 4 hours in order to test accuracy, and serum potassium level is checked 12-hourly, intravenous potassium chloride being given if the level falls below 3.6 mmol/l. The insulin infusion rate is increased in patients in severe left ventricular failure or cardiogenic shock (Killip grades C and D [46]) because of our observations on the high levels of catecholamines and cortisol in these patients [113]. The algorithm also allows for the insulin resistance of obesity by a 50% increase in starting infusion rates in patients in excess of 120% of ideal body weight.

This regimen has been applied to 27 patients with confirmed myocardial infarction admitted over the last year. The results are shown in

Table 3 Insulin infusion regimen for diabetic patients admitted after acute myocardial infarction

1. Insulin infusion given by diluting 50 U human soluble insulin in 50 ml isotonic saline in an intravenous infusion pump
2. Blood glucose checked on reflectance meter in accident and emergency department
3. Clinical status of patient assessed

   Group A

   Patients without cardiac failure (Killip grade A)
   Patients with mild cardiac failure, e.g. elevated JVP, third heart sound, basal rales (Killip grade B)

   Group B

   Patients in severe left ventricular failure with clinical or radiological pulmonary oedema (Killip grade C)
   Patients in cardiogenic shock with systolic blood pressure < 90 mmHg, oliguria, cold clammy periphery (Killip grade D)
4. Select insulin infusion rate as follows:

Blood glucose (mmol/l)	Insulin infusion rate (U/h)	
	Group A	Group B
< 4	0	0
4–6.9	1	2
7–10.9	2	3
11–12.9	3	5
> 13	6	9

Increase dosage by 50% if patient is greater than 120% of ideal body weight

5. Check blood glucose level hourly on bedside reflectance meter until stable at 4–6 mmol/l for 3 consecutive hours, then 2-hourly for 4 hours, and 4-hourly for 12 hours
6. Check serum potassium level 12-hourly. Add potassium to infusion (5–10 mmol/h) if level < 3.6 mmol/l
7. Check results of bedside blood glucose estimation against laboratory sample every 4 hours
8. Call diabetic doctor if blood glucose is still more than 10 mmol/l after 4 hours or if symptomatic hypoglycaemia occurs

Figure 4, where it is seen that the mean blood glucose level was reduced to 9.3 mmol/l after 6 hours and remained stable at levels between 6.8 mmol/l and 9.1 mmol/l between 9 hours and 48 hours. The mean blood glucose level between 6 hours and 48 hours was 8.04 (SD 0.74) mmol/l. The regimen was as effective in 4 patients with pulmonary oedema or cardiogenic shock, who were severely hyperglycaemic on admission, as in the remaining 23 patients. Only 4 patients had blood glucose levels recorded below 3.0 mmol/l and only 2 of these experienced any symptoms.

Other Therapy in Diabetic Patients with Acute Myocardial Infarction

Thrombolytic agents such as streptokinase [68, 114] or tissue plasminogen activator [115] administered intravenously following acute myocardial infarction have become components of routine therapy. The major studies of these agents after myocardial infarction have included diabetic patients, but to date only one detailed analysis has been presented on the efficacy of these drugs in such patients. The ISIS-II study [116] employed intravenous streptokinase 1.5 MU over 1 hour, plus 160 mg of enteric-coated aspirin daily for 1 month, in 1287 diabetic and 15 694 non-diabetic patients. Whereas the benefits of streptokinase were similar in diabetic and non-diabetic patients (31% versus 23% reduction in 35-day mortality), aspirin showed no benefit in diabetic patients (0% versus 23% reduction in non-diabetic patients). Although this may be a subgroup effect, it is also possible that aspirin therapy in diabetic patients may require larger or more frequent doses (see below). The efficacy of other approaches [117], such as early intervention with β-blockers [45], intravenous nitrates, calcium-channel blockers, or anticoagulants, have not been systematically studied in diabetic patients. A subgroup analysis of the ISIS-I study, employing intravenous atenolol 5–10 mg followed by 100 mg orally for 7 days, showed a 19.8% reduction in 7-day vascular mortality in 958 diabetic patients, compared with a 13.9% reduction in non-diabetic patients [45]. However, even with nearly 1000 diabetic patients, the reduction in mortality was far from significant ($\chi^2 = 0.9$, $P < 0.4$). The high risk of thromboembolism might imply that the diabetic patient should receive subcutaneous heparin, although such therapy could further elevate levels of NEFA. Moreover, heparin may have proaggregatory effects on platelets in patients with vascular disease, a property that may not be shared by low molecular weight heparinoids [118].

Several studies have suggested that a reduction in long-term mortality after myocardial infarction may be produced by β-adrenergic blocking agents [119] and by antiplatelet drugs [120]. A separate analysis of the diabetic patients admitted to the timolol study showed a 63% benefit in reducing total mortality over 1–3 years and parallel reductions in cardiac deaths and non-fatal reinfarctions in these patients [121]. Two other reports have also suggested that the benefits of β-blockade may be greater in diabetic than in non-diabetic subjects [122, 123]. A meta-analysis of the studies of treatment with

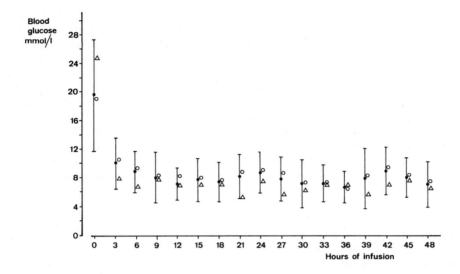

Figure 4 Blood glucose levels in the initial 48 hours following admission after myocardial infarction in 27 diabetic patients treated with the insulin infusion regimen in Table 3. Values shown are means and 1 standard deviation. Four patients were classified as Killip grade C or D (triangles), and 23 patients were classified as Killip grade A or B (circles)

antiplatelet agents in patients following myocardial infarction suggests that such drugs may produce around 12% reduction in long-term vascular mortality [120], 29% reduction in non-fatal myocardial infarcts and 23% reduction in all vascular events. A dose of aspirin of 300 mg daily is as effective as higher doses, and no additional benefit accrues from the use of other drugs, either alone or in combination with aspirin [120]. The benefits of aspirin in diabetic patients have not been studied, although it is possible that the higher rate of platelet turnover would require a more frequent dosage interval, or an enteric-coated preparation, to maintain effective antiaggregatory action [124].

Stopping cigarette smoking would seem logical advice for a diabetic (as for a non-diabetic) patient who has sustained a myocardial infarction. Studies of angioplasty or coronary artery bypass in diabetic subjects following infarction have not been published, although the results of coronary artery surgery in diabetic patients as a whole are rather worse than those in non-diabetic patients [125]. There is a clear association between elevated levels of cholesterol and recurrence of myocardial infarction, and secondary prevention studies suggest that outcome after infarction is improved by lipid-lowering regimens [126, 127]. Secondary prevention studies in non-diabetic subjects have shown that

progression of atheroma can be slowed, or even reversed, by cholesterol-lowering drugs [128–130], and because diabetic patients after myocardial infarction are at such high risk of further coronary events, it would seem logical to investigate and treat elevated levels of total or low-density lipoprotein cholesterol, using target levels and therapeutic regimens similar to those that have been recommended for non-diabetic subjects [131, 132].

HYPERGLYCAEMIA FOLLOWING MYOCARDIAL INFARCTION AND THE CONTRIBUTION OF UNDIAGNOSED DIABETES

Hyperglycaemia is often present in patients admitted to hospital following myocardial infarction. Depending on the criteria, as many as 1 patient in 3 admitted with myocardial infarction may have an elevated blood glucose concentration [133–136]. In this unit, among 248 patients without known diabetes who had admission plasma glucose levels measured before administration of glucose or adrenergic drugs, 49 (19.8%) had a plasma glucose level of over 11 mmol/l [137, 138]. The hospital case fatality among these patients was 55%, compared with 18% among those patients with admission plasma glucose levels of under 11 mmol/l. The major cause of death in these patients, as in patients with known diabetes, was cardiogenic shock. Moreover, the relationship between hyperglycaemia and mortality remained significant even when age, gender, and infarct size as estimated by peak levels of aspartate transaminase, were included in the analysis [113].

Several series have attempted to define the contribution of undiagnosed diabetes to acute hyperglycaemia after myocardial infarction. Glucose tolerance following myocardial infarction is frequently abnormal, but the proportion showing such abnormal tolerance decreases with time [134–136, 139]: although up to 70% of patients with myocardial infarction show abnormal glucose tolerance within the first 3 days, only 6–15% of these patients have clinically apparent diabetes at follow-up. This may imply that these numbers had pre-existing diabetes, but could also be explained by the possibility that diabetes had been precipitated by the acute event.

A new approach to investigating this question has been provided by the advent of the glycated haemoglobin assay. We have demonstrated that the level is unaffected for 24 hours following a major vascular event [54], and can therefore assume that the assay reflects blood glucose levels over a period of several weeks preceding the infarct. In our unit we have validated the use of glycated haemoglobin assay, employing an isoelectric focusing technique with removal of the pre-A_{1c} band, against follow-up glucose tolerance tests at 3 months in 110 survivors of myocardial infarction [138]. This enabled us to define a level of glycated haemoglobin which was 100% sensitive and 99% specific for overt diabetes mellitus with fasting hyperglycaemia at follow-up. Employing these criteria, we have estimated that 4.3% of all patients admitted with myocardial infarction had previously undiagnosed overt diabetes mellitus, and these patients contributed 9.6% of hospital deaths [138]. Moreover, when these criteria were applied to the 49 patients without known diabetes mellitus, admitted with plasma glucose levels of over 11 mmol/l, only 9 (18.4%) had levels of glycated haemoglobin suggesting undiagnosed diabetes. There were only 3 patients of the 110 survivors with diabetic glucose tolerance tests at 3 months, but normal admission levels of glycated haemoglobin and non-diabetic glucose tolerance tests within 10 days of the infarct. All 3 patients had normal fasting blood glucose levels, and all were in chronic heart failure and on large doses of diuretics [138]. This would suggest that the phenomenon of diabetes being precipitated by myocardial infarction per se is a rare event.

Previous estimates of the proportion of hyperglycaemic patients with undiagnosed diabetes, as indicated by elevated glycated haemoglobin levels, have varied from 5% to 63% [136, 140, 141], but these studies did not validate the cut-off levels of glycated haemoglobin for defining diabetes against follow-up glucose tolerance tests. Three more recent studies, in Indian patients admitted to hospital in Durban, South Africa [142], in Denmark [143] and in New Zealand [144], have performed follow-up glucose tolerance tests. In the South African series, 53% of surviving patients admitted with plasma glucose levels exceeding 8 mmol/l had diabetes mellitus at 3 months follow-up. However, the levels of glycated haemoglobin and admission plasma glucose in the patients who died were not reported [142]. In the Danish series, 9 of 15 patients (60%) with admission blood glucose levels over 9 mmol/l had diabetic glucose tolerance tests at 2 months follow-up, and of these, 6 had elevated levels of glycated haemoglobin on admission, but glycated haemoglobin estimates were not performed on those with lower levels of blood glucose [143]. The New Zealand study suggested that the fructosamine assay was both sensitive (78%) and specific (95%) for diabetes at follow-up [144]. It is clear that the proportion of hyperglycaemic subjects with undiagnosed diabetes will vary according to the prevalence of diabetes in the population, and will also depend on the cut-off level used, and on the delay between onset of symptoms and time of admission or blood sampling.

The Determinants and Importance of Stress Hyperglycaemia

The relationship between admission hyperglycaemia and poor outcome from myocardial infarction has been well recognised. We analysed the hospital case fatality from myocardial infarction in 248 subjects without known diabetes and 75 known diabetics in whom both admission plasma glucose and glycated haemoglobin levels were available [137]. Table 4 shows the relationship between mortality and admission plasma glucose levels. It is seen that,

Table 4 Case fatality of myocardial infarction according to admission levels of plasma glucose and glycated haemoglobin in non-diabetic subjects

Admission plasma glucose	Glycated haemoglobin level			Non-diabetic patients: total	Known diabetes
	< 6.9%	6.9–7.8%	> 7.8%		
< 8 mmol/l	12/112 (11%)	0/12 (0%)	–	12/124 (10%)	1/4 (25%)
8–11 mmol/l	13/52 (25%)	8/20 (40%)	2/3 (67%)	23/75 (31%)	2/10 (20%)
> 11 mmol/l	13/21 (62%)	9/19 (47%)	5/9 (56%)	27/49 (55%)	28/61 (46%)
Total	38/185 (21%)	17/51 (33%)	7/12 (58%)	62/248 (25%)	31/75 (41%)

From reference 137, with permission.

regardless of previous tolerance status, there is an increasing mortality with elevation of plasma glucose. Moreover, there was no significant effect of glycated haemoglobin level on mortality when plasma glucose level was taken into account, the mortality being similar in non-diabetic and diabetic subjects at the same level of admission plasma glucose [137]. A study in Asian patients in Durban, South Africa, also suggested that stratification of subjects by blood glucose concentration demonstrates similar mortality rates in diabetic and non-diabetic subjects [40]. This might suggest that hyperglycaemia, rather than previous glucose intolerance, is the mediating factor for morbidity and mortality following myocardial infarction. Three other studies have demonstrated that hyperglycaemia, in the presence of normal levels of glycated haemoglobin, is associated with poor outcome [136, 140, 145], with hyperglycaemia frequently being associated with congestive cardiac failure or cardiogenic shock [145].

Using the cut-off levels for glycated haemoglobin defined by our follow-up studies [138], 4.3% of all patients admitted to hospital with myocardial infarction have undiagnosed overt diabetes, but because of the substantially increased mortality rate in such patients, these represent 9.6% of all hospital deaths [138]. This implies that in our unit patients with both known and previously undiagnosed diabetes comprised 18% of admissions with myocardial infarction, and represent 28% of hospital deaths. Moreover, if the patients with admission hyperglycaemia (> 11 mmol/l) and known diabetes are considered together, such patients represented 32% of all admissions with myocardial infarction but contributed 55% of hospital deaths [137]. Figure 5 shows the relationship between admission levels of glycated haemoglobin and of plasma glucose and outcome of

hospital stay in patients without known diabetes admitted with myocardial infarction over a 2-year period [138].

We have studied the determinants of hyperglycaemia in patients with normal levels of glycated haemoglobin admitted after myocardial infarction [113]. There is only a weak relationship between levels of plasma glucose and infarct size (Figure 6), with 7 of the 12 patients with admission plasma glucose levels above 11 mmol/l having peak levels of aspartate transaminase in the lower 50% of the distribution; 6 of these 7 patients either developed left ventricular failure or died, predominantly from cardiogenic shock. Thus, infarct size is a weak determinant of admission hyperglycaemia, and the poor outcome of hyperglycaemic patients from cardiogenic shock and left ventricular failure cannot be explained on the basis of their sustaining larger infarcts.

We studied 27 patients with normal levels of glycated haemoglobin in order to assess the determinants of admission plasma glucose levels [113]. This study demonstrated that approximately 75% of the variance of admission plasma glucose could be explained by levels of cortisol, adrenaline and noradrenaline, but infarct size and glycated haemoglobin levels did not further contribute in this model (Figures 7–9) [113]. In these patients there was a weak relationship between infarct size and levels of adrenaline ($r = 0.48$, $P < 0.02$), but the relationships between infarct size and cortisol and noradrenaline levels were not significant.

These findings do not provide any indication as to cause and effect in the relationship between hyperglycaemia and poor outcome. It is possible that patients with a small infarct but with premorbid abnormalities of left ventricular function develop left ventricular failure or cardiogenic shock and that this increases the levels

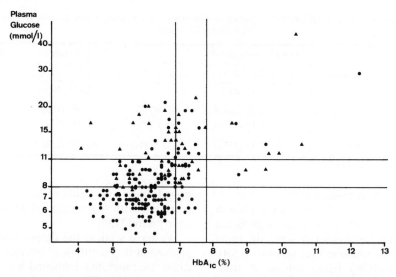

Figure 5 The relationship between admission plasma glucose levels and those of glycated haemoglobin in patients admitted with acute myocardial infarction. Patients who died are indicated by triangles, and those who survived by circles

of cortisol and catecholamines [146, 147]. In this case, hyperglycaemia might merely be an indicator of the presence of left ventricular failure. However, an alternative hypothesis is that hyperglycaemia, or a parallel metabolic abnormality, is the mediating agent in poor outcome after myocardial infarction. The relationship between elevated levels of free fatty acids [92, 94,

95] and the effects of hyperglycaemia on platelet function after myocardial infarction [84] have been discussed above. We have reported that non-diabetic patients developing cardiogenic shock with acute hyperglycaemia after myocardial infarction show marked elevation of plasma levels of platelet α-granule proteins, and that these correlate with levels of glucose and

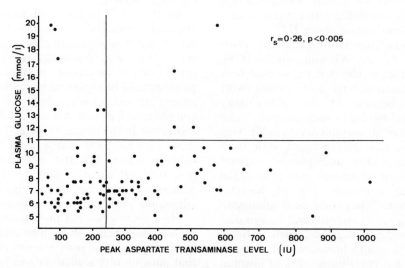

Figure 6 Plasma glucose levels on admission and peak aspartate transaminase levels in 101 consecutive patients with myocardial infarction with levels of glycated haemoglobin below 6.9%. Lines indicate the median value for aspartate transaminase activity and a plasma glucose concentration of 11 mmol/l (from reference 113, with permission)

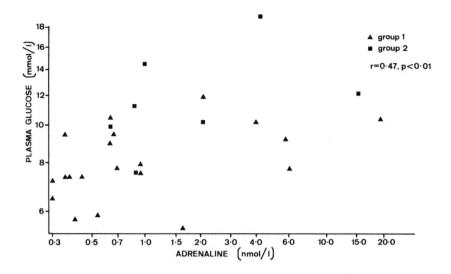

Figure 7 Log/log plot of adrenaline and plasma glucose levels in 26 non-diabetic patients with myocardial infarction. Group 1 (triangles), glycated haemoglobin levels below 6.9%; group 2 (squares), glycated haemoglobin levels 6.9–7.8% (from reference 113, with permission)

adrenaline and with the presence of pump failure [84]. Thus it is possible that the metabolic abnormalities in these patients are associated with an increase in platelet aggregation and the consequent risk of failure of coronary artery recanalisation.

Management of Hyperglycaemia in Patients Without Known Diabetes after Myocardial Infarction

It was noted above that only approximately 20% of patients with admission hypergly-

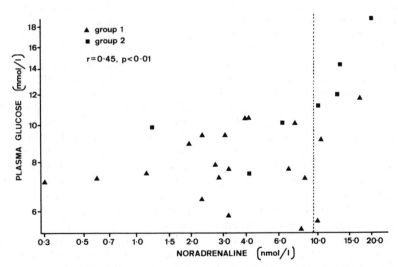

Figure 8 Log/log plot of noradrenaline and plasma glucose levels in 27 non-diabetic patients with myocardial infarction. The vertical dotted line is the threshold concentration for metabolic effects of noradrenaline in the basal state (from reference 113, with permission). Group 1 (triangles), glycated haemoglobin levels below 6.9%; group 2 (squares), glycated haemoglobin levels 6.9–7.8% (from reference 113, with permission)

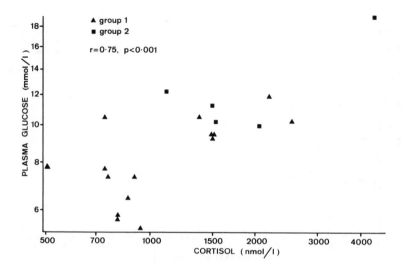

Figure 9 Log/log plot of cortisol and plasma glucose levels in 20 non-diabetic patients with myocardial infarction. Group 1 (triangles), glycated haemoglobin levels below 6.9%; group 2 (squares), glycated haemoglobin levels 6.9–7.8% (from reference 113, with permission)

caemia (admission plasma glucose levels above 11 mmol/l) have previously undiagnosed diabetes [138]. These patients share with known diabetic patients the excess risk of cardiogenic shock and left ventricular failure following myocardial infarction, with the hospital mortality being similar in both groups [44, 54, 113]. It is clear, however, that the benefits of treatment with intravenous insulin in these patients, and in those with stress hyperglycaemia, are even less clear than in patients with previously known diabetes. Moreover, the assessment of a glycated haemoglobin level, which would separate patients with undiagnosed diabetes from those with stress hyperglycaemia, is unlikely to be available in the acute phase of treatment, so that approximately 4 patients with stress hyperglycaemia would be treated for each patient with undiagnosed diabetes. Such patients require much larger doses of insulin to induce normoglycaemia than patients with previously undiagnosed diabetes, presumably as a result of the marked elevation in levels of cortisol and catecholamines. Nevertheless, despite the observation that levels of catecholamines in patients with acute myocardial infarction remain elevated and relatively constant over the first 48 hours following admission [148], we have found that around 50% of patients with stress hyperglycaemia and normal levels of glycated haemoglobin show a reduction in plasma glucose levels

over the subsequent 24 hours, and no longer require insulin infusion to maintain normoglycaemia.

ACUTE STROKE IN PATIENTS WITH DIABETES MELLITUS

The risk of thromboembolic stroke is increased in patients with diabetes mellitus [2], and this excess risk remains after controlling for age, obesity, hypertension, cholesterol level and cigarette smoking [5, 149]. There does not appear to be an increased risk of haemorrhagic stroke in patients with diabetes [149].

Diabetic patients represent between 7% and 25% of all patients with stroke in different series [150–159], and as well as the increased incidence of stroke, patients with diabetes mellitus may have a higher case fatality following an acute stroke. Asplund et al reported a 30% increase in hospital case fatality after a stroke in patients with known diabetes mellitus [150], and other studies reported a twofold [151] and a sevenfold excess [152]. However, in these reports, some 8–20% of the diabetic patients were so characterised during their hospital stay on the basis of persistently elevated blood-glucose levels, and bearing in mind the relationship between hyperglycaemia and poor outcome which is discussed below, the effect of diabetes on outcome is still obscure. In a series of 392 patients admitted to hospital in Israel between 1969 and 1975, mortality among the patients known to have diabetes was no greater than that in the non-diabetic subjects [153]. Long-term prognosis has been reported as being significantly worse in diabetic patients, with greater residual disability [151, 152], an excess risk of recurrent stroke [154] and of mortality in the first 6 months [154, 155].

Stress Hyperglycaemia or Undiagnosed Diabetes in Patients Following Acute Stroke

Acute hyperglycaemia, variously defined, has been found in 12–41% of non-diabetic patients with an acute stroke [153, 155, 158–160]. There is some controversy in the literature as to the proportion of these patients who have undiagnosed diabetes, and few studies have validated the cut-off levels of glycated haemoglobin employed to define previous glucose intolerance, against follow-up glucose tolerance tests. Thus, elevated levels of glycated haemoglobin were found in 5.3% [158], 30% [159] and 52% [156] of non-diabetic patients admitted with acute stroke. In our unit we have used our previously validated cut-off levels of glycated haemoglobin to define undiagnosed diabetes among 100 patients admitted with acute stroke [157]. Among these patients, 8 had known diabetes and 6 had levels of glycated haemoglobin indicating undiagnosed diabetes with fasting hyperglycaemia. We found no significant difference in overall 3-month mortality among the diabetic and non-diabetic groups—9 out of 14 (64%) versus 33 out of 86 (38%)—although all deaths in the diabetic group, but only 42% of those in the non-diabetic group, had occurred by 7 days following admission [157]. Gray et al [155, 159], by contrast, found no significant difference in total mortality at 4 weeks between those with raised glycated haemoglobin and those with normal levels, although by 12 weeks the mortality was greater among patients aged 65 years and older with elevated concentrations of glycated haemoglobin [155]. A Yugoslavian study found increased 3-week mortality in both known diabetic patients and those with elevated glycated haemoglobin levels on admission [160].

Acute Hyperglycaemia and Outcome of Stroke

Melamed [153] found a threefold increased mortality among stroke patients without known diabetes but with initial fasting serum glucose levels above 6.8 mmol/l, but no significant increase in mortality in known diabetic patients. Two groups [155, 158, 159] suggest that patients with normal levels of glycated haemoglobin, but who are hyperglycaemic on admission following acute stroke, have a worse outcome than patients remaining normoglycaemic. Thus Cox and Lorains [158] reported a mortality of 80% in patients with stress hyperglycaemia compared with 31% in those admitted with normal levels of glucose. Gray et al [155, 159] reported a 4-week mortality of 48% among those with admission blood-glucose levels of 8 mmol/l and above (including known diabetics), compared with 23% in those with normal levels of blood glucose on admission. This relationship was stronger in patients younger than 65 years. These authors also noted that 4 weeks after the acute stroke, no patients admitted with acute hyperglycaemia had regained full functional use of their limbs [159]. It appears from these observations that stress hyperglycaemia is a more reliable predictor of adverse outcome after stroke than is previous diabetes, although these findings are not universal [160, 161]. However, there was a significant difference in the distribution and type of cerebral injury in the hyperglycaemic and normoglycaemic patients in two of these studies, with brain-stem infarcts [153, 159] and haemorrhagic stroke [153] more commonly associated with hyperglycaemia.

Benefits of Tight Blood Glucose Control in Diabetic and Hyperglycaemic Patients after Acute Stroke

As is the situation with acute myocardial infarction, there is little scientific evidence on which to base therapeutic regimens in diabetic and hyperglycaemic patients following acute stroke. There appears to be a clear association between hyperglycaemia in both diabetic and non-diabetic subjects, and poor outcome from stroke; furthermore, animal studies have demonstrated that acute hyperglycaemia at the time of cerebral ischaemia results in greater metabolic abnormalities in brain tissue and poorer clinical outcome than in normoglycaemic controls [162–164]. This may result from an increase in anaerobic metabolism and local production of lactic acid. Siemkowicz demonstrated that correcting the blood glucose in hyperglycaemic rats after induction of cerebral ischaemia reduced the degree of functional damage [165]. However, a prospective study would be necessary in order to apply such conclusions to patients with acute stroke, as the severity of hyperglycaemia may be a consequence, rather than a cause, of cerebral damage [161].

As is the case with diabetic patients with acute myocardial infarction, the relative numbers of stroke patients with known or previously undiagnosed diabetes make the task of therapeutic trials in such subjects prohibitively difficult. Moreover, the state of the art regarding therapeutic intervention after stroke is much less developed than that after acute myocardial infarction, so that firm recommendations concerning the management of these patients cannot be made. For acute phase therapy, several agents are currently on trial; but apart from careful control of severe hypertension and correcting hypoxia, no convincing evidence of benefit from any intervention is apparent [166, 167]. Further trials of tissue plasminogen activator, of haemodilution with dextran, of anticoagulation with heparin in progressing thrombosis, or of calcium channel blockade or β-blockade, may provide future guidelines for improved care [167]. Numerous studies have shown a convincing reduction in cerebrovascular mortality and other vascular events by the use of antiplatelet agents in patients with transient ischaemic attacks or minor strokes, and a recent review [120] suggests that aspirin at a daily dose of 300 mg is as effective as larger doses, with no added benefits from other antiplatelet drugs.

REFERENCES

1. Pell S, D'Alonzo CA. Factors associated with long-term survival of diabetics. JAMA 1970; 214: 1833-40.
2. Garcia MJ, McNamara PM, Gordon T, Kannel WB. Morbidity and mortality in diabetics in the Framingham population. Sixteen year follow-up study. Diabetes 1974; 23: 105-11.
3. Herman JB, Medalie JH, Goldbourt U. Differences in cardiovascular morbidity and mortality between previously known and newly diagnosed adult diabetics. Diabetologia 1977; 13: 229-34.
4. Fuller JH, Shipley MJ, Rose G, Jarrett RJ, Keen H. Coronary-heart-disease risk and impaired glucose tolerance. The Whitehall Study. Lancet 1980; i: 1373-6.
5. Kannel WB, McGee DL. Diabetes and glucose tolerance as risk factors for cardiovascular disease: the Framingham Study. Diabetes Care 1979; 2: 120-6.
6. Jarrett RJ, McCartney P, Keen H. The Bedford Survey: ten year mortality rates in newly diagnosed diabetics, borderline diabetics and normoglycaemic controls and risk indices for coronary heart disease in borderline diabetics. Diabetologia 1982; 22: 79-84.
7. Entmacher PS, Root HF, Marks HH. Longevity of diabetic patients in recent years. Diabetes 1964; 13: 373-7.
8. Kannel WB, McGee DL. Diabetes and cardiovascular disease: the Framingham Study. JAMA 1979; 241: 2035-8.
9. Jarrett RJ. Type 2 (non-insulin dependent) diabetes mellitus and coronary heart disease—chicken, egg or neither? Diabetologia 1984; 26: 99-102.
10. Borch-Johnsen K, Kreiner S. Proteinuria: value as prediction of cardiovascular mortality in insulin dependent diabetes mellitus. Br Med J 1987; 294: 1651-4.
11. Mogensen CE. Microalbuminuria predicts clinical proteinuria and early mortality in maturity-onset diabetes. New Engl J Med 1984; 310: 356-60.
12. Robertson WB, Strong JP. Atherosclerosis in persons with hypertension and diabetes mellitus. Lab Invest 1968; 18: 538-51.
13. Sternby NH. Atherosclerosis in a defined population. An autopsy survey in Malmö, Sweden. Acta Pathol Microbiol Scand 1968; suppl. 194: 152-64.
14. Mustard JF, Packham MA. Platelets and diabetes mellitus. New Engl J Med 1984; 311: 665-7.
15. Fuller JH, Keen H, Jarrett RJ et al. Haemostatic variables associated with diabetes and its complications. Br Med J 1979; 2: 964-6.
16. McMillan DE. The effect of diabetes on blood flow properties. Diabetes 1983; 32 (suppl. 2): 56-63.
17. Partamian JO, Bradley RF. Acute myocardial infarction in 258 cases of diabetes. Immediate mortality and five-year survival. New Engl J Med 1965; 273: 455-61.
18. McGuire LB, Kroll MS. Evaluation of cardiac care units and myocardial infarction. Arch Int Med 1972; 130: 677-81.
19. Soler NG, Bennett MA, Lamb P, Pentecost BL, FitzGerald MG, Malins JM. Coronary care for myocardial infarction in diabetics. Lancet 1974; i: 475-7.

20. Soler NG, Bennett MA, Pentecost BL, Fitz-Gerald MG, Malins JM. Myocardial infarction in diabetics. Quart J Med 1975; 44: 125–32.

21. Henning R, Lundman T. Swedish Cooperative CCU Study, part A: a description of the early stage. Acta Med Scand 1975; suppl 586: 1–64.

22. Harrower ADB, Clarke BF. Experience of coronary care in diabetes. Br Med J 1976; i: 126–8.

23. Lichstein E, Kuhn LA, Goldberg E, Mulvihill MN, Smith H, Chalmers TC. Diabetic treatment and primary ventricular fibrillation in acute myocardial infarction. Am J Cardiol 1976; 38: 100–2.

24. Kvetny J. Diabetes mellitus and acute myocardial infarction. Acta Med Scand 1976; 200: 151–3.

25. Tansey MJB, Opie LH, Kennelly BM. High mortality in obese women diabetics with acute myocardial infarction. Br Med J 1977; 1: 1624–6.

26. Maempel JVZ. Effect of diabetes on the course of acute myocardial infarction in Malta. Israel J Med Sci 1978; 14: 424–31.

27. Czyżyk A, Królewski AS, Szablowska S, Alot A, Kopczyński J. Clinical course of myocardial infarction among diabetic patients. Diabetes Care 1980; 3: 526–9.

28. Weitzman S, Wagner GS, Heiss G, Haney TL, Slome C. Myocardial infarct site and mortality in diabetes. Diabetes Care 1982; 5: 31–5.

29. Jaffe AS, Spadaro JJ, Schechtman K, Roberts R, Geltman EM, Sobel BE. Increased congestive heart failure after myocardial infarction of modest extent in patients with diabetes mellitus. Am Heart J 1984; 108: 31–7.

30. Gwilt DJ, Petri M, Lamb P, Nattrass M, Pentecost BL. Effect of intravenous insulin infusion on mortality among diabetic patients after myocardial infarction. Br Heart J 1984; 51: 626–30.

31. Rytter L, Troelsen S, Beck-Nielsen H. Prevalence and mortality of acute myocardial infarction in patients with diabetes. Diabetes Care 1985; 8: 230–4.

32. Yudkin JS, Oswald GA. Determinants of hospital admissions and case fatality in diabetic patients with myocardial infarction. Diabetes Care 1988; 11: 351–8.

33. Mølstad P, Nastad M. Acute myocardial infarction in diabetic patients. Acta Med Scand 1988; 222: 433–7.

34. Malmberg K, Rydén L. Myocardial infarction in patients with diabetes mellitus. Eur Heart J 1988; 9: 259–64.

35. Kouvaras G, Cokkinos D, Spyropoulou M. Increased mortality of diabetics after acute myocardial infarction attributed to diffusely impaired left ventricular performance as assessed by echocardiography. Jap Heart J 1988; 29: 1–9.

36. Savage MP, Krolewski AS, Kenien GG, Lebeis MP, Christlieb R, Lewis SM. Acute myocardial infarction in diabetes mellitus and significance of congestive heart failure as a prognostic factor. Am J Cardiol 1988; 62: 665–9.

37. Day JJ, Bayer AJ, Chadha JS, Pathy MSJ. Myocardial infarction in old people. The influence of diabetes mellitus. J Am Geriat Soc 1988; 36: 791–4.

38. Herlitz J, Malmberg K, Karlson BW, Rydén L, Hjalmarson Å. Mortality and morbidity during a five-year follow-up of diabetics with myocardial infarction. Acta Med Scand 1988; 224: 31–8.

39. Stone PH, Muller JE, Hartwell T et al. The effect of diabetes mellitus on prognosis and serial left ventricular function after acute myocardial infarction: contribution of both coronary disease and diastolic left ventricular dysfunction to the adverse prognosis. Am J Cardiol 1989; 14: 49–57.

40. Sewdarsen M, Vythilingum S, Jialal I, Becker PJ. Prognostic importance of admission plasma glucose in diabetic and non-diabetic patients with acute myocardial infarction. Quart J Med 1989; 71: 461–6.

41. Singer DE, Moulton AW, Nathan DM. Diabetic myocardial infarction. Interaction of diabetes with other preinfarction risk factors. Diabetes 1989; 38: 350–7.

42. Gwilt DJ. Why do diabetic patients die after myocardial infarction? Pract Diabetes 1984; 1(2): 36–9.

43. Eschwège E, Ducimetière P, Papoz L, Claude JR, Richard JL. Blood glucose and coronary heart disease. Lancet 1980; ii: 472–3.

44. Yudkin JS, Oswald GA, McKeigue PM, Forrest RD, Jackson CA. The relationship of hospital admission and fatality from myocardial infarction to glycohaemoglobin level. Diabetologia 1988; 31: 201–5.

45. ISIS-I. Randomised trial of intravenous atenolol among 16 027 cases of suspected acute myocardial infarction: ISIS-I. Lancet 1986; ii: 57–66.

46. Killip T, Kimball JT. Treatment of myocardial infarction in a community care unit. A two-year experience with 250 patients. Am J Cardiol 1967; 20: 457–64.

47. Mathewson ZM, McCloskey BG, Evans AE, Russell CJ, Wilson C. Mobile coronary care and community mortality from myocardial infarction. Lancet 1985; i: 441–4.

48. Tunstall Pedoe H, Clayton D, Morris JN, Brigden W, McDonald L. Coronary heart-attacks in East London. Lancet 1975; ii: 833–8.

49. Kannel WB. Role of diabetes in cardiac disease: conclusions from population studies. In Zoneraich S (ed.) Diabetes and the heart. Springfield: Thomas, 1978: pp 97–112.

50. University Group Diabetes Program. A study of the effects of hypoglycemic agents on vascular complications in patients with adult-onset diabetes. 2. Mortality results. Diabetes 1970; 19 (suppl. 2): 785–830.

51. University Group Diabetes Program. Effects of hypoglycemic agents on vascular complications in patients with adult-onset diabetes. 4. A preliminary report on phenformin results. JAMA 1971; 217: 777–84.

52. Barrett-Connor E, Orchard TJ. Insulin-dependent diabetes mellitus and ischemic heart disease. Diabetes Care 1985; 8 (suppl. 1): 65–70.

53. Keen H, Jarrett RJ. The WHO Multinational Study of vascular disease in diabetes. 2. Macrovascular disease prevalence. Diabetes Care 1979; 2: 187–95.

54. Oswald GA, Corcoran S, Yudkin JS. Prevalence and risks of hyperglycaemia and undiagnosed diabetes in patients with acute myocardial infarction. Lancet 1984; i: 1264–7.

55. Bradley RF, Shonfeld A. Diminished pain in diabetic patients with acute myocardial infarction. Geriatrics 1962; 17: 322–6.

56. Niakan E, Harati Y, Rolak LA, Comstock JP, Rokey R. Silent myocardial infarction and diabetic cardiovascular autonomic neuropathy. Arch Int Med 1986; 146: 2229–30.

57. Faerman I, Faccio E, Milei J, Nuñez R, Jadzinski M, Fox D, Rapaport M. Autonomic neuropathy and painless myocardial infarction in diabetic patients. Histological evidence of their relationship. Diabetes 1977; 26: 1147–58.

58. Kannel WB, Abbott RD. Incidence and prognosis of unrecognised myocardial infarction: an update on the Framingham study. New Engl J Med 1984; 311: 1144–7.

59. Margolis JR, Kannel WB, Feinleib M, Dawber TR, McNamara PM. Clinical features of unrecognised myocardial infarction—silent and symptomatic. Eighteen year follow-up: the Framingham Study. Am J Cardiol 1973; 32: 1–7.

60. Gwilt DJ, Petri M, Lewis PW, Nattrass M, Pentecost BL. Myocardial infarct size and mortality in diabetic patients. Br Heart J 1985; 54: 466–72.

61. Vatner S, Baig H, Manders WT, Maroko PR. Effects of coronary artery reperfusion on myocardial infarct size calculated from creatine kinase. J Clin Invest 1978; 61: 1048–56.

62. Blanke H, von Hardenberg D, Cohen M et al. Patterns of creatine kinase release during acute myocardial infarction after nonsurgical reperfusion: comparison with conventional treatment and correlation with infarct size. J Am Coll Cardiol 1984; 3: 675–80.

63. Ong L, Reiser P, Coromilas J, Scherr L, Morrison J. Left ventricular function and rapid release of creatine kinase-MB in acute myocardial infarction: evidence for spontaneous reperfusion. New Engl J Med 1983; 309: 1–6.

64. Rennert G, Saltz-Rennert H, Wanderman K, Weitzman S. Size of acute myocardial infarcts in patients with diabetes mellitus. Am J Cardiol 1985; 55: 1629–30.

65. Takahashi N, Iwasaka T, Sugiura T et al. Left ventricular regional function after acute myocardial infarction in diabetic patients. Diabetes Care 1989; 12: 630–5.

66. Oswald GA, Corcoran JS, Patterson DLH, Yudkin JS. The extent of coronary artery disease in diabetic patients with myocardial infarction: an ECG study. Diabet Med 1986; 3: 541–4.

67. Waller BF, Palumbo PJ, Lie JT, Roberts WC. Status of the coronary arteries at necropsy in diabetes mellitus with onset after age 30 years. Analysis of 229 diabetic patients with and without clinical evidence of coronary heart disease and comparison to 183 control subjects. Am J Med 1980; 69: 498–506.

68. White HD, Norris RM, Brown MA et al. Effect of intravenous streptokinase on left ventricular function and early survival after acute myocardial infarction. New Engl J Med 1987; 317: 850–5.

69. De Wood MA, Spores J, Notske R et al. Prevalence of total coronary occlusion during the early hours of transmural myocardial infarction. New Engl J Med 1980; 303: 897–902.

70. Falk E. Unstable angina with fatal outcome: dynamic coronary thrombosis leading to infarction and/or sudden death. Autopsy evidence of recurring mural thrombosis with peripheral embolization culminating in total vascular occlusion. Circulation 1985; 71: 699–708.

71. Haines AP, Howarth D, North WRS et al. Haemostatic variables and the outcome of myocardial infarction. Thromb Haemost 1983; 50: 800–3.

72. Meade TW, Brozovic M, Chakrabarti RR et al. Haemostatic function and ischaemic heart disease: principal results of the Northwick Park Heart Study. Lancet 1986; ii: 533–7.

73. Hamsten A, Wiman B, de Faire U, Blombäck M. Increased plasma levels of a rapid inhibitor of tissue plasminogen activator in young survivors of myocardial infarction. New Engl J Med 1985; 313: 1557–63.

74. Hamsten A, de Faire U, Walldius G et al. Plasminogen activator inhibitor in plasma: risk factor for recurrent myocardial infarction. Lancet 1987; ii: 3–9.

75. Auwerx J, Bouillon R, Collen D, Geboers J. Tissue-type plasminogen activator antigen and plasminogen activator inhibitor in diabetes mellitus. Arteriosclerosis 1988; 8: 68–72.

76. Small M, Kluft C, MacCuish AC, Lowe GDO. Tissue plasminogen activator inhibition in diabetes mellitus. Diabetes Care 1989; 12: 655–8.

77. Juhan-Vague I, Roul C, Alessi MC, Ardissone JP, Heim M, Vague P. Increased plasminogen activator inhibitor activity in non insulin dependent diabetic patients—relationship with plasma insulin. Thromb Haemost 1989; 61: 370–3.

78. Nagi DK, Jain S, Garvey S, Walji S, Yudkin JS. Defective fibrinolysis in non-insulin-dependent diabetics relates to plasma insulin concentrations. Clin Sci 1990; 79 (suppl. 24): 25P.

79. Alessi MC, Juhan-Vague I, Kooistra T, Declerck PJ, Collen D. Insulin stimulates the synthesis of plasminogen activator inhibitor-1 by human hepatocellular cell line Hep G$_2$. Thromb Haemost 1988; 60: 491–4.

80. Nagi DK, Hendra TJ, Ryle AJ et al. The relationships of concentrations of insulin, intact proinsulin and 32,33 split proinsulin with cardiovascular risk factors in type 2 (non-insulin-dependent) diabetic subjects. Diabetologia 1990; 33: 532–7.

81. Gray R, Yudkin JS, Patterson D. Impaired fibrinolytic activity relates to glycaemia in patients with acute myocardial infarction. Clin Sci 1990; 79 (suppl. 24): 23P.

82. Barbash GI, Hod H, Roth A et al. Correlation of baseline plasminogen activator inhibitor activity with patency of the infarct artery after thrombolytic therapy in acute myocardial infarction. Am J Cardiol 1989; 64: 1231–5.

83. Lucore CL, Fujii S, Sobel BE. Dependence of fibrinolytic activity on the concentration of free rather than total tissue-type plasminogen activator in plasma after pharmacologic administration. Circulation 1989; 79: 1204–13.

84. Oswald GA, Smith CCT, Delamothe AP, Betteridge DJ, Yudkin JS. Elevated levels of glucose and adrenaline after myocardial infarction are associated with increased in-vivo platelet activation. Br Heart J 1988; 59: 663–71.

85. Swan HJC. Acute myocardial infarction: a failure of timely, spontaneous thrombolysis. J Am Coll Cardiol 1989; 13: 1435–7.

86. Trip MD, Cats VM, van Capelle FJL, Vreeken J. Platelet hyperactivity and prognosis in survivors of myocardial infarction. New Engl J Med 1990; 322: 1549–54.

87. Regan TJ, Lyons MM, Ahmed SS, Levinson GE, Oldewurtel HA, Ahmad MR, Haider B. Evidence for cardiomyopathy in familial diabetes mellitus. J Clin Invest 1977; 60: 885–99.

88. van Hoeven KH, Factor SM. A comparison of the pathological spectrum of hypertensive, diabetic and hypertensive-diabetic heart disease. Circulation 1990; 82: 848–55.

89. Factor SM, Okun EM, Minase T. Capillary microaneurysms in the human diabetic heart. New Engl J Med 1980; 302: 384–8.

90. Yudkin JS, Cooper MB, Gould BJ, Oughton J. Glycosylation and cross-linking of cardiac myosin in diabetic subjects—a post mortem study. Diabet Med 1988; 5: 338–42.

91. Ganguly PK, Thliveris JA, Mehta A. Evidence against the involvement of non-enzymatic glycosylation in diabetic cardiomyopathy. Metabolism 1990; 39: 769–73.

92. Opie LH. Metabolism of free fatty acids, glucose and catecholamines in acute myocardial infarction. Relation to myocardial ischemia and infarct size. Am J Cardiol 1975; 36: 938–53.

93. Taegtmeyer H, Passmore JM. Defective energy metabolism of the heart in diabetes. Lancet 1985; i: 139–41.

94. Liedtke AJ, Nellis S, Neely JR. Effects of excess free fatty acids on mechanical and metabolic function in normal ischemic myocardium in swine. Circ Res 1978; 43: 652–61.

95. Kjekshus JK, Mjøs OD. Effect of free fatty acids on myocardial function and metabolism in the ischemic dog heart. J Clin Invest 1972; 51: 1767–76.

96. McCord JM. Oxygen-derived free radicals in postischemic tissue injury. New Engl J Med 1985; 312: 159–63.

97. Davies SW, Ranjadayalan K, Wickens DG, Dormandy TL, Timmis AD. Lipid peroxidation associated with successful thrombolysis. Lancet 1990; 335: 741–3.

98. Davies SW, Wickens DG, Ranjadayalan K, Dormandy TL, Timmis AD. Oxidative stress on reperfusion of myocardial infarction in man. Clin Sci 1990; 79 (suppl. 24): 25P.

99. Jennings PE, Jones AF, Florkowski CM, Lunec J, Barnett AH. Increased diene conjugates in diabetic subjects with microangiopathy. Diabet Med 1987; 4: 452–6.

100. Wickens DG, Griffin JF, Maher ER, Curtis JR, Dormandy TL. The effect of systemic heparinisation and haemodialysis on plasma octadeca-9,11-dienoic acid (9,11-LA'). Free Rad Res Comm 1987; 3: 99–106.

101. Hendra TJ, Wickens DG, Dormandy TL, Yudkin JS. Platelet function and conjugated diene concentrations in diabetic and non-diabetic survivors of acute myocardial infarction. Cardiovasc Res 1991; 25: 676–83.

102. Hilsted J, Madsbad S, Krarup T, Sestoft L, Christensen NJ, Tronier B, Galbo H. Hormonal, metabolic and cardiovascular responses to hypoglycemia in diabetic autonomic neuropathy. Diabetes 1981; 30: 626–33.

103. White NH, Skor DA, Cryer PE, Levandoski LA, Bier DM, Santiago JV. Identification of type I diabetic patients at increased risk for

hypoglycemia during intensive therapy. New Engl J Med 1983; 308: 485–91.

104. Smith JW, Marcus FI, Serokman R. Prognosis of patients with diabetes mellitus after acute myocardial infarction. Am J Cardiol 1984; 54: 718–21.

105. Ulvenstam G, Åberg A, Bergstrand R et al. Long term prognosis after myocardial infarction in men with diabetes. Diabetes 1985; 34: 787–92.

106. Abbott RD, Donahue RP, Kannel WB, Wilson PWF. The impact of diabetes on survival following myocardial infarction in men vs women. The Framingham Study. JAMA 1988; 260: 3456–60.

107. Frier BM, Hilsted J. Does hypoglycaemia aggravate the complications of diabetes? Lancet 1985; ii: 1175–7.

108. Trovati M, Anfossi G, Cavalot F et al. Studies on mechanisms involved in hypoglycemia-induced platelet activation. Diabetes 1986; 35: 818–25.

109. Grant JA, Scrutton MC. Positive interaction between agonists in the aggregation response of human blood platelets: interaction between ADP, adrenaline and vasopressin. Br J Haem 1980; 44: 109–25.

110. Gwilt DJ, Nattrass M, Pentecost BL. Use of low-dose insulin infusions in diabetes after myocardial infarction. Br Med J 1982; 285: 1402–4.

111. Husband DJ, Alberti KGMM, Julian DG. Methods for the control of diabetes after acute myocardial infarction. Diabetes Care 1985; 8: 261–7.

112. Clark RS, English M, McNeill GP, Newton RW. Effect of intravenous infusion of insulin in diabetics with acute myocardial infarction. Br Med J 1985; 291: 303–5.

113. Oswald GA, Smith CCT, Betteridge DJ, Yudkin JS. Determinants and importance of stress hyperglycaemia in non-diabetic patients with myocardial infarction. Br Med J 1986; 293: 917–22.

114. ISAM Study Group. A prospective trial of intravenous streptokinase in acute myocardial infarction (ISAM): mortality, morbidity and infarct size at 21 days. New Engl J Med 1986; 314: 1465–71.

115. TIMI Study Group. The thrombolysis in myocardial infarction (TIMI) trial. Phase I findings. New Engl J Med 1985; 312: 932–6.

116. Second International Study of Infarct Survival Collaborative Group. Randomised trial of intravenous streptokinase, oral aspirin, both, or neither among 17187 cases of suspected acute myocardial infarction: ISIS-2. Lancet 1988; ii: 349–60.

117. Evans AE. Secondary prevention after myocardial infarction. Lancet 1986; ii: 150–1.

118. Mikhailidis DP, Fonseka VA, Barradas MA, Jeremy JY, Dandona P. Platelet activation following injection of a conventional heparin: absence of effect with a low molecular weight heparinoid (Org 10172). Br J Clin Pharm 1987; 24: 415–24.

119. Yusuf S, Peto R, Lewis J, Collins R, Sleight P. Beta blockade during and after myocardial infarction: an overview of the randomised trials. Prog Cardiovasc Dis 1985; 27: 335–71.

120. Anti-Platelet Trialists Collaboration. Secondary prevention of vascular disease by prolonged anti-platelet therapy. Br Med J 1988; 296: 320–31.

121. Gundersen T, Kjekshus J. Timolol treatment after myocardial infarction in diabetic patients. Diabetes Care 1983; 6: 285–90.

122. Malmberg K, Herlitz J, Hjalmarson Å, Rydén L. Effects of metoprolol on mortality and late infarction in diabetics with suspected acute myocardial infarction. Retrospective data from two large studies. Eur Heart J 1989; 10: 423–8.

123. Kjekshus J, Gilpin E, Cali G, Blackey AR, Henning H, Ross J. Diabetic patients and beta-blockers after acute myocardial infarction. Eur Heart J 1990; 11: 43–50.

124. Di Minno G, Silver MJ, Cerbone AM, Murphy S. Trial of repeated low dose aspirin in diabetic angiopathy. Blood 1986; 68: 886–91.

125. Lawrie GM, Morris GC, Glaeser DH. Influence of diabetes mellitus on the results of coronary artery bypass surgery. Follow-up of 212 diabetic patients 10 to 15 years after surgery. JAMA 1986; 256: 2967–71.

126. Oliver MF. Why measure cholesterol after myocardial infarction, and when? Br Med J 1984; 289: 1641–2.

127. Rossouw JE, Lewis B, Rifkind BM. The value of lowering cholesterol after myocardial infarction. New Engl J Med 1990; 323: 1112–19.

128. Nikkilä EA, Viikinkoski P, Valle M, Frick MH. Prevention of progression of coronary atherosclerosis by treatment of hyperlipidaemia: a seven year prospective angiographic study. Br Med J 1984; 289: 220–3.

129. Blankenhorn DH, Nessim SA, Johnson RL, Sanmarco ME, Azen SP, Cashin-Hemphill L. Beneficial effects of combined colestipol-niacin therapy on coronary atherosclerosis and coronary venous bypass grafts. JAMA 1987; 257: 3233–40.

130. Brown G, Albers JJ, Fisher LD et al. Regression of coronary artery disease as a result of intensive lipid-lowering therapy in men with high levels of apoliproprotein B. New Engl J Med 1990; 323: 1289–98.

131. Consensus Conference Development Panel. Lowering blood cholesterol to prevent heart disease. JAMA 1985; 253: 2080–6.

132. Shepherd J, Betteridge DJ, Durrington P et al. Strategies for reducing coronary heart disease and desirable limits for blood lipid concentrations; guidelines of the British Hyperlipidaemia Association. Br Med J 1987; 295: 1245–6.

133. Ellenberg M, Osserman KE, Pollack H. Hyperglycemia in coronary thrombosis. Diabetes 1952; 1: 16–20.

134. Datey KK, Nanda NC. Hyperglycemia after acute myocardial infarction. Its relation to diabetes mellitus. New Engl J Med 1967; 276: 262–5.

135. Ravid M, Berkowicz M, Sohar E. Hyperglycemia during acute myocardial infarction—a six-year follow-up study. JAMA 1975; 233: 807–9.

136. Soler NG, Frank S. Value of glycosylated hemoglobin measurements after acute myocardial infarction. JAMA 1981; 246: 1690–3.

137. Yudkin JS, Oswald GA. Hyperglycaemia, diabetes and myocardial infarction. Diabet Med 1987; 4: 13–18.

138. Oswald GA, Yudkin JS. Hyperglycaemia following acute myocardial infarction: the contribution of undiagnosed diabetes. Diabet Med 1987; 4: 68–70.

139. Sowton E. Cardiac infarction and the glucose-tolerance test. Br Med J 1962; i: 84–6.

140. Lakhdar A, Stromberg P, McAlpine SG. Prognostic importance of hyperglycaemia induced by stress after acute myocardial infarction. Br Med J 1984; 288: 288.

141. Husband DJ, Alberti KGMM, Julian DG. Stress induced hyperglycaemia during acute myocardial infarction: an indicator of pre-existing diabetes. Lancet 1983; ii: 179–81.

142. Sewdarsen M, Jialal I, Vythilingum S, Govender G, Rajput MC. Stress hyperglycaemia is a predictor of abnormal glucose tolerance in Indian patients with acute myocardial infarction. Diabetes Res 1987; 6: 47–9.

143. Madsen JK, Haunsøe S, Helquist S et al. Prevalence of hyperglycaemia and undiagnosed diabetes mellitus in patients with acute myocardial infarction. Acta Med Scand 1986; 220: 329–32.

144. Kyle C, Johnson R, Baker J, Norris R, Metcalf P. Serum fructosamine as a screening method for diabetes mellitus in patients with suspected acute myocardial infarction. Aust NZ J Med 1987; 17: 467–71.

145. Bellodi G, Manicardi V, Malavasi V et al. Hyperglycemia and prognosis of acute myocardial infarction in patients without diabetes mellitus. Am J Cardiol 1989; 64: 885–8.

146. Cohn JN, Levine TB, Olivari MT et al. Plasma norepinephrine as a guide to prognosis in patients with chronic congestive heart failure. New Engl J Med 1984; 311: 819–23.

147. Prakash R, Parmley WW, Horvat M, Swan HJC. Serum cortisol, plasma free fatty acids, and urinary catecholamines as indicators of complications in acute myocardial infarction. Circulation 1972; 45: 736–45.

148. Videbaek J, Christensen NJ, Sterndorff B. Serial determination of plasma catecholamines in myocardial infarction. Circulation 1972; 46: 846–55.

149. Abbott RD, Donahue RP, MacMahon SW, Reed DM, Yano K. Diabetes and the risk of stroke. The Honolulu Heart Program. JAMA 1987; 257: 949–52.

150. Asplund K, Hägg E, Helmers C, Lithner F, Strand T, Wester P-O. The natural history of stroke in diabetic patients. Acta Med Scand 1980; 207: 417–24.

151. Lithner F, Asplund K, Eriksson S, Hägg E, Strand T, Wester P-O. Clinical characteristics in diabetic stroke patients. Diabète Métab 1988; 14: 15–19.

152. Pulsinelli WA, Levy DE, Sigsbee B, Scherer P, Plum F. Increased damage after ischemic stroke in patients with hyperglycemia with or without established diabetes mellitus. Am J Med 1983; 74: 540–4.

153. Melamed E. Reactive hyperglycaemia in patients with acute stroke. J Neurol Sci 1976; 29: 267–75.

154. Olsson T, Viitanen M, Asplund K, Eriksson S, Hägg E. Prognosis after stroke in diabetic patients. A controlled prospective study. Diabetologia 1990; 33: 244–9.

155. Gray CS, French JM, Bates D, Cartlidge NEF, Venables GS, James OFW. Increasing age, diabetes mellitus and recovery from stroke. Postgrad Med J 1989; 65: 720–4.

156. Riddle MC, Hart J. Hyperglycemia, recognised and unrecognised, as a risk factor for stroke and transient ischaemic attacks. Stroke 1982; 13: 356–9.

157. Oppenheimer SM, Hoffbrand BI, Oswald GA, Yudkin JS. Diabetes mellitus and early mortality from stroke. Br Med J 1985; 291: 1014–15.

158. Cox NH, Lorains JW. The prognostic value of blood glucose and glycosylated haemoglobin estimation in patients with stroke. Postgrad Med J 1986; 62: 7–10.

159. Gray CS, Taylor R, French JM et al. The prognostic value of stress hyperglycaemia and previously unrecognised diabetes in acute stroke. Diabet Med 1987; 4: 237–40.

160. Topić E, Pavliček I, Brinar V, Koršić M. Glycosylated haemoglobin in clarification of the origin of hyperglycaemia in acute cerebrovascular accident. Diabet Med 1989; 6: 12–15.

161. Stout RW. Hyperglycaemia and stroke. Quart J Med 1989; 73: 997–1004.

162. Ginsberg MD, Welsh FA, Budd WW. Deleterious effects of glucose pretreatment on recovery from diffuse cerebral ischemia in the cat. 1. Local cerebral blood flow and glucose utilization. Stroke 1980; 11: 347–54.

163. Venables GS, Miller SA, Gibson G, Hardy JA, Strong AJ. The effects of hyperglycaemia on changes during reperfusion following focal cerebral ischaemia in the cat. J Neurol Neurosurg Psychiat 1985; 48: 663–9.

164. Siemkowicz E, Gjedde A. Post-ischemic coma in rat: effect of different pre-ischemic blood glucose levels on cerebral metabolic recovery after ischemia. Acta Phys Scand 1980; 110: 225–32.

165. Siemkowicz E. Hyperglycemia in the reperfusion period hampers recovery from cerebral ischemia. Acta Neurol Scand 1981; 64: 207–16.

166. Grotta JC. Current medical and surgical therapy for cerebrovascular disease. New Engl J Med 1987; 317: 1505–16.

167. Lowe GDO. Drugs in cerebral and peripheral arterial disease. Br Med J 1990; 300: 524–8.

Chronic Complications of Diabetes

Specific Complications
Macrovascular Disease
Other Complications

52

Complications of Diabetes: the Changing Scene

Knut Borch-Johnsen and Torsten Deckert

Steno Memorial Hospital, Gentofte, Denmark

More than 60 years have passed since Banting and co-workers [1] made the breakthrough in the treatment of insulin dependent diabetes mellitus (IDDM). Their discovery of insulin remains the most important factor influencing the life expectancy of IDDM patients. Before 1922 diabetic children had a life expectancy of 2–3 years, and 90% died from keto-acidosis [2]. However, the introduction of insulin unmasked the second consequence of diabetes—the late diabetic complications. Kimmelstiel and Wilson were the first to suggest the existence of a renal disease specific to diabetes in 1936 [3]. Diabetic renal disease has been systematically described in the preinsulin era by Hirschberg [4], but together with macroangiopathic complications it is now recognized as an element in the late diabetic syndrome [5].

Since 1922 things have changed. Improved insulin preparations and multiple injection regimens are now daily practice in the diabetes clinic, and the diabetic patient has been integrated in the diabetic 'team'. The primary aim of these efforts is to prolong life expectancy and to decrease the risk of developing late diabetic complications. The question is, however, whether the prognosis has actually improved during the past 60 years with insulin, or whether this is nothing but wishful thinking.

MORTALITY OF IDDM PATIENTS—HAS IT DECLINED?

In his 1984 review of the epidemiological data on excess mortality and life expectancy in IDDM, Panzram concluded, 'Whether the prognosis of IDDM has improved within the last decades remains uncertain' [6]. Panzram probably reached this disillusioned conclusion mainly because of methodological deficiencies in the reported studies. Several studies included IDDM as well as NIDDM patients and, furthermore, crude mortality rates were employed rather than relative mortality rates.

In 1967 Hirohata et al [7] published the first estimates of relative survival rates in 1004 IDDM patients, diagnosed from 1939 to 1959, and admitted to the Joslin Clinic. In patients diagnosed before the age of 20 years no change was found in relative survival, whereas patients diagnosed after that age experienced a constantly increasing relative survival with diabetes onset over the period 1939 to 1959.

In a more recent study from Pittsburg [8] of 1966 IDDM patients diagnosed between 1950

International Textbook of Diabetes Mellitus. Edited by K.G.M.M. Alberti, R.A. DeFronzo, H. Keen and P. Zimmet
© 1992 John Wiley & Sons Ltd

and 1981 and before the age of 17 years, a significant decrease in cumulative mortality was found when comparing patients diagnosed in the period 1966–71 with patients diagnosed before this period (1.4% and 4.1%, respectively).

Deckert [9] in 1980 presented the relative survival of 1451 IDDM patients diagnosed prior to 1953, before the age of 31 years, and admitted to the Steno Memorial Hospital (SMH). When subdividing the population into three groups according to the year of diagnosis (before 1933, 1933–42 and 1943–52), he found the lowest relative survival in patients diagnosed between 1933 and 1942. No difference was found between the first and the last cohorts. However, the first cohort including 307 patients may have been less representative of all Danish IDDM patients than the latter two groups, as the patients had to survive the very early insulin era and until 1932 to be included in the study. Thus, this study does not answer the question whether the prognosis has really improved. Two recent Danish studies have focused on this problem.

In a study including IDDM patients admitted to the SMH, diagnosed before 1953, and all prevalent cases of IDDM patients diagnosed before the age of 31 years and living in Funen County in 1973 [10], a consistently decreasing trend in the relative mortality with increasing calendar year of diagnosis was found. This finding was re-evaluated by including another 1767 patients diagnosed before the age of 31 years and in the period between 1953 and 1972 [11]. The study confirmed the observation of a decreasing relative mortality with increasing calendar year of diagnosis, the major decrease occurring between 1941 and 1955. The overall decrease in relative mortality from 1933 to 1972 was 40%. Thus, there is substantial evidence for a decreasing relative mortality.

The distribution of causes of death has changed significantly during the observation period (Table 1). The major change is that the fraction dying with or from uraemia has decreased. However, an alarming increase in the fraction dying from suicide has been observed. In patients diagnosed after 1953 a total of 17 suicides were observed, 10 of these (17% of 58 patients) were in patients with diabetes of short duration, and without any major, late diabetic complications.

These epidemiological studies give limited information regarding factors influencing the relative mortality. However, low age at diagnosis was found to be associated with increased relative mortality. Relative mortality was consistently highest in the group aged 30–45 years. The bell-shaped correlation between age and relative mortality (Figure 1) suggests that IDDM is a disease with two different potential outcomes: either the patient has a poor prognosis and dies before the age of 45 years, or the disease runs a much more benign course leading to a relatively good prognosis. It is therefore of interest to identify factors predicting high or low relative mortality. Proteinuria seems to be one of these factors.

PROTEINURIA AND MORTALITY

The term 'proteinuria' is used here synonymously with the term 'clinical diabetic nephropathy'— i.e. the appearance of persistent proteinuria (more than three consecutive samples, of over 0.5 g per 24 hours) in diabetic patients without cardiac insufficiency, urinary tract infection or other renal disease. The definition is based on clinical observations *only* and does not indicate the degree of morphological change. The reason for using the clinical definition is not only convenience. Several studies have shown that the correlation between functional measures (e.g. proteinuria, glomerular filtration rate, serum creatinine) and morphological changes is relatively poor, except from patients already approaching end-stage renal failure [12, 13]. Furthermore, in 1972 Watkins et al [14] showed that the level of proteinuria was more strongly correlated with mortality than with the degree of glomerulosclerosis.

In a cohort of 1030 IDDM patients diagnosed between 1933 and 1952, patients *not* developing proteinuria had a low but constant relative mortality, whereas patients with proteinuria had a 40 times higher relative mortality [15]. Relative mortality was highest in females but independent of age, diabetes duration and age at diagnosis. Patients with proteinuria showed a characteristic bell-shaped relationship between age and relative mortality, with the maximum in the age interval 34–38 years. The crude mortality rate was identical in males and females (10–15% per year) from 5 years after the onset of proteinuria.

The mortality pattern in patients with proteinuria seems to explain the bell-shaped relationship

Table 1 Cause of death according to year of diagnosis and diabetes duration in a cohort of 2930 Danish IDDM patients

	Diabetes duration				
	0–15 years		16–30 years		31 + years
Year of diagnosis	1933–52 (n = 66) %	1953–72 (n = 58) %	1933–52 (n = 365) %	1953–72 (n = 148) %	1933–52 (n = 199) %
Uraemia	27	5	56	42	15
Myocardial infarction	6	12	16	18	36
Cardiovascular disease (others)	5	9	8	6	20
Hypoglycaemia	3	9	3	3	2
Ketoacidosis	18	17	2	3	3
Diabetes	2	2	1	2	1
Infections	0	5	2	5	4
Suicide	0	17	2	5	3
Others	18	19	6	12	9
	$p < 0.0001$		$p < 0.02$		

n = number of deaths in age group for that 20-year period.
From reference 11, with permission.

between relative mortality and age seen in the diabetic population. If this is true, the decreasing relative mortality among IDDM patient's should be associated with a decline of incidence in proteinuria during the last 50 years. This is in fact the case.

Among 2930 IDDM patients diagnosed between 1933 and 1972, before the age of 31 years, and admitted to the SMH [16], 525 patients developed proteinuria. During the observation period the cumulative incidence decreased by 30% (Figure 2). The pattern of the incidence curve was unchanged, with a maximal rate of increase of incidence after 15–20 years which then decreased. This indicates that development of proteinuria has not only been

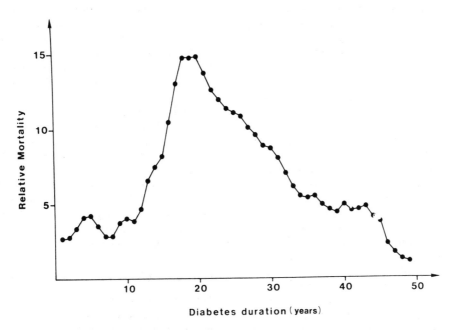

Figure 1 Relative mortality as a function of diabetes duration in 2930 IDDM patients (from reference 11, reproduced with permission from Springer-Verlag)

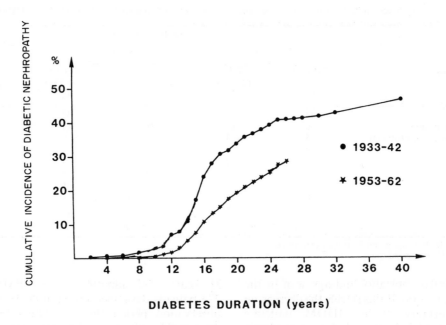

DIABETES DURATION (years)

Figure 2 Cumulative incidence of persistent proteinuria (DN) in IDDM patients diagnosed 1933 to 1942 (closed circles) and 1953 to 1962 (asterisks). $N = 2890$, $P < 0.001$

postponed but seems to have been prevented in 10–15% of the IDDM patients. These results are in agreement with those from the study by Krolewski et al [17], who also showed a significantly lower incidence of proteinuria in patients diagnosed in 1959 compared with patients diagnosed in 1939. Thus, the decrease in the incidence of proteinuria explains the decreasing relative mortality observed during the past 50 years.

PROTEINURIA AND CAUSE OF DEATH

In IDDM patients as well as in NIDDM patients the predominant causes of death are cardiovascular and renal disease, accounting for 50–80% of deaths [18–20]. As development of proteinuria in IDDM patients is followed by a progressive loss in glomerular filtration rate, it is not surprising that the majority of these patients die from, or with, uraemia. However, 15–25% still die from cardiovascular disease, despite the relatively low age at death [15, 21, 22]. In 1984 Braun et al [23] published a study of 100 diabetic patients admitted for renal transplantation. They found severe cardiac disease (i.e. greater than 70% occlusion of the coronary arteries and/or moderate to severe left ventricular dysfunction) in 38% of the patients, and of the

remaining patients 34% had cardiomegaly, angina or previous myocardial infarction.

As these studies indicated an association between development of proteinuria and cardiovascular disease, we studied the relative mortality from cardiovascular disease in 722 IDDM patients with proteinuria and 1920 patients without proteinuria [24]. As seen in Figure 3, patients without proteinuria had a low and constant relative cardiovascular mortality, independent of age and diabetes duration. In patients with proteinuria the picture was distinctly different. The bell-shaped relationship between diabetes duration and relative mortality was found again here, with the highest relative mortality after 25 years of diabetes duration, and the relative cardiovascular mortality was 5 to 15 times higher than in the non-proteinuric patients. Thus, the study suggests that development of proteinuria is a marker of generalized vascular lesions, not confined to the kidneys.

THE RENAL–RETINAL SYNDROME

Retinopathy is the second major cause of disability in IDDM patients, and it is still the leading cause of acquired blindness below the age of 60 years. Development of diabetic retinopathy is

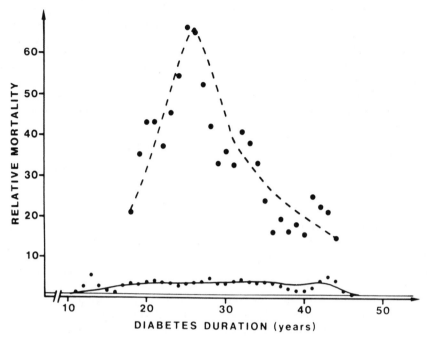

Figure 3 Relative mortality of cardiovascular disease in patients with proteinuria (pecked line) and without proteinuria (solid line) as a function of diabetes duration (from reference 24, reproduced with permission from Martinus Nijhoff Publishing)

closely related to diabetes duration. Even in patients surviving with IDDM for very long periods, retinopathy is the most frequently registered complication [25, 26]. Recent data from the Joslin Clinic [27] indicate that after 10 years of diabetes there is a linear relationship between diabetes duration and the risk of developing proliferative retinopathy. This linear correlation was independent of whether the patient was diagnosed in 1939, 1949 or 1959, and by 40 years of diabetes duration 60% of the patients had developed proliferative retinopathy. However, development of proliferative retinopathy is also closely correlated with development of persistent proteinuria. This has been observed in a number of cross-sectional studies [28–30], showing that the prevalence of proliferative retinopathy is consistently higher in patients with persistent proteinuria than in patients without this condition.

This correlation was confirmed in a study from the Joslin Clinic [27] which showed that in patients developing persistent proteinuria, 80% also developed proliferative retinopathy, whereas the corresponding figure for patients not developing persistent proteinuria was only 25%. This observation was confirmed in a case-control study including 110 IDDM patients developing persistent proteinuria and 110 IDDM patients matched for gender, age, age at diagnosis and diabetes duration not developing proteinura [31]. In the patients not developing proteinuria, a low (< 1% per year) but constant incidence of proliferative retinopathy was observed, whereas in patients developing proteinuria the incidence started to increase 3–4 years *before* development of proteinuria, and by the time of onset of proteinuria the incidence was 10–15% per year. This study, together with previous studies [32, 33], indicates that even patients with microalbuminuria have an increased risk of developing proliferative retinopathy. Thus, in conclusion it appears that retinopathy of the simplex type is related to diabetes duration, whereas the development of proliferative retinopathy is closely associated with the development of proteinuria.

TWO TYPES OF ANGIOPATHY IN IDDM PATIENTS?

As outlined above, patients developing persistent proteinuria are characterized by a high excess mortality, attributable not only to renal failure but also to cardiovascular disease. The same association between persistent proteinuria and cardiovascular morbidity was found in a case-control study of 59 IDDM patients developing persistent proteinuria [34]. Within 6 years of onset of proteinuria the cumulative incidence of coronary heart disease was 8 times higher than in the non-proteinuric patients. Furthermore, as described above, there is a close association between development of proteinuria and proliferative retinopathy.

However, patients developing persistent proteinuria are also characterized by a clustering of different risk factors for cardiovascular disease as well as for retinopathy. Patients with proteinuria have higher blood pressures [35], higher and more atherogenic blood lipid levels [36] and higher fibrinogen levels [36] than patients without proteinuria. These differences are not present at the onset of diabetes [26, 35] but develop concomitantly with the development of proteinuria. However, these differences in risk factor levels are too small to account for the tenfold increase in cardiovascular morbidity and mortality and the tenfold increase in incidence of retinopathy in patients developing proteinuria. Therefore, another link between microangiopathy and macroangiopathy must be sought. This link may be associated with increased endothelial permeability [37]. Thus, as (a) microangiopathic and macroangiopathic complications develop simultaneously, (b) a non-renal pathogenetic link seems to exist between these complications, and (c) patients with proteinuria suffer not only from impaired renal function but also from widespread non-renal lesions, we prefer to characterize patients developing persistent proteinuria as having a malignant angiopathy. On the other hand, as patients *not* developing microalbuminuria and persistent proteinuria have normal blood pressure, lower risk of developing proliferative retinopathy and lower risk of developing microvascular disease, we prefer to characterize the vascular lesions in these patients as benign diabetic angiopathy.

FUTURE ASPECTS—HOW TO IMPROVE THE PROGNOSIS?

As the high relative mortality in IDDM patients is almost entirely confined to patients develop-

ing persistent proteinuria, and as the decreasing mortality so far can be explained through a decreasing incidence of proteinuria, it is evident that the only way of obtaining a further increase in life expectancy in IDDM patients is through prevention of persistent proteinuria. Thus the question of how to improve the prognosis could equally well be how to prevent persistent proteinuria in IDDM patients?

Metabolic Regulation

It is tempting to assume that the risk of developing late diabetic complications is related to the degree of hyperglycaemia. Formal scientific evidence for this hypothesis is, however, still lacking because of the practical and ethical implications of a long-term controlled clinical trial aimed at solving this complex problem.

However, several epidemiological studies have indicated that good metabolic control is related to life expectancy [26] as well as to the risk of developing persistent proteinuria [17, 38]. Two recent trials have focused on the possibility of secondary prevention (i.e. prevention of further deterioration of an already established renal disorder). Both studies include patients with an urinary albumin excretion rate (UAER) above the normal range, but without persistent proteinuria. The study by Feldt-Rasmussen et al [39] randomly allocated 36 patients either to continuous subcutaneous insulin infusion (CSII) or to conventional insulin treatment. The two groups were matched for age, diabetes duration, gender, degree of metabolic regulation and UAER. The patients treated with CSII had significantly lower mean blood glucose levels during the 2-year follow-up period. In the CSII group the UAER remained constant and no further increase in blood pressure was observed in the follow-up period, whereas patients treated with conventional therapy experienced an increase in UAER of 15–20% per year and also showed an increase in blood pressure. This study thus indicated that strict metabolic control is of major importance, even in patients who already have microalbuminuria. Similar observations were made in a Norwegian study. When pooling data from two studies at the SMH, it was found that in the conventionally treated group 10 of 25 patients progressed to persistent proteinuria, whereas only 1 of 26 CSII-treated patients developed persistent proteinuria [40]. Thus, strict metabolic control in patients with persistent microalbuminuria seems to be able to decrease further the incidence of clinical nephropathy.

Hypertension

Hypertension is closely related to retinopathy as well as to proteinuria [41, 42]. In patients with proteinuria it has been shown that the rate of decline of the glomerular filtration rate (GFR) may be influenced by antihypertensive treatment [43]. Without antihypertensive therapy the rate of decline in GFR was 0.91 ml/min per month. With antihypertensive treatment the rate of decline in GFR was reduced to 0.39 ml/min per month. This decrease in rate of decline of GFR corresponds to an increase in 'renal life expectancy' from 7 years to 13.1 years. This observation has not been confirmed by controlled clinical trials, but the observations are so convincing that antihypertensive treatment is now a routine part of the treatment of IDDM patients with persistent proteinuria. Recent data from our own clinic comparing the survival of patients with proteinuria either with or without antihypertensive treatment strongly supports the observations by Parving et al [43], as we found a significantly lower mortality in the patients receiving antihypertensive treatment as a part of the clinical routine [52]. Thus, antihypertensive treatment in patients with IDDM and proteinuria seems not only to reduce the rate of decline of GFR but also the high mortality in these young patients. A reasonable treatment strategy therefore will probably lead to a further improvement in the prognosis of IDDM. Recently, there has also been discussion of whether antihypertensive therapy should be given to patients with persistent microalbuminuria where the blood pressure is slightly but significantly elevated [44–47]. It is possible that antihypertensive therapy in these patients would lead to a delay in the decline of GFR and a reduction in the incidence of proliferative retinopathy and cardiovascular disease.

Susceptibility

Epidemiological studies have shown that fewer than 50% of all IDDM patients will ever develop persistent proteinuria [16, 17, 21, 48]. Furthermore, low age at diagnosis and male sex confer an increased risk of developing persistent proteinuria [16, 21]. These studies indicate that heterogeneity with respect to susceptibility for development of proteinuria exists within the diabetic population. Identification of markers for susceptibility would enable intensified treatment of 'at risk' individuals, resulting in better prognosis. However, genetic markers for the development of proteinuria have not yet been identified [49]. Familial predisposition to essential hypertension [53, 54] and increased red cell sodium/lithium countertransport [54–56] have both been suggested as markers of increased susceptibility. However, recent data from a family study have been unable to confirm these two hypotheses [57]. The family study data suggest that hypertension and increased sodium/lithium countertransport may be consequences of—rather than risk markers for—development of persistent proteinuria.

Familial clustering of persistent proteinuria does, however, occur in some multiplex families with IDDM, indicating that as yet unidentified genetic factors are involved in defining susceptibility [58, 59].

PRACTICAL CONSEQUENCES

The introduction of insulin in 1922–23 still represents the major breakthrough in the treatment of IDDM patients. However, epidemiological studies have demonstrated that during the last 50 years IDDM patients have experienced a 15-year to 30-year increase in life expectancy, and the risk of developing the most life-threatening complication—diabetic nephropathy—has decreased by 20–30%. This improvement in the prognosis is not only a positive item of information to impart to the individual diabetic patient, it also suggests that the current discrimination against IDDM patients, for example when applying for life-insurance, should be revised.

In 1975 Goodkin [50] reported survival data on more than 10 000 IDDM and NIDDM patients applying for life-insurance between 1951 and 1970. He concluded that 'the age of onset of diabetes is the most significant factor in mortality' and he also found the mortality of patients diagnosed before the age of 15 years so high that 'it is doubtful that he can qualify for insurance'. As shown in this chapter, the prognosis has improved considerably since these early years, and we have also shown that the prognosis for the individual patient is primarily related to whether he or she develops persistent proteinuria. In Denmark the present life-insurance practice for IDDM patients has taken the improved prognosis of IDDM patients into account. By comparing the mortality of Danish IDDM patients with the expected mortality based on the 'substandard life tables' used by the Danish life-insurance companies, we found that the life-insurance premiums paid by IDDM patients were generally too high. It was also found that the only factors necessary for estimating the insurance premiums were age at diagnosis, gender and presence or absence of persistent proteinuria [51]. On the basis of these facts it was accepted that insurance premiums should be based on gender and age at diagnosis. Today, all patients without persistent proteinuria can be offered life-insurance, and subsequently all patients without persistent proteinuria by the age of 50 years will be offered a reduction in the premium.

Life-insurance is, however, only one of the areas where action should be taken in view of the documented improvement in prognosis. Other areas include, for example, adoption regulations and pension funds.

CONCLUSION

The prognosis of IDDM has improved considerably during the last 30 years. However, the mortality rate of IDDM patients is still higher than that of the general population. As high mortality is confined almost entirely to patients developing diabetic renal disease, as diagnosed by development of persistent proteinuria, the major challenge today and in the future is how to prevent renal disease. Unfortunately, relatively little is known about the factors causing the development of proteinuria. It appears that only 30–50% of patients are susceptible, but a method of identification of these patients is still being sought. A wide spectrum of factors involving increased susceptibility to development of proteinuria has been suggested, but very little hard evidence is available. Metabolic control is probably of major importance, but what is the 'safe' level—if it exists? Dietary habits regarding lipids as well as proteins may also be of importance, as well as physical activity and abstinence from smoking. In advising the diabetic patient it is necessary to consider the restrictions in lifestyle involved in any advice given, and to make the diabetic patient understand that he or she is the only person responsible for the final evaluation of costs and benefits of following such advice. It is, however, also necessary to encourage the person to follow the advice, as it is clear that the prognosis for the individual patient can be influenced thereby.

REFERENCES

1. Banting FG, Best CH, Collip JB, Campbell WR, Fletsher AA. Pancreatic extracts in the treatment of diabetes mellitus. Can Med Ass J 1922; 2: 141–6.
2. Joslin EP. The treatment of diabetes mellitus 4th edn. Philadelphia: Lea & Febiger, 1928.
3. Kimmelstiel P, Wilson C. Intercapillary lesions in glomeruli of the kidney. Am J Pathol 1936; 12: 82–97.
4. Hirschberg J. Über diabetische Netzhautentzundung. Dtsch Med Wschr 1890; 51: 1181–238.
5. Lundbæk K. Long-term diabetes. Thesis, Copenhagen, 1953.
6. Panzram G. Epidemiologic data on excess mortality and life expectancy in insulin-dependent diabetes mellitus—critical review. Exp Clin Endocrinol 1984; 83: 93–100.
7. Hirohata T, MacMahon B, Root HF. The natural history of diabetes. 1. Mortality. Diabetes 1967; 16: 875–81.
8. Dorman JS, LaPorte RE, Kuller LH et al. The Pittsburgh insulin dependent diabetes mellitus (IDDM) morbidity and mortality study. Mortality results. Diabetes 1984; 33: 271–6.
9. Deckert T. The influence of supervision and endogenous insulin secretion on the course of insulin dependent diabetes mellitus. Acta Endocrinol 1980; 94 (suppl. 238): 31–8.
10. Green A, Borch-Johnsen K, Andersen PK, Hougaard P, Keiding N, Kreiner S, Deckert T. Relative mortality of Type 1 (insulin-dependent) diabetes in Denmark: 1933–1981. Diabetologia 1985; 28: 339–42.
11. Borch-Johnsen K, Kreiner S, Deckert T. Mortality of Type 1 (insulin-dependent) diabetes mellitus in Denmark. Diabetologia 1986; 29: 767–72.
12. Thomsen AC. The kidney in diabetes mellitus. Copenhagen: Munksgaard, 1965.
13. Deckert T, Parving HH, Thomsen OF, Jørgensen HE, Brun C, Thomsen ÅC. Renal structure and function in type 1 (insulin-dependent) diabetic patients: a study of 44 kidney biopsies. Diabet Nephr 1985; 4: 163–8.
14. Watkins PJ, Blainey JD, Brewer DB, Fitzgerald MG, Malins JM, O'Sullivan JO, Pinto JA. The

natural history of diabetic renal disease. Quart J Med 1972; 164: 437–56.

15. Borch-Johnsen K, Andersen PK, Deckert T. The effect of proteinuria on relative mortality in Type 1 (insulin-dependent) diabetes mellitus. Diabetologia, 1985; 28: 590–6.

16. Kofoed-Enevoldsen A, Borch-Johnsen K, Kreiner S, Nerup J, Deckert T. Declining incidence of persistent proteinuria in Type 1 (insulin-dependent) diabetic patients in Denmark. Diabetes 1987; 36: 205–9.

17. Krolewski AS, Warram JH, Christlieb AR, Busick EJ, Kahn CR. The changing natural history of nephropathy in Type 1 diabetes. Am J Med 1985; 78: 785–94.

18. Marble A. Insulin—clinical aspects: the first fifty years. Diabetes 1972; 21 (suppl. 2): 632–6.

19. Krolewski AS, Warram JH, Christliet AR. Onset, course, complications, and prognosis of diabetes mellitus. In Joslin's Diabetes mellitus, 12th edn. Philadelphia: Lea & Febiger, 1985: pp 251–77.

20. Jarret RJ. The epidemiology of coronary heart disease and related factors in the context of diabetes mellitus and impaired glucose tolerance. In Jarret RJ (ed.) Diabetes and heart disease. Amsterdam: Elsevier, 1984: pp 1–23.

21. Andersen AR, Christiansen JS, Andersen JK, Kreiner S, Deckert T. Diabetic nephropathy in Type 1 (insulin-dependent) diabetes: an epidemiological study. Diabetologia 1983; 25: 496–501.

22. Moloney A, Tunbridge WMG, Ireland JT, Watkins PJ. Mortality from diabetic nephropathy in the United Kingdom. Diabetologia 1983; 25: 26–30.

23. Braun WE, Phillips DF, Vidt DG et al. Coronary artery disease in 100 diabetics with end stage renal failure. Transpl Proc 1984; 16: 603–7.

24. Borch-Johnsen K, Kreiner S. Proteinuria: value as predictor of cardiovascular mortality in insulin-dependent diabetes mellitus. Br Med J 1987; 294: 1651–4.

25. Paz-Gouevara AT, Tah-Hsiung H, White P. Juvenile diabetes after forty years. Diabetes 1975; 24: 559–65.

26. Borch-Johnsen K, Nissen H, Henriksen E, Kreiner S, Salling N, Deckert T, Nerup J. The natural history of insulin-dependent diabetes mellitus in Denmark. Diabet Med 1987; 4: 201–17.

27. Krolewski AS, Warram JH, Rand LI, Christlieb AR, Busick EJ, Kann CR. Risk of proliferative diabetic retinopathy in juvenile-onset type I diabetes: a 40-year follow-up study. Diabetes Care 1986; 9: 443–52.

28. Klein R, Klein BEK, Moss SE, Davis ME, DeMetz DL. The Wisconsin epidemiology study of diabetic retinopathy: proteinuria and retinopathy in a population of diabetic persons diag-

nosed prior to 30 years of age. In Friedman EA, L'Esperance FA (eds) Diabetic renal–retinal syndrome 3. New York: Grune & Stratton, 1986: pp 245–64.

29. Deckert T, Poulsen JE, Larsen M. Prognosis of diabetics with diabetes onset before the age of thirty-one. I. Survival, causes of death and complications. Diabetologia 1978; 14: 363–70.

30. Agardth E, Tallroth G, Bauer B, Cavallin-Sjöberg U, Agardt CD. Retinopathy and nephropathy in insulin-dependent diabetics: an inconsistent relationship. Diabet Med 1987; 4: 248–50.

31. Kofoed-Enevoldsen A, Jensen T, Borch-Johnsen K, Deckert T. Incidence of retinopathy in Type 1 (insulin-dependent) diabetes: association with clinical nephropathy. Diabet Comp 1987; 1: 96–9.

32. Barnett AH, Dallinger K, Jennings R, Fletcher J, Obdubesan O. Microalbuminuria and diabetic retinopathy. Lancet 1985; i: 53–4.

33. Vigstrup J, Mogensen CE. Proliferative diabetic retinopathy: at risk patients identified by early detection of microalbuminuria. Acta Ophthalmol 1985; 63: 530–4.

34. Jensen T, Borch-Johnsen K, Kofoed-Enevoldsen A, Deckert T. Coronary heart disease in young Type 1 (insulin-dependent) diabetic patients with and without diabetic nephropathy: incidence and risk-factors. Diabetologia 1987; 30: 144–8.

35. Jensen T, Borch-Johnsen K, Deckert T. Changes in blood pressure and renal function in patients with Type 1 (insulin-dependent) diabetes mellitus prior to clinical diabetic nephropathy. Diabetes Res 1987; 4: 159–162.

36. Valdorf-Hansen F, Jensen T, Borch-Johnsen K, Deckert T. Cardiovascular risk factors in Type 1 (insulin-dependent) diabetic patients with and without proteinuria. Acta Med Scand 1987; 222: 439–44.

37. Feldt-Rasmussen B. Increased transcapillary escape rate of albumin in Type 1 (insulin-dependent) diabetic patients with microalbuminuria. Diabetologia 1986; 29: 282–6.

38. Pirart J. Diabetes mellitus and its degenerative complications: a prospective study of 4400 patients observed between 1947 and 1973. Diabetes Care 1978; 1: 168–88.

39. Feldt-Rasmussen B, Mathiesen ER, Deckert T. Effect of two years strict metabolic control on the progression of incipient nephropathy in insulin-dependent diabetes. Lancet 1986; ii: 1300–4.

40. Deckert T, Feldt-Rasmussen B, Borch-Johnsen K, Jensen T, Bent-Hansen L, Kofoed-Enevoldsen A. Proteinuria, an indicator of malignant angiopathy. In Andreani D (ed.) Diabetic complications, early diagnosis and treatment. New York: John Wiley, 1987: pp 257–61.

41. Hasslacher CH, Stech W, Wahl P, Ritz E. Blood pressure and metabolic control as risk factors for

nephropathy in Type 1 (insulin-dependent) diabetes. Diabetologia 1985; 28: 6–11.

42. Parving HH, Andersen AR, Smidt UM, Oxenbøll B, Edsberg B, Christiansen JS. Diabetic nephropathy and arterial hypertension. Diabetologia 1983; 24: 10–12.

43. Parving HH, Andersen AR, Smidt UM, Svendsen PA. Early aggressive anti-hypertensive treatment reduces rate of decline in kidney function in diabetic nephropathy. Lancet 1983 i: 1175–9.

44. Viberti GJ, Jarret RJ, Mahmud U, Hill RD, Argyropoulos A, Keen H. Microalbuminuria as a predictor of clinical nephropathy in insulin dependent diabetes mellitus. Lancet 1982; i: 1430–2.

45. Mogensen CE. Microalbuminuria predicts clinical proteinuria and early mortality in maturity-onset diabetes. New Engl J Med 1984; 310: 356–60.

46. Mathiesen ER, Oxenbøll B, Johansen K, Svendsen PA, Deckert T. Incipient nephropathy in Type 1 (insulin-dependent) diabetes. Diabetologia 1984; 26: 406–10.

47. Christensen CK, Mogensen CE. The course of incipient diabetic nephropathy: studies of albumin excretion and blood pressure. Diabet Med 1985; 2: 97–102.

48. Lestradet H, Papoz L, Hellouin de Meibus C et al. Long-term study of mortality and vascular complications in juvenile-onset (type 1) diabetes. Diabetes 1981; 30: 175–9.

49. Barbosa J, Saner B. Do genetic factors play a role in the pathogenesis of diabetic microangiopathy? Diabetologia 1984; 27: 487–92.

50. Goodkin G. Mortality factors in diabetes. J Occup Med 1975; 17: 716–21.

51. Ramlau-Hansen H, Bang Jespersen NC, Andersen PK, Borch-Johnsen K, Deckert T. Life insurance for insulin-dependent diabetics. Scand Actuarial J 1987; 19–36.

52. Mathiesen ER, Borch-Johnsen K, Jensen DV, Deckert T. Improved survival in patients with diabetic nephropathy. Diabetologia 1989; 32: 884–6.

53. Viberti GC, Keen H, Wiseman HJ. Raised arterial pressure in parents of proteinuric insulin-depenent diabetics. Br Med J 1987; 295: 515–7.

54. Krolewski AS, Canessa H, Warram JH et al. Predisposition to hypertension and susceptibility to renal disease in insulin-dependent diabetes mellitus. N Engl J Med 1988; 318: 140–5.

55. Mangili R, Bending JJ, Scott G, Lai LK, Gupta A, Viberti GC. Increased sodium–lithium counter transport activity in red cells of patients with insulin dependent diabetes and nephropathy. N Engl J Med 1988; 318: 146–50.

56. Walker JD, Tariq T, Viberti GC. Sodium–lithium counter transport activity in red cells of patients with insulin-dependent diabetes and nephropathy and their parents. Br Med J 1990; 301: 635–8.

57. Jensen JS, Mathiesen ER, Nørgaard K et al. Increased blood pressure and red cell sodium–lithium counter transport are not inherited in diabetic nephropathy. Diabetologia 1990; 33: 619–24.

58. Seaquist ER, Goetz FC, Rich S, Barbasa J. Familial clustering of diabetic kidney disease. N Engl J Med 1989; 320: 1161–5.

59. Borch-Johnsen K, Nørgaard K, Hommel E et al. Diabetic nephropathy: an inherited complication. Kidney Int 1991 (in press).

Specific Complications

53

The Genesis of Diabetes Complications: Blood Glucose and Genetic Susceptibility

Philip Raskin and Julio Rosenstock

University of Texas Southwestern Medical Center at Dallas, Texas, USA

Although the value of glycemic control has long been taken as an article of faith by the diabetes community, the clinical evidence linking blood glucose control with diabetic complications remains far from proven. At present, the data relating these two can only be interpreted at best, as *suggestive*. There are those who consider that the relationship between hyperglycemia and diabetic complications is no longer a debatable issue. In a recent report, the Scandinavians have gone so far as to state: 'We think that the question to be addressed in the future is not in essence *why* but *how* to maintain good metabolic control' [1].

However, we believe that the question of *why* has not yet been answered. It is conceivable that hyperglycemia is a necessary prerequisite for the development of diabetic microvascular complications, but there are individual genetic differences in the susceptibility to respond to the metabolic derangement. It seems clear that, regardless of blood glucose control, 15–20% of patients with diabetes mellitus do not develop complications involving the small blood vessels. Thus, some genetic predisposition or protection from the damaging effects of hyperglycemia may also be involved [2–4].

As hyperglycemia is the only potentially correctable variable, intensive diabetes management is being offered to increasing numbers of diabetic patients with the idea of delaying or preventing diabetic complications. Achievement of near-normoglycemia for prolonged periods of time is theoretically possible with the current use of more effective insulin delivery strategies and frequent self-monitoring of blood glucose [5, 6]. However, it is increasingly recognized that for most patients, despite a considerable investment in effort, time and money, glycemic control cannot be improved to the normal or even the near-normal range. More importantly, the risk of clinically significant hypoglycemia is a major consideration and, indeed, it is 2–3 times greater in intensively treated patients [7, 8].

International Textbook of Diabetes Mellitus. Edited by K.G.M.M. Alberti, R.A. DeFronzo, H. Keen and P. Zimmet
© 1992 John Wiley & Sons Ltd

As discussed below, given the uncertainty about the relationship between blood glucose control and complications, it is inappropriate to insist on intensive control in all patients. For some, such a regimen will be too psychologically and financially burdensome; moreover, it exposes them to a significant risk of hypoglycemia. It is neither accurate nor advisable to imply that non-adherence to the diabetes regimen will inevitably result in the development of complications. On the other hand, the incompleteness of our information should not be used as an excuse for casual diabetes control. In this chapter, evidence is reviewed suggesting that, in the majority of patients, better diabetes control can be expected to lessen or delay later complications involving small blood vessels, but the degree of improvement required and the real impact on complications remain unknown. Within the wide range between poor and intensive control, patients should be encouraged to aim for the best blood glucose control they can realistically attain.

To review the issue of glycemic control, genetic susceptibility and diabetic complications, we have analyzed pertinent epidemiological and experimental evidence, as well as the most recent clinical information bearing on these issues.

EPIDEMIOLOGICAL EVIDENCE

Cross-sectional, population-based studies provide important information as to the prevalence of diabetic complications and the possible relationship with some potential risk factors (duration of disease, sex, blood pressure, glucose control, etc.). However, these data have limitations and need to be interpreted cautiously. Furthermore, the assumption that retinopathy, nephropathy and neuropathy respond to the same pathogenic mechanisms, or may be influenced by the same factors, may not necessarily be correct. Indeed, there are marked differences in temporal patterns of occurrence and incidence rate, suggesting that retinopathy and nephropathy may evolve as two distinct processes influenced in different ways by some genetic or metabolic determinants.

The careful ophthalmological prevalence surveys by Palmberg et al [9] from St Louis, Missouri and Klein et al [10] from Madison, Wisconsin are landmark studies discerning the complex natural history of retinopathy in insulin

dependent diabetes mellitus (IDDM). Both studies clearly demonstrated an increased frequency of retinopathy with increasing duration of diabetes. Palmberg et al [9] showed that the ascertainment of diabetic retinopathy was increased with the use of fundus photography (similar to fluorescein angiography) as opposed to using the ophthalmoscope only (Figure 1). They analyzed 461 IDDM patients attending specialized diabetic centers: it is possible, therefore, that severe forms of diabetic retinopathy may be overrepresented. They found that, after a lag period, the prevalence of background diabetic retinopathy rose in sigmoidal fashion, reaching 50% by 7 years duration, and asymptomatically approaching 90% at 17–50 years. The Wisconsin survey [10] is probably a better-designed study, respresenting a larger, unselected population of 996 IDDM patients. Using standardized fundus photography, Klein et al found some degree of retinopathy in 17% of patients with diabetes of less than 5 years' duration, and a prevalence of 97.5% in those with diabetes of 15 or more years' duration.

At first glance, these data appear to indicate that almost all patients will develop diabetic retinopathy if they live long enough. However, if one looks at the type of severity of retinopathy, another interpretation of these data can be offered. In the St Louis study, proliferative retinopathy was first seen at 13 years' duration and its prevalence rose to 20% at 26–50 years. In Wisconsin, the frequency of proliferative retinopathy increased from 4% in those who had had diabetes for 10 years, to 25% in those who had had diabetes for 15 years and to 67% in those who had had it for 35 years. This last figure coincides with the Joslin Clinic report, showing a cumulative risk for proliferative retinopathy of 62% after 40 years of diabetes [11]. Thus it can be concluded that regardless of diabetes duration, approximately 40% of diabetic patients will not develop proliferative retinopathy. Furthermore, careful reanalysis of the degrees of retinopathy found in the Wisconsin study indicate that, after 15 years of diabetes, 20% of the patients are persistently found to have very mild retinopathy at level 2 or less (microaneurysms only). Thus, a second conclusion is that, regardless of the long-term exposure to diabetes, approximately 20% of the patients will develop only minimal or negligible diabetic retinopathy. This may be due either to

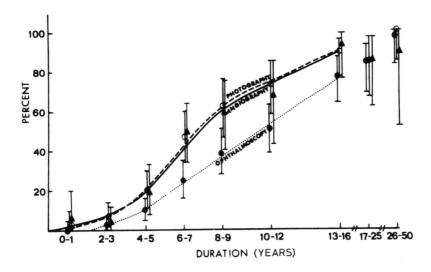

Figure 1 The prevalence of retinopathy given for the diagnostic modalities of ophthalmoscopy (solid circles), fundus photography (open circles) and fluorescein angiography (triangles) at each duration of disease (published courtesy of *Ophthalmology* (1981; 88: 613–618))

a lack of genetic susceptibility for the development of diabetic microvascular complications or to some unknown protective factors. Patients who have survived diabetes for more than 30–40 years with no or minimal complications have indeed been reported [12–14], and they may represent a special subset of patients who, if investigated further, might shed some light on this issue.

Initial studies, from the Steno Hospital in Denmark and the Joslin Clinic in Boston, analyzing data collected over many years of follow-up, indicated that 35–40% of IDDM patients developed nephropathy [14, 15]. Diabetic nephropathy, as defined by persistent proteinuria (protein excretion exceeding 0.5 g per 24 hours), was found in 41% of the 1303 patients who were followed at the Steno Hospital until death, or for at least 25 years after the onset of diabetes [15]. The highest prevalence of diabetic nephropathy was seen after 20–25 years of diabetes, and it declined subsequently to about 10% in patients who had suffered from diabetes for 40 years or more. The onset of proteinuria had two incidence peaks, the first after 16 years' duration of diabetes, and the second after 32 years. In addition, a significant difference was observed when the pattern of annual incidence rates in 1933 and in the periods 1933–42 and 1943–52 were compared. This last observation prompted

a second, more extensive analysis of the Steno population that demonstrated a declining incidence of persistent proteinuria in IDDM patients in Denmark [16]. They reviewed the data on 2658 patients who represented approximately 30% of all Danish IDDM subjects diagnosed between 1933 and 1972. When comparing patients diagnosed between 1933 and 1942 with those diagnosed between 1953 and 1962 the incidence of proteinuria decreased by 30%. The peak incidence of proteinuria was still found to occur at around 15–17 years of diabetes duration. The declining incidence resulted in a decrease in cumulative incidence after 25 years, from 41% in patients diagnosed between 1933 and 1942 to 27% in patients diagnosed between 1953 and 1962.

Similar data are available from the Joslin Clinic group whose first report was the analysis of 112 IDDM patients listed in the death registry of the Joslin Clinic between 1962 and 1972, as well as patients diagnosed as having diabetic nephropathy from 1966 to 1967. They also found that persistent proteinuria occurred after an average of 17–19 years and death ensued 5–6 years thereafter [14]. More recently, they reported on a cohort of 292 IDDM patients who were followed for 20–40 years [17]. These data also suggested that the natural history of diabetic nephropathy may be changing in later decades.

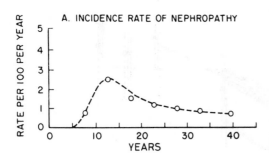

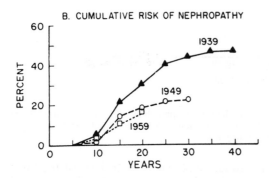

Figure 2 (A) The incidence rate of diabetic nephropathy in patients with insulin-dependent diabetes mellitus. (B) The cumulative risk according to the decade of diagnosis (reprinted, by permission of *The New England Journal of Medicine* (317; 1395, 1987))

Figure 2 shows that the cumulative risk of diabetic nephropathy in patients with IDDM diagnosed in 1959 and 1949 is around half of that found in patients with diabetes diagnosed in 1939 [18]. Once persistent proteinuria occurs, the average survival is 10 years, and end-stage renal failure develops in approximately 25% of the patients within 6 years, in 50% within 10 years and in 75% within 15 years. The overall cumulative risk for the development of diabetic nephropathy was 35% after 40 years of diabetes duration [17].

These careful epidemiological data indicate that around 60–65% of all IDDM patients do not develop nephropathy even after very long-term follow-up periods. Furthermore, the Steno and Joslin data indicate that the risk for overt proteinuria starts after a lag period of 5 years; the incidence rate peaks in the second decade and declines thereafter, suggesting that this complication occurs mainly in a subset of susceptible patients. A very attractive (although speculative) interpretation of the decline in the inci-

dence rate after 20–25 years of diabetes is that the pool of genetically susceptible nephropathic patients has been exhausted over time [18].

Multiple suggestions have been made attempting to identify risk or protective factors by use of sophisticated statistical analysis of the above retinopathy and nephropathy studies. Interpretation of these data has limitations and can only provide associations that do not necessarily imply causality. For example, the Wisconsin study found that after 10 years of diabetes the Cox regression model related the severity of retinopathy to longer duration, higher levels of glycated hemoglobin (one single determination per patient), higher diastolic blood pressure, the presence of proteinuria and male sex [10]. Variables associated with higher incidence of proteinuria in the large Steno study were only male sex and a higher body mass index [16]. The lowest incidence of nephropathy was found in patients developing diabetes after age 20 years. The role of blood pressure or glycemic control was not analyzed. The Joslin Clinic study, using an arbitrary index or hyperglycemia, seemed to indicate that the incidence rate of proteinuria increased in the interval 10 through 24 years of diabetes, as the frequency of severe hyperglycemia increased. Only the patients in the highest quartile of hyperglycemia had a risk of persistent proteinuria that was 4.5 times greater than that for those with hyperglycemia in the lowest quartile. It appears that the analysis of intermediate hyperglycemic quartiles did not reach statistical significance. More importantly, the index of hyperglycemia had no relation to the rate of progression from proteinuria to end-stage renal failure [17].

DIABETIC COMPLICATIONS: THE HYPOTHESES

As clearly demonstrated in the above epidemiological studies, not all patients with diabetes develop microvascular complications. Some patients with long-term IDDM never develop severe complications, regardless of their glycemic control. This subset of 'protected' patients comprises approximately 20% of all IDDM patients. At the opposite extreme is a far smaller proportion of patients in whom severe complications develop quite early, often with only mild elevations in blood glucose levels.

Because there are such widespread differences

in the appearance of diabetic complications, two major hypotheses have arisen to explain their pathogenesis. The genetic hypothesis suggests that the microvascular complications of diabetes are not directly related to the metabolic abnormalities of the disorder, but are genetically predetermined as part of the diabetic syndrome. Persons with diabetes, therefore, will develop diabetic complications because of some genetic susceptibility to do so. The metabolic hypothesis, however, suggests that diabetic complications develop as a direct consequence of the hyperglycemia of diabetes. Normalize blood glucose, the theory goes, and complications will not occur; improve blood glucose, and slow the progression of—or reverse—existing complications.

We favor a less polarized interpretation of available evidence that suggests that susceptibility to develop diabetic complications may differ significantly from patient to patient. Hyperglycemia appears to be a prerequisite, but may not be sufficient for the development of complications. Depending on the extent of genetic predisposition, the impact of the metabolic milieu may be more or less influential. We believe that three broad levels of susceptibility may exist. A small proportion of patients, perhaps 5%, seems to be virtually destined to develop complications, given even a relatively brief, mild rise in blood glucose levels. A larger group, perhaps 20%, seems able to tolerate prolonged hyperglycemia with relative impunity. The remaining three-quarters of patients with diabetes have varying moderate degrees of susceptibility; in such patients, intensive glycemic control and/or aggressive blood-pressure lowering may, indeed, prevent or favorably retard the progression of the microvascular diabetic complications.

Basement Membranes and HLA Antigens: The Possibility of a Hypertensive rather than a Genetic Cause

The hallmark of the microangiopathic lesion of diabetes is represented by a thickened capillary basement membrane, in association with disturbances in membrane permeability, and occlusion of small blood vessels. Although major clinical consequences occur in the retina, kidney and nerve, such morphologic alterations are found throughout the body, notably in capillaries of skeletal muscle which is accessible for human studies.

The original and most controversial argument in support of the genetic hypothesis and against the theory that diabetic microangiopathy is the consequence of the metabolic abnormalities of the disease was proposed by Siperstein and colleagues [19]. Using a simple morphometric method for measuring the basement membrane thickness of quadriceps muscle capillaries, these authors demonstrated that more than 90% of adult diabetic patients had a thickened capillary basement membrane. The skeletal muscle capillary width in the diabetic patients was compared with that in a group of normoglycemic controls who had no family histories of diabetes. In addition, they showed that 53% of 30 adults genetically predisposed to diabetes, who were offspring of two overt diabetic parents but who had normal glucose tolerance, had thickened capillary basement membranes compared with those in the control group. No correlation could be found between the severity or duration of the diabetes and the thickness of the basement membrane. Lastly, they showed that in 8 patients with 'secondary' diabetes due to chronic pancreatitis, some of whom had longstanding fasting hyperglycemia, only 1 patient had a thickened skeletal muscle capillary basement membrane.

Over the years these data have been the subject of considerable debate. Although there has been disagreement about the prevalence of the lesion in patients with diabetes, as well as its relationship to the age of the patient or the duration of the disease, a thickened basement membrane in skeletal muscle capillaries has often been found in diabetic patients [20–26]. Kilo, Williamson and colleagues [20, 21] have worked extensively in this area. Although their work has been critical of that of Siperstein and co-workers [19], differences between these two groups are more quantitative than qualitative. The reason for the differences in results obtained by these two groups is not completely clear, but may be attributable to differences in both fixative and measurement techniques [25].

The fundamental issue of whether a thickened capillary basement membrane represents a genetic marker or a tissue reponse to chronic hyperglycemia can now be considered resolved. We have demonstrated prospectively that intensive insulin treatment resulting in long-term, near-normoglycemic control causes a significant reduction of skeletal capillary basement membrane thickness in IDDM patients [27, 28]. Furthermore, Siperstein's group [29] recently had the unique opportunity to study individuals with secondary diabetes caused by the ingestion of the rodenticide, Vacor. In contrast with the previous findings in secondary diabetes, they demonstrated thickening of the skeletal capillary basement membrane probably caused by the drug-induced chronic hyperglycemia.

Additional support for the genetic hypothesis is based on some studies suggesting an increased frequency of the antigen HLA-DR4 in patients with diabetic microvascular complications. Dornan and colleagues [30] related the prevalence of retinopathy in a group of 127 patients with IDDM to their HLA haplotypes. They found that HLA-DR4 was present in 89 patients (70%) with background or proliferative retinopathy and in only 69 (54%) with no retinopathy. They also found that the retinopathy was more common in patients with 'poor diabetic control'. The combination of poor diabetic control and presence of HLA-DR4 increased the probability of having retinopathy to 33.3%. The authors concluded that genetically determined factors appear to influence susceptibility to retinopathy. This relationship between HLA-DR4 and a seemingly increased susceptibility to retinopathy has not been confirmed by other investigators, however [31–33].

Marks and associates [34] have provided additional evidence about the influence of genetic factors on the development of microvascular disease. They measured basement membrane thickness of skeletal muscle capillaries in 38 unaffected parents (those with normal oral glucose tolerance tests) of children with IDDM, and found a striking relationship between the presence of the antigen HLA-DR4 and the thickness of the basement membrane.

Recently, in an attempt to identify genetic markers that might be associated with an increased susceptibility to diabetic complications, we measured HLA-DR, glycemic control and capillary basement membrane width in 60 IDDM patients [35]; 42 subjects were a special subset of patients with longstanding diabetes (more than 25 years' duration) without microvascular complications. A matched group of 18 patients with advanced diabetic complications served as controls. The patients free of complications had a mean age of 13 years at diagnosis and had had the disease for an average of 32 years. Those with complications had a similar age of onset but a shorter duration of diabetes (16 years). There were no differences between the groups in terms of the percentage of patients with HLA-DR3, DR4 or both (88% versus 83%). Hypertension was more common in patients with advanced complications. Although in the hyperglycemic range, glycated hemoglobin values were lower in the patients with no complications (9.5 ± 0.3% versus 10.8 ± 0.6%). These findings are summarized in Table 1, indicating also that those patients with complications had a thicker capillary basement membrane. These data indicate that genetic factors at the HLA-DR locus do not appear to identify patients who are at a greater risk of developing diabetic complications. Patients with no complications after more than 25 years of diabetes had lower glycated hemoglobin levels than those with advanced complications. However, in both groups these levels were clearly in the hyperglycemic range (9.5% versus 10.8%). It would be naïve to interpret these data by simply saying that the relative absence of diabetic complications is probably due to the better diabetes control. What this study probably indicates is that the role of glycemic control in the pathogenesis of diabetic complications is intrinsically related to the degree of genetic susceptibility to develop these complications. It is conceivable that some protective determinants that confer reduced susceptibility to complications may also allow improved glycemic control to be achieved more easily. Alternatively, differences in glycemic thresholds could determine a specific level at which some tissues might respond to chronic hyperglycemia.

Of interest are the recent reports proposing an explanation for the frequency of diabetic nephropathy occurring in only one-third of all patients with IDDM. The susceptibility to develop diabetic nephropathy may be determined by a genetic predisposition to hypertension in this subset of patients [36, 37]. Krolewski et al [36] studied possible markers for the genetic predisposition to hypertension by comparing the frequency of a history of parental hypertension and the maximal velocities for sodium transport systems in red blood cells. They found that in 33 patients with diabetic nephropathy the maximal velocity of lithium–sodium countertransport in red cells was significantly higher than that in 56 diabetic control patients without nephropathy.

Table 1 Type 1 (insulin dependent) diabetes mellitus: absent versus advanced complications

| Complications | n | HLA-DR type | | | | Glycated hemoglobin (HbA$_1$) (%) | Capillary basement membrane width (nm) |
		3/x	4/x	3/4	Other		
Absent	42	5	12 88% NS	15	5	9.5 ± 0.3 *	169.6 ± 13.8 **
Advanced	18	5	3 83%	6	1	10.8 ± 0.6	243.7 ± 18.0

* $P < 0.02$ absent versus advanced; ** $P < 0.001$ absent versus advanced.

Having a parent with hypertension tripled the risk of developing diabetic nephropathy. The excess risk associated with both these indicators of a predisposition to hypertension was evident mainly in patients with poor glycemic control during the first decade of diabetes. Mangili et al [37] confirmed these findings by demonstrating higher rates of sodium–lithium countertransport in patients with diabetic nephropathy when compared with diabetic patients without renal disease and with non-diabetic patients with other kinds of renal diseases.

Testing the Metabolic Hypothesis in Experimental Diabetes and Transplantation Studies

Models of experimental diabetes in animals have the fundamental limitation of not developing the classic advanced lesions of proliferative diabetic retinopathy or those of end-stage renal failure as seen in humans [38]. Despite these limitations, a legion of studies indicate that improving or normalizing the metabolic milieu in experimental diabetes may prevent, slow or reverse some microvascular lesions similar to those found in human diabetes.

The classic study of the role of glycemic control and the development of retinopathy in animals is from Engerman et al [39]. They randomly assigned alloxan-induced diabetic dogs to one of two groups according to the level of glucose control to be achieved. In one group chronic hyperglycemia was maintained and the animals had a mean plasma glucose level that averaged between 350 mg/dl and 400 mg/dl. The other group of dogs received twice-daily insulin injections and their blood glucose levels averaged between 90 mg/dl and 180 mg/dl. After 2–3 years the poorly controlled group showed signs of early diabetic retinopathy. By the end of the study, after 5 years of follow-up, the differences between the two groups of dogs were striking. The hyperglycemic group showed saccular microaneurysms, pericyte ghosts and retinal hemorrhages, in contrast to the near-normoglycemic dogs whose retinas were similar to those of the non-diabetic control animals.

Renal and pancreatic transplantations provide ideal means of examining the effects of normalized blood glucose on the kidney. More than merely improving diabetes control, transplants test the effects of true physiological normoglycemia.

Studies using immunohistochemical techniques have added considerable information on renal lesions in patients with diabetes. Miller and Michael [40] performed a comprehensive immunofluorescent analysis on renal tissue from three groups of patients. Group 1 consisted of 24 normal living renal allograft donors, and 2 infants who were less than 1 week old. Group 2 included 24 patients with severe nephropathy who had had diabetes mellitus for 16–30 years; their ages ranged from 20 years to 47 years. Group 3 consisted of 33 patients who had chronic renal failure of diverse causes other than diabetes; ages ranged from 5 years to 63 years. Renal sections from patients with diabetes were easily distinguished from those of the other patients and normal controls by the intense linear staining of extracellular membranes. The most specific reaction was the presence of IgG and albumin lining the tubular basement membrane. With the exception of some minimal staining of the glomerular basement membrane in the patients with normal kidneys, practically no overlap occurred among these three groups. Thus, something about the diabetic milieu appears to result in the accumulation of immunofluorescence material in the kidneys of diabetic patients who have diabetic nephropathy but not in those who have renal disease from other causes. Experimental studies of diabetes in rats have yielded data on the role of hyperglycemia in diabetes. Immunofluorescent staining for rat IgG and complement C3 occur after 4–6 months of hyperglycemia in kidneys from rats made diabetic experimentally. If kidneys from diabetic rats are transplanted into normal rats, the characteristic immunofluorescent lesion disappears in 2 months, and if kidneys from non-diabetic rats are transplanted into diabetic rats the lesion appears after 2 months [41]. If diabetic rats become normoglycemic following islet cell transplantation, regression of the immunofluorescent changes occurs, as well as reductions in glomerular volume and percentage of the mesangial volume occupied by the matrix component [42].

In humans, similar experiments have given results remarkably similar to those obtained from the experimental studies of diabetes in animals. Mauer and co-workers [43] examined kidney tissue obtained from 12 diabetic and 17 non-diabetic patients 2–12 years after renal transplantation. The frequency and intensity of IgG and albumin stains of the tubular and glomerular basement membranes and Bowman's capsule were significantly greater in the diabetic than in the non-diabetic patients. With the exception of some staining of the glomerular basement membranes in the non-diabetic kidneys, practically no overlap occurred between the two groups. The significance of these immunofluorescence changes remains speculative, however. Mauer's group also studied vascular changes in renal transplant tissue from 12 diabetic and 28 non-diabetic patients who had had renal grafts for at least 2 years [44]. Ten of the 12 kidneys from diabetic patients showed arteriolar hyalinosis; in 6 of the 10, the hyaline changes involved both the afferent and efferent limbs of glomerular arterioles. One diabetic patient developed typical nodular glomerulosclerosis 35 months after transplantation. Of the 28 kidneys from the transplant recipients without diabetes, 3 showed hyaline vascular changes. These changes occurred only rarely in vessels, did not appear until 5 years after transplantation, and never involved both afferent and efferent limbs of the arterioles. At transplantation, none of the blood-vessel changes was present in the kidneys given to the 12 dia-

betic recipients, although 10 had received living-related-donor grafts.

A rare opportunity to study the effect of normalizing blood glucose on the diabetic human kidney came about because of a Kuwaiti transplantation center's urgent need for functioning kidneys [45]. The kidneys from a brain-dead IDDM victim were transplanted into two non-diabetic recipients. The donor had been diabetic for 17 years, pretransplantation urine was positive for both glucose and protein, and renal biopsy revealed diffuse histologic changes of established glomerulosclerosis with increased mesangial matrix, and thickening of the glomerular capillary basement membrane. Seven months after transplantation a repeat renal biopsy showed complete resolution of the abnormalities; 14 months after transplantation, kidneys continued to function well and there was no evidence of proteinuria.

The Minnesota group recently reported that successful pancreatic transplantation in 8 patients with longstanding IDDM was associated with an amelioration of the renal lesions of the native kidneys 24 months after transplantation [46]. They found significant reductions in mean glomerular volume and in the average mesangial volume per glomerulus. The rate of increase of mean glomerular basement membrane width was significantly less than in control patients on conventional therapy. However, creatinine clearance declined from 96 ± 22 ml/min in the initial post-transplant period to 60 ± 15 ml/min; this decline probably was related to the cyclosporine treatment.

Hyperglycemia and Complications: What Is the Mechanism?

One additional issue of great importance needs to be discussed. Given that hyperglycemia is required for the development of complications involving small blood vessels in those diabetic individuals susceptible to its damaging effects, what are the mechanisms by which hyperglycemia damages tissues? This point is still under active investigation, and an in-depth discussion is beyond the scope of this review. However, there are at least three possible explanations. The first relates to the possibility that prolonged hyperglycemia may lead to widespread post-translational glycation of tissue proteins [47]. Once glycated, the function of the proteins may be altered, thus resulting in tissue damage.

Another potential explanation is related to the polyol–inositol pathway [48]. In the presence of hyperglycemia the polyol pathway is activated by the enzyme aldose reductase, catalyzing the conversion of glucose to sorbitol. This enzymatic reaction is coupled to a series of biochemical reactions in many tissues of the body affected by the complications of diabetes, resulting in depletion of myo-inositol and decrease in Na^+-K^+-ATPase activity. This series of biochemical changes that result from activation of the polyol pathway may be a mechanism by which hyperglycemia causes tissue damage. Finally, there is the possibility that the hemodynamic changes resulting from hyperglycemia may be an important factor [49].

We consider it naïve to think that only a single mechanism is reponsible for the potential damaging effects of hyperglycemia; it is more likely that a combination of some or all of the factors discussed above is responsible. Furthermore, it is likely that what occurs in one target tissue (the retina) differs from what happens in another (the kidney). Clearly, more research is needed before this is understood.

THE CLINICAL ARENA

In ascertaining the metabolic influences on the development of diabetic microvascular disease, some fundamental questions need to be addressed. If we control hyperglycemia in patients with diabetes, can we also prevent the complications of diabetes, reverse established complications and/or slow the progression of established complications? There may well be separate answers to these three questions. For example, it may be possible to prevent diabetic complications in patients by long-term normoglycemia, but it may not be possible to reverse established complications. In addition, the effect of hyperglycemia may differ in different tissues.

Retrospective Studies

The Malmö Study

Johnsson [50] reviewed the cases of all patients in Malmö, Sweden, who had their diabetes diagnosed between 1922 and 1945 and who were less than 40 years old at the onset of disease. The patients were separated into two groups. Series 1 consisted of 56 patients who were diagnosed between 1922 and 1935. All received initial treatment of strict diet control and multiple daily injections of insulin in an attempt to keep the urine free of glucose. Series 2 consisted of 104 patients whose disease was diagnosed between 1935 and 1945. These patients were treated with long-acting insulin and a much less regimented diet. The patients in series 2 had a much greater incidence of vascular complications than did those in series 1. Although the mean duration of diabetes for patients in series 1 was 10 years longer than in patients in series 2, only 18 of 56 (32%) had nephropathy as compared with 58 of 104 (56%) in series 2. The difference becomes more pronounced when comparing the incidence of nephropathy in patients who have had this disease for more than 15 years. Only 5 of 56 (9%) patients in series 1 had nephropathy, compared with 63 of 104 (61%) in series 2. Similar striking differences were seen when the incidence of retinopathy was compared. Hypoglycemia was more frequent in patients in series 1, reflecting attempts to achieve normoglycemia and the use of multiple daily insulin injections.

The Pirart Study

This monumental study is perhaps the largest of its kind. Pirart followed 4400 patients with diabetes from 1947, of whom a cohort of 2795 patients had been followed since the inital diagnosis of their diabetes [51]. Despite the obvious limitation of this study, that of the inability to assess long-term diabetes control accurately, Pirart's data suggest a strong relationship between the level of diabetic control and the development of diabetic complications. Some of the data can be seen in Figure 3, which demonstrates the prevalence of retinopathy as related to the level of diabetic control over the years of follow-up. It appears that the higher the level of diabetic control, the greater the prevalence of diabetic retinopathy. Of note, however, is the fact that almost 30% of Dr Pirart's patients, despite many years of poor diabetes control, had essentially no diabetic retinopathy as assessed by conventional means.

Controlled Prospective Trials

The Job Study

The controversial French study by Job et al attempted to assess the effect of glycemic control on retinopathy [52]. Diabetic patients were randomly assigned either to a group receiving single

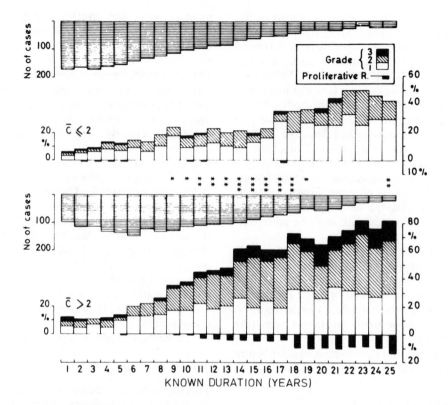

Figure 3 Varying degrees of retinopathy as function of the duration of diabetes in patients with good (top) or poor (bottom) glycemic control (from reference 51, with permission)

insulin injections or to a group receiving multiple insulin injections (three times daily). Both groups were followed for a mean duration of 3 years. The progression of retinopathy was evaluated by fluorescein angiography and funduscopic examination. The authors reported a significantly greater increase in the number of microaneurysms in the single-injection group compared with the multiple-injection group. Unfortunately, this study suffered from an important defect, which makes the results difficult to evaluate: of those 21 patients whose data were analyzed from the single-injection group, only 16 received one daily insulin injection for the entire period of the study; the other 5 were changed either to two or three injections per day after the study began. In the multiple-injection group only 5 of 21 patients analyzed had three insulin injections daily for the entire period of the study; the others either initially accepted only two injections (4 patients) or some only one (4 patients). Nine of the 13 who originally accepted three injections daily were reduced

to two injections after 1 year. The small number of patients initially studied, coupled with the many crossovers in the protocol, make this study invalid, despite the fact that the authors contend that fewer microaneurysms developed in the multiple-injection group.

The Steno Studies

The Danish have carefully assessed the effects of near-normoglycemia on established background retinopathy [53, 54] and early diabetic nephropathy [55, 56]. In their initial study, 30 IDDM patients with background retinopathy were randomly assigned to groups receiving either unchanged conventional treatment (UCT) with two daily injections of insulin or treatment with continuous subcutaneous insulin infusion (CSII). The study was originally designed for 1 year, but because of the disappointing results showing that 1 year of near-normoglycemia could not prevent the development of proliferative retinopathy [53] the study was extended to

Table 2 The Steno study: fundus photographic findings in thirty patients with insulin dependent diabetes retinopathy

	Conventional treatment	Continuous subcutaneous insulin infusion
After 1 year		
Improved	3	3
No change	7	2
Worse	5	10
After 2 years		
Improved	2	7
No change	2	2
Worse	10	6

From reference 54, with permission

a 2-year follow-up [54]. Retinal examinations were done at 6-month intervals. Mean blood glucose levels and hemoglobin A_{1c} values were significantly lower in the insulin infusion treatment group than in the conventional treatment group. Retinal morphology deteriorated during the first year in both groups and no significant differences were seen between the two groups. The frequency of deterioration was higher, however, in the group treated with CSII, especially among the patients with the best glycemic control. Fundus photographs showed that despite the apparent (although not statistically significant) progression of retinopathy after the first year of the study, a plateau appears to have been reached after 2 years of follow-up, with improvement of retinopathy more frequently seen in the CSII group than among the conventionally treated patients (Table 2). However, by the end of the study, 4 patients in the CSII group and 5 patients in the conventional group had developed proliferative retinopathy. In this same study the effect of diabetic control on glomerular filtration rate and urinary albumin excretion rate was also evaluated [55]. The authors showed that glomerular filtration rate can be decreased and frequently returned to normal with improved metabolic control. Urinary albumin excretion rates remained stable in the group receiving continuous insulin infusions.

Long-term prospective studies have suggested that microalbuminuria, as defined by a persistent elevation of urinary albumin excretion in otherwise healthy IDDM patients without overt proteinuria, predicts future development of overt diabetic nephropathy [56–59]. The Steno Memorial Hospital conducted a study specifically designed to assess the impact of strict glycemic control on kidney function in IDDM patients with persistent microalbuminuria [60, 61]. Patients selected for the study had two of three 24-hour (Albustix-negative) urine collections with an albumin excretion rate between 30 mg and 300 mg per 24 hours (20–200 μg/min). Thirty-six patients were matched in pairs according to albumin excretion rate, sex and HbA_{1c} level before random assignment to either usual conventional treatment or CSII. The first report after 1 year showed that despite a significant reduction in HbA_{1c} values (from 9.5% to 7.3%) in the CSII group, the albumin excretion rate remained constant in both groups [60]. Glomerular filtration rate was unchanged, and kidney size was significantly reduced in the CSII group. However, in another report after 2 years of follow-up, clinical diabetic nephropathy (urinary albumin excretion rate greater than 300 mg per 24 hours) developed in 5 patients in the conventionally treated group but in none of the CSII group [61]. More careful analysis within the conventionally treated group revealed that the 5 patients who progressed had a mean baseline microalbuminuria considerably higher (189 $\pm$ 61 mg per 24 hours) than those who remained stable in the same treatment group (51 $\pm$ 24 mg per 24 hours). Near-normoglycemia had an overall beneficial effect on the annual increase in urinary albumin excretion. Mean glycosylated hemoglobin values and diastolic blood pressure levels correlated positively with the annual change in albumin excretion rate.

The Kroc Study

The Kroc prospective multicenter trial [62] had 70 patients with non-proliferative diabetic retinopathy and absent C peptide, randomly assigned to receive either pump therapy ($n = 35$) or conventional therapy ($n = 35$). Subsequently, glycemic control and retinopathy (determined by fundus photography and fluorescein angiography) were periodically assessed over a 8-month follow-up period as originally designed. At the start of the study, age, duration of diabetes, insulin dosage, glycemic control and degree of retinopathy were similar in the two groups. After randomization, mean blood glucose and glycated hemoglobin levels remained elevated in the conventional treatment group, but fell to near-normal values during the entire period of pump treatment. The frequency of biochemically determined hypoglycemia was similar in both groups, but ketoacidosis occurred only in those receiving pump therapy. The level of retinopathy, assessed from fundus photographs, progressed in both groups. Continuous subcutaneous insulin infusion was associated with slightly more deterioration compared with conventional treatment, primarily because of the appearance of soft exudates and intraretinal microvascular abnormalities. The authors concluded that the establishment of near-normal blood glucose levels for 8 months does not retard progression of, and may initially worsen, pre-existing retinopathy. Similarly to the Steno studies and with the same limitations (lack of planning for study extension), the Kroc group has also reported results of a 2-year follow-up [63]. Although the data contain serious flaws from 8 months forward (a high percentage of patients switched to the other treatment group), the results at 2 years showed that the retinopathy in the insulin infusion group had stabilized; in the conventional treatment group, the retinopathy tended to progress. The authors then concluded that, after 2 years, no benefits accrued to patients receiving pump therapy, nor did risk increase in terms of progression of retinopathy. Both the Steno and Kroc studies reported a tendency toward transient acceleration of diabetic retinopathy in patients treated intensively to achieve near-normoglycemia. As discussed below, this phenomenon appears to be transient and reversible.

The Kroc multicenter study also found a beneficial effect of near-normoglycemia on microalbuminuria. Complete 24-hour urine collections were obtained throughout the 8-month study in 59 of the 68 IDDM patients. At baseline, the urinary albumin excretion rate was normal (below 12 μg/min) in 39 patients (20 receiving conventional insulin treatment and 19 on CSII), and above normal in the other 20 patients (10 patients in each group). In the patients with normoalbuminuria, the albumin excretion rate was relatively constant regardless of the type of treatment. However, patients on CSII with an elevated albumin excretion rate had a progressive decline in albumin excretion from 48 $\pm$ 18 μg/min at entry to 19 $\pm$ 6 μg/min at 4 months and to 16 $\pm$ 5 μg/min at 8 months. In contrast, the elevated albumin excretion rate in the conventional treatment group remained unchanged. The main objection to this study is

that baseline urinary albumin consisted of only a single sample, which could have reflected the poor glycemic control before the CSII treatment. Several urine samples are usually required to define persistent microalbuminuria characteristic of early diabetic nephropathy [64].

The Oxford Study

In the study by Homan et al [65] conducted in diabetes clinics at Oxford and Aylesbury in the UK, 74 patients with IDDM and background retinopathy were randomly assigned to continue with usual diabetic care (group U) or to receive a more intensive program (group A) using ultralente insulin as basal coverage and soluble insulin before meals. In addition, group A patients attended the clinic more frequently, received closer dietary supervision and were taught how to self-monitor blood glucose levels. Group A had significantly lower mean glycated hemoglobin levels during the study, although the mean levels also fell in group U toward the end of the second year. The rate of progression of retinopathy was similar in both groups and by the end of the study, 6 patients in the intensive treatment program developed new retinal vessels compared with only 2 patients in the conventionally treated group.

The Aarhus Study

The Danish Aarhus study reported the effects of improved glycemic control in 24 normoalbuminuric IDDM patients with minimal or no background retinopathy [66]. Again, at the end of the 1-year study, no differences were found in the rate of progression of retinopathy between the conventional treatment group and the CSII group. Urinary albumin excretion rate remained basically unchanged in both treatment groups. Only the glomerular filtration rate was significantly reduced, from 130 $\pm$ 18 ml/min to 116 $\pm$ 15 ml/min in the CSII group.

The Oslo Study

Two different modalities of intensive diabetes management—either multiple insulin injections (MDI) or CSII—were compared with conventional treatment in the 2-year Oslo study [67, 68]. Fifteen IDDM patients were allocated to each treatment group. They were carefully followed by fundus photography and fluorescein angiograms at baseline and then at 3, 6, 12 and 24 months. As previously seen in the Steno and Kroc studies, an early transient deterioration of retinopathy was found in the intensively treated patients [67]. During the initial 3–6 months of treatment, 50% of all patients on either CSII or MDI developed cotton-wool exudates, whereas none was found in the conventional hyperglycemic group. These retinal findings regressed in all but 4 patients by 12 months of therapy. Those patients who developed cotton-wool spots had larger reductions in glycated hemoglobin levels, a longer duration of diabetes and had more advanced retinopathy at onset. It has been suggested that this transient worsening of retinopathy may be due to increased retinal ischemia resulting from a reduction of the glucose-related enhanced retinal blood flow [69].

By the second year, the Oslo study reported slightly more optimistic findings [68]. Diabetic retinopathy appeared to continue progressing only in the hyperglycemic group. Microaneurysm counts increased only in the conventionally treated group, whereas in the two intensively treated groups they remained unchanged. Of note, however, was that the evaluation of retinopathy status by fluorescein angiograms failed to reveal any differences in progression between the three treatment groups. Glomerular hyperfiltration was reduced with CSII, but the urinary albumin excretion rate remained unchanged.

The Dallas Study

For the past several years, Raskin and co-workers [70–78] have been conducting a long-term, prospective, non-randomized trial on the effect of an experimental, intensive treatment program on diabetic complications in patients with IDDM diabetes (C-peptide negative). This treatment program includes intensive dietary instruction, self-monitoring of blood glucose levels and CSII delivered by portable insulin infusion devices. Data from a group of 30 patients have been compared with those from a similar group of 24 patients with type 1 IDDM who preferred to continue on a more conventional treatment regimen rather than to enter into the above intensive treatment program. Over the years, the intensive treatment program has shown considerable short-term advantage over conventional treatment with respect to many metabolic variables such as plasma glucagon profiles [70], lipid and lipoprotein levels [71–73, 77, 78] and motor nerve conduction [74]. The long-term changes induced by near-normoglycemia in lipid and lipoprotein levels are directed towards a reduction in risk factors for atherosclerosis [77].

The authors also have followed the progression of early diabetic retinopathy and measured basement membrane width of skeletal muscle capillaries in those patients in whom observations have been made from 1 to 3 years [75, 76]. During the 3 years of improved diabetes control, reflected by decrease in glycated hemoglobin levels, patients participating in the intensive treatment program had significant reductions in the width of basement membrane in skeletal muscle capillaries. This reduction was not seen in the group of diabetic patients treated more conventionally, who showed a stable though unimproved level of diabetic control. In addition, they [76] recently reported that near-normoglycemic patients in the intensive treatment group had significantly less progression of diabetic retinopathy than those patients in the conventional treatment group. Masked assessment of retinopathy was carefully done using two separate grading systems and each method showed similar findings (Table 3). Furthermore, patients whose diabetic retinopathy progressed during the treatment period showed a tendency for thickening of skeletal muscle capillary basement membranes, irrespective of the treatment group (Figure 4).

The Minnesota Study

Theoretically, pancreatic transplantations resulting in physiological normoglycemia would be the ideal setting to study the impact of glucose control on microvascular complications. However, very disappointing (but perhaps not unexpected) findings were recently reported by researchers from Minnesota. In this study, 22 IDDM patients rendered normoglycemic by successful pancreas transplantation were compared with 16 similar hyperglycemic patients in whom pancreas transplantation had been unsuccessful [79]. After a mean follow-up of 24 months, no significant differences in the rate of progression of retinopathy were found between the two groups. Most of the patients in both groups had advanced proliferative retinopathy,

Table 3 The Dallas study: effect of diabetes control on progression of retinopathy

	Modified early treatment diabetic retinopathy study criteria		Macular microaneurysm count	
	Experimental treatment*	Conventional treatment	Experimental treatment*	Conventional treatment
Better	4	0	1	0
Stable	23	18	28	19
Worse	3	6	1	5

* $P < 0.05$, experimental treatment versus conventional treatment (log-likelihood chi-squared).

but progression to retinopathy was observed more commonly in patients with less advanced forms of retinopathy. The authors concluded that pancreatic transplantation and subsequent normoglycemia can neither reverse nor prevent the progression of established diabetic retinopathy. It is thus conceivable that, once a certain degree of retinopathy is reached, it may be irreversible.

The DCCT Study

All the above data, particularly the Oslo and Dallas studies [68, 76], can at best be interpreted as only *suggestive* that improved glycemic control may have a role in changing the progression rate of diabetic microvascular complications. These data do not justify the rigid attitude and heavy burden that are imposed on many patients with diabetes by their health care providers when their diabetes control does not achieve 'ideal goals'. These data also emphasize the need

to acquire the definitive information that only an expensive, long-term, carefully designed study such as the Diabetes Control and Complications Trial (DCCT) can provide [80]. This multicenter trial [81], the largest and most ambitious clinical trial to date, involves 28 clinical centers, 26 in the USA and 2 in Canada. The study plans to follow two large groups of patients with IDDM for as long as 8–10 years. More than 1400 patients have been randomly assigned to one of two specific treatment regimens. One group will receive conventional treatment, and the other group an intensive treatment designed to achieve euglycemia. The major end-point will be the development of early diabetic retinopathy in the primary intervention trial (that is, patients without retinopathy at entry), and the rate of progression of the retinal lesions will be assessed in the secondary intervention trial.

Those patients in the secondary intervention trial constitute a highly homogeneous population

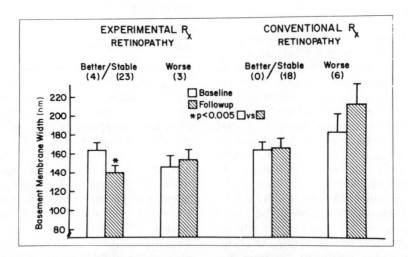

Figure 4 Skeletal muscle capillary basement membrane width (baseline, open bars; follow-up, crosshatched bars) in patients treated with either an experimental or conventional treatment as a function of the status of their retinopathy (from reference 76, with permission)

Table 4 The DCCT study: severe hypoglycemia and coma

	Subjects		Events	
	n	%	n	Per 100 subject-years
Total severe reactions				
Experimental	38	26.0*	79	54.1
Standard	13	9.8	23	17.4
Coma				
Experimental	29	19.9†	49	33.6
Standard	8	6.1	16	12.1
Single episode of coma				
Experimental	17	11.6‡	17	11.6
Standard	5	3.8	5	3.8
Multiple episodes of coma				
Experimental	12	8.2§	32	21.9
Standard	3	2.3	11	2.3

Total experimental subjects, 146; total standard subjects, 132. * $P = 0.0009$, † $P = 0.00013$, ‡ $P = 0.028$, § $P = 0.05$ (standard versus experimental chi-squared).
Reproduced from reference 82, with permission from the American Diabetes Association, Inc.

with minimal background retinopathy ($< P_2$ by modified Airlie House criteria) with or without associated microalbuminuria (below 200 mg per 24 hours of urinary albumin). The decision to follow these 1400 patients for a mean duration of 7 years was based on statistical analysis of the data generated by the Wisconsin and St Louis studies reviewed above [9, 10]. It was estimated that both the primary prevention and the secondary intervention cohorts, with 700 patients each, will have a power or more than 91% to detect a 33% reduction in the annual hazard rate for the onset and progression of diabetic retinopathy. So far some important contributions have emerged from this trial and can be summarized as follows:

(1) Intensive diabetes management can be a dangerous therapeutic strategy. Results of the first 2-year feasibility study revealed a threefold increase in severe hypoglycemia in the intensively treated group [82] (Table 4).
(2) It is possible to achieve and maintain difference in glycemic control between large groups of conventionally and intensively treated IDDM patients. However, the goal of normal glycated hemoglobin levels is extremely difficult to achieve and perhaps unrealistic for most patients (Figure 5).
(3) Despite the excellence of the diabetes research centers involved, utilizing unlimited resources with no preoccupation for the enormous cost of sophisticated care, the

DCCT has shown that it is probably impossible to obtain mean normal HbA_{1c} in large groups of patients

There are obviously patients in whom the HbA_{1c} levels can be normalized and others who continue in the near-normal or mild hyperglycemic range. Most of the time this reflects the desire and motivation of the patients to comply with the dietary and insulin regimens. We are intrigued by those patients who, with minimal efforts, maintain normal HbA_{1c} and by those patients in whom, despite enormous dedication to the management of their diabetes, the glycated hemoglobin levels cannot be reduced to normal levels. We wonder if this 'easily controllable' diabetes with lower HbA_{1c} may be genetically determined by some unknown factors which may also be involved in the genesis of diabetic complications. If this is true, then the finding of a lower complication rate in the better-controlled groups may not necessarily indicate causality with the metabolic control, but rather a suggestion that perhaps some individuals achieve a lower HbA_{1c} as part of the spectrum of decreased genetic susceptibility to complications.

CONCLUSION

Which hypothesis on the causes of microvascular complications of diabetes—the genetic or the metabolic—is better supported? Choosing between the two remains difficult. Alternatively, we propose that the complications of diabetes

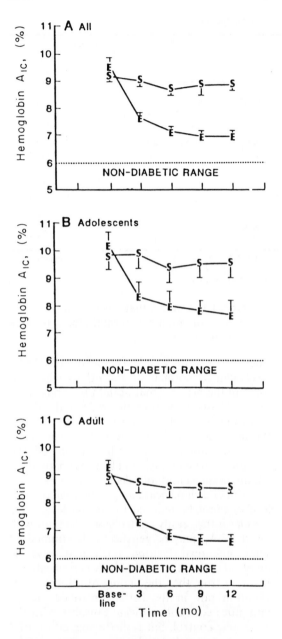

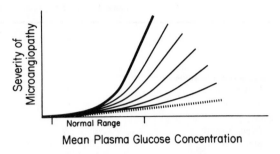

Figure 6 The influence of genetic predisposition on the severity of diabetic microangiopathy. Thick line indicates a strong predisposition; dotted line, minimal (reproduced, with permission, from Raskin P, Rosenstock J. Blood glucose control and diabetic complications. *Ann. Intern. Med.* 1986; 105: 254–63)

Figure 5 Glycated hemoglobin values from the DCCT 2-year feasibility study. A, all patients; B, adolescent only; C, adults only. S = standard therapy; E = experimental (intensive) therapy (reproduced from reference 82, with permission from the American Diabetes Association, Inc.)

is not a sufficient cause in itself: in addition to hyperglycemia, some 'genetic predisposition' is also required. A theoretical model regarding the interrelationship between genetic and metabolic factors in the development of diabetic complications is shown diagrammatically in Figure 6.

In approximately 20% of diabetic patients, the genetic predisposition to develop diabetic complications is very low. Thus, regardless of the severity of the metabolic abnormality (how much hyperglycemia occurs for the duration of their illness), the patients rarely develop significant complications. If we could identify this subset of patients at the onset of disease, our treatment recommendations would be simple: keep them free of symptoms and avoid hypoglycemia, severe hyperglycemia and ketoacidosis. These patients would not need expensive, intensive diabetes management that would significantly affect their life-styles. In another 5% of patients, the genetic predisposition to develop microvascular complications is so great that even a slight degree of hyperglycemia results in severe microvascular complications. Unfortunately, present treatment techniques may not have the capacity to normalize the blood glucose level sufficiently to help this group of patients. Finally, we have the majority of diabetic patients who have varying degrees of the genetic predisposition to develop microvascular complications. We believe that, in this group, improved diabetes control resulting in lowering of the overall blood glucose level might reduce the severity or progression of the microvascular complications. It may well be that there is a blood glucose threshold for the development of

involving the small blood vessels are related to both genetic and metabolic influences. Although hyperglycemia is needed for the microvascular complications of diabetes to develop, it complications. The ideal situation would be to reduce HbA$_{1c}$ levels below this threshold without necessarily achieving normoglycemia. Although the data appear to support our hypothesis, it has yet to be proven.

Regarding the three questions posed earlier, it may well be that intensive diabetes treatment with resultant long-term near-normoglycemia or normo-glycemia should be considered preventive. We believe the data eventually will prove that we can only prevent diabetic complications; once significant diabetic complications have occurred, no degree of normoglycemia will cause a reversal, although some slowing of the progression is probably possible.

However, we do not recommend giving intensive treatment to all patients with IDDM in the absence of a definitive answer to this question. We would recommend it only if no detractions existed to this form of treatment. Intensive treatment is very expensive, both to the patient and to the health care system. The ever-present danger of insulin-induced hypoglycemia with potentially lethal consequence also exists. Thus, given both the risks of aggressive insulin therapy and the considerable ambiguity of the evidence presented here, we strongly believe that results of a large-scale clinical trial are needed to define these issues more clearly. The Diabetes Control and Complications Trial [80–82] is such a trial, and it is well under way. Until the results of this trial are known, we must make careful decisions about which patients to enroll in intensive diabetes treatment programs.

REFERENCES

1. Hanssen KF, Dahl-Jorgensen K, Lauritzen T, Feldt-Rasmussen B, Brinchmann-Hanssen O, Deckert T. Diabetic control and microvascular complications: the near-normoglycaemic experience. Diabetologia 1986; 29: 677–85.
2. Raskin P. Diabetic regulation and its relationship to microangiopathy. Metabolism 1978; 27: 235–51.
3. Barbosa J, Sone B. Do genetic factors play a role in the pathogenesis of diabetic microangiopathy? Diabetologia 1984; 27: 487–92.
4. Raskin P, Rosenstock J. Blood glucose control and diabetic complications. Ann Intern Med 1986; 105: 254–63.
5. Raskin P. Treatment of insulin-dependent diabetes with portable insulin infusions devices. Med Clin North Am 1982; 66: 1269–83.
6. Rosenstock J, Strowig S, Raskin P. Insulin pump therapy. A realistic appraisal. Clin Diabetes 1985; 3: 25–31.
7. Unger RH. Meticulous control of diabetes: benefits, risks and precautions. Diabetes 1982; 31: 479–83.
8. DCCT Research Group. Diabetes Control and Complications Trial (DCCT): results of feasibility study. Diabetes Care 1987; 10: 1–19.
9. Palmberg P, Smith M, Waltman S et al. The natural history of retinopathy in insulin-dependent juvenile-onset diabetes. Ophthalmology 1981; 88: 613–18.
10. Klein R, Klein BEK, Moss SE, Davis ME, DeMets DL. The Wisconsin epidemiologic study of diabetic retinopathy. II. Prevalence and risk of diabetic retinopathy when age at diagnosis is less than 30 years. Arch Ophthalmology 1984; 102: 520–6.
11. Krolewski AS, Warram JH, Rand LI, Christlieb AR, Busick EJ, Kahn CR. Risk of proliferative diabetic retinopathy in juvenile-onset type I diabetes: a 40 year follow-up study. Diabetes Care 1986; 9: 443–52.
12. Oakley WG, Pyke DA, Tattersall RB, Watkins PJ. Long-term diabetes: a clinical study of 92 patients after 40 years. Quart J Med 1974; 43: 145–56.
13. Paz-Guevara AT, Hsu TH, White P. Juvenile diabetes mellitus after forty years. Diabetes 1975; 24: 559–65.
14. Kussman MJ, Goldstein HH, Gleason RE. The clinical course of diabetic nephropathy. JAMA 1976; 236: 1861–3.
15. Anderson AK, Christiansen JS, Andersen JK, Kreiner S, Deckert T. Diabetic nephropathy in type I (insulin-dependent) diabetes: an epidemiological study. Diabetologia 1983; 25: 496–501.
16. Kofoed-Enevoldsen A, Borch-Johnsen K, Kreiner S, Nerup J, Deckert T. Declining incidence of persistent proteinuria in type I (insulin-dependent) diabetic patients in Denmark. Diabetes 1987; 36: 2056–9.
17. Krolewski AS, Warram JH, Christlieb AR, Busick EJ, Kahn DR. The changing natural history of nephropathy in Type I diabetes. Am J Med 1985; 78: 785–94.
18. Krolewski AS, Warram JH, Rand LI, Kahn CR. Epidemologic approach to the etiology of Type I diabetes mellitus and its complications. New Engl J Med 1987; 317: 1390–8.
19. Siperstein MD, Unger RH, Madison LL. Studies of muscle capillary basement membranes in normal subjects, diabetic, and prediabetic patients. J Clin Invest 1968; 47: 1973–99.
20. Kilo C, Vogler N, Williamson JR. Muscle capillary basement membrane changes related to aging and to diabetes mellitus. Diabetes 1972; 21: 881–905.

21. Williamson JR, Rowold E, Hoffman P, Kilo CL. Influence of fixation and morphometric technics on capillary basement-membrane thickening prevalence data in diabetes. Diabetes 1976; 25: 604–13.

22. Vracko RL. Skeletal muscle capillaries in diabetics; a quantitative analysis. Circulation 1970; 41: 271–83.

23. Pardo V, Perez-Stable E, Alzamora DB, Cleveland WW. Incidence and significance of muscle capillary basal albumina thickness in juvenile diabetes. Am J Pathol 1972; 68: 67–80.

24. Danowski TS, Fisher ER, Khurana RC, Nolan S, Stephan TL. Muscle capillary basement membrane in juvenile diabetes mellitus. Metabolism 1972; 21: 1125–32.

25. Siperstein MD, Raskin P, Burns H. Electron microscopic quantification of diabetic microangiopathy. Diabetes 1973; 22: 514–27.

26. Raskin P, Marks JF, Burns H Jr, Plumer MD, Siperstein MD. Capillary basement membrane width in diabetic children. Am J Med 1975; 58: 365–72.

27. Raskin P, Pietri A, Unger R, Shannon WA Jr. The effect of diabetic control on skeletal muscle capillary basement membrane width in patients with type I diabetes mellitus. New Engl J Med 1983; 309: 1546–50.

28. Rosenstock J, Challis P, Strowig S, Raskin P. Improved diabetes control reduces skeletal muscle capillary basement membrane width in insulin-dependent diabetes mellitus. Diabetes Res Clin Pract 1988; 4: 167–75.

29. Feingold KR, Lee TH, Chung MY, Siperstein MD. Muscle capillary basement membrane width in patients with Vacor-induced diabetes mellitus. J Clin Invest 1986; 78: 102–7.

30. Dornan TL, Ting A, McPherson CK, Peckar CO, Mann JI, Turner RC, Morris PJ. Genetic susceptibility to the development of retinopathy in insulin-dependent diabetics. Diabetes 1982; 31: 226–31.

31. Christy M, Nerup J, Platz P, Thomsen M, Ryder LP, Svejgaard A. A review of HLA antigens in longstanding IDDM with and without severe retinopathy. Horm Metab Res 1981; 11 (suppl.): 73–7.

32. Johnston PB, Kidd M, Middleton D, Greenfield AA, Archer DB, Maguire CJF, Kennedy L. Analysis of HLA antigen association with proliferative diabetic retinopathy. Br J Ophthalmol 1982; 66: 277–9.

33. Gray RS, Starkey IR, Rainbow S et al. HLA antigens and other risk factors in the development of retinopathy in type 1 diabetes. Br J Opthalmol 1982; 66: 280–5.

34. Marks JR, Raskin P, Stastny P. İncrease in capillary basement membrane width in parents of

children with type I diabetes mellitus: association with HLA-DR4. Diabetes 1981; 30: 475–80.

35. Rosenstock J, Marks J, Stastny P, Raskin P. The relationship of HLA-DR4 locus to diabetic microvascular complications: Genes or glycemia. Diabetes 1988; 32 (suppl. 1): 24A.

36. Krolewski AS, Canessa M, Warram JH, Laffel LMB, Christlieb AR, Knowles WC, Rand LI. Predisposition to hypertension and susceptibility to renal disease in insulin-dependent diabetes mellitus. New Engl J Med 1988; 318: 140–5.

37. Mangili R, Bending JJ, Scott G, Li LK, Gupta A, Viberti GC. Increased sodium–lithium countertransport activity in red cells of patients with insulin-dependent diabetes and nephropathy. New Engl J Med 1988; 18: 146–50.

38. Engerman R, Finkelstein D, Aguirre G, Diddie KR, Fox RR, Frank RN, Varma SD. Ocular complications. Diabetes 1982; 31 (suppl. 1): 82–8.

39. Engerman R, Bloodworth JMB, Nelson S. Relationship of microvascular disease in diabetes to metabolic control. Diabetes 1977; 26: 760–9.

40. Miller K, Michael AF. Immunopathology of renal extracellular membranes in diabetes mellitus: specificity of tubular basement membrane immunofluorescence. Diabetes 1976; 25: 701–8.

41. Lee CS, Mauer SM, Brown DM, Sutherland DER, Michael AF, Najarian JS. Renal transplantation in diabetes mellitus in rats. J Exp Med 1974; 139: 793–800.

42. Mauer SM, Steffes MW, Sutherland DER, Najarian JS, Michael AF, Brown DM. Studies of the rate of regression of the glomerular lesions in diabetic rats treated with pancreatic islet transplantation. Diabetes 1975; 24: 280–5.

43. Mauer SM, Miller K, Goetz FC, Barbosa J, Simmons RL, Najarian JS, Michael AF. Immunopathology of renal extracellular membranes in kidneys transplanted into patients with diabetes mellitus. Diabetes 1976; 25: 709–12.

44. Mauer SM, Barbosa J, Vernier RL et al. Development of diabetic vascular lesions in normal kidneys transplanted into patients with diabetes mellitus. New Engl J Med 1976; 295: 916–20.

45. Abouna GM, Al-Adnani MS, Kremer GD, Kumar SA, Daddah SK, Kusma G. Reversal of diabetic nephropathy in human cadaveric kidneys after transplantation into nondiabetic recipients. Lancet 1983; ii: 1274–6.

46. Bilous RW, Steffer MW, Guetz FC, Sutherland DER, Mauer SM. Pancreas transplantation for more than two years ameliorates glomerular pathology in insulin-dependent diabetic patients. Diabet Med 1987; 4: 554A.

47. Cerami A, Stevens VJ, Mannier VM. Role of nonenzymatic glycosylation in the development of the sequelae of diabetes mellitus. Metabolism 1979; 28 (suppl. 1): 431–2.

48. Greene DA, Lattimer SA, Simon AAF. Sorbitol, phosphoinositides and sodium potassium-ATPase in the pathogenesis of diabetic complications. New Engl J Med 1987; 316: 599–606.
49. Zatz R, Meyer TW, Rennke HG, Brenner BM. Predominance of hemodynamic rather than metabolic factors in the pathogenesis of diabetic glomerulopathy. Proc Natl Acad Sci USA 1985; 82: 5963–7.
50. Johnsson SL. Retinopathy and nephropathy in diabetes mellitus: comparison of the effect of two forms of treatment. Diabetes 1960; 9: 1–8.
51. Pirart J. Diabetes mellitus and its degenerative complications: a prospective study of 4400 patients observed between 1947 and 1973. Diabète Métab 1977; 3: 97–107.
52. Job D, Eshwège E, Guyot-Argenton C, Aubry JP, Tchobbroutsky G. Effect of multiple daily insulin injections on the course of retinopathy. Diabetes 1976; 25: 463–9.
53. Lauritzen T, Frost-Larsen K, Larsen HW, Deckert T. Effect of 1 year of near-normal blood glucose levels on retinopathy in insulin-dependent diabetics. Lancet 1983; i: 200–4.
54. Lauritzen T, Frost-Larsen K, Larsen HW, Deckert T. Steno Study Group: two-year experience with continuous subcutaneous insulin infusion in relation to retinopathy and neuropathy. Diabetes 1985; 34 (suppl. 3): 74–9.
55. Deckert T, Lauritzen T, Parving H, Christensen JS. Steno Study Group: effect of two years of strict metabolic control on kidney function in long-term insulin-dependent diabetics. Diabet Nephr 1983; 2: 6–10.
56. Parving HH, Oxenboll B, Svendsen PA, Sandahl-Christiansen J, Anderson AR. Early detection of patients at risk of developing diabetic nephropathy. A longitudinal study of urinary albumin excretion. Acta Endocrinol 1982; 100: 550–5.
57. Viberti GC, Jarrett RJ, Mahmuc U, Hill RD, Argyropoulos A, Keen H. Microalbuminuria as a predictor of clinical nephropathy in insulin-dependent diabetes mellitus. Lancet 1982; i: 1430–2.
58. Morgensen DE, Christiansen CK. Predicting diabetic nephropathy in insulin-dependent patients. New Engl J Med 1984; 311: 89–93.
59. Mathiesen ER, Oxenboll B, Johansen K, Svendsen PA, Deckert T. Incipient nephropathy in Type I (insulin-dependent) diabetes. Diabetologia 1984; 26: 406–10.
60. Feldt-Rasmussen B, Mathiesen ER, Hegedus L, Deckert T. Kidney function during 12 months of strict metabolic control in insulin-dependent diabetic patients with incipient nephropathy. New Engl J Med 1986; 314: 665–70.
61. Feldt-Rasmussen B, Mathiesen ER, Deckert T. Effect of two years of strict metabolic control on progression of incipient nephropathy in insulin-dependent diabetes. Lancet 1986; ii: 1300–4.
62. Kroc Collaborative Study Group. Blood glucose control and the evolution of diabetic retinopathy and albuminuria: a preliminary multicenter trial. New Engl J Med 1984; 311: 365–72.
63. Kroc Collaborative Study Group. The Kroc study patients at two years: a report on further retinal changes (abstr.). Diabetes 1985; 34 (suppl. 1): 39A.
64. Rosenstock J, Raskin P. Early diabetic nephropathy. Assessment and potential therapeutic interventions. Diabetes Care 1986; 9: 529–45.
65. Homan RR, Dorman TL, Mayon-White V et al. Prevention of deterioration of renal and sensory-nerve function by more intensive management of insulin-dependent diabetic patients: a two-year randomized prospective study. Lancet 1983; i: 204–8.
66. Beck-Neilsen H, Rickelsen B, Mogensen CE, Olsen T, Ehlers N, Nielsen CB, Charles P. Effect of insulin pump treatment for one year on renal function and retinal morphology in patients with IDDM. Diabetes Care 1985; 85: 585–9.
67. Dahl-Jorgensen K, Brichmann-Hanssen O, Hanssen KF, Sandvik L, Aagenaes O. Aker diabetes group. Rapid tightening of blood glucose control leads to transient deterioration of retinopathy in insulin-dependent diabetes mellitus: the Oslo study. Br Med J 1985; 290: 811–15.
68. Dahl-Jorgensen K, Brichmann-Hanssen O, Hanssen KF, Ganes T, Kierulf P, Smeland E, Sandvik L, Aagenaes O. Effect of near normoglycemia for two years on progression of early diabetic retinopathy, nephropathy, and neuropathy: the Oslo study. Br Med J 1986; 293: 1195–9.
69. Kohner EM, Sleightholm M, Fallon T. Why does retinopathy deteriorate when diabetic control is improved? Invest Ophthalmol Vis Sci 1987; 28 (suppl.): 244 (abstr.).
70. Raskin P, Pietri A, Unger RH. Changes in glucagon levels after four to five weeks of glucoregulation by portable insulin infusion pumps. Diabetes 1979; 28: 1033–4.
71. Pietri A, Dunn FL, Raskin P. The effect of improved diabetic control on plasma lipid and lipoprotein levels: a comparison of conventional therapy and continuous subcutaneous insulin infusion. Diabetes 1980; 29: 1001–5.
72. Dunn FL, Pietri A, Raskin P. Plasma lipid and lipoprotein levels with continuous subcutaneous insulin infusion in type I diabetes. Ann Intern Med 1981; 95: 426–31.
73. Pietri A, Dunn FL, Grundy SM, Raskin P. The effect of continuous subcutaneous insulin infusion on very-low-density lipoprotein triglyceride

metabolism in type I diabetes mellitus. Diabetes 1983; 32: 75–81.

74. Pietri A, Ehli AL, Raskin P. Changes in nerve conduction velocity after six weeks of glucoregulation with portable insulin infusion pumps. Diabetes 1980; 29: 668–71.

75. Friberg TR, Rosenstock J, Sanborn G, Vaghefi A, Raskin P. The effect of long-term near-normal glycemic control on mild diabetic retinopathy. Ophthalmology 1985; 92: 1051–8.

76. Rosenstock J, Friberg T, Raskin P. The effect of glycemic control on the microvascular complications in patients with Type I diabetes mellitus. Am J Med 1986; 81: 1012–18.

77. Rosenstock J, Strowig S, Cercone S, Raskin P. Reduction in cardiovascular risk factors with intensive diabetes treatment in Type I insulin-dependent diabetes mellitus. Diabetes Care 1987; 10: 729–34.

78. Rosenstock J, Vega G, Raskin P. The effect of intensive diabetes treatment on low density lipoprotein apo B kinetics in insulin dependent diabetes mellitus. Diabetes 1988; 37: 393–7.

79. Ramsay RC, Goetz FC, Sutherland DER et al. Progression of diabetic retinopathy after pancreas transplantation for insulin dependent diabetes mellitus. New Engl J Med 1988; 318: 208–14.

80. DCCT Research Group. Are continuing studies of metabolic control and microvascular complications in insulin-dependent diabetes mellitus justified? New Engl J Med 1988; 318: 246–9.

81. DCCT Research Group. The Diabetes Control and Complications Trial (DCCT); design and methodologic considerations for the feasibility phase. Diabetes 1986; 35: 530–45.

82. DCCT Research Group. Diabetes Control and Complications Trial (DCCT): results of feasibility study. Diabetes Care 1987; 10: 1–19.

54

Basement Membrane Physiology and Pathophysiology

Joseph R. Williamson and Charles Kilo

Washington University School of Medicine, St Louis, Missouri, USA

The ultrastructural, biochemical and immunocytochemical characteristics of capillary basement membranes of diabetic humans and animals have been extensively investigated in the hope that such information may provide a better understanding of the pathogenesis of the vascular complications of diabetes. Although discrepancies in some of the early morphological observations and biochemical analyses reported by different investigators were the source of considerable confusion and controversy [1–4], more recent investigations in humans are in better agreement on key issues regarding the primacy of relative or absolute insulin deficiency versus hereditary factors in the pathogenesis of diabetic microangiopathy [5–7]. In addition, recent studies in diabetic humans and in animal models of diabetes have provided important new insights into the nature of the metabolic imbalances and hormones that mediate and modulate diabetes-induced vascular changes, including those affecting capillary basement membranes [8].

Investigators have long been perplexed by the apparent discrepancy between the increasing prevalence and severity of all forms of diabetic microangiopathy (including capillary basement membrane changes, retinopathy and nephropathy) with increasing duration and increasing severity of diabetes on the one hand, and the fact that the presence of one manifestation of microangiopathy (i.e. capillary basement membrane thickening) is not a reliable predictor of the presence of other forms of microangiopathy.

The disparate observations and controversies associated with earlier ultrastructural and biochemical studies have been dealt with in previous reviews [1–4] and are considered only briefly in this chapter. More attention is focused here on (a) recent observations that have yielded important new insights into pathogenetic mechanisms of diabetic vascular disease and which have potentially important therapeutic implications, and (b) discussion of structural relationships and functional specialization of vessels in different tissues which may predispose them to injury in diabetes and which may also determine the nature of the clinical manifestations of injury.

International Textbook of Diabetes Mellitus. Edited by K.G.M.M. Alberti, R.A. DeFronzo, H. Keen and P. Zimmet
© 1992 John Wiley & Sons Ltd

NORMAL STRUCTURE AND FUNCTION

Morphological and Anatomical Aspects

Virtually all cells that line body surfaces produce a 'basement membrane' which serves to anchor them to underlying connective tissue extracellular matrix. These basement membranes are found only on the (basal) cell surface facing connective tissue. Examples of such cells are those forming the inner lining of vessels (endothelium), cells that line mucosal surfaces (respiratory tract, gastrointestinal tract and genitourinary tract), and cells that line body cavities (peritoneum, pericardium and pleura). A variety of mesenchymal cells (fat cells, pericytes, smooth muscle cells and skeletal muscle cells) form basement membranes over their entire surface.

When tissues are prepared by conventional methods for examination by electron microscopy, the basement membrane of most cells appears as a moderately electron-dense meshwork (lamina densa) about 70–100 nm in thickness (Figure 1A) and is composed of an interlacing network of fine fibrils about 7–10 nm in diameter. An electron-lucent (lamina rara) layer is usually evident between the lamina densa and the plasma membrane of the cell.

The basement membrane of glomerular capillaries differs from that of other capillaries in that it is a composite membrane, formed and lined by endothelial cells on one side and by epithelial cell foot processes (podocytes) on the other; it also is much thicker than that of most other capillaries. Thus, the glomerular capillary basement membrane consists of a thick central lamina densa, lined by a lamina rara interna on its endothelial surface and a lamina rara externa on its abluminal epithelial side (Figure 2).

Composition

Multidisciplinary studies have revealed that the basement membrane is a composite structure comprising several different species of macromolecules (Table 1), the spatial distribution of which differs within the membrane [8–12].

The major structural component of basement membrane is type IV collagen which constitutes about 98% of the dry weight of glomerular capillary basement membrane. It appears that four triple helical monomers of type IV collagen are linked to each other via their terminal disulfide-rich (7S collagen) domain. The opposite end of each monomer in the tetrad connects with a monomer of another tetrad to form a network of interlacing fibers [13]. The 7S domain is readily solubilized by proteases and antigenically intact portions of it are released into the circulation during normal basement membrane metabolism. Recent studies with monoclonal antibodies indicate that intact chains of type IV collagen are also present in serum of normal subjects [92]. Two additional molecular species, heparan sulfate proteoglycan and laminin, also are considered to be intrinsic basement membrane constituents. They appear to be asymmetrically distributed within the membrane, i.e. in the lamina rara interna and externa of glomerular basement membrane and on the abluminal aspect of basement membranes in other capillaries (Figure 3). Heparan sulfate proteoglycans are relatively highly sulfated, negatively charged molecules which are believed to contribute to the charge permselectivity characteristics of the capillary wall. Laminin is a high molecular weight sialoprotein which is believed to facilitate adhesion and attachment of cells to basement membrane. As sialic acid residues account for 4–6% of the dry weight of laminin, this molecule also contributes to the negative charge characteristics of basement membrane.

Fibronectin and entactin are two additional glycoproteins present in basement membrane. Fibronectin also is rich in sialic acid (2% by weight), tends to be localized in the lamina rara and participates in cell–cell and cell–substrate adhesion. It is at present not clear how much of the fibronectin in basement membrane is derived from plasma and how much is intrinsic to the basement membrane. Mohan and Spiro [11] have suggested that the proportion of fibronectin (about 17%) in bovine glomerular basement membrane that can be solubilized only under reducing conditions is likely to be of local origin. Entactin is a sulfated glycoprotein (which also contains sialic acid residues) with a molecular weight of about 150 000; it is localized, in glomerular capillaries, to the lamina rara externa of the basement membrane and the adjoining podocytes of epithelial cells, and is probably of local origin.

Function

Capillary basement membranes serve at least

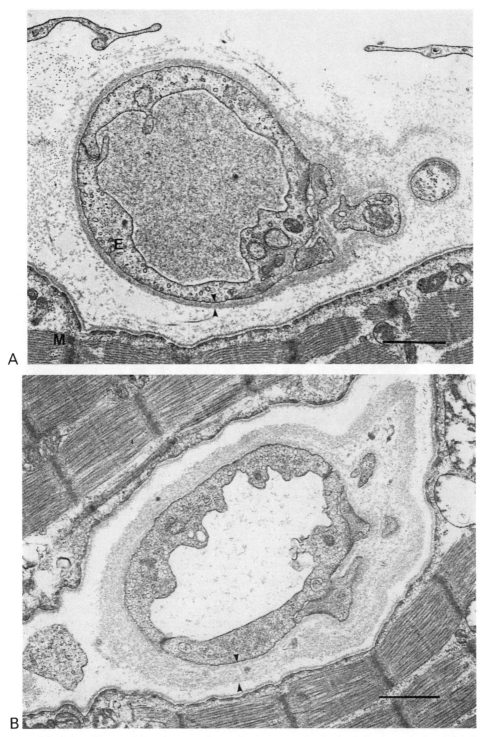

Figure 1 (A) Normal capillary and basement membrane (between arrowheads) in skeletal muscle. E, endothelial cell; M, muscle cell. (B) Skeletal muscle capillary from a diabetic patient demonstrating marked thickening of basement membrane (between arrows); scale bar 1μm. From reference 8, copyright John Wiley & Sons Inc.

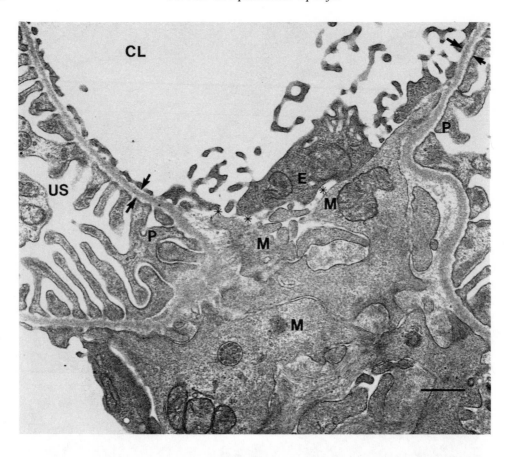

Figure 2 Electron micrograph of a portion of a glomerulus from a normal rat. The mesangium occupies most of the lower portion of the micrograph while the lumen of the glomerular capillary occupies the upper portion. The basement membrane (shown between the arrowheads) of the glomerular capillary stays with the foot processes rather than with the endothelium at the point where they intersect the margins of the mesangium. Note the absence of basement membrane (asterisks) between glomerular capillary endothelium (E) and mesangial cells (M). P, podocytes; US, urinary space; CL, capillary lumen; scale bar 0.25 μm

three functions: (a) they provide structural support or rigidity to the vessel wall; (b) they serve as a scaffolding—support for the endothelial cell lining of the capillary—and (c) they function as a coarse sieve or filter to retain cellular and particulate components of the blood. The contributions of each of the major components of basement membrane to these functions are summarized in Table 2.

The scaffolding and sieving functions, especially the latter, have been investigated in considerable detail. After endothelial cells have been injured, they may disintegrate or detach from the underlying basement membrane. When this happens, platelets may adhere to, and spread on, the exposed basement membrane,

providing a temporary replacement for the endothelial lining of the capillary. Alternatively (or later) adjacent viable endothelial cells spread over the denuded basement membrane, reconstituting a normal capillary lining without forming significant amounts of new basement membrane. Following more severe vascular injury with denudation of extensive areas of basement membrane, provided that the basement membrane remains intact, regenerating endothelial cells may utilize the basement membrane as a scaffolding and they may also synthesize an additional layer of new basement membrane. Vracko and Benditt [14] have shown that regenerating capillaries may acquire multiple lamellae of basement membrane in this way.

Table 1 Characteristics of major glomerular basement membrane constituents

	Approximate molecular weight	Approximate percentage dry weight*	Charge†	Change in diabetes
Type IV collagen				
α_1(IV)	210 000‡	98	115$^+$ basic amino acid	↑
α_2(IV)	190 000‡		96$^-$ free carboxyl	
Heparan sulfate proteoglycan	350 000‡	0.6	2$^-$ hexuronic acid	↓
	210 000‡		2$^-$ sulfate	
Laminin	900 000	0.15	5$^-$ sialic acid	↓
Fibronectin	450 000	0.29	4$^-$ sialic acid§	?
Entactin	150 000	?¶	? sulfate	?

* Percentage dry weight of human glomerular basement membrane, from Shimomura and Spiro [5].
† Charged groups per 1000 amino acid residues (bovine glomerular basement memebrane), from Spiro and Parthasarathy [4] except fibronectin (see footnote §).
‡ From Shimomura and Spiro [5].
§ Estimate based on 2% sialic acid content of fibronectin.
¶ Identified as present, but not quantified, by Shimomura and Spiro [5].

The contribution of basement membrane to the charge/size permselectivity characteristics of capillaries has been examined in many tissues, most extensively in glomerular capillaries. In most capillary beds the endothelial lining is the major barrier to permeation of the vessel wall by water, electrolytes and plasma macromolecules. Impaired endothelial barrier function is associated with an increase in hydraulic conductance as well as an outpouring of plasma proteins across the vessel wall. At such sites, plasma lipoproteins (very low-density lipoproteins and

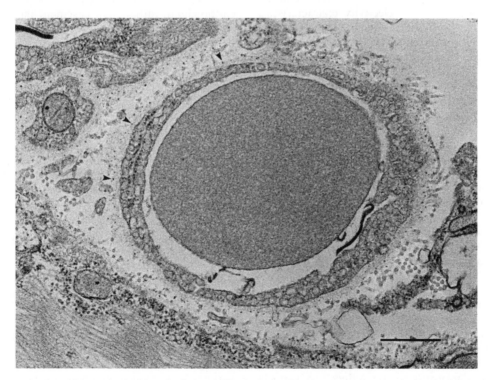

Figure 3 Muscle capillary stained with ruthenium red. The dark granules (arrow) on the abluminal surface of the basement membrane illustrate the typical asymmetrical distribution of heparan sulfate proteoglycans in basement membrane; scale bar 0.5 μm. From reference 8, copyright John Wiley & Sons Inc.

Table 2 Determinants of functional characteristics and physical properties of capillary basement membrane

	Function
Type IV collagen	Structural stability Size permselectivity
Heparan sulfate proteoglycan	Charge permselectivity
Laminin	Adhesion of endothelial cells and podocytes to basement membrane Charge permselectivity
Fibronectin	Cell adhesion Charge permselectivity
Entactin	Cell adhesion

chylomicrons) and large electron-dense particulate tracers such as colloidal carbon are filtered out and retained by the basement membrane, whereas macromolecules the size of ferritin or smaller readily pass through the basement membrane.

The structure of glomerular capillaries is much more complex than that of other capillaries and the anatomical determinants of its charge and size permselectivity characteristics have not been fully elucidated. Although many investigations have demonstrated that reductions in glomerular basement membrane heparan sulfate proteoglycans and sialoproteins occur in association with experimentally induced proteinuria (i.e. aminonucleoside nephrosis, perfusion with neuraminidase or heparatinase) [9, 15, 16], such observations do not document a causal relationship and must be viewed in the context of evidence that proteoglycans and sialoproteins in glomerular basement membrane constitute a small fraction of the total glomerular content of these substances. Indeed, heparan sulfate proteoglycans and sialoproteins account for only about 2 and 5%, respectively, of total anionic groups in glomerular basement membrane [12, 17]; furthermore, the glomerular basement membrane content of these constituents is less than 10% of the total glomerular content [18, 19]. The few investigations in which changes in sialoproteins have been assessed in whole glomeruli and in glomerular epithelial cells in rats with aminonucleoside nephrosis indicate that the sialic acid content of foot processes is reduced to a much greater extent than that of basement membrane [20, 21].

Electron-microscopic studies of glomerular capillaries of rats with proteinuria induced by aminonucleoside or by perfusion with neuraminidase indicate that the leakage of plasma proteins and tracer molecules occurs primarily at sites of detachment of podocytes from the glomerular basement membrane [15, 22–24]. On the basis of these and other investigations [8] it would appear that the sum total of anionic charges in glomerular basement membrane may contribute importantly to both the size and charge permselectivity characteristics of the glomerular capillary. On the other hand, in the authors' view, experimentally induced proteinuria is more likely to be attributable to impaired podocyte barrier function than to impaired basement membrane barrier function. This interpretation is, nevertheless, consistent with the possibility that barrier functional integrity of podocytes is dependent on normal attachment to basement membrane, which may be defective as a consequence of compositional changes in basement membrane and/or podocyte surface membranes.

In the light of these considerations it is noteworthy that in retinal capillaries (in which endothelium, rather than basement membrane, is widely accepted as the site of the blood–retinal barrier), perfusion with heparatinase (which degrades heparan sulfate proteoglycans) is associated with an increased rate of permeation of tracer protein (hemoglobin) across the endothelial lining into basement membrane and extravascular spaces [25]. These observations attest to the importance of (endothelial) surface membrane-bound heparan sulfate proteoglycans as determinants of capillary permeability and are consistent with a comparable role for podocyte surface membrane-bound heparan sulfate proteoglycan in glomerular capillaries.

BASEMENT MEMBRANE CHANGES IN DIABETES

A variety of qualitative and quantitative changes have been described in basement membrane constituents of diabetic humans and animals [2, 8, 26]. The most readily quantifiable change, thickening of microvascular basement membrane (see Figure 1b), is widely accepted as the ultrastructural hallmark of diabetic microangiopathy as it has been documented by numerous investigators in many tissues including the retina, glomerular capillaries, choriocapillaris, skin,

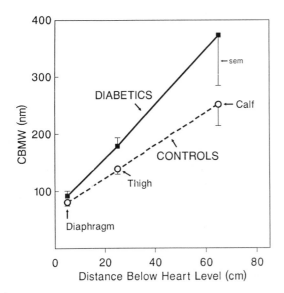

Figure 4 Relationship between muscle capillary basement membrane width (CBMW) and distance below heart level in controls and diabetic subjects. From reference 8, copyright John Wiley & Sons Inc.

skeletal muscle, heart and peripheral nerve [2, 8, 26]. Interestingly, basement membrane thickening in diabetes is not restricted to the vasculature: it also affects several types of epithelium including that of the ciliary body, perineurium and proximal convoluted tubules of the kidney. On the other hand, basement membrane of fat cells and skeletal muscle cells is unaltered in diabetes. The magnitude of capillary basement membrane thickening varies considerably in different tissues: it is especially prominent in tissues that are sites of clinically significant microangiopathy such as ocular tissues (retina, ciliary process epithelium and choriocapillaris) and glomerular capillaries. In skeletal muscle capillaries, basement membrane thickening increases with increasing distance below heart level, not only in the diabetic subject, but also in non-diabetics (Figure 4). These observations indicate that local (environmental) factors or conditions, independent of the diabetic milieu, modulate diabetes-induced capillary basement membrane thickening.

Collagen Changes

The only tissue in which accumulation of excess basement membrane has been confirmed biochemically is the glomerulus. Increased amounts

(1.5–3 times normal) of type IV collagen, the dominant collagen of basement membrane, have been demonstrated by numerous investigators in isolated glomeruli obtained from diabetic humans and animals. Recent studies have demonstrated a threefold increase in type IV collagen in glomeruli of diabetic humans [93]. Studies in rodent models of diabetes indicate that synthesis of type IV collagen is increased and degradation is impaired [8]. It is of interest in this regard that mRNA levels for type IV collagen are increased in glomeruli isolated from diabetic mice [94]. Elevated plasma levels of 7S collagen have been observed in diabetic humans and rats and have been correlated with increased glomerular basement membrane synthesis in diabetic rats [27, 28, 92].

Several investigators have reported that increased amounts of glucose are bound (non-enzymatically) to glomerular basement membrane collagen isolated from kidneys of diabetic humans and animals [8, 26, 29]. In addition, non-enzymatic glycation of basement membrane of bovine retinal capillary pericytes and of intact bovine retinal capillaries is increased by incubation in glucose-enriched media. On the other hand, whereas some investigators have reported an increase in hydroxylysine-linked glucosylgalactosyl disaccharide units (in association with an increase in hydroxylysine residues and a corresponding decrease in lysine residues) this finding has not been confirmed by others [8, 26, 29].

In view of evidence of increased crosslinking of type I collagen in many tissues of diabetic patients [26, 29], it is of interest that LePape et al [30] have reported a decrease in crosslinking in association with increased non-enzymatic glycation of type IV collagen in glomeruli of diabetic rats. This observation is consistent with the report of Li et al [31] that basement membrane produced by retinal capillary pericytes cultured in vitro is more soluble (i.e. less crosslinked) when the cells are cultured in glucose-enriched media.

An apparent change in the distribution and/or antigenicity of type IV collagen in glomerular capillary basement membrane of diabetic rats has been reported by Bendayan [32]. Using the protein A–gold technique and specific antibodies to type IV collagen (obtained from the mouse EHS tumor), Bendayan reported that in normal rats the gold particles labelled the central lamina densa of glomerular capillary basement membrane. In rats with streptozotocin diabetes of 7–15 months' duration, and with thickening of glomerular capillary basement membrane, gold labelling was restricted to the subendothelial aspect of the lamina densa. In the light of evidence that (a) non-enzymatic glycation of type I collagen has been reported to alter its antigenicity [33], and (b) the finding of LePape et al [30] that increased non-enzymatic glycation of glomerular basement membrane is associated with decreased crosslinking of type IV collagen in diabetic rats, the observations of Bendayan may reflect increased non-enzymatic glycation and/or decreased crosslinking of type IV collagen synthesized after induction of diabetes.

In view of immunocytochemical evidence that the distribution of extracellular matrix constituents differs in mesangial matrix and glomerular capillary basement membrane, it is noteworthy that the collagen analyses described above (and analyses discussed below) are performed on glomerular preparations that contain both mesangial matrix and capillary basement membranes. Some of the discrepancies in basement membrane composition and changes in diabetes reported by different investigators may be accounted for by differences in the proportions of mesangial matrix versus glomerular basement membrane constituents recovered by the different isolation and purification procedures employed.

Heparan Sulfate Proteoglycans

The content of heparan sulfate proteoglycan in glomerular basement membrane isolated from diabetic humans and rats is markedly reduced. Shimomura and Spiro [12] reported that the level was reduced by 70% in basement membrane isolated from human diabetic subjects. Studies in vitro of proteoglycan metabolism in diabetic rats demonstrating a marked decrease in ^{35}S incorporation into glomerular basement proteoglycans are consistent with these observations [8].

Laminin

Falk et al [34] reported that the intensity of immunofluorescence staining for laminin was increased in the mesangium, glomerular basement membrane and renal tubular basement membrane in subjects with early and moderately advanced stages of diabetic nephropathy, but was decreased in advanced stages of glomerulosclerosis. The latter observation in advanced glomerulosclerosis is consistent with the finding of Shimomura and Spiro [12] that the laminin content of isolated human glomerular basement membrane was reduced by 40%. As laminin is rich in sialic acid, this finding could account for the significant reduction in sialic acid residues in glomerular basement membrane isolated from human diabetic subjects reported by some (but not all) investigators. Plasma levels of laminin are reported to be increased in diabetes; however, it is not known whether this change reflects increased synthesis, decreased degradation or increased turnover [28].

Fibronectin

Relatively little information is available regarding fibronectin changes in vascular basement membrane in diabetes. Falk et al [34] reported that the intensity of immunofluorescence staining for fibronectin was increased in the mesangium (but not in glomerular basement membrane) of diabetics with early and moderately advanced stages of diabetic nephrosclerosis, but was decreased in subjects with advanced nephropathy. These observations are basically consistent with those of Shimomura and Spiro [12] who found no significant decrease in the quantity of fibronectin extractable from glomeruli of diabetics with varying degrees of nephropathy. The intensity of immunofluorescence staining of fibronectin has been reported to be increased in the skin of diabetics [35].

Abnormal Binding of Plasma Proteins

Michael and Brown and their associates [34, 36] used immunofluorescence techniques to demonstrate increased binding of several plasma proteins (IgG, albumin, αl-acid glycoprotein, amyloid-P, and αl-antitrypsin) to glomerular capillary basement membranes, mesangial matrix, basement membranes of renal tubules and skeletal muscle, and capillary basement membranes in skin and skeletal muscle in diabetic humans and animals. They have confirmed the increased albumin content of glomerular and tubular basement membranes of human subjects by use of radioimmunoassay techniques. It is of particular interest that, of all of the subclasses of

IgG, it is only IgG_4 (which has the lowest isoelectric point and is present in lowest concentration in the plasma) that binds to basement membrane in diabetes [36]. Thus, these investigators have suggested that their studies 'are consistent with the hypothesis that circulating anionic plasma proteins are electrostatically bound in vivo to positively charged moieties in normal and especially diabetic basement membranes'. Kern and Engerman [37] have confirmed the increased immunofluorescence staining for IgG and albumin in the mesangium and in glomerular basement membrane of diabetic dogs. Cohen et al [38] have reported that increased amounts of fibronectin bind to glomerular basement membrane isolated from diabetic versus control rats. Whereas Jeraj et al [39] have shown that nonenzymatic glycation of albumin has no effect on its binding to basement membrane, non-enzymatic glycation of fibronectin does impair its binding to basement membrane [40, 41]. The mechanism responsible for the selective increased binding of anionically charged plasma proteins to basement membranes in diabetic subjects remains to be elucidated; it has been postulated to be a consequence of either nonenzymatic glycation of basement membrane or a reduction in the content of negatively charged proteoglycans and sialoproteins.

An increase in the intensity of immunofluorescence staining for type V collagen in the mesangium, glomerular basement membrane and tubular basement membrane has been reported in human diabetic subjects [34].

PATHOPHYSIOLOGICAL CONSEQUENCES OF BASEMENT MEMBRANE CHANGES IN DIABETES

Despite the demonstration of marked diabetes-induced changes in capillary basement membranes, the pathophysiological significance of these changes remains, for the most part, obscure. This situation is largely attributable to two problems: (a) virtually nothing is known about corresponding diabetes-induced changes in proteoglycans and sialoproteins in endothelial cell and (epithelial) podocyte plasma membranes which might have a similar effect to that of basement membrane changes on microvascular-barrier function; and (b) in view of the intimate structural relationships between basement mem-

brane and endothelial cells and glomerular podocytes (and the lack of information regarding diabetes-induced changes in endothelium and podocytes) it is virtually impossible to document that basement membrane changes are responsible for size and charge permselectivity changes in glomerular capillary barrier function in diabetes. Thus, the discussion in this section is, of necessity, largely speculative in nature.

Effects on Capillary Barrier Function

Just as capillary basement membrane thickening is widely accepted as the ultrastructural hallmark of diabetic microangiopathy, increased vascular permeability is the hallmark of impaired vascular functional integrity in diabetes. Both phenomena have been demonstrated in a wide variety of tissues in diabetic patients and are, perhaps, most marked in the eyes and kidneys [8]. Although numerous investigators have attributed diabetes-induced increased vascular permeability to alterations in capillary basement membrane composition, there is, in fact, little evidence in support of this hypothesis. Indeed, as is discussed in the section on pathogenesis of basement membrane changes in diabetes, the authors feel that it is more likely that basement membrane thickening may be a consequence of increased vascular permeability or that both are merely closely associated phenomena, but not causally related.

In view of the fact that, in most tissues, permeation of the microvasculature by plasma macromolecules is limited by endothelium rather than by basement membrane, it is more likely that diabetes-induced increased vascular permeability in such tissues is the consequence of impaired barrier functional integrity of vascular endothelium rather than of altered barrier function of basement membrane.

The structure of glomerular capillaries is more complex and, in the authors' view, the epithelial foot processes (podocytes) probably limit the permeation of glomerular capillaries by plasma macromolecules (as well as by water and electrolytes) into the urinary space. This view is supported by recent studies in animal models of proteinuria (i.e. aminonucleoside nephrosis, removal of heparan sulfate proteoglycan by perfusion with heparatinase) in which the loss of glomerular basement membrane anionic constituents is similar to that observed in diabetes

[15, 16, 20]. The development of proteinuria in these animal models, however, appears to be more closely linked to detachment of foot processes from basement membrane than to alterations in basement membrane composition and barrier function [15, 22–24]. Indeed, the loss of anionic sialoproteins from basement membrane in aminonucleoside nephrosis is much smaller than the loss of sialoproteins from foot processes [20, 21].

As over 90% of total glomerular sialoproteins and proteoglycans are associated with podocyte membranes, and virtually nothing is known about changes in these constituents (in podocytes) in diabetes, it is premature (in the authors' opinion) to attribute changes in charge permselectivity characteristics of glomerular capillaries in diabetes to decreases in basement membrane content of proteoglycan, laminin, etc.

Effects on Adhesion of Endothelial Cells and Podocytes to Basement Membrane

On the other hand, a decrease in basement membrane-associated anchoring proteins (and/or chemical changes in such proteins) such as laminin, which are important in mediating adhesion of podocytes to basement membrane, could lead to focal detachment of foot processes from basement membrane and impairment of podocyte barrier function. Although subtle changes of this kind could be difficult, if not impossible, to detect by electron microscopy, it is noteworthy that focal detachment of podocytes from basement membrane, similar to that described in animal models of proteinuria discussed above, has been observed in kidneys of human diabetic patients [24, 42].

In like manner, if endothelial cell barrier functional integrity is critically dependent upon adherence of endothelial cells to basement membrane, then a decrease in basement membrane content of anchoring proteins such as laminin or fibronectin (or impairment of their anchoring function) could contribute to the increase in vascular permeability in tissues such as retina, sciatic nerve, etc.

Impact of Increased Non-enzymatic Glycation and Decreased Crosslinking of Type IV Collagen

In view of the likelihood that structural support

(rigidity) provided to the walls of capillaries and venules by basement membrane is a function of the extent of lysyl oxidase-mediated crosslinking of type IV collagen, the observation (discussed above) that type IV collagen solubility (an index of crosslinking) is inversely related to non-enzymatic glycation in glomerular and ocular vessels suggests that the walls of these vessels may be more distensible than normal. This could contribute, or predispose, to vasodilation and development of microaneurysms, which have been described in glomerular capillaries as well as in the retina. The positive association between increased non-enzymatic glycation of collagen and increased collagen solubility (indicative of decreased crosslinking) is presumably the consequence of competition between glucose and the enzyme lysyl oxidase for lysine, and is unrelated to the glucose-derived protein crosslinks caused by non-enzymatic glycation [43] discussed elsewhere in this book.

Non-enzymatic glycation of laminin and type IV collagen in vitro markedly alters the association of these basement membrane constituents to each other and to heparin [95].

Impact of Excess Accumulation of Basement Membrane

Perhaps the most important adverse consequence of accumulation of excess basement membrane material is the expansion of mesangium, which eventually encroaches on the glomerular capillary lumen (reducing the surface area available for filtration of waste products) and culminates in renal failure. Indeed as this loss of filtration function, rather than proteinuria, is the cause of renal failure, it is not surprising that renal failure is much more strongly correlated with mesangial hypertrophy than with glomerular capillary basement membrane thickening [44, 45].

Although it seems reasonable to expect that marked thickening of capillary basement membranes might impede emigration of leukocytes across vessel walls into sites of infection, there is, in fact, little evidence to suggest that capillary basement membrane thickening is a risk factor for increased susceptibility to infections in diabetes.

PATHOGENESIS OF BASEMENT MEMBRANE CHANGES IN DIABETES

Thickening of capillary basement membrane is, in the authors view, the mildest form of a spectrum of vasoproliferative responses to diabetes-induced vascular injury. It is probably primarily attributable to increased synthesis by endothelial cells in general, and by podocytes and endothelial cells in the glomerulus. At the other end of the spectrum is neovascularization of the retina and optic disc, i.e. formation of complete new vessels including endothelial cells and associated basement membranes. Retinal capillary microaneurysms, atherosclerotic plaques and mesangial hypertrophy with hyperplasia of mesangial cells appear to reflect hyperplasia of vascular cells plus accumulation of basement membrane collagen (scar tissue), but without new vessel formation, and therefore fit into the middle of the spectrum.

The proliferation of collagen-producing cells and production of scar tissue are typical responses of cells and tissues to injury. On the other hand, the decreased content of heparan sulfate proteoglycans and laminin probably reflect impaired synthesis of these constituents attributable to diabetes-associated metabolic and hormonal imbalances. This view is consistent with evidence that metabolism of heparan sulfate proteoglycans by hepatocytes is impaired [46] and the sialic acid content of hepatocyte and red blood cell plasma membranes is decreased in diabetes [47], independent of collagen synthesis.

Although the nature of the putative metabolic and hormonal imbalances responsible for the decreased basement membrane content of heparan sulfate proteoglycan and laminin remains enigmatic, significant progress has been made in recent years in identifying risk factors for increased accumulation of capillary basement membrane (presumably primarily type IV collagen).

Hyperglycemia

Hyperglycemia per se, independent of other hormonal and metabolic imbalances associated with diabetes, appears to be the most important risk factor for capillary basement membrane thickening and other vascular complications of diabetes. Hyperglycemia may affect basement membrane metabolism and structure by three independent mechanisms.

Increased Polyol Metabolism

Several lines of evidence indicate that increased metabolism of glucose by the polyol pathway is associated not only with capillary basement membrane thickening but also with diabetes-induced hemodynamic and vascular permeability changes [8]. Metabolism of glucose by this pathway occurs in two steps (Figure 5). In the first reaction, glucose is reduced to its sugar alcohol, sorbitol, by the enzyme aldose reductase using NADPH as a hydrogen donor. In the second reaction, sorbitol is oxidized to fructose by the enzyme sorbitol dehydrogenase using NAD^+ as the hydrogen acceptor. Enough sorbitol accumulates in the lens to create an osmotic imbalance [48]; however, in most cells and tissues it would appear that the increased rate of glucose metabolism via the polyol pathway, rather than increased intracellular sorbitol levels, leads to impaired cellular function [49–51]. It is postulated that the increased rate of metabolism of glucose through the polyol pathway results in imbalances in the redox state of the pyridine nucleotide co-factors (NAD and NADP) which modulate a variety of cell functions including Na^+-K^+-ATPase activity [51, 52].

A reduction in intracellular myo-inositol levels appears to have an important role in mediating peripheral nerve functional impairment associated with increased polyol metabolism. Supplementation of the diet with myo-inositol prevents the loss of Na^+-K^+-ATPase activity and impairment of electrophysiological function in sciatic nerve of diabetic rats, without normalizing nerve sorbitol levels or plasma glucose levels [52]. Myo-inositol supplemented diets also significantly attenuate diabetes-induced vascular dysfunction in the eyes, peripheral nerve, aorta, and kidney in rats [96].

Galactose (as well as a number of other sugars) also is metabolized by the polyol pathway: animals fed galactose-enriched diets develop diabetes-like cataracts, neuropathy and vascular changes including basement membrane thickening of retinal and glomerular capillaries, and retinal capillary microaneurysms with relatively normal glycemia and plasma insulin levels.

The first evidence implicating increased polyol metabolism in the pathogenesis of diabetic vascular complications was the demonstration that retinal capillary basement membrane thick-

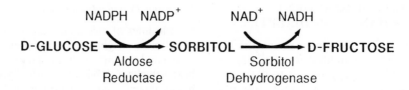

Figure 5 Sorbitol pathway. The first step in the sorbitol pathway of glucose metabolism involves the reduction of glucose by the enzyme aldose reductase which uses NADPH as the hydrogen donor. The second step is the oxidation of sorbitol to fructose by the enzyme sorbitol dehydrogenase which uses NAD^+ as the hydrogen acceptor. From reference 8, copyright John Wiley & Sons Inc.

ening in diabetic rats and in rats fed galactose-enriched diets was prevented by inhibitors of aldose reductase (Sorbinil, Alcon-1576, and tolrestat) which had no effect on plasma glucose levels [53–55].

Subsequent studies have demonstrated that increased vascular permeability and blood flow in ocular tissues (retina, anterior uveal vessels and choroid), sciatic nerve and kidney, as well as increased glomerular filtration rates in diabetic rats and in rats fed galactose-enriched diets, are prevented by several structurally different inhibitors of aldose reductase [49, 50, 56–58]. It is particularly noteworthy that vascular permeability and blood flow are not increased in all tissues of diabetic and galactose-fed rats, and are most pronounced in tissues that are sites of vascular complications in human diabetic subjects.

The observations that vascular permeability and hemodynamic changes in diabetic rats and in rats fed galactose-enriched diets are demonstrable as early as 3 weeks after the onset of diabetes or galactose feeding [49, 50], whereas retinal and glomerular capillary basement membrane thickening are not demonstrable for several months to several years [37, 54, 55, 59], coupled with evidence that acute hyperglycemia of only a few hours' duration leads to hemodynamic changes in non-diabetic humans and animals [60, 61], strongly suggest that diabetes-induced increases in vascular permeability and blood flow precede capillary basement membrane changes. These observations and interpretations are consistent with the hypothesis that capillary basement membrane thickening may be the consequence of increased vascular permeability and/or hemodynamic changes.

A variety of observations in non-diabetic as well as in diabetic humans and animals is consistent with the possibility that diabetes-induced increased synthesis of capillary basement membrane may be contributed to by cleavage products of fibrinogen which would be expected to permeate vessel walls at an increased rate, as demonstrated for albumin labelled with iodine 125 [8, 50, 56, 57]. Fibrinogen and its cleavage products induce a variety of changes in human endothelial cells cultured in vitro, that are virtually identical to endothelial cell changes associated with angiogenesis in vivo [8]. Indeed, the propensity of fibrin clots to become vascularized and transformed into granulation and scar tissue in vivo is well known.

Direct Stimulation of Basement Membrane Synthesis

The possibility that hyperglycemia per se may promote increased protein synthesis (in general) including basement membrane proteins in cells freely permeable to glucose, is supported by observations of Li et al [62, 63] who found that bovine retinal pericytes synthesized more protein in general, including basement membrane collagen, when maintained in culture media containing 20 or 40 mmol/l glucose than in media containing 5 mmol/l glucose. Several investigators have recently reported that mRNA levels for basement membrane constituents (i.e. type IV collagen and fibronectin) are increased in cultured vascular cells exposed to elevated glucose levels [97–99]. Preferential accumulation of basement membrane collagen (versus other cellular proteins) might be predicted because of the relatively slow rate of turnover of basement membrane collagen compared with non-structural cellular proteins.

Non-enzymatic Glycation

Although non-enzymatic glycation of basement membrane collagen has been well documented in tissues from diabetic humans and animals [8, 29, 43], the pathophysiological consequences of this change, and whether it has a significant role in the accumulation of excess basement membrane in diabetes, are at present unknown.

As lysine is a favored site for non-enzymatic binding of glucose to collagen, the non-enzymatic glycation reaction competes with the enzyme lysyl oxidase for its substrate. This means that an excess of glucose bound non-enzymatically to lysine residues will result in a corresponding decrease in lysyl oxidase-mediated crosslinking of collagen molecules. Whereas many studies have demonstrated that interstitial (type I) collagen from diabetic humans and animals is more crosslinked than normal [29], and studies in experimental animals suggest that these are lysyl oxidase-mediated crosslinks [64], assessment of crosslinking of basement membrane (type IV) collagen in animal models of diabetes indicates that type IV collagen crosslinking is reduced [30, 31]. These observations argue against increased protein crosslinking associated with advanced glycated end-products [43] in type IV collagen. In view of these observations, and the fact that aldose reductase inhibitors prevent retinal capillary basement membrane thickening associated with diabetes and with galactose ingestion (without affecting glycemia or non-enzymatic glycation of hemoglobin and granulation tissue proteins), it is difficult at present to attribute a significant role to non-enzymatic glycation in the pathogenesis of capillary basement membrane thickening in diabetes. These observations, however, do not preclude a role for non-enzymatic glycation in end-stage diabetic vascular disease.

Hemodynamic Factors

Studies in non-diabetic and diabetic humans and in identical twins discordant for type 1 diabetes indicate that increased blood pressure, alone and in combination with diabetes, plays an important part in capillary basement membrane thickening [65–68]. Thus, muscle capillary basement membrane width is correlated linearly with hydrostatic pressure in non-diabetics and the slope of the regression line is increased in diabetics (Figure 4). These observations are consistent with a large body of evidence supporting the importance of hemodynamic changes in the pathogenesis of diabetic vascular disease in general [8, 69–71] and with evidence that hypertension stimulates vascular synthesis of collagen in small as well as in large arteries in nondiabetic animals [100, 101]. Although the mechanism by which an increase in vascular pressure leads to capillary basement membrane thickening remains obscure, the authors suggest that increased vascular wall tension and/or increased permeation of vessel walls by macromolecules (i.e. fibrinogen, as discussed earlier) may stimulate synthesis of basement membrane by vascular cells in general.

The likelihood that the correlation between vascular pressure and muscle capillary basement membrane thickening is linked to venous pressure rather than to arterial pressure is supported by two lines of evidence. First, muscle capillary basement membrane width is increased in non-diabetic subjects with longstanding congestive heart failure in whom venous pressure is increased but arterial pressure and muscle blood flow are decreased [72]. Second, no association is demonstrable between systolic or diastolic blood pressure and muscle capillary basement membrane width in diabetic humans [73]. The demonstration of increased capillary basement membrane width in muscles of the distal lower extremity compared with proximal muscles in non-diabetics as well as in diabetics [65–68], coupled with the absence of regional differences in muscle capillary basement membrane width at birth [65], attests to the importance of increased vascular pressure (independent of glycemia) in the pathogenesis of capillary basement membrane thickening.

These observations in non-diabetic subjects also support the hypothesis that capillary basement membrane thickening in diabetes is mediated by effects of metabolic and hormonal imbalances (associated with diabetes) on vascular permeability and hemodynamics in addition to direct effects of the diabetic milieu on vascular basement membrane metabolism. Further support for this hypothesis is evident in studies of identical twins discordant for type 1 diabetes [67]. In the diabetic twins, capillary basement membrane width in gastrocnemius muscle was significantly thicker than that in quadriceps muscle, in addition to being thicker than that of gastrocnemius muscle in the non-diabetic twins; in the non-diabetic twins, capillary basement membrane widths of quadriceps and gastrocnemius muscle did not differ significantly.

Hormonal Modulation

Numerous cross-sectional epidemiological studies have demonstrated an increase in the prevalence and severity of diabetic retinopathy and nephropathy in postpubertal versus prepubertal type 1 diabetics with disease of comparable duration and severity [8, 50, 74]. Recent studies by Sosenko et al [5] and by Rogers et al [6] in type 1 diabetics have shown that muscle capillary basement membrane width is significantly correlated with glycemia in pubertal and postpubertal subjects, but not in prepubertal subjects. Rogers et al [6] also observed a significant correlation between bone age and muscle capillary basement membrane width independent of glycemia in postpubertal but not in prepubertal subjects. As bone age in postpubertal individuals with normal thyroid and growth hormone function is primarily related to sex steroid levels, the observations by Rogers et al suggest that sex steroids may modulate vascular metabolism of glucose in tissues that are sites of diabetic vascular disease.

Clues to the mechanisms by which sex steroids modulate glucose metabolism as well as the onset and progression of diabetic vascular disease have been revealed by recent studies in animal models of diabetes [8, 50, 74]. Castration of male diabetic rats significantly reduces tissue polyol levels and vascular permeability increases in several complication-prone tissues, including retina and sciatic nerve, and also reduces glomerular filtration rate. Thus, diabetes-induced increases in vascular permeability and polyol metabolism (which are closely linked to retinal and glomerular capillary basement membrane thickening, as discussed earlier) in animal models of diabetes are sex steroid-modulated phenomena. The likelihood that polyol metabolism in humans also is modulated by sex steroids is supported by the observation that red blood cell polyol levels double after puberty in non-diabetic as well as in diabetic males [75].

Genetic Factors

The possibility that genetic factors, independent of those implicated in the susceptibility to develop diabetes, may be important determinants of the susceptibility to develop vascular complications of diabetes has been extensively examined by many investigators [1, 8, 76]. Although the results of some investigations are consistent with genetic modulation of vascular complications of diabetes, others are not. Perhaps the most significant recent investigation attesting to the primacy of the diabetic milieu versus genetic factors in the pathogenesis of muscle capillary basement membrane thickening is that of Feingold et al [7]. These investigators found that the prevalence and magnitude of muscle capillary basement membrane thickening (as well as retinopathy and proteinuria) were virtually the same in subjects (with no family history of diabetes) with secondary diabetes induced by ingestion of Vacor (a diabetogenic rodenticide), as they were in genetic diabetic subjects with positive family histories of diabetes matched for age, sex and duration of disease. These observations, together with the evidence discussed above regarding hormonal modulation of vascular complications and polyol metabolism in diabetic humans and animals, provide strong evidence for the primacy of metabolic and hormonal imbalances associated with diabetes in the pathogenesis of capillary basement membrane thickening and other vascular complications of diabetes.

On the other hand, the implication of the polyol pathway in the pathogenesis of vascular complications of diabetes raises the possibility that genetic modulation of enzyme levels and co-factors involved in metabolism of glucose by the polyol pathway could modulate the onset and progression of capillary basement membrane thickening and other vascular complications associated with diabetes.

RELATIONSHIP OF CAPILLARY BASEMENT MEMBRANE CHANGES TO CLINICAL NEPHROPATHY AND RETINOPATHY

In view of the evidence linking basement membrane thickening of retinal and glomerular capillaries (as well as increased vascular permeability and hemodynamic changes in the eyes, kidneys and other tissues) in animal models of diabetes to increased metabolism of glucose to sorbitol, it might be predicted that the detection of changes in one organ, i.e. capillary basement membrane thickening in skeletal muscle or kidney, might be predictive of corresponding changes in other tissues such as the retina. Indeed, numerous investigators have examined the relationship between muscle capillary basement membrane thickening, retinopathy and nephropathy [1, 7, 8, 45]; as might be expected, significant associations have been demonstrated in some studies but not in others. Although significant correlations have been demonstrated between muscle capillary basement membrane thickening and glomerular capillary basement membrane thickening in three different studies [45, 77, 78], neither muscle capillary basement membrane thickening nor glomerular capillary basement membrane thickening appear to be reliable predictors of clinical nephropathy [45, 78] or of basement membrane accumulation in the mesangium, the glomerular structural change that appears to correlate best with clinical nephropathy [44]. Similarly, only about 50% of diabetic subjects with retinopathy have evidence of nephropathy [79], while about 75% of subjects with nephropathy have evidence of retinopathy.

These observations suggest that risk factors (independent of glycemia per se) for capillary basement membrane thickening (and other forms of diabetic vascular disease) differ in different tissues within the same individual and between individuals. The likelihood that these risk factors (and the apparent predilection of some tissues such as the eyes, kidneys and nerves to develop complications) are related to unusual structural and functional characteristics and anatomical relationships of the vasculature in these tissues is supported by several lines of evidence.

Nephropathy

The functional changes in the kidney associated with renal failure are a progressive decrease in glomerular filtration rate and increasing proteinuria. Whereas the proteinuria is attributable to loss of barrier functional integrity of the glomerular capillary wall, the loss of filtration function appears to be caused by mesangial hypertrophy which encroaches on the capillary lumen, reducing the capillary surface area available for filtration of waste products. In view of the absence of a blood–mesangial barrier, it is not clear why the development of proteinuria should be predictive of mesangial hypertrophy unless (a) they are simply associated phenomena with impairment of capillary barrier function developing in parallel with mesangial hypertrophy, or (b) both share a common pathogenetic factor.

An important point to be made from the standpoint of pathogenesis is that it would appear that mesangial hypertrophy cannot be attributed to compromised glomerular capillary barrier function (including changes in basement membrane composition) as there is no continuous basement membrane between glomerular capillary endothelium and the mesangium (Figure 2), and the endothelial pores pose no barrier to the permeation of plasma proteins and particulate tracers into the mesangium [8, 80]. In the absence of a podocyte–basement membrane barrier at the mesangial–capillary interface, diabetes-induced increases in glomerular capillary pressure [81, 82] will increase the permeation of plasma macromolecules into the mesangium (in addition to increasing permeation of plasma macromolecules across the glomerular capillary into the urinary space). The impact of an increase in glomerular capillary pressure on permeation of plasma macromolecules into the mesangium is, therefore, equivalent to an increase in vascular permeability in glomerular capillaries and capillaries of other tissues. Thus, the lack of a blood–mesangial barrier (rather than changes in basement membrane and epithelium) may be the Achilles' heel of the glomerulus in diabetes.

In view of the fact that glomerular capillary pressure may be influenced by many factors that modulate glomerular filtration rate [71], without affecting blood flow or vascular pressure in skeletal muscle or retina, it is not surprising that muscle capillary basement membrane thickening (or retinopathy) in a diabetic subject is not a reliable predictor of diabetic nephropathy.

Retinopathy

As in the kidney, a number of factors may contribute to the failure of muscle capillary basement membrane thickening to predict retinopathy accurately [8]. Several lines of evidence are consistent with the likelihood that the absence of blood–retinal and blood–optic nerve barriers at the margins of the optic nerve head [83–85], coupled with hemodynamic changes in the choroidal circulation and the placement of the retinal vein within the optic nerve, are important risk factors that conspire to produce retinopathy in diabetes. Several clinical observations are consistent with this hypothesis: the optic disc and adjoining retina are favored sites for diabetes-induced angiogenesis, and neovascularization occurring at these sites carries a poorer prognosis than neovascularization occurring elsewhere in the retina [86–89]. These observations suggest that the conditions (environment) in and around the optic nerve head favor angiogenesis. Although many factors may contribute to the marked dilation of retinal veins which is evident early in the course of poorly controlled diabetes, the most relevant factors in the context of the present discussion would be increased blood flow and compression of the retinal vein as it enters the optic nerve head. Furthermore, some investigators have noted an association between dilation of retinal veins and the subsequent development of proliferative retinopathy [70, 90].

Several morphological and physiological studies utilizing fluorescein or horseradish peroxidase as vascular tracers indicate that, following intravenous injection, the tracers diffuse from the choriocapillaris via connective tissue spaces [91] into the optic nerve head in normal monkeys and in humans [83–85]. In view of the marked increase in blood flow and vascular permeability in the choroidal vessels in diabetic rats [50, 57], if corresponding changes occur in diabetic humans it is reasonable to predict that permeation of plasma constituents from choriocapillaris into the optic nerve head and around the retinal pigment epithelium into adjoining retina would be increased in diabetic subjects. These events could result in (a) the presence of increased amounts of plasma-derived angiogenic factors in and around the optic nerve head, and (b) edema of the optic nerve head which would tend to compress the retinal vein. Thus, the normal absence of a plasma–optic nerve barrier between the choriocapillaris and the optic nerve head and the placement of the retinal vein within the optic nerve (where it is at high risk of compression by edema of the optic nerve head), coupled with diabetes-induced increased blood flow and vascular permeability in the choroidal (and retinal) vessels, would accentuate the effects of diabetes on the retinal vasculature, culminating in vasoproliferative changes (including capillary basement membrane thickening and angiogenesis) in vessels in the optic nerve head and adjoining retina.

It is probably not a coincidence that microvascular changes associated with retinopathy and nephropathy, the two most important microvascular complications of diabetes, have two important risk factors in common. The significant vascular changes in both tissues occur in close juxtaposition to (a) vessels that have the highest blood flow in the body (the choriocapillaris and the glomerular capillaries), and (b) anatomical defects in blood–tissue barriers, i.e. the absence of anatomical–structural barriers at the mesangial–glomerular capillary interface and between the choriocapillaris and the optic nerve head and adjacent retina.

CONCLUSION

From the preceding discussion it is evident that the pathogenesis of capillary basement membrane thickening and the nature of its relationship to other manifestations of diabetic vascular disease remain somewhat enigmatic. On the other hand, recent studies in diabetic humans and animals have yielded several important new insights into the mechanisms by which metabolic and hormonal imbalances associated with diabetes lead to functional and structural vascular changes, including capillary basement membrane thickening. These new insights are the product of a combination of morphological, biochemical and pathophysiological investigations. An integrated view of these new findings is depicted schematically in Figure 6. The solid arrows indicate associations and causal relationships which, in the authors' opinion, are supported by substantial experimental evidence. The dotted arrows and question marks, on the other hand, indicate potential effects or interactions for which the authors consider the experimental evidence to be weak at present.

According to the proposed sequence of events, relative or absolute insulin deficiency—of whatever cause—that results in hyperglycemia will, in turn, lead to increased intracellular glucose levels in cells that do not require insulin for glucose uptake. Such cells include vascular endothelium. The increased intracellular levels of free glucose increase the availability of substrate for the aldo–keto-reductase family of enzymes, which then metabolize the glucose to sorbitol. Before puberty the activity of the sorbitol pathway is so low that not enough glucose is metabolized to sorbitol to cause vascular injury. Increased sex steroid levels (presumably primarily androgens) at the time of puberty increase sorbitol pathway activity so that the rate of glucose metabolism to sorbitol is sufficient to impair vascular function, resulting in

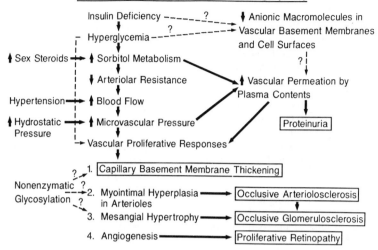

Figure 6 Sequence of events and interrelationships of risk factors in the pathogenesis of diabetic microangiopathy. Dashed lines represent alterations and interactions, the functional consequences of which are obscure. From reference 8, copyright John Wiley & Sons Inc.

decreased arteriolar resistance (presumably due to impaired contractile function of arteriolar smooth muscle) and increased vascular permeability (presumably due to impaired endothelial cell barrier functional integrity in most tissues and impaired podocyte–basement membrane barrier function in the kidney).

The increase in vascular permeation by macromolecules in the kidney is manifested by proteinuria, and in the eyes by increased leakage of intravenously injected dyes across retinal vessels. The decrease in arteriolar resistance results in increased blood flow in the affected tissues and transmission of arterial blood pressure further downstream into the microvasculature. This increase in microvascular pressure, in turn, increases the rate of permeation of vessels by plasma constituents which normally permeate these vessels, without any increase in pore size or number. The increase in vascular permeability and the increased permeation of vessels (and mesangium) by angiogenic factors derived from plasma (possibly cleavage products of fibrinogen) and/or produced locally by the vasculature itself stimulate vasoproliferative responses manifested by (a) capillary basement membrane thickening in many different tissues, (b) myointimal hyperplasia in arterioles, (c) mesangial hypertrophy and (d) angiogenesis in the eye. Progression of the latter three phenomena culminates in occlusive arteriolosclerosis, occlusive glomerulosclerosis and proliferative retinopathy.

An increase in arterial blood pressure will further increase blood flow and increase microvascular pressure in the eyes and kidneys, and perhaps in selected other tissues, but will have minimal effect on microvascular pressure in skeletal muscle [8]. An increase in venous hydrostatic pressure, on the other hand, will increase pressure in capillaries and venules of skeletal muscle.

Studies currently in progress in many different laboratories should provide additional important new insights into the pathogenesis of diabetic microangiopathy in the next few years.

REFERENCES

1. Dornan TL, Tattersall RB. Muscle capillary basement membrane thickening: marker of microvascular complications or false prophet. Diabet Med 1986; 3: 413–18.
2. Williamson JR, Kilo C. Current status of capillary basement membrane disease in diabetes mellitus. Diabetes 1977; 26: 65–75.
3. Siperstein MD, Feingold KR, Bennett PH. Hyperglycaemia and diabetic microangiopathy. Diabetologia 1978; 15: 365–7.
4. Williamson JR, Kilo C. A common sense

approach resolves the basement membrane controversy and the NIH Pima Indian study. Diabetologia 1979; 17: 129–31.

5. Sosenko JM, Miettinen OS, Williamson JR et al. Muscle capillary basement membrane thickness and long-term glycemia in type I diabetes mellitus. New Engl J Med 1984; 311: 694–8.

6. Rogers DG, White NH, Santiago JV et al. Glycemic control and bone age are independently associated with muscle capillary basement membrane width in diabetic children after puberty. Diabetes Care 1986; 9: 453–9.

7. Feingold KR, Lee TH, Chung MY et al. Muscle capillary basement membrane width in patients with Vacor-induced diabetes mellitus. J Clin Invest 1986; 78: 102–7.

8. Williamson JR, Tilton RG, Chang K et al. Basement membrane abnormalities in diabetes mellitus: relationship to clinical microangiopathy. Diabetes Metab Rev 1988; 4: 339–370.

9. Farquhar MG. The glomerular basement membrane: a selective macromolecular filter. In Hay ED (ed.) Cell biology of extracellular matrix. New York: Plenum Press, 1981: pp 335–78.

10. Scott PG. Macromolecular constituents of basement membranes: a review of current knowledge on their structure and function. Can J Biochem Cell Biol 1983; 61: 942–8.

11. Mohan PS, Spiro RG. Macromolecular organization of basement membranes: characterization and comparison of glomerular basement membrane and lens capsule components by immunochemical and lectin affinity procedures. J Biol Chem 1986; 261: 4328–36.

12. Shimomura H, Spiro RG. Studies on macromolecular components of human glomerular basement membrane and alterations in diabetes: decreased levels of heparan sulfate proteoglycan and laminin. Diabetes 1987; 36: 374–81.

13. Timpl R, Wiedemann H, Van Delden V et al. A network model for the organization of type IV collagen molecules in basement membranes. Eur J Biochem 1981; 120: 203–11.

14. Vracko R, Benditt EP. Capillary basal lamina thickening. Its relationship to endothelial cell death and replacement. J Cell Biol 1970; 47: 281–5.

15. Kanwar YS, Farquhar MG. Detachment of endothelium and epithelium from the glomerular basement membrane produced by kidney perfusion with neuraminidase. Lab Invest 1980; 42: 375–84.

16. Rosenzweig LJ, Kanwar YS. Removal of sulfated (heparan sulfate) or nonsulfated (hyaluronic acid) glycosaminoglycans results in increased permeability of the glomerular basement membrane to ^{125}I-bovine serum albumin. Lab Invest 1982; 47: 177–84.

17. Spiro RG, Parthasarathy N. Studies on the proteoglycan of basement membranes. In Kuhn K, Schoene H, Timpl R, (eds) New trends in basement membrane research. New York: Raven Press, 1982: pp 87–98.

18. Brown DM, Michael AF, Oemega TR. Glycosaminoglycan synthesis by glomeruli in vivo and in vitro. Biochem Biophys Acta 1981; 674: 96–104.

19. Kerjaschki D, Sharkey DJ, Farquhar MG. Identification and characterization of podocalyxin—the major sialoprotein of the renal glomerular epithelial cell. J Cell Biol 1984; 98: 1591–6.

20. Blau EB, Michael AF. Rat glomerular glycoprotein composition and metabolism in aminonucleoside nephrosis. Proc Soc Exp Biol (NY) 1972; 141: 164–72.

21. Kerjaschki D, Vernillo AT, Farquhar MG. Reduced sialylation of podocalyxin—the major sialoprotein of the rat kidney glomerulus—in aminonucleoside nephrosis. Am J Pathol 1985; 118: 343–9.

22. Kanwar YS. Biophysiology of glomerular filtration and proteinuria. Lab Invest 1984; 51: 7–21.

23. Olson JL, Rennke HG, Venkatachalam MA. Alterations in the charge and size selectivity barrier of the glomerular filter in aminonucleoside nephrosis in rats. Lab Invest 1981; 44: 271–9.

24. Messina A, Davies DJ, Dillane PC et al. Glomerular epithelial abnormalities associated with the onset of proteinuria in aminonucleoside nephrosis. Am J Pathol 1987; 126: 220–9.

25. Pino RM. Perturbation of the blood–retinal barrier after enzyme perfusion: a cytochemical study. Lab Invest 1987; 56: 475–80.

26. Sternberg M, Cohen-Forterre L, Peyroux J. Connective tissue in diabetes mellitus: biochemical alterations of the intercellular matrix with special reference to proteoglycans, collagens, and basement membranes. Diabète Métab 1985; 11: 27–50.

27. Hasslacher CH, Reichenbacher R, Fechter F et al. Glomerular basement membrane synthesis and serum concentration of type IV collagen in streptozotocin-diabetic rats. Diabetologia 1984; 26: 150–4.

28. Hogemann B, Voss B, Altenwerth FJ et al. Concentrations of 7S collagen and laminin P1 in sera of patients with diabetes mellitus. Klin Wochenschr 1986; 64: 382–5.

29. Williamson JR, Kilo C. Extracellular matrix changes in diabetes mellitus. In Scarpelli DG, Migaki G (eds) Comparative pathobiology of major age-related diseases: current status and research frontiers. New York: Alan R. Liss, 1984: pp 269–88.

30. LePape A, Guitton JD, Muh JP. Modifications of glomerular basement membrane cross-links in experimental diabetic rats. Biochem Biophys Res Comm 1981; 100: 1214–21.

31. Li W, Shen S, Robertson GA et al. Increased solubility of newly synthesized collagen in retinal capillary pericyte cultures by nonenzymatic glycosylation. Ophthalm Res 1984; 16: 315–21.

32. Bendayan M. Alteration in the distribution of type IV collagen in glomerular basal laminae in diabetic rats as revealed by immunocytochemistry and morphometrical approach. Diabetologia 1985; 28: 373–8.

33. Bassiouny AR, Rosenberg H, McDonald TL. Glucosylated collagen is antigenic. Diabetes 1983; 32: 1182–4.

34. Falk RJ, Scheinman JI, Mauer SM et al. Polyantigenic expansion of basement membrane constituents in diabetic nephropathy. Diabetes 1983; 32 (suppl. 2): 34–9.

35. Leutenegger M, Birembaut P, Poynard JP et al. Distribution of fibronectin in diabetic skin. Path Biol 1983; 31: 45–8.

36. Melvin T, Kim Y, Michael AF. Selective binding of IgG4 and other negatively charged plasma proteins in normal and diabetic human kidneys. Am J Pathol 1984; 115: 443–6.

37. Kern TS, Engerman RL. Kidney morphology in experimental hyperglycemia. Diabetes 1987; 36: 244–9.

38. Cohn R, Mauer M, Barbosa J et al. Immunofluorescence studies of skeletal muscle extracellular membranes in diabetes mellitus. Lab Invest 1978; 39: 13–16.

39. Jeraj KP, Michael AF, Mauer SJ et al. Glucosylated and normal human or rat albumin do not bind to renal basement membranes of diabetic and control rats. Diabetes 1983; 32: 380–2.

40. Cohen MP, Ku L. Inhibition of fibronectin binding to matrix components by nonenzymatic glycosylation. Diabetes 1984; 33: 970–4.

41. Tarsio JF, Wigness B, Rhode TD et al. Nonenzymatic glycation of fibronectin and alterations in the molecular association of cell matrix and basement membrane components in diabetes mellitus. Diabetes 1985; 34: 477–84.

42. Cohen AH, Mampaso F, Amboni L. Glomerular podocyte degeneration in human renal disease. An ultrastructural study. Lab Invest 1977; 37: 40–2.

43. Brownlee M, Vlassara H, Kooney A et al. Aminoguanidine prevents diabetes-induced arterial wall protein cross-linking. Science 1986; 232: 1629–32.

44. Mauer SM, Steffes MW, Ellis EN et al. Structural–functional relationships in diabetic nephropathy. J Clin Invest 1984; 74: 1143–55.

45. Steffes MW, Sutherland DER, Goetz FC et al. Studies of kidney and muscle biopsy specimens from identical twins discordant for type I diabetes mellitus. New Engl J Med 1985; 312: 1282–7.

46. Kjellen L, Bielefeld D, Hook M. Reduced sulfation of liver heparan sulfate in experimentally diabetic rats. Diabetes 1983; 32: 337–42.

47. Chandramouli V, Carter JR. Cell membrane changes in chronically diabetic rats. Diabetes 1975; 24: 257–62.

48. Kinoshita JH, Kador PF, Datiles M. Aldose reductase in diabetic cataracts. JAMA 1981; 246: 257–61.

49. Chang K, Tomlinson M, Jeffrey JR et al. Galactose ingestion increases vascular permeability and collagen solubility in normal male rats. J Clin Invest 1987; 79: 367–3.

50. Williamson JR, Chang K, Tilton RG et al. Increased vascular permeability in spontaneously diabetic BB/W rats and in rats with mild versus severe streptozotocin-induced diabetes: prevention by aldose reductase inhibitors and castration. Diabetes 1987; 36: 813–21.

51. Barnett PA, Gonzalez RG, Chylack LT Jr et al. The effect of oxidation on sorbitol pathway kinetics. Diabetes 1986; 35: 426–32.

52. Greene DA, Lattimer S, Ulbrecht J et al. Glucose-induced alterations in nerve metabolism: current perspective on the pathogenesis of diabetic neuropathy and future directions for research and therapy. Diabetes Care 1985; 8: 290–9.

53. Chandler ML, Shannon WA, DeSantis L. Prevention of retinal capillary basement membrane thickening in diabetic rats by aldose reductase inhibitors. Invest Ophthalmol Vis Sci 1984; 25: 159.

54. Frank RN, Keirn RJ, Kennedy A et al. Galactose-induced retinal capillary basement membrane thickening: prevention by sorbinil. Invest Ophthalmol Vis Sci 1983; 24: 1519–24.

55. Robison WG Jr, Kador PF, Akagi Y et al. Prevention of basement membrane thickening in retinal capillaries by a novel inhibitor of aldose reductase, tolrestat. Diabetes 1986; 35: 295–9.

56. Tilton RG, Chang K, Pugliese G et al. Prevention of hemodynamic and vascular albumin filtration changes in diabetic rats by aldose reductase inhibitors. Diabetes 1989; 38: 1258–70.

57. Williamson JR, Chang K, Tilton RG et al. Increased ocular blood flow and ^{125}I-albumin permeation in diabetic rats are aldose reductase-linked phenomena. Invest Ophthalmol Vis Sci 1987; 28: 69.

58. Lightman S, Rechthand E, Terubayashi H et al. Permeability changes in blood–retinal barrier of galactosemic rats are prevented by aldose reductase inhibitors. Diabetes 1987; 36: 1271–5.

59. Engerman RL, Kern TS. Experimental galactosemia produces diabetic-like retinopathy. Diabetes 1984; 33: 97–100.

60. Atherton A, Hill DW, Keen H et al. The effect of acute hyperglycaemia on the retinal circulation of the normal cat. Diabetologia 1980; 18: 233–7.

61. Christiansen JS, Frandsen M, Parving H-H. Effect of intravenous glucose infusion on renal function in normal man and in insulin-dependent diabetics. Diabetologia 1981; 21: 368–73.

62. Li W, Shen S, Khatami M et al. Stimulation of retinal capillary pericyte protein and collagen synthesis in culture by high-glucose concentration. Diabetes 1984; 33: 785–9.

63. Li W, Khatami M, Rockey JH. The effects of glucose and an aldose reductase inhibitor on the sorbitol content and collagen synthesis of bovine retinal capillary pericytes in culture. Exp Eye Res 1985; 40: 439–44.

64. Chang K, Uitto J, Rowold EA et al. Increased collagen cross-linkages in experimental diabetes: reversal by β-aminopropionitrile and D-penicillamine. Diabetes 1980; 29: 778–81.

65. Williamson JR, Vogler N, Kilo C. Regional variations in the width of the basement membrane of muscle capillaries in man and giraffe. Am J Pathol 1971; 63: 359–70.

66. Tilton RG, Hoffmann PL, Kilo C et al. Pericyte degeneration and basement membrane thickening in skeletal muscle capillaries of human diabetics. Diabetes 1981; 30: 326–34.

67. Ganda OP, Williamson JR, Soeldner JS et al. Muscle capillary basement membrane width and its relationship to diabetes mellitus in monozygotic twins. Diabetes 1983; 32: 549–56.

68. Tilton RG, Faller AM, Burkhardt JK et al. Pericyte degeneration and acellular capillaries are increased in the feet of human diabetic patients. Diabetologia 1985; 28: 895–900.

69. Parving H-H, Viberti GC, Keen H et al. Hemodynamic factors in the genesis of diabetic microangiopathy. Metabolism 1983; 32: 943–9.

70. Stefansson E, Landers MB III, Wolbarsht ML. Oxygenation and vasodilatation in relation to diabetic and other proliferative retinopathies. Ophthalm Surg 1983; 14: 209–26.

71. Zatz R, Brenner BM. Pathogenesis of diabetic microangiopathy: the hemodynamic view. Am J Med 1986; 80: 443–53.

72. Longhurst J, Capone RJ, Zelis R. Evaluation of skeletal muscle capillary basement membrane thickness in congestive heart failure. Chest 1975; 67: 195–8.

73. Kilo C, Miller JP, Williamson JR. Capillary basement membrane (CBM) thickening (CBMT) and risk factors for vascular disease in University Group Diabetes Program (UGDP) subjects. Diabetes 1982; 31 (suppl. 2); 26A.

74. Williamson JR, Rowold E, Chang K et al. Sex steroid dependency of diabetes-induced changes in polyol metabolism, vascular permeability, and collagen cross-linking. Diabetes 1986; 35: 20–7.

75. Rogers DG, Deren S, Sherman WR et al. Sex and puberty-related differences in red blood cell polyol levels (RBC-P) in type I diabetics. Diabetes 1986; 35 (suppl. 1): 105A.

76. Barbosa J, Saner B. Do genetic factors play a role in the pathogenesis of diabetic microangiopathy? Diabetologia 1984; 27: 487–92.

77. Williamson JR, Kilo C. The relationship between glomerular and skeletal muscle capillary basement membrane. Diabetes 1978; 27: 513.

78. Ellis EN, Mauer SM, Goetz FC et al. Relationship of muscle capillary basement membrane to renal structure and function in diabetes mellitus. Diabetes 1986; 35: 421–5.

79. Sterky G, Wall S. Determinants of microangiopathy in growth-onset diabetes: with special reference to retinopathy and glycaemic control. Acta Pediatr Scand 1986; suppl. 327: 6–45.

80. Latta H, Maunsbach AB, Madden SC. The centrolobular region of the renal glomerulus studied by electron microscopy. Ultrastruct Res 1960; 4: 455–72.

81. Hostetter TH, Troy JL, Brenner BM. Glomerular hemodynamics in experimental diabetes mellitus. Kidney Int 1981; 19: 410–15.

82. Jensen PK, Christiansen JS, Steven K et al. Renal function in streptozotocin-diabetic rats. Diabetologia 1981; 21: 409–14.

83. Grayson MC, Laties AM. Ocular localization of sodium fluorescein. Arch Ophthalmol 1971; 85: 600–9.

84. Tso MOM, Shih C-Y, McLean IW. Is there a blood–brain barrier at the optic nerve head? Arch Ophthalmol 1975; 93: 815–25.

85. Flage T. A defect in the blood–retina barrier in the optic nerve head region in the rabbit and the monkey. Acta Ophthalmol 1980; 58: 645–51.

86. Garner A. Pathology of diabetic retinopathy. Br Med Bull 1970; 26: 137–42.

87. Cunha-Vaz JG. Diabetic retinopathy. Human and experimental studies. Trans Ophthalmol Soc UK 1972; 92: 111–24.

88. Kohner EM, Oakley NW. Diabetic retinopathy. Metabolism 1975; 24: 1085–92.

89. Valone JA, McMeel JW. Severe adolescent-onset proliferative diabetic retinopathy. Arch Ophthalmol 1978; 96: 1349–53.

90. Root HF, Mirsky S, Ditzel J. Proliferative retinopathy in diabetes mellitus. JAMA 1959; 169: 903–9.

91. Cohen AI. Is there a potential defect in the blood–retinal barrier at the choroidal level of

the optic nerve canal? Invest Ophthalmol 1973; 12: 513–19.

92. Matsumoto E, Matsumoto G, Ooshima A et al. Serum type IV collagen concentrations in diabetic patients with microangiopathy as determined by enzyme immunoassay with monoclonal antibodies. Diabetes 1990; 39: 885–90.

93. Mohan PS, Carter WG, Spiro RG. Occurrence of type VI collagen in extracellular matrix of renal glomeruli and its increase in diabetes. Diabetes 1990; 39: 31–7.

94. Ledbetter S, Copeland EJ, Noonan D et al. Altered steady-state mRNA levels of basement membrane proteins in diabetic mouse kidneys and thromboxane synthase inhibition. Diabetes 1990; 39: 196–203.

95. Tarsio JF, Reger LA, Furcht LT. Molecular mechanisms in basement membrane complications of diabetes: alterations in heparin, laminin, and type IV collagen association. Diabetes 1988; 37: 532–9.

96. Pugliese G, Tilton RG, Speedy A et al. Modulation of hemodynamic and vascular filtration changes in diabetic rats by dietary myo-inositol. Diabetes 1990; 39: 312–22.

97. Cagliero E, Roth T, Roy JS et al. Characteristics and mechanisms of high-glucose-induced overexpression of basement membrane components in cultured human endothelial cells. Diabetes 1991; 40: 102–10.

98. Berman A, Ledbetter S. Regulation of type IV collagen mRNA in retinal capillary endothelial cells and pericytes by glucose levels and aldose reductase inhibitor, sorbinil. Diabetes 1988; 37 (suppl. 1): 96A.

99. Tan EML, Glassberg E, Unger GA et al. Glucose stimulates gene expression of basement membrane matrix proteins in human microvascular endothelial cells. Diabetes 1988; 37 (suppl. 1): 96A.

100. Ooshima A, Fuller G, Cardinale G et al. Collagen biosynthesis in blood vessels of brain and other tissues of the hypertensive rat. Science 1975; 190: 989–90.

101. Iwatsuki K, Cardinale GJ, Spector S et al. Hypertension: increase of collagen biosynthesis in arteries but not in veins. Science 1977; 198: 403–5.

55

Diabetic Nephropathy

G.C. Viberti*, J.D. Walker† and J. Pinto‡

*Unit for Metabolic Medicine, Guy's Hospital, London, UK, †St Bartholomew's Hospital, London, UK, and ‡Santa Maria University Hospital, Lisbon, Portugal

Diabetic nephropathy is a relatively common microvascular complication of both insulin dependent diabetes mellitus (IDDM) and non-insulin dependent diabetes mellitus (NIDDM). It is clinically defined by the presence of persistent proteinuria (more than 0.5 g per 24 hours) in a diabetic patient with concomitant retinopathy and elevated blood pressure, but without urinary tract infection, other renal disease or heart failure.

Although proteinuria had been noted in patients with diabetes since the eighteenth century [1, 2] it was not until the late 1830s that it was postulated that albuminuria could reflect a serious renal disease specific to diabetes [3, 4]. In 1936, Kimmelstiel and Wilson [5] described the nodular glomerular intercapillary lesions in the diabetic kidney, and related them to the clinical syndrome of profuse proteinuria and renal failure accompanied by arterial hypertension.

The size of the problem of diabetic kidney disease became clear in the 1950s following the longer survival afforded to IDDM patients after the discovery of insulin in 1921. Recent studies indicate that approximately 600 cases of end-stage diabetic renal failure occur every year in the UK (about 10 cases per million population) [6], and in the USA in 1985 about one-third of all patients beginning renal replacement therapy were diabetic. The cost of caring for these diabetic patients in renal failure approached $1 billion (US) in 1985 [7].

EPIDEMIOLOGY

The epidemiology of diabetic nephropathy has been predominantly, although not exclusively, studied in IDDM patients and the largest studies are from Denmark and the Joslin Clinic (Table 1). NIDDM patients have been less investigated, but within this type of diabetes major differences exist between ethnic groups. At present, it is prudent to treat the epidemiology of nephropathy separately in the two types of diabetes.

Insulin Dependent Diabetes

Two major cohort studies have described the prevalence and incidence of diabetic nephropathy, as defined by persistent clinical proteinuria, in IDDM patients who developed diabetes before the age of 31 years [8–10]. The *prevalence* (number of cases at a given time) of nephropathy increases with duration of diabetes to a peak of 21% after 20–25 years, after which it declines to about 10% in those who have diabetes for 40 years or more. After 5 years of diabetes, the annual *incidence* (number of cases per given time) of nephropathy rises rapidly over the next 10 years to a peak after 15–17 years at about 3% per year. It then declines to around 1% per year

---

International Textbook of Diabetes Mellitus. Edited by K.G.M.M. Alberti, R.A. DeFronzo, H. Keen and P. Zimmet
© 1992 John Wiley & Sons Ltd

Table 1　The epidemiology of diabetic nephropathy. A comparison of three studies

	Steno Hospital, Copenhagen [8]	Joslin Clinic, Boston [9]	Steno Hospital, Copenhagen [10]
No of patients	1384	292	2890
Peak incidence	16 years	10–14 years	15–17 years
Cumulative incidence	45% after 40 years	35% after 40 years	34% after 25 years
Sex difference	M : F = 1.8 : 1	No difference	M : F = 1.5 : 1
Calendar year effect	Present	Present	Present
Associations	Domicile Insulin dose	Glycaemia	High body mass index
Prognosis	50% dead after 7 years of proteinurea	End-stage renal failure in 75% within 15 years	Not stated

in those with 40 years or more of diabetes [11] (Figure 1).

This pattern of risk indicates that accumulation of exposure to diabetes (i.e. intensity times duration) is not sufficient to explain the development of clinically manifest kidney disease, and suggests that only a subset of patients are susceptible to renal complications. The paucity of new cases of nephropathy among long-standing diabetic patients supports the view that this complication occurred in most of the susceptible individuals earlier in the course of diabetes. During the first 10 years of diabetes only about 4% of patients develop nephropathy. The cumulative incidence increases thereafter to a plateau after about 25 years. Nephropathy develops in only 4% of patients with more than 35 years of diabetes. This indicates that only a proportion of juvenile diabetic patients ever develop neph-

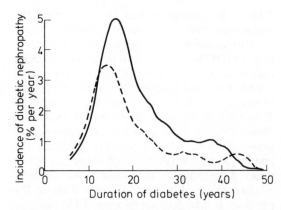

Figure 1　The annual incidence of clinical proteinuria in IDDM patients as a function of diabetes duration (broken line, women; solid line, men). From reference 11 with permission

ropathy. This proportion has changed over the years [9, 10]; in cohorts of patients diagnosed before 1942, the cumulative risk up to 25–30 years' duration was approximately 41%, but it has declined to around 25% in patients diagnosed after 1949 (the so-called 'calendar effect'). The reason for the lower frequency of diabetic nephropathy in recent decades is not entirely clear. Cohort differences may be related to changes in diabetes care and control, to more intensive and early treatment of concomitant conditions such as hypertension, or, less probably, to dietary changes. An alternative explanation is that before 1942 persistent proteinuria in diabetic patients may have been, in a proportion of cases, the manifestation of some other form of renal disease, particularly glomerulonephritis, the incidence of which has declined during this century [12]. This interpretation would explain why a sharp decrease in incidence occurred in patients diagnosed in the late 1940s, but not since.

There is a male preponderance in the development of proteinuria, with a male-to-female ratio of around 1.7. The cumulative incidence is 46% in male but only 32% in female diabetic patients in cohort studies that have followed patients for 40 years or more. This sex difference in the incidence of renal disease is also found in non-diabetic subjects [13, 14]. Interestingly, a male preponderance has also been reported by some authors [15, 16] in the development of proliferative diabetic retinopathy. It has been suggested that sex steroids may be of importance, because castrated diabetic rats seem less prone to late diabetic complications than non-castrated control animals [17].

Age at diagnosis significantly influences the risk of nephropathy. The time to development of microvascular complications is not influenced by prepubertal duration of the disease [18], and nephropathy develops more slowly in individuals with diabetes of onset before the age of 10 years than in those diagnosed after puberty [9]. The highest cumulative incidence of 44% is seen in subjects who developed diabetes between 11 years and 20 years of age [10], while after the age of 20 years the cumulative incidence of nephropathy is around 35%. Current age has been found by some authors [9] but not by others [10] to influence the incidence of proteinuria, with a maximal risk in the age interval of 18–35 years and a rapid decline in incidence after the age of 35 years, regardless of duration of diabetes [19]. This discrepancy in findings may be partly related to the different age groups of the cohorts studied.

In one study the level of hyperglycaemia during the first 15 years of diabetes was found to be positively related to the risk of persistent proteinuria [9]. However, the incidence of nephropathy rapidly declined after 15 years duration of diabetes, even though there was no improvement in the control of glycaemia, suggesting that susceptibility to this condition is related to non-metabolic factors, most probably genetic. The complex metabolic disturbances of diabetes appear, therefore, to be necessary, but not sufficient, for the clinical manifestation of nephropathy.

The development of *end-stage renal failure* and the mortality associated with it are closely related to the occurrence of persistent proteinuria [9]: 25% of the patients develop end-stage renal failure within 6 years and 75% within 15 years of onset of proteinuria. Progression to end-stage renal failure seems to take longer in those diabetic patients diagnosed before puberty. Median time between onset of persistent proteinuria and development of end-stage renal failure was 14 years in the group of subjects with onset of diabetes before age 12, and 8 years in those with onset of diabetes between the ages of 12 years and 20 years [9]. The range of survival after the onset of persistent proteinuria is wide, varying between 1 year and 24 years. Median survival has been reported to be around 7–10 years [8, 9].

The ominous significance of renal involvement in IDDM is clearly shown by the comparison of long-term outcome in patients with and without nephropathy. After 40 years of diabetes, only 10% of patients with proteinuria are alive, in contrast to more than 70% of those without proteinuria [8]. Almost all of the latter have normal renal function, and up to about 70% are clinically well in all respects, only about 10% being seriously disabled by virtue of amputation, or visual or cardiovascular complications [20].

When renal replacement therapy was not widely available, the main cause of death (approximately 60%) in insulin dependent patients with diabetic nephropathy was uraemia, but a substantial proportion died before terminal renal failure from ischaemic heart disease (19%) or stroke (5%). The proportion of cardiovascular deaths increases significantly to around 40% in patients who develop proteinuria after more than 20 years of diabetes [8]. The advent of renal replacement therapy, which has postponed uraemic death, has by the same token increased the pool of cardiovascular deaths, which now usually occur after institution of treatment for end-stage renal disease. The development of persistent proteinuria in IDDM patients increases early mortality from cardiovascular disease approximately ninefold [21, 22]. The risk of developing coronary artery disease is estimated to be 15 times higher in those with proteinuria than in those without [23], and its cumulative incidence 5 years after onset of proteinuria is 8 times higher than in matched controls without renal involvement [22]. Whatever the cause, mortality from all causes by age 45 years in IDDM patients with proteinuria has been reported to be 20–40 times higher than that in patients without proteinuria, who experience a relative mortality only double that of the non-diabetic population [11]. Recent studies suggest that more effective antihypertensive treatment during the past decade has significantly improved the prognosis in patients with diabetic nephropathy. Ten-year survival after onset of persistent proteinuria has risen from 30–50% [8, 9] to about 80% [24, 25].

Non-insulin Dependent Diabetes

Data on the prevalence and incidence of nephropathy in NIDDM patients, as indicated by persistent proteinuria, have been relatively scarce until recent years. The overall prevalence of proteinuria in excess of 500 mg per 24 hours has been reported to be approximately 16% in one study of European diabetic patients diagnosed after age 40 years [26]. Other studies in slightly different selected populations have reported lower prevalences of 12–14%, with males being affected more frequently (19%) than females (4%) [27, 28]. The prevalence of proteinuria increases steadily with duration of diabetes, from 7–10% in patients with diabetes diagnosed less than 5 years before, to 20–35% in patients who have had diabetes diagnosed for more than 20–25 years [26, 27].

In non-European NIDDM patients the lowest prevalence of proteinuria of 2.4% has been reported in patients in Hong Kong [29], but prevalences higher than those in European patients have been found in Native Americans [29–31] Mexican-Americans [32], American blacks [33], Japanese [29], Nauruans from central Pacific islands [34], and Asian Indians in the UK [35], in whom an increased prevalence of microalbuminuria has also been described [36]. In some non-European ethnic groups there is also a tendency for the prevalence to increase with duration of diabetes.

A male preponderance in the prevalence of proteinuria has been reported by some authors [37]. Both blood glucose control and level of arterial pressure have been related to prevalence of proteinuria in a number of ethnic groups. Of European NIDDM patients, 62% maintain normal protein excretion after 16 years of diabetes. Those who develop proteinuria have a higher prevalence of hypertension before onset of persistent proteinuria than those who do not [38]. These findings suggest that cumulative exposure to diabetes and to raised arterial pressure are both important determinants of renal involvement in NIDDM.

Incidence data in NIDDM patients of European origin in a population-based study in the USA showed a cumulative risk of persistent proteinuria of 25% after 20 years of diabetes [37]. Recent data from Europe shows a 57% cumulative risk of proteinuria after 25 years of diabetes duration [39]. Reports on NIDDM patients of Japanese [40] and of Pima Indian [41] origin indicate that the incidence rate of nephropathy, as measured by persistent proteinuria, rises with duration of diabetes, with a cumulative risk of proteinuria of about 50% after 20 years of diabetes. Of particular importance are the recent observations in the Pima that blood

pressure elevation before the onset of diabetes predicts abnormal albuminuria [42], and that the risk of development of diabetic nephropathy in the offspring of a diabetic parent is markedly increased when the parent also has diabetic renal disease [43]. Thus in NIDDM as in IDDM, susceptibility factors, either genetic or shared environmental, appear to be critical in the pathogenesis of nephropathy.

Progression to end-stage renal failure in proteinuric NIDDM patients is variable, and has been reported to be infrequent in individuals of European origin [26]. In a period prevalence survey of diabetic end-stage renal failure (defined as a serum creatinine value greater than 500 μmol/l and/or serum urea value greater than 25 mmol/l) in the UK in 1985, only 3.5 cases per million total population were found, and some of these patients were of non-European origin. This figure compares with 6.5 cases per million for IDDM patients [6]. Given the approximately tenfold higher prevalence of NIDDM, this observation suggests that end-stage renal failure is about 20 times less frequent in NIDDM than in IDDM of European origin. However, this view is not supported by the finding of a cumulative risk of chronic renal failure of 12% by 15 years in NIDDM patients who had persistent proteinuria at the time of diagnosis. In those patients developing proteinuria after the diagnosis of diabetes, the cumulative risk was 17%, 15 years after the onset of persistent proteinuria [44]. In another longitudinal study in European patients followed for a median time of 20 years, the cumulative risk of renal failure (diagnosed by a serum creatinine value greater than 124 μmol/l) 3 and 5 years after onset of persistent proteinuria was even higher, at 41% and 63%, respectively, but this may reflect the less stringent criterion for renal failure [39].

The discrepancy between frequency of proteinuria and frequency of end-stage renal disease in some studies of European subjects may arise for different reasons. Many IDDM patients are taking insulin by the time they reach terminal renal failure, which may lead to misclassification of type of diabetes. Many of these patients are old and have associated cardiovascular disease, and they may simply not be considered for renal replacement therapy [45], or may die before reaching end-stage renal failure. Proteinuria of non-diabetic origin, which occurs in close to

30% of proteinuric NIDDM patients [28, 46], may also contribute to this disparity.

In a prospective study of a cohort of 503 NIDDM subjects, 10-year survival was significantly worse (around 30%) in patients with elevated urinary albumin excretion ranging from microalbuminuria to clinical proteinuria, compared with 55% in patients with normal albumin excretion rates. The majority of deaths (58%) were due to cardiovascular causes, only 3% being ascribed to uraemia [47]. These data agree with previous findings from prospective studies of European NIDDM patients, in whom microalbuminuria markedly increased the risk of cardiovascular death [48, 49].

In NIDDM affecting non-European ethnic groups, the incidence of end-stage renal failure is strongly associated with the presence of proteinuria. In diabetic Pima Indians, the incidence of end-stage renal failure increases with duration of diabetes to about 41 cases per 1000 person-years at risk after 20 years of diabetes, when the cumulative risk of this complication reaches 15% [50]. Compared with European NIDDM patients, an excess incidence of end-stage renal disease (ESRD) has also been reported in Mexican-Americans (Mexican-American/white ratio of about 6) [51] and in black diabetic subjects [33, 52]. In the UK, an excess of Afro-Caribbean and Asian patients has been found among NIDDM patients treated for ESRD [46], and its incidence has been reported to be higher in NIDDM in African countries [53, 54].

In diabetic Pima Indians, proteinuria confers a 3.5 times higher risk of premature mortality, and the concomitant presence of arterial hypertension increases this relative risk to 7.1 [55]. The mortality rate of the diabetic Pima Indians without proteinuria is similar to that of the non-diabetic subjects. Of the excess mortality associated with NIDDM in this population, 97% is found in patients with proteinuria: 16% of deaths were ascribed to uraemia, while 22% were due to cardiovascular disease. These mortality data are slightly higher than the twofold to threefold excess of early mortality observed in the European NIDDM patients with proteinuria [47, 56] (Figure 2).

CLINICAL COURSE AND NATURAL HISTORY

The natural history of renal involvement has been better defined in IDDM than in NIDDM,

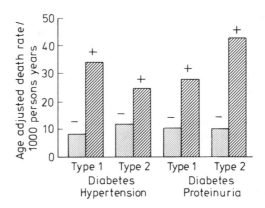

Figure 2 Age-adjusted death rates in insulin dependent and non-insulin dependent patients with (+) and without (−) hypertension (left panel) and proteinuria (right panel). From reference 56 with permission

partly because the usual relatively acute onset of diabetes in the former allows a more precise timing of observed clinical and physiological events.

Early Phase: Glomerular Hyperfiltration and Microalbuminuria

After diagnosis of diabetes a clinically silent phase of variable duration occurs. During this period, however, important abnormalities of renal function and structure develop.

Glomerular Hyperfiltration

Glomerular filtration rate (GFR) is found to be elevated on average by 20–40% above that of age-matched normal subjects in both adults and children with IDDM [57–61]. Data are controversial in NIDDM, with some groups reporting normal and others supranormal GFR values [62–65]. Approximately 25% of patients with IDDM have a GFR exceeding the upper limit of the normal range [66]. Hyperfiltration is related to the degree of blood glucose control, at least within the range of moderate hyperglycaemia (i.e. to about 14 mmol/l), whereas higher blood glucose values tend to be associated with normal or low GFR [66]. Intensified insulin treatment and good metabolic control reduce the GFR toward normal levels after a period of weeks to months in both IDDM [67, 68] and NIDDM [69]. Renal plasma flow (RPF) has been reported as elevated, normal or reduced in IDDM [61, 70–72], although more recent work shows an elevation of RPF ranging between 9% and 14% [73].

The increased GFR and RPF are accompanied by an approximately 20% increase in kidney size, and a good correlation between GFR and kidney volume has been described in IDDM patients [71, 74–76]. Approximately 40% of IDDM patients have kidneys larger than normal. A large kidney is a prerequisite for the occurrence of a GFR above the upper limit of the normal range, but normal GFRs can be found in patients with large kidneys [76]. In one autopsy study of NIDDM subjects, increased kidney volumes were found only in those patients with normal serum creatinine [77]. The relationship of kidney size to glycaemic control is less clear-cut than that of GFR. In newly diagnosed IDDM [78] and NIDDM [69] patients, 3 months of insulin treatment has been claimed to reduce kidney size. This observation has, however, not been confirmed in longer-term IDDM subjects treated by intensified insulin treatment for periods of up to 1 year. In these patients, in spite of a reduction in GFR, kidney volume remained unchanged [67, 68, 79]. Nephromegaly in the animal model can also be reversed only if insulin treatment is started soon after induction of diabetes [80], whereas correction of hyperglycaemia after 4 weeks fails to normalize kidney volume [81]. Indeed, contrary to most forms of renal disease, in diabetes large kidneys can persist even in the presence of advanced renal failure [82, 83]. It is not known why renal enlargement becomes irreversible, but it has been speculated that this irreversibility may have prognostic implications for the development of clinically significant renal damage [84]. If hydronephrosis and duplex kidneys are excluded, diabetes is the most common cause of nephromegaly associated with renal disease [85].

The prognostic significance of glomerular hyperfiltration in humans remains uncertain. A positive correlation between initial hyperfiltration and subsequent increase in albuminuria and development of clinical nephropathy was described in two retrospective studies [86, 87], but these findings were not confirmed by a more recent study spanning an observation period of 18 years [88]. In all these reports, a number of potentially important confounding variables, such as levels of albumin excretion rate, blood pressure or protein intake, which can all affect outcome, were not controlled for. The 5-year results of an ongoing prospective case-control study of IDDM patients with and without hyperfiltration [89] seem to suggest that diabetic patients with hyperfiltration, although showing a faster rate of GFR decline (Figure 3), do not show an increased frequency rate of rising albuminuria or blood pressure.

Microalbuminuria

Although in this silent phase patients do not, by definition, demonstrate clinically detectable proteinuria, the use of a sensitive radioimmunoassay for urinary albumin has shown that in several circumstances a proportion of patients with relatively early diabetes have elevated supranormal rates of albumin excretion. A significant increase in albumin excretion rate to 3–4 times above the normal level was first demonstrated in NIDDM patients newly detected in a population survey [90]. Young, newly diagnosed IDDM subjects, or short-term diabetic subjects in poor control, often demonstrate an elevated albumin excretion rate [91–93]. Subclinical elevations of both albumin and IgG excretion rates are also found in longer-term IDDM patients [94]. These abnormal, though subclinical, increases in albumin excretion rate have been termed *microalbuminuria*. Albumin excretion in healthy individuals ranges between $1.5\,\mu g/min$ and $20\,\mu g/min$, with a geometric mean around $6.5\,\mu g/min$. These levels have been termed *normoalbuminuria*. The wide use of chemical reagent dipsticks has led to the definition of *persistent* or *clinical proteinuria* in patients whose urine is positive to these tests. Such patients generally have albumin excretion rates in excess of $200\,\mu g/min$. 'Microalbuminuria' thus defines the wide subclinical range of albumin hyperexcretion ranging between $20\,\mu g/min$ and $200\,\mu g/min$.

Albumin excretion rate in both normal individuals and diabetic patients tends to be about 25% higher during the day than during the night, and has an average day-to-day variation of about 40% [91, 95–99]. Similar coefficients of variation are found for albumin/creatinine ratios, suggesting that this variability is a true biological phenomenon and not due to inadequate urine collection [91, 96–98]. An important practical implication of this variability is that the

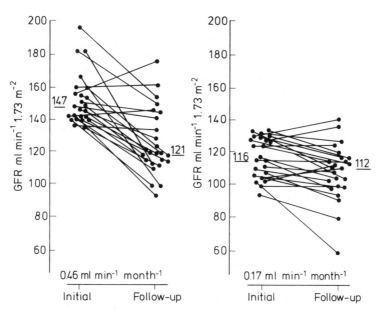

Figure 3   Initial and 5-year follow-up glomerular filtration rates (GFR) in 25 hyperfiltering (left panel) and 25 normofiltering (right panel) IDDM patients. From reference 89, with permission

accurate classification of albumin excretion rates should depend on measurements in at least three collections over a 6-month period. The prevalence of microalbuminuria in IDDM has been reported to vary from 5% to 37% in different population-based and diabetic clinic-based studies [100–105]. These rather large differences in prevalance are probably ascribable to patient selection. No correlation is found between albumin excretion rate and age, but there is a male preponderance among IDDM microalbuminuric patients, who also tend to have an earlier onset and longer duration of diabetes than normoalbuminuric patients [104, 105]. Persistent elevations in albumin excretion rate are exceptional in the first 5 years of diabetes [101, 105] (Figure 4), and microalbuminuria has not been detected in children less than 15 years old [100]. The phase of persistent microalbuminuria has been termed by some authors 'incipient nephropathy' [106]. Albumin excretion rate is influenced by glycaemic control, and correction of hyperglycaemia can reduce microalbuminuria, not only in short-term IDDM but also in IDDM of long duration [92–94, 96, 107]. Moderately strenuous exercise is also capable of provoking an exaggerated rise in albumin excretion rate in diabetic patients with normal resting values

[108, 109]. The severity of the exercise-induced albuminuria seems related to the duration of diabetes, and is modulated by the level of blood glucose control [110–112].

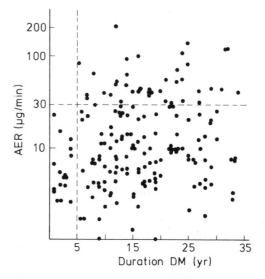

Figure 4   Albumin excretion rates (AER) as a function of disease duration in 164 IDDM patients. From reference 101, with kind permission from the author

In NIDDM, prevalences of microalbuminuria between 8% and 46% have been reported in Europeans [26, 47, 103, 105, 113], and prevalences of 47% in the Pima Indians [31]. Its correlation with glycaemic levels is apparent not only in diabetic patients, but also in patients with impaired glucose tolerance [31, 90, 113]. No correlation is found with sex, but significant positive associations are found with diastolic blood pressure and resting heart rate [114].

The prognostic significance of microalbuminuria for development of persistent proteinuria and overt nephropathy has been demonstrated by four longitudinal studies of cohorts of IDDM patients [86, 96, 115, 116]. These investigations have all suggested the existence of a threshold of albumin excretion above which the risk of progression to clinical nephropathy increases by about 20 times. The overall findings of these studies are remarkably similar, the differences in methods of urine collection and length of follow-up probably being responsible for the different risk levels of AER. Microalbuminuria is unlikely to be a marker of susceptibility to the development of clinical nephropathy as it is undetectable in the first 5 years of diabetes, but is more likely to be a sign of early disease. This interpretation has recently been corroborated by the finding that patients with persistent microalbuminuria have more severe renal histological lesions than those with normal albumin excretion rates [117]. There is no evidence, at present, that exercise-induced microalbuminuria improves the predictive power of resting microalbuminuria. A good correlation has been found between albumin excretion rate and albumin/creatinine ratios, particularly in first morning urine samples, and albumin excretion rates greater than 30 μg/min correspond to albumin/creatinine ratios greater than 2.5 [98].

Three retrospective studies have also examined the prognostic value of microalbuminuria in cohorts of NIDDM patients [47–49]. Over an interval of 10–14 years, they have all shown an increased risk of cardiovascular death in these patients. A recent prospective study of 3 years' duration has confirmed the greater incidence of cardiovascular events in NIDDM patients with microalbuminuria [118]. Moreover, microalbuminuria has been found to be predictive of risk of cardiovascular events in the non-diabetic population [119].

Late Phase: Clinical Nephropathy

The onset of the clinical phase of diabetic nephropathy is signalled, by convention, by the appearance of persistent proteinuria (total daily protein excretion of 0.5 g or more), which corresponds to an albumin excretion rate greater than about 200 μg/min (i.e. about 300 mg per day). A phase of intermittent dipstick-positive urine for protein precedes persistent proteinuria [120], but this probably corresponds to the late phases of high microalbuminuria, with values intermittently breaking through the clinical threshold [121, 122]. The value of the term and concept of intermittent proteinuria is limited to being an indication for quantitative measurements of urinary albumin; its use as a description of a specific phase of disease should be abandoned. In patients in whom persistent proteinuria develops, there is a progressive decline of the glomerular filtration rate to end-stage renal failure [123–126]. Whether the fall in GFR starts at the time of, or after, the appearance of the microalbuminuric phase, is a matter for debate [121, 127]. The fall in GFR appears to be linear with time in all patients, but the rate of decline varies over an approximately fivefold range between individual patients.

The reasons for these different speeds of progression are not entirely clear and do not seem to be related to age, sex, duration of diabetes or degree of proteinuria at onset. Adequacy of blood glucose control has only a limited impact on progression [128, 129], even though some (but not all) authors have reported a correlation between glycated haemoglobin levels and rate of fall of GFR [130, 131]. The level of diastolic blood pressure has been found to be correlated with the rate of progression of established diabetic nephropathy, and serum creatinine concentrations have been reported to rise sooner in proteinuric patients who have higher blood pressure levels [123, 129, 132]. The failure by other authors [124–126] to confirm the relationship with blood pressure may result from the current, more widepread treatment of mild hypertension in these patients. In evaluating the rate and magnitude of fall of GFR, caution must be applied when serum creatinine levels or creatinine clearance are used as indices of glomerular function [133]. Because of the asymptotic relationship between serum creatinine and GFR, a rise in serum creatinine levels may not occur before more than 50% of the GFR has been lost. A linear decline in the inverse of the creatinine concentration is not seen for serum creatinine concentrations below 200 μmol/l [124]. Moreover, the use of creatinine clearance tends to overestimate GFR because of the enhanced tubular secretion of creatinine which takes place in advanced renal failure [134].

In the past, end-stage renal failure occurred on average 7 years after the onset of persistent proteinuria. In recent years, this interval has probably more than doubled, with early and more intensive treatment of hypertension [24, 25] and early restriction of dietary protein [135, 136].

Arterial pressure is almost invariably elevated in diabetic patients with established nephropathy. A small proportion (about 25%) of patients may still have blood pressures within the so-called normal range at the onset of persistent proteinuria, although it may have risen within the normal range from previous lower preproteinuric levels [96, 137, 138]. With progression to renal insufficiency, virtually all patients become hypertensive [24, 120, 129]. Several studies suggest that the excess of arterial hypertension described in IDDM patients is almost entirely accounted for by patients with persistent proteinuria [129, 139, 140]. Long-term IDDM patients without proteinuria have blood pressures that are, indeed, lower than those of age-matched controls [142]. The degree of proteinuria in diabetic patients is usually in the subnephrotic range, but heavy protein excretion and nephrotic syndrome may occur, and this has been related to a poorer renal outcome [142]. The level of proteinuria is roughly related to the degree of severity of the glomerular lesions, but glomerular histological damage has been reported in patients without proteinuria [142, 143]. The clinical significance of this finding remains obscure. In our personal experience of follow-up of more than 90 IDDM patients with diabetic nephropathy, we have not met a single case of progressive renal failure in the absence of some degree of proteinuria.

Non-renal Complications

Diabetic retinopathy is present in virtually all IDDM patients with nephropathy [104, 143–145]. In advanced renal disease, retinopathy is usually severe with new vessel formation. Indeed, the absence of retinopathy should lead to more than usually careful consideration of other non-diabetic causes for proteinuria and renal disease (see below). Whereas all patients with nephropathy have retinopathy, the reverse is not true: retinopathy, even of the proliferative kind, may occur in the absence of proteinuria and renal disease [146]. Up to one-third of patients with proliferative retinopathy may be free of proteinuria [147, 148]. The exact reasons for this discrepancy in manifestations of microvascular disease are not clear, but epidemiological evidence suggests that retinopathy and nephropathy recognize different environmental determinants. The cumulative risk of retinopathy approaches 100% after 15 years of diabetes [149], demonstrating a close relationship to a history of poor blood glucose control; in contrast, levels of blood pressure are stronger determinants of the development of nephropathy. In NIDDM patients with persistent proteinuria, retinopathy is present in 47–63% [28, 47, 150], consistent with the observation that about 30% of proteinuria in NIDDM is of non-diabetic origin.

Urinalysis in proteinuric diabetic patients shows, in a substantial number of cases, the presence of *microhaematuria*. A recent study has demonstrated that in proteinuric diabetic patients with microhaematuria there is a higher prevalence of concomitant non-diabetic renal disease [151]. However, microhaematuria can occur in proteinuric diabetic patients in the absence of other renal conditions as part of the diabetic nephropathy syndrome. It has been reported in 66% of all cases in a large series of 136 consecutive renal biopsies in IDDM and NIDDM patients, and it has been claimed to be of little use in distinguishing non-diabetic renal disease [152]. Red cell casts are unusual in diabetic nephropathy and call for further evaluation. Although this is still a matter for debate, the presence of red cells in the urinary sediment must alert the physician to the possibility of another renal disease.

End-stage Renal Failure

The development of uraemia in diabetic patients is compounded by a number of other complications. Fluid retention and oedema occur relatively early in the development of renal failure, in the absence of hypoalbuminaemia [153]. The variable contributions, particularly in older patients, of cardiac insufficiency and of vasomotor defects secondary to neuropathy and peripheral vascular disease were recognized long ago [154–156]. Depressed renal function further compromises disposal of water and solutes and impairs osmotic diuresis, especially in the face of rapid compartmental shifts of fluid secondary to variations in glycaemia [157]. Pulmonary oedema may follow and the prognosis at this stage is poor. Hyperkalaemia may develop, partly due to the hyporeninaemic hypoaldosteronism common in patients with advanced diabetic nephropathy [158], which may itself aggravate the metabolic acidosis of chronic renal failure.

Peripheral neuropathy affects the majority of diabetic patients with renal failure. Uraemia, itself a cause of neuropathy, is likely to contribute to the severity of symptoms in a number of cases. Foot sepsis leading to amputation may occur, due probably to a combination of neural and arterial disease. This can be a major cause of incapacity and morbidity in these patients, but it can be prevented by good patient education and active involvement of the chiropodist. Autonomic neuropathy, notably postural hypotension, can make treatment of arterial hypertension particularly troublesome. Good control of blood pressure in the supine position is often accompanied by an unacceptable postural drop in standing blood pressures. Diabetic diarrhoea [144] and gastroparesis [159] causing nausea and vomiting are sometimes hard to distinguish from the gastrointestinal symptoms of uraemia. Impotence and profuse sweating are also common manifestations of autonomic neuropathy in uraemic patients [160]. Neurogenic bladder, a particularly serious problem, may necessitate long-term urinary catheterization with the inevitable sequelae of urinary sepsis which may render the patient unsuitable for renal transplantation.

Arterial disease and medial calcification of larger arteries (Mönckeberg's sclerosis) is present in almost all diabetic patients with advanced renal disease [161]. Disturbances of lipid metabolism of diabetes and uraemia combined with arterial hypertension all contribute to the development of severe sclerotic damage. Coronary artery disease is the major cause of death in these patients, and peripheral artery disease may contribute to gangrene and amputation, both

Table 2 Type and frequency of complications in insulin treated and non-insulin treated diabetic patients with renal failure

Complications	Insulin treated number (%)	Non-insulin treated number (%)
Disabling stroke	2/112 (1.8)	6/62 (9.7)
Leg amputation	8/113 (7.1)	3/62 (4.8)
Myocardial infarct	19/111 (17.1)	11/62 (17.7)
Severe bilateral vision loss	41/111 (36.9)	19/63 (30.2)

From reference 6, with permission.

before and particularly after renal replacement therapy (Table 2).

PATHOGENESIS OF DIABETIC NEPHROPATHY

Hyperglycaemia and Non-enzymatic Glycation

There is no doubt that a positive relationship between the abnormal glycaemic milieu of diabetes and microvascular complications does exist. The view that small vessel disease and, in particular, abnormalities in capillary basement membrane thickness are primarily an inherited phenomenon [162] has been negated by an overwhelming body of evidence linking hyperglycaemia to diabetic complications [163, 164]. Small vessel complications can be found in secondary diabetes in humans [165, 166] and in a variety of types of chemically induced and genetic diabetes in the animal model [167]. In the kidney, histological lesions such as mesangial expansion may be reversed by the transplantation of a diabetic kidney into a normal animal [168] or by curing diabetes with islet cell transplantation [169–171]. Moreover, in the rat model renal histological lesions [80, 172] and albuminuria [173] can be prevented by near-normalization of blood glucose levels with intensified insulin treatment from induction of diabetes.

There are, however, two important aspects to consider. The animal model most frequently used for the study of diabetic nephropathy is the rat. This animal does not develop advanced renal failure and the severe histological lesions seen in the human diabetic subject, and there are considerable species differences in the glomerular haemodynamic responses to different glycaemic levels, making extrapolation of data to humans difficult [167, 174]. In addition, the rats used as models of chemically induced or genetic diabetes are highly inbred strains of animals, a condition which is unrepresentative of the genetic heterogeneity of human diabetes. In humans the evidence of a straightforward causal relationship between hyperglycaemia and renal disease is less compelling. The development of clinically overt renal disease is not linearly related to the duration of diabetes, and affects only between 35% and 50% of patients. The majority of diabetic patients escape renal failure and, although some histological damage occurs in their kidneys, their renal function remains essentially normal until death. Kidneys from non-diabetic human donors develop typical lesions of diabetic glomerulopathy when they are transplanted into a diabetic recipient [175], but the rate of development of the lesions varies greatly, independently of the blood glucose control over the years [176]. It therefore appears that in humans hyperglycaemia is necessary, but not alone sufficient, to cause the renal damage that leads to kidney failure, and that other (possibly non-environmental) factors are needed for the manifestation of the clinical syndrome.

Non-enzymatic Glycation

The reaction between glucose and the lysine amino terminal of circulating and structural proteins gives rise to glycation products by a non-enzymatic process [177] (see also Chapter 24). Two major classes of glycated products have been identified, depending on the half-life of the protein involved. Relatively short-lived proteins form a Schiff base which undergoes an Amadori rearrangement, with the formation of a stable, but still chemically reversible, sugar–protein adduct. Structural proteins with a slower turnover, such as collagen, myelin, crystallins and elastin, accumulate different products derived from slow reactions of dehydration, degradation and rearrangement of the Amadori adducts, to form chemically irreversible advanced glycation end-products [177, 178]. Non-enzymatic glycation is thus likely to affect the glomerular basement membrane (GBM) and other matrix components in the glomerulus.

The pathophysiological consequences of this process are unsettled, but several possibilities have been suggested. Excess GBM glycation, as seen in diabetes, may lead to an increase in the degree of disulphide bridge cross-linking

between collagen components via increased oxidation of sulphydryl groups. This process may induce molecular rearrangement and has been implicated in cataract formation in the lens [179]. Similar crosslinking by disulphide bonds might affect the assembly and architecture of GBM and mesangial matrix. It has also been shown that advanced glycation end-products are capable of extensive crosslinking throughout the collagen molecule. Rotary shadowing electron microscopy of glycated basement membrane components has revealed increased collagen IV crosslinking and altered molecular morphology [178]. It is noteworthy that the compound aminoguanidine, which blocks the formation of advanced glycation end-products, has been shown to prevent, in Lewis alloxan-diabetic rats, both the increased aortic collagen crosslinking and the crosslinking of collagen to lipoproteins, as well as the thickening of GBM and the glomerular trapping of IgG molecules [178].

However, the pathogenic consequences of enhanced crosslinking in the kidney remain obscure. The reaction of glycation may theoretically enhance the binding of circulating plasma proteins to structural components in the GBM and mesangial matrix by the presence of the reactive carbonyl group on the glucose attached to these structures. It has been suggested that this increased binding may account for the linear deposition of albumin and IgG observed along glomerular and tubular basement membranes in diabetes [180]. Glycation of structural proteins or of circulating proteins trapped in the glomerular structures may interfere with their degradation. Degradation of fibrin by plasmin has been found to be reduced by glycation [181]. Reduced degradation of glomerular components may result in mesangial matrix and GBM accumulation and expansion. Other glycoproteins, such as fibronectin, which are found in the mesangial matrix and are involved in the control of cell growth, replication and adhesion, are also susceptible to non-enzymatic glycation. This process has been shown to interfere, in vitro, with the binding characteristics of fibronectin, inhibiting its adhesion to matrix components [182] and enhancing its binding to GBM [183]. In vivo this phenomenon may result in alterations in the integrity and adhesive properties of the matrix and promote the development of selectivity defects in the capillary barrier. It has been claimed that an alteration of the charge distribution of glycated albumin could provide a mechanism for the abnormal flux of modified albumin across the glomerular membrane [184]. However, these results have not been confirmed by Nakamura and Myers [185], who were unable to show differences in the isoelectric point distribution of glycated and non-glycated albumin. Recently, a membrane-associated macrophage receptor that specifically recognizes advanced glycation end-products in proteins has been identified [186]. This receptor enables the selective removal of senescent crosslinked denatured proteins. The binding of this receptor to protein with advanced glycation end-products induces macrophage monokine (interleukin 1 and tumour necrosis factor) synthesis, which in turn stimulates nearby mesenchymal cells to synthesize extracellular proteases. These monokines also initiate a cascade of stimuli and interactions, the end result of which is an increased protein synthesis and cell proliferation, and, in the endothelium, an increased vascular permeability [178].

In conclusion, excessive formation of glycation products in the glomerulus may lead to enhanced deposition of GBM-like material and circulating proteins in the mesangium, interfere with mesangial clearance mechanisms and alter the macrophage removal system, and so contribute to mesangial expansion and glomerular occlusion.

The Polyol Pathway

Sorbitol is produced in cells from glucose by a reaction catalysed by aldose reductase. In the normal kidney, aldose reductase is present in the papilla, glomerular epithelial cells, distal tubular cells, and probably mesangial cells [187, 188]. The physiological significance of aldose reductase is difficult to define in many tissues, but in the renal medullary cells of the kidney its primary role seems to be the generation of sorbitol, and organic osmolyte, in response to the high salinity in the medullary interstitium. Sorbitol would aid in preventing osmotic stress [189]. It has been argued that, in tissues in which glucose entry into cells is insulin independent, more glucose becomes available for reduction by aldose reductase, resulting in an increased sorbitol and/or a reduced intracellular myo-inositol concentration. These changes might contribute

to diabetic complications, via an upset of cellular osmoregulation [190, 191]. Depletion of tissue myo-inositol has been observed in association with enhanced activity of the polyol pathway in sciatic nerve, lens, retina and glomeruli of humans and animals [192].

A series of trials has been carried out with various aldose reductase inhibitors, with the aim of blocking the intracellular conversion of glucose to sorbitol and thus preventing some complications of diabetes. In glomeruli obtained from diabetic rats, the increased flux through the polyol pathway, with accumulation of sorbitol, depletion of myo-inositol and reduced Na^+-K^+-ATPase activity, has been shown to be preventable by the administration of the aldose reductase inhibitor sorbinil. The increased GFR and proteinuria in rats with streptozotocin-induced diabetes have also been reported to be reduced by inhibitors of aldose reductase or by supplementation of myo-inositol [193–195]. These studies, however, were not confirmed by a more recent report, and have been criticized because large volumes of saline were infused during clearance studies, kidney haemodynamics were factored for body weight, diabetes was of short duration, and total urinary protein rather than albumin was measured [196]. There is some evidence that renal clearance of low molecular weight proteins may be affected to a greater degree by sorbinil than the clearance of proteins the size of albumin or larger, which more directly reflect glomerular barrier permeability function [195]. It has also been suggested that sorbinil may act as a vasoconstrictor [197, 198] and may lower renal prostaglandin synthesis [199], thereby modifying renal haemodynamics independently of the aldose reductase pathway. It is of interest that sulindac, a potent inhibitor of prostanoid synthesis, also blocks aldose reductase, suggesting that certain aldose reductase inhibitors may have similarity of action with non-steroidal anti-inflammatory drugs [200]. Although sorbinil has been shown to prevent renal hypertrophy in galactose-fed rats [201], all authors concur that aldose reductase inhibitors have no effect on the increased kidney weight of streptozotocin-induced diabetes. Moreover, the histological lesions of glomerular disease after 6 months of diabetes in the rat were unaffected by the administration of statil, another aldose reductase inhibitor [202].

In contrast to these data of relative inefficacy

of statil on renal function and structure, Tilton et al [203] reported, using three different aldose reductase inhibitors, a reduction in the clearance of ethylenediaminetetraacetic acid (EDTA) labelled with chromium 51 in albuminuria and in the permeation of ^{125}I-labelled bovine serum albumin into the vascular wall in the streptozotocin-diabetic Sprague-Dawley rat. These authors concluded that 'virtually all of the early functional and structural renal and vascular changes associated with diabetes in animals are aldose reductase-linked phenomena'. The same group has also shown that myo-inositol-supplemented diets that raise plasma myo-inositol levels fivefold, reduce or normalize GFR, renal blood flow, urinary protein excretion and serum albumin permeation of blood vessels [192].

This diversity of effects of aldose reductase inhibitors persists in the few studies carried out in humans. Reductions of GFR [204] and albumin excretion rates [205] have been claimed in IDDM patients, but no effects have been reported in a controlled study of microalbuminuric NIDDM subjects [206].

Biochemical Abnormalities of Extracellular Matrix

Diabetic glomerulopathy is characterized by an excessive accumulation of glomerular basement membrane and mesangial matrix. Studies in diabetic animals suggest that the rates of matrix and GBM synthesis are significantly accelerated. Collagen represents a major component of extracellular membranes, and its biosynthesis, measured by the incorporation of radiolabelled amino acids, has been shown to be increased in diabetic rats [207]. The activity of protocollagen lysyl hydroxylase, an enzyme involved in the hydroxylation of peptide-bound lysine during collagen biosynthesis [208], has been found to be increased in the glomeruli of diabetic rats. These abnormalities can be prevented by insulin therapy started at the time of induction of diabetes.

Synthesis of the non-collagenous moieties of the GBM and GBM-like material can be measured by the rate of glucosamine, galactose and sulphate incorporation into GBM sialoglycoproteins and glycosaminoglycans, its two major carbohydrate constituents. Glycosaminoglycan polysaccharides account for approximately 90% of the total carbohydrate component of GBM, with sialoproteins constituting the remainder. The principal glycosaminoglycan in the GBM is heparan sulphate which, together with sialic acid, contributes to the negative charge of the glomerular capillary wall, and thereby the charge-selectivity properties of the filtration barrier [209, 210]. In diabetes there is reduced de novo synthesis of glomerular heparan sulphate, and the total glycosaminoglycan content in the glomerulus and GBM is reduced [211–215]. The heparan sulphate content of the GBM has been found to be decreased in IDDM patients with nephropathy [216]. Moreover, findings in studies of both diabetic humans and experimental diabetic animals have also consistently reported a reduction in sialic acid components [217–219]. Sialoglycoproteins are highly negatively charged and coat glomerular epithelial cells, their foot processes and the epithelial slit diaphragm. A loss of negative charge of the glomerular membrane may be responsible for foot-process fusion with consequent obliteration of the slit diaphragm, and could partly explain the albuminuria of diabetic nephropathy (see pathology section).

Abnormalities in carbohydrate components of the GBM in diabetes remain more controversial. An increase in the hydroxylysine content of the GBM, as well as in the glucose and galactose disaccharide units attached to hydroxylysine residues, has been described. Elevated activity of the enzyme glycosyltransferase, responsible for the attachment of glucose to the glycoprotein, has also been reported. A number of other studies, however, have failed to confirm these findings [217–222].

Glucotoxicity

Direct pathogenetic effects of glucose itself have only recently been described. Lorenzi et al [223, 224] have demonstrated convincingly that cultured human endothelial cells after prolonged, although not acute, exposure to high ambient glucose concentrations display consistent alterations in cell replication and maturation, which cannot be ascribed to abnormalities of the polyol pathway [225]. These abnormalities in cultured endothelial cells are associated with evidence of damage to DNA [226], which has also been demonstrated in peripheral blood lymphocytes from poorly controlled diabetic patients, but not from those with better control

[227]. Furthermore, high glucose can be shown to enhance the expression in cultured endothelial cells of those glycoproteins characteristically increased in diabetic basement membrane [228]. Similarly, cultured human endothelial cells show abnormal expression of tissue factor mRNA in response to thrombin and interleukin 1 after prolonged exposure to high glucose concentrations [229].

Whether glucose exerts a direct toxic effect on human endothelial cells in vivo is currently unknown, but it is of interest that abnormalities of endothelial cell function have been implicated in the increased frequency of cardiovascular disease which is a feature of diabetic nephropathy. It has been shown that such abnormalities, evidenced by raised plasma von Willebrand factor [230] and decreased release of tissue plasminogen activator in response to exercise [231], are present even before overt nephropathy develops.

Haemodynamic and Hypertrophic Pathways

Glomerular haemodynamic disturbances with an elevation of flows and pressures occur early in the course of diabetes. These alterations have been suggested to be directly responsible for the development of glomerulosclerosis and its attendant proteinuria [232]. The notion that increments in GFR, renal plasma flow (RPF) and glomerular capillary hydraulic pressure produce diabetic glomerular injury is based on several observations. Mesangial expansion and mesangial accumulation of circulating plasma proteins were found to be greater in uninephrectomized diabetic rats, in whom abnormalities of renal haemodynamics are known to occur, compared with control animals without unilateral nephrectomy [233], suggesting that altered microcirculatory dynamics may affect the rate of development of glomerular lesions. The induction of systemic hypertension in the diabetic rat, by the two-kidney one-clip Goldblatt hypertension model, resulted in the development of much more severe glomerular lesions in the unclipped kidney than in the kidneys of normotensive diabetic control animals [234]. The clipped kidney showed lesser degrees of glomerular damage than the kidney of diabetic control rats. Autopsy findings in two diabetic men with hypertension and unilateral renal artery stenosis showed nodular glomerulosclerotic lesions to be confined to the kidney with the patent renal artery, while the contralateral kidney was spared [235, 236]. Finally, in the diabetic animal model, manoeuvres that lessen disturbed renal haemodynamics, such as low-protein diet or converting-enzyme inhibition, have been shown to prevent the increase in urinary albumin excretion and the glomerular histological lesions that occur in the untreated diabetic control animal [237, 238].

How alterations in the set of glomerular haemodynamic forces lead to mesangial expansion, GBM thickening and, eventually, sclerosis, is uncertain, but several suggestions have been made. Elevated intraglomerular pressure may lead to an increase in mesangial cells and in matrix production, and to GBM thickening via an increase in arteriolar or capillary wall tension, as described in smooth muscle cells exposed to higher pressures [232, 239, 240]. Physical stress and shear forces may damage endothelial and epithelial surfaces and disrupt the normal glomerular barrier, again by analogy to what is believed to occur at sites of turbulence in larger arteries in systemic hypertension [241–243]. The proteinuria associated with disruption of the normal glomerular barrier would lead to accumulation and deposition of plasma proteins and lipoproteins in the mesangial area. Their persistence because of reduced clearance in diabetes [244] might act as a local stimulus for more mesangial matrix production and accumulation [245–247].

The evidence that alterations in local physical forces within the glomerulus lead to later sclerotic changes in diabetes is, however, debatable and has been recently questioned [248]. A dissociation between the haemodynamic changes and the subsequent sclerosis has been reported in a number of studies. Severely hyperglycaemic rats develop renal sclerotic changes, even though they have no evidence of raised pressures and flows early in the course of diabetes [170, 249]. Bank et al [250], in a study of two strains of diabetic rats, found no relationship between levels of glomerular hyperfiltration and pressure and subsequent degree of glomerular sclerosis. Lowering high lipid levels in the Zucker rat model has been reported to protect against renal sclerosis without affecting haemodynamics [251]. Moreoover, manoeuvres which affect renal haemodynamics also have marked effects on other cell functions. Unilateral nephrectomy, for instance, is a potent stimulus for glomerular hypertrophy and hyperplasia [252], and Gold-blatt hypertension leads to (compensatory) hypertrophy in the unclipped kidney [253]. Hypertrophic changes in the glomerulus have been shown to be invariably related to subsequent glomerular sclerosis [248]. It is of interest that marked renal hypertrophy is a very early event in diabetes. Treatments that modify renal haemodynamics and the degree of glomerular sclerosis also affect the accompanying glomerular hypertrophy. Low-protein diets and angiotensin converting enzyme inhibitors significantly attenuate the renal hypertrophy associated with nephrectomy or streptozotocin-induced diabetes [254–256]. In certain animal models of renal disease, reduction of hypertrophic and sclerotic changes has been obtained independently of modification of renal haemodynamics; and agents that affect glomerular and mesangial cell proliferation but are not known to have haemodynamic effects have been shown to ameliorate glomerular sclerosis [257–264]. It has been argued that hyperplastic and hypertrophic changes in the diabetic kidney precede the haemodynamic abnormalities [265]. Hypertrophic factors in diabetes may activate mesangial cell proliferation and augment mesangial matrix formation or suppress matrix degradation, giving rise to the histological alterations that are pathognomonic of diabetic glomerulopathy. Perhaps one of the clearest demonstrations linking glomerular hypertrophy to subsequent sclerosis has been obtained using transgenic mice with chronic overexpression of growth hormone and growth hormone releasing factor; these animals develop early enlargement of the glomerulus which is followed by glomerulosclerosis [266].

Familial and Genetic Pathways

In human diabetic renal disease, however, a central question remains to be answered. Why do only a proportion of diabetic patients develop renal failure? If a diabetes-induced abnormality in systemic or local growth promoters, or in haemodynamic forces, were sufficient to cause renal damage, all patients would develop overt renal disease given time. However, this is *not* the case.

Diabetes induces important metabolic, hormonal and growth factor changes. These changes, which are partly related to the degree of glycaemic control, occur in virtually all patients,

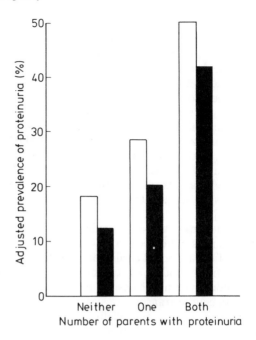

Figure 5 Prevalence of proteinuria in diabetic offspring of diabetic parents with and without proteinuria (open bars, males; solid bars, females). From reference 43, with permission

but to date it has been impossible to isolate a subset of individuals in whom the severity of these environmental perturbations is convincingly linked to the development of renal complications. On the contrary, there is ever-growing evidence that the degree of diabetic control is only a necessary component but is not linearly related to the development of renal failure. Moreover, there is the consistent observation in humans that early renal hypertrophic and haemodynamic changes occur only in a subgroup of subjects. To explain the susceptibility to renal failure in this subgroup it is therefore necessary to formulate an alternative hypothesis which takes into account the host response to diabetes-induced environmental disturbances.

Familial clustering of diabetic kidney disease has been reported. In IDDM, 83% of diabetic siblings of probands with diabetic nephropathy have evidence of nephropathy, compared with only 17% of diabetic siblings of probands without nephropathy, a significant fivefold difference [267]. A familial influence on development of nephropathy has similarly been described in Pima Indians with NIDDM [43] (Figure 5). The findings of these studies are consistent with the postulate that inherited factors play an important part in determining susceptibility to diabetic nephropathy, but do not provide insight into the nature of these factors. A familial predisposition to raised arterial pressure has been suggested by two independent reports as a possible contributing factor to the susceptibility to nephropathy in diabetes. Parents of IDDM subjects with proteinuria were found to have significantly higher arterial pressure than matched parents of non-proteinuric diabetic patients, by some authors [268, 269] but not by all [270].

Further insight into the predisposition to (and mechanisms of) diabetic renal disease and possibly of the attendant cardiovascular disease has come from studies of cell-membrane cation transport systems. Rates of red cell sodium–lithium countertransport, a system of which the activity is largely genetically determined and associated with the risk of essential hypertension [271, 272], have been found to be higher in proteinuric diabetic patients and their parents than in matched, long-term normoalbuminuric controls [269, 273, 274] (Figure 6). The risk of nephropathy seems to be magnified by the combination of a previous history of poor glycaemic control and the possession of a high sodium–lithium countertransport activity [269]. Micro-albuminuric diabetic patients, a group at increased risk of overt nephropathy, have also been found to have higher rates of sodium–lithium countertransport [275]. Moreover, an association has been described between plasma lipoprotein levels and sodium–lithium counter-transport activity in insulin dependent patients without persistent clinical proteinuria. Higher rates of sodium–lithium countertransport were associated with elevated LDL cholesterol, total and VLDL triglycerides and with reduced HDL_2 cholesterol concentrations [276]. The mechanisms of the association between sodium–lithium countertransport activity, hypertension and lipid abnormalities in the context of susceptibility to diabetic renal and vascular disease are obscure, but could be related to factors involved in the control of insulin sensitivity [277]. In a study of short-term, non-clinically proteinuric diabetic patients with arterial hypertension (blood pressure greater than 140/90 mmHg), the hypertensive patients with higher rates of sodium–lithium countertransport were more insulin resistant, and

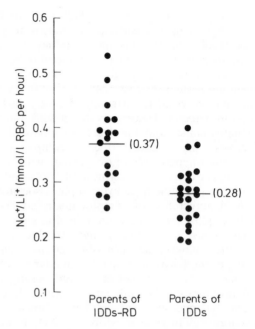

Figure 6 Red blood cell sodium–lithium countertransport rates in parents of insulin-dependent diabetic patients with and without diabetic nephropathy. Mid-parental values of 40 parents in each group are shown. IDDs, insulin dependent diabetic patients; IDDs-RD, insulin dependent diabetic patients with renal disease. From reference 274, with permission

in addition had higher albumin excretion rates, increased total-body exchangeable sodium, enlarged kidneys and left ventricular hypertrophy [278]. These associations were independent of the actual level of blood pressure or the duration of arterial hypertension. These findings suggest that it is the diabetic hypertensive patient with high sodium–lithium countertransport who displays those features (i.e. albuminuria, left ventricular and renal hypertrophy, and insulin resistance) that have been related to renal and vascular injury [117, 279–281]. This combination of risk factors may not be confined to the diabetic population but may be a manifestation of a syndrome also described in the general population [282].

It is believed that sodium–lithium countertransport is one mode of operation of the physiological sodium–hydrogen antiport, a system crucial in the control of intracellular pH, cell growth and the renal reabsorption of sodium, and thus in the regulation of blood pressure [283]. Recently, leukocytes and cultured skin fibroblasts from IDDM patients with albuminuria have been reported to have elevated sodium–hydrogen antiport activity [284, 285]. Moreover, an increased [³H]thymidine incorporation into DNA of skin fibroblasts of diabetic patients with nephropathy has been documented [284]. These findings are consistent with the view that cells of diabetic patients who develop nephropathy have an intrinsic enhanced capacity to proliferate, and that this phenomenon is associated with high rates of sodium–hydrogen exchanger activity. Of note is that phases of growth of the whole body, such as puberty in humans, are associated with insulin resistance [286]. Thus the activity of the sodium–hydrogen antiport seems to act as an indicator of some mechanism, possibly genetically determined, controlling cell growth and hypertrophy on the one hand, and intracellular sodium homeostasis on the other. The environmental changes brought about by diabetes could lead to dysregulation of these mechanisms in susceptible individuals, and induce cell hypertrophy and hyperplasia contributing in the kidney to glomerular hypertrophy and mesangial expansion, as well as tubular hypertrophy and hyperplasia. An increased renal sodium reabsorption would augment systemic and renal perfusion pressure to maintain sodium balance. The increased perfusion pressure would be readily transmitted to the glomerular capillaries because of the general vasodilation present in diabetes [287]. This would lead to increased intraglomerular pressure which determines, at least in part, the increase in GFR, and may be responsible for the disruption of glomerular membrane permeability properties generating proteinuria. On the other hand, progressive mesangial expansion would lead to glomerulosclerosis and further disruption of GBM membrane permselective properties. The insulin resistance associated with excessive growth and the consequent hyperinsulinaemia may cause lipid abnormalities that, in the setting of the vascular hyperpermeability characteristic of diabetic microvascular disease [288], would further aggravate the renal histological damage [289] and contribute, in combination with hypertension, to the accelerated atherosclerosis of diabetic renal failure. That insulin resistance is associated with increased cardiovascular events has been reported in the general population [290]. The sequence of phenomena just described could trigger a vicious cycle of events producing reduction in renal function, more hypertension, more proteinuria, more severe glomerulosclerosis, more hyperlipidaemia and eventually renal failure and cardiovascular death (Figure 7).

PATHOPHYSIOLOGY OF DIABETIC NEPHROPATHY

Pathophysiology of Glomerular Hyperfiltration

Several studies using accurate techniques for estimating GFR have confirmed that in subjects with IDDM, GFR is elevated by 20–40% above normal. The investigation of the intrarenal haemodynamic basis for hyperfiltration is easier in animal models of IDDM that in humans because of the ability to make direct measurements in single nephrons of the major determinants of GFR: renal plasma flow, transglomerular hydraulic pressure gradient (P) with a filtration coefficient (K_F), and oncotic pressure. Both sources of data are used in this chapter.

Renal plasma flow (RPF), one of the major determinants of GFR, has been reported as elevated, normal or reduced in human IDDM [61, 70, 72]. However, most recent work shows an elevation of RPF between 9% and 14% [73], which is less than the elevation of GFR. Several studies have demonstrated a good correlation between the increases in RPF and GFR in diabetic patients [71, 75, 78]. These findings suggest that at least part of the increased GFR is accounted for by elevation of the RPF.

Increased renal plasma flow, however, does not explain the whole rise in GFR. In human studies where GFR and RPF were measured simultaneously, RPF accounted for about 50–60% of the GFR increase [71, 74]. Increased filtration fraction, sometimes associated with elevated urinary albumin excretion, in short-term IDDM patients, is compatible with the suggestion that intraglomerular pressure may be elevated under these circumstances [70, 92].

Direct measurements of *hydraulic filtration pressure* cannot be obtained in humans, but micropuncture studies in moderately hyperglycaemic rats have shown a significant increase in the transglomerular pressure gradient [237, 255], although this has not always been confirmed [291, 292]. Severely hyperglycaemic rats show no elevation in intraglomerular pressure [255, 291, 293]. In the rat model, analysis of the arteriolar vasculature has shown that increases in both

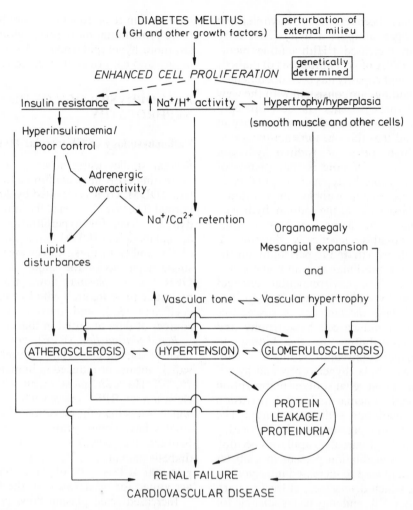

Figure 7 Hypothetical sequence of events leading to renal and cardiovascular disease in a subset of diabetic patients

flow and pressure are achieved by a reduction of total arteriolar vascular resistance, more marked at the afferent than at the efferent end of the arteriole [255]. These findings have a counterpart in diabetic humans with glomerular hyperfiltration, whose calculated renal vascular resistance is reduced [294]. However, the renal lesion in the rat model is that of focal segmental glomerular sclerosis, not of diabetic nephropathy, and not all strains of rats develop hyperfiltration and increased glomerular pressure (see pathogenesis). The elevation in glomerular transcapillary hydraulic pressure difference appears, therefore, to account for a further proportion of the rise in GFR, estimated at approximately 25%.

A third determination of GFR is the *glomerular ultrafiltration coefficient*, the product of the capillary hydraulic conductivity and the capillary surface area available for filtration. Although in animal studies the calculated glomerular ultrafiltration coefficient did not account for the increased filtration rate [255, 291, 292], filtration surface area has been found to be increased in IDDM patients [295] as well as in diabetic rats [171], and a significant correlation has been described between GFR and filtration surface area in young IDDM patients [296]. Thus, an increase in the surface area available for filtration (a component of the ultrafiltration coefficient) may be a determinant of the elevation of the GFR. Changes in GFR can occur with changes in metabolic control [67, 93, 294], within a time period that might not appear sufficient to alter the filtration surface area as assessed by conventional morphological techniques [295]. However, filtration surface area may dynamically be affected by mesangial contraction in response to vasoactive stimuli such as angiotensin II. A reduction of angiotensin II receptor density has been demonstrated in diabetic rats [297]. A close correlation has been found between GFR and kidney size. Kidney size, which is enlarged in 40% of IDDM patients, has been found to be related to changes in transglomerular pressure gradient and filtration surface area [298].

A fourth determinant of GFR is *systemic oncotic pressure*, which has been reported to be normal both in human [299] and animal diabetes [255].

Metabolic and Hormonal Mediators of GFR Elevation

Glucose and Ketone Bodies

The elevation of GFR appears to be multifactorial. Hyperfiltration is a phenomenon that occurs under conditions of moderate hyperglycaemia, as severe hyperglycaemia exceeding 14–16 mmol/l is associated, not with an elevated GFR, but with normal or reduced glomerular filtration [66, 255, 300]. In unselected groups of IDDM patients with baseline GFR ranging from normal to high, increasing blood glucose concentration to an average of 16 mmol/l by intravenous glucose infusion leads to an average GFR rise of approximately 5% [299]. Other studies show that only those diabetic patients with baseline glomerular hyperfiltration increase their GFR significantly (on average by 12%) in response to intravenous glucose [294]. In normal individuals, blood glucose elevations are associated with either an increase [299, 301, 302] or no change in the GFR [294]. These differences may depend at least in part on the level of glycaemia achieved. High blood glucose levels may induce vasodilation, and this has been shown to occur in the retinal circulation [303]. A similar mechanism might apply to the glomerular arterioles. In rats, hyperglycaemia and glycosuria, both separately and additively, affect the tubuloglomerular feedback mechanism by blunting the GFR reduction in response to increased proximal tubular flow through a reduced sodium flux across the macula densa, thus producing relative hyperfiltration [304]. An increase in glucose-coupled reabsorption of sodium and water in the proximal tubule may also cause an increase in GFR [305]. Recently, infusion of ketone bodies in supraphysiological doses in diabetic patients has been shown to cause an increase of GFR of about 33%, the single most powerful effect so far described. This effect was accompanied by a concomitant rise of about 16% in renal plasma flow and a 14% increase in the filtration fraction [306].

Insulin, Growth Hormone and Glucagon

In addition to the altered level of glucose and other metabolites found in diabetes, a number of changes in circulating levels as well as in vascular responsiveness to metabolic fuel-related and vasoactive hormones may be seen in diabetes. Acute reduction of blood glucose level in diabetic patients by insulin infusion reduces the GFR within 30–60 minutes, but the effect is small (about 6%) [307]. This reduction of the elevated GFR and RPF by insulin infusion does not occur if blood glucose is maintained at euglycaemic levels by concomitant glucose infusion [308]. Euglycaemic insulin infusion in normal humans is not associated with changes in either GFR or RPF [309, 310]. These findings have been interpreted as indicating that insulin per se has no effect on GFR and RPF. Daily administration of growth hormone for some days, although not by acute infusion [311], increases GFR and RPF in normal subjects [312, 313] and in IDDM patients [314] by 7% and 6% respectively in the face of unchanged glycaemic control. However, a correlation between plasma growth hormone concentration and GFR has not been found in unselected diabetic patients [315], and hyperfiltering diabetic subjects have diurnal profiles of growth hormone not dissimilar from those of diabetic subjects with a normal GFR [316]. Intravenous infusion of glucagon to reach plasma levels found in poorly controlled diabetics raises GFR both in normal [317] and diabetic [318] subjects. In diabetic patients, this increase is accompanied by an equivalent rise in RPF, with a significant relationship between RPF and GFR. However, circulating levels of glucagon were found to be no higher throughout the day in hyperfiltering diabetic patients than in patients with a normal GFR [316]. It is controversial whether glucagon infused into the renal artery causes consistent modification of GFR, but intraportal infusion of the hormone induces a significant rise [319, 320]. Recent evidence suggests that the glucagon effect on renal haemodynamics may be mediated through renal prostaglandin production [321].

Prostaglandins

Small elevations of plasma renin activity, coupled with increased urinary excretion of 6-keto $PGF_{1\alpha}$, have been described recently in IDDM patients wtih glomerular hyperfiltration [322]. Other authors, however, have found in similar patients significantly lower levels of plasma renin activity and normal levels of urinary prostaglandin excretion [323]. In streptozotocin-diabetic rats, both the circulating levels of renin and the glomeruli angiotensin II receptor density were found to be reduced [297], suggesting that the expected upregulation of receptors with suppression of renin did not occur. Other workers have provided evidence in the animal model that renal prostaglandin production may be important in the genesis of glomerular hyperfiltration. In the isolated perfused kidney, the increased GFR and the vasodilation in response to hyperglycaemia have been found to be blocked by indomethacin infusion, implicating renal prostanoids as possible mediators of this effect [324]. Administration of indomethacin to diabetic animals has been found to cause a significant reduction in GFR and RPF [325], and an increased synthesis of prostaglandins in isolated glomeruli taken from diabetic rats has been described [326]. Aspirin administration to streptozotocin-diabetic rats prevented early hyperfiltration as well as the decrease in GFR and accompanying increase in GBM thickness at 16 weeks in the control animals [327].

The predominance of the prostaglandin system is further supported by the finding that inhibition of prostaglandin production by acetyl-salicylate reduces GFR in hyperfiltering IDDM patients [323]. However, short-term administration of indomethacin to recently diagnosed patients has been reported not to affect GFR [328]. A reduction in GFR in response to indomethacin administration was, however, found in persistently proteinuric IDDM patients

[329], as has been reported for other non-diabetic renal disease.

Glomerulopressin and Atrial Natriuretic Peptide

Some authors have postulated that an hepatic product could be responsible for the increased GFR. This substance, which has been named *glomerulopressin*, is thought to be a glucuronic acid conjugate [330], and has been reported to be increased in dogs with diabetes [320]. In diabetic rats, raised levels of *atrial natriuretic peptide* (ANP) have been found to be associated with glomerular hyperfiltration and intraglomerular hypertension. Reduction of plasma ANP levels by antibody blockade led to a parallel fall in GFR. It has been postulated that diabetes-induced volume expansion (as seen on average in these animals) may mediate the rise in ANP levels, which in turn could elevate the GFR [331]. Atrial natriuretic peptide levels have been reported to be higher in hyperfiltering diabetic patients [332–334], but these findings were not confirmed by other authors [335]. Conflicting results in patients with microalbuminuria and persistent proteinuria have also been produced [333, 334, 336]. Similarly, extracellular fluid volume has been found by different authors to be normal or expanded [335–338].

In conclusion, metabolic and hormonal mechanisms acting both systemically and locally are likely to be involved in the GFR alteration of diabetes. The effects of a number of mediators, themselves small, may combine to induce the observed GFR elevations. These disturbances are not only related to the diabetic state, but seem specifically to affect the function of susceptible kidneys in diabetes.

Pathophysiology of Renal Hypertrophy

Patients with IDDM have on average larger kidneys than control subjects, and animals made diabetic develop kidney enlargement within days of the induction of diabetes. Whole kidney weight increases by an average of 15% within the first 3 days of diabetes, and parallel increases in protein and RNA content of the kidney are observed. DNA synthesis remains stable for the first 3 days but increases thereafter [81, 265]. Insulin treatment started soon after the induction of diabetes is capable of preventing the increment in kidney weight [80], but if insulin treatment is started after 28 days the enlargement of the kidney is not reversed [81]. When near-normoglycaemia is achieved by islet transplantation after 4 weeks of diabetes, a partial reduction in kidney size and normalization of RNA/DNA ratio is obtained [171]. This situation resembles the findings in human diabetic patients, in whom good metabolic control at onset of diabetes appears capable of reducing kidney size [74], whereas chronic strict metabolic control for up to 1 year in longer-term diabetic patients with established kidney enlargement does not seem to have any effect on kidney volume [67, 68, 79]. In the animal model, glomerular growth is prominent during the first 4 days following induction of diabetes. Tubular growth then catches up and eventually exceeds the glomerular growth over the first 6 weeks after onset of diabetes [339]. Glomerular capillary length appears to be the earliest change, and is followed in the succeeding weeks by increases in the radial cross-sectional area of the capillary loop, which eventually becomes the dominant change for the increased glomerular size [340]. Both proximal and distal tubule lengths increase by about 20%, but whereas proximal tubular cells retain their normal appearance, the distal cells in the cortex and outer medullary stripe appear laden with glycogen-like granules, and show a marked reduction in the number of organelles and basal infoldings [341]. Some authors believe that these morphological changes precede the early haemodynamic alterations and in fact may be contributory to them [265, 342].

Pathophysiology of Microalbuminuria

In a percentage of IDDM patients, urinary albumin excretion rate is increased above the upper limit of normal but is still undetectable by current routine clinical tests. Exaggerated excretion of albumin can also be induced by periods of poor metabolic control [93] or by moderately strenuous exercise [108, 109]. In these situations microalbuminuria is not accompanied by an increase in the excretion rate of β_2-microglobulin, a protein that is freely filtered across the glomerular capillary barrier and almost entirely reabsorbed by proximal tubular cells, so reflecting proximal tubular function [343, 344]. The consistency of normal β_2-microglobulin excretion rate in the face of augmented albumin excretion rate suggests that the excess albuminuria is not the result of

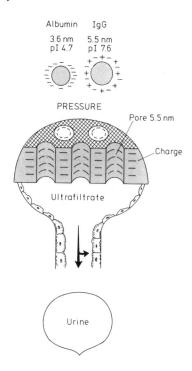

Figure 8 Glomerular filter showing contribution of pore size and charge to the filtration of circulating protein macromolecules

a change in tubular reabsorption of the protein, but more probably derives from increased glomerular leakage.

Glomerular Filter

The glomerular capillary blood–urine barrier can be regarded functionally as a membrane perforated by pores of an average size of 5.5 nm and uniformly coated by a negative electrical charge [209, 345–348] (Figure 8). Therefore, both the size and charge of the circulating molecule, as well as the set of haemodynamic forces operating across the capillary wall, determine the passage of proteins and other molecules across the glomerular membrane. In microalbuminuric diabetic patients, the fractional clearances of albumin, a polyanion with molecular radius of about 3.6 nm, and of IgG, a larger but electrically neutral molecule with radius of around 5.5 nm, are both increased [349, 350]. These early increases are likely to be the consequence of alterations in glomerular haemodynamics and, in particular, of transglomerular pressure gradient which is elevated in moderately hyperglycaemic diabetic rats [237, 255, 325]. This is consistent with the findings in humans of an increased filtration fraction in poorly controlled diabetic patients [70, 78, 93] and of a raised absolute urinary clearance of neutral dextran over a wide range of molecular weights in parallel with the elevated glomerular filtration rate [351].

As microalbuminuria becomes persistent and increases in degree, the selectivity index—the clearance of IgG as a proportion of the clearance of albumin—starts to fall, reaching its lowest values when albumin excretion is around 90 µg/min or higher. This is due to a disproportionate increase in the filtration of albumin compared with that of IgG, and it marks a new selective stage of glomerular leakage of anionic albumin [349, 350]. Experiments with clearances of neutral dextrans have shown that medium-size pores are unchanged at this stage [70, 348]. A probable reason for the increased glomerular filtration of albumin is a loss of the fixed negative electrical charge on the membrane [211, 217, 352, 353]. This would permit increased permeation of anionic albumin, with its smaller molecular weight, but would have little influence on IgG, a larger neutral molecule, the filtration of which is regulated by pore radius or number, and by glomerular pressures and flows. The mechanism of this transition from low to high levels of microalbuminuria is unknown, but may result from a combination of haemodynamic abnormalities with the cumulative derangement of synthesis of the electronegative membrane glycosialoproteins and proteoglycans [212, 232, 350, 354]. Recent studies suggest, however, that preferential filtration on the basis of charge discrimination due to loss of glomerular polyanion does not entirely explain the facilitated clearance of anionic proteins. Permeation of both large and medium-sized molecules through a shunt pathway that is not size-discriminatory could account for the observed renal clearances of albumin, IgG and dextrans [185]. An alternative suggestion is that the facilitated clearance of anionic proteins, including IgG_4 [355], may reflect an increased expression of cationic sites on the glomerular filter, rather than a loss of glomerular polyanion [356]. This would be compatible with the consistent finding of a linear deposition of anionic albumin and IgG_4 in the diabetic glomerular basement membrane [357].

Glycation and Filtration

Exposure of structural and circulating proteins to high glucose concentrations increases the rate of their non-enzymatic glycation [358, 359]. Recent studies indicate that microvessels isolated from rat epididymal fat pads preferentially take up glycated rat albumin by endocytosis; glycation of endothelial membrane components seems to enhance this process of pinocytosis even further [360]. Two recent reports seem to indicate that glycated proteins (including albumin) may undergo preferential transport across the glomerular barrier [184, 361]. The reason for this facilitated flux of glycated macromolecules through the glomerular membrane barrier remains unknown, but it is possible that conformational changes such as those induced by glycation are important [362].

The transition to high-selectivity proteinuria signals the advent of heavier proteinuria. This may indicate the critical importance of the loss of the charge barrier in the unfolding sequence of pathogenic events.

The Concomitants of Microalbuminuria

The positive association between urine flow and albumin excretion [363, 364] has led to the suggestion that glucose-induced diuresis could impair proximal tubular reabsorption of albumin, as it does for several other solutes. However, rat albumin excretion by the kidney is unaffected by osmotic diuresis, whereas it is increased after volume expansion, probably through a change in the GFR [365]. In the diabetic human, there is no correlation between glycosuria and urinary albumin excretion [91, 366]. The transient microalbuminuria seen in normal subjects after water loading is likely to be mediated, as in the volume-expanded rat, by transient changes in glomerular filtration rate [367]. Whether acute worsening of glycaemia by glucose ingestion or infusion increases albumin excretion rate remains somewhat controversial. Glucose ingestion has been reported to increase albuminuria in normal subjects but not in diabetic patients [366]. A number of other studies have failed to show any acute effect of either oral or intravenous glucose on urinary albumin excretion [299, 368]. Mild metabolic acidosis has no effect on urinary albumin excretion but increases the excretion of β_2-microglobulin [306].

Table 3 Associations of microalbuminuria in diabetic patients

Variable	Effect
Sex	More frequent in males 2 : 1 ratio
Duration of diabetes	Very rare in first 5 years
Arterial pressure	Raised compared with matched normoalbuminuric IDDM patients but may be still within 'normal' range
Serum lipoproteins	'Atherogenic' profile
Exercise	May increase albumin excretion rate
Poor glycaemic control	May increase albumin excretion rate
Transcapillary escape rate of albumin	Increased
Red blood cell Na^+/Li^+ countertransport activity	Increased in IDDM patients with microalbuminuria as a group
Diabetic retinopathy	Associated

Although a bolus intravenous injection of insulin was reported to increase urinary albumin excretion [307], these findings have not been reproduced [308, 369]. Neither glucagon nor growth hormone affects urinary albumin excretion in normal or in diabetic subjects [313, 314, 317, 318].

A consistent association of microalbuminuria is with higher levels of arterial pressure. A positive, linear and independent correlation between arterial pressure and albumin excretion rate has been confirmed by several investigators [96, 137]. This association is much closer than that between albumin excretion rate and blood glucose level, and is independent of a number of other variables including age, duration of diabetes, body mass index, sex and blood glucose concentration itself. The observation of higher arterial pressures in microalbuminuric patients without reduced GFR speaks against the assumption that the higher blood pressure is a consequence of renal dysfunction, and argues in favour of a more complex relationship. This raises the possibility either that the rise in blood pressure could be contributory to the renal disease, or alternatively, that microalbuminuria and high blood pressure may both recognize a common determinant. It is of interest that microalbuminuric patients with elevated arterial pressure show significantly more marked mesangial expansion than do patients with a similar duration of diabetes but with lower levels of albumin excretion rate and arterial pressure [117]. Table 3 summarizes some of the clinical and laboratory associations of microalbuminuria.

Pathophysiology of Tubular Function

Changes in tubular function take place early in IDDM diabetes and are related to the degree of metabolic control. Both the maximum rates of glucose reabsorption and absolute rates of sodium reabsorption are elevated in these patients [300]. The increase in sodium reabsorption is probably attributable, at least in part, to its proximal tubular cotransport with glucose [370]. It has been suggested that enhanced proximal tubular reabsorption could diminish distal sodium delivery, and thereby trigger tubuloglomerular feedback mechanisms, which would lead to an increase in glomerular filtration rate [371]. A direct effect of insulin, increasing distal sodium reabsorption, has been shown in both normal [309] and diabetic patients [310]. A number of tubular proteins, such as N-acetyl-β-D-glucosaminidase (NAG), have also been found to be increased in IDDM patients, their elevation being related to the degree of glycaemic control [372, 373]. On the other hand, tubular phosphate absorption is diminished in IDDM patients. The defect in phosphate reabsorption also appears to be related to blood glucose concentration. It has been proposed that there is a competition between these two solutes for tubular reabsorption [374]. Insulin has been shown to reduce the renal clearance of phosphate by stimulating its proximal reabsorption [309, 310]. These abnormalities are rapidly corrected by improvement of blood glucose control and their prospective significance for renal function outcome is largely unknown.

Pathophysiology of the Decline of Glomerular Filtration Rate

In established diabetic nephropathy, GFR declines relentlessly towards end-stage renal failure. The reduction in GFR is accompanied by a reduction in renal plasma flow, filtration fraction remaining relatively constant [352]. Advancing renal disease is associated with progressive mesangial expansion and capillary occlusion. This process, by reducing filtering surface area, would be compatible with the suggestion that a reduction in the ultrafiltration coefficient contributes to the decline in GFR [375]. Although direct measurements of these variables are not possible in humans, indirect calculations, using neutral dextran-sieving curves, support this view [352, 376]. It is believed that in established renal disease the surviving glomeruli filter at or near their maximal capacity. This assumption is consistent with findings that administration of an oral protein load did not induce a further expansion of GFR over baseline values in diabetic patients with impaired renal function [377]. This loss of 'renal functional reserve' has been suggested as one of the possible deleterious mechanisms that would lead to further renal damage. However, it seems more likely that this is a result, not of a general loss of renal reserve, but of a more specific defect in the renal response to protein loading, as other stimuli have been shown to have profound effects on the GFR in patients with diabetic renal failure. Hyperglycaemia, for instance, has been shown to induce a GFR rise of about 50% in these patients [378]. This glucose-induced effect seems to be mediated by changes in renal prostaglandin production, as it can be significantly blunted by cyclo-oxygenase inhibition [379]. Whether, in the setting of renal failure, the higher GFR that accompanies hyperglycaemia represents an advantage or a disadvantage in the long term remains an open question. It is worth noting that correction of hyperglycaemia at this advanced stage of renal disease has no significant impact on the progression of renal failure [121, 128].

As the degree of proteinuria progresses, a change from high-selectivity to low-selectivity proteinuria takes place. When GFR is below 10–20 ml/min, more IgG relative to albumin is filtered, the selectivity index rising from 0.12 to approximately 0.6 [349]. Studies with neutral dextran-sieving curves have demonstrated that the proteinuria of the late stages of overt nephropathy is probably the result of a defect in size-selectivity properties of the glomerular membrane. The fractional clearance of neutral molecules with radii greater than 4.6 nm is elevated, and mathematical analysis indicates that this increase is consistent with the appearance of a 'shunt pathway' within the glomerular capillary wall. The development of a small population of unselective pores would allow the unrestricted movement of very large plasma proteins into the urine. Whether the size-selectivity defect totally explains the proteinuria of advanced nephropathy remains to be established [185, 348, 376]. It is likely that charge selectivity defects, as well as abnormal renal haemodynamics, persist at this stage of advanced nephropathy. It is of interest that the sialic acid component of the glomerular barrier has been found to be reduced in patients with long-standing diabetes [217–219]. Moreover, a reduction in the synthesis of heparan sulphate within the glomerular basement membrane has been described in diabetic animals [211–215], and a loss of heparan sulphate has been demonstrated in the GBM of IDDM patients with nephropathy [216]. This glycosaminoglycan is a major contributor of the fixed negative charge of the glomerular capillary wall.

With advancing renal failure, proteinuria becomes of mixed tubular and glomerular origin. At GFR of 40 ml/min or less, a significant increase in the urinary excretion of β_2-microglobulin is noted [350]. This may represent tubular damage or could be the consequence of saturation of proximal tubular reabsorption capacity for β_2-microglobulin, as a consequence of a greater filtered load per functioning nephron.

Hyperlipidaemia

With advancing renal disease, clear disturbances of plasma lipoproteins take place. Increases in cholesterol, LDL cholesterol, total triglycerides, VLDL triglyceride and apolipoprotein B1 have been described, and HDL_2 cholesterol has been found to be decreased [380–382]. The pathogenic role of these lipid disturbances in the progression of renal failure remains uncertain in human diabetes. However, studies in the diabetic animal model suggest that hyperlipidaemia may contribute to late glomerular sclerotic changes [251].

Recent findings suggest that these lipid changes may not entirely be secondary to heavy proteinuria and advancing renal disease: both micro-albuminuric IDDM [383, 384] and NIDDM [385] patients with normal renal function have also been found to have a similar pattern of lipid abnormalities, although of a lesser degree. It is clearly important now to establish the potential of early correction of the lipid disturbances for prevention of deteriorating renal function as well as of histological damage.

PATHOLOGY

The renal morphological changes associated with diabetes mellitus were first described in 1936 by Kimmelstiel and Wilson [5]. In the early 1940s these findings were confirmed and extended by other workers [386, 387]. Both the early autopsy and biopsy series and later studies [152, 388] have shown that the histological findings in kidneys of IDDM and NIDDM patients are similar.

Light Microscopy

The *nodular lesion* described by Kimmelstiel and Wilson [5] has for a long time been considered virtually specific for diabetes [155, 156]. Reports that it could be found in the absence of diabetes have not stood critical review [389], and some patients may have had the nodular form of light-chain nephropathy.

The nodules are well-demarcated hard masses, eosinophilic and PAS-positive, located in the central regions of peripheral glomerular lobules. When not acellular they contain pyknotic nuclei, and not infrequently foam cells can be seen to surround them. They are relatively homogeneous when stained with haematoxylin, but their structure is laminated when viewed on PAS or reticulin stains. They are characteristically irregular in size and distribution, both within and between glomeruli, and located *away* from the hilus. A rim of mesangial cells can sometimes be seen between them and the adjoining capillary, which is often distended. The location and the morphogenesis of the nodules has been the subject of long dispute, as reflected by the use of both the terms 'intracapillary' and 'intercapillary' to describe them. Recent evidence [390] seems to establish the mesangium as their site of origin, and extends the original sug-gestion that mesangial disruption and lysis of the lobule centre was related to previous micro-aneurysmal dilatation of the associated capillary, followed by a laminar reorganization of the mesangial debris [391].

Although, when present, this lesion is path-ognomonic for diabetes, it is a far from universal finding. Its incidence varies considerably from 12% to 46% in different series which included both IDDM and NIDDM cases, probably due to differences in selection [392]. Nodules have been found in 55% of an autopsy series of Pima NIDDM patients [388]. Nodules are not seen in the absence of the diffuse lesion, and this reflects their appearance only after a long period of disease (14 years in the series of Gellman et al [156]).

The *diffuse glomerular lesion* comprises an increase of the mesangial area and capillary wall thickening, with the mesangial matrix extending to involve the capillary loops. The accumulated material has staining properties similar to that of the nodules. In its early stages it may be difficult to distinguish the minor mesangial expansion from changes present with aging or other glomerular pathology [142]. In more severe cases, the capillary wall thickening and the mesangial expansion lead to capillary narrowing and eventual complete hyalinization. In this advanced state, periglomerular fibrosis is often present. As with the nodules, the distribution of the diffuse lesion is non-uniform, both among lobules of the same glomerulus and between different glomeruli, leading to appearances sug-gestive of transition to nodule formation. The thickening of the capillary walls tends also to be non-uniform, and this is particularly evident when the histological changes are not very severe. This lesion is more frequent than the nodular one, but again its incidence varies in different series [392]. In a large autopsy study, however, changes compatible with diabetic glomerulosclerosis were found in as many as 90% of IDDM patients with disease duration of more than 10 years [143]. In NIDDM patients, the reported prevalences of these changes varies between 25% and 51% [77, 155, 392].

The *exudative lesions* are highly eosinophilic, rounded, homogeneous structures seen in the capsular space, overlying a capillary loop (fibrin cap) or lying on the inside of Bowman's capsule (capsular drop). They are non-specific, contain-ing various proteins and sometimes lipid material, and similar lesions are seen in a variety of other renal conditions.

In IDDM patients, increases in glomerular volume and in luminal volume are noted 1–6 years after diagnosis [393]. Whereas the initial glomerular enlargement is not accompanied by hyperplasia, the number of nuclei in patients with 16 and more years of disease is increased, and the volume of the patient glomeruli becomes even larger. This late hypertrophy has been considered to be distinct from the early one, and may be an expression of compensatory growth in the face of progressive glomerular loss [394, 395]. Although atrophic ischaemic glomeruli are present, some of the non-functioning obsolete glomeruli seem to be filled up with solid PAS-positive material, and preserve their increased dimension. This hypertrophy has not been found in subjects with NIDDM [396], although hyalinized non-atrophic glomeruli can be seen in these patients [143].

Arteriolar lesions are prominent in diabetes, with hyaline material progressively replacing the entire wall structure. Bell [155] first underlined the fact that both afferent *and* efferent arterioles could be affected. He also pointed out that these lesions were often present in the absence of hypertension, and that involvement of the efferent vessel was highly specific for diabetes. These arteriolar changes may be the first detectable change by light microscopy in the diabetic kidney, as judged by their recurrence at 2 years in non-diabetic kidneys transplanted into diabetic patients [397].

The *tubules* and *interstitium* may show a variety of changes which are non-specific and similar to those seen in other forms of progressive renal disease. The *Armanni–Ebstein lesion* is the result of accumulation of glycogen in tubular cells of the corticomedullary region in patients with profound glycosuria, and was common in IDDM before the advent of insulin. More subtle tubular changes, consisting of vacuolization, a decrease in the intercellular spaces normally present between the macula densa cells, and a significant increase in the contact area between them and the extraglomerular mesangial cells of Goormaghtigh, have been described at the ultrastructural level in the streptozotocin-diabetic rat. It was suggested that these changes may represent a morphological counterpart to disturbed tubuloglomerular feedback which might contribute to hyperfiltration in diabetes [398].

Immunopathology

Westberg and Michael [217] confirmed previous observations of thin linear staining of the glomerular basement membrane for IgG, IgM, albumin and fibrinogen in kidneys of IDDM patients, and concluded that it represented a non-specific consequence of increased permeability rather than an expression of immunologic binding. Their findings were later extended, and the presence of thin linear positivity for IgG and albumin, along not only the GBM but also the Bowman's capsule and especially the outer aspect of the tubular basement membrane, was considered specific for diabetes [399]. This assertion has been supported by the demonstration of similar staining in kidneys from non-diabetic donors transplanted into IDDM patients [397].

Immunofluorescence techniques have shown increased mesangial amounts of types IV and V collagen, laminin and fibronectin, and the presence of antigens normally expressed in fetal glomeruli only [400]. Immunochemical analysis has confirmed the increase in type IV collagen, but showed reduced laminin levels and markedly decreased content of the heparan sulphate proteoglycan, whereas fibronectin levels were no different from those in normal controls [216]. Collagens type I [401] and type VI, but not type III [402], have also been described in the diabetic mesangium. Type VI collagen, which is probably synthesized only by mesangial cells and therefore is absent from the basement membrane, has been found to be increased about threefold in longstanding diabetic kidneys when compared with non-diabetic controls [403]. The possibility of anomalies in the contractile properties of the mesangium has been considered following the demonstration of increased amounts of actomyosin [404]. Fibrin products as well as IgG and complement components have also been found in the exudative lesions of the glomerulus and of the arterioles [392], suggesting a role for coagulation processes in the genesis of glomerulosclerosis [217, 405].

Electron Microscopy

Glomerular basement membrane thickening is a prominent finding in the kidneys of patients with diabetes. It has been studied particularly in IDDM subjects, in whom it is absent at diagnosis [406], becoming detectable after 2–5 years of disease [407]. The increased synthesis taking place during this period is reflected in the 80% increase of peripheral capillary wall area found in young IDDM subjects within months of diagnosis [295]. In advanced stages of the disease, the basement membrane can become very thick, particularly so in association with nodular lesions [408]. Whereas in early disease the increase in thickness is even, marked irregularity in its width appears later [409]. Localized areas of electron-lucent material can make up to 10% of total basement membrane volume, and between 1% and 6% of the capillary length is lined by abnormally thin membrane [395]. Throughout all the stages up to sclerosis, features suggestive of immune deposits are absent, although subendothelial fibrilar electron-dense material interpreted as fibrin–fibrinogen products has been described [405].

The foot processes of the epithelial cells in diabetes remain discrete soon after proteinuria has become persistent [410] and until renal function has declined to 20% of normal [395]. At this stage, epithelial cell cytoplasm preserves a healthy appearance and contains prominent organelles (rough endoplasmic reticulum, mitochondria, Golgi vesicles) that may be the expression of continued basement membrane synthesis. However, with further disease progression, the foot processes appear wider in cross-section, and the length of the filtration slits tends to decrease [411]. Aspects suggestive of degenerative changes have also been noted, accompanied by detachment from the underlying basement membrane that is left exposed [412]. Eventually, podocyte effacement and fusion are noted [408].

Although it is normal at diagnosis of IDDM [413], an increase of the fractional volume of the mesangium, initially involving an expansion of the matrix component, follows the thickening of the glomerular basement membrane [414]. Its delicate strands anastomose and widen, and collagen fibrils become detectable with progression of the disease. The core of the typical nodules seems to correspond to local accumulation of these components [415, 416], while their laminated periphery may derive from expanded and folded basement membrane [402]. In more advanced stages of the disease, the number of mesangial nuclei is sometimes increased, and the fractional volume of the mesangium can become more than double the value found in normal controls [375].

The exudative lesions appear on electron

Table 4 Histological lesions characteristically found in patients with diabetic nephropathy

Light microscopy	Electron microscopy
Diffuse glomerular sclerotic lesions with mesangial expansion	Glomerular basement membrane thickening
Nodular lesions	Epithelial foot process widening and detachment
Exudative lesions (capsular drop)	Mesangial expansion
Arteriolar hyalinosis	

microscopy as finely granular electron-dense material. In the arterioles, this material spreads from an initial subintimal location towards the media, sometimes to its near replacement. The 'capsular drop' corresponds to accumulation of this material betwen the epithelial cells and Bowman's capsule basement membrane, whereas the 'fibrin cap' represents its presence along the endothelial side of the glomerular basement membrane [392].

Endothelial cell changes are not prominent in diabetes.

Table 4 summarizes the light- and electron-microscopic changes most commonly found in patients with diabetic nephropathy.

Relationship of Structure and Function

Understanding the relationship between abnormal morphological appearances and altered function may help to clarify the pathogenesis of diabetic kidney disease. Information concerning this important issue is almost totally restricted to patients with IDDM.

Increased glomerular volume is a salient feature in the kidneys of IDDM patients, and is part of a generalized hypertrophic process which also involves the tubules and results in increased kidney volume. Larger glomeruli are probably a necessary condition for the early hyperfiltration of IDDM. Unlike most other renal diseases, relatively large kidneys persist with advancing renal failure in diabetes mellitus.

More than thirty years ago, Gellman et al [156] were the first to show that the nodular lesions are of little functional significance, and that it is the degree of *diffuse glomerulosclerosis*, encompassing changes in the glomerular capillary and the mesangial region, that correlates with the clinical manifestations of worsening renal function. In the early phases of IDDM, the

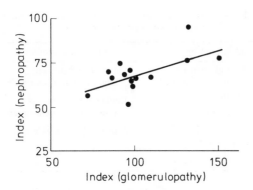

Figure 9 Relationship between an index of glomerular structure [(basement membrane thickness/10) + $100V_v$ (matrix/glom) + % occluded glomeruli] and an index of nephropathy [(100/GFR) + 10(log urinary albumin excretion) + BP/4] in IDDM patients with renal disease. V_v(matrix/glom), volume fraction of mesangial matrix with glomerulus (glom: circumscribed polygon) as reference space; BP, mean blood pressure. Reprinted with permission from R. Osterby et al, *Diabetes*, Vol. 39, No. 9, September 1990. Copyright © 1990 by the American Diabetes Association

increase in luminal volume and filtering surface area shown by light and electron microscopic studies offers a structural counterpart to the higher GFR [295]. With advancing renal disease a close association has been reported between an index of glomerulopathy and an index of glomerular function [417] (Figure 9). A fractional mesangial volume in excess of 37% has been claimed to characterize patients with clinical proteinuria [375]. Mesangial expansion also correlates inversely with the capillary filtering area, a variable closely associated with glomerular filtration rate, from levels of hyperfiltration to markedly reduced renal function [418, 419]. It has therefore been suggested that it is the expansion of the mesangium, with the attendant reduction in glomerular filtration surface area, that is responsible for the progressive loss of renal function in IDDM. However, it should be remembered that there is overlap of fractional mesangial volume between patients with and without proteinuria [420, 421], making the prognostic significance of this variable open to question.

In IDDM patients, morphometric parameters did not correlate with albumin excretion rate up to 40 mg/day (about 30 μg/min). In patients with higher albumin excretion rates, however, the fractional volume of mesangium was on average

significantly increased, and a minor reduction in creatinine clearance and elevation in blood pressure were observed [117]. Similar findings have recently been reported in NIDDM patients [422]. These data confirm the reliability of persistent microalbuminuria and the attendant blood pressure elevation as clinical markers of significant renal damage [137].

Indications for Renal Biopsy in Diabetic Patients

It can be argued that if a patient has diabetes and also shows urinary abnormalities, there is no need to do a renal biopsy, which will almost certainly show changes consistent with diabetic nephropathy. Although it is true that in the great majority of patients with clinical diabetes proteinuria and/or haematuria are the result of diabetic nephropathy, this is not always the case.

The first step in the investigation of a proteinuric diabetic patient is to obtain information on the number, size and position of the kidneys by ultrasonography. Should there be a suspicion of papillary necrosis or tuberculosis of the renal tract—conditions that have an increased incidence in diabetic patients and may be associated with modest proteinuria—a full radiological assessment of the urinary tract should be performed.

Several clues may suggest that the patient has disease other than diabetic nephropathy. Retinopathy is almost invariably present in patients with diabetic nephropathy. A concordance rate varying between 63% in NIDDM [28] and up to 85–99% in IDDM [104, 143–145] makes the absence of retinopathy a strong argument for performing a biopsy.

The frequency of haematuria has been variably reported depending on the type of diabetes studied and on the definition of haematuria. In a large series of 136 consecutive biopsies in IDDM and NIDDM patients, Taft et al [152] found haematuria in excess of 10 000 cells per ml to be present in 66% of patients and to be of little help in distinguishing diabetic and non-diabetic renal disease. In a smaller biopsy series, Hommel et al [151] reported that of 13 IDDM patients with proteinuria and haematuria, 69% had a concomitant non-diabetic renal disease. Red cell casts have been noted in 4% of cases of biopsy-proven diabetic disease [423]. Although it is still controversial, the presence of haematuria, especially when accompanied by red cell casts, should alert one to the possibility of other renal disease.

In IDDM, proteinuria develops in only 4% of patients within 10 years of onset of diabetes. Thus, early onset of proteinuria is likely to indicate a disease other than diabetic nephropathy [424]. Conversely, the likelihood that a diabetic patient with onset in childhood who develops proteinuria 20 years later has diabetic nephropathy, approaches 100%.

In NIDDM, proteinuria can be present at diagnosis in as many as 8% of patients [105], and the number presenting with proteinuria increases with increasing age at presentation [144]. Moreover, in these older patients the duration of diabetes is uncertain, and the presence of other renal disease more likely [424]. Thus, early proteinuria is of lesser value in differentiating between renal injury of diabetic and non-diabetic origin.

The diagnosis of a coincident glomerular disease by renal biopsy may be helpful from both the therapeutic and prognostic standpoints. Besides detecting a potentially treatable non-diabetic renal disease, renal biopsy may be useful in the future for monitoring the effect of treatment of the early, potentially reversible, phases of diabetic nephropathy.

Other Glomerular Diseases in Diabetic Patients

Almost every form of glomerular disease has been shown to occur in diabetic patients, and this is not surprising considering that approximately 3% of the general population is diabetic.

IgA nephropathy and other forms of mesangial glomerulonephritis, acute glomerulonephritis, lupus, amyloidosis, mesangiocapillary glomerulonephritis types I and II, crescentic glomerulonephritis and steroid-responsive minimal-change disease in both children and adults [152, 425–427] have all been reported in diabetic patients. In a few patients, *two* additional glomerulopathies have been noted, as well as diabetic nephropathy [428].

The overall incidence of non-diabetic glomerular disease was 8% of 50 biopsied diabetic subjects [429], 9% of 122 patients [425], 22% of 164 patients [427] and 10% of 136 patients [152]. When NIDDM patients only were examined, 27% of 33 were found to have non-diabetic renal disease [28]. In a retrospective study of renal biopsies in diabetic subjects 12% of 49 IDDM patients and 28% of 60 NIDDM patients were found to have another disease [424]. These figures will undoubtedly be an overestimate of the true rate, since in most units routine renal biopsy of proteinuric diabetics is not practised, and those submitted to biopsy will, becuase of selection bias, contain a greater proportion of patients with non-diabetic glomerulopathies.

Membranous nephropathy is the glomerular disease that has most often been reported in association with diabetes. Since the first description by Churg's group [416] at least 60 cases have been reported, and many other similar patients seen more recently have not been reported because the association is now well recognized (see references 425, 426, 429 and 430 for reviews of published cases). The most common age at presentation was 40–60 years, similar to that of membranous nephropathy without diabetes, as well as that of NIDDM itself. However, patients as young as 13 years and several in their twenties have been reported. In most cases, duration of diabetes was 10 years or more and two-thirds of the patients were using insulin. Only 25% of the patients had retinopathy, although not all had fluorescein angiography. Most of the patients were nephrotic, with proteinuria as high as 35 g per 24 hours. Histological appearances ranged from typical membranous nephropathy to an almost typical diabetic glomerulosclerosis complicated by mild or occasional membranous changes.

It is difficult to be sure if this association is simply the coincidence of one of the more common glomerulopathies in middle age with diabetes of either type, or whether it represents a specific association. Certainly, the excess of membranous cases over other glomerular pathologies noted in nephrotic patients aged 30–60 years is striking.

Although the superimposition of Heymann membranous nephropathy on streptozotocin-induced diabetes in rats has been found to lead to a more severe nephrotic syndrome and a higher mortality than either disease alone [431], Chihara et al [427] reported that coincidence of membranous nephropathy and diabetes did not affect the prognosis for kidney function in humans.

TREATMENT OF DIABETIC NEPHROPATHY

Blood Pressure Control

Up to ten years ago, hypertension was viewed as a late phenomenon of diabetic nephropathy in IDDM, and was thought to be a consequence of it [120]. In NIDDM no consensus was achieved regarding its frequency or pathogenic importance [432].

It has, however, become apparent that rises in blood pressure take place in proteinuric IDDM even in the face of normal, although declining, GFR [125]. Moreover, micro-albuminuric IDDM patients have also been shown to have higher arterial pressures than matched normoalbuminuric patients [96, 137]. These observations, coupled with evidence for a central role of blood pressure level in the progression of diabetic renal disease [129], have led to a different perception of the importance of arterial hypertension.

Mogensen [123] was the first to show, in a small number of IDDM patients with established nephropathy, that reduction in blood pressure slowed the rate of loss of GFR and checked the increasing albuminuria. A prospective self-controlled study of 6 years' duration [433] demonstrated that effective blood pressure treatment reduced the rate of fall of GFR, from 0.94 ml/min per month before therapy to 0.29 ml/min per month during the first 3 years, and to 0.1 ml/min per month by 6 years of effective blood pressure treatment. This change was attended by 50% reduction in albuminuria, from 1038 μg/min to 504 μg/min. Despite the small number of patients and the lack of a randomized controlled design, these results were taken as evidence of the significant impact of antihypertensive treatment on the progression of diabetic kidney disease. The authors speculated that, should the slowing of progression be maintained, the renal survival of these patients might be extended from the current 7–10 years to more than 20 years. Recent longitudinal cohort studies seem to support this prediction, as a remarkable reduction in cumulative mortality —from over 50% at 10 years to only 18%—has been noted in patients receiving antihypertensive treatment [24, 25].

In the earlier studies, multiple drug therapy for hypertension was used, including a β-blocker, a diuretic and a vasodilator. During the last few years, great interest has surrounded the use of angiotensin converting-enzyme (ACE) inhibitors, not only in established diabetic nephropathy but also in non-hypertensive patients with micro-albuminuria. Studies in experimentally diabetic animals [238, 434], by implicating glomerular hypertension as a determinant of glomerular damage, have led to the suggestion that ACE inhibitors may be specifically protective of renal function because of their ability to reduce efferent arteriolar vasoconstriction, and thus to reduce intraglomerular hypertension. This 'specific' effect has been claimed to be separate from any effect on systemic blood pressure.

A reduction in proteinuria and in the rate of fall of GFR was shown to occur independently of significant blood pressure changes in two uncontrolled studies by Taguma et al [435] and by Bjørck et al [436]. In more recent controlled trials, however, the proteinuria-lowering effect and the effect on the rate of GFR decline were found to be associated with a reduction of systemic blood pressure, even when non-hypertensive proteinuric patients were investigated [437–439]. The decrease in the rate of fall of GFR obtained with treatment with ACE inhibitors does not appear to be of greater magnitude than that achieved with conventional antihypertensive therapy. A physiological approach to the study of the antiproteinuric effect of converting enzyme inhibitors has employed the fractional clearance of graded-size neutral dextrans. Three studies using different designs [440–442] have demonstrated that treatment of proteinuric diabetic patients with ACE inhibitors significantly reduces the augmented clearance of large dextrans (molecular radii 5.6–7.4 nm) and of large, essentially neutral plasma proteins such as IgG. This improvement in glomerular membrane size-selective properties seems to be unique to ACE inhibitors and independent of systemic blood pressure changes, as other antihypertensive drugs (such as diuretics or clonidine) are not followed by the same effect in spite of similar reductions in systemic arterial pressure. The prognostic significance of these membrane changes on selectivity remains unknown, however.

The effect of ACE inhibition has also been studied prospectively in non-hypertensive IDDM patients with microalbuminuria. In a randomized study, Marre et al [443] showed a reduction in albumin excretion rate, with normalization in 50% of cases, after 1 year of enalapril treatment. Mean blood pressure was reduced by about 10 mmHg throughout the study and GFR remained unchanged. By contrast, in the placebo group mean blood pressure rose and GFR decreased significantly, with 30% of the patients becoming persistently proteinuric by 1 year. A decrease in the fractional clearance of albumin, in the absence of changes in GFR or RPF, was also found in a short-term crossover study of the effects of enalapril on patients with normal albumin excretion rates [444].

Antihypertensive treatment appears, therefore, to delay the progression of established diabetic nephropathy and, if started at the stage of microalbuminuria, may even prevent or at least retard the onset of clinically overt renal disease. Caution must be applied in the extrapolation of data primarily based on reduction of urinary protein excretion, and long-term trials are needed to establish a definite effect on the rate of deterioration of glomerular function.

Dietary Treatment

A reduction of protein intake has long been advocated for the treatment of chronic renal failure [445], and diabetic nephropathy is no exception. Early studies by Attman et al [446] provided no evidence of a beneficial effect of protein restriction (as low as 0.3 g/kg per day) on the progression of renal disease in IDDM patients, but the lack of a therapeutic effect in this study may have been due to the advanced stage of the disease, as indicated by serum creatinine levels at entry of about 800 μmol/l. Recent data in diabetic patients with less severe impairment of renal function seem more encouraging. Barsotti et al [447] and Evanoff et al [448] claimed that the administration of a diet reduced in protein retards the progression of diabetic nephropathy in IDDM patients. These studies have been criticized, however, because assessment of renal function was made by creatinine clearance or the reciprocal of serum creatinine levels, two indices that are unreliable markers of renal function in advanced renal disease and especially in patients given a low-protein diet [126, 133, 134]. Other important potentially confounding variables such as blood pressure were also not controlled for.

Two long-term longitudinal studies have used reliable markers of glomerular function. Walker et al [135], in a 5-year self-controlled study of 19 IDDM patients with moderate renal failure at entry (mean GFR about 60 ml/min), showed that the mean rate of decline of GFR, measured as plasma clearance of ^{51}Cr-EDTA, was reduced from 0.61 ml/min per month on a diet with a daily protein content of 1.13 g/kg body weight, to 0.14 ml/min per month on a diet of 0.67 g/kg. The individual response to the low-protein diet was, however, heterogeneous, with 4 patients failing to respond and 7 showing a non-significant reduction in the rate of GFR fall. The low-protein diet reduced albuminuria from 467 mg to 340 mg per 24 hours, and was able to check the progressive rise in the fractional clearance of albumin. The effects of the diet seemed to be independent of blood pressure changes, which contributed only 11% to the decreased rate of loss of GFR.

Zeller et al [136], in a controlled 5-year prospective study of 35 IDDM patients with nephropathy, in whom GFR was assessed by iothalamate clearance, found that the rate of GFR decline in the group on a diet with restricted protein and phosphorus was 0.26 ml/min per month. By contrast, the control group on normal protein intake lost GFR at a significantly faster rate of 1.01 ml/min per month. A remarkable finding in this study was that 50% of the patients on dietary therapy showed no decline in GFR during a 31-month follow-up period. Blood pressure was similarly controlled in both groups. Table 5 illustrates the effect of protein restriction on the fall of GFR in these two studies.

Diets with protein restricted to 0.5–0.6 g/kg body weight daily seem to have no long-term detrimental effects on nutritional status. Anthropometric measurements such as mid-arm muscle circumference were not affected by such diets, and several authors noted an increase in serum albumin during protein restriction [135, 447, 448].

Short-term studies in diabetic humans with nephropathy on the physiological mechanisms of action of low-protein diets indicate that they lead to a reduction in the fractional clearance of albumin, IgG and broad-sized neutral dextrans, and thus to an improvement of glomerular membrane permselectivity, while not affecting GFR or RPF [449, 450]. Micropuncture studies in the streptozotocin-diabetic Munich-Wistar rat sug-

Table 5 Dietary protein restriction in diabetic nephropathy

Study	Rate of decline of GFR on normal protein diet (ml/min month)	Rate of decline of GFR on low-protein diet (ml/min month)
Walker et al, 1989 [135]	0.61	0.14
Zeller et al, 1991 [136]	1.01	0.26

gest that the antiproteinuric effect of a severely protein-restricted diet may be modulated by changes in intraglomerular pressure [237]. However, the mode of action of a low-protein diet is complex, unlikely to be mediated simply by haemodynamic changes [248, 377], and probably involving the effects of changes in other nutritional components such as phosphorus and lipids [135].

Reduction of dietary protein by approximately 50% has also been shown to reduce the fractional clearance of albumin in patients with microalbuminuria [451] and to lower GFR in patients with hyperfiltration [452], independently of changes in glucose control and blood pressure.

The prognostic significance of these changes remains at present obscure as no long-term studies are available in patients with early renal involvement. It also remains to be determined if the contributions of good blood-pressure control and of a low-protein diet may have an additive sparing effect on renal function. It is of interest that renal functional changes similar to those obtained by a low-protein diet can be induced in normal individuals by the administration of a vegetarian diet with normal protein content. The mediators of this effect are not entirely understood but may involve changes in glucagon secretion and the production of renal prostaglandins [453].

Glycaemic Control

Blood glucose control appears to have only limited impact on the progression of diabetic renal failure. A positive correlation between levels of HbA_{1c} and rate of decline of GFR reported by some authors [130] has not been confirmed subsequently by others [131]. In a study of strict blood glucose control by continuous subcutaneous insulin infusion, long-term correction of hyperglycaemia for nearly 2 years did not affect the rate of fall of GFR or the increasing rates of albumin and IgG fractional clearances in IDDM patients with persistent

proteinuria [128]. Similarly, poor results of intensified insulin treatment have been obtained in a controlled study of intermittently proteinuric patients [121]. It would appear that there is a point beyond which the diabetic metabolic abnormality is no longer necessary for progression of disease.

More encouraging are the effects of reducing elevated blood glucose levels at earlier stages of renal disease. The exaggerated albuminuric response to exercise in IDDM patients is corrected by a relatively short period of better diabetic control [110–112]. A significant correlation between indices of blood glucose control and albumin excretion rate have been reported by several authors in IDDM patients without persistent proteinuria [94, 127, 137]. In patients with microalbuminuria, strict metabolic control by continuous subcutaneous insulin infusion has been effective in reducing the albumin excretion rate [107, 454, 455] and in preventing the progressive increase in the fractional clearance of albumin in the long term [127]. In the Steno study over a 2-year period, 28% of conventionally treated patients progressed to clinical nephropathy, whereas no progression was seen in the group given intensified insulin treatment [127]. Similar reductions in albumin excretion rate can be obtained by multiple injection therapy, provided that similar levels of blood glucose control are achieved, suggesting that it is the blood glucose concentration attained rather than the modality of treatment that matters [456] (Table 6). Improvement of blood glucose control by diet or oral therapy also reduced microalbuminuria in NIDDM patients [69, 457].

The results of these studies are consistent with the epidemiological observation of a fourfold increase in the risk of developing nephropathy in IDDM patients with a track record of poor glycaemic control [9, 269, 458], and suggest a beneficial effect of tight glucose control on progression of microalbuminuria. Whether this effect may be translated to prevention of end-stage renal failure remains to be established.

Table 6 Studies investigating improved glycaemic control in insulin-dependent diabetic patients with microalbuminuria

Study	Type/number of patients		Glycated haemoglobin	Duration of study	Outcome
Kroc	39 NA	20 CIT	9.9 → 9.9	8 months	No change in AER in either group
		19 CSII	10.2 → 8.0		
	20 MA	10 CIT	11.5 → 11.8		AER (μg/min): 34 → 26
		10 CSII	11.3 → 8.2		30 → 10
Steno	36 MA	18 CIT	9.3 → 8.6	2 years	θ ALB: 160 → 360
		18 CSII	9.5 → 7.2		170 → 160
Oslo	30 'low' MA	15 CIT	9.5 → 10.5	4 years	AER (mg/24 h): 21 → 22
		15 CSII	10.1 → 9.0		26 → 16

NA, normoalbuminuria; MA, microalbuminuria; AER, urinary albumin excretion rate; θ ALB, fractional clearance of albumin; CIT, conventional insulin treatment; CSII, continuous subcutaneous insulin infusion.

Correction of hyperglycaemia shortly after diagnosis of IDDM induces a decrease in GFR, which in some [78] but not all [67] studies was accompanied by a reduction in the increased kidney size. Recent evidence suggests that the increased kidney size is associated with an exaggerated renal response to amino acid infusion, and that both can be corrected by 3 weeks of intensified insulin therapy [459]. With disease of longer duration, however, near-normoglycaemia lowers GFR although not affecting kidney hypertrophy. Cessation of strict glycaemic control in these patients with large, hyperfiltering kidneys leads to a prompt return of GFR to previous levels [68]. It has been suggested that the establishment of the irreversibility of kidney enlargement signals the onset of a phase of progressive renal disease in which overproduction of intrarenal growth factors perpetuates renal damage [84].

Other Treatment Modalities

Although there is a substantial amount of experimental data on the renal effect of aldose reductase inhibitors in rats, only a small number of studies have been reported in humans. Whereas a reduction of GFR [204] and a decrease in albumin excretion rate [205] were noted in IDDM patients with either normal albumin excretion rate or microalbuminuria, a controlled study on NIDDM subjects with microalbuminuria failed to show any effects on renal function, blood pressure or glucose control after a short period of treatment [206]. Longer-term studies will probably be needed to clarify the role of this class of compounds in human disease.

It has been claimed that a therapeutic regimen with aspirin and dipyridamole may delay the progression of chronic renal failure in some patients with diabetic nephropathy [460]. However, this study was uncontrolled and did not allow for the confounding effect of other variables.

OTHER MANIFESTATIONS OF DIABETIC RENAL DISEASE

Renal Papillary Necrosis

Diabetes has long been associated with renal papillary necrosis (RPN), which has an average prevalence in autopsy cases of 4.4% [461]. This figure may be an underestimation as diabetes has been found in up to 50% of cases of RPN [462–464].

In a recent prospective series of 76 consecutive IDDM patients with normal serum creatinine in whom urography was performed, RPN was diagnosed in 24% [465]. It tends to occur in patients with longstanding disease, and affects both kidneys in up to 65% of cases [461]. When unilateral, it has been shown to involve the contralateral kidney in the ensuing years. It is more frequent in women, particularly those with recurrent urinary tract infection.

Renal papillary necrosis has been viewed in the past as an acute devastating condition, often leading to sepsis and death; it has now become clear that it can be nearly asymptomatic and follow a more indolent course, with bouts of urinary infection and/or renal colic. Microscopic haematuria has been reported to be more frequent when this condition is present, and pyuria will often be present even in the absence of documented infection, a finding that should alert one to the possibility of underlying silent papillary necrosis [464, 465]. Proteinuria is often present but is usually modest (less than 2 g per 24 hours), and patients with persistent proteinuria do not seem to have an incidence of RPN in excess of that in patients without proteinuria [465]. The urographic appearances of 'moth-eaten' calices and the 'ring shadow' image of the necrotic papilla are highly suggestive of this condition.

The management of the acute form of renal papillary necrosis in the diabetic patient is compounded by the need to maintain adequate metabolic control. If obstruction is present, its relief is urgent and will often condition the success of associated antibiotic therapy. In the chronic, indolent form, the use of non-steroidal anti-inflammatory agents may further compromise medullary circulation, and should therefore be avoided.

Autonomic Neuropathy and the Bladder

It is difficult to ascertain the true prevalence of autonomic neuropathy of the bladder in diabetes because of the insidious onset of the condition. In the older literature, this uncertainty is reflected by prevalence figures that range from 1% to 26% [466, 467], whereas more recent studies, where diagnosis was based on urodynamic criteria, report prevalence of bladder autonomic dysfunction in longstanding diabetes of about 40% [468].

The first abnormality, usually detected in asymptomatic patients, is impairment of sensation with decreased awareness of bladder distention, due to involvement of proprioceptive afferent fibres. As a result, micturition occurs at progressively larger bladder volumes, and this, together with progressive damage of the parasympathetic innervation of the detrusor, leads to weaker bladder contraction, incomplete emptying, and increasing residual volume. Involvement of the efferent sympathetic innervation to the trigone may lead to functional incompetence of the vesicoureteric junction and to incomplete relaxation of the internal sphincter during micturition [469, 470].

Patients are often unaware of the extent of their bladder abnormality. Symptoms are scarce and, at the initial stages, may be confined to disappearance of previous nocturia, with less frequent daytime voiding of large volumes of urine. These changes may go unnoticed for a long time. Later, a weaker stream produced only on straining, terminal dribbling, and involuntary stream interruption or overflow incontinence due to detrusor–urethral sphincter dyssynergia, may become apparent. From the early stages, recurrent and/or persistent urinary tract infections may set in as a consequence of incomplete emptying and/or reflux [471, 472].

Recognition of the insidious course assists early diagnosis. Proper consideration given to recurring urinary infections in a longstanding diabetic patient may lead to detection of an unsuspected enlarged bladder by physical examination, or alternatively to disclosure of residual urine by ultrasound scanning. Diabetic patients are capable of developing other conditions (e.g. prostatic hypertrophy, asymptomatic stone) that may interfere with bladder function, and overt symptoms may occur due to associated treatment with anticholinergic drugs [473, 474]. Urodynamic studies with uroflowmetry (mictiography) [475] and cystometrogram study [476] can characterize the bladder dysfunction, and may be invaluable for accurate prognosis and decisions about treatment.

Detection of autonomic bladder involvement in a diabetic patient should lead to adoption of a policy of voluntary, regular voiding performed by the patient even in the absence of subjective urge. Suprapubic manual pressure will help complete emptying. Intermittent or temporary catheterization, and its association with parasympathomimetic drug treatment with bethanechol chloride, may lead to reduction of bladder distention and recovery of detrusor function [477]. The effect of the drug seems unpredictable, however, and may be limited by side-effects [478]. In the presence of detrusor–urethral dyssynergia, centrally acting muscle relaxants or an α-adrenergic blocking agent (depending on whether dysfunction involves the external or the internal sphincter, respectively) may be of help. Bladder neck resection is sometimes very successful. More complex operations to reduce bladder capacity are sometimes performed. Long-term catheterization may be the only solution in severely disabled patients. The most serious complication of neurogenic bladder is an intractable urinary infection, which may render the patient unsuitable for renal transplantation.

Pregnancy in Diabetic Nephropathy

Up to the 1980s, pregnancy in women with diabetic nephropathy was discouraged, and therapeutic abortion was recommended because of the very poor fetal outcome [479]. During the last decade, more than 100 pregnancies in IDDM patients with nephropathy have been reported [480–484]. Both the impact of pregnancy on nephropathy and the outcome of gestation appear to be more encouraging.

The increase in creatinine clearance, which takes place in normal gestation, occurs in only about 56% of pregnant women with diabetic nephropathy during the first trimester [481, 482]. In proteinuric patients with initial creatinine clearances of 50 ml/min or more, elevated blood pressure (140/90 mmHg or over) is present in approximately one-third during the first trimester, rising to just over one-half at the end of pregnancy. In women with more reduced renal function, these proportions increase to about 80%.

Pre-eclampsia is reported to occur in 26% of all diabetic nephropathic pregnancies. Its diagnosis is dependent upon the detection of an acute rise in blood pressure, serum creatinine and proteinuria. Other signs of deranged hepatic and central nervous system function, and thrombocytopenia with elevated fibrin-split products, may coexist. Changes in serum uric acid have been found to be of no pathognomonic significance in the context of diabetic nephropathy [480].

A common finding in pregnancy in diabetic nephropathy is an increase in proteinuria, sometimes of massive proportions. Among patients with more than 50 ml/min of creatinine clearance, 16% in the first trimester and 71% in the third trimester excrete more than 3 g of protein per 24 hours. Pooled data suggest that about 50% of patients reach 24-hour proteinuria greater than 5 g, and 17% greater than 10 g [480–484].

Anaemia was found to relate significantly to the decreased renal function, and haematocrits of 28% of below and/or haemoglobin 10 g/dl or below were seen in 42% [480, 484].

The natural history of nephropathy does not appear to be adversely affected by pregnancy.

Following delivery, a marked reduction in proteinuria is common, and in the 27 patients in whom it was measured within 1 year, it had returned to or below preconception values in 67%. The rate of decline of creatinine clearance was calculated in 23 patients followed for 6–35 months after delivery, and was found to be 0.85 ml/min per month [480]. A reduction in renal function after pregnancy was more likely in patients with more severe proteinuria or hypertension during the first trimester. Overall, the impact of pregnancy on the kidney seemed not to be different from that observed in other renal diseases [485, 486].

Fetal survival in a pooled series of five studies was 91.3% [480–484]. The unacceptably high rates of spontaneous abortions and of congenital malformations seen in women with diabetic nephropathy before the 1980s [479, 487] have been considerably reduced, to around 9.5%. There is ample evidence that normalization of HbA_{1c} *before* conception reduces the frequency of malformations in diabetic pregnancies in general [488–492], and the same may apply to women with diabetic nephropathy [481, 491, 492]. Increases in blood pressure, fetal distress and premature labour are responsible for a high rate (about 55%) of preterm deliveries, which is similar to that reported in women with non-diabetic renal disease and depressed renal function [486].

Pregnancy in a woman with diabetic nephropathy should be carefully considered and planned. Its outcome depends to a great extent on the joint efforts of the patient and of a team of experts in a specialized centre. The ultimate decision should consider the long-term prognosis for the patient with diabetic nephropathy and the increased risk to the fetus.

Urinary Tract Infections

Urinary tract infections have been considered to be more frequent in patients with diabetes, probably due to reports of renal histological evidence of interstitial inflammation and scarring in 10–40% of diabetics [26, 156, 392, 425, 493, 494]. These histological aspects could arise from other conditions like ischaemia, reflux nephropathy or renal papillary necrosis, and are difficult to distinguish from those of 'chronic pyelonephritis' [143, 152, 392]. Indeed, several surveys have failed to show an increased incidence of urinary infection in diabetic patients when compared with control populations [495–497]. However, some workers have reported that women with diabetes have an incidence of bacteriuria that is approximately double that of non-diabetic controls [497–500]. Diabetic nephropathy seems to be associated with an increased frequency of infection only in pregnant diabetic patients [501, 502]. A high proportion of urinary tract infections are asymptomatic, and their pathogenic role is not clear. However, in patients with diabetic nephropathy even asymptomatic infection may be associated with worsening renal function, and every effort should be directed to its eradication.

Urinary tract infections can lead to severe complications in the diabetic patient when such infections involve the upper urinary tract. *Perinephric abscesses*, which can be bilateral [503], are more frequent in diabetic patients, and may have an insidious onset followed by persistent fever and rigors. Urinary cultures are frequently negative, and a tender flank mass can sometimes be felt [504]. Computerized tomography (CT) may establish the diagnosis [505]. Prolonged antibiotic therapy is usually needed.

Infections of the kidney with anaerobic gas-forming organisms are distinctly more common in diabetic patients, and have recently been reviewed by Evanoff et al [506]. More than 90% of cases of *emphysematous pyelonephritis* occur in patients with diabetes. This condition of parenchymal infection is more frequent in women and is in the majority of cases attributable to *Escherichia coli*, but *Candida* sp. and *Cryptococcus neoformans* have also been reported. Fever, abdominal pain, nausea and vomiting in an ill-appearing patient are common presenting features. Elevated white blood cell count and creatinine serum and grossly elevated blood glucose are common, and frank pyuria is usually present. The infection is bilateral in about 10% of cases. Plain abdominal radiographic examination, an intravenous urogram or ultrasound scanning are diagnostic in about 85% of cases, showing gas bubbles extending along the renal pyramids and collecting under the perirenal fascia, or after its rupture extending into the adjoining retroperitoneal space. A CT scan will be needed in the remaining cases, and will define more precisely the location of the gas. Emphysematous pyelonephritis has a guarded prognosis. Medical treatment alone results in a mor-

tality of about 60% when gas is confined to the kidney, and of over 80% when it has extended to the perirenal spaces. Nephrectomy can be a life-saving procedure and should not be delayed, but is still fraught with a mortality of about 20%.

Emphysematous pyelitis refers to the presence of gas within the collecting system only, and 50% of cases occur in diabetic patients, particularly women. Its clinical presentation is similar to that of emphysematous pyelonephritis, although renal failure may be absent and glucose control remain adequate. Radiographic examination by plain film, intravenous urogram or ultrasound shows gas outlining the pelvicaliceal system, and sometimes the ureters. Obstruction and dilatation are not uncommon associated features needing urgent correction. Medical supportive treatment and antibiotic therapy are usually effective, although the overall mortality is still about 20%.

RENAL REPLACEMENT THERAPY

Not all patients with diabetic nephropathy will ultimately require renal replacement therapy (RRT) for end-stage renal failure (ESRF) since many will die from non-renal causes, usually cardiovascular, before they need renal support [21]. However, the number of patients receiving RRT is increasing in most developed countries due, in the main, to an increased willingness of physicians to refer patients to renal centres and a changing policy in most renal centres.

The treatments offered to diabetic patients are often determined by national and local policies, resources and experience, with renal transplantation being increasingly recognised as the treatment of choice. The prognosis for diabetic patients on renal replacement is generally less favourable than for non-diabetic patients, although this varies for the type of replacement and is mainly due to non-renal causes of morbidity and mortality.

This section of the chapter discusses the size of the problem, the indications for renal replacement and the options available, together with the merits and disadvantages of each treatment modality. Mention is made of the concomitant complications seen in diabetic patients on RRT.

The Size of the Problem

In the two decades since the first diabetic

patients suffering from end-stage renal failure were treated with haemodialysis, the number of patients now on renal replacement programmes has expanded to such an extent that uraemia, in many countries, in insulin dependent and non-insulin dependent patients is the most prevalent cause of renal failure treated by maintenance haemodialysis or renal transplantation [507–509]. In 1981 diabetic patients accounted for 25% of all patients treated for ESRF in the USA, and in 1985 between 20% and 45% of new dialysis patients had a diagnosis of diabetic nephropathy in the Medicare records of the USA and Canada [508, 510]. In Europe, where less is spent generally on health care, diabetic patients represented only 10% of new patients starting on replacement therapy in 1984 [509]. There are marked national differences within Europe, with the Scandinavian countries reporting up to a quarter of all patients starting on renal replacement programmes as having diabetic nephropathy.

In Europe there is a relation between the total number of patients taken on to renal replacement programmes per million population per year and the number of new diabetic patients being treated for ESRF [509]. Thus different take-on rates between countries may not only reflect different prevalences of ESRF due to diabetes but also the general availability of renal replacement in the country concerned. The increased availability of renal replacement in the UK has benefited diabetic patients in ESRF, in that in 1976 only 1.4% of new ESRF patients taken on to renal replacement programmes were diabetic yet by 1984 this had risen to 11.1% [509]. However, it is likely that as many as 200 diabetic patients in the UK who are considered as suitable candidates for renal replacement by their physicians are not receiving such treatment, and this shortfall is likely to be similar in other European countries [6]. The excess costs of treating diabetic patients in ESRF in terms of financial expense and increased medical and paramedical personnel time are difficult to quantify, but the evidence does suggest that these patients require greater resources than do similar non-diabetic patients [511, 512].

When to Initiate Renal Replacement Therapy

The diabetic patient with nephropathy is identified by the presence of persistent proteinuria, retinopathy and arterial hypertension. Serial assessments of renal function, either using serum creatinine or its inverse, or more accurately using isotopic clearances, will enable the physician to predict when ESRF is likely to occur. The rate of decline in renal function varies considerably between individuals but is thought to be constant in any one individual [124, 126].

Diabetic nephropathy is usually clinically silent throughout most of its course, although occasionally punctuated by episodes of urinary infection or nephrosis. Glycaemic control may well become erratic as renal function deteriorates; hypoglycaemia may more frequently occur on fixed doses of insulin as catabolism by the kidney is reduced with declining glomerular filtration rate (GFR) and renal plasma flow [513]. Insulin is catabolised by the kidney after filtration and uptake into proximal tubule cells where it is proteolytically degraded [514]. When renal function declines the half-life of exogenously administered insulin increases, and in the latter stages of chronic renal failure if anorexia supervenes hypoglycaemia is a common and serious event, as many of these patients have lost the warnings of the impending hypoglycaemia. In patients with non-insulin dependent diabetes mellitus (NIDDM) frequent, unexplained hypoglycaemia may herald declining renal function as the majority of sulphonylurea drugs are renally excreted. Hypoglycaemic comas due to glibenclamide accumulation in patients with renal impairment ran a more serious course than in patients with normal renal function [515]. Glipizide, which is metabolised in the liver to two non-hypoglycaemic metabolites, and gliquidone, which is excreted by the liver, are the sulphonylureas of choice in renal failure [516]. Metformin, also renally excreted, will accumulate in chronic renal failure, necessitating a commensurate reduction in dosage.

Hyperkalaemic hyperchloraemic acidosis, a so-called normal ionic gap acidosis, may be encountered in diabetic patients with a GFR less than 40 ml/min [158]. This is due, in some patients, to reduced levels of plasma renin and aldosterone; the reasons for this are obscure, but in practical terms any potassium-sparing drugs in these patients should be administered with even more care than is usually exercised when prescribing in renal impairment [517, 518].

During the time of the final deterioration of

renal function the diabetic patient will require careful treatment of blood pressure and plasma volume. Access for dialysis, arteriovenous fistula or peritoneal catheter placement (or both) and tissue typing should be planned well in advance of dialysis being necessary. The point at which dialysis is initiated shows local variation and depends to some extent on the treatment being offered. Our practice is to provide access when the GFR is approximately 15 ml/min (serum creatinine levels around 500 μmol/l) and to initiate dialysis just before the symptoms of uraemia are likely to become manifest. Diabetic patients tolerate uraemia less well than do non-diabetic patients and often need renal support at a GFR of 10 ml/min [510].

Before renal replacement is initiated all patients should be fully aware of the treatment options and introduced to other patients already on the form of renal replacement they are to be offered. In centres that encourage live related donation the family will need careful explanation before reaching their decision.

As cardiovascular mortality is such a major problem in all diabetic patients on renal replacement programmes the question of cardiac assessment before dialysis or transplantation has been brought into focus. This is especially pertinent in the case of the patient receiving a live related donor renal graft. In 25 consecutive diabetic recipients scheduled for live related transplants, 5 were found to have asymptomatic life-threatening coronary artery disease following investigation using stress testing, Muga scan and cardiac catheterisation [519]. The precise investigation for the diagnosis of coronary disease in these patients is still under debate, but thallium stress testing in a prospective study failed to provide useful prognostic information [520]. The stress test or exercise electrocardiogram has limited diagnostic value in the non-diabetic subject, and it is likely that coronary arteriography is necessary to determine precisely the need for coronary revascularization prior to dialysis or transplant [521].

The Treatment Options

As with any patient in ESRF, the diabetic subject can be offered haemodialysis, peritoneal dialysis, renal transplantation or, very occasionally, haemofiltration (Table 7). These options are considered below.

Haemodialysis

Haemodialysis is the form of renal replacement therapy used most frequently in diabetic patients with ESRF in the USA and in some European countries. The Regional Kidney Disease Program based in Minneapolis has one of the largest experiences in treating insulin dependent diabetes mellitus (IDDM) and NIDDM patients with ESRF using haemodialysis [522]. In reviewing this experience it was found that an increasing number of NIDDM patients of increasing age were taken on to the programme throughout an 18-year follow-up. There was also a trend to initiate dialysis at a time when renal function was less impaired. In contrast, in IDDM patients with ESRF the annual number of patients starting haemodialysis has remained static and the mean serum creatinine level at the time of initiation has decreased only minimally. Cumulative survival rates for diabetic and non-diabetic patients on haemodialysis were 55% and 70% respectively at 3 years. These figures are comparable to those from other centres in North America and Europe [523, 524]. When considering survival data for diabetic subjects, an age correction is mandatory as patients aged 60 years or over have a much poorer prognosis, especially in the insulin dependent cohort [522, 525, 526]. Recent long-term dialysis data from Minneapolis, where 95% of diabetic patients are treated by haemodialysis, reveal that on this treatment 30% of patients survive 5 years and 10% survive 9 years. No difference is seen in survival between IDDM and NIDDM patients [527].

Cardiovascular and cerebrovascular events account for the majority of the excess deaths seen in diabetic patients on haemodialysis. These two causes account for over half of the deaths and most occur within 2 years of the commencement of dialysis [522, 524, 526]. Uraemic deaths, including cachexia, caused 10% of deaths in the European experience and nearly 20% in the USA. Age, particularly if over 60 years, is an important indicator of survival in patients with IDDM and less so for those with NIDDM [522, 528]. The presence of severe coronary artery disease, documented by coronary angiography, has been shown to be associated with a much higher incidence of coronary deaths [529, 530]. Interestingly, the increased levels of cholesterol and triglycerides seen in dialysed diabetic

Table 7 Advantages and disadvantages of forms of renal replacement therapies for diabetic patients

	Haemodialysis	CAPD
Advantages	Widespread availability Frequent monitoring by staff	Stable control of volume and blood pressure Intraperitoneal insulin giving stable glycaemia Patient freedom Lower cost Less staff intensive
Disadvantages	Acute dialysis morbidity: hypoglycaemia, hyperglycaemia hyperkalaemia hypotension, hypertension nausea, vomiting headache cramps Poor rehabilitation	Risk of peritonitis Finite life of peritoneum

patients when compared with non-diabetic patients on dialysis do not correlate with the presence of coronary artery occlusion [531].

Particular problems posed by diabetics on haemodialysis. Vascular access in the diabetic patient is generally more difficult than in the non-diabetic patient of similar age, and this is of paramount importance when considering the optimum form of vascular access for haemodialysis. The arteriovenous Scribner shunt (cannula) has yielded poor results in diabetic subjects, and evidence suggests that bovine or PTFE grafts survive for the longest duration [532, 533]. Shunts are more prone to infection in diabetic compared with non-diabetic patients, and many renal units use the arteriovenous fistula utilising native vessels, despite previous reports of their high failure rate [532, 533]. For emergency access a subclavian line is most often employed.

Owing to pre-existing, although asymptomatic, coronary artery disease and autonomic impairment, episodes of hypotension and hypertension are more common in diabetic patients while undergoing haemodialysis [534]. Angina during haemodialysis should alert the physician to the need for coronary arteriography. The metabolic consequences of intermittent dialysis can become a problem for the non-diabetic patient, but for the diabetic patient the acute variations in blood glucose and plasma potassium levels can have more serious or even fatal consequences [535–538]. Hyperkalaemia during the first 18 months of treatment is common and in one series caused nearly 4% of deaths, as many as

were attributable to sepsis [537]. Hyperkalaemia coupled with coronary artery disease and autonomic neuropathy may contribute to the sudden deaths seen in some patients during dialysis.

With respect to other diabetic complications, patients on haemodialysis have a low incidence of lower limb amputations compared with patients on continuous ambulatory peritoneal dialysis (CAPD) or who have undergone transplantation [522].

Up to 40% of patients presenting for haemodialysis are blind, yet the incidence of new blindness while on dialysis has declined over an 18-year period [522], despite no significant change in the anticoagulation regimen used. Control of blood pressure, careful ophthalmological assessment and prompt treatment may have more bearing on the visual outcome than the dialysis procedure itself. The best renal treatment with regard to maintenance of visual function is renal transplantation [539].

Quality of life for diabetic patients on haemodialysis. In 1982 in the USA, 26% of 7300 diabetic patients on haemodialysis were employed [540]; this figure corresponds to the numbers of patients employed while on CAPD or after transplantation, taking into account the effect of age, other complications and family support on the mode of therapy offered to an individual patient. Loss of visual acuity accounts for most of the problems with employment, and as this complication has declined over the years for patients on haemodialysis the expectation is that more patients on this treatment will have adequate vision and hence employment. A happy and fulfilling life is certainly feasible on chronic haemodialysis. Of 24 patients who have survived more than 4 years on dialysis, 16 felt themselves to be very happy and led active lives [527]. Time spent in hospital especially once the patient is established on dialysis (after the first year) may not be markedly different from that for patients not on dialysis [527]. In contrast, some diabetic patients have a miserable time and 14% of one series died owing to termination of dialysis, which was, presumably, a joint decision between physician and patient. Blindness or amputation was no more common in those who terminated dialysis [541].

Continuous Ambulatory Peritoneal Dialysis

Over the last decade CAPD has gained acceptance in many centres for treating ESRF of varying aetiologies, and it offers specific benefits for the diabetic patient [542–544]; these benefits include a steady state control of uraemia without marked swings of volume, control of hypertension, improvement of anaemia and a smooth control of blood glucose concentration using intraperitoneal insulin added to the dialysate [543]. The lack of need for vascular access has a further advantage in the diabetic subject. Although in our centre patients receiving CAPD also have a fistula fashioned, a subclavian line provides vascular access in an emergency in the majority of cases.

Peritonitis, a perennial risk for all CAPD patients, appears to be no more frequent in diabetic than non-diabetic patients, although the patient selection, learning curve of the patient, the centre and the methods used to express incidence rates will all influence these rates. The organisms responsible for peritonitis in diabetic patients are not substantially different from those found in non-diabetic patients and comprise mainly skin flora. In non-diabetic patients some CAPD delivery systems have proved preferable to others in reducing the rate of peritonitis but, again, methods are usually governed by local practice [545, 546]. The introduction of insulin into the dialysate bag does not appear to alter significantly the risk of introducing infection. For blind diabetic patients, aids are available for the injection of insulin into the dialysate bag—visual handicap is not a contraindication to CAPD [547]. All commercially available dialysate solutions contain glucose at various concentrations. Although these concentrations will permit the removal of sodium and water through a dialysing peritoneum, glucose as an osmotic agent does have some disadvantages. Glucose readily diffuses through the peritoneum into the blood stream, resulting in a considerable glucose load [548]. For diabetic patients this usually involves an increase in their insulin requirement, with the concomitant risk of weight gain and hypertriglyceridaemia which may act as a further cardiovascular risk factor [542, 549, 550]. New osmotic agents are under observation, but the long-term effects of these agents on the peritoneum are unknown.

The dose of insulin is usually higher than previously needed due, in part, to the glucose in the dialysate [543]. Glycaemic control in uraemic patients should be assessed by regular home blood glucose monitoring rather than by measurement of glycated haemoglobin, which may be inaccurate in uraemia owing to hydrolysis of urea to cyanate and hence to carbamino-haemoglobin which can falsely elevate the HbA_{1C} level [551]. This effect may be related to the method used for measuring glycated haemoglobin and the level of uraemia [552, 553]. Furthermore, shortened red-cell survival times, commonly seen in patients on haemodialysis or patients in chronic renal failure, may lead to falsely low levels of glycated haemoglobin [554]. The use of serum fructosamine to assess short-term glycaemic control may be a useful alternative. In early renal failure we have found a good correlation between serum fructosamine values and serum fructosamine/serum albumin ratio with fasting plasma glucose and diurnal 2-hourly glucose profiles [555].

Prognosis for patients on CAPD. Compared with haemodialysis, CAPD offers specific advantages for the diabetic patient in terms of the progression of other diabetic complications. Given that probably 10% of patients starting CAPD will have severe visual impairment, the progression of retinopathy seems little affected by this form of treatment [543]. The blood pressure swings and heparinisation of haemodialysis are avoided with CAPD; the improved glycaemic control, implicated in a transient worsening of retinopathy in previous studies, does not appear to be a problem in this group of patients [454, 556]. Despite adequate dialysis, little beneficial effect has been seen on peripheral or autonomic neuropathy [557]. Similarly, peripheral vascular disease is not notably affected by CAPD, and data collected between 1976 and 1983 showed the lower limb amputation rate to be higher for patients on CAPD than for those on haemodialysis [522]. Successful pregnancy has been reported in a patient on CAPD [558]. Cardiovascular events dominate the causes of death in patients on CAPD. In a series of 81 patients on CAPD for nearly 2 years, 24 died during a 7-year follow-up: 40% of these deaths were due to cardiovascular causes [544]. Cardiovascular events determine to a large extent the duration of survival on CAPD [559]. Patient survival rates vary around the range of 80% at 1 year and 50% at 3 years for IDDM patients and are slightly more for NIDDM patients [544, 560–563]. Technique survival tends to be 10–20% less than the patient survival.

The clinical status of diabetic patients on CAPD is often reasonable and most feel well. There is relief from uraemic symptoms and the steady levels of urea, creatinine and phosphate plus the higher haemoglobin levels may add to the sense of well-being [564]. Most insulin-requiring patients quickly master the technique of intraperitoneal insulin administration and achieve a smooth control of glycaemia.

Transplantation

Since the first renal transplants in diabetic patients were reported at the beginning of the 1980s, the results of this treatment have improved markedly. In the view of many practitioners this form of therapy is the treatment of choice in insulin dependent patients with ESRF, and a living related donor graft produces the highest patient and graft survival rates and the best rehabilitation prospects [519, 565]. The addition of cyclosporin to the immunosuppressive regimens has further improved graft survival in diabetic patients as in other patients receiving renal graft [529, 566, 567]. In a 9-year experience at the University of Minnesota during which 865 diabetic patients received a renal transplant, 65% survived 5 years and 45% survived 10 years [529]. The 3-year survival rate has improved in the more recent cyclosporin era for HLA identical, HLA non-identical and cadaver donor kidneys. An

actuarial survival rate at 3 years of 49% has been recorded in Europe [509].

As far as other diabetic complications are concerned, amputations are a major problem in diabetic patients after transplantation. Approximately 15% of such patients have had an amputation at 3 years and 30% at 10 years [524, 568–570]. In contrast, visual acuity is well preserved after kidney transplantation [539]. Whether this is due to the method of RRT or to improved and more careful detection, follow-up and treatment of proliferative retinopathy is not known. Initially, 70% of patients receiving transplants achieve a high level of rehabilitation, but this decreases with time, due possibly to amputations or failure of the graft [571, 572].

Recently, simultaneous combined kidney and pancreas grafts have been performed; although initial experience has highlighted significant technical problems to be overcome, there is evidence that a successful pancreatic graft protect the grafted kidney from the development of diabetic nephropathy [573–575].

Haemofiltration

Haemofiltration is a relatively new method of blood filtration that has become an accepted method for treating renal failure, often in the acute setting [576]. It is of particular use in cases of acute volume overload, and it uses relatively simple equipment. The urea clearance of the system is comparable to that of CAPD [577]. Experience in diabetic patients is limited: one report suggests that CAPD and haemofiltration achieve similar results [578].

An Overview of Dialysis and Transplantation

It is not possible to make a direct comparison, in terms of patient survival and morbidity, of the various forms of dialysis or transplantation in diabetic patients. Patients who are selected for transplantation tend to be younger and healthier, certainly in North America, and the remainder continue on dialysis. The rationale behind this is to make the best use of a scarce resource. Occasionally a 'high-risk' patient may be given a renal transplant in preference to a more suitable recipient, simply because the high-risk patient may be unable to cope with the rigours of managing a dialysis programme.

Referring to data from Minnesota, which has

one of the largest experiences in the world, the within-age group survival rates at 5 years for haemodialysis and cadaver transplants are similar [527]. The same is true for the European experience, which concludes that survival rates in the groups treated with CAPD, haemodialysis or transplantation are similar [509].

Recent data from the EDTA Registry has again highlighted the markedly increased relative risk of ischaemic heart disease in diabetic patients on renal replacement regimens [579]. The rate of death from myocardial infarction was ten times higher in diabetic patients than in non-diabetic patients. This sobering statistic is a warning to the clinician to be aware that renal failure is not the only aspect of the diabetic patient's management that requires full attention.

REFERENCES

1. Cotunnius D. De ischiade nervosa commentarius. Naples: Simonios, 1764.
2. Rollo J. Cases of diabetes mellitus (2nd edn). London: Dilly, 1798.
3. Bright R. Cases and observations illustrative of renal disease accompanied with the secretion of albuminous urine. Guy's Hosp Rep 1836; 1: 338–400.
4. Rayer P. In Traité des maladies du rein, vol. 2. Paris: Bailliére, Tindall and Cox, 1840.
5. Kimmelstiel P, Wilson C. Intercapillary lesions in glomeruli of kidney. Am J Path 1936; 12: 83–97.
6. Joint Working Party on Diabetic Renal Failure. Renal failure in diabetics in the UK: deficient provision of care in 1985. Diabet Med 1988; 5: 79–84.
7. Eggers PW. Effect of transplantation on the Medicare end-stage renal disease program. New Engl J Med 1988; 318: 223–9.
8. Andersen AR, Christiansen JS, Andersen JK, Kreiner S, Deckert T. Diabetic nephropathy in type 1 (insulin-dependent) diabetes: an epidemiological study. Diabetologia 1983; 25: 496–501.
9. Krolewski AS, Warram JH, Chriestlieb AR, Busick EJ, Kahn CR. The changing natural history of nephropathy in type 1 diabetes. Am J Med 1985; 78: 785–94.
10. Kofoed-Enevoldsen A, Borch-Johnsen K, Kreiner S, Nerup J, Deckert T. Declining incidence of persistent proteinuria in type 1 (insulin-dependent) diabetic patients in Denmark. Diabetes 1987; 36: 205–9.
11. Borch-Johnsen K, Andersen PK, Deckert T. The effect of proteinuria on relative mortality in type 1 (insulin-dependent) diabetes mellitus. Diabetologia 1985; 28: 590–6.
12. Cameron JS. The natural history of glomerulonephritis. In Kincaid-Smith P, d'Apice AJ, Atkins RC (eds) Progress in glomerulonephritis. New York: Wiley, 1979: pp 1–25.
13. Finn R, Harmer D. Etiological implications of sex ratio in glomerulonephritis. Lancet 1979; ii: 1194.
14. Pasternack A, Kasanen A, Sourander L, Kaarsalo E. Prevalence and incidence of moderate and severe clinical renal failure in South Western Finland. Acta Med Scand 1985; 218: 173–80.
15. Danielsen R, Helgason T, Jonasson F. Prognostic factors and retinopathy in type 1 diabetics in Iceland. Acta Med Scand 1983; 213: 323–36.
16. Klein R, Klein BEK, Moss SE, Davis MD, DeMets DL. The Wisconsin epidemiology study of diabetic retinopathy: proteinuria and retinopathy in a population of diabetic persons diagnosed prior to 30 years of age. In Friedman EA, L'Esperance FA (eds) Diabetic renal–retinal syndrome, vol. 3. New York: Grune & Stratton, 1986: pp 245–64.
17. Williamson JR, Rowald E, Chang K et al. Sex steroid dependency of diabetes-induced changes in polyol metabolism, vascular permeability and collagen cross-linking. Diabetes 1986; 35: 20–7.
18. Kostraba JN, Dorman JS, Orchard TJ et al. Contribution of diabetes duration before puberty to development of microvascular complications in IDDM subjects. Diabetes Care 1989; 12: 686–93.
19. Derby L, Laffel LBM, Krolewski AS. Risk of diabetic nephropathy declines with age in type 1 (insulin-dependent) diabetes. Diabetologia 1988; 31: 485A.
20. Deckert T, Poulsen JE, Larsen M. Prognosis of diabetics with diabetes onset before the age of thirty-one. Diabetologia 1978; 14: 363–70.
21. Borch-Johnsen K, Kreiner S. Proteinuria: value as predictor of cardiovascular mortality in insulin-dependent diabetes. Br Med J 1987; 294: 1651–4.
22. Jensen T, Borch-Johnsen K, Kofoed-Enevoldsen A, Deckert T. Coronary heart disease in young type 1 (insulin-dependent) diabetic patients with and without diabetic nephropathy: incidence and risk factors. Diabetologia 1987; 30: 144–8.
23. Krolewski AS, Kosinski EJ, Warram JM et al. Magnitude and determinants of coronary artery disease in juvenile-onset, insulin-dependent diabetes mellitus. Am J Cardiol 1987; 59: 750–5.
24. Parving HH, Hommel E. Prognosis in diabetic nephropathy. Br Med J 1989; 29; 230–3.
25. Mathiesen ER, Borch-Johnsen K, Jensen DV, Deckert T. Increased survival in patients with

diabetic nephropathy. Diabetologia 1989; 32: 884–6.

26. Fabre J, Balant LP, Dayer PG, Fox HM, Vernet AT. The kidney in maturity onset diabetes mellitus: a clinical study of 510 patients. Kidney Int 1982; 21: 730–8.

27. Klein R, Klein BEK, Moss S, DeMets DL. Proteinuria in diabetes. Arch Int Med 1988; 148: 181–6.

28. Parving HH, Gall MA, Skøtt P, Jørgensen HE, Jørgensen F, Larsen S. Prevalence and causes of albuminuria in non-insulin-dependent diabetic (NIDDM) patients. Kidney Int 1990; 37: 243.

29. WHO Multinational Study of Vascular Disease in Diabetes. Prevalence of small vessel and large vessel disease in diabetic patients from 14 centres. Diabetologia 1985; 28: 615–40.

30. Rate RG, Knowler WC, Morse HG et al. Diabetes mellitus in Hopi and Navajo Indians. Diabetes 1983; 32: 894–9.

31. Nelson RG, Kunzelman CL, Pettitt DJ, Saad MF, Bennett PH, Knowler WC. Albuminuria in type 2 (non-insulin-dependent) diabetes mellitus and impaired glucose tolerance in Pima Indians. Diabetologia 1989; 32: 870–6.

32. Haffner SM, Mitchell BD, Pugh JA et al. Proteinuria in Mexican Americans and Non-Hispanic Whites with NIDD. Diabetes Care 1989; 12: 530–6.

33. Cowie CC, Port FK, Wolfe RA, Savage PJ, Moll PP, Hawthorne VM. Disparities in incidence of end-stage renal disease according to race and type of diabetes. New Eng J Med 1989; 321: 1074–9.

34. Collins VR, Dowse GK, Finch CF, Zimmet PZ, Linnane AW. Prevalence and risk factors for micro- and macroalbuminuria in diabetic subjects and entire population of Naura. Diabetes 1989; 38: 602–10.

35. Samanta A, Burden AC, Freehally J, Walls J. Diabetic renal disease: differences between Asian and White patients. Br Med J 1986; 293: 366–7.

36. Allawi J, Rao PV, Gilbert R et al. Microalbuminuria in non-insulin-dependent diabetes: its prevalence in Indian compared with Europid patients. Br Med Journal 1988; 296: 462–4.

37. Ballard DJ, Humphrey LL, Melton J et al. Epidemiology of persistent proteinuria in type 2 diabetes mellitus. Population based study in Rochester, Minnesota. Diabetes 1988; 37: 405–12.

38. Hasslacher C, Ritz E, Tschøpe W, Gallasch G, Mann JFE. Hypertension in diabetes mellitus. Kidney Int 1988; 34 (S25): S133–7.

39. Hasslacher C, Ritz E, Wahl P. Michael C. Similar risks of nephropathy in patients with type 1 or type 2 diabetes mellitus. Nephrol Dial Transplant 1989; 4: 859–63.

40. Sasaki A, Horiuchi N, Hasegawa K, Uehara M. Risk factors related to the development of persistent albuminuria among diabetic patients observed in a long-term follow-up. J Japan Diab Soc 1986; 29: 1017–23.

41. Kunzelman CL, Knowler WC, Pettitt DJ, Bennett PH. Incidence of proteinuria in type 2 diabetes mellitus in the Pima Indians. Kidney Int 1989; 35: 681–7.

42. Knowler WC, Bennett PH, Nelson RG. Prediabetic blood pressure predicts albuminuria after development of NIDDM. Diabetes 1988; 37 (suppl. 1): 120A.

43. Pettitt DJ, Saad MF, Bennett PM, Nelsen RG, Knowler WC. Familial predisposition to renal disease in two generations of Pima Indians with Type 2 (non-insulin dependent) diabetes mellitus. Diabetologia 1990; 33: 438–43.

44. Humphrey LL, Ballard DJ, Frohnest PP, Chu C-P, O'Fallon M, Pallumbo PJ. Chronic renal failure in non-insulin-dependent diabetes mellitus. Ann Int Med 1989; 111: 788–96.

45. Joint Working Party on Diabetic Renal Failure. Treatment and mortality of diabetic renal failure patients identified in the 1985 UK survey. Br Med J 1989; 299: 1135–6.

46. Grenfell A, Bewick M, Parsons V, Snowden S, Taube D, Watkins PJ. Non-insulin-dependent diabetes and renal replacement therapy. Diabet Med 1988; 5: 172–6.

47. Schmitz A, Vaeth M. Microalbuminuria: a major risk factor in non-insulin dependent diabetes. A 10 year follow-up study of 503 patients. Diabet Med 1988; 5: 126–34.

48. Jarrett RJ, Viberti GC, Argyropoulos A, Hill RD, Mahmud U, Murrells TJ. Microalbuminuria predicts mortality in non-insulin-dependent diabetes. Diabet Med 1984; 1: 17–19.

49. Mogensen CE. Microalbuminuria predicts clinical proteinuria and early mortality in maturity onset diabetes. New Eng J Med 1984; 310: 356–60.

50. Nelson RG, Newman JM, Knowler WC et al. Incidence of end-stage renal disease in type 2 (non-insulin-dependent) diabetes mellitus in Pima Indians. Diabetologia 1988; 31: 730–6.

51. Pugh JA, Stern MP, Haffner SM, Eifler CW, Zapata M. Excess incidence of treatment of end-stage renal disease in Mexican Americans. Am J Epidemiol 1988; 127: 135–44.

52. Rostand SG, Kirk KA, Rutsky EA, Pate BA. Racial differences in the incidence of treatment for end-stage renal disease. New Engl J Med 1982; 306: 1276–9.

53. Abdullah MS. Diabetic nephropathy in Kenya. E Afr Med J 1978; 55: 513–18.

54. Adetuyibi A. Diabetes in the Nigerian African: 1. Review of long-term complications. Trop Geogr Med 1976; 28: 155–9.

55. Nelson RG, Pettitt DJ, Carraher JM, Naird HR, Knowler WC. Effect of proteinuria on mortality in NIDDM. Diabetes 1988; 37: 1499–504.

56. Morrish NJ, Stevens LK, Head J, Fuller JH, Jarrett RJ, Keen H. A prospective study of mortality among middle-aged diabetic patients (the London cohort of the WHO multinational study of vascular disease in diabetics). II: associated risk factors. Diabetologia 1990; 33: 542–8.

57. Cambier P. Application de la théorie de Rehberg à l'étude clinique des affections rénales et du diabète. Ann Méd 1934; 35: 273–99.

58. Fiaschi E, Grassi B, Andres G. La funzione renale nel diabete mellito. Rassegna Fisiopatol Clin Terapeut 1952; 4: 373–410.

59. Stalder G, Schmid R. Severe functional disorders of glomerular capillaries and renal haemodynamics in treated diabetes mellitus during childhood. Ann Paediatr 1959; 193: 129–38.

60. Ditzel J, Schwartz M. Abnormal glomerular filtration and short-term insulin-treated diabetic subjects. Diabetes 1967; 16: 264–7.

61. Mogensen CE. Glomerular filtration rate and renal plasma flow in short-term and long-term juvenile diabetes mellitus. Scand J Clin Lab Invest 1971; 28: 91–100.

62. Schmitz A, Christensen T, Jensen FT. Glomerular filtration rate and kidney volume in normo-albuminuric non-insulin-dependent diabetics—lack of glomerular hyperfiltration and renal hypertrophy in uncomplicated NIDDM. Scand J Clin Lab Invest 1989; 49: 103–8.

63. Palmisano JJ, Lebowitz HE. Renal function in Black Americans with type 2 diabetes. J Diabet Compl 1989; 3: 40–4.

64. Vora J, Thomas DM, Dean J, Peters J, Owens D, Williams JD. Renal function and albumin excretion rate in 62 newly presenting non-insulin dependent diabetics (NIDDM). Kidney Int 1990; 37: 245.

65. Loon N, Nelson R, Myers BD. Glomerular barrier abnormality in new onset NIDDM in Pima Indians. Kidney Int 1990; 37: 513.

66. Wiseman MJ, Viberti GC, Keen H. Threshold effect of plasma glucose in the glomerular hyperfiltration in diabetes. Nephron 1984; 38: 257–60.

67. Christiansen JS, Gammelgaard J, Tronier B, Svendsen PA, Parving H-H. Kidney function and size in diabetics before and during initial insulin treatment. Kidney Int 1982; 21: 683–8.

68. Wiseman MJ, Saunders AJ, Keen H, Viberti GC. Effect of blood glucose on increased glomerular filtration rate and kidney size in insulin-dependent diabetes. New Engl J Med 1985; 312: 617–21.

69. Schmitz A, Hansen HH, Christensen T. Kidney function in newly diagnosed type 2 (non-insulin-dependent) diabetic patients, before and during treatment. Diabetologia 1989; 32: 434–9.

70. Mogensen CE. Kidney function and glomerular permeability to macromolecules in early juvenile diabetes. Scand J Clin Lab Invest 1971; 28: 79–90.

71. Christiansen JS, Gammelgaard J, Frandsen M, Parving H-H. Increased kidney size, glomerular filtration rate and renal plasma flow in short-term insulin-dependent diabetics. Diabetologia 1981; 20: 451–6.

72. Ditzel J, Junker K. Abnormal glomerular filtration rate, renal plasma flow, and renal protein excretion in recent and short-term diabetics. Br Med J 1972; 2: 13–19.

73. Christiansen JS. On the pathogenesis of the increased glomerular filtration rate in short-term insulin-dependent diabetics. Thesis, University of Copenhagen, 1984.

74. Mogensen CE, Andersen MJF. Increased kidney size and glomerular filtration rate in early juvenile diabetes. Diabetes 1973; 22: 706–12.

75. Puig JG, Mateos Anton F, Grande C et al. Relation of kidney size to kidney function in early insulin-dependent diabetes. Diabetologia 1981; 21: 363–7.

76. Wiseman M, Viberti GC. Kidney size and GFR in type 1 (insulin-dependent) diabetes mellitus revisited. Diabetologia 1983; 25: 530.

77. Dumler F, Kumar V, Romanski NM, Cortes R, Levin N. Renal involvement in type 2 diabetes mellitus: a clinicopathologic study of the Henry Ford Hospital experience. Henry Ford Hosp Med J 1987; 35: 221–5.

78. Mogensen CE, Andersen MJF. Increased kidney size and glomerular filtration rate in untreated juvenile diabetics: normalization by insulin treatment. Diabetologia 1975; 11: 221–4.

79. Christensen CK, Christiansen JS, Christensen T, Hermansen K, Mogensen CE. The effect of six months continuous subcutaneous insulin infusion on kidney function and size in insulin-dependent diabetics. Diabet Med 1986; 3: 29–32.

80. Rasch R. Prevention of diabetic glomerulopathy in streptozotocin diabetic rats by insulin treatment. Kidney size and glomerular volume. Diabetologia 1979; 16: 125–8.

81. Seyer-Hansen K. Renal hypertrophy in streptozotocin-diabetic rats. Clin Sci Molec Med 1976; 51: 551–5.

82. Kahn CB, Paman PG, Zic, Z. Kidney size in diabetes mellitus. Diabetes 1974; 23: 788–92.

83. Ellis EN, Steffes MW, Gøetz FC, Sutherland

DER, Mauer SM. Relationship of renal size to nephropathy in type 1 (insulin-dependent) diabetes. Diabetologia 1985; 28: 12–15.

84. Kleinman KS, Fine LG. Prognostic implications of renal hypertrophy in diabetes mellitus. Diabetes Metab Rev 1988; 4: 179–89.

85. Segel MC, Lecky JW, Slasky BS. Diabetes mellitus: the predominant cause of bilateral renal enlargement. Radiology 1984; 153: 341–2.

86. Mogensen CE, Christensen CK. Predicting diabetic nephropathy in insulin-dependent diabetic patients. New Eng J Med 1984; 311: 89–93.

87. Mogensen CE. Early glomerular hyperfiltration in insulin-dependent diabetics and late nephropathy. Scand J Clin Lab Invest 1986; 46: 201–6.

88. Lervang H-H, Jensen S, Brøchner-Mortensen J, Ditzel J. Early glomerular hyperfiltration and the development of late nephropathy in type 1 (insulin-dependent) diabetes mellitus. Diabetologia 1988; 31: 723–9.

89. Jones SL, Wiseman MJ, Viberti GC. Glomerular hyperfiltration as a risk factor for diabetic nephropathy: five year report of a prospective study. Diabetologia 1991; 34: 59–60.

90. Keen H, Chlouverakis C, Fuller JH, Jarrett RJ. The concomitants of raised blood sugar: studies in newly detected hyperglycaemics. II. Urinary albumin excretion, blood pressure and their relation to blood sugar levels. Guy's Hosp Rep 1969; 118: 247–52.

91. Mogensen CE. Urinary albumin excretion in early and long term juvenile diabetes. Scand J Clin Lab Invest 1971; 28: 183–93.

92. Mogensen CE. Renal function changes in diabetes. Diabetes 1976; 25: 872–9.

93. Parving H-H, Noer I, Deckert T et al. The effect of metabolic regulation on microvascular permeability to small and large molecules in short-term juvenile diabetics. Diabetologia 1976; 12: 161–6.

94. Viberti GC, Mackintosh D, Bilous RW, Pickup JC, Keen H. Proteinuria in diabetes mellitus: role of spontaneous and experimental variation of glycaemia. Kidney Int 1982; 21: 714–20.

95. Feldt-Rasmussen B, Mathiesen ER. Variability of urinary albumin excretion in incipient diabetic nephropathy. Diabet Nephropathy 1984; 3: 101–3.

96. Mathiesen ER, Øxenboll B, Johansen K, Svendsen PA, Deckert T. Incipient nephropathy in type 1 (insulin-dependent) diabetes. Diabetologia 1984; 26; 406–10.

97. Rowe DJF, Bagga H, Betts PB. Normal variation in the rate of albumin excretion and albumin to creatinine ratios in overnight and daytime urine collections in non-diabetic children. Br Med J 1985; 291: 693–4.

98. Cohen DL, Close CF, Viberti GC. The variability of overnight urinary albumin excretion in insulin-dependent diabetic and normal subjects. Diabet Med 1987; 4: 437–40.

99. Chachati A, von Frenckell R, Foidart-Willems J, Godon JP, Lefèbvre PJ. Variability of albumin excretion in insulin-dependent diabetics. Diabet Med 1987; 4: 441–5.

100. Mathiesen ER, Saurbrey N, Hommel E, Parving H-H. Prevalence of microalbuminuria in children with type 1 (insulin-dependent) diabetes mellitus. Diabetologia 1986; 29: 640–3.

101. Close CF, on behalf of the MCS group. Sex, diabetes duration and microalbuminuria in type 1 (insulin-dependent) diabetes mellitus. Diabetologia 1987; 30: 508A.

102. Gardete LM, Silva-Graça A, Boavida JM, Cruz M, Carreiras F, Nunes-Correa J. Microalbuminuria—an early marker of developing microangiopathy. Diabetologia 1986; 29: 539A.

103. Gatling W, Knight C, Mullee MA, Hill RD. Microalbuminuria in diabetes: a population study of the prevalence and an assessment of three screening tests. Diabet Med 1988; 5: 343–7.

104. Parving H-H, Hommel E Mathiesen E et al. Prevalence of microalbuminuria, arterial hypertension, retinopathy and neuropathy in patients with insulin-dependent diabetes. Br Med J 1988; 296: 156–60.

105. Marshall SM, Alberti KGMM. Comparison of the prevalence and associated features of abnormal albumin excretion in insulin-dependent and non-insulin-dependent diabetes. Quart J Med 1989; 70: 61–71.

106. Mogensen CE, Christensen CK, Vittinghus E. The stages in diabetic renal disease with emphasis on the stage of incipient diabetic nephropathy. Diabetes 1983; 32 (Suppl. 2): 64–78.

107. Viberti GC, Pickup JC, Jarrett RJ, Keen H. Effect of control of blood glucose on urinary excretion of albumin and beta-2 microglobulin in insulin-dependent diabetes. New Engl J Med 1979; 300: 638–41.

108. Mogensen CE, Vittinghus, E. Urinary albumin excretion during exercise in juvenile diabetes: a provocation test for early abnormalities. Scand J Clin Lab Invest 1975; 35: 295–300.

109. Viberti GC, Jarrett RJ, McCartney M, Keen H. Increased glomerular permeability to albumin induced by exercise in diabetic subjects. Diabetologia 1978; 14: 293–300.

110. Koivisto VA, Huttenen NP, Vierikko P. Continuous subcutaneous insulin infection corrects exercise-induced albuminuria in juvenile diabetes. Br Med J 1981; 282: 778–9.

111. Viberti GC, Pickup JC, Bilous RW, Keen H, Mackintosh D. Correction of exercise-induced microalbuminuria in insulin-dependent diabet-

ics after 3 weeks of subcutaneous insulin infusion. Diabetes 1981; 30: 818–23.

112. Vittinghus E, Mogensen CE. Graded exercise and protein excretion in diabetic man and the effect of insulin treatment. Kidney Int 1982; 21: 725–9.

113. Damsgaard EM, Mogensen CE. Microalbuminuria in elderly hyperglycaemic patients and controls. Diabet Med 1986; 3: 430–5.

114. Allawi, J, Jarrett RJ. Microalbuminuria and cardiovascular risk factors in Type 2 diabetes mellitus. Diabet Med 1990; 7: 115–18.

115. Viberti GC, Hill RD, Jarrett RJ, Argyropoulos A, Mahmud U, Keen H. Microalbuminuria as a predictor of clinical nephropathy in insulin-dependent diabetes mellitus. Lancet 1982; i: 1430–2.

116. Parving H-H, Øxenboll B, Svendsen PA, Christiansen JS, Andersen AR. Early detection of patients at risk of developing diabetic nephropathy. A longitudinal study of urinary albumin excretion. Acta Endocrinol 1982; 100: 550–5.

117. Chavers BM, Bilous RW, Ellis EN, Steffes MW, Mauer SM. Glomerular lesions and urinary albumin excretion in type 1 diabetes without overt proteinuria. New Engl J Med 1989; 320: 966–70.

118. Mattock M et al. Microalbuminuria as a predictor of mortality in type 2 (non-insulin-dependent) diabetic patients: results from a three-year prospective study. Diabetologia 1990; 33 (S): 49A.

119. Yudkin JS, Forrest RD, Jackson CA. Microalbuminuria as a predictor of vascular disease in non-diabetic subjects. Lancet 1988; ii: 530–3.

120. Ireland JT, Viberti GC, Watkins PJ. The kidney and renal tract. In Keen H, Jarrett J (eds) Complications of diabetes (2nd edn). London: Edward Arnold, 1982: pp 137–78.

121. Bending JJ, Viberti GC, Watkins PJ, Keen H. Intermittent clinical proteinuria and renal function in diabetes: evolution and the effect of glycaemic control. Br Med J 1986; 292: 83–6.

122. Jerums J, Cooper ME, Seeman E, Murray RML, McNeil JJ. Spectrum of proteinuria in type 1 and type 2 diabetes. Diabetes Care 1987; 10: 419–27.

123. Mogensen CE. Progression of nephropathy in long-term diabetics with proteinuria and effect of initial anti-hypertensive treatment. Scand J Clin Lab Invest 1976; 36: 383–8.

124. Jones RH, Hayakawa H, Mackay JD, Parsons V, Watkins PJ. Progression of diabetic nephropathy. Lancet 1979; i: 1105–6.

125. Parving H-H, Smidt UM, Friisberg B, Bonnevie-Nielsen V, Andersen AR. A prospective study of glomerular filtration rate and arterial blood pressure in insulin-dependent diabetics with diabetic nephropathy. Diabetologia 1981; 20: 457–61.

126. Viberti, GC, Bilous RW, Mackintosh D, Keen H. Monitoring glomerular function in diabetic nephropathy. Am J Med 1983; 74: 256–64.

127. Feldt-Rasmussen B, Mathiesen ER, Deckert T. Effect of two years of strict metabolic control on progression of incipient nephropathy in insulin-dependent diabetes. Lancet 1986; ii: 1300–4.

128. Viberti GC, Bilous RW, Mackintosh D, Bending JJ, Keen H. Long term correction of hyperglycaemia and progression of renal failure in insulin-dependent diabetes. Br Med J 1983; 286: 598–602.

129. Hasslacher C, Stech W, Wahl P, Ritz E. Blood pressure and metabolic control as risk factors for nephropathy in type 1 (insulin-dependent) diabetes. Diabetologia 1985; 28: 6–11.

130. Nyberg G, Blohne G, Norden G. Impact of metabolic control in progression of diabetic nephropathy. Diabetologia 1987; 30: 82–6.

131. Viberti GC, Keen H, Dodds R, Bending JJ. Metabolic control and progression of diabetic nephropathy. Diabetologia 1987; 30: 481–2.

132. Laffel LMB, Krolewski AS, Rand LI, Warram JH, Chriestlieb AR, D'Elia JA. The impact of blood pressure on renal function in insulin-dependent diabetes. Kidney Int 1987; 31: 207.

133. Walser M, Drew HH, LaFrance ND. Creatinine measurements often yield false estimates of progression in chronic renal failure. Kidney Int 1988; 34: 412–18.

134. Shemesh O, Golbetz H, Kriss JP, Myers BD. Limitations of creatinine as a filtration marker in glomerulopathic patients. Kidney Int 1985; 28: 830–8.

135. Walker JD, Bending JJ, Dodds RA et al. Restriction of dietary protein and progression of renal failure in diabetic nephropathy. Lancet 1989; ii: 1411–14.

136. Zeller K, Whittaker E, Sullivan L, Raskin P, Jacobsen HR. Effect of restricting dietary protein on renal failure in patients with insulin-dependent diabetes mellitus. New Engl J Med 1991; 324: 78–84.

137. Wiseman MJ, Viberti GC, Mackintosh D, Jarrett RJ, Keen H. Glycaemia, arterial pressure and micro-albuminuria in type 1 (insulin-dependent) diabetes mellitus. Diabetologia 1984; 2: 401–5.

138. Jensen T, Borch-Johnsen K, Deckert T. Changes in blood pressure and renal function in patients with type 1 (insulin-dependent) diabetes mellitus prior to clinical diabetic nephropathy. Diabetes Res 1987; 4: 159–62.

139. Keen H, Track NS, Sowry GSC. Arterial pressure in clinically apparent diabetics. Diabete Métabolisme 1975; 1: 159–78.

140. Drury PL. Diabetes and arterial hypertension. Diabetologia 1983; 24: 1–9.

141. Borch-Johnsen K, Nissen RN, Nerup J. Blood pressure after 40 years of diabetes. Diabet Nephropathy 1985; 4: 11–12.

142. Watkins PJ, Blainey JD, Brewer DB et al. The natural history of diabetic renal disease. A follow-up study of series of renal biopsies. Quart J Med 1972; 41; 437–56.

143. Thomsen AC. The kidney in diabetes mellitus. PhD Thesis Copenhagen: Munksgaard, 1965.

144. Malins J. Clinical diabetes mellitus. London: Eyre & Spottiswoode 1968: pp 170.

145. Deckert T, Poulsen JE. Prognosis for juvenile diabetics with late diabetic manifestations. Acta Med Scand 1968; 183: 351–6.

146. Bilous RW, Viberti GC, Christiansen JS, Parving H-H, Keen H. Dissociation of diabetic complications in insulin-dependent diabetes: a clinical report. Diabet Nephropathy 1985; 4: 73–6.

147. Root HF, Mirsky S, Ditzel J. Proliferative retinopathy in diabetes mellitus; review of eight hundred forty-seven cases. JAMA 1959; 169: 903–9.

148. Feldman JN, Hirsch SR, Beyer MB, James WA, L'Esperance FA, Friedman EA. Prevalence of diabetic nephropathy at time of treatment for diabetic retinopathy. In Friedman EA, L'Esperance FA. (eds) Diabetic renal–retinal syndrome, vol. 2. New York: Grune & Stratton, 1982: pp 9–20.

149. Krolewski AS, Warram JH, Rand LI, Khan CR. Epidemiologic approach to the etiology of type 1 diabetes mellitus and its complications. New Engl J Med 1987; 317: 1390–8.

150. West KM, Erdreich LJ, Stober JA. A detailed study of risk factors for reinopathy and nephropathy in diabetes. Diabetes 1980; 29: 501–8.

151. Hommel E, Carstensen H, Skøtt P, Larsen S, Parving H-H. Prevalence and causes of microscopic haematuria in type 1 (insulin-dependent) diabetic patients with persistent proteinuria. Diabetologia 1987; 30: 627–30.

152. Taft JL, Billson VR, Nankervis A, Kincaid-Smith P, Martin FIR. A clinical–histological study of individuals with diabetes mellitus and proteinuria. Diabet Med 1990; 7: 215–21.

153. Hatch FE Jr, Parrish AE. Apparent remission of a severe diabetic on developing the Kimmelstiel–Wilson syndrome. Ann Intern Med 1961; 54: 544–9.

154. Rifkin H, Parker JG, Polin EB, Berkman JI, Spiro D. Diabetic glomerulosclerosis. Medicine 1948; 27: 429–57.

155. Bell ET. Renal vascular disease in diabetes mellitus. Diabetes 1953; 2: 376–89.

156. Gellman DD, Pirani CL, Soothill JF, Muehrcke RC, Kark RM. Diabetic nephropathy: a clinical and pathologic study based on renal biopsies. Medicine (Baltimore) 1959; 38: 321–67.

157. Axelroth L. Response of congestive heart failure to correction of hyperglycaemia in the presence of diabetic nephropathy. New Engl J Med 1975; 293: 1243–5.

158. DeFronzo RA. Hyperkalaemia and hyporeninaemic hypo-aldosteronism. Kidney Int 1980; 17: 118–34.

159. Campbell IW, Heading RC, Totill P et al. Gastric emptying in diabetic autonomic neuropathy. Gut 1977; 18: 462–7.

160. Watkins PJ. Facial sweating after food: a new sign of autonomic diabetic neuropathy. Br Med J 1973; 1: 583–7.

161. White P, Graham CA. The child with diabetes. In Marble A, White P, Bradley RF, Krall LP (eds) Joslin's Diabetes Mellitus (11th edn). Philadelphia: Lea & Febiger, 1971: pp 539–60.

162. Siperstein MD, Unger RH, Madison LL. Studies of muscle capillary basement membranes in normal subjects, diabetic, and prediabetic patients. J Clin Invest 1968; 47: 1973–99.

163. Williamson JR, Kilo C. Current status of capillary basement-membrane disease in diabetes mellitus. Diabetes 1977; 26: 65–73.

164. Steffes MW, Sutherland DER, Gøetz FC, Rich SS, Mauer SM. Studies of kidney and muscle biopsy specimens from identical twins discordant for type 1 diabetes mellitus. New Engl J Med 1985; 312: 1282–7.

165. Becker D, Miller M. Presence of diabetic glomerulosclerosis in patients with haemochromatosis. New Engl J Med 1960; 263: 367–73.

166. Ireland JT, Patnaik BK, Duncan LJP. Glomerular ultrastructure in secondary diabetics and normal subjects. Diabetes 1967; 16: 628–35.

167. Brown DM, Andres GA, Hostetter TH, Mauer SM, Price R, Venkatachalam MA. Proceedings of a task force on animals appropriate for studying diabetes mellitus and its complications. Kidney complications. Diabetes 1982; 31 (suppl. 1): 71–81.

168. Lee CS, Mauer SM, Brown DM, Sutherland DER, Michael AF, Najarian JS. Renal transplantation in diabetes mellitus in the rat. J Exper Med 1974; 139: 793–800.

169. Mauer SM, Steffes MW, Sutherland DER, Najarian JS, Michael AF, Brown DM. Studies of the rate of regression of the glomerular lesions in diabetic rats treated with pancreatic islet transplantation. Diabetes 1975; 24: 280–5.

170. Steffes MW, Brown DM, Basgen JM, Mauer, SM. Amelioration of mesangial volume and surface alterations following islet transplantation in diabetic rats. Diabetes 1980; 29: 509–15.

171. Gøtzsche O, Gundersen HJG, Østerby R. Irreversibility of glomerular basement membrane accumulation despite reversibility of renal hypertrophy with islet transplantation in early experimental diabetes. Diabetes 1981; 30: 481–5.

172. Rasch R. Prevention of diabetic glomerulopathy in streptozotocin diabetic rats by insulin treatment. The mesangial regions. Diabetologia 1979; 17: 243–8.

173. Rasch R. Prevention of diabetic glomerulopathy in streptozotocin diabetic rats. Albumin excretion. Diabetologia 1980; 18: 413–16.

174. O'Donnell MP, Kasiske BL, Keane WF. Glomerular haemodynamics and structural alterations in experimental diabetes mellitus. FASEB 1988; 2: 2339–47.

175. Mauer SM, Steffes MW, Connet J, Najarian JS, Sutherland DER, Barbosa J. The development of lesions in the glomerular basement membrane and mesangium after transplantation of normal kidneys into diabetic patients. Diabetes 1983; 32: 948–52.

176. Mauer SM, Goetz FC, McHugh LE et al. Long-term study of normal kidneys transplanted into patients with type 1 diabetes. Diabetes 1989; 38: 516–23.

177. Brownlee M, Vlassara H, Cerami A. Non-enzymatic glycosylation and the pathogenesis of diabetic complications. Ann Intern Med 1984; 101: 527–37.

178. Brownlee M, Cerami A, Vlassara H. Advanced glycosylation end-product in tissue and the biochemical basis of diabetic complications. New Engl J Med 1988; 318: 1315–21.

179. Stevens VJ, Rouzer CA, Monnier VM, Cerami A. Diabetic cataract formation: potential role of glycosylation of lens crystallins. Proc Nat Acad Sci USA 1978; 75: 2918–22.

180. Brownlee M, Pongor S, Cerami A. Covalent attachment of soluble proteins by nonenzymatically glycosylated collagen: role in the in situ formation of immune complexes. J Exper Med 1983; 158: 1739–44.

181. Brownlee M, Vlassara H, Cerami A. Nonenzymatic glycosylation reduces the susceptibility of fibrin to degradation by plasmin. Diabetes 1983; 32: 680–4.

182. Cohen MP, Ku L. Inhibition of fibronectin binding to matrix components by non-enzymatic glycosylation. Diabetes 1984; 33: 970–4.

183. Cohen MP, Saini R, Klepser H, Vasanthi LG. Fibronectin binding to glomerular basement membrane is altered in diabetes. Diabetes 1987; 36: 758–63.

184. Ghiggeri GM, Candiano G, Delfino G, Queirolo C. Electrical charge of serum and urinary albumin in normal and diabetic humans. Kidney Int 1985; 28: 168–77.

185. Nakamura Y, Myers BD (1988). Charge selectivity of proteinuria in diabetic glomerulopathy. Diabetes 1988; 37: 1202–11.

186. Vlassara H, Brownlee M, Cerami A. Novel macrophage receptor for glucose-modified proteins is distinct from previously described scavenger receptors. J Exper Med 1986; 164: 1301–9.

187. Ludvigson MA, Sorenson RL. Immunohistochemical localization of aldose reductase. II. Rat eye and kidney. Diabetes 1980; 29: 450–9.

188. Kikkawa R, Umemura K, Haneda M, Arimura T, Ebata K, Shigeta Y. Evidence for existence of polyol pathway in cultured rat mesangial cells. Diabetes 1987; 36: 240–3.

189. Burg MB. Role of aldose reductase and sorbitol in maintaining the medullary intracellular milieu. Kidney Int 1988; 33: 635–41.

190. Cogan DG. Aldose reductase and complications of diabetes. Ann Intern Med 1984; 101: 82–91.

191. Kador PF, Robinson WG Jr, Kinoshita JH. The pharmacology of aldose reductase inhibitors. Ann Rev Pharmacol Toxicol 1985; 25: 691–714.

192. Pugliese G, Tilton RG, Speedy A et al. Modulation of haemodynamics and vascular filtration changes in diabetic rats by dietary myo-inositol. Diabetes 1990; 39: 312–22.

193. Beyer-Mears A, Ku L, Cohen MP. Glomerular polyol accumulation in diabetes and its prevention by oral sorbinil. Diabetes 1984; 33: 604–7.

194. Goldfarb S, Simmons DA, Kern EFO. Amelioration of glomerular hyperfiltration in acute experimental diabetes mellitus by dietary myo-inositol supplementation and aldose reductase inhibition. Trans Assoc Amer Phys 1986; 99: 67–72.

195. Beyer-Mears A, Cruz E, Edelist T, Varagianuis E. Diminished proteinuria in diabetes mellitus by sorbinil, an aldose reductase inhibitor. Pharmacology 1986; 32: 52–60.

196. Daniels BS, Hostetter TH. Aldose reductase inhibitors and glomerular abnormalities in diabetic rats. Diabetes 1989; 38: 981–6.

197. Coco M, Aynedjian HS, Bank N. Effect of galactose and aldose reductase inhibition on renal haemodynamics. Clin Res 1988; 36: 626A.

198. Mower P, Aynedjian H, Silverman S, Wilkes B, Bank N. Sorbinil prevents glomerular hyperperfusion in diabetic rats. Kidney Int 1989; 35: 433.

199. Frey J, Zager P, Jackson J, Eaton P, Scavini M. Aldose reductase activity mediates renal prostaglandin production in streptozotocin diabetic rats. Kidney Int 1989; 35: 292.

200. Jacobson M, Sharma YR, Cotlier E, Hollander JD. Diabetic complications in lens and nerve and their prevention by sulindac or sorbinil: two novel aldose reductase inhibitors. Invest Ophthalmol Vis Sci 1983; 24: 1426–9.

201. Beyer-Mears A, Cruz E, Dillon P, Tanis D, Roche M. Diabetic renal hypertrophy diminished by aldose reductase inhibition (abstr). Fed Proc 1983; 42: 505.

202. Rasch R, Østerby R. Lack of influence of aldose reductase inhibitor treatment for 6 months on the glycogen nephrosis in streptozotocin diabetic rats. Diabetologia 1989; 32: 532A.

203. Tilton RG, Chang K, Pugliese G et al. Prevention of haemodynamic and vascular albumin filtration changes in diabetic rats by aldose reductase inhibitors. Diabetes 1989; 38: 1258–70.

204. Pedersen MM, Christiansen JS, Mogensen CE. Renal effects of an aldose reductase inhibitor (Statil) during 6 months treatment in type 1 (insulin-dependent) diabetic patients. Diabetologia 1989; 32: 516A.

205. Blohmé G, Smith U. Aldose reductase inhibition reduces urinary albumin excretion rate in incipient diabetic nephropathy. Diabetologia 1989; 32: 467A.

206. Cohen DL, Allawi J, Brophy K, Keen H, Viberti GC. Tolerance safety and effects of Statil, an aldose reductase inhibitor in type 2 (non-insulin-dependent) diabetic patients with microalbuminuria. Diabetologia 1989; 32: 477A.

207. Brownlee M, Spiro MG. Glomerular basement membrane metabolism in the diabetic rat. In vivo studies. Diabetes 1979; 28: 121–5.

208. Khalifa A, Cohen MP. Glomerular protocollagen lysil hydroxylase activity in streptozotocin diabetes. Biochim Biophys Acta 1975; 386: 322–9.

209. Brenner BM, Hostetter TH, Humes HD. Molecular basis of proteinuria of glomerular origin. New Engl J Med 1978; 298: 826–33.

210. Farquhar MG. The glomerular basement membrane: a selective macromolecular filter. In Hay ED (ed.) Cell biology of extracellular matrix. New York: Plenum, 1981: pp 335–78.

211. Parthasarathy N, Spiro RG. Effect of diabetes on the glycosaminoglycan component of the human glomerular basement membrane. Diabetes 1982; 31: 738–41.

212. Kanwar YS, Rosenzweig LJ, Linker A, Jakubowski ML. Decreased de novo synthesis of glomerular proteoglycans in diabetes: biochemical and autoradiographic evidence. Proc Nat Acad Sci USA 1983; 80: 2272–5.

213. Rohrbach DH, Wagner CW, Star VL, Martin GR, Brown KS. Reduced synthesis of basement membrane heparan sulfate proteoglycan in streptozotocin-induced diabetic mice. J Biol Chem 1983; 258: 11676–7.

214. Cohen MP, Surma ML. Effect of diabetes on in vivo metabolism of ^{35}S-labeled glomerular basement membrane. Diabetes 1984; 33: 8–12.

215. Wu V-Y, Wilson B, Cohen MP. Disturbances in glomerular basement membrane glycosaminoglycans in experimental diabetes. Diabetes 1987; 36: 679–83.

216. Shimomura H, Spiro RG. Studies on the macromolecular components of human glomerular basement membrane and alterations in diabetes: decreased levels of heparan sulfate proteoglycan and laminin. Diabetes 1987; 36: 374–81.

217. Westberg NG, Michael AF. Human glomerular basement membrane: chemical composition in diabetes mellitus. Acta Med Scand 1973; 194: 39–47.

218. Kefalides NA. Biochemical properties of human glomerular basement membrane in normal and diabetic kidneys. J Clin Invest 1974; 53: 403–7.

219. Wahl P, Deppermann D, Hasslacher C. Biochemistry of glomerular basement membrane of the normal and diabetic human. Kidney Int 1982; 21: 744–9.

220. Spiro RG, Spiro MJ. Effect of diabetes on the biosynthesis of the renal glomerula basement membrane: studies on the glucosyltransferase. Diabetes 1971; 20: 641–8.

221. Beisswenger PJ, Spiro RG. Studies on the human glomerular basement membrane: composition, nature of the carbohydrate units and chemical changes in diabetes mellitus. Diabetes 1972; 22: 180–93.

222. Beisswenger PJ. Glomerular basement membrane. Biosynthesis and chemical composition in the streptozotocin diabetic rat. J Clin Invest 1976; 58: 844–52.

223. Lorenzi M, Cagliero E, Toledo S. Glucose toxicity for human endothelial cells in culture: delayed replication, disturbed cell cycle, and accelerated death. Diabetes 1985; 34: 621–7.

224. Lorenzi M, Nordberg J, Toledo S. High glucose prolongs cell-cycle tranversal of cultured human endothelial cell. Diabetes 1987; 36: 1261–7.

225. Lorenzi M, Toledo S, Boss GR, Lane MJ, Montisano DF. The polyol pathway and glucose-6-phosphate in human endothelial cells cultured in high glucose concentrations. Diabetologia 1987; 30: 222–7.

226. Lorenzi M, Montisano D, Toledo S, Barrieux A. High glucose induces DNA damage in cultured human endothelial cells. J Clin Invest 1986; 77: 322–5.

227. Lorenzi M, Montisano DF, Toledo S, Wong, H-CH. Increased single strand breaks in DNA of lymphocytes from diabetic subjects. J Clin Invest 1987; 79: 653–6.

228. Cagliero E, Maiello M, Boeri D, Roy S, Lorenzi M. Increased expression of basement membrane components in human endothelial cells cultured in high glucose. J Clin Invest 1988; 82: 735–8.

229. Boeri D, Almus FE, Maiello M, Cagliero E, Rao LVM, Lorenzi M. Modification of tissue-factor

mRNA and protein response to thrombin and interleukin 1 by high glucose in cultured human endothelial cells. Diabetes 1989; 38: 312–8.

230. Jensen T. Increased plasma level of von Willebrand factor in type 1 (insulin-dependent) diabetic patients with incipient nephropathy. Br Med J 1989; 298: 27–8.

231. Jensen T, Feldt-Rasmussen B, Bjerre-Knudsen J, Deckert T. Features of endothelial dysfunction in early diabetic nephropathy. Lancet 1989; i: 461–3.

232. Hostetter TH, Rennke HG, Brenner BM. The case for intrarenal hypertension in the initiation and progression of diabetic and other glomerulopathies. Am J Med 1982; 72: 375–80.

233. Steffes MW, Brown DM, Mauer SM. Diabetic glomerulopathy following unilateral nephrectomy in the rat. Diabetes 1978; 27: 35–41.

234. Mauer SM, Steffes MW, Azar S, Sandberg SK, Brown DM. The effects of Goldblatt hypertension on development of the glomerular lesions of diabetes mellitus in the rat. Diabetes 1978; 27: 738–44.

235. Berkman J, Rifkin H. Unilateral nodular diabetic glomerulosclerosis (Kimmelstiel–Wilson). Report of a case. Metabolism 1973; 22: 715–22.

236. Béroniade VC, Lefèbvre R, Falardeau P. Unilateral diabetic glomerulosclerosis: recurrence of an experiment of nature. Am J Nephrol 1987; 7: 55–9.

237. Zatz R, Meyer TW, Rennke HG, Brenner BM. Predominance of haemodynamic rather than metabolic factors in the pathogenesis of diabetic glomerulopathy. Proc Nat Acad Sci USA 1985; 82: 5963–7.

238. Anderson S, Rennke HG, Brenner BM. Therapeutic advantages of conveting-enzyme inhibitors in arresting progressive renal disease associated with systemic hypertension in the rat. J Clin Invest 1986; 77: 1925–30.

239. Ausiello DA, Kreisberg JI, Roy C, Karnovsky MJ. Contraction of cultured rat glomerular cells of apparent mesangial origin after stimulation with angiotensin II and arginine vasopressin. J Clin Invest 1980; 65: 754–60.

240. Webb RC, Bohr DF. Recent advances in the pathogenesis of hypertension: consideration of structural, functional, and metabolic vascular abnormalities resulting in elevated arterial resistance. Am Heart J 1981; 102: 251–64.

241. Leung DYM, Glagov S, Mathews MB. Cyclic stretching stimulates synthesis of matrix components by arterial smooth muscle cells in vitro. Science 1976; 191: 475–7.

242. Ross R, Glomset JA. The pathogenesis of atherosclerosis. New Engl J Med 1976; 295: 369–77.

243. Olson JL, Hostetter TH, Rennke HG, Brenner

BM, Venkatachalam MA. Altered glomerular permselectivity and progressive sclerosis following extreme ablation of renal mass. Kidney Int 1982; 22: 112–26.

244. Mauer SM, Steffes MW, Chern M, Brown DM. Mesangial uptake and processing of macromolecules in rats with diabetes mellitus. Lab Invest 1979; 41: 401–6.

245. Velosa JA, Glasser RJ, Nevins TE, Michael AF. Experimental model of focal sclerosis. II. Correlations with immunopathologic changes, macromolecular kinetics, and polyanion loss. Lab Invest 1977; 36: 527–34.

246. Mauer SM, Steffes MW, Brown DM. The kidney in diabetes. Am J Med 1981; 70: 603–12.

247. Grond J, Schilthuis MS, Koudstaal J, Elema J. Mesangial function and glomerular sclerosis in rats after unilateral nephrectomy. Kidney Int 1982; 22: 338–43.

248. Fogo A, Ichikawa I. Evidence for the central role of glomerular growth promoters in the development of sclerosis. Semin Nephrol 1989; 9: 329–42.

249. Orloff MJ, Yamanaka N, Greenleaf GE, Huang Y-T, Huang D-G, Leng X-S. Reversal of mesangial enlargement in rats with long-standing diabetes by whole pancreas transplantation. Diabetes 1986; 35: 347–54.

250. Bank N, Klose R, Aynedjian HS, Nguyen D, Sablay LB. Evidence against increased glomerular pressure initiating diabetic nephropathy. Kidney Int 1987; 31: 898–905.

251. Kasiske BL, O'Donnell MP, Cleary MP, Keane WF. Treatment of hyperlipidaemia reduces glomerular injury in obese Zucker rats. Kidney Int 1988; 33: 667–72.

252. Yoshida Y, Fogo A, Shiraga H, Glick AD, Ichikawa I. Serial micropuncture analysis of single nephron function in subtotal renal ablation. Kidney Int 1988; 33: 851–5.

253. Neugarten J, Feiner HD, Schacht RG, Gallo GR, Baldwin DS. Aggravation of experimental glomerulonephritis by superimposed clip hypertension. Kidney Int 1982; 22: 257–63.

254. Halliburton IW, Thomson RY. Chemical aspects of compensatory renal hypertrophy. Cancer Res 1965; 25: 1882–7.

255. Hostetter TH, Troy JC, Brenner BM. Glomerular haemodynamics in experimental diabetes mellitus. Kidney Int 1981; 19: 410–5.

256. Anderson S, Meyer TW, Rennke HG, Brenner BM. Control of glomerular hypertension limits glomerular injury in rats with reduced renal mass. J Clin Invest 1985; 76: 612–9.

257. Purkerson ML, Hoffsten PE, Klahr S. Pathogenesis of the glomerulopathy associated with renal infarction in rats. Kidney Int 1976; 9: 407–17.

258. Purkerson ML, Joist JH, Greenberg JM, Kay D, Hoffsten PE, Klahr S. Inhibition by anticoagulant drugs of the progressive hypertension and uraemia associated with renal infarction in rats. Thrombosis Res 1982; 26: 227–40.

259. Purkerson ML, Joist JH, Yates J, Valdes A, Morrison A, Klahr S. Inhibition of thromboxane synthesis ameliorates the progressive kidney disease of rats with subtotal renal ablation. Proc Nat Acad Sci USA 1985; 82: 193–7.

260. Purkerson ML, Tollefsen DM, Klahr S. N-desulfated/acetylated heparin ameliorates the progression of renal disease in rats with subtotal renal ablation. J. Clin Invest 1988; 81: 69–74.

261. Olson JL. Role of heparin as a protective agent following reduction of renal mass. Kidney Int 1984; 25: 376–82.

262. Castellot JJ, Hoover RL, Harper PA, Karnovsky MJ. Heparin and glomerular epithelial cell-secreted heparin-like species inhibit mesangial cell proliferation. Am J Path 1985; 120: 427–35.

263. Fogo A, Yoshida Y, Ichikawa I. Angiotensin converting enzyme inhibitor suppresses accelerated growth of glomerular cells in vivo and in vitro. Kidney Int 1988; 33: 296.

264. Ichikawa I, Yoshida Y, Fogo A, Purkerson ML, Klahr S. Effect of heparin on the glomerular structure and function of remnant nephrons. Kidney Int 1988; 34: 638–44.

265. Cortes P, Dumler F, Goldman J, Levin NW. Relationship between renal function and metabolic alterations in early streptozotocin-induced diabetes in rats. Diabetes 1987; 36: 80–7.

266. Doi T, Striker LJ, Quaife C et al. Progressive glomerular sclerosis develops in transgenic mice chronically expressing growth hormone and growth hormone releasing factor but not in those expressing insulin-like growth factor-1. Am J Path 1988; 131: 398–403.

267. Seaquist ER, Gœtz FC, Rich S, Barbosa J. Familial clustering of diabetic kidney disease. Evidence for genetic susceptibility to diabetic nephropathy. New Engl J Med 1989; 320: 1161–5.

268. Viberti GC, Keen H, Wiseman MJ. Raised arterial pressure in parents of proteinuric insulin-dependent diabetics. Br Med J 1987; 295: 515–17.

269. Krolewski AS, Canessa M, Warram JM et al. Predisposition to hypertension and susceptibility to renal disease in insulin-dependent diabetes mellitus. New Engl J Med 1988; 318: 140–5.

270. Jensen JS, Mathiesen ER, Norgaard K et al. Increased blood pressure and erythrocyte sodium–lithium countertransport activity are not inherited in diabetic nephropathy. Diabetologia 1990; 33: 619–25.

271. Dadone MM, Hasstedt SJ, Hunt SC, Smith JB, Ash KO, Williams RR. Genetic analysis of sodium–lithium countertransport in ten hypertension-prone kindreds. Am J Med 1984; 17: 565–77.

272. Boerwinkle E, Turner ST, Weinshilboum R, Johnson M, Richelson E, Sing CF. Analysis of the distribution of sodium lithium countertransport in a sample representative of the general population. Gen Epidemiol 1986; 3; 365–78.

273. Mangili R, Bending JJ, Scott G, Li LK, Gupta A, Viberti GC. Increased sodium–lithium countertransport activity in red cells of patients with insulin-dependent diabetes and nephropathy. New Engl J Med 1988; 318: 146–50.

274. Walker JD, Tariq T, Viberti GC. Sodium–lithium countertransport activity in red cells of patients with insulin dependent diabetes and nephropathy and their parents. Br Med J 1990; 301: 635–8.

275. Jones SL, Trevisan R, Tariq T et al. Sodium–lithium countertransport in microalbuminuric insulin-dependent diabetic patients. Hypertension 1990; 15: 570–5.

276. Jones SL, Faria J, Tariq T, Mattock MB, Viberti GC. Sodium–lithium countertransport activity and serum lipoproteins in insulin-dependent diabetic patients. Diabet Med 1989; 6 (suppl. 2): 28A.

277. Bunker CH, Mallinger AG. Sodium-lithium countertransport, obesity, insulin and blood pressure in healthy premenopausal women. Circulation 1985; 72 (S3): III-296.

278. Nosadini R, Viberti GC, Doria A et al. Increased Na^+/H^+ countertransport activity is associated with cardiac hypertrophy and insulin resistance in hypertensive type 1 (insulin-dependent) diabetic patients. Diabetologia 1989; 32: 523A.

279. Foster DW. Insulin resistance—a secret killer? New Engl J Med 1989; 320: 733–4.

280. Silberberg JS, Barre PE, Prichard SS, Sniderman AD. Impact of left ventricular hypertrophy on survival in end-stage renal disease. Kidney Int 1989; 36: 286–90.

281. Sampson MJ, Chambers J, Sprigings D, Drury PL. Intraventricular septal hypertrophy in type 1 diabetic patients with microalbuminuria or early proteinuria. Diabet Med 1990; 7: 126–31.

282. Reaven GM, Hoffman BP. A role for insulin in the aetiology and course of hypertension? Lancet 1987; ii: 435–7.

283. Mahnensmith RL, Aronson PS. The plasma membrane sodium–hydrogen exchanger and its role in physiological and pathological processes. Circulation Res 1985; 56: 773–88.

284. Li LK, Trevisan R, Walker JD, Viberti GC. Overactivity of Na^+/H^+ antiport and enhanced

cell growth in fibroblasts of type 1 (insulin-dependent) diabetics with nephropathy. Kidney Int 1990; 37: 199.

285. Ng LL, Simmons D, Frigh V, Garrido MC, Bomford J. Effect of protein kinase C modulators on the leucocyte Na^+-H^+ antiport in type 1 (insulin-dependent) diabetic subjects with albuminuria. Diabetologia 1990; 33: 278–84.

286. Amiel SA, Sherwin RS, Simonson DC, Lauritano AA, Tamborlane WV. Impaired insulin action in puberty. A contributing factor to poor glycaemic control in adolescents with diabetes. New Engl J Med 1986; 315: 215–19.

287. Parving H-H, Viberti GC, Keen H, Christiansen JS, Lassen NA. Haemodynamic factors in the genesis of diabetic microangiopathy. Metabolism 1983; 32: 943–9.

288. Feldt-Rasmussen B. Increased transcapillary escape rate of albumin in type 1 (insulin-dependent) diabetic patients with microalbuminuria. Diabetologia 1986; 29: 282–6.

289. Moorhead JF, Chan MK, El-Nahas M, Varghese Z. Lipid nephrotoxicity in chronic progressive glomerular and tubulo-interstitial disease. Lancet 1982; ii: 1309–11.

290. Zavaroni I, Bonora E, Pagliara M et al. Risk factors for coronary artery disease in healthy persons with hyperinsulinaemia and normal glucose tolerance. New Engl J Med 1989; 320: 702–6.

291. Michels LD, Davidman M, Keane WF. Determinants of glomerular filtration and plasma flow in experimental diabetic rats. J Lab Clin Med 1981; 98: 869–85.

292. Jensen PK, Christiansen JS, Steven K, Parving H-H. Renal function in streptozocin-diabetic rats. Diabetologia 1981; 21: 409–14.

293. O'Donnell MP, Kasiske BL, Daniels FX, Keane WF. Effects of nephron loss on glomerular haemodynamics and morphology in diabetic rats. Diabetes 1986; 35: 1011–15.

294. Wiseman MJ, Mangili R, Alberetto M, Keen H, Viberti GC. Glomerular response mechanisms to glycaemic changes in insulin-dependent diabetics. Kidney Int 1987; 31: 1012–18.

295. Kroustrup JP, Gundersen HJG, Østerby R. Glomerular size and structure in diabetes mellitus. III. Early enlargement of the capillary surface. Diabetologia 1977; 13: 207–10.

296. Hirose K, Tsuchida H, Østerby R, Gundersen HJG. A strong correlation between glomerular filtration rate and filtration surface area in diabetic kidney hyperfunction. Lab Invest 1980; 43: 434–7.

297. Ballerman BJ, Skorecki KL, Brenner BM. Reduced glomerular angiotensin II receptor density in early untreated diabetes mellitus in the rat. Am J Physiol 1984; 247: F110–16.

298. Viberti GC, Wiseman MJ. The kidney in diabetes: significance of the early abnormalities. Clin Endocrinol Metab 1986; 15: 753–82.

299. Christiansen JS, Frandsen M, Parving H-H. Effect of intravenous glucose infusion on renal function in normal man and in insulin-dependent diabetics. Diabetologia 1981; 21: 368–73.

300. Mogensen CE. Maximum tubular reabsorption capacity for glucose and renal haemodynamics during rapid hypertonic glucose infusion in normal and diabetic subjects. Scand J Clin Lab Invest 1971; 28: 101–9.

301. Fox M, Thier S, Rosenberg L, Segal S. Impaired renal tubular function induced by sugar infusion in man. J Clin Endocrinol Metab 1964; 24: 1318–27.

302. Brøchner-Mortensen J. The glomerular filtration rate during moderate hyperglycaemia in normal man. Acta Med Scand 1973; 194: 31–7.

303. Atherton A, Hill DW, Keen H, Young S, Edwards EJ. The effect of acute hyperglycaemia on the retinal circulation of the normal cat. Diabetologia 1980; 18: 233–7.

304. Blantz RC, Peterson OW, Gushwa L, Tucker BJ. Effect of modest hyperglycaemia on tubulo-glomerular feedback activity. Kidney Int 1982; 22 (S12): S202–12.

305. Leyssac PP. The renin angiotensin system and kidney function. A review of contributions to a new theory. Acta Physiol Scand 1976; 442 (S): 1–52.

306. Trevisan R, Nosadini R, Fioretto P et al. Ketone bodies increase glomerular filtration rate in normal man and in patients with type 1 (insulin-dependent) diabetes mellitus. Diabetologia 1987; 30: 214–21.

307. Mogensen CE, Christensen NJ, Gundersen HJG. The acute effect of insulin on renal haemodynamics and protein excretion in diabetics. Diabetologia 1978; 15: 153–7.

308. Christiansen JS, Frandsen M, Parving H-H. The effect of intravenous insulin infusion on kidney function in insulin-dependent diabetes mellitus. Diabetologia 1981; 20: 199–204.

309. DeFronzo RA, Cooke CR, Andres R, Faloona GR, Davis PJ. The effect of insulin on renal handling of sodium, potassium, calcium and phosphate in man. J Clin Invest 1975; 55: 845–55.

310. Skøtt P, Hother-Nielsen O, Bruun N et al. Effects of insulin on kidney function and sodium excretion in healthy subjects. Diabetologia 1989; 32: 694–9.

311. Parving H-H, Noer I, Mogensen CE, Svendsen PA. Kidney function in normal man during short-term growth-hormone infusion. Acta Endocrinol 1978; 89: 796–800.

312. Corvilain J, Abramow M. Some effects of

human growth hormone on renal haemodynamics and on tubular phosphate transport in man. J Clin Invest 1962; 41: 1230–5.

313. Christiansen JS, Gammelgaard J, Ørskov H, Andersen AR, Telmer S, Parving H-H. Kidney function and size in normal subjects before and during growth hormone administration for one week. Eur J Clin Invest 1981; 11: 487–90.

314. Christiansen JS, Gammelgaard J, Frandsen M, Ørskov H, Parving H-H. Kidney function and size in type 1 (insulin-dependent) diabetic patients before and during growth hormone administration for one week. Diabetologia 1982; 22: 333–7.

315. Lundbaek K, Christensen NJ, Jensen VA et al. Diabetic angiopathy and growth hormone. Lancet 1970; ii: 131–3.

316. Wiseman MJ, Redmond S, House F, Keen H, Viberti GC. The glomerular hyperfiltration of diabetics is not associated with elevated levels of glucagon and growth hormone. Diabetologia 1985; 28: 718–21.

317. Parving H-H, Noer I, Kehlet H, Mogensen CE, Svendsen PA, Heding LG. The effect of short-term glucagon infusion on kidney function in normal man. Diabetologia 1977; 13: 323–5.

318. Parving H-H, Christiansen JS, Noer I, Tronier B, Mogensen CE. The effect of glucagon infusion on kidney function in short-term type 1 (insulin-dependent) juvenile diabetics. Diabetologia 1980; 19: 350–4.

319. Ueda J, Nakanishi H, Miyazaki M, Abe Y. Effects of glucagon on the renal haemodynamics of dogs. Eur J Pharmacol 1977; 41: 209–12.

320. Uranga J, Frenzalida R, Rapoport AL, Del Castillo E. Effect of glucagon and glomerulopressin on the renal function of the dog. Horm Metab Res 1979; 11: 275–9.

321. Fioretto P, Trevisan R, Valerio A et al. Impaired renal response to a meat meal in insulin-dependent diabetes: role of glucagon and prostaglandins. Am J Physiol 1990; 258: F675–83.

322. Viberti GC, Benigni A, Bognetti E, Remuzzi G, Wiseman MJ. Glomerular hyperfiltration and urinary prostaglandins in type 1 diabetes mellitus. Diabet Med 1989; 6: 219–23.

323. Esmatjes E, Fernandez MR, Halperin I et al. Renal haemodynamic abnormalities in patients with short-term insulin-dependent diabetes mellitus: role of renal prostaglandins. J Clin Endocrinol Metab 1985; 60: 1231–6.

324. Kasiske BL, O'Donnell MP, Keane WP. Glucose induced increases in renal haemodynamic function. Possible modulation by renal prostaglandins. Diabetes 1985; 34: 360–4.

325. Jensen PK, Steven K, Blæhr H, Christiansen JS, Parving H-H. Effects of indomethacin on glomerular haemodynamics in experimental diabetes. Kidney Int 1986; 29: 490–5.

326. Schambelan M, Blake S, Sraer J, Bens M, Nivez M-P, Wahbe F. Increased prostaglandin production by glomeruli isolated from rats with streptozotocin-induced diabetes mellitus. J Clin Invest 1985; 75: 404–12.

327. Moel DI, Safirstein RL, McEvoy RC, Hsueh W. Effect of aspirin on experimental diabetic nephropathy. J Lab Clin Med 1987; 110: 300–7.

328. Christiansen JS, Feldt-Rasmussen B, Parving H-H. Short-term inhibition of prostaglandin synthesis has no effect on the elevated glomerular filtration rate of early insulin-dependent diabetes. Diabet Med 1985; 2: 17–20.

329. Hommel E, Mathiesen E, Arnold-Larssen S, Edsberg B, Olsen UB, Parving H-H. Effect of indomethacin on kidney function in type 1 (insulin-dependent) diabetic patients with diabetic nephropathy. Diabetologia 1987; 30: 78–81.

330. Del Castillo E, Fuenzalida R, Uranga J. Increased glomerular filtration rate and glomerulopressin activity in diabetic dogs. Horm Metab Res 1977; 9: 46–53.

331. Ortola FV, Ballerman BJ, Anderson S, Mendez RE, Brenner BM. Elevated plasma atrial natriuretic peptide levels in diabetic rats. Potential mediators of hyperfiltration. J Clin Invest 1987; 80: 670–4.

332. Rave K, Heinemann L, Sawicki P, Hohmann A, Berger M. Increased concentration of atrial natriuretic peptide in type 1 (insulin-dependent) diabetic patients with glomerular hyperfiltration. Diabetologia 1987; 30: 573A.

333. Sawiki PT, Heineman L, Rave K, Hohmann A, Berger M. Atrial natriuretic factor in various stages of diabetic nephropathy. J Diabet Comp 1988; 2: 207–9.

334. Solerte SB, Fioravanti M, Spriano P, Aprile C, Patti AL, Ferrari E. Plasma atrial natriuretic peptide, renal haemodynamics and microalbuminuria in short-term type 1 (insulin-dependent) diabetic patients with hyperfiltration. Diabetologia 1987; 30: 584A.

335. Jones SL, Perico N, Benigni A, Remuzzi G, Viberti GC. Glomerular filtration rate, extracellular fluid volume and atrial natriuretic factor in insulin-dependent diabetics. Kidney Int 1988; 33: 268.

336. Hommel E, Mathiesen ER, Giese J, Nielsen MD, Schutten HJ, Parving H-H. On the pathogenesis of arterial pressure elevation early in the course of diabetic nephropathy. Scand J Clin Lab Invest 1989; 49: 537–44.

337. Brøchner-Mortensen J, Ditzel J. Glomerular filtration rate and extracellular fluid volume in

insulin-dependent patients with diabetes mellitus. Kidney Int 1982; 21: 696–8.

338. Feldt-Rasmussen B, Mathiesen ER, Deckert T et al. Central role for sodium in the pathogenesis of blood pressure changes independent of angiotensin, aldosterone and catecholamines in type 1 (insulin-dependent) diabetes mellitus. Diabetologia 1987; 30: 610–17.

339. Seyer-Hansen K, Hansen J, Gundersen HJG. Renal hypertrophy in experimental diabetes. A morphometric study. Diabetologia 1980; 18: 501–5.

340. Østerby R, Gundersen HJG. Fast accumulation of basement membrane material and the rate of morphological changes in acute experimental diabetic glomerular hypertrophy. Diabetologia 1980; 18: 493–500.

341. Rasch R. Tubular lesions in streptozotocin-diabetic rats. Diabetologia 1984; 27: 32–7.

342. Seyer-Hansen K. Renal hypertrophy in experimental diabetes mellitus. Kidney Int 1983; 23: 643–6.

343. Peterson PA, Evrin PE, Berggård I. Differentiation of glomerular, tubular, and normal proteinuria: determinations of urinary excretion of β_2-microglobulin, albumin, and total protein. J Clin Invest 1969; 48: 1189–98.

344. Wibell L. Studies of β_2-microglobulin in human serum, urine and amniotic fluid (thesis). Abstracts of Dissertations from the Uppsala Faculty of Medicine 1974: p 183.

345. Pappenheimer JR, Renkin EM, Barrero LM. Filtration diffusion and molecular sieving through peripheral capillary membranes. A contribution to the pore theory of capillary permeability. Am J Physiol 1951; 167: 13–46.

346. Venkatachalam MA, Rennke HG. The structural and molecular basis of glomerular filtration. Circulation Res 1978; 43: 337–47.

347. Deen WM, Satvat B. Determinants of glomerular filtration of proteins. Am J Physiol 1981; 241: F162–70.

348. Myers BD, Winetz JA, Chui F, Michaels AS. Mechanisms of proteinuria in diabetic nephropathy: a study of glomerular barrier function. Kidney Int 1982; 21: 633–41.

349. Viberti GC, Mackintosh D, Keen H. Determinants of the penetration of proteins through the glomerular barrier in insulin-dependent diabetes mellitus. Diabetes 1983; 32 (suppl. 2): 92–5.

350. Viberti GC, Keen H. The patterns of proteinuria in diabetes mellitus. Relevance to pathogenesis and prevention of diabetic nephropathy. Diabetes 1984; 33: 686–92.

351. Parving H-H, Rutili F, Granath K et al. Effect of metabolic regulation on renal leakiness to dextran molecules in short-term insulin-dependent diabetics. Diabetologia 1979; 17: 157–60.

352. Winetz JA, Golbetz HV, Spencer RJ, Lee JA, Myers BD. Glomerular function in advanced human diabetic nephropathy. Kidney Int 1982; 21: 750–6.

353. Schober E, Pollack A, Coradello H, Lubec G. Glycosylation of glomerular basement membrane in type 1 (insulin-dependent) diabetic children. Diabetologia 1982; 23: 485–7.

354. Brenner BM. Nephron adaptation to renal injury or ablation. Am J Physiol 1985; 249: F234–337.

355. Deckert T, Feldt-Rasmussen B, Djurup R, Deckert M. Glomerular size and charge selectivity in insulin-dependent diabetes mellitus. Kidney Int 1988; 33: 100–6.

356. Bertolatus JA, Abuyousef M, Hunsicker LG. Glomerular sieving of high molecular weight proteins in proteinuric rats. Kidney Int 1987; 31: 1257–66.

357. Melvin T, Kim Y, Michael AF. Selective binding of IgG_4 and other negatively charged plasma proteins in normal and diabetic human kidney. Am J Pathol 1984; 115: 443–6.

358. Guthrow CE, Morris MA, Day JF, Thorp SR, Baynes JW. Enhanced non-enzymatic glycosylation of human serum albumin in diabetes mellitus. Proc Nat Acad Sci USA 1979; 76: 4258–61.

359. Cohen MP, Urdanivia E, Surma M, Ciborowski C. Non-enzymatic glycosylation of basement membranes in in vitro studies. Diabetes 1981; 30: 367–71.

360. Williams SK, Devenny JJ, Bitensky MW. Micropinocytic ingestion of glycosylated albumin by isolated microvessels: possible role in pathogenesis of diabetic microangiopathy. Proc Nat Acad Sci USA 1981; 78: 2393–7.

361. Williams SK, Siegel RK. Preferential transport of non-enzymatically glycosylated ferritin across the kidney glomerulus. Kidney Int 1985; 28: 146–52.

362. Shaklai N, Garlick RL, Bunn HF. Nonenzymatic glycosylation of human serum albumin alters its conformation and function. J Biol Chem 1984; 259: 3812–17.

363. Pillay VKG, Gandhi VC, Sharma BK, Smith EC, Dunea G. Effect of hydration and frusemide given intravenously on proteinuria. Arch Int Med 1972; 130: 90–2.

364. Jarrett RJ, Verma NP, Keen H. Urinary albumin excretion in normal and diabetic subjects. Clin Chim Acta 1976; 71: 55–9.

365. First MR, Patel VB, Pesce RJ, Bramlage RJ, Pollack VE. Albumin excretion by the kidney. The effect of osmotic diuresis. Nephron 1978; 20: 171–5.

366. Hegedüs L, Christensen NJ, Mogensen CE, Gundersen HJG. Oral glucose increases urinary albumin excretion in normal subjects but not in insulin-dependent diabetics. Scand J Clin Lab Invest 1980; 40: 479–82.

367. Viberti GC, Mogensen CE, Keen H, Jacobsen RJ, Jarrett RJ, Christiansen CK. Urinary excretion of albumin in normal man: the effect of water loading. Scand J Clin Lab Invest 1982; 42: 147–51.

368. Viberti GC, Strakosch CR, Keen H, Mackintosh D, Dalton N, Home PD. The influence of glucose-induced hyperinsulinaemia on renal glomerular function and circulating catecholamines in normal man. Diabetologia 1981; 21: 436–9.

369. Viberti GC, Haycock GB, Pickup JC, Jarrett RJ, Keen H. Early functional and morphologic vascular renal consequences of the diabetic state. Diabetologia 1980; 18: 173–5.

370. Kokko JP. Proximal tubule potential difference. Dependence on glucose, HCO_3, and aminoacids. J Clin Invest 1973; 52: 1362–7.

371. Ditzel J, Brøchner-Mortensen J, Kawahara R. Dysfunction of tubular phosphate reabsorption related to glomerular filtration and blood glucose control in diabetic children. Diabetologia 1982; 23: 406–10.

372. Watanabe Y, Nunoi K, Maki Y, Nakamura Y, Fujishima M. Contribution of glycaemic control to the levels of N-acetyl-β-D-glucosaminidase and serum NAG in type 1 (insulin-dependent) diabetes mellitus without proteinuria. Clin Nephrol 1987; 28: 227–31.

373. Gibb DM, Tomlinson PA, Dalton NR, Turner C, Shah V, Barratt TM. Renal tubular proteinuria and microalbuminuria in diabetic patients. Arch Dis Child 1989; 64: 129–34.

374. Ditzel J, Brøchner-Mortensen J. Tubular reabsorption rates as related to glomerular filtration in diabetic children. Diabetes 1983; 32 (suppl. 2): 28–33.

375. Mauer SM, Steffes MW, Ellis EN, Sutherland DER, Brown DM, Gøetz FC. Structural-functional relationships in diabetic nephropathy. J Clin Invest 1984; 74: 1143–55.

376. Tomlanovich S, Deen WM, Jones HW, Schwartz HC, Myers BD. Functional nature of glomerular injury in progressive diabetic glomerulopathy. Diabetes 1987; 36: 556–65.

377. Pinto JR, Bending JJ, Dodds R, Viberti GC. Failure of low-protein diet to restore the physiological response to protein ingestion in proteinuric type 1 (insulin-dependent) diabetic patients. Diabetologia 1988; 31: 531A.

378. Remuzzi A, Viberti GC, Ruggenenti P, Battaglia C, Pagni R, Remuzzi G. Glomerular response to

hyperglycaemia in human diabetic nephropathy. Am J Physiol 1990; 259: F545–52.

379. De Cosmo S, Ruggenenti P, Walker JD, Remuzzi G, Viberti GC. Mechanisms of glucose induced glomerular haemodynamic changes in diabetic nephropathy. Diabetologia 1989; 32: 480A.

380. Vannini P, Ciavarella A, Flammini M et al. Lipid abnormalities in insulin-dependent diabetic patients with albuminuria. Diabetes Care 1984; 7: 151–4.

381. Winocour PH, Durrington PN, Ishola M, Anderson DC, Cohen H. Influence of proteinuria on vascular disease, blood pressure, and lipoproteins in insulin dependent diabetes mellitus. Br Med J 1987; 294: 1648–51.

382. Jensen T, Stender S, Deckert T. Abnormalities in plasma concentrations of lipoproteins and fibrinogen in type 1 (insulin-dependent) diabetic patients with increased albumin excretion. Diabetologia 1988; 31: 142–5.

383. Jones SL, Close CE, Mattock MB, Jarrett RJ, Keen, H, Viberti GC. Plasma lipid and coagulation factor concentrations in insulin dependent diabetics with microalbuminuria. Br Med J 1989; 298: 487–90.

384. Dullaart RPF, Dikkeschei LD, Doorenbos HH. Alterations in serum lipids and apolipoproteins in male type 1 (insulin-dependent) diabetic patients with microalbuminuria. Diabetologia 1989; 32: 685–9.

385. Mattock MB, Keen H, Viberti GC et al. Coronary heart disease and albumin excretion rate in type 2 (non-insulin-dependent) diabetic patients. Diabetologia 1988; 31: 82–7.

386. Fahr T. Über Glomerulosklerose. Virchows Archiv Pathol Anat Physiol 1942; 309: 16–33.

387. Spühler O, Zollinger HU. Direfe diabetische Glomerulosklerose. Dtsch Arch Klin Med 1943; 190: 321–79.

388. Kamenetzky SA, Bennet P, Dippe SE, Miller M, LeCompte PM. A clinical and histologic study of diabetic nephropathy in the Pima Indians. Diabetes 1974; 23: 61–8.

389. Tchobroutsky G. Prevention and treatment of diabetic nephropathy. In Hamburger J, Crosnier J, Grunfeld J-P, Maxwell MH. (eds) Advances in nephrology. Chicago: Year Book, 1979: pp 63–86.

390. Saito Y, Kida H, Takeda S et al. Mesangiolysis in diabetic glomeruli; its role in the formation of nodular lesions. Kidney Int 1988; 34: 389–96.

391. Bloodworth JMB. A re-evaluation of diabetic glomerulosclerosis 50 years after the discovery of insulin. Hum Path 1978; 9: 439–53.

392. Heptinstall RH. Diabetes mellitus and gout. In Heptinstall RH (ed.) Pathology of the kidney (3rd edn). Boston: Little, Brown, 1983: pp 1397–1453.

393. Østerby R, Gundersen HJG. Glomerular size and structure in diabetes mellitus. I. Early abnormalities. Diabetologia 1975; 11: 225–9.

394. Gundersen HJG, Østerby R. Glomerular size and structure in diabetes mellitus. II. Late abnormalities. Diabetologia 1977; 13: 43–8.

395. Østerby R, Gundersen HJG, Nyberg G, Aurell M. Advanced diabetic glomerulopathy. Quantitative structural characterization of non-occluded glomeruli. Diabetes 1987; 36: 612–19.

396. Schmitz A, Gundersen HJG, Østerby R. Glomerular morphology by light microscopy in non-insulin-dependent diabetes mellitus—lack of glomerular hypertrophy. Diabetes 1988; 37: 38–43.

397. Mauer SM, Barbosa J, Vernier RL et al. Development of diabetic vascular lesions in normal kidneys transplanted into patients with diabetes mellitus. New Engl J Med 1976; 295: 916–20.

398. Rasch R, Holck P. Ultrastructure of the macula densa in streptozotocin diabetic rats. Lab Invest 1988; 59: 666–72.

399. Miller K, Michael AF. Immunopathology of renal extracellular membranes in diabetes mellitus. Specificity of tubular basement membrane immunofluorescence. Diabetes 1976; 25: 701–8.

400. Falk RJ, Scheinman JI, Mauer SM, Michael AF. Polyantigenic expansion of basement membrane constituents in diabetic nephropathy. Diabetes 1983; 32 (suppl. 2): 34–9.

401. Glick AD, Jacobson HR, Haralson MA. Evidence for type I collagen synthesis in diabetic glomerulosclerosis. Kidney Int 1990; 37: 507.

402. Ikeda K, Kida H, Oshima A. Participation of type VI collagen fibres in formation of diabetic nodular lesions. Kidney Int 1990; 37: 252.

403. Mohan PS, Carter WG, Spiro RG. Occurrence of type VI collagen in extracellular matrix of renal glomeruli and its increase in diabetes. Diabetes 1990; 39: 31–7.

404. Scheinman JI, Fish AJ, Michael AF. The immunohistopathology of glomerular antigens. The glomerular basement membrane, collagen, and actomyosin antigens in normal and diseased kidneys. J Clin Invest 1974; 54: 1144–54.

405. Farquhar A, MacDonald MK, Ireland JT. The role of fibrin deposition in diabetic glomerulosclerosis: a light, electron and immunofluorescence microscopy study. J Clin Pathol 1972; 25: 657–67.

406. Østerby-Hansen R. A quantitative estimate of the peripheral glomerular basement membrane in recent juvenile diabetes. Diabetologia 1965; 1: 97–100.

407. Østerby R. Early phases in the development of diabetic glomerulopathy. A quantitative electron microscopy study. Acta Med Scand 1975; S574: 1–82.

408. Kimmelstiel P, Osawa G, Beres J. Glomerular basement membrane in diabetics. Am J Pathol 1966; 45: 21–31.

409. Østerby R, Gundersen HJG, Hørlyck A, Kroustrup JP, Nyberg G, Westberg G. Diabetic glomerulopathy. Structural characteristics of the early and advanced stages. Diabetes 1983; 32 (suppl. 2): 79–82.

410. Ireland JT, Patnaik BK, Duncan LJP. Effect of pituitary ablation on the renal arteriolar and glomerular lesions in diabetes. Diabetes 1967; 16: 636–42.

411. Ellis EN, Steffes MW, Chavers B, Mauer SM. Observations of glomerular epithelial cell structure in patients with type 1 diabetes mellitus. Kidney Int 1987; 32: 736–41.

412. Cohen AH, Mampaso F, Zamboni L. Glomerular podocyte degeneration in human renal disease. An ultrastructural study. Lab Invest 1977; 37: 30–4.

413. Ireland JT. Diagnostic criteria in the assessment of glomerular capillary basement membrane lesions in newly diagnosed juvenile diabetics. Adv Metab Dis 1970; 1: 273.

414. Østerby R. A quantitative electron microscopic study of mesangial regions in glomeruli from patients with short-term juvenile diabetes mellitus. Lab Invest 1973; 29: 99–110.

415. Kimmelstiel P, Kim OJ, Beres J. Studies on renal biopsies specimens with the aid of the electron microscope. I. Glomeruli in diabetes. Am J Pathol 1962; 38: 270–7.

416. Dachs S, Churg J, Mautner W, Grishman E. Diabetic nephropathy. Am J Pathol 1964; 44: 155–68.

417. Østerby R, Parving H-H, Hommel E, Jorgensen HE, Lokkegaard, H. Glomerular structure and function in diabetic nephropathy. Early to advanced stages. Diabetes 1990; 39: 1057–63.

418. Ellis EN, Steffes MW, Gøetz FC, Sutherland DER, Mauer SM. Glomerular filtration surface in type 1 diabetics mellitus. Kidney Int 1986; 29: 889–94.

419. Østerby R, Parving H-H, Nyberg G et al. A strong correlation between glomerular filtration rate and filtration surface in diabetic nephropathy. Diabetologia 1988; 31: 265–70.

420. Thomsen OF, Andersen AR, Christiansen JS, Deckert T. Renal changes in long-term type 1 (insulin-dependent) diabetic patients with and without clinical nephropathy; a light microscopic, morphometric study of autopsy material. Diabetologia 1984; 26: 361–5.

421. Steffes MW, Østerby R, Chavers B, Mauer SM. Mesangial expansion as a central mechanism for

loss of kidney function in diabetic patients. Diabetes 1989; 38: 1077–81.

422. Inomata S, Nakamoto Y, Inoue M, Itoh M, Ohsawa Y, Masamune O. Relationship between urinary albumin excretion and renal histology in non-insulin-dependent diabetes mellitus: with reference to the clinical significance of micro-albuminuria. J Diabet Comp 1989; 3: 178–88.

423. Kincaid-Smith P, Whitworth JA. Haematuria and diabetic nephropathy. In Mogensen CE (ed.) The kidney and hypertension in diabetes mellitus. Boston: Nijhoff, 1988: pp 81–9.

424. Amoah E, Glickman JL, Malchoff CD. Sturgill BC, Kaiser DL, Bolton WK. Clinical identification of non-diabetic renal disease in diabetic patients with type 1 and type 2 disease presenting with renal dysfunction. Am J Nephrol 1988; 8: 204–11.

425. Kasinath BS, Musais SK, Spargo BH, Katz AI. Non diabetic renal disease in patients with diabetes mellitus. Am J Med 1983; 75: 613–17.

426. Silva FG, Pace EH, Burns DK, Krous H. The spectrum of diabetic nephropathy and membranous glomerulopathy: report of two cases and review of the literature. Diabet Nephr 1983; 2: 28–32.

427. Chihara J, Takebayashi S, Taguchi T, Yokoyama K, Harada T, Naito S. Glomerulonephritis in diabetic patients and its effect on prognosis. Nephron 1986; 43: 45–9.

428. Bertani T, Olesnicky L, Abu-Regiaba S, Glasberg S, Pirani CL. Concomitant presence of three different glomerular diseases in the same patient. Nephron 1983; 34: 260–6.

429. Rao KV, Crosson JT. Idiopathic membranous glomerulonephritis in diabetic patients. Report of three cases and review of the literature. Arch Int Med 1980; 140: 624–7.

430. Kobayashi K et al. Idiopathic membranous glomerulo-nephritis associated with diabetes mellitus. Nephron 1981; 28: 163–8.

431. Okuda S, Oh Y, Onoyama K, Fujimi S, Omae T. Autologous immune-complex nephritis in streptozotocin-induced diabetic rats. Nephron 1984; 37: 166–73.

432. Jarrett RJ, Keen H, Chakrabarthi R. Diabetes hyperglycaemia, and arterial disease. In Keen H, Jarrett J (eds) Complications of diabetes (2nd edn). London: Edward Arnold, 1982: pp 179–204.

433. Parving H-H, Andersen AR, Smidt UM, Hommel E, Mathiesen ER, Svendsen PA. Effect of antihypertensive treatment on kidney function in diabetic nephropathy. Br Med J 1987; 294: 1443–7.

434. Zatz R, Dunn BR, Meyer TW, Anderson S, Rennke HG, Brenner BM. Prevention of diabetic glomerulopathy by pharmacologic amelioration of glomerular capillary hypertension. J Clin Invest 1986; 77: 1925–30.

435. Taguma Y, Kitamoto Y, Futaki G et al. Effect of captopril on heavy proteinuria in azotemic diabetics. New Engl J Med 1985; 313: 1617–20.

436. Bjørck S, Nyberg G, Mulec H, Granerus G, Herlitz H, Aurell M. Beneficial effects of angiotensin converting enzyme inhibition on renal function in patients with diabetic nephropathy. Br Med J 1986; 293: 471–4.

437. Hommel E, Parving H-H, Mathiesen E, Edsberg B, Nielsen MD, Giese J. Effect of captopril on kidney function in insulin-dependent diabetic patients with nephropathy. Br Med J 1986; 293: 467–70.

438. Parving H-H, Hommel E, Smidt UM. Protection of kidney function and decrease in albuminuria by captopril in insulin-dependent diabetics with nephropathy. Br Med J 1988; 297: 1086–91.

439. Parving H-H, Hommel E, Nielsen MD, Giese J. Effect of captopril on blood pressure and kidney function in normotensive insulin dependent diabetics with nephropathy. Br Med J 1989; 299: 533–6.

440. Pinto JR, Walker JD, Turner CD, Beesley M. Viberti GC. Renal response to lowering of arterial pressure by angiotensin converting enzyme inhibitor or diuretic therapy in insulin-dependent diabetic patients with nephropathy. Kidney Int 1990; 37: 516.

441. Ruggenenti P, Viberti GC, Battaglia C, Perticucci E, Remuzzi G, Remuzzi A. Low-dose enalapril and glomerular selective function in insulin-dependent diabetics. Kidney Int 1990; 37: 519.

442. Morelli E, Loon N, Meyer T, Peters W, Myers BD. Effects of converting-enzyme inhibition on barrier function in diabetic glomerulopathy. Diabetes 1990; 39: 76–82.

443. Marre M, Chatellier G, Leblanc H, Guyene TT, Menard J, Passa P. Prevention of diabetic nephropathy with enalapril in normotensive diabetics with microalbuminuria. Br Med J 1988; 297: 1092–5.

444. Pedersen MM, Schmitz A, Pedersen EB, Danielsen H, Christiansen JS. Acute and long-term renal effects of angiotensin converting-enzyme inhibition in normotensive, normoalbuminuric insulin-dependent diabetic patients. Diabet Med 1988; 5: 562–9.

445. Bergstrom J. Discovery and rediscovery of low-protein diet. Clin Nephrol 1984; 21: 29–35.

446. Attman PO, Bucht H, Larsson O, Uddebom G. Protein reduced diet in diabetic renal failure. Clin Nephrol 1983; 19: 217–20.

447. Barsotti G, Morelli E, Giannoni A, Guiducci A, Lupetti S, Giovannetti S. Restricted phosphorus and nitrogen intake to slow the progression of

chronic renal failure: a controlled trial. Kidney Int 1983; 24 (S16): S278–84.

448. Evanoff GV, Thompson CS, Brown J, Weinman EJ. The effect of dietary protein restriction on the progression of diabetic nephropathy. A 12 month follow-up. Arch Int Med 1987; 147: 492–5.

449. Bending JJ, Dodds RA, Keen H, Viberti GC. Renal response to restricted protein intake in diabetic nephropathy. Diabetes 1988; 37: 1641–6.

450. Rosenberg ME, Swanson JE, Thomas BL, Hostetter TH. Glomerular and hormonal responses to dietary protein intake in human renal disease. Am J Physiol 1987; 253: F1083–90.

451. Cohen D, Dodds R, Viberti GC. Effect of protein restriction in insulin-dependent diabetics at risk of nephropathy. Br Med J 1987; 294: 795–8.

452. Wiseman MJ, Bognetti E, Dodds R, Keen H, Viberti GC. Changes in renal function in response to protein restricted diet in type 1 (insulin-dependent) diabetic patients. Diabetologia 1987; 30: 154–9.

453. Kontessis PS, Dodds RA, Jones SJ, Pinto JR, Trevisan R, Viberti GC. Renal, metabolic and hormonal responses to ingestion of protein of different sources in normal man. Kidney Int 1989; 35: 470.

454. Kroc Collaborative Study Group. Blood glucose control and the evolution of diabetic retinopathy and albuminuria. A preliminary multicentre trial. New Engl J Med 1984; 311: 365–72.

455. Bending JJ, Viberti GC, Bilous RW, Keen H. Eight-month correction of hyperglycaemia in IDDM is associated with a significant and sustained reduction of urinary albumin excretion rates in patients with microalbuminuria. Diabetes 1985; 34 (suppl. 3): 69–73.

456. Dahl-Jørgensen K, Hanssen KF, Kierulf P, Bjøro T, Sandvik L, Aagenæs Ø. Reduction of urinary albumin excretion after 4 years of continuous subcutaneous insulin infusion in insulin-dependent diabetes mellitus. The Oslo study. Acta Endocriniol (Copenh) 1988; 117: 19–25.

457. Vasquez B, Flock EV, Savage PJ et al. Sustained reduction of proteinuria in type 2 (non-insulin-dependent) diabetes following diet-induced reduction of hyperglycaemia. Diabetologia 1984; 26: 127–33.

458. Warram J, Derby L, Laffel L, Krolewski AS. Role of mean arterial pressure in the development of persistent proteinuria. Kidney Int 1990; 37: 404.

459. Tuttle K, Perusek M, DeFronzo R, Kunau R. Increased renal reserve and size regress with strict glycaemic control in insulin-dependent diabetes mellitus. Kidney Int 1990; 37: 261.

460. Donadio JV, Ilstrup DM, Holley KE, Romero JC. Platelet-inhibitor treatment of diabetic nephropathy: a 10-year prospective study. Mayo Clin Proc 1988; 63: 3–15.

461. Mujais SK. Renal papillary necrosis in diabetes mellitus. Semin Nephrol 1984; 4: 40–7.

462. Mandel EE. Renal medullary necrosis. Am J Med 1952; 13: 322–7.

463. Lauler DP, Schreiner GE, David A. Renal medullary necrosis. Am J Med 1960; 29: 132–56.

464. Eknoyan G, Quinibi WY, Grissom RT, Tuma SN, Ayus JC. Renal papillary necrosis: an update. Medicine 1982; 61: 55–73.

465. Groop L, Laasonen L, Edgren J. Renal papillary necrosis in patients with IDDM. Diabetes Care 1989; 12: 198–202.

466. Rundles RW. Diabetic neuropathy: general review with report of 125 cases. Medicine 1945; 24: 111–60.

467. Martin MM. Diabetic neuropathy. A clinical study of 125 cases. Brain 1953; 76: 594–624.

468. Frimodt-Møller C. Diabetic cystopathy. I. A clinical study of the frequency of bladder dysfunction in diabetes. Dan Med Bull 1976; 23: 267–78.

469. Mahony DJ, Laferte RO, Blais DJ. Integral storage and voiding reflexes. Neurophysiologic concept of continence and micturition. Urology 1977; 9: 95–106.

470. deGroat WC, Booth AM. Physiology of the urinary bladder and urethra. Ann Intern Med 1980; 92: 312–15.

471. Ellenberg M. Diabetic neurogenic vesical dysfunction. Arch Int Med 1966; 117: 348–54.

472. Kahan M, Goldberg PD, Mandell EE. Neurogenic vesical dysfunction and diabetes mellitus. NY State J Med 1970; 2: 2448–55.

473. Gibberd FB. The neurogenic bladder. Clin Obster Gynecol 1981; 8: 149–60.

474. Rubinow DR, Nelson JC. Tricyclic exacerbation of undiagnosed diabetic uropathy. J Clin Psych 1982; 943: 210–12.

475. Ewing DJ, Clark F. Autonomic neuropathy: its diagnosis and prognosis. Clin Endocrinol Metab 1986; 15: 855–88.

476. Bradley WE. Diagnosis of urinary bladder dysfunction in diabetes mellitus. Ann Intern Med 1980; 92: 323–6.

477. Frimodt-Møller C, Mortensen S. Treatment of diabetic cystopathy. Ann Intern Med 1980; 92: 327–8.

478. Ellenberg M. Development of urinary bladder dysfunction in diabetes mellitus. Ann Intern Med 1980; 92: 321–3.

479. Pedersen J. The pregnant diabetic and her newborn. (2nd edn) Copenhagen: Munksgaard, 1977.

480. Kitzmiller JL, Brown ER, Phillippe M et al. Diabetic nephropathy and perinatal outcome. Am J Obstet Gynecol 1981; 141: 741–5.

481. Jovanovic R, Jovanovic L. Obstetric management when normoglycaemia is maintained in diabetic pregnant women with vascular compromise. Am J Obstet Gynecol 1984; 149: 617–23.

482. Dicker D, Feldberg D, Peleg D, Karp M, Goldman JA. Pregnancy complicated by diabetic nephropathy. 1986; 14: 299–307.

483. Grenfell A, Brudenell JM, Doddridge MC, Watkins PJ. Pregnancy in diabetic women who have proteinuria. Quart J Med 1986; 59: 379–86.

484. Reece EA, Constan DR, Hayslett JP et al. Diabetic nephropathy: pregnancy performance and fetomaternal outcome. Am J Obstet Gynecol 1988; 159: 56–66.

485. Katz AI, Davison JM, Hayslett JP, Singson E, Lindheimer MD. Pregnancy in women with kidney disease. Kidney Int 1980; 18: 192–206.

486. Hou SH, Grossman SD, Madias NE. Pregnancy in women with renal disease and moderate renal insufficiency. Am J Med 1985; 78: 185–94.

487. Hare JW, White P. Pregnancy in diabetes complicated by vascular disease. Diabetes 1977; 26: 953–5.

488. Fuhrmann K, Reiher H, Semmler K, Fischer F, Fischer M, Glöckner E. Prevention of cogenital malformations in infants of insulin-dependent diabetic mothers. Diabetes Care 1983; 6: 219–23.

489. Buschard K, Hougaard P, Mølsted-Pedersen L, Kühl C. Type 1 (insulin-dependent) diabetes mellitus diagnosed during pregnancy: a clinical and prognostic study Diabetologia 1990; 33: 31–5.

490. Hanson U, Persson B, Thunell S. Relationship between haemoglobin A_{1c} in early type 1 (insulin-dependent) diabetic pregnancy and the occurrence of spontaneous abortion and fetal malformation in Sweden. Diabetologia 1990; 33: 100–4.

491. Peterson CM, Jovanovic L. Natural history of the diabetic renal–retinal syndrome during pregnancy. In Friedman EA, L'Esperance FA (eds.) Diabetic renal–retinal syndrome, vol. 3. New York: Grune & Stratton, 1986: pp 471–80.

492. Miodovnik M et al. Major malformations in infants of IDDM mothers. Vasculopathy and early first-trimester poor glycaemic control. Diabetes Care 1988; 11: 713–18.

493. Young KR, Clancy CF. Symposium on diabetes and obesity. Urinary tract infections complicating diabetes mellitus. Med Clin North Am 1955; 39: 1665–70.

494. Ditscherlein G. Renal histopathology in hypertensive diabetic patients. Hypertension 1985; 7 (suppl. 2): 29–32.

495. Huvos A, Rocha H. Frequency of bacteriuria in patients with diabetes mellitus. A controlled study. New Engl J Med 1959; 261: 1213–16.

496. O'Sullivan DJ, Fitzgerald MG, Meynell MJ, Malins JM. Urinary tract infection. A comparative study in the diabetic and general populations. Br Med J 1961; 1: 786–8.

497. Vejlsgaard R. Studies on urinary infections in diabetics. I. Bacteriuria in patients with diabetes mellitus and in control subjects. Acta Med Scand 1966; 179: 173–82.

498. Pometta D, Rees SB, Younger D, Kass EH. Asymptomatic bacterium in diabetes mellitus. New Engl J Med 1967; 276: 1118–21.

499. Vejlsgaard R. Studies on urinary infections in diabetics. III. Significant bacteriuria in pregnant diabetics and in matched controls. Acta Med Scand 1973; 193: 337–41.

500. Forland M, Thomas V, Shelokov A. Urinary tract infections in patients with diabetes mellitus. JAMA 1977; 238: 1924–6.

501. Vejlsgaard R. Studies on urinary infections in diabetics. II. Significant bacteriuria in relation to long-term diabetic manifestations. Acta Med Scand 1966; 179: 183–8.

502. Vejlsgaard R. Studies on urinary infections in diabetics. IV. Significant bacteriuria in pregnancy in relation to age of onset, duration of diabetes, angiopathy and urologic symptoms. Acta Med Scand 1973; 193: 343–6.

503. Bevan JS, Griffiths GJ, Williams JD, Gibby OM. Bilateral renal cortical abscesses in a young woman with type 1 diabetes. Diabet Med 1989; 6: 454–7.

504. Thorley JD, Jones SR, Sanford JP. Perinephric abscess. Medicine 1974; 53: 441–51.

505. Bova JG, Potter JL, Arevalos E, Hopens T, Goldstein HM, Radwin HM. Renal and perirenal infection: the role of computerized tomography. J Urology 1985; 133: 539–43.

506. Evanoff GV, Thompson CS, Foley R, Weinman EJ. Spectrum of gas within the kidney. Emphysematous pyelonephritis and emphysematous pyelitis. Am J Med 1987; 83: 149–54.

507. Avram MM. Use of special haemodialysis methods in diabetic uraemia. Conference on Dialysis by the National Dialysis Committee. New York: National Union Catalogue, 1966: 15.

508. Avram MM. Diabetic renal failure. Nephron 1982; 31: 285–8.

509. Cameron JS, Challah S. Treatment of end-stage renal failure due to diabetes in the United Kingdom, 1975–84. Lancet 1986; ii: 962–6.

510. Friedman EA. Clinical strategy in diabetic nephropathy. In Friedman EA, L'Esperance FA Jr (eds) Diabetic renal–retinal syndrome, vol. 3: Therapy. New York: Grune & Stratton, 1986: pp 311–32.

511. Shyh T-P, Butt KH, Beyer MM, Friedman EA.

Excess costs of diabetic renal transplants. Diabet Nephr 1983; 2: 23–7.

512. Butt KH, Hanson P, Emmett L et al. Total patient care in diabetic kidney transplants: cyclosporine era. In Friedman EA, L'Esperance FA Jr (eds) Diabetic renal–retinal syndrome, vol. 13: Therapy. New York: Grune & Stratton, 1986: pp. 311–32.

513. Bending JJ, Pickup JC, Viberti GC, Keen H. Glycaemic control in diabetic nephropathy. Br Med J 1984; 288: 1187–91.

514. Bourdeau JE, Chen ER, Carone EA. Insulin uptake in the renal proximal tubule. Am J Physiol 1973; 225: 1399–404.

515. Asplund K, Wiholm B-E, Lithner F. Glibenclamide-associated hypoglycaemia: a report on 57 cases. Diabetologia 1983; 24: 412–17.

516. Skillman TG, Feldman JM. The pharmacology of sulphonylureas. Am J Med 1981; 70: 361–72.

517. De Leiva A, Christlieb AR, Melby JC. Big renin and biosynthetic defect of aldosterone in diabetes mellitus. New Engl J Med 1979; 295: 639–43.

518. Christlieb AR. Renin–angiotensin–aldosterone system in diabetes mellitus. Diabetes 1976; 25 (suppl. 2): 820–5.

519. Belzer FO, Miller DT, Sollinger HW, Glass NR. Simplified kidney transplants in insulin dependent diabetics. In Friedman EA, L'Esperance FA Jr (eds) Diabetic renal–retinal syndrome, vol. 3: Therapy. New York: Grune & Stratton, 1986: pp 413–20.

520. Morrow CE, Schwartz JS, Sutherland DER et al. Predictive value of thallium stress testing for cardiovascular events in uraemic diabetics before renal transplantation. Am J Surg 1983; 146: 331–5.

521. Philipson JD, Carpenter BJ, Itzkoff J et al. Evaluation of cardiovascular risk for renal transplantation in diabetic patients. Am J Med 1986; 81: 630–4.

522. Whitley KY, Shapiro FL. Haemodialysis for end-stage diabetic nephropathy. In Friedman EA, L'Esperance FA Jr (eds) Diabetic renal–retinal syndrome, vol. 3: Therapy. New York: Grune & Stratton, 1986: pp 349–62.

523. Kraukauer H, Grauman MS, McMullan MR, Creede CC. The recent US experience in the treatment of end-stage renal disease by dialysis and transplantation. New Engl J Med 1983; 308: 1558–63.

524. Jacobs C, Brunner FP, Brynger H, Shallah S, Kramer P, Selwood NH, Wing AJ. The first five thousand diabetics treated by dialysis and transplantation in Europe. Diabet Nephr 1983; 2: 12–16.

525. Vollmer WM, Wahl P, Blagg CR. Survival with dialysis and transplantation in patients with end-stage renal disease. New Engl J Med 1983; 308: 1553–8.

526. Kjellstrand CM. A comparison of dialysis and transplantation in patients with end-stage renal failure of diabetes. In Friedman EA, L'Esperance FA Jr (eds) Diabetic renal–retinal syndrome, vol. 3: Therapy. New York: Grune & Stratton, 1986; pp 333–49.

527. Jacobson SH, Fryd D, Sutherland DER, Kjellstrand CM. Treatment of the diabetic patient with end-stage renal failure. Diabetes Metab Rev 1988; 4: 191–200.

528. Kjellstrand CM, Whitley K, Comty CM, Shapiro FL. Dialysis in patients with diabetes mellitus. Diabet Nephr 1983; 2: 5–17.

529. Weinrauch LA, D'Elia JA, Healy RW et al. Asymptomatic coronary artery disease: angiography in diabetic patients before renal transplantation. Ann Int Med 1978; 88: 346–8.

530. Bennett WM, Kloster F, Rosch J, Barry J, Porter GA. Natural history of asymptomatic coronary arteriographic lesions in diabetic patients with end-stage renal disease. Am J Med 1978; 65: 779–84.

531. Braun WE, Phillips D, Vidt DG et al. Coronary arteriography and coronary artery disease in 99 diabetic and non-diabetic patients on chronic haemodialysis or renal transplant programmes. Transplant Proc 1981; 13: 128–35.

532. Shapiro FL, Comty CM. Haemodialysis in diabetics—1979 update. In Friedman EA, L'Esperance FA Jr (eds) Diabetic renal–retinal syndrome, vol. 1. New York: Grune & Stratton, 1980: pp 333–43.

533. Aman LC, Le Vin NW, Smith DW. Haemodialysis access site morbidity. Proc Clin Dial Transplant Forum 1980; 10: 277–84.

534. Shideman JR, Buselmeier TJ, Kjellstrand CM. Haemodialysis complications in insulin dependent diabetics accepted for transplantation. Arch Int Med 1976; 136: 1126–30.

535. Legrain M, Rottembourg J, Bentchikou A et al. Dialysis treatment of insulin dependent diabetic patients. A ten year experience. Clin Nephrol 1984; 21: 72–81.

536. Shapiro FL, Comty CM. Haemodialysis in diabetics—1981 update. In Friedman EA, L'Esperance FA Jr (eds) Diabetic renal–retinal syndrome, vol. 2: Prevention and management. New York: Grune & Stratton, 1982: pp 309–20.

537. Popp D, Achtenberg JF, Cryer PE. Hyperkalaemia and hyperglycaemia increments in plasma potassium in diabetes mellitus. Arch Int Med 1980; 140: 1617–21.

538. Nicholi GL, Kahn T, Sanchez A et al. Glucose induced hyperkalaemia in diabetic subjects. Ann Intern Med 1981; 141: 49–53.

539. Ramsay RC, Goetz FC, Sutherland DER et al. Progression of diabetic retinopathy after pancreatic transplantation for insulin-dependent diabetes mellitus. New Engl J Med 1988; 318: 208–14.

540. Schreiber MJ, Vidt DG. Rehabilitation of Type 1 uraemic diabetics according to therapy. In Friedman EA, L'Esperance FA Jr (eds) Diabetic renal–retinal syndrome, vol. 3: Therapy. New York: Grune & Stratton, 1986: pp 429–42.

541. Matson M, Kjellstrand CM. Long-term follow-up of 369 diabetic patients undergoing dialysis. Arch Int Med 1988; 148: 600–4.

542. Harrington JT. Chronic ambulatory peritoneal dialysis. New Engl J Med 1982; 306: 670–1.

543. Amair P, Khanna R, Leibel B et al. Continuous ambulatory peritoneal dialysis in diabetics with end-stage renal disease. New Engl J Med 1982; 306: 625–30.

544. Khanna R, Wu G, Prowant B et al. Continuous ambulatory peritoneal dialysis in diabetics with end-stage renal disease: a combined experience of two North American centres. In Friedman EA, L'Esperance FA Jr (eds) Diabetic renal–retinal syndrome, vol. 3: Therapy. New York: Grune & Stratton, pp 363–81.

545. Mairoca R, Caraluppi A, Carcarini GC et al. Prospective controlled trial of a Y-connector and disinfectant to prevent peritonitis in continuous ambulatory peritoneal dialysis. Lancet 1983; ii: 642–4.

546. Parsons FM, Ahmed-Jushuf IH, Brownjohn AM et al. Preventing CAPD peritonitis. Lancet 1983; ii: 907–8.

547. Clayton S. Training the diabetic patient on continuous ambulatory peritoneal dialysis. Perit Dial Bull 1982; 2: 538–9.

548. Grodstein GP, Blumenkrantz MJ, Kopple JD et al. Glucose absorption during continuous ambulatory peritoneal dialysis. Kidney Int 1981; 19: 564–7.

549. Kurtz SB, Wong VH, Anderson CF et al. Continuous ambulatory peritoneal dialysis. Three years experience at the Mayo Clinic. Mayo Clin Proc 1983; 58: 633–9.

550. Ramos JM, Gokal R, Siamopolous K, Ward MK, Wilkinson R, Kerr DNS. Continuous ambulatory peritoneal dialysis: three years' experience. Quart J Med 1983; 206: 165–86.

551. Fluckiger R, Harmon W, Meier W, Loo S, Gabbay KH. Haemoglobin carbamylation in uraemia. New Engl J Med 1981; 304: 823.

552. Boer MJ, Miedema K, Caspaie AF. Glycosylated haemoglobin in renal failure. Diabetologia 1980; 18: 437–40.

553. Paisley R, Banks R, Holton R, Young K, Hopton M, White D, Harlog M. Glycosylated haemoglobin in uraemia. Diabet Med 1986; 3: 445–8.

554. Freedman D, Dandona P, Fernando O, Moorhead JF. Glycosylated haemoglobin in chronic renal failure and after renal transplantation. J Clin Pathol 1982; 35: 737–9.

555. Collins ACG, Bending JJ, Viberti GC, Keen H. Serum fructosamine measurement in diabetic nephropathy. Diabet Med 1987; 4: 369A.

556. Dahl-Jorgensen K, Brinchmann-Hansen O, Hanssen KF, Sandvik L, Aagenaes O. Rapid tightening of blood glucose control leads to transient deterioration of retinopathy in insulin-dependent diabetes mellitus: the Oslo Study. Br Med J 1985; 290: 811–15.

557. Legrain M, Rottembourg J, Benthikou A et al. Dialysis treatment of insulin-dependent diabetic patients: ten years experience. Clin Nephrol 1984; 21: 72–81.

558. Kioko EM, Shaw KM, Clarke AD, Warren DJ. Successful pregnancy in a diabetic patient treated with continuous ambulatory peritoneal dialysis. Diabetes Care 1983; 6: 298–300.

559. Zimmerman SV, Johnson CA, O'Brien M. Long term survival on peritoneal dialysis. Am J Kidney Dis 1987; 10: 241–9.

560. Wing AF, Broyer M, Brunner FP et al. Combined report on regular dialysis and transplantation in Europe. Proc EDTA ERA 1983; 20: 1–78.

561. Grefberg N, Danielson BG, Nilsson P. Continuous ambulatory peritoneal dialysis in the treatment of end-stage diabetic nephropathy. Acta Med Scand 1984; 215: 427–31.

562. Nolph KD, Cutler SJ, Steinberg SM, Nowak WJ. Continuous ambulatory peritoneal dialysis in the United States: a three-year study. Kidney Int 1985; 28: 198–205.

563. Legrain M, Gahl GM, Boudjeman A, Rottenbourg J. The case for dialysis in diabetics. Transport Proc 1986; 18: 1693–7.

564. Oreopoulos DG, Kharna R, Williams P et al. Continuous ambulatory dialysis 1981. Nephron 1982; 30: 293–303.

565. Sagalowsky AI, Gailiunas P, Helderman JH et al. Renal transplantation in diabetic patients: the end result does justify the means. J Urol 1982; 129: 253–5.

566. Najarian JS, Strand M, Fryd DS et al. Comparison of cyclosporine versus azathioprine antilymphocyte globulin in renal transplantation. In Kahan B (ed.) Cyclosporine. New York: Grune & Stratton, 1984: pp 247–52.

567. Ferguson RM, Rynasiewicz JJ, Sutherland DER, Simmons RL, Najarian JS. Cyclosporine A in renal transplantation: a prospective randomised trial. Surgery 1982; 92: 175–82.

568. Parfrey PS, Hutchinson TA, Harvey C, Gutt-

man RD. Transplantation versus dialysis in diabetic patients with renal failure. Am J Kidney Dis 1985; 5: 112–16.

569. Butt KMH, Arshad GA, Chandhy M et al. Total surgical care in uraemic diabetics. In Friedman EA, L'Esperance FA Jr (eds) Diabetic renal–retinal syndrome, vol. 2: Prevention and management. New York: Grune & Stratton, 1982: pp 361–71.

570. Bentley FR, Sutherland DER, Mauer SM et al. The status of renal allograft recipients who survived for 10 or more years after transplantation. Transplant Proc 1985; 17: 1573–6.

571. Simmons RG, Kanistra-Hennen L, Thompson CR. Psychosocial adjustment five to nine years post transplant. Transplant Proc 1981; 14: 40–3.

572. Johnson JP, McCauley CR, Copley JB. The quality of life of haemodialysis and transplantation patients. Kidney Int 1985; 22: 284–91.

573. Garvin PJ, Castanda M, Carney K. Simultaneous cadaver renal and pancreas transplantation in type 1 diabetes. Arch Surg 1986; 122: 274–8.

574. Bohman SO, Tyden G, Wilczeh M et al. Prevention of kidney graft diabetic nephropathy by pancreas transplantation in man. Diabetes 1985; 34: 306–8.

575. Bilous RW, Mauer SM, Sutherland DER, Najarian JS, Goetz FC, Steffes MW. The effects of pancreas transplantation on the glomerular structure of renal allografts in patients with insulin-dependent diabetes. New Engl J Med 1989; 321: 80–5.

576. Kramer P, Scrader J, Bohnsack W, Grieben G, Grone MJ, Scheler F. Continuous arteriovenous haemofiltration. A new kidney replacement therapy. Proc Eur Dial Transplant Assoc 1981; 18: 743–9.

577. Pattison ME, Lee SM, Ogden DA. Continuous arteriovenous haemodiafiltration: an aggressive approach to the management of acute renal failure. Am J Kidney Dis 1988; 11: 43–7.

578. Quellhurst EA, Schuenmann B, Hildebrand U. Morbidity and mortality in long-term haemofiltration. ASAIO J 1983; 6: 185–91.

579. Raine AEG, MacMahon SM, Selwood NH, Wing AJ, Brunner FP. Mortality from myocardial infarction in patients on renal replacement therapy in the UK. Nephrol Dial Transpl (in press).

56
Diabetic Retinopathy

Matthew D. Davis* and Lawrence I. Rand†

**Department of Ophthalmology, University of Wisconsin-Madison, USA,
and †West Newton, Massachusetts, USA*

NATURAL COURSE OF DIABETIC RETINOPATHY

The natural course of diabetic retinopathy has been described in some detail, and is best understood in relation to five fundamental pathologic processes: (a) formation of retinal capillary microaneurysms, (b) excessive vascular permeability, (c) vascular occlusion, (d) proliferation of new blood vessels and accompanying fibrous tissue on the surface of the retina and optic disc, and (e) contraction of these fibrovascular proliferations and the vitreous [1–7]. The clinical picture of diabetic retinopathy in an individual patient depends on the relative contributions of these five processes. Microaneurysm formation, unless accompanied by excessive vascular permeability or capillary occlusion, is a benign process with no visual consequences. When microaneurysms and/or retinal capillaries become excessively permeable, the resulting clinical picture is that of retinal edema and hard exudate formation, often involving the center of the macula and leading to moderate impairment of vision. Vascular occlusion appears to begin in the capillary bed and initially is of little clinical importance. As the vaso-occlusive process worsens, involvement of terminal arterioles becomes apparent and larger patches of capillaries become occluded, presumably causing

elaboration of one or more growth factors [7–13]. Vasoproliferation follows, first within the retina and then on its anterior surface. The resulting preretinal new vessels are the principal source of the vitreous hemorrhage that is a characteristic feature of the proliferative stage of diabetic retinopathy (PDR) and a common cause of severe visual loss. Equally characteristic are the fibrous proliferations that accompany the new vessels. Contraction of these proliferations is the principal mechanism leading to distortion or detachment of the retina, also common causes of visual loss in PDR. These processes and the clinical pictures resulting from them are discussed in more detail below.

Microaneurysms

The retinal capillary microaneurysm, although seen in many other conditions as well (such as branch retinal vein occlusion, hyperviscosity syndromes and idiopathic telangiectasis of the retinal vessels), is the hallmark of diabetic retinopathy and its earliest reliable sign. Histologically, microaneurysms appear initially as hypercellular saccular outpouchings from the capillary wall, seen best with the trypsin digest technique of Kuwabara and Cogan, in which retinal tissue is digested away from the vascular

International Textbook of Diabetes Mellitus. Edited by K.G.M.M. Alberti, R.A. DeFronzo, H. Keen and P. Zimmet

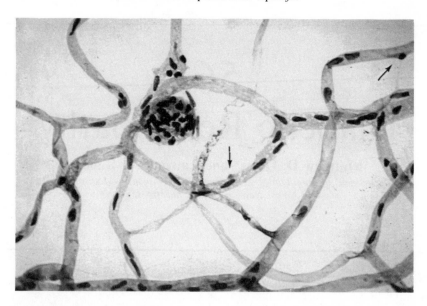

Figure 1 Saccular capillary microaneurysm in a trypsin digest preparation of dog retinal vessels after 60 months of alloxan diabetes. Most capillaries are hypocellular and some are acellular. Oblique arrow indicates pericyte nucleus, vertical arrow a pericyte ghost. Oval nuclei are those of endothelial cells (courtesy of R.L. Engerman)

network, which can then be stained and examined as a flat mount [14]. Studies with this technique have shown that loss of the intramural pericytes of the capillaries, development of acellular (non-perfused) capillaries and microaneurysm formation are the earliest morphologic abnormalities (Figure 1) [15–19]. The sequence of these changes is not clear, some observers suggesting that pericyte loss occurs first, others that capillary closure may be the earlier event [15, 20]. Few human autopsy eyes with very early retinopathy have been studied, but in experimental diabetic retinopathy in dogs it appears that pericyte loss usually precedes the development of microaneurysms and acellular capillaries [19]. Angiographically, microaneurysms appear to precede capillary non-perfusion [21], but the resolution of angiography is probably not sufficient to recognize capillary loss at its earliest stage. At the ultrastructural level another early morphologic finding is thickening of the basement membrane of retinal capillaries, but the pathogenetic importance of this abnormality is obscure [22, 23, 24]. Mechanisms suggested for microaneurysm formation have included vasoproliferation, weakness of the capillary wall (perhaps from loss of pericytes), abnormalities of the adjacent retina and increased intraluminal

pressure, but there is no convincing evidence for any of these alternatives [9, 15, 23].

Early in their evolution microaneurysms are seen with direct ophthalmoscopy as tiny dots of the same deep-red color as the retinal veins. At this stage the wall of the microaneurysm is completely transparent and only the blood within its lumen is visible, as is the case for normal retinal vessels. Ophthalmoscopically visible microaneurysms commonly vary in diameter from about $15\,\mu m$ to $60\,\mu m$, i.e. from one-eighth to one-half the diameter of a normal retinal vein at the disc margin, but occasionally may be larger (the dimensions used here are based on the commonly used clinical convention of considering the diameter of the average optic disc to be $1500\,\mu m$, although 1800–$1900\,\mu m$ may be a better estimate) [25, 26]. It is sometimes difficult to determine ophthalmoscopically whether a given red spot is a microaneurysm or a punctate hemorrhage. Most round, red dots with smooth edges fill during fluorescein angiography, proving that they are microaneurysms; some that do not fill can be shown by clinico-histopathologic correlation to be microaneurysms packed with red blood cells [27]. When only occasional microaneurysms are present, a careful, unhurried search may be required for their detection, preferably through a dilated pupil with the bright light of a halogen bulb ophthalmoscope powered by a transformer or rechargeable battery handle. The major retinal vessels should be followed out for 4–5 disc diameters from the optic disc in all directions, methodically scanning the retina between them. Because it is a common location for the first microaneurysms, special attention should be paid to the posterior pole, a roughly circular area bounded above and below by the usual location of the major temporal vascular arcades and nasally by the disc. Pupillary dilation is of special importance for this area, particularly if lens opacities are present.

When only one or two microaneurysms are present in one or both eyes, a patient may readily be misclassified as free of retinopathy. Clinically, little or no harm is done by such an error, because follow-up of patients with only occasional microaneurysms differs little from that of patients free of any retinal abnormality (a careful ophthalmoscopic examination every year or so). For this same reason, there is little point in using fluorescein angiography clinically for early detection of retinopathy in patients free of it on ophthalmoscopic examination. Microaneurysms are certainly more easily seen by angiography, because they appear as bright dots against the darker choroidal background rather than as red dots against an orange background, and usually more microaneurysms are visible in any given retinal area with angiography than with color photography or ophthalmoscopy (Figure 2). However, patients free of microaneurysms by ophthalmoscopy or color photography, but in whom they are found on angiography, usually have only one or two microaneurysms in only one eye, a clinically unimportant finding [21].

Microaneurysms may show little change over periods of several years, or their walls may become thickened, sometimes sufficiently to occlude their lumens [27]. As the wall of a microaneurysm thickens it becomes less transparent and its color changes from the bluish-red of venous blood through shades of orange, offering little contrast with the fundus background, to the yellowish-white color of hard exudate. During the reddish-orange stage the wall of the microaneurysm, seen on edge, may be visible as a white ring surrounding the blood in its lumen (Figure 3).

Excessive Vascular Permeability

When the number of microaneurysms in an eye exceeds 10, fluorescein angiography usually demonstrates retinal capillary abnormalities, consisting of focal fluorescein leakage from microaneurysms or more diffuse leakage from capillaries, capillary dilation, and/or capillary non-perfusion (capillary dropout) (Figure 4) [21]. By ophthalmoscopy, such eyes can usually be seen to have progressed beyond the microaneurysm-only stage, with development of retinal hemorrhages and/or hard exudates, or more advanced lesions (see below). Hard exudates are made up mainly of lipid, most of which has presumably leaked from the plasma across the excessively permeable walls of microaneurysms and adjacent leaky capillaries. Hard exudates may be sprinkled across the fundus in no particular pattern, but more often are arranged in partial or complete rings, each ring marking the circumference of a roughly circular zone of thickened (edematous) retina that surrounds one or more microaneurysms (Figures 3 and 5). The lipid appears to remain dispersed within the retina in the edematous zones and to become deposited at their edges, as water and other small molecules are resorbed across the walls of surrounding, more normal, capillaries. Retinal edema is not easy to recognize with direct ophthalmoscopy, because the thickened retina maintains normal or near-normal transparency and its increased thickness is difficult to appreciate without a stereoscopic examining method, such as slit-lamp biomicroscopy or stereoscopic fundus photography. Fluorescein leakage, although characteristically most prominent in areas of thickened retina, particularly those within hard exudate rings, may also be seen to a lesser degree in areas where the retina does not appear thickened. *Thus fluorescein leakage alone does not indicate retinal edema.*

The posterior pole is the most common location of retinal edema and hard exudates, and when the retina within a disc diameter or two of the center of the macula is involved (macular edema), visual acuity is threatened, although it does not actually become impaired until the center of the macula is involved (Figure 5). If the center is not involved by a plaque of hard exudate and thickening here is mild, visual loss may be slight and may go unnoticed by the

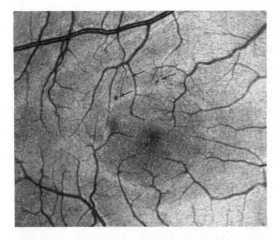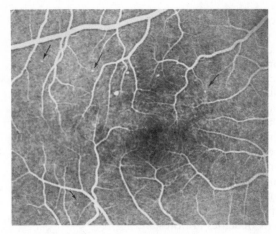

Figure 2 (A) Black and white print from a color photograph showing one large and two small definite microaneurysms (arrows) in the right eye of a patient with type 1 diabetes. (B) Early phase fluorescein angiogram showing the same three microaneurysms and four more (arrows), some of which could be detected in the original color stereo photograph as tiny red dots. The capillary network adjacent to the foveal avascular zone was intact and there was no fluorescein leakage in the late phase (courtesy of DCCT Research Group)

patient for a long time, if vision in the fellow eye is good. Because retinal thickening is often difficult to recognize, patients with hard exudates or other obvious retinal lesions in the posterior pole should be referred for ophthalmologic consultation, as should patients with any impairment of visual acuity uncorrected by glasses. Photocoagulation has been found capable of

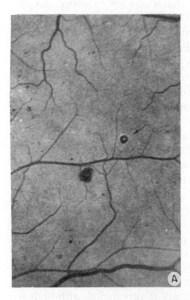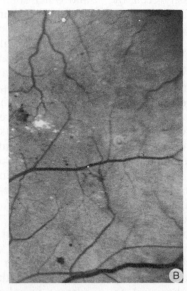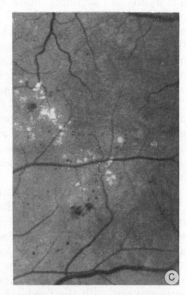

Figure 3 Evolution of a very large microaneurysm in the left eye of a patient with type 2 diabetes. (A) The microaneurysm (arrow) has a central light reflex and its wall is mostly invisible (except from 9 to 12 o'clock) and does not obscure the blood in its lumen. (B) Fifteen months later the wall of the microaneurysm is apparent as a ring around its lumen and the blood in the lumen is obscured by the wall. (C) Two years later the microaneurysm is an opaque white spot, its lumen presumably closed. Partial hard exudate rings surround groups of smaller microaneurysms below the large microaneurysm and at the left side of the figure (courtesy of Fundus Photo Reading Center, University of Wisconsin)

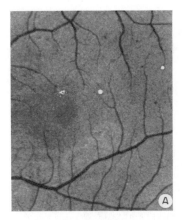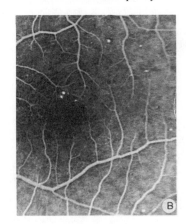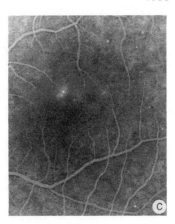

Figure 4 (A) Fundus photograph showing about 6 of the more than 20 small microaneurysms that were present in the left eye of a patient with type 1 diabetes. There appear to be several tiny hard exudates above the center of the macula. No retinal thickening was visible. (B) Early phase fluorescein angiogram showing two large microaneurysms at the edge of the foveal avascular zone at 11 o'clock, in the location of the hard exudates, with a small area of capillary dropout adjacent to them. Most, but not all, of the microaneurysms visible in the color photo are visible. (C) Late phase of the angiogram showing a little fluorescein leakage, principally adjacent to the large microaneurysms (courtesy of the DCCT Research Group)

reducing macular edema and slowing or preventing visual loss, but is not very effective in restoring visual acuity already lost [28]. Thus it is important to recognize macular edema early so that treatment can be initiated while vision is still reasonably good.

Vaso-obliteration

As already mentioned, individual acellular capillaries are usually visible histologically in the earliest stages of diabetic retinopathy. As retinopathy becomes more severe, larger patches of acellular capillaries are seen. Frequently it is evident that such patches were supplied by terminal arterioles that have become occluded. Adjacent to patches of acellular capillaries, clusters of microaneurysms and tortuous, hypercellular vessels are often present (Figure 6). It is difficult to determine whether these vessels are dilated pre-existing capillaries or intraretinal new vessels; the term intraretinal microvascular abnormalities (IRMA) is used to include both possibilities [29]. The ophthalmoscopic counterpart of capillaries that have recently closed following occlusion of a terminal arteriole is the cotton-wool spot (soft exudate). In diabetic retinopathy these lesions are characteristically less intensely white and fade less rapidly (often over a period of many months) than is the case in hypertensive retinopathy. IRMA are often seen adjacent to cotton-wool spots, but may be seen elsewhere as well (Figure 7). As capillary closure becomes extensive it is common to see many dark-red blot hemorrhages and/or segmental

Figure 5 A hard exudate ring about 1.5 disc diameters in diameter is centered about 1.0 disc diameter superotemporal to the center of the macula in this right eye. Part of the ring is a plaque of hard exudate just above the center of the macula. Within the ring many large microaneurysms can be seen, some with visible walls. They are slightly out of focus because the retina here is thickened (edematous) and the camera is focused on the surrounding retina. With stereoscopic viewing retinal thickening was obvious and could be seen to extend into the center of the macula (courtesy of the ETDRS Research Group)

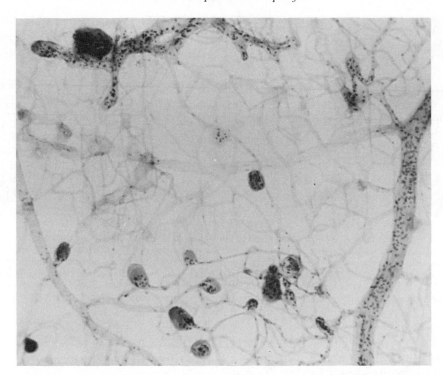

Figure 6 Trypsin digest preparation of human diabetic retina. A central zone of acellular vessels is bordered by microaneurysms below and a large hypercellular vessel above (courtesy of R.L. Engerman)

dilation of retinal veins (venous beading) (Figures 7 and 8). In trypsin digest preparations both beaded veins and IRMA appear hypercellular, the pathogenetic mechanism for their development (and that of preretinal new vessels as well) presumably being endothelial proliferation in response to partial ischemia of the inner retinal layers caused by capillary closure. When these lesions (cotton-wool spots, IRMA, venous beading and retinal hemorrhages) are prominent, non-proliferative diabetic retinopathy (NPDR) is considered *severe*, or *preproliferative*, and new vessels are likely to appear soon on the surface of the retina or optic disc. Recently it has been emphasized that, of these four lesions, cotton-wool spots are the least predictive of the subsequent development of PDR [30]. Small, subtle spots may be seen very early in NPDR, when microaneurysms are only occasionally evident, or not at all [31]. When capillary closure becomes very extensive, these intraretinal lesions tend to disappear, leading to a *featureless* appearance (Figure 9B).

A great deal of thought has been devoted to attempts to understand the basic mechanisms leading to capillary closure, with limited success [19, 20, 23, 24, 32]. One of the more appealing hypotheses currently under investigation proposes that retinal vascular cells are damaged by an increased flux of glucose through the polyol pathway, which may occur within them during periods of hyperglycemia, and that this damage leads to loss of autoregulation and perhaps increased blood flow, followed by capillary closure [33–38]. In the polyol pathway the conversion of glucose to sorbitol (and of galactose to galactitol) is catalyzed by the enzyme aldose reductase. Sorbitol is then converted to fructose by sorbitol dehydrogenase, to some extent in some cells (see also Chapter 53). Aldose reductase has low substrate affinity for glucose and thus during normoglycemia this pathway is inactive, but during hyperglycemia might become important in retinal vascular cells (assuming that they contain aldose reductase), because they do not require insulin for glucose penetration. Sorbitol does not readily cross cell membranes, and may accumulate within the cells to damaging

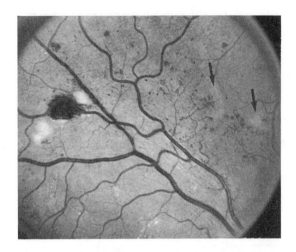

Figure 7 Severe NPDR. On the left side of the figure there are two prominent cotton-wool spots with a large blot hemorrhage between them. Venous beading is prominent where the superior branch of the superior temporal vein passes by the upper spot. On the right side of the figure there are two faint cotton-wool spots (arrows) and many prominent IRMA (courtesy of the ETDRS Research Group)

concentrations. This hypothesis is supported by the demonstration of aldose reductase in human retinal pericytes [39], by the production of retinopathy indistinguishable from that of diabetes by feeding a galactose-enriched diet to normal

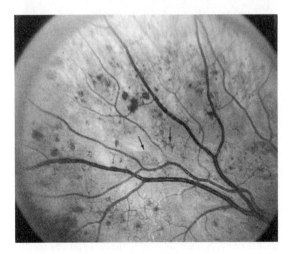

Figure 8 Transition from severe NPDR to PDR. There are extensive retinal hemorrhages, venous beading, and several large faint cotton-wool spots (just to the left of the center of the figure). Arrows indicate tortuous small vessels that could be either IRMA or early new vessels on the surface of the retina (courtesy of the ETDRS Research Group)

dogs [40], and by the prevention of basement membrane thickening in retinal capillaries of galactosemic and diabetic rats treated with aldose reductase inhibitors [41–43]. Recently, high doses of aldose reductase inhibitors have been reported to slow the development of retinal capillary pericyte loss and microaneurysm formation in dogs after 2–3 years of galactose feeding [44]. However, in another laboratory no inhibition of pericyte ghosts or microaneurysm formation was observed after 42 months of galactosemia, in dogs given the aldose reductase inhibitor sorbinil in doses sufficient to prevent 93% of the increase in red blood cell hexitol that occurred in the control group [45]. In a randomized clinical trial in insulin dependent patients, sorbinil has recently been reported to show no beneficial effect in slowing the development or progression of retinopathy [46].

Proliferation of New Vessels and Fibrous Tissue

When new vessels appear on the surface of the retina or optic disc, diabetic retinopathy is said to have entered the proliferative stage. New vessels arise most frequently posteriorly, within 45 degrees of the optic disc, and are particularly common on the disc itself [4, 47]. Eyes with new vessels on the disc are at greater risk of visual loss [48–51], and new vessels here (on or within one disc diameter of the disc, or in the vitreous cavity anterior to this area) are commonly designated NVD and considered separately from new vessels elsewhere (NVE) [29, 52, 53]. NVD begin typically as fine loops or networks lying on the surface of the disc or adjacent retina, or bridging across the physiologic cup. In their earliest stages, they may easily be mistaken for normal vessels during ophthalmoscopy, but can usually be correctly identified by stereoscopic examination with slit-lamp and contact lens, or by their characteristic leakage on fluorescein angiography (Figure 9C). When well established, NVD are easily identified using direct ophthalmoscopy (Figure 10). In a puzzling condition easily mistaken for papilledema, diabetic papillopathy, it may be difficult to distinguish NVD from dilated small vessels within the swollen disc and adjacent retina. This condition occurs typically before the age of 30 years in patients with good vision and mild NPDR, but NVD are present in some cases [54]. Spontaneous resolution of the disc edema within several months is the rule,

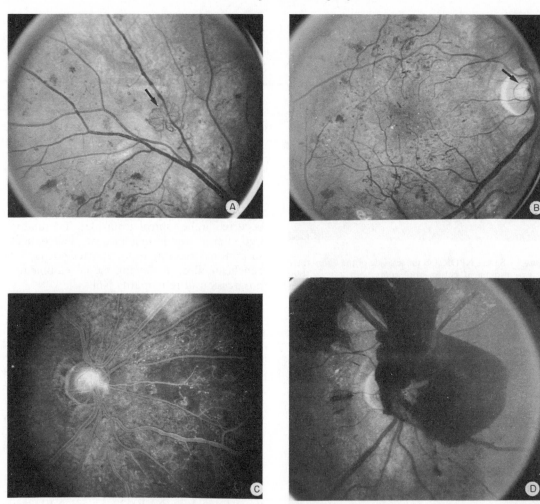

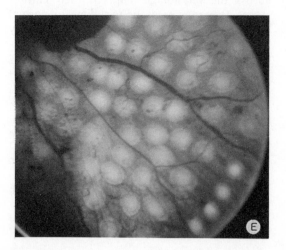

Figure 9 (A) New vessels forming a wheel-like network (arrow) in the superior temporal quadrant of an eye with venous beading, cotton-wool spots, IRMA and blot hemorrhages. (B) Posterior pole of the same eye showing IRMA and retinal hemorrhages centrally and featureless retina near the left edge of the figure. With stereoscopic examination the vascular loop on the disc (arrow) could be seen to bridge the physiologic cup and was clearly a new vessel. (C) In the late-stage angiogram the position of new vessels on the disc is marked by fluorescein leakage. Fluorescein leakage along the superior nasal vein at the upper edge of the figure is from new vessels here. There is an area of capillary dropout nasal to the disc. (D) Ten months later, preretinal and vitreous hemorrhage occurred from the new vessels. (E) Lower nasal quadrant showing fresh burns of the first episode of scatter photocoagulation, carried out on the same day. After repeated photocoagulation almost all new vessels regressed and good vision was maintained (courtesy of the ETDRS Research Group)

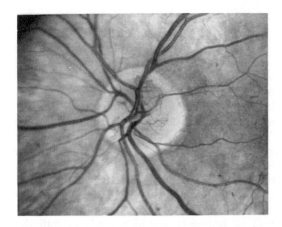

Figure 10 Standard Photograph 10A of the Modified Airlie House Classification [52]. New vessels cover about a quarter of the area of this disc, which is a little larger than average. New vessels equalling or exceeding those in this photograph are sufficient to place an eye in the high-risk category (without regard to the size of the disc) (courtesy of the DRS Research Group)

and when NVD are present they sometimes regress concurrently (Figure 11).

Early NVE are easily overlooked and may be difficult to distinguish from IRMA (Figure 8). As they become larger, NVE are easily iden-

tified, either by their tendency to form networks (Figures 9A and 13) or by their course across both arterial and venous branches of the underlying retinal vessels, a pattern never occurring in the normal vasculature (Figure 12). The most striking networks are roughly circular patches resembling carriage wheels, with vessels radiating like spokes from the center of the patch to a circumferential vessel bounding its periphery. The centers of such patches often lie over retinal veins, from which the vessels appear to arise.

The rate of growth of new vessels is extremely variable. In some patients a patch of vessels may remain essentially unchanged for many months, while in others a definite increase may be seen in as little as a week or two. New vessels characteristically follow a cycle of proliferation and regression [3, 4]. Early in their evolution new vessels appear bare, but later translucent fibrous tissue often appears adjacent to them and becomes increasingly opaque as regression of the new vessels occurs (Figure 13). Usually regression is incomplete, but occasionally blood-filled new vessels may disappear altogether, being replaced by tufts of white tissue or networks of white lines, or occasionally leaving no trace at all. These fibrovascular proliferations

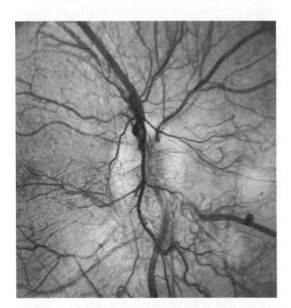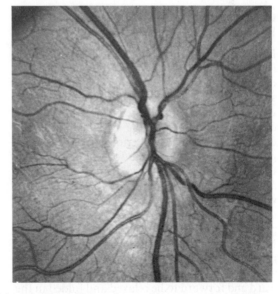

Figure 11 Optic disc swelling. This 20-year-old man, whose diabetes had been diagnosed at age 14 years, sought ophthalmologic attention because of the sudden onset of floaters, first in the left eye and several days later in the right. (A) The disc is swollen, has blurred margins, and is partially obscured by extensive new vessels arising on it and extending onto the retina in all quadrants. (B) Five months later, disc swelling had resolved and all new vessels had regressed spontaneously. Vision remained 20/15 (courtesy of the DRS Research Group)

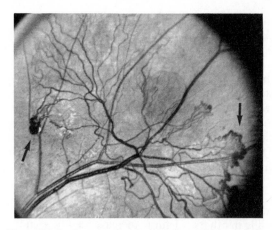

Figure 12 In the upper temporal quadrant of this eye extensive new vessels extend for several disc diameters across the retina without prominent network formation. Large aneurysmal dilations are present at the end of a long new vessel loop (left arrow) and at the circumference of a partial wheel-like network (right arrow) (courtesy of the DRS Research Group)

characteristically become adherent to the vitreous framework and such adhesions remain even after the new vessels regress. As long as neither vitreous contraction nor contraction of the fibrous tissue associated with the new vessels occurs, the new vessels usually remain asymptomatic.

Contraction of Vitreous and Fibrovascular Proliferations

Posterior vitreous detachment is a process occurring in most normal eyes during or after the sixth or seventh decade. Its mechanism, apparently, is shrinkage of the posterior surface of the vitreous, a zone that has more collagen fibers than does the central part of the vitreous. Shrinkage in the plane of the posterior vitreous surface produces a vector of force forward away from the retina (conveniently explained to patients and students by comparison with a bowl lined with a piece of cloth that is adherent to the edges of the bowl; shrinkage of the cloth will lead it to move upwards toward the top of the bowl). Normally the vitreous is not adherent to the retina, so that its posterior surface can pull away without causing retinal tears and can fall downward and forward to lie relaxed and folded in the anterior and inferior part of the vitreous cavity, with fluid vitreous occupying the remainder of this cavity, an appearance designated posterior vitreous detachment with collapse.

Posterior vitreous detachment tends to occur at an earlier age in patients with PDR. In areas free of fibrovascular proliferations the posterior vitreous surface pulls away from the retina. Where proliferations are present, they are pulled forward, and with them the retina from which they arise, often producing localized areas of tractional retinal detachment (Figure 14). The fibrovascular proliferations themselves also play an important part in the contraction process, particularly when they are extensive. In addition to producing a vector of force that tends to pull the retina forward away from the retinal pigment epithelium and choroid, contraction of a sheet of fibrous tissue also tends to pull the surrounding retina towards the center of the sheet (tangential traction). As fibrovascular membranes are usually centered on or near the optic disc, tangential traction often leads to displacement ('dragging') of the macula nasally toward the disc (Figure 15) [55].

As contraction begins, traction is exerted upon the new vessels [4, 5]. Vitreous hemorrhage often occurs concomitantly, probably in part because of the traction. The severity of visual symptoms varies with the extent of vitreous hemorrhage, from a few floating specks lasting only an hour or two (until the blood disperses or settles inferiorly) to loss of all but hand movement or light perception vision. It is unusual for the first vitreous hemorrhage that occurs in an eye to be massive, but a large hemorrhage often follows an initial small one within a few days or weeks; thus, even a very small vitreous

Figure 13 (*opposite*) (A) Severe NPDR in a patient with newly diagnosed type 2 diabetes (superior temporal quadrant of the right eye). There are many microaneurysms, hemorrhages and hard exudates, as well as extensive retinal edema and venous beading. Most of the tortuous small vessels appeared to be within the retina (large IRMA), but some may have been on its surface (NVE). (B) Eight months later there had been marked improvement in the intraretinal abnormalities, but a wheel-like network of new vessels had appeared on the surface of the retina. (C) Three months later the new vessel patch had enlarged and a second patch had developed above it. During the next 2 years the new vessels continued to grow slowly at the edges of the patches, while regressing at their centers. (D) Three years after they had appeared, most of the new vessels had regressed, although there was still one dilated loop at the upper edge of the upper patch. No contraction of fibrous proliferations or vitreous had occurred, there had been no vitreous hemorrhage, and vision remained good (courtesy of Fundus Photo Reading Center, University of Wisconsin)

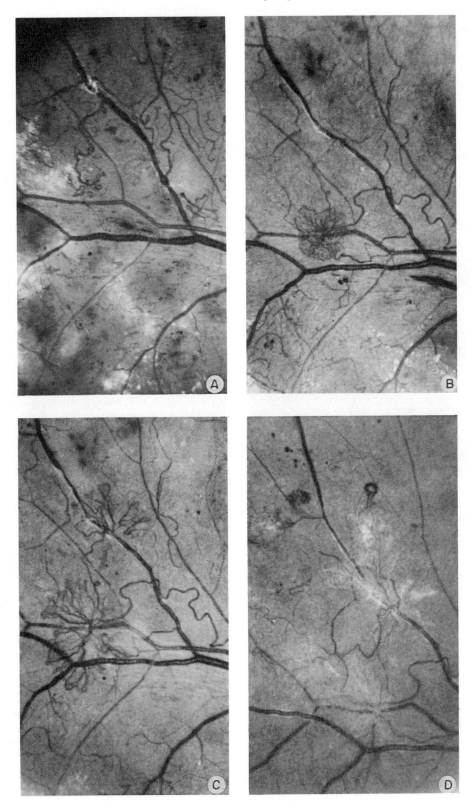

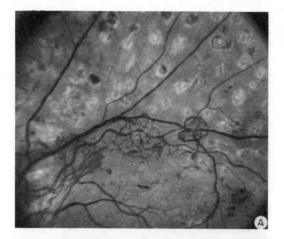

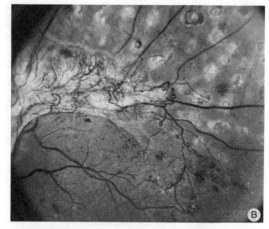

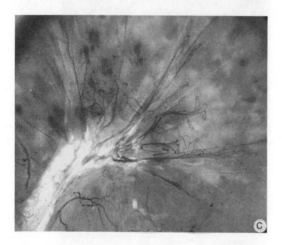

Figure 14 (A) Networks of new vessels extend over the surface of the retina along the superior temporal vein. Scars are typical of initial scatter photocoagulation, with ample room for additional treatment (in retrospect, this probably would have been advisable). (B) Four months later, new vessels had increased and dense fibrous tissue had appeared. (C) Seven months later, fibrous proliferations had contracted. Broad adhesions prevented them from pulling away from the retina; instead, the retina has been pulled forward (detached) throughout the area included in the figure. The photocoagulation scars are blurred by the overlying detached retina (and are also out of focus) (courtesy of DRVS Research Group)

hemorrhage is an urgent indication for prompt ophthalmologic attention. The rate at which hemorrhages clear is highly variable, from a few weeks when they are small to months, years or never, when they are large. Hemorrhages tend to recur periodically, usually without any obvious precipitating event and often during sleep [56, 57].

RETINOPATHY AND TYPE AND DURATION OF DIABETES

PDR has generally been considered to be a more important problem in type 1 (insulin dependent) diabetes and macular edema more important in type 2 (non-insulin dependent). Accurate comparisons have been difficult, because of uncertainties in the clinical assessment of diabetes type, the paucity of studies that have evaluated patients of both types with the same methods, and the even greater rarity of population-based studies. Figures 16 and 17 from a study by Klein and co-workers summarize the prevalence of any degree of retinopathy and of PDR, respectively, in a population-based sample of diabetic individuals in southwestern Wisconsin [58]. Retinopathy severity was assessed in stereoscopic color fundus photographs graded according to the Modified Airlie House Classification [52, 53]. In the younger-onset group, which was made up of individuals whose age at diagnosis of diabetes was less than 30 years and who were taking insulin at the time of examination (nearly all presumably had type 1 diabetes), prevalence of retinopathy (Figure 16) rose steeply from about 13% in persons with less than 5 years' duration of diabetes to 90% in those with durations of 10–15 years. Retinopathy was more common in the older-onset individuals with diabetes of less than 5 years' known duration, and prevalence rose less rapidly with increasing

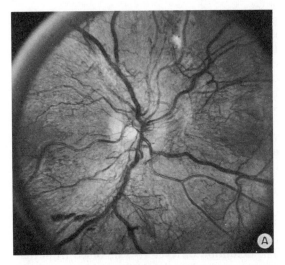
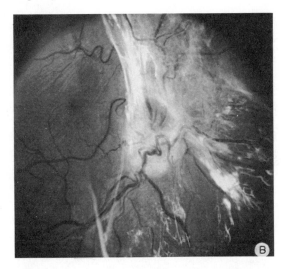

Figure 15 (A) There are extensive new vessels on the surface of the disc and retina in this right eye as well as many dilated intraretinal vessels (IRMA). There is a cotton-wool spot about 1 disc diameter superonasally to the disc and several small preretinal hemorrhages near the bottom of the figure to the left. The macula is in its normal position, centered at or just temporal to the left edge of the figure. Fibrous tissue accompanying the new vessels is visible adjacent to the temporal vascular arcades and in a small area 0.5 disc diameter superonasal to the disc. Fibrous proliferations were actually much more extensive, but were transparent and difficult to detect. Visual acuity was 20/20. Contraction of the fibrous proliferations occurred within the next several months, dragging the retina nasally and superiorly, and new vessels regressed. (B) Four years later, the center of the macula was about 1.5 disc diameters superotemporal to the disc margin. The first major bifurcation of the inferior temporal vein had been pulled upward to the disc margin from its previous position. New vessels had regressed completely, some of them now appearing as networks of fine white lines. Visual acuity was 20/30 (courtesy of the DRVS Research Group)

duration, both in the group taking insulin (a mixture of type 1 and type 2 diabetes) and in the group not taking insulin (type 2).

Prevalence of PDR (Figure 17) in the younger-onset group was 0% when duration of diabetes was less than 5 years, 2% in the 5–10 years' duration interval, and then rose rapidly to more than 50% in persons with 20 or more years of diabetes. In the older-onset group taking insulin, prevalence rose fairly steadily from 2% in

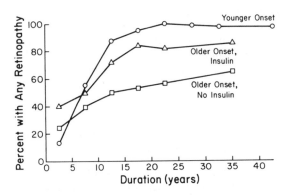

Figure 16 Percentage of persons with diabetic retinopathy by duration of diabetes in each of three groups classified by age at diagnosis and insulin use. The number of persons in each duration interval in each group was at least 70, with the following exceptions — younger-onset group: interval 30–34 years, 43, interval 35 years and over, 44; non-insulin-taking group: interval 20–24 years, 41, interval 25 years and over, 15 (from reference 62)

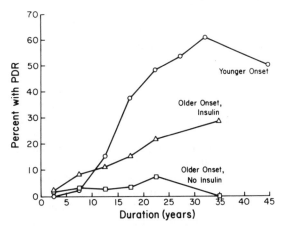

Figure 17 Percentage of persons with PDR by duration of diabetes in each of the three groups (from reference 62)

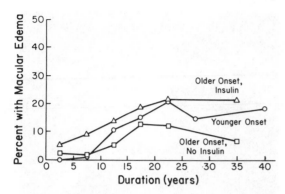

Figure 18 Percentage of persons with macular edema by duration of diabetes in each of the three groups (from reference 62)

persons with less than 5 years of diabetes to more than 25% in those with 20 years or more. In the group not taking insulin, prevalence remained about 2–5%, regardless of duration. Among individuals with PDR, its severity did not appear to differ between the younger-onset and the combined older-onset groups; in each case in the worse eye about 25% of individuals had Diabetic Retinopathy Study (DRS) high-risk characteristics and 15% had retinopathy severity ungradable because of extensive vit-reous hemorrhage, or phthisis bulbi or enuclea-tion secondary to complications of diabetic retinopathy.

Prevalence of macular edema did not vary as widely by diabetes type (Figure 18), but PDR was significantly more common in younger-onset individuals with macular edema (65%, versus 36% and 19%, respectively, in both the older-onset groups) and moderately extensive hard exudate was significantly less common (2%, 9% and 18% in the three groups, respect-ively).

Because diabetes with onset after the age of 30 years is more common than the younger-onset type, however, in the population from which Klein and co-workers drew their sample these older-onset individuals comprised a majority of the total number with either macular edema or PDR. Of all subjects with macular edema, 20% were estimated to belong to the younger-onset group, 59% to the older-onset group taking insulin and 21% to the older-onset group not taking insulin. Of all subjects with PDR, 43% belonged to the younger-onset

group, 42% to the older-onset group taking insulin, and 15% to the older-onset group not taking insulin [58]. Among patients with PDR entering the DRS [59] or attending the Eye Unit of the Joslin Clinic [60], the percentage belong-ing to the younger-onset group appeared to be somewhat higher, in the range of 50–65%.

The risk of progression to PDR among patients with NPDR is related both to retinopathy severity and diabetes type, more strongly to the former (Table 1) [61, 62]. The retinopathy severity scale used in Table 1, which is modified slightly from previous proposals [63, 64], is shown in Table 2 (see also Figures 19 and 20) for *individual eyes*. The definition for each severity level assumes that the definition for a higher level is not met. The definition of level 51 is modified from that used for group 3 in the DRS and for group P2 in the Early Treatment Diabetic Retinopathy Study (ETDRS) in order to give more weight to presence of venous beading and severity of reti-nal hemorrhages, and less to cotton-wool spots [30, 51]. The definition of level 70 is that developed in the DRS for eyes at high risk of severe visual loss without treatment [65]. After 2 years of follow-up about 25% of untreated eyes in this group had visual acuity of less than 5/200. When this scale is used for *persons*, as in Table 1, two steps are provided for each step on the eye severity scale (except for the first step), one for individuals with the specified level in each eye and one for those with a less severe level in the second eye. In Table 1, particularly in the younger-onset group, patients with a given severity level in both eyes were at higher risk of progression than those with the same level in one eye and a milder level in the other. Overall, the 4-year rate of PDR increased from near 0% in patients free of retinopathy to around 50% in those with level 51 in one or both eyes.

DIABETIC RETINOPATHY AND BLOOD GLUCOSE CONTROL

The relationship between control of diabetes and its chronic complications has been a subject of intense interest [66]. There is little doubt that retinopathy tends to be more prevalent and more severe in groups of patients who have higher blood glucose levels, i.e. more severe or less well-controlled diabetes, but it has been dif-ficult to determine whether poorer control causes more severe retinopathy, or whether both

Table 1 Four-year rates of progression to PDR by baseline severity of NPDR

Baseline retinopathy level	Percentage with progression to PDR (no. at risk)					
	yo-i		oo-i		oo-ni	
	%	(n)	%	(n)	%	(n)
10/10	0.4	(271)	0.0	(154)	0.6	(320)
21/< 21	3.0	(66)	0.0	(49)	1.5	(65)
21/21	4.8	(105)	0.0	(23)	0.0	(24)
31/< 31	10.3	(58)	8.1	(37)	0.0	(27)
31/31	20.3	(74)	2.0	(49)	10.5	(19)
41/< 41	18.3	(60)	16.3	(43)	6.2	(16)
41/41	42.4	(59)	19.4	(36)	25.0	(4)
51/< 51 or 51/51	50.0	(20)	48.1	(27)	36.4	(11)

yo-i, younger-onset patients treated with insulin; oo-i, older-onset patients treated with insulin; oo-ni, older-onset patients not treated with insulin.
Data from Klein et al [61, 62].

more severe retinopathy and greater difficulty in achieving good control are parallel effects of more severe diabetes [67–75].

The best means for differentiating between these two possibilities is a clinical trial, in which the randomization process establishes (if the trial is large enough) two groups that are essentially the same in diabetes severity and in all other respects except the treatment to which they are assigned. If the trial is large enough and participants are followed long enough, and if the assigned treatments are adhered to and produce substantial differences in glycemic control, a firm answer to the question may be anticipated. The University Group Diabetes Program (UGDP) was such a trial [76]. Non-insulin dependent patients entered this study within

1 year of diagnosis of diabetes between 1961 and 1965. During a follow-up period of 9–13 years, diabetic retinopathy developed in 43% of 127 individuals in the placebo group, 45% of 117 in the insulin standard group, and 43% of 118 in the insulin variable group. The placebo group was treated with diet plus a placebo matching the oral hypoglycemic agents used in several other groups; the insulin standard group received a standard dose of insulin based on body weight; the insulin variable group received insulin in the manner that was conventional then, attempting to achieve good blood glucose control (in most patients with once-a-day insulin). Control was not ideal, but was better in the insulin variable group, particularly during the first 4 years, as shown in Figure 21. However,

Table 2 Classification of retinopathy severity

Severity level	Lesions present
10 No retinopathy	No microaneurysms or other lesions
21 Microaneurysms only	No lesions other than microaneurysms (rarely, eyes with retinal hemorrhage or cotton-wool spot, but without microaneurysms)
31 Mild NPDR	Microaneurysms plus retinal hemorrhage, hard exudate and/or venous loops (or questionable cotton-wool spots, IRMA or venous beading)
41 Moderate NPDR	Microaneurysms plus cotton-wool spots and/or IRMA
51 Severe NPDR	Microaneurysms plus venous beading definitely present and/or H/Ma $\geqslant$ Standard Photograph 2A (Figure 19); or IRMA present in 4 quadrants and $\geqslant$ Standard Photograph 8A (Figure 20) in at least 2 of them
65 PDR without HRC	New vessels and/or fibrous proliferations; or preretinal and/or vitreous hemorrhage
70 PDR with HRC	NVD $\geqslant$ Standard Photograph 10A (Figure 10); or less extensive NVD, if vitreous or preretinal hemorrhage is present; or NVE $\geqslant \frac{1}{2}$ disc area, if vitreous or preretinal hemorrhage is present
80 Advanced PDR	Extensive vitreous hemorrhage precluding grading, retinal detachment involving the macula, or phthisis bulbi or enucleation secondary to a complication of diabetic retinopathy.

IRMA, intraretinal microvascular abnormalities; H/Ma, hemorrhages and/or microaneurysms (graded as one lesion); NVD, new vessels on or within one disc diameter of the optic disc, or in the vitreous cavity anterior to this area; NVE, new vessels elsewhere; NPDR, non-proliferative diabetic retinopathy; PDR, proliferative diabetic retinopathy; HRC, high-risk characteristics.

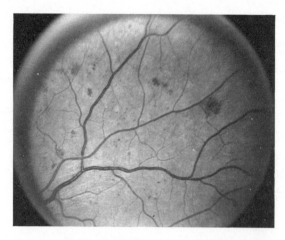

Figure 19   Standard Photograph 2A of the Modified Airlie House Classification, defining lower margin of moderately severe category for retinal hemorrhages and/or micro-aneurysms (from reference 52)

there was no suggestion of a reduction in the incidence of retinopathy in this group. The number of patients completing this study provided about 80% power for detection of a reduction from the observed rate of 43% to 25%. There have been many criticisms of the UGDP, but none seems sufficient to invalidate this result [77].

Several small, randomized clinical trials in patients with type 1 diabetes have compared intensive treatment, i.e. home blood glucose

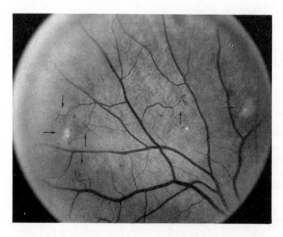

Figure 20   Standard Photograph 8A of the Modified Airlie House Classification. Four areas show definite IRMA (arrows) (from reference 52)

monitoring combined with either continuous subcutaneous insulin infusion (CSII) or multiple daily insulin injections, with conventional treatment, generally two insulin injections per day without home blood glucose monitoring [78–86]. In each of the four studies summarized in Table 3, patients were allocated randomly and analyzed according to that assignment, assessment of retinopathy status was masked, compliance was good, follow-up was nearly complete, and the difference in mean glycated hemoglobin between intensively and conventionally treated groups was about 1.5 to 2.0 percentage points. All of these studies suffer from small numbers of patients and brief periods of observation. There were differences between studies with regard to severity of retinopathy and duration of diabetes in the patients enrolled. Duration of diabetes was shortest and retinopathy mildest in the Århus study: 50% of patients had no retinopathy and the remainder had fewer than five microaneurysms. From comparisons of baseline and 1-year follow-up photographs and fluorescein angiograms, two ophthalmologists masked to treatment group found progression of retinopathy (mainly an increase in numbers of microaneurysms in the angiograms) in 3 of 12 patients in the CSII group and 4 of 12 in the conventional treatment group. Neither in the photographs nor in an ophthalmoscopic examination at the 6-month follow-up visit were cotton-wool spots seen to develop in any patient.

About 75% of the patients in the Oslo study had at least some retinopathy at the baseline examination. In the intensive treatment group, cotton-wool spots had developed at the 3-month or 6-month visit in 15 of 28 patients free of them at the beginning of the study, compared with none of 12 such patients in the conventional treatment group. All but 1 of the patients developing spots belonged to the subgroup with some degree of retinopathy on enrollment. One intensively treated patient developed proliferative retinopathy that regressed without photocoagulation. Retinopathy had improved again at the 1-year visit, with disappearance of the cotton-wool spots in all but 4 cases. After 41 months of follow-up there was a trend toward more frequent progression in the conventionally treated group.

Mild to moderate NPDR (severity level 2/ < 2 to 4/4 inclusive) was required for entry into the

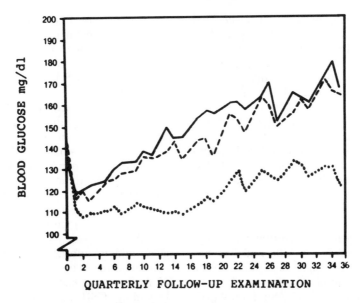

Figure 21 Mean fasting blood glucose levels at each quarterly visit for groups of patients assigned to insulin variable (dotted line), insulin standard (dashed line), and placebo (solid line) in the University Group Diabetes Program (from reference 72)

Kroc study. After 8 months of follow-up, 13 of the 32 patients in the CSII group showed retinopathy progression of at least one level, compared with 9 of 33 patients in the conventional treatment group. Development of cotton-wool spots and/or IRMA accounted for the worsening in most cases. This trend for an adverse effect of CSII was of borderline statistical significance at 8 months and had reversed direction at the 24-month visit.

About 60% of patients entering the Steno study had retinopathy level 4 in the worse eye, about 27% had level 5 or 6. At 12 months there was a trend toward more frequent progression in the CSII group, but at 24 months the trend had reversed. Progression was mainly development of cotton-wool spots, but occasional eyes developed proliferative retinopathy.

Verrillo and co-workers briefly reported a study similar to those summarized in Table 3, in

Table 3 Summary of four randomized trials comparing intensive and conventional insulin treatment in individuals with type 1 diabetes

	Trial							
	Århus [82]	Oslo [81, 83, 86]			Kroc [79, 84]		Steno [78, 80]	
Patient characteristics								
Mean duration of diabetes (yr)	10	13			17		19	
Retinopathy severity	50% none	24% none			Level 2/ < 2 to 4/4		Worse eye:	
	50% < 5 Ma	27% 1–3 Ma					13% level 3	
		33% ⩾ 4 Ma					60% level 4	
		16% exudates					27% level 5 or 6	
HbA₁ difference between groups (percentage points)	2.1	1.5			2.0		1.6	
Number of patients with retinopathy progression/number at risk								
Follow-up (months)	12	3–6	12	41	8	24*	12	24
Intensive treatment	3/12	15/28	4/28	15/28	13/32	4/29	10/15	6/15
Conventional treatment	4/12	0/12	0/12	12/15	9/33	7/31	5/15	10/15

* At this visit progression was defined as ⩾ 2 levels worse, rather than ⩾ 1 as at the 8-month visit. The analysis was by original randomization, ignoring several crossovers that occurred after the 8-month visit.
Level designations (from references 63 and 79) correspond closely to those in Table 2 (2 = 21, 3 = 31, 4 ≈ 41, 5 ≈ 51, 6 = 65 + 70).
Ma, microaneurysm.

which 44 insulin-taking patients (of unspecified age at diagnosis), were randomly assigned to treatment that was intensified (three insulin injections per day and home blood glucose monitoring) or conventional (one or two injections per day). A difference in glycated hemoglobin of about 2 percentage points was maintained for 5 years in the 38 patients remaining in the study. Retinopathy progression occurred with about equal frequency in the two groups (8 of 18 intensively treated patients progressed, 3 to PDR, versus 11 of 20 conventionally treated patients, 3 to PDR) [87].

The Oslo study found the degree to which control improved to be important: within the intensively treated group the average fall in glycated hemoglobin between baseline and 3-month follow-up visits was 3.3 percentage points in the 15 patients who developed cotton-wool spots, 1.3 percentage points in the 13 who did not [81]. In 11 of the 15 patients, cotton-wool spots had disappeared at the 12-month visit and did not seem to be of clinical importance, leading to the term *transient worsening* for this phenomenon. Possible mechanisms that have been suggested are decrease in nutrient substrate, decrease in retinal blood flow and increase in growth factors [36, 38, 81].

Of the randomized trials discussed above, only the Steno study included patients with severe NPDR or PDR, in whom worsening of retinopathy following rapid improvement in control might not be expected to be so mild or transient, but several uncontrolled case series including such patients have been published. Following two isolated case reports of remarkable improvement of retinopathy shortly after CSII was begun in such patients [88, 89], three small case series appeared that reported continued, perhaps accelerated, progression of retinopathy in similar cases [90–92]. In these three studies combined there were 12 patients who had severe NPDR in one or both eyes and had substantial improvement in glycated hemoglobin maintained for 6–22 months. Progression to PDR occurred within 4 months of beginning CSII in 6 patients, and during the next 5 months in 3 more. No patient improved. Six of these cases apparently underwent rapid and dramatic worsening, with development of macular edema, extensive new vessels and/or vitreous hemorrhage, and are reminiscent of reports (mostly concerning pubertal children) of rapid

development of PDR or severe NPDR soon after improvement of long-standing poor control in patients with mild or absent retinopathy [93–95]. The best comparison groups are provided by the DRS and the ETDRS, in which about 50% of untreated eyes with severe NPDR developed PDR within the first 15 months of follow-up [30, 49], and the recent study by Klein and co-workers, in which about 40–50% of patients with severe NPDR developed PDR during a 4-year period (Table 1).

Two of the three reports mentioned above [90, 91] included 12 patients who had PDR in at least one eye and had substantial improvement of glycated hemoglobin maintained for 4–23 months. In 5 patients new vessels continued to grow and in another 4 vitreous hemorrhages continued to occur while on CSII. Eight of the 12 patients had had photocoagulation prior to beginning CSII and this was repeated in 6 because of retinopathy progression while receiving CSII. Three patients had photocoagulation for the first time while on CSII, for increasing new vessels. Although none of these cases apparently had the dramatic progression described in the patients with NPDR, the authors' conclusions that CSII was, at best, of no benefit seem justified. Reports of retinopathy progression following successful pancreatic transplantation [96] and in diabetic women brought rapidly under good control as a part of prenatal care [97] provide additional support for the probable clinical importance of the 'transient worsening' concept.

On the basis of the reports cited above it would appear desirable to proceed cautiously when improvement of longstanding poor control is undertaken in patients with severe NPDR or active PDR, maintaining careful ophthalmologic monitoring during this period and perhaps aiming for gradual rather than rapid improvement. Photocoagulation of at least one eye of such patients before initiating better control would seem prudent.

More than 10 years ago Engerman and co-workers presented impressive evidence that good control, when initiated within a few weeks of the onset of diabetes, can almost completely inhibit the retinopathy that regularly develops after 5 years of poorly controlled alloxan diabetes in dogs [98]. More recently, Engerman and Kern found that when 30 months of good control were preceded by 30 months of poor

Table 4 Inhibition of retinopathy in alloxan diabetic dogs by good glycemic control: impaired effectiveness following poor control (mean $\pm$ SEM)

	Group				
	Poor control $(n = 8)$	Good control $(n = 7)$	Poor improving to good $(n = 6)$		Non-diabetic subjects $(n = 14)$
Duration	5	5	$2\frac{1}{2}$*	5†	5
Plasma glucose (mmol/l)					
8:00 a.m.	21 ± 0.7	5.9 ± 0.5	19 ± 0.7	5.7 ± 0.7	4.4 ± 0.1
8:00 p.m.	21 ± 0.9	3.9 ± 0.3	21 ± 2.3	3.4 ± 0.3	4.3 ± 0.2
Glycosuria (g/day)	104 ± 8	< 2	107 ± 7	< 2	0
Sugar-free days (%)	0	65	0	64	100
Hemoglobin A$_1$(%)	11.1 ± 0.4	6.6 ± 0.3	11.2 ± 0.9	6.7 ± 0.3	6.5 ± 0.2
Retinopathy					
Microaneurysms per eye	42 ± 10	2 ± 1.3	0 ± 0.3	29 ± 16	1 ± 0.2
Capillary atrophy‡	264 ± 25	80 ± 20	48 ± 8	224 ± 29	39 ± 6
Pericyte loss	$+++$	0 to $+$	0 to $+$	$++$	0
Hemorrhage	$++$	0	0	$+$	0
Basement membrane thickness (nm)	319 ± 34	186 ± 14	164 ± 12	227 ± 14	168 ± 8

SEM, standard error of the mean.
* Left eye obtained surgically (after $2\frac{1}{2}$ years of poor control).
† Right eye obtained at autopsy (after 5 years: $2\frac{1}{2}$ years of poor control followed by $2\frac{1}{2}$ years of good control).
‡ Acellular capillaries/11 mm^2 of trypsin-digested vasculature.
Data from Engerman and Kern [99].

control, retinopathy was almost as severe as it was in dogs under poor control for the entire 5-year period, even though retinopathy was not yet present when the switch from poor to good control was made (Table 4) [99]. To the extent that these results may apply to human diabetes they suggest that good control may be effective only if instituted early in the course of diabetes, as suggested earlier by Constam [100] and Caird [101], or that if improving control after several years of poor control is of benefit, there may be a considerable delay before beneficial effects become apparent. On the other hand, Klein and co-workers recently reported a strong association between glycated hemoglobin levels at entry into their population-based study and progression of retinopathy 4 years later, a relationship that appeared quite uniform across all severity levels of NPDR and durations of diabetes. In each of their three groups classified by age at diagnosis and insulin use there was a steady increase in the percentage of patients with retinopathy progression across ten deciles of glycated hemoglobin values (Figure 22) [102]. This study suggests that improved control may be beneficial even in patients with established retinopathy, and that there may be no threshold level of control that must be reached before such an effect is observed.

The Diabetes Control and Complications Trial (DCCT), in which patients with type 1 diabetes are randomly assigned to either intensive or conventional insulin treatment, has now been under way for several years [103]. It includes both primary prevention and secondary intervention components: the former enrolls patients with diabetes duration of 1–5 years and no retinopathy; the latter, patients with 1–15 years of diabetes and mild to moderate NPDR.

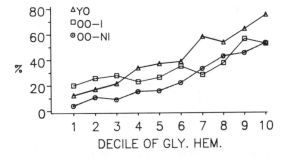

PROGRESSION OF RETINOPATHY

Figure 22 Percentage of patients with NPDR at baseline showing progression of retinopathy by two or more levels (Table 1) 4 years later, by decile of glycated hemoglobin at baseline. YO, younger-onset patients; OO-I, older-onset patients treated with insulin; OO-NI, older-onset patients not treated with insulin (courtesy of R. Klein and co-workers)

This study has reached its enrollment goal of 1400 patients, some of whom have now been followed for more than 5 years, and should provide reliable information on the possible value of improved control from intensive insulin treatment.

OTHER RISK FACTORS

Other factors have been reported to be associated with prevalence, severity or progression of retinopathy, but the evidence is much less clear than that concerning type and duration of diabetes and level of hyperglycemia, and in some reports lack of adjustment for these latter factors makes interpretation difficult Moreover, comparisons between studies are hazardous because of different methods used to detect retinopathy and classify its severity and to assess other variables. Several studies of individuals with insulin dependent diabetes have found PDR to be more prevalent in men [67, 71, 104]. This observation, and the finding that risk of retinopathy increases after the age of puberty [105–107], suggest a possible pathogenetic role for hormonal factors [108]. There is also some evidence that pregnancy accelerates progression of retinopathy, but the mechanism is uncertain [97, 109, 110]. HLA studies seeking evidence of genetic factors have given conflicting results [72, 111]. A positive association between retinopathy and blood pressure has been reported in several studies, particularly in subjects with type 1 diabetes, but whether this relationship is causal or reflects parallel effects of underlying vascular disease is not clear [67, 68, 112–113].

Retinopathy is also positively associated with nephropathy, in part because these complications share close associations with diabetes duration and type and level of hyperglycemia [67, 68, 114, 115].

TREATMENT OF DIABETIC RETINOPATHY

This section is concerned mainly with the principal modalities currently in use, photocoagulation and vitreous surgery, which have been shown to be highly effective and have replaced earlier treatments of uncertain value (such as vitamins, lipid-lowering agents and various agents postulated to have favorable effects on capillary walls [116–118]) or having serious side-

effects (pituitary ablation). Recent clinical trials of aspirin, which has been advocated for its antiplatelet effects, are mentioned briefly at the end of this section. Brief comments on pituitary ablation are included for historical interest.

Pituitary Ablation

Building on the fundamental discovery of Houssay [119] that hypophysectomy reduced the severity of diabetes in pancreatectomized dogs, Luft and co-workers carried out hypophysectomy in the hope of ameliorating the vascular complications of diabetes [120]. Further impetus was provided by Poulsen's report of remission of diabetic retinopathy in a woman with postpartum anterior pituitary insufficiency (Sheehan's syndrome) [121, 122]. Over the next 25 years various types of pituitary suppression were used, ranging from external irradiation to transfrontal hypophysectomy, and consensus developed among advocates of these procedures that complete or nearly complete suppression of anterior pituitary function (pituitary ablation) produced rapid improvement in eyes that had both the intraretinal lesions characteristic of severe NPDR and actively growing new vessels not yet accompanied by extensive fibrous proliferations. Although only two randomized trials have been reported [123, 124], both small and neither in itself compelling, the weight of evidence supports the strongly held opinion of those most experienced with this procedure that it is of benefit. Particularly persuasive are comparisons between patients in whom transsphenoidal implantation of radioactive yttrium was followed by complete, or nearly complete, anterior pituitary suppression, and similar patients in whom little or no suppression was achieved; substantially better outcome was observed in the former group [125]. Additional support is provided by a non-randomized comparison of eyes with extensive new vessels and IRMA in which outcome was better in the eyes of patients undergoing pituitary ablation than in similar eyes receiving photocoagulation or no treatment [126]. Pituitary ablation is now of only theoretical and historical interest, because photocoagulation is probably at least equally effective and is free of the many substantial disadvantages of achieving and living with the hypopituitary state. However, the influence of pituitary suppression on retinopathy is a finding that may eventually prove to be a key factor in the development of our understanding of the pathogenesis of diabetic retinopathy.

Photocoagulation

Photocoagulation can favorably influence the course of diabetic retinopathy in two ways: firstly, by inducing regression of new vessels (or preventing their development), and secondly by reducing macular edema. After its introduction in 1960 by Meyer-Schwickerath [127], xenon-arc (white light) photocoagulation was initially used to destroy directly patches of new vessels on the surface of the retina. Large (1000–1500 μm), slow (0.2–1.0 seconds), moderately intense exposures were required, because most of the light is absorbed in the retinal pigment epithelium and the resulting burn must spread forward through the full thickness of the transparent sensory retina to reach the new vessels on its inner surface. New vessels on the optic disc or in the vitreous cannot be treated directly with this technique because they are too far from the retinal pigment epithelium, because blood within them is flowing too rapidly to be coagulated directly, and because the minimum burn size that is technically feasible is too large to treat the new vessels while sparing adjacent structures. A major stimulus for the development of the argon laser was the hope that its smaller (50–500 μm), more intense, blue-green beam could deliver enough energy rapidly enough to stop blood flow, so that the vessels could then be destroyed by heat generated from the absorption of light by the blood trapped within them. This hope proved false, because new vessels apparently destroyed in this way had a strong tendency to recur within several weeks. By this time, however (late 1960s), it was becoming apparent that extensive photocoagulation seemed to have a beneficial *indirect* effect, as it was sometimes followed by regression of new vessels and diminution of retinal edema and vascular congestion in areas of the retina not directly treated [128]. Such indirect treatment, in which hundreds of burns are scattered throughout the fundus in a pattern that leaves about one-half to one burn width between burns (*scatter* or *panretinal* photocoagulation) is now the principal way in which photocoagulation is used when the aim is to induce regression or prevent growth of new vessels (Figure 23) [129]. This scatter treatment can be carried out with either the xenon arc photocoagulator or any of several lasers.

Shortly after its introduction, xenon arc photocoagulation was also used to treat macular edema [127, 130, 131]. The anatomic arrangement most amenable to treatment with its large burns (minimum useful size about 500 μm) is a clump of large, leaking microaneurysms at least 1 mm from the center of the macula with a surrounding zone of retinal thickening that extends, or threatens to extend, into the center of the macula (see Figure 5). Such a favorable anatomic arrangement is seen in a minority of eyes with diabetic macular edema. Most such eyes have microaneurysms closer to the center of the macula and, in many, microaneurysms are scattered diffusely throughout the posterior pole. In such eyes, individual microaneurysms can be treated with the much smaller (50 μm) burns and more convenient delivery system (a slit-lamp biomicroscope) of the argon laser, and in the USA this instrument has almost entirely replaced the xenon arc apparatus for treatment of macular edema (Figure 24) [28, 132–136]. The small burn size of the laser also makes it possible to apply grid treatment when macular edema appears to be caused by a diffusely leaking capillary bed rather than by individual microaneurysms. Grid treatment consists of scattering many 50-μm or 100-μm burns throughout zones of thickened retina, leaving about one burn width between burns and sparing the area within 500 μm of the center of the macula (Figure 25).

Mechanisms of Action of Photocoagulation

Clinical trials (discussed below) have documented the efficacy of scatter photocoagulation in PDR, but its mechanism is not clear. One theory proposes that areas of the inner retina that have become partially ischemic from capillary loss produce a factor that stimulates new vessels, which is capable of diffusing through the vitreous to other areas of the retina and into the anterior chamber, where formation of new vessels and fibrous tissue in the anterior chamber angle can lead to angle closure and in intractable form of glaucoma (*neovascular glaucoma*) [8–12]. It is suggested that scatter photocoagulation may reduce production of the factor by destroying some of the ischemic retina [10, 137]. A second theory suggests that photocoagulation

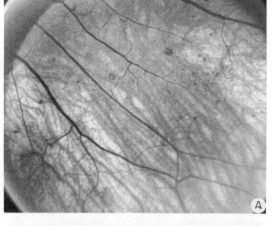

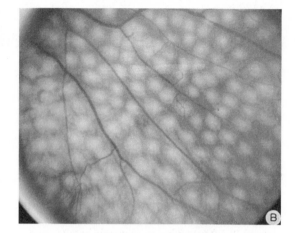

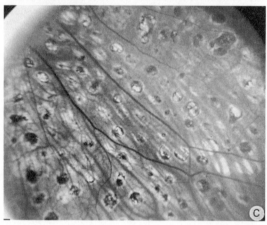

Figure 23 (A) Lower nasal quadrant of the left eye of a patient with NVE in several quadrants, showing patch of NVE in lower left corner. (B) The same eye shortly after application of ETDRS full scatter photocoagulation. New vessels regressed promptly. (C) At the 5-year visit there had been no recurrence of NVE (courtesy of the ETDRS Research Group)

improves oxygenation of the ischemic inner retinal layers by destroying some of the metabolically highly active photoreceptor cells and allowing the oxygen normally diffusing from the choriocapillaris to supply these cells to continue on into the inner layers of the retina [138–140]. The latter theory is appealing because it is principally the photoreceptor cells that are destroyed by mild argon laser burns, but fails to explain why stronger burns sometimes seem more effective clinically. This theory is supported by reports that retinal blood flow decreases, and autoregulatory response to breathing 100% oxygen improves, following scatter photocoagulation, as might be expected if more oxygen were reaching the inner retina from the choroid [141]. An additional possibility is that the cells of the retinal pigment epithelium may produce a factor that *inhibits* new vessels, and that the response of

these cells to photocoagulation injury may favor production of this factor [142].

It has also been demonstrated in controlled trials that photocoagulation reduces macular edema [28, 131–136]. One mechanism seems obvious: obliteration of leaky microaneurysms by focal treatment. It is not as clear how grid treatment reduces edema. Improved oxygenation of the inner retina by the same mechanism described above, in conjunction with scatter photocoagulation, is one possibility; modification of fluid transit across the retinal pigment epithelium, or facilitation of endothelial cell renewal by growth factors reaching the capillaries via the altered retinal pigment epithelial cells, are others [143–145].

Photocoagulation for PDR

The efficacy of photocoagulation for PDR has

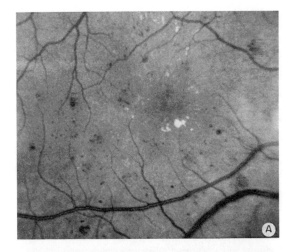

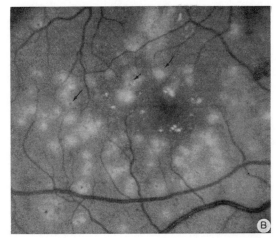

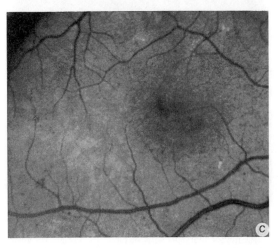

Figure 24 (A) Microaneurysms are scattered throughout the posterior pole of this right eye. There is a faint, hard exudate ring surrounding the center of the macula and perhaps another fainter one above the first. The retina was mildly thickened throughout the area within 1.5 disc diameters of the center of the macula, including the center itself. Visual acuity was 20/25. (B) The same eye shortly after focal photocoagulation. Arrows indicate some of the treated microaneurysms that have had their color changed by treatment (turned brown or white). (C) One year later the retina was no longer thickened and most of the microaneurysms and hard exudates had disappeared. Photocoagulation scars were faint. Visual acuity remained 20/25 (courtesy of the ETDRS Research Group)

been demonstrated in three randomized clinical trials, each of which found that treatment reduced the rate of blindness to less than 50% of the rate observed in untreated eyes [49, 50, 65, 146, 147].

The largest of these trials was the DRS, conducted from 1971 to 1979 by the National Eye Institute of the United States Public Health Service. The DRS enrolled patients with unequivocal new vessels in at least one eye or severe NPDR in both eyes, and visual acuity of 20/100 or better in each eye. Patients were randomly assigned to either the argon laser or xenon arc treatment group; one eye of each patient was randomly assigned to photocoagulation treatment and the other to indefinite deferral of treatment (i.e. no treatment ever, unless the protocol

were to be modified because of evidence that treatment was beneficial). Patients were followed at 4-month intervals according to a protocol that provided for measurement of best corrected visual acuity, with different charts for each eye, by specially trained and certified examiners who did not know the identity of the treated eye or type of treatment, and who attempted to reduce patient bias by urging the patient to read as far down the chart as possible with each eye, guessing at letters until more than one in a line was missed. All patients gave written informed consent and understood that the information being collected would be analyzed at frequent intervals and used, if possible, for their benefit.

Both photocoagulation techniques included scatter treatment extending from the posterior

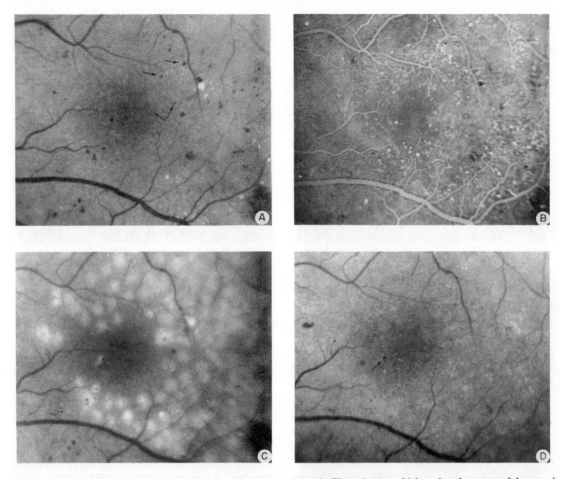

Figure 25 (A) Microaneurysms and hard exudates in the posterior pole. The retina was thickened at the center of the macula and temporally for about 2 disc diameters. Arrows indicate fairly large microaneurysms with visible walls. Visual acuity was 20/40. (B) Early-phase fluorescein angiogram showing many dilated capillaries and early diffuse leakage. (C) Because most of the leakage came from dilated capillaries, photocoagulation was applied mainly in a grid pattern (but three of the four microaneurysms indicated by arrows in the upper left part of the figure were treated focally, all but the one closest to the center of the macula). (D) Four months later most of the microaneurysms and hard exudates had disappeared. The retina was no longer thickened. Photocoagulation scars were inconspicuous. Arrow indicates moderately large microaneurysm that was incompletely treated focally and remains patent. Visual acuity had improved to 20/25 (courtesy of the ETDRS Research Group)

pole to the equator and often completed in a single sitting. The argon technique specified 800–1600 500-μm scatter burns of 0.1 seconds duration and direct treatment of new vessels on the disc and elsewhere, whether flat or elevated. Direct treatment was also applied to microaneurysms or other lesions thought to be causing macular edema. Follow-up treatment was applied as needed at 4-month intervals. The xenon technique was similar, but burns were fewer, of longer duration and stronger, and direct treatment was not applied to elevated new vessels or to those on the surface of the disc.

The DRS chose as its principal outcome variable visual acuity of less than 5/200 at each of two consecutively completed follow-up visits, using for this the term *severe visual loss*. Visual acuity of less than 5/200 was chosen as the level at which vision becomes too poor to be useful for walking about and other self-care activities; the 'two consecutive visits' requirement was included because the rate of recovery to better

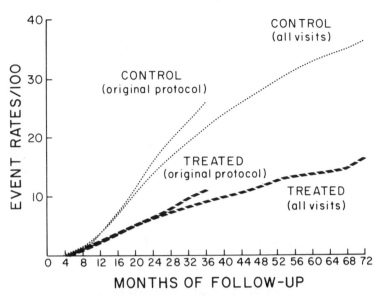

Figure 26 Cumulative rates of severe visual loss, including and excluding observations made after the 1976 protocol change, argon and xenon groups combined (from reference 61)

visual acuity after a single visit at the less than 5/200 level was 29% in the control group and 49% in the treated group, whereas after two visits it was 12% and 29%, respectively (and after three visits 8% and 21%) [146]. Because recovery was more frequent in treated eyes, the end-point chosen tends to underestimate treatment benefit.

Figures 26, 27 and 28 depict cumulative rates of severe visual loss for eyes assigned to treatment and control groups [65]. In Figure 26 the argon and xenon groups are combined, and separate analyses are shown including and excluding visits made after the protocol was changed in 1976 (on the basis of analyses similar to those to be discussed shortly) to encourage treatment of control group eyes that were then at high risk of severe visual loss. All eyes were classified in the group to which they were originally randomly assigned, ignoring treatment of control group eyes. In the analysis including visits after the protocol change, 43% of the 2-year visits and all of the 4-year visits were carried out after this change occurred; by the 2-year visit, 12% of control group eyes had been treated, and by the 4-year visit 35% had been treated. The two curves for control group eyes are very similar over the first 20 months of follow-up and those for treated eyes are similar

over at least the first 28 months. The difference between the two control group curves is probably due, at least in part, to the beneficial effect of treatment experienced by some of these eyes after the protocol change, and the long-term analysis probably slightly underestimates treatment effect. In each of these analyses, treatment reduced the risk of severe visual loss by 50% or more, at and after the 16-month visit.

In Figure 27, the Figure 26 analysis including all visits is presented separately for the argon and xenon groups. The treatment effect, i.e. the difference between treatment and control groups, appears to be slightly greater in the xenon group, but this difference is small, its statistical significance borderline, and its clinical importance outweighed by the greater harmful effects of the xenon treatment used in the DRS (Table 5).

In Figure 28, the Figure 26 analysis including all visits is presented for three subgroups defined by retinopathy severity in baseline stereoscopic fundus photographs. These three groups correspond approximately to levels 51, 65 and 70 in Table 2. In each group, treatment reduced the risk of severe visual loss to about one-half that observed in control group eyes, but this effect became apparent later and the percentage of eyes treated that benefited (the arithmetic

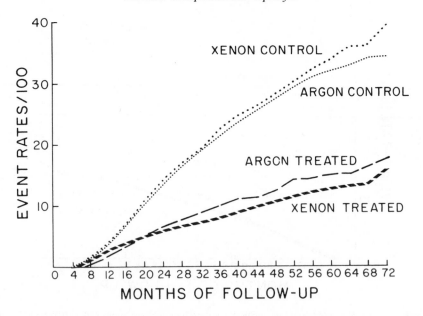

Figure 27 Cumulative rates of severe visual loss for argon and xenon groups separately (from reference 61)

treatment difference) became smaller as retinopathy severity decreased. On the basis of this analysis and the harmful effects of treatment summarized in Table 5, the DRS confirmed its earlier conclusion that, for eyes with high-risk characteristics, the chance of benefit from treatment (for example, reduction of the 2-year risk of severe visual loss from about 26% to 11%) clearly outweighed its risks of harm, and recommended prompt photocoagulation for most such eyes.

When the DRS first reported strong evidence of a beneficial treatment effect and modified its protocol to encourage treatment of those control group eyes that were then at the high-risk stage, it also modified its treatment protocol. Because the harmful effects of argon treatment

were less, it was given preference and, in the hope of further reducing these effects, treatment was more often divided between two or more episodes several days apart [65]. However, because the beneficial effect observed with the xenon protocol (in which focal treatment of NVD and elevated NVE was not used) had been the same or greater than that with the argon protocol, these technically difficult parts of the argon protocol were dropped. This modified technique was very much like the argon laser panretinal photocoagulation advocated by Little and co-workers [137], and similar to the extensive milder xenon treatment advocated by Meyer-Schwickerath and co-workers [148] and Okun and co-workers [149]. A very similar technique was specified for the ETDRS: 1200–1600 500-μm argon laser burns lasting 0.1 second and placed about one-half burn diameter apart, extending from the posterior pole to or beyond the equator, and applied in two or more episodes (see Figure 23). In the ETDRS this scatter treatment is combined with moderate direct treatment of new vessels on the surface of the retina [129], but many experienced observers use scatter treatment alone. New vessels usually regress substantially within a few weeks following photocoagulation. When they do not, or when they recur after initial regression, there is generally ample room between the

Table 5 Estimated percentages of eyes with harmful effects attributable to diabetic retinopathy study treatment

	Argon (%)	Xenon (%)
Constriction of visual field (Goldmann IVe4 test object) to an average of		
⩽ 45°, > 30° per meridian	5	25
⩽ 30° per meridian	0	25
Decrease in visual acuity		
1 line	11	19
⩾ 2 lines	3	11

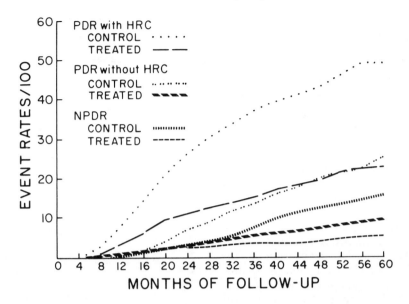

Figure 28 Cumulative rates of severe visual loss for eyes classified by presence of proliferative retinopathy (PDR) and high-risk characteristics (HRC) in baseline fundus photographs, argon and xenon groups combined. NPDR, non-proliferative diabetic retinopathy (from reference 61)

scars of the initial treatment to add more, and this is usually effective [148, 150–154]. Eyes with small patches of residual new vessels often do well without additional treatment, remaining free of serious vitreous hemorrhage for many years.

For eyes with severe NPDR or PDR without high-risk characteristics, the DRS concluded that either of two approaches was satisfactory, and that DRS results were not helpful in choosing between them: (a) prompt treatment, or (b) careful follow-up with prompt treatment if high-risk characteristics develop. In the ETDRS these alternatives were compared in eyes with severe NPDR or PDR without high-risk characteristics and in eyes with mild to moderate NPDR as well. Rates of severe visual loss were low in both the early treatment and deferral groups (at 5 years, 2.6% and 3.7% respectively). Some harmful effects of scatter treatment were observed: an early decrease in visual acuity (a doubling or more of the visual angle at the 4-month visit in about 10% of treated eyes, compared to about 5% in the deferral group) and some decrease in visual field. It was recommended that scatter treatment should not be used in eyes with mild to moderate NPDR, but that it be considered in eyes approaching the high-risk stage, i.e. eyes with very severe NPDR or PDR without high-

risk characteristics, and that it usually should not be delayed when the high-risk stage is present [155].

In its early stages, before the anterior chamber angle is completely closed, neovascular glaucoma can be arrested by scatter photocoagulation, or by peripheral retinal cryocoagulation, if the media are too cloudy for photocoagulation, and this is an urgent indication for such treatment, regardless of the severity of retinopathy [156, 157].

Photocoagulation for Diabetic Macular Edema

In the ETDRS, eyes with mild to moderate NPDR and macular edema were randomly assigned either to a combination of focal and grid photocoagulation for macular edema (scatter treatment was withheld unless severe NPDR or PDR developed) or to no photocoagulation unless PDR with high-risk characteristics developed. The principal outcome variable was a decrease of three lines on a specially designed eye chart, on which a three-line decrease in any part of the chart amounts to a doubling of the visual angle, for example, a change from 20/20 to 20/40, or from 20/50 to 20/100. After 3 years of follow-up, 24% of 526 control group eyes had experienced such a loss, compared with 12% of 268 treated eyes. Among eyes entering the study with visual acuity of worse than 20/40, about 40% of treated eyes showed visual improvement of one line or more, compared with 20% of control group eyes, but few eyes in either group improved by as much as three lines [28]. No adverse effects of focal and grid photocoagulation on visual acuity, visual field or color vision were detected.

Clinically significant macular edema was defined as retinal thickening, or hard exudates adjacent to thickened retina, within 500 μm of the center of the macula, or a zone of retinal thickening at least as large as the optic disc, any part of which was within one disc diameter of the center of the macula. At the baseline examination about 74% of eyes with clinically significant macular edema had involvement of the center of the macula (in both treated and control groups). At the 3-year follow-up visit this percentage had decreased to 24% for treated eyes and to 54% for control group eyes [28].

Figure 29 shows the percentages of treated and control group eyes with a visual acuity decrease of three or more lines at each follow-up visit for three subgroups defined by macular edema severity in baseline stereoscopic fundus photographs [134]. In the mildest subgroup, eyes with less than clinically significant macular edema (upper panel), there was little difference between treated and control groups, but in the other two subgroups treatment reduced visual loss by more than 50% at most visits. The risk of visual loss in untreated eyes was greater when the center of the macula was involved (lowest panel). Prompt photocoagulation is usually indicated for such eyes. When the center is not involved, visual acuity is usually good and either prompt treatment or deferral of treatment with careful follow-up may be appropriate. If major leakage sites are close to the center, increasing the risk that it may be damaged directly during treatment or indirectly by the spread of retinal pigment epithelial degeneration into it from nearby scars some years later, deferral may be preferable. If a large plaque of hard exudate threatens the center by its close proximity, prompt treatment may be the wiser course, particularly if the principal leakage sites are more than 500 μm from the center. Such decisions may be difficult, and it is helpful if the ophthalmologist who will be responsible for treatment (when

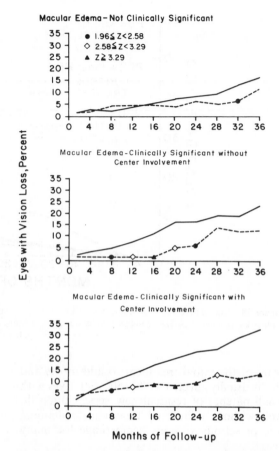

Figure 29 Comparison of percentages of eyes that experienced visual loss of three or more lines (equivalent to at least doubling of the initial visual angle) in eyes classified by severity of macular edema in baseline fundus photographs and assigned either to immediate photocoagulation for macular edema (broken line) or to deferral of photocoagulation unless high-risk characteristics develop (solid line) (from reference 126)

and if it is carried out) has been able to follow the patient for some time before a decision is necessary.

Vitrectomy

The principal indication for pars plana vitrectomy, when initially developed by Machemer in 1970, was longstanding vitreous hemorrhage due to diabetic retinopathy [158]. The importance of this technical breakthrough can hardly be overestimated, certainly not by the thousands of patients to whom it was first made available —those who had waited for many months hoping for spontaneous clearing of vitreous hemorrhage so extensive that vision had been reduced to light perception or hand movements. In the two decades that have elapsed since its introduction, pars plana (closed) vitrectomy has undergone many improvements [159]. These include better instrumentation (e.g. smaller instruments, more versatile scissors for cutting membranes, and adaptation of the argon laser to allow photocoagulation during surgery) and improved techniques (e.g. multiple incisions to allow use of two instruments simultaneously, use of intraocular air or other gas to push the detached retina back into place, and improvement of irrigating solutions so that they do not cause clouding of the lens necessitating its removal during vitrectomy). The risks of serious complications (chiefly retinal detachment secondary to retinal breaks occurring during surgery and postoperative neovascular glaucoma) have been reduced from 20% or more to about 10% [160, 161].

Indications have also expanded. Extensive vitreous hemorrhage that fails to clear spontaneously after 6 months or more, and retinal detachment involving the center of the macula, remain the two principal indications, but today vitrectomy is often advised soon after the occurrence of severe hemorrhage, particularly when new vessels and fibrous proliferations behind the hemorrhage are known from a previous examination to be extensive or are considered likely to be so on the basis of type (and possibly duration) of diabetes. The Diabetic Retinopathy Vitrectomy Study (DRVS), a randomized clinical trial, found that for patients with type 1 diabetes (under 20 years old at diagnosis and taking insulin) the chance of recovering good vision (20/40 or better at the 2-year follow-up visit) in eyes with recent severe vitreous hemorrhage was greater (36% of 101 eyes versus 12% of 103) when vitrectomy was carried out early (1–6 months after the onset of the hemorrhage) than when it was deferred, unless retinal detachment involving the center of the macula occurred or the hemorrhage failed to clear spontaneously during a 1-year period of observation [162]. This effect was thought to be related to the more extensive new vessels, fibrous proliferations, and vitreoretinal adhesions characterizing PDR in type 1 diabetes, and the substantial risk that distortion, dragging or detachment of the macula would occur while waiting for the hemorrhage to clear. In the subgroup of type 1 patients whose severe vitreous hemorrhage

occurred when diabetes had been present for less than 20 years, deferral of vitrectomy appeared to be particularly disadvantageous, and this subgroup tended to have the most severe PDR (34% of 50 eyes in the early group recovered good vision, versus 2% of 53 in the deferral group). In patients over 20 years old at diagnosis, early vitrectomy did not improve the outlook for good vision (about 17% in both early and deferral groups), probably in part because fibrovascular proliferations were less severe and in part because the potential of the macula for near-normal function was less in these older patients.

Other current indications for prompt vitrectomy are traction on the disc, peripapillary retina, or macula that distorts these structures and leads to substantial reduction in visual acuity, opaque fibrous proliferations in front of the macula, and extensive preretinal hemorrhage [161, 163, 164].

The DRVS has also provided information supporting the use of early vitrectomy in eyes with very severe PDR and good vision, eyes in which contraction of extensive fibrovascular proliferations threatens (but has not yet caused) loss of vision from retinal detachment. When such eyes had severe NVD and/or NVE (Figure 30), the chance of visual acuity of 20/40 or better at the 4-year follow-up visit was greater when vitrectomy was carried out promptly than when it was deferred, unless retinal detachment involving the center of the macula developed or severe vitreous hemorrhage occurred and failed to clear during a 6-month period (40.6% of 64 eyes versus 17.6% of 68) [165, 166].

Aspirin

Three multicenter, randomized clinical trials of antiplatelet agents in the treatment in diabetic retinopathy have recently been reported. In the Dipyridamole Aspirin Microangiopathy of Diabetes (DAMAD) study, 475 patients with at least five microaneurysms visible on fluorescein angiography within 10 degrees of the center of the macula in at least one eye, but without macular edema, proliferative lesions or previous photocoagulation, were randomly assigned to one of three treatment groups: aspirin 990 mg per day, aspirin 990 mg plus dipyridamole 225 mg per day, or placebo [167]. Patients were recruited during a 5-year period (1976–81) and followed for 3 years. There was little difference

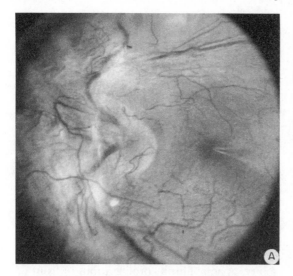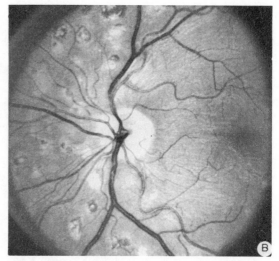

Figure 30   (A) Fibrous proliferations have contracted, pulling the retina in the posterior pole towards the disc. The center of the macula is about 1 disc diameter from the temporal disc margin. Scatter photocoagulation has been carried out previously. Visual acuity was 20/60. This eye was randomly assigned to early vitrectomy in the DRVS. (B) At vitrectomy it was possible to remove almost all of the fibrovascular proliferations, restoring the retina to normal or near-normal position, as shown in this 1-year follow-up photograph. Visual acuity was 20/40. Photocoagulation scars are quite far apart; if there had been an opportunity to apply additional scatter photocoagulation before fibrous proliferations developed, they might have been prevented (courtesy of DRVS Research Group)

between the three treatment groups in regard to change in retinopathy severity as judged by visual acuity measurements or ophthalmoscopy, but a difference was observed in counts of micro-aneurysms in the angiograms. The mean yearly increase in number of definite (greater than $33\,\mu m$) microaneurysms was 1.44 (SD 4.49) in the placebo group, 0.69 (SD 5.09) in the aspirin group, and 0.34 (SD 3.01) in the aspirin plus dipyridamole group. Comparison of these rates, which were based on slopes of microaneurysm counts weighted for angiographic quality, yielded a P value of 0.02 (one-tailed) for the comparison of placebo versus the two aspirin groups combined ($P = 0.06$ without weighting). Counts of total microaneurysms (all lesions larger than $25\,\mu m$) showed twofold to fivefold larger annual rates of increase with similar, but statistically non-significant, differences between groups. These small differences were of borderline statistical significance and uncertain clinical importance, and it is unfortunate that the patients were not followed longer.

Similar results were reported in a very similar study of ticlopidine, an antiplatelet agent, in which 435 patients were enrolled and followed for 3 years [168]. The mean yearly increase in

definite microaneurysms counted by the same technique was 1.44 (SD 4.67) in the placebo group and 0.48 (SD 5.79) in the ticlopidine group ($P = 0.03$, one-tailed; $P = 0.06$ without weighting for angiographic quality). There was a similar, statistically non-significant difference for mean yearly increase in counts of total micro-aneurysms, 2.60 (SD 14.02) and 0.81 (SD 10.36) respectively, in the two groups. In this study, trends of borderline statistical significance favoring ticlopidine were also observed in over-all retinopathy severity (worsening in 19.5% of placebo versus 13.4% of ticlopidine patients) and in development of proliferative retinopathy (4% versus 1.4%, respectively). There was a suggestion that treatment benefit was limited to insulin-treated patients. In this study also, it is very unfortunate that patients were not followed longer. They were recruited over a 6-year period (1979–85), so that if followed to a common termination date many patients would have had 5 or more years of follow-up.

In the ETDRS, 3711 patients with mild to severe NPDR or early PDR were randomly assigned to aspirin 650 mg daily or placebo and followed for 4–8 years [169]. No difference was observed in rate of development of high-risk

PDR in eyes assigned to deferral of photocoagulation between the placebo and aspirin groups (life-table rates at 5 years, 41.0% and 40.5% respectively). The power of the study, with losses to follow-up and compliance taken into consideration, was estimated to be about 90% for detection of a reduction of a 40% rate to 30% or less (with $\alpha = 0.01$, two-sided). Patients with the least severe retinopathy included in the trial, who had mild to moderate hemorrhages and/or microaneurysms and hard or soft exudates, but no more severe lesions, were analyzed for retinopathy progression, as assessed in stereoscopic color fundus photographs taken at yearly intervals, and again no significant difference was found. The 5-year life-table rates of progression of two or more steps on a scale similar to that shown in Table 2 (but with one additional step in the moderate NPDR range) were 71.5% in the placebo group and 66.3% in the aspirin group. There was also no evidence that aspirin increased the risk of vitreous hemorrhage in eyes with PDR. It was concluded that aspirin could be used for cardiovascular indications in diabetic patients with retinopathy without increasing the risk of vitreous hemorrhage, but that it was unlikely to have a clinically important effect in slowing retinopathy progression, at least for patients at or beyond the stage of moderate NPDR.

Acknowledgment

This work is supported in part by an unrestricted grant from Research to Prevent Blindness, Inc. to the University of Wisconsin.

REFERENCES

1. Larsen HW. Diabetic retinopathy. An ophthalmoscopic study with a discussion of the morphologic changes and the pathogenetic factors in this disease. Acta Ophthalmol (Copenh) 1960; 60: 1–89.
2. Beetham WP. Visual prognosis of proliferating diabetic retinopathy. Br J Ophthalmol 1963; 47: 611–19.
3. Dobree JH. Proliferative diabetic retinopathy: evolution of the retinal lesions. Br J Ophthalmol 1964; 48: 637–49.
4. Davis MD. Vitreous contraction in proliferative diabetic retinopathy. Arch Ophthalmol 1965; 74: 741–51.
5. Tolentino FI, Lee PF, Schepens CL. Biomicroscopic study of vitreous cavity in diabetic retinopathy. Arch Ophthalmol 1966; 75: 238–46.
6. Davis MD. The natural course of diabetic retinopathy. In Kimura SJ, Caygil WM (eds) Vascular complications of diabetes mellitus. St Louis: CV Mosby, 1967: pp 139–69.
7. Davis MD, Myers FL, Engerman RL et al. Clinical observations concerning the pathogenesis of diabetic retinopathy. In Goldberg MF, Fines SL (eds) Symposium on the treatment of diabetic retinopathy. Public Health Service publ. no. 1890. Washington, DC: US Govt Printing Office, 1969: pp 569–92.
8. Michaelson IC. The mode of development of the vascular system of the retina, with some observations on its significance for certain retinal diseases. Trans Ophthalmol Soc UK 1948; 68: 137–80.
9. Wise GN. Retinal neovascularization. Trans Am Ophthalmol Soc 1956; 54: 729–826.
10. Patz A. Clinical and experimental studies on retinal neovascularization. Am J Ophthalmol 1982; 94: 715–43.
11. Shimizu K, Kobayashi Y, Murako K. Mid-peripheral fundus involvement in diabetic retinopathies. Ophthalmology 1981; 88: 601–12.
12. Glaser BM, D'Amore PA, Michels RG, Patz A, Fenselau A. Demonstration of vasoproliferative activity from mammalian retina. J Cell Biol 1980; 84: 298–304.
13. Schreiber AB, Kenney J, Kowalski J et al. A unique family of endothelial cell polypeptide mitogens: the antigenic and receptor cross-reactivity of bovine endothelial cell growth factor, brain-derived acidic fibroblast growth factor, and eye-derived growth factor II. J Cell Biol 1985; 101: 1623–6.
14. Kuwabara T, Cogan DG. Retinal vascular patterns. I. Normal architecture. Arch Ophthalmol 1960; 64: 904–11.
15. Cogan DG, Toussaint D, Kuwabara T. Retinal vascular patterns. IV. Diabetic retinopathy. Arch Ophthalmol 1961; 66: 366.
16. Kuwabara T, Cogan DG. Retinal vascular patterns. VI. Mural cells of the retinal capillaries. Arch Ophthalmol 1963; 69: 492–502.
17. Speiser P, Gittelsohn AM, Patz A. Studies on diabetic retinopathy. III. Influence of diabetes on intramural pericytes. Arch Ophthalmol 1968; 80: 332–7.
18. Addison DJ, Garner A, Ashton N. Degeneration of intramural pericytes in diabetic retinopathy. Br Med J 1970; 1: 264–6.
19. Engerman RL. Pathogenesis of diabetic retinopathy. Diabetes 1989; 38: 1203–6.
20. Ashton N. Pathogenesis of diabetic retinopathy. In Little HL, Jack RL, Patz A, Forsham PH (eds) Diabetic retinopathy. New York: Thieme-Stratton, 1983: pp 85–106.
21. DCCT Research Group. Color photography

versus fluorescein angiography in the detection of diabetic retinopathy in the Diabetes Control and Complication Trial. Arch Ophthalmol 1987; 105: 1344–51.

22. Bloodworth JMB. Fine structure of retina in human and canine diabetes mellitus. In Kimuara SJ, Caygill WM (eds) Vascular complications of diabetes mellitus. St Louis: CV Mosby, 1967: pp 73–86

23. Frank RN. Etiologic mechanisms in diabetic retinopathy. In Ryan SJ (ed.) Retina. Vol. 2: Schachat AP, Murphy RP, Patz A (eds) Medical retina. CV Mosby: St Louis, 1989: pp 301–326.

24. Frank RN. On the pathogenesis of diabetic retinopathy—a 1990 update. Ophthalmology (in press).

25. Jonas JB, Gusek GC, Guggenmoos-Holzmann I, Naumann GOH. Variability of the real dimensions of normal human optic discs. Graefes Arch Clin Exp Ophthalmol 1988; 226: 332–6.

26. Mansour AM, Walsh JB, Henkind P. Optic disc size in central vein occlusion. Ophthalmology 1990; 97: 165–6.

27. de Venecia G, Davis M, Engerman R. Clinicopathologic correlations in diabetic retinopathy. I. Histology and fluorescein angiography of microaneurysms. Arch Ophthalmol 1976; 94: 1766–73.

28. Early Treatment Diabetic Retinopathy Study Research Group. Photocoagulation for diabetic macular edema. Early Treatment Diabetic Retinopathy Study Report 1. Arch Ophthalmol 1985; 103: 1796–806.

29. Davis MD, Norton EWD, Myers FL. Airlie classification of diabetic retinopathy. In Goldberg M, Fine SL (eds) Symposium on the treatment of diabetic retinopathy. Washington, DC: US Govt Printing Office, 1969: pp 7–22.

30. Early Treatment Diabetic Retinopathy Study Research Group. Fundus photographic risk factors for progression of diabetic retinopathy. Early Treatment Diabetic Retinopathy Study Report 12. Ophthalmology (in press).

31. Roy MS, Rick ME, Higgins KE, McCulloch JC. Retinal cotton-wool spots: an early finding in diabetic retinopathy? Br J Ophthalmol 1986; 70: 772–8.

32. Kohner EM. Pathogenic mechanisms in the development of diabetic retinopathy. In Andreani D, Crepaldi G, Di Mario U, Pozza G (eds) Diabetic complications: early diagnosis and treatment. New York: John Wiley, 1987: pp 55–63.

33. Kinoshita JH. Aldose reductase in the diabetic eye. Am J Ophthalmol 1986; 102: 685–92.

34. Kennedy A, Frank RN, Varma SD. Aldose reductase activity in retinal and cerebral microvessels and cultured vascular cells. Invest Ophthalmol Vis Sci 1983; 24: 1250–8.

35. Atherton A, Hill DW, Keen H, Young S, Edwards EJ. The effect of acute hyperglycaemia on the retinal circulation of the normal cat. Diabetologia 1980; 18: 233–7.

36. Ernest JT, Goldstick TK, Engerman RL. Hyperglycemia impairs retinal oxygen autoregulation in normal and diabetic dogs. Invest Ophthalmol Vis Sci 1983; 24: 985–9.

37. Grunwald JE, Riva CE, Martin DB, Quint AR, Epstein PA. Effect of an insulin-induced decrease in blood glucose on the human diabetic retinal circulation. Ophthalmology 1987; 94: 1614–20.

38. Kohner EM, Sleightholm M, Fallon T. Why does retinopathy deteriorate when diabetic control is improved? Invest Ophthalmol Vis Sci 1987; 29 (suppl.): 244.

39. Akagi Y, Kador PF, Kuwabara T, Kinoshita JH. Aldose reductase localization in human retinal mural cells. Invest Ophthalmol Vis Sci 1983; 24: 1516–19.

40. Engerman RL, Kern TS. Experimental galactosemia produces diabetic-like retinopathy. Diabetes 1984; 33: 97–100.

41. Frank RN, Keirn RJ, Kennedy A, Frank KW. Galactose-induced retinal capillary basement membrane thickening: prevention by sorbinil. Invest Ophthalmol Vis Sci 1983; 24: 1519–24.

42. Robison WG, Kador PF, Akagi Y et al. Prevention of basement membrane thickening in retinal capillaries by a novel inhibitor of aldose reductase, Tolrestat. Diabetes 1986; 35: 195–199.

43. Chandler ML, Shannon WA, DeSantis L. Prevention of retinal capillary basement membrane thickening in diabetic rats by aldose reductase inhibitors. Invest Ophthalmol Vis Sci 1984; 25: 159.

44. Kador PF, Akagi Y, Takahashi Y et al. Prevention of retinal vessel changes associated with diabetic retinopathy in galactose-fed dogs by aldose reductase inhibitors. Arch Ophthalmol 1990; 108: 1301–9.

45. Engerman RL, Kern TS. Determinants of experimental diabetic retinopathy. Proceedings of the International Diabetes Federation (in press).

46. Sorbinil Retinopathy Trial Research Group. A randomized trial of sorbinil, an aldose reductase inhibitor, in diabetic retinopathy. Arch Ophthalmol 1990; 108: 1234–44.

47. Taylor E, Dobree JH. Proliferative diabetic retinopathy: site and size of initial lesions. Br J Ophthalmol 1970; 54: 11–18.

48. Deckert T, Simonsen SE, Poulsen JE. Prognosis of proliferative retinopathy in juvenile diabetes. Diabetes 1967; 16: 728–33.

49. Diabetic Retinopathy Study Research Group. Photocoagulation treatment of proliferative

diabetic retinopathy. The second report of Diabetic Retinopathy Study findings. Ophthalmology 1978; 85: 82–106.

50. British Multicenter Study Group. Photocoagulation for proliferative diabetic retinopathy: a randomized controlled clinical trial using the xenon arc. Diabetologia 1984; 26: 109–115.

51. Rand LI, Prud'homme GJ, Ederer F, Canner PL. Diabetic Retinopathy Study Research Group. Factors influencing the development of visual loss in advanced diabetic retinopathy. Invest Ophthalmol Vis Sci 1985; 26: 893–991.

52. Diabetic Retinopathy Study Research Group. A modification of the Airlie House classification of diabetic retinopathy. Diabetic Retinopathy Study Report no. 7. Invest Ophthalmol Vis Sci 1981; 21: 210–26.

53. Early Treatment Diabetic Retinopathy Research Group. Grading diabetic retinopathy from stereoscopic color fundus photographs: an extension of the modified Airlie House classification. Early Treatment Diabetic Retinopathy Study Report no. 10. Ophthalmology 1991; 98 (suppl): 786–806.

54. Schwartz JS, Pavan PR. Optic disc edema. Int Ophthalmol Clin 1984; 24: 83–91.

55. Bresnick GH, Haight B, de Venecia G. Retinal wrinkling and macular heterotopia in diabetic retinopathy. Arch Ophthalmol 1979; 97: 1890–5.

56. Tasman W. Diabetic vitreous hemorrhage and its relationship to hypoglycemia. Mod Probl Ophthalmol 1979; 20: 413–14.

57. Anderson B. Activity and diabetic vitreous hemorrhages. Ophthalmology 1980; 87: 173–5.

58. Klein R, Davis MD, Moss SE, Klein BEK, DeMets DL. The Wisconsin Epidemiologic Study of Diabetic Retinopathy: a comparison of retinopathy in younger and older onset diabetic persons. In Vranic M, Hollenberg C and Steiner G (eds) Comparison of type I and type II diabetes. New York: Plenum, 1985: pp 321–5.

59. Diabetic Retinopathy Study Research Group. Design, methods, and baseline results. Diabetic Retinopathy Study Report 6. Invest Ophthalmol Vis Sci 1981; 21: 149–209.

60. Aiello LM, Rand LI, Briones JC et al. Diabetic retinopathy in Joslin Clinic patients with adult-onset diabetes. Ophthalmology 1981; 88: 619–23.

61. Klein R, Klein BEK, Moss SE et al. The Wisconsin Epidemiologic Study of Diabetic Retinopathy. IX. Four-year incidence and progression of diabetic retinopathy when age at diagnosis is less than 30 years. Arch Ophthalmol 1989; 107: 237–43.

62. Klein R, Klein BEK, Moss SE et al. The Wisconsin Epidemiologic Study of Diabetic Retinopathy. X. Four-year incidence and progression of diabetic retinopathy when age at diagnosis is 30 years of age or more. Arch Ophthalmol 1989; 107: 244–9.

63. Klein BEK, Davis MD, Segal P et al. Diabetic retinopathy. Assessment of severity and progression. Ophthalmology 1984; 91: 10–17.

64. Davis MD, Hubbard LD, Trautman J, Klein R. Studies of retinopathy. Methodology for assessment and classification with fundus photographs. Diabetes 1985; 34 (suppl. 3): 42–9.

65. Diabetic Retinopathy Study Research Group. Photocoagulation treatment of proliferative diabetic retinopathy. Clinical application of DRS findings. Diabetic Retinopathy Study Report 8. Ophthalmology 1981; 88: 583–600.

66. DCCT Research Group. Design and methodologic considerations for the feasibility phase. Diabetes 1986; 35: 530–45.

67. Klein R, Klein BEK, Moss SE, Davis MD, DeMets DL. The Wisconsin Epidemiologic Study of Diabetic Retinopathy. II. Prevalence and risk of diabetic retinopathy when age at diagnosis is less than 30 years. Arch Ophthalmol 1984; 102: 520–6.

68. Klein R, Klein BEK, Moss SE, Davis MD, DeMets DL. The Wisconsin Epidemiologic Study of Diabetic Retinopathy. III. Prevalence and risk of diabetic retinopathy when age at diagnosis is 30 or more years. Arch Ophthalmol 1984; 102: 527–32.

69. Howard-Williams J, Hillson RM, Bron A, Awdry P et al. Retinopathy is associated with higher glycemia in maturity-onset type diabetes. Diabetologia 1984; 27: 198–202.

70. Doft BH, Kingsley LA, Orchard IJ, Kuller L, Drash A, Becker D. The association between long term diabetic control and early retinopathy. Ophthalmology 1984; 91: 763–8.

71. Bodansky HJ, Cudworth AG, Drury PL, Kohner EM. Risk factors associated with severe proliferative retinopathy in insulin-dependent diabetes mellitus. Diabetes Care 1982; 5: 97–100.

72. Rand LI, Krolewski AS, Aiello LM et al. Multiple factors in the prediction of risk of proliferative diabetic retinopathy. New Engl J Med 1985; 313: 1433–7.

73. Dornan T, Mann JI, Turner R. Factors protective against retinopathy in insulin-dependent diabetics free of retinopathy for 30 years. Br Med J 1982; 285: 1073–7.

74. Krolewski AS, Warram JH, Rand LI, Christlieb AR, Busick EJ, Kahn CR. Risk of proliferative diabetic retinopathy in juvenile-onset type I diabetes: a 40-yr follow-up study. Diabetes Care 1986; 9: 443–52.

75. Krolewski AS, Rand LI, Warram JH, Aiello LM. Proliferative diabetic retinopathy (PDR)

risk is closely related to hemoglobin A_{1c} (A1C) level. Diabetes 1985; 34 (suppl. 1): 71A.

76. Knatterud GL, Klimt CR, Levin ME, Jacobson ME, Goldner MG. Effects of hypoglycemic agents on vascular complications in patients with adult-onset diabetes. VII. Mortality and selected nonfatal events with insulin treatment. JAMA 1978; 240: 37–42.

77. Kilo C, Miller JP, Williamson JR. The crux of the UGDP. Diabetologia 1980; 18: 179–85.

78. Lauritzen T, Frost-Larsen K, Larsen HW, Deckert T. Steno Study Group. Effect of one year of near-normal blood glucose levels on retinopathy in insulin-dependent diabetics. Lancet 1983; i: 200–4.

79. Kroc Collaborative Study Group. Blood glucose control and the evolution of diabetic retinopathy and albuminuria. New Engl J Med 1984; 311: 365–72.

80. Lauritzen T, Frost-Larsen K, Larsen HW et al. Two-year experience with continuous subcutaneous insulin infusion in relation to retinopathy and neuropathy. Diabetes 1985; 34: 74–9.

81. Dahl-Jorgensen K, Brinchmann-Hansen O, Hanssen KF, Sandvik KF, Aagenaes O, Aker Diabetes Group. Rapid tightening of blood glucose control leads to transient deterioration of retinopathy in insulin-dependent diabetes mellitus: the Oslo Study. Br Med J 1985; 290: 811–15.

82. Beck-Nielsen H, Rickelsen B, Mogensen CE et al. Effect of insulin pump treatment for one year on renal function and retinal morphology in patients with IDDM. Diabetes Care 1985; 8: 585–9.

83. Brinchmann-Hansen O, Dahl-Jorgensen K, Hanssen KF, Sandvik L. Oslo Study Group. Effects of intensified treatment on various lesions of diabetic retinopathy. Am J Ophthalmol 1985; 100: 644–53.

84. Kroc Collaborative Study Group. The Kroc Study patients at two years: a report on further retinal changes. Diabetes 1985; 34: 39.

85. Dahl-Jorgensen K, Brinchmann-Hansen O, Hanssen KF, Ganes T, Kierulf P, Smeland E, Sandvik KF, Aagenaes O. Effects of near normoglycaemia for two years on progression of early diabetic retinopathy, nephropathy, and neuropathy: the Oslo Study. Br Med J 1986; 293: 1195–9.

86. Brinchmann-Hanssen O, Dahl-Jorgensen K, Hanssen KF, Sandvik L. The response of diabetic retinopathy to 41 months of multiple insulin injections, insulin pumps, and conventional insulin therapy. Arch Ophthalmol 1988; 106: 1242–6.

87. Verrillo A, de Teresa A, Martino C et al. Long-

term improvement of metabolic control does not affect progression of background retinopathy. Transplant Proc 1986; XVIII: 1569–70.

88. Irsigler K, Kritz H, Najemnik C. Reversal of florid diabetic retinopathy. Lancet 1979; ii: 1068.

89. White MC, Kohner EM, Pickup JC, Keen H. Reversal of diabetic retinopathy by continuous subcutaneous insulin infusion: a case report. Br J Ophthalmol 1981; 65: 307–11.

90. Pucklin JE, Tamborlane WV, Felig P et al. Influence of long-term insulin infusion pump treatment of type I diabetes on diabetic retinopathy. Ophthalmology 1982; 89: 735–47.

91. Lawson PM, Champion MC, Canny C et al. Continuous subcutaneous insulin infusion does not prevent progression of proliferative and preproliferative retinopathy. Br J Ophthalmol 1982; 66: 762–6.

92. van Ballegooie E, Hooymans JM, Timmerman Z et al. Rapid deterioration of diabetic retinopathy during treatment with continuous subcutaneous insulin infusion. Diabetes Care 1984; 7: 236–42.

93. Daneman D, Drash AL, Lobes LH et al. Progressive retinopathy with improved control in diabetic dwarfism (Mauriac's syndrome). Diabetes Care 1981; 4: 360–5.

94. Lawrence JR, Bedford GJ, Thomson R. Rapid development during puberty of proliferative retinopathy after strict control. Lancet 1985; ii: 322.

95. Dandona P, Bolger JP, Boag F, Fonesca V, Abrams JD. Rapid development and progression of proliferative retinopathy after strict diabetic control. Br Med J 1985; 290: 895–6.

96. Ramsay RC, Goetz FC, Sutherland DER et al. Progression of diabetic retinopathy after pancreas transplantation for insulin-dependent diabetes mellitus. New Engl J Med 1988; 318: 208–14.

97. Phelps RL, Sakol P, Metzker BE et al. Changes in diabetic retinopathy during pregnancy: corrections with regulation of hyperglycemia. Arch Ophthalmol 1986; 104: 1806–10.

98. Engerman RL, Bloodworth JMB, Nelson S. Relationship of microvascular disease in diabetes to metabolic control. Diabetes 1977; 26: 760–9.

99. Engerman RL, Kern TS. Progression of incipient diabetic retinopathy during good glycemic control. Diabetes 1987; 36: 808–12.

100. Constam GR. Zur Spätprognose des Diabetes mellitus. Helv Med Acta 1965; 32: 287.

101. Caird FI. Diabetes and the eye. Oxford: Blackwell, 1968: p 84.

102. Klein R, Klein BEK, Moss SE, Davis MD, DeMets DL. Glycosylated hemoglobin predicts the incidence and progression of diabetic retinopathy. JAMA 1988; 260: 2864–71.

103. DCCT Research Group. Diabetes Control and Complications Trial (DCCT): update. Diabetes Care 1990; 13: 427–33.

104. Danielson R, Jonarson F, Helgason T. Prevalence of retinopathy and proteinuria in type I diabetics in Iceland. Acta Med Scand 1982; 212: 277.

105. Starup K, Larsen H, Enk B et al. Fluorescein angiography in diabetic children. Acta Ophthalmol 1980; 58: 347.

106. Frank RN, Hoffman WH, Podgor MJ et al. Retinopathy in juvenile-onset diabetes of short duration. Ophthalmology 1980; 87: 1–9.

107. Klein R, Klein BEK, Moss SE et al. Retinopathy in younger-onset diabetic patients. Diabetes Care 1985; 8: 311.

108. Grant M, Russell B, Fitzgerald C, Merimee TJ. Insulin-like growth factors in vitreous. Studies in control and diabetic subjects with neovascularization. Diabetes 1986; 35: 416–20.

109. Moloney JBM, Drury MI. The effect of pregnancy on the natural course of diabetic retinopathy. Am J Ophthalmol 1982; 93: 745.

110. Klein BE, Moss SE, Klein R. Effect of pregnancy on progression of diabetic retinopathy. Diabetes Care 1990; 13: 34–40.

111. Dornan TL, Ting A, McPherson CK et al. Genetic susceptibility to the development of retinopathy in insulin-dependent diabetes. Diabetes 1982; 31; 226.

112. Stersky G, Wall S. Determinants of microangiopathy in growth-onset diabetes. Acta Paediatr Scand 1986; 327 (suppl.): 1–45.

113. Janka HU, Warram JH, Rand LI et al. Risk factors for progression of background retinopathy in long-standing insulin-dependent diabetes mellitus. Diabetes 1989; 38: 460–4.

114. Deckert T, Parving HH, Anderson AR et al. Diabetic nephropathy. In Eschwège E (ed.) Advances in diabetes epidemiology. New York: Elsevier, 1982: pp 235–43.

115. Klein R, Klein BEK, Moss SE, Davis MD, DeMets DL. The Wisconsin Epidemiologic Study of Diabetic Retinopathy. V. Proteinuria and retinopathy in a population of diabetic persons diagnosed prior to 30 years of age. Diabetic Renal–Retinal Syndrome 1986; 3: 245–64.

116. Cullen JF, Town SM, Campbell CJ. Double-blind trial of Atromid-S in exudative diabetic retinopathy. Trans Ophthalmol Soc UK 1974; 94: 554.

117. Larsen HW, Sander E, Hoppe R. The value of calcium dobesilate in the treatment of diabetic retinopathy. A controlled clinical trial. Diabetologia 1977; 13: 105.

118. Stamper RL, Smith ME, Aronson SB et al. The effect of calcium dobesilate on nonproliferative diabetic retinopathy. A controlled study. Ophthalmology (Rochester, Minn) 1978; 85: 594.

119. Houssay BA, Biasotti A. La diabetes pancreatica de los perros hipofisoprivos. Rev Soc Argent Biol 1930; 6: 251–96.

120. Luft R, Olivecrona H, Sjogren B. Hypophysectomy in man. Nord Med 1952; 47: 351–4.

121. Poulsen JE. The Houssay phenomenon in man: recovery from retinopathy in a case of diabetes with Simmonds' disease. Diabetes 1953; 2: 7–12.

122. Poulsen JE. Diabetes and anterior pituitary insufficiency. Final course and postmortem study of a diabetic patient with Sheehan's syndrome. Diabetes 1966; 15: 73–7.

123. Kohner EM, Joplin GF, Blach RK, Cheng H, Fraser TR. Pituitary ablation in the treatment of diabetic retinopathy. Trans Ophthalmol Soc UK 1972; 42: 79–90.

124. Lundaek K, Malmros R, Andersen HC et al. Hypophysectomy for diabetic angiopathy: a controlled clinical trial. In Goldberg MF Fine SL (eds) Symposium on the treatment of diabetic retinopathy. Public Health Service Publ. no. 1890. Washington, DC: US Govt Printing Office, 1969: pp 291–311.

125. Panisset A, Kohner EM, Cheng H, Fraser TR. Diabetic retinopathy: new vessels arising from the optic disc. II. Response to pituitary ablation by yttrium 90 implant. Diabetes 1971; 20: 824–33.

126. Kohner EM, Hamilton AM, Joplin GF, Fraser TR. Florid diabetic retinopathy and its response to treatment by photocoagulation or pituitary ablation. Diabetes 1976; 25: 104–10.

127. Meyer-Schwickerath G. Light coagulation (trans. Drance SM). St Louis: CV Mosby, 1960.

128. Beetham WP, Aiello JM, Balodimos MC, Koncz L. Ruby laser photocoagulation of early diabetic neovascular retinopathy. Trans Am Ophthalmol Soc 1969; 67: 39–67.

129. Early Treatment Diabetic Retinopathy Study Research Group. Techniques for scatter and local photocoagulation treatment of diabetic retinopathy. Early Treatment Diabetic Retinopathy Study Report 3. Int Ophthalmol Clin 1987; 27: 254–64.

130. Rubinstein K, Myska V. Pathogenesis and treatment of diabetic maculopathy. Br J Ophthalmol 1974; 58: 76–84.

131. British Multicenter Study Group. Photocoagulation for diabetic maculopathy. Diabetes 1983; 32: 1010–16.

132. Patz A, Schatz H, Berkow JW et al. Macular edema—an overlooked complication of diabetic retinopathy. Trans Am Acad Ophthalmol Otol 1973; 77: 34–42.

133. Ferris FL, Patz A. Macular edema. A complication of diabetic retinopathy. Surv Ophthalmol 1984; 28 (suppl.): 452–61.

134. Early Treatment Diabetic Retinopathy Study Research Group. Photocoagulation for diabetic macular edema. Early Treatment Diabetic Retinopathy Study Report 4. Int Ophthalmol Clin 1987; 27: 265–73.

135. Early Treatment Diabetic Retinopathy Study Research Group. Treatment techniques and clinical guidelines for photocoagulation of diabetic macular edema. Early Treatment Diabetic Retinopathy Study Report 2. Ophthalmology 1987; 94: 761–74.

136. Olk RJ. Modified grid argon (blue-green) laser photocoagulation for diffuse diabetic macular edema. Ophthalmology 1986; 93: 938–50.

137. Little HL, Zweng C, Jack RL, Vassiliadis A. Techniques of argon laser photocoagulation of diabetic disk new vessels. Am J Ophthalmol 1976; 82: 675–83.

138. Wolbarsht ML, Landers MB. The rationale of photocoagulation therapy for proliferative diabetic retinopathy: a review and a model. Ophthalmic Surg 1980; 11: 235–45.

139. Weiter JJ, Zuckerman R. The influence of the photoreceptor–RPE complex on the inner retina; an explanation for the beneficial effects of photocoagulation. Ophthalmology 1980; 87: 1133–9.

140. Molnar J, Poitry S, Tsacopoulos M et al. Effect of laser photocoagulation on oxygenation of the retina in miniature pigs. Invest Ophthalmol Vis Sci 1985; 26: 1410–14.

141. Grunwald JE, Riva CE, Bruckner AJ et al. Altered vascular response to 100% oxygen breathing in diabetes mellitus. Ophthalmology 1984; 91: 1447–52.

142. Glaser BM, Campochiaro PA, Davis DL Jr, Sato M. Retinal pigment epithelial cells release an inhibitor of neovascularization. Arch Ophthalmol 1985; 103: 1870–5.

143. Peyman GA, Bok D. Peroxidase diffusion in the normal and laser-photocoagulated primate retina. Invest Ophthalmol 1972; 11: 35–45.

144. Marshall J, Clover G, Rothery S. Some new findings on retinal irradiation by krypton and argon lasers. Doc Ophthalmol 1984; 36: 21–37.

145. Bresnick GH. Diabetic macular edema. Ophthalmology 1986; 93: 989–97.

146. Diabetic Retinopathy Study Research Group. Preliminary report on the effects of photocoagulation therapy. Am J Ophthalmol 1976; 81: 383–96.

147. Hercules BL, Gayed II, Lucas SB, Jeacock J. Peripheral retinal ablation in the treatment of proliferative diabetic retinopathy: a three-year interim report of a randomised, controlled study using the argon laser. Br J Ophthalmol 1977; 61: 555–63.

148. Meyer-Schwickerath G, Gerke E. Bjerrum lecture. Treatment of diabetic retinopathy with photocoagulation. Results of photocoagulation therapy of proliferative retinopathy in childhood-onset and maturity-onset diabetes and an approach to the dosage of photocoagulation. Acta Ophthalmol (Copenh) 1983; 61: 756–68.

149. Okun E, Johnston GP, Boniuk I, Arribas NP, Escoffery RF, Grand MG. Xenon arc photocoagulation of proliferative diabetic retinopathy. Ophthalmology 1984; 91: 1458–63.

150. Doft BH, Blankenship GW. Retinopathy risk factor regression after laser panretinal photocoagulation for proliferative diabetic retinopathy. Ophthalmology 1984; 91: 1453–7.

151. Blankenship GW. A clinical comparison of central and peripheral argon laser panretinal photocoagulation for proliferative diabetic retinopathy. Trans Am Ophthalmol Soc 1987; 85: 176–94; Ophthalmology 1988; 95: 170–7.

152. Rogell GD. Incremental panretinal photocoagulation: results in treating proliferative diabetic retinopathy. Retina 1983; 3: 308–11.

153. Vine AK. The efficacy of additional argon laser photocoagulation for persistent, severe proliferative diabetic retinopathy. Ophthalmology 1985; 92: 1532–7.

154. Early Treatment Diabetic Retinopathy Study Research Group. Case reports to accompany Early Treatment Diabetic Retinopathy Study Reports 3 and 4. Int Ophthalmol Clin 1987; 27: 273–333.

155. Early Treatment Diabetic Retinopathy Study Research Group. Early photocoagulation for diabetic retinopathy. Early Treatment Diabetic Retinopathy Study Report 9. Ophthalmology 1991; 98 (suppl.) 766–85.

156. Jacobson DR, Murphy RP, Rosenthal AR. The treatment of angle neovascularization with panretinal photocoagulation. Ophthalmology 1979; 86: 1270–5.

157. May DR, Bergstrom TJ, Parmet AJ et al. Treatment of neovascular glaucoma with transscleral panretinal cryotherapy. Ophthalmology 1980; 87: 1106–11.

158. Machemer R, Buettner H, Norton EWD, Parel JM. Vitrectomy: a pars plana approach. Ophthalmology 1971; 75: 813.

159. Michels RG, de Bustros S. Vitreous surgery for visual loss from proliferative diabetic retinopathy. In Friedman EA, L'Esperance FA (eds) The retinal–renal syndrome. New York: Grune & Stratton, 1986: pp 265–82.

160. Rice TA, Michels RC, Maguire MG, Rice EF. The effect of lensectomy on the incidence of iris

neovascularization and neovascular glaucoma after vitrectomy for diabetic retinopathy. Am J Ophthalmol 1963; 95: 1–11.

161. de Bustros S, Thompson JT, Michels RG, Rice TA. Vitrectomy for progressive proliferative diabetic retinopathy. Arch Ophthalmol 1987; 105: 196–9.

162. Diabetic Retinopathy Vitrectomy Study Research Group. Early vitrectomy for severe vitreous hemorrhage in diabetic retinopathy. Two-year results of a randomized trial. Diabetic Retinopathy Vitrectomy Study Report 2. Arch Ophthalmol 1985; 103: 1644–52.

163. O'Hanley GP, Canny CLB. Diabetic dense premacular hemorrhage. A possible indication for prompt vitrectomy. Ophthalmology 1985; 92: 507–11.

164. Ramsay RC, Knoblock WH, Cantrill HL. Timing of vitrectomy for active proliferative diabetic retinopathy. Ophthalmology 1986; 93: 283–9.

165. Diabetic Vitrectomy Study Research Group. Early vitrectomy for severe proliferative diabetic retinopathy in eyes with useful vision. Results of a randomized trial. Diabetic Retinopathy Vitrectomy Study Report 3. Ophthalmology 1988; 95: 1307–20.

166. Diabetic Vitrectomy Study Research Group. Early vitrectomy for severe proliferative diabetic retinopathy in eyes with useful vision. Clinical application of results of a randomized trial. Diabetic Retinopathy Vitrectomy Study Report 4. Ophthalmology 1988; 95: 1321–34.

167. Dipyridamole Aspirin Microangiopathy of Diabetes Study Group. Effect of aspirin alone and aspirin plus dipyridamole in early diabetic retinopathy. A multicenter randomized controlled clinical trial. Diabetes 1989; 38: 491–8.

168. Ticlopidine Microangiopathy of Diabetes Study Group. Ticlopidine treatment reduces the progression of nonproliferative diabetic retinopathy. Arch Ophthalmol 1990; 108: 1577–83.

169. Early Treatment Diabetic Retinopathy Study Research Group: Effects of aspirin treatment on diabetic retinopathy. Early Treatment Diabetic Retinopathy Study Report 8. Ophthalmology 1991; 98 (suppl): 757–65.

57

Diabetic Effects on Non-retinal Ocular Structures

Lawrence I. Rand*, Jerry D. Cavallerano† and Lloyd M. Aiello†
* *West Newton, Massachusetts, USA, and † Joslin Diabetes Center, Boston, Massachusetts, USA*

Diabetic eye disease is not limited to diabetic retinopathy: all structures of the eye are susceptible to the deleterious effects of diabetes. Some of these effects are of little consequence, and go unnoticed by both the patient and the doctor. Other effects, while not sight-threatening, result in uncomfortable vision or other symptoms interfering with normal visual function. Still other effects, while perhaps most prevalent with diabetes, must be fully evaluated to rule out potentially life-threatening underlying causes other than diabetes. This chapter reviews some of the more common non-retinal complications of diabetes mellitus.

OPHTHALMOPLEGIA

Mononeuropathy of the third, fourth or sixth cranial nerves is an uncommon (0.4%) but dramatic complication of diabetes [1]. Presentation of such neuropathy, however, is of serious concern to the patient, because the presenting symptom is usually frank diplopia sometimes accompanied by eye pain. The mononeuropathies also present a serious clinical challenge for the examiner, as a misdiagnosis may result in an overlooked cranial neoplasm or aneurysm. On the other hand, complete neurological evaluation proves time-consuming, costly and sometimes uncomfortable for the patient.

In the diabetic mononeuropathies, the third nerve (oculomotor) is most commonly affected, followed by the sixth (abducens) cranial nerve. Infrequently the fourth nerve (trochlear) may be involved alone or in combination with one of the other nerves. The presenting complaint is usually diplopia and may be associated with ipsilateral headache or eye pain which can precede the onset of diplopia. Bilateral nerve palsies are not rare.

Third nerve palsies usually result in a ptosis of the eyelid on the affected side. The eye is directed down and out, and supraorbital pain may precede or be associated with the palsy. The pupil is generally spared, although pupillary evaluation may be compromised either by the diabetic condition itself or by previous panretinal laser photocoagulation [2–8]. Patients with sixth nerve palsies usually have the affected eye turned inward toward the nose. Movement of the eye laterally past the midline is restricted or absent. The sixth nerve has a long intracranial course and multiple causes are responsible for sixth nerve palsies, necessitating careful neurologic evaluation. Weakness of the fourth nerve

International Textbook of Diabetes Mellitus. Edited by K.G.M.M. Alberti, R.A. DeFronzo, H. Keen and P. Zimmet
© 1992 John Wiley & Sons Ltd

results in a combination of vertical and lateral diplopia, and the patient may present with a head tilt or a complaint of tilting images. Fourth nerve palsies are comparatively rare.

Complete recovery of function usually occurs in 1–9 months. Recurrence may develop, but aberrant regeneration of the nerve is not seen. Particularly important in third nerve palsies of diabetic origin is the sparing of the pupillary fibers, which distinguishes these third nerve palsies from those due to intracranial aneurysms and tumors which affect the pupil in 80–90% of the cases. Nevertheless, ocular palsies in a diabetic patient should prompt a thorough medical and neurological evaluation, as 42% of such palsies seen in diabetics in one series were of non-diabetic origin [9]. Other diagnoses includes myasthenia gravis, Graves' disease, herpes zoster, demyelinating disease, primary and metastatic brain tumor, and hypoglycemia.

Treatment of ophthalmoplegia is symptomatic to relieve diplopia, and usually consists of temporary occlusion of one eye, together with a mild analgesic if needed. Severe pain is not characteristic, so the need for strong analgesics should arouse suspicion that an intracranial aneurysm may be present. Diabetic nerve palsies are usually self-limited, with resolution occurring in a few weeks to up to 6–9 months later. Nerve palsies that have not begun to resolve after approximately 6 months are most probably not of diabetic origin.

THE DIABETIC CORNEA

Diabetes affects the cornea in a variety of fashions. The cornea of a person with diabetes injures more easily and heals more slowly than the cornea of a person who does not have diabetes. One significant factor is reduced corneal sensitivity related to diabetes, compared with age-matched non-diabetic individuals [10]. This reduction was symmetrical in each patient, and the thresholds increased with the duration of diabetes, although diabetic patients did not exhibit more clinically significant corneal disease than non-diabetic patients. Furthermore, in a separate study, impairment of corneal sensitivity was found to correlate significantly with duration of diabetes in experiments conducted on diabetic dogs [11].

Corneal nerve alterations in diabetic rats have been demonstrated in the basal lamina of Schwann cells, as well as occasional axonal degenerations [12]. Such alterations are probably implicated in the development of neurotrophic corneal ulcerations with diabetes [13]. Another aspect involves histological studies of the endothelial cells of the diabetic cornea. The endothelial cells clearly show morphological abnormalities resulting in a less stable and more vulnerable cell layer [14]. Minute folds in Descemet's membrane probably represent an alteration in the tissue fluid level of the cornea [1].

The corneal epithelium and its basement membrane have also been implicated in corneal disease associated with diabetes. As the human corneal epithelium contains significant levels of both sorbitol and fructose, it is likely that the sorbitol pathway operates in this tissue [15]. Poor adhesion of epithelial cells to its basement membrane is probably the result of osmotic changes within the cornea.

Such corneal changes pose numerous clinical problems. The patient with diabetes may be a poor candidate for contact lenses, as discomfort from a poorly fitting or damaged lens may be absent because of reduced corneal sensitivity. Corneal abrasions or minor erosions which may be detected early in an otherwise healthy cornea may develop into significant ulcerations. Corneal erosions may also be more likely to become recurrent because of slow or poor wound healing. Minor infections, which might otherwise be of little or no consequence, may become sight-threatening in the presence of diabetes.

Another complication of compromised corneal integrity relates to the treatment for diabetic retinopathy. In order to perform a thorough ocular evaluation of the anterior segment or of the retina of the eye, a contact lens for examining purposes is frequently necessary. The mechanical action of the lens, although cushioned by a solution, may be enough to damage the cornea. Furthermore, similar types of contact lenses are required for laser treatments, and the mechanical action of the lens, in conjunction with the length of time that the lens must be placed on the eye, may result in an iatrogenic corneal abrasion; this also applies to vitrectomy surgery.

The tendency for corneal abrasion may necessitate the use of an artificial tear, particularly in dry environments. Patients with diabetes should be alerted to the potential side-effects of contact lenses, and follow-up evaluations need to be frequent and thorough. The use of extended-wear contact lenses should be discouraged. The necessity for safety glasses and goggles should be emphasized for appropriate work and sport environments. For ocular examination and treatment, a soft contact lens may be used between the cornea and the examining or treating lens, particularly if the patient has had a corneal abrasion in the past.

GLAUCOMA

Primary open angle glaucoma is reported to be more common among individuals with diabetes (4.0%) than it is among those without it (1.8%); in addition, diabetes has been found to be more common among glaucoma patients (4–18%) than in the general population (2%) [16]. Why this should be the case is not well understood, as the pathogenesis of primary open angle glaucoma remains unknown. Glaucoma or elevated intraocular pressure has been proposed as protecting an eye from developing severe diabetic retinopathy, based on studies of patients with diabetes and unilateral glaucoma. As the intraocular pressure is the main component of tissue pressure in the eye, and retinal venous pressure usually just barely exceeds intraocular pressure, it would not be surprising if alterations in the regulation of intraocular pressure and its relationship with vascular resistance could play a major part in the pathogenesis of diabetic retinopathy.

Treatment of open angle glaucoma in diabetic individuals must be influenced by their general medical condition. Caution must be exercised with the use of topical β-blockers in masking hypoglycemic symptoms or affecting frequently occurring cardiovascular disease. Acetazolamide or other carbonic anhydrase inhibitors may be used if needed, but as these medications can cause a metabolic acidosis, more frequent electrolyte monitoring should be done. The presence of renal disease may influence how these and other pressure-lowering drugs may be used, and close cooperation between the internist and eye doctor is important.

Narrow angle glaucoma or acute angle closure glaucoma is comparatively rare. Narrow angle glaucoma does not seem to be more common in persons with diabetes than in the general population, but recent investigations suggest that the shallower the anterior chamber of the eye, the more likely a person is to have an abnormal response to an oral glucose tolerance test [17]. The postulated mechanism for this association is the autonomic dysfunction within the anterior segment of the eye, resulting in a hypersensitivity to both sympathetic and parasympathetic autonomic mediators, with the iris–lens diaphragm moving forward and closing the angle.

In acute angle closure glaucoma, the outflow angle in the anterior chamber of the eye formed by the iris plane and the posterior corneal surface becomes closed, blocking outflow to the outflow channels of the trabecular meshwork. The result is a dramatic and rapid rise in intraocular pressure with ocular pain, decreased vision, colored halos around lights, and frequently nausea and vomiting. Angle closure glaucoma should be considered as part of the differential diagnosis for a diabetic patient presenting with nausea and vomiting.

Angle closure glaucoma is considered to be a medical emergency. Treatment consists of attempting to break the angle closure medically with miotic drops and to lower the pressure with either systemic or topical medications. A peripheral iridectomy or laser iridotomy can restore the normal aqueous outflow in the eye if the angle closure is broken. As pupil dilation can trigger an angle closure attack, care needs to be exercised before any pupil is dilated.

Another type of glaucoma that is most common in diabetic individuals is neovascular glaucoma, in which a proliferation of new blood vessels grows in the angle of the anterior chamber, blocking normal aqueous outflow. This rubeosis iridis seems to be related to the vascular proliferation on the retina of the eye, and is probably the result of the same poorly understood mechanism that results in proliferative retinopathy.

Rubeosis iridis usually is first seen around the pupillary margin, although the vessels can grow initially in or near the filtration angle. Evaluation with a slit-lamp biomicroscope is necessary to observe and evaluate these vessels. The development of neovascular glaucoma in one eye is strongly correlated to the development of the same condition in the patient's other eye. Prognosis for the eye is usually guarded if neovascular glaucoma is present [1].

Treatment with panretinal laser photocoagulation has been shown to be beneficial in the management of rubeosis iridis [18, 19]. Neovascular glaucoma also can be treated by goniophotocoagulation if the surgeon is unable to dilate the pupil, or if cloudy media or vitreous hemorrhage prevents visualization of the fundus [20]. In this procedure, discrete laser applications are applied directly to the new vessels as they arborize in the angle, resulting in angle synechiae. Frequently, a combination of pan-retinal photocoagulation and goniophotocoagulation is used to treat neovascular glaucoma. Adjunct medical therapy may include β-adrenergic blocking agents or carbonic anhydrase inhibitors to depress aqueous formation and thereby lower the intraocular pressure. Cycloplegic agents and topical steroid drops may reduce local ocular inflammation and relieve some of the associated pain. YAG contact laser ablation of the ciliary body appears to be a promising new mode of controlling high pressures when medical therapy fails. Filtration surgery has, in general, had poor results but new techniques are being developed.

DIABETES AND CATARACT

Opacification of the crystalline lens or cataract is another important ocular manifestation of diabetes [21]. Three types of cataract have been noted [1]: these are the 'snowflake' or metabolic cataract, the senile cataract and the cataracta complicata or secondary cataract.

Snowflake cataracts are seen primarily in young diabetic patients with uncontrolled diabetes [22]; the name is derived from the snow-flake or flocculent appearance, which starts in the subcapsular regions of the lens. The cataract may progress rapidly, and total opacification of the lens resulting in a mature cataract can occasionally occur over a period of a few days. Institution of aequate diabetic control has been reported to stop or to reverse these lens opacities when they are discovered in their incipient stages.

Development of a metabolic cataract occurs in most animal models of diabetes. Investigation of this cataract led to the discovery of the sorbitol pathway, an alternative route for glucose metabolism requiring the enzyme aldose reductase and in which sorbitol, a sugar alcohol, is the byproduct. Inhibition of sorbitol production by use of an aldose reductase inhibitor prevents the development of cataract in these diabetic experimental animals and in galactosemia as well. Recently, the possible role of sugar alcohol accumulation as an underlying factor in other diabetic complications, including neuropathy and possibly retinopathy, has received much attention. Aldose reductase inhibitors are currently under investigation in both of these complications, but their clinical efficacy is still uncertain.

Senile cataract is the most common form of cataract seen in diabetes, and cannot be distinguished from the senile cataract of non-diabetic individuals. With diabetic patients, however, the senile changes of nuclear sclerosis and cortical and subcapsular opacification develop at an earlier age than in non-diabetic patients (in 59% of older-onset diabetic individuals at 30–54 years of age, compared with 12% of age-matched non-diabetic individuals) [21]. The cataracts also may progress to a vision-impairing level more rapidly, necessitating cataract extraction.

The indications for cataract extraction are, in general, similar for those with diabetes and those without, but the retinopathy status of the patient may influence the surgical procedure performed. In the past, the insertion of an intraocular lens was not recommended in patients with diabetes, particularly those with any significant diabetic retinopathy, because of reports of difficulty in visualizing the retina in order to examine or to treat retinopathy following surgery. Advent of the posterior chamber intraocular lens and YAG laser capsulotomy, and additional experience with lens implant surgery, has reduced these concerns, and most diabetic patients may now receive the benefits of this major advance in visual rehabilitation. Individual judgement, however, is still needed in deciding whether to insert an intraocular lens in a patient with advanced retinopathy, particularly if laser treatment has not been applied or the eye has not responded well to previous laser treatments. The incidence of rubeosis iridis and neovascular glaucoma in these eyes following cataract extraction is reported to be significant [22, 23].

Cataracta complicata, or cataracts associated with other ocular disease such as iridocyclitis chorioretinitis, high myopia or retinal detachment, were seen in 6% of a large group of diabetic patients examined by Waite and Beetham, a figure not significantly different from that seen in the non-diabetic group [1].

REFRACTIVE ERRORS

Diabetic individuals have the same range of refractive errors as the general population [1]. The effects of blood glucose level on refractive error, however, have been well documented and investigators now have a better understanding of the relationship of refractive changes to the effects of the sorbitol pathway [24–27]. Hyperglycemia is usually recognized as resulting in a myopic shift, and Waite and Beetham [1] measured shifts of up to 10.0 dioptres. A lowering of blood glucose level is similarly recognized as causing a reduction in myopia and an increase in hyperopia. The mechanism remains open to debate, but it is suggested that, in a hyperglycemic state, glucose enters the intracellular spaces of the lens, resulting in lens swelling and an associated increase in myopia [27].

Sudden refractive shifts are frequently the presenting symptom for a person with new diabetes. Patients who could see clearly at distance, either with or without their glasses, may complain that their distance vision is now blurred. On the other hand, those who required reading glasses or who were experiencing difficulty with near work may now find they can read more easily without their glasses, misinterpreting the change as 'an improvement' in their eyes. Patients with uncontrolled or poorly controlled blood glucose levels should be encouraged to postpone spectacle purchase until their blood glucose levels have stabilized; this stabilization may take 4–6 weeks to occur, although the effects of a rise in blood glucose on refractive state are generally recognized as being more sudden. Any coexisting physical condition that affects blood glucose level, such as infection, cold or even stress, should be considered a reason not to prescribe glasses if a patient recognizes recent or sudden changes in vision.

MISCELLANEOUS OCULAR EFFECTS

There are other non-retinal effects of diabetes that, while not frequently reported by patients, may have an impact on their vision or visual function. Because of autonomic nervous system abnormalities, pupil size is frequently smaller in a diabetic person than in an age-matched and sex-matched individual without diabetes. Pupil size has been shown to be related to duration of diabetes and metabolic control [1–7]: studies have shown that there is a smaller pupil size and a loss of spontaneous fluctuation of pupil diameter with increased duration or poor control. These abnormalities, once believed to be related to stiffness of iris tissues, are probably related to autonomic neuropathy predominantly affecting the sympathetic innervation to the iris dilator muscle, with the parasympathetic innervation to the iris sphincter muscle being relatively spared. Laser injury to the short ciliary nerves as they course anteriorly on the inner surface of the retina can, similarly, result in pupillary abnormalities and reduced amplitude of accommodation [8]. Reduction in accommodative ability can also occur, especially in the young, newly diagnosed diabetic individual [28].

CONCLUSION

Diabetic eye disease is not restricted to diabetic retinopathy alone. As with all aspects of diabetic care, interaction with the patient and other health care providers is necessary to assist patients properly in managing their diabetic condition.

REFERENCES

1. Waite JH, Beetham WP. Visual mechanism in diabetes mellitus: comparative study of 2002 diabetics and 457 non-diabetics for control. New Engl J Med 1935; 212: 367–429.
2. Hreidarsson AB. Pupil size in insulin-dependent diabetes: relationship to duration, metabolic control, and long-term manifestations. Diabetes 1982; 31: 442–8.
3. Hreidarsson AB. Acute, reversible autonomic nervous system abnormalities in juvenile insulin-dependent diabetes. Diabetologia 1981; 20: 475–81.
4. Hreidarsson AB. Pupil motility in long-term diabetes. Diabetologia 1979; 17: 145–50.
5. Smith SE, Smith SA, Brown PM, Fox C, Sonksen PH. Pupillary signs in diabetic autonomic neuropathy. Br Med J 1978; 2: 924–7.
6. Clapp CA. Diabetic iridopathy. Am J Ophthalmol 1945; 28: 617–23.
7. Gundersen HJG. An abnormality of the central autonomic nervous system in long-term diabetes: absence of hippus. Diabetologia 1974; 10: 346.
8. Rogell GD. Internal ophthalmoplegia after argon laser panretinal photocoagulation. Arch Ophthalmol 1979; 97: 904–5.

9. Zorrilla C, Kozak GP. Ophthalmoplegia in diabetes mellitus. Ann Intern Med 1967; 67: 968.

10. Schwartz DE. Corneal sensitivity in diabetics. Arch Ophthalmol 1974; 91: 174–8.

11. MacRae SM, Engerman RL, Hatchell DL, Hyndiuk RA. Corneal sensitivity and control of diabetes. Cornea 1982; 1: 223–6.

12. Ishida N, Rao GN, del Cerro M, Aquavella JV. Corneal nerve alterations in diabetes mellitus. Arch Ophthalmol 1984; 102: 1380–4.

13. Hyndiuk RA, Kazarian EL, Schultz RO, Seideman S. Neurotrophic corneal ulcers in diabetes mellitus. Arch Ophthalmol 1977; 95: 2193–6.

14. Schultz RO, Matsuda M, Yee RW, Edelhauser HF, Schultz KJ. Corneal endothelial changes in type I and type II diabetes mellitus. Am J Ophthalmol 1984; 98: 401–10.

15. Foulks GN, Thoft RA, Perry HD, Tolentino FI. Factors related to corneal epithelial complications after closed vitrectomy in diabetics. Arch Ophthalmol 1979; 97: 1076–8.

16. Armstrong JR, Daily RK, Dobson HL, Gerard LJ. The incidence of glaucoma in diabetes mellitus. A comparison with the incidence in the general population. Am J Ophthalmol 1960; 50: 55.

17. Mapstone R, Clark CV. Prevalence of diabetes in glaucoma. Br Med J 1985; 291: 9395.

18. Wand M, Dueker DK, Aiello LM, Grant WM. Effects of panretinal photocoagulation on rubeosis iridis, angle neovascularization, and neovascular glaucoma. Am J Ophthalmol 1978; 86: 332–9.

19. Pavan PR, Folk JC, Weingeist TA, Hermsen VM, Watzke RC, Montague PR. Diabetic rubeosis and panretinal photocoagulation: a prospective, controlled, masked trial using iris fluorescein angiography. Arch Ophthalmol 1983; 101: 882–4.

20. Simmons RJ, Dueker DK, Kimbrough RI, Aiello LM. Goniophotocoagulation for neovascular glaucoma. Trans Am Acad Ophthalmol Otol 1977; 83: 80–9.

21. Klein BEK, Klein R, Moss S. Prevalence of cataracts in a population based study of persons with diabetes mellitus. Ophthalmology 1985; 92: 1191–6.

22. Aiella LM, Wand M, Liang G. Neovascular glaucoma and vitreous hemorrhage following cataract surgery in patients with diabetes mellitus. Ophthalmology 1983; 90: 814–20.

23. Aiello LM, Rand LI, Weiss JN, Sebestyen JG, Wafai MZ, Bradbury M, Briones JC. The eye and diabetes. In Marble A, Krall L, Bradley RF et al (eds) Joslin's Diabetes mellitus. Philadelphia: Lea & Febiger, 1985: pp 600–34.

24. Duke-Elder WS. Changes in refraction in diabetes mellitus. Br J Ophthalmol 1925: 9: 167–87.

25. Kinoshita JH, Merola LO, Satoh K, Dikmak E. Osmotic changes caused by the accumulation of dulcitol in the lenses of rats fed with galactose. Nature 1962; 194: 1085–7.

26. Gabbay KH. The sorbitol pathway and the complications of diabetes. New Engl J Med 1962; 194: 831–6.

27. Gwinup G, Villarreal A. Relationship of serum glucose concentration to changes in refraction. Diabetes 1976; 25: 29–31.

28. Marmor MF. Transient accommodative paralysis and hyperopia in diabetes. Arch Ophthalmol 1973; 89: 419–20.

58

Visual Impairment and Diabetes

Ronald Klein and Scot E. Moss

Department of Ophthalmology, University of Wisconsin Medical School, Madison, Wisconsin, USA

Diabetes mellitus is a major cause of visual impairment in the USA [1]. Diabetes has been estimated to cause approximately 5000 new cases of legal blindness each year (visual acuity of 20/200 or worse in the better eye). Blindness is 25 times more common in diabetic than in non-diabetic people [2, 3]. The purpose of this chapter is to review the epidemiology of visual impairment associated with diabetes mellitus and to examine preventive and rehabilitative strategies for dealing with this complication.

EPIDEMIOLOGY

Prevalence

Data about blindness due to diabetes come mainly from the Health Interview Study (HIS) [4], the Framingham Eye Study (FES) [5], a few population-based studies [3, 6], registries [7, 8], clinical trials on photocoagulation [9, 10] and specialty clinics [11–13]. The data from these sources are limited by the size of the sample, the select nature of the group studied or by the measure of visual impairment. For these reasons, data from a large population-based cohort study in southern Wisconsin, the Wisconsin Epidemiological Study of Diabetic Retinopathy (WESDR), are presented here.

From 1980 to 1982, 2366 subjects were examined; they were classified as younger-onset, i.e. diagnosed at less than 30 years of age and taking insulin (YO-I, $n = 996$), or older-onset, i.e. diagnosed at or after 30 years of age, and either taking insulin (OO-I, $n = 674$) or not taking insulin (OO-NI, $n = 696$) [14, 15]. The examinations and procedures consisted of standardized measurements of the best corrected visual acuity (using the Early Treatment Diabetic Retinopathy Study protocol [10]), intraocular pressure, lens examination, and grading of stereoscopic fundus photographs of the seven standard Diabetic Retinopathy Study (DRS) fields for presence and severity of diabetic retinopathy and clinically significant macular edema (CSME) [10].

The prevalence of any visual impairment (20/40 or worse in the better eye) was highest in subjects in the OO-I group (18.4%) and lowest in subjects in the YO-I group (7.9%) at the time of the WESDR baseline examination (Table 1). The YO-I group had the highest prevalence (3.2%) of legal blindness (20/200 or worse in the better eye), and the OO-NI group had the lowest (2.3%).

International Textbook of Diabetes Mellitus. Edited by K.G.M.M. Alberti, R.A. DeFronzo, H. Keen and P. Zimmet
© 1992 John Wiley & Sons Ltd

Table 1   Percentage distribution of visual impairment as measured by visual acuity in the better eye by sex in the Wisconsin Epidemiologic Study of Diabetic Retinopathy (WESDR), 1980–82

Group and sex	No.	> 20/40	20/40 to 20/63	20/80 to 20/160	20/200 or worse	Not determined
Younger onset						
Male	512	91.2	3.7	1.6	3.1	0.4
Female	484	92.1	2.9	1.2	3.3	0.4
Total	996	91.7	3.3	1.4	3.2	0.4
Older onset, taking insulin						
Male	321	84.4	9.3	4.4	1.6	0
Female	353	78.8	11.0	6.5	3.7	0
Total	674	81.6	10.2	5.5	2.7	0
Older onset, not taking insulin						
Male	315	89.5	6.0	1.6	2.2	0.6
Female	381	85.8	9.2	2.6	2.4	0
Total	696	87.5	7.8	. 2.2	2.3	0.3

A negative association was found between age at examination and visual function (Tables 2–4). Legal blindness was not found in subjects younger than 25 years of age (Table 2). The frequency of legal blindness increased with age in both males and females, reaching peaks of 13% and 20% respectively in the YO-I group. Similarly, a strong association between increasing age and prevalence of visual impairment was found in older onset patients diagnosed to have diabetes after age 30 (Tables 3 and 4). Age-specific prevalence of visual impairment was generally higher in people in the OO-I group compared with those in the OO-NI group. The higher prevalence of legal blindness found for females compared with males in both the WESDR older-onset groups has also been described for other diabetic and non-diabetic populations [3, 5, 8]. It may reflect a higher survival rate of visually impaired females compared with visually impaired males.

Age-specific prevalence of legal blindness was found to be significantly higher in diabetic than in non-diabetic subjects (Figure 1) [3]. The frequency of blindness was higher in younger-onset diabetic subjects than in older-onset subjects. In older-onset diabetic participants, the prevalence of blindness increased with increasing current age, but was nearly parallel to the prevalence in non-diabetic people until about 70 years of age.

Table 2   Percentage distribution of visual impairment as measured by visual acuity in the better eye by sex and age at examination in younger-onset diabetic patients in the WESDR, 1980–82

Age at examination (years)	No.	> 20/40	20/40 to 20/63	20/80 to 20/160	20/200 or worse	Not determined
Males						
0–17	110	96.4	1.8	0	0	1.8
18–24	113	96.5	2.7	0.9	0	0
25–34	151	91.4	3.3	2.0	3.3	0
35–44	71	87.3	1.4	4.2	7.0	0
45–54	39	76.9	7.7	2.6	12.8	0
55+	28	78.6	17.9	0	3.6	0
Total	512	91.2	3.7	1.6	3.1	0.4
Females						
0–17	87	97.7	2.3	0	0	0
18–24	123	95.1	3.3	1.6	0	0
25–34	138	94.2	2.2	0.7	2.9	0
35–44	66	89.4	1.5	3.0	4.5	1.5
45–54	40	82.5	7.5	0	7.5	2.5
55+	30	73.3	3.3	3.3	20.0	0
Total	484	92.1	2.9	1.2	3.3	0.4

From reference 3, reproduced with permission from *Ophthalmology*.

Table 3 Percentage distribution of visual impairment as measured by visual acuity in the better eye by sex and age at examination in older-onset diabetic patients taking insulin in the WESDR, 1980–82

Age at examination (years)	No.	> 20/40	20/40 to 20/63	20/80 to 20/60	20/200 or worse
Males					
30–44	14	100.0	0	0	0
45–54	48	97.9	0	0	2.1
55–64	92	93.5	3.3	3.3	0
65–74	108	87.0	10.2	2.8	0
75–84	44	63.6	15.9	13.6	6.8
85+	15	20.0	60.0	13.3	6.7
Total	321	84.7	9.3	4.4	1.6
Females					
30–44	14	100.0	0	0	0
45–54	53	92.5	7.5	0	0
55–64	85	88.2	3.5	4.7	3.5
65–74	129	73.6	14.0	7.0	5.4
75–84	63	65.1	19.0	12.7	3.2
85+	9	44.4	22.2	22.2	11.1
Total	353	78.8	11.0	6.5	3.7

From reference 3, reproduced with permission from *Ophthalmology*.

However, in younger-onset diabetic people, the frequency of legal blindness increased dramatically after 25 years of age.

Visual impairment was also found to be strongly associated with increasing duration of diabetes (Figures 2 and 3) and increasing severity of retinopathy (Tables 5 and 6) in the younger-onset and older-onset groups with diabetes at the time of the WESDR baseline examination [3]. In the younger-onset group, after 30 years of diabetes, 22% of the population had some degree of visual impairment. In this group, legal blindness was first found to begin with persons with 15 or more years of diabetes, irrespective of their current age. The proportion legally blind increased from 3% in patients with 15–19 years' duration of diabetes to 12% in people with 30 or more years of diabetes. Older-onset subjects were more likely to have visual impairment and legal blindness earlier in the course of their

Table 4 Percentage distribution of visual impairment as measured by visual acuity in the better eye by sex and age at examination in older-onset diabetic patients not taking insulin in the WESDR, 1980–82

Age at examination (years)	No.	> 20/40	20/40 to 20/63	20/80 to 20/160	20/200 or worse	Not determined
Males						
30–44	8	100.0	0	0	0	0
45–54	34	97.1	0	0	0	2.9
55–64	83	96.4	0	2.4	1.2	0
65–74	112	93.8	4.5	0.9	0.9	0
75–84	66	77.3	15.2	0	6.1	1.5
85+	12	41.7	33.3	16.7	8.3	0
Total	315	89.5	6.0	1.6	2.2	0.6
Females						
30–44	13	100.0	0	0	0	0
45–54	26	88.5	7.7	0	3.8	0
55–64	98	98.0	1.0	1.0	0	0
65–74	119	92.4	5.9	0.8	0.8	0
75–84	97	73.2	17.5	5.2	4.1	0
85+	28	50.0	28.6	10.7	10.7	0
Total	381	85.8	9.2	2.6	2.4	0

From reference 3, reproduced with permission from *Ophthalmology*.

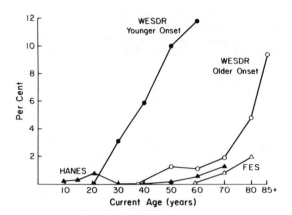

Figure 1 Percentage of subjects with visual acuity of 20/200 or worse in the better eye in the Wisconsin Epidemiologic Study of Diabetic Retinopathy (WESDR), in the Health and Nutrition Examination Survey (HANES) and in the Framingham Eye Study (FES) by current age (reprinted with permission from Klein R, Klein BEK, Moss SE. Visual impairment in diabetes. *Ophthalmology* 1984; 91: 1–9)

diabetes, but the frequencies were lower after 15 or more years of diabetes than in younger-onset persons. Both increasing current age as well as increasing duration of diabetes were associated with an increased risk of legal blindness in the older-onset groups.

Although the overall frequency of legal blindness was highest in insulin dependent younger-onset persons, the actual number of diabetic

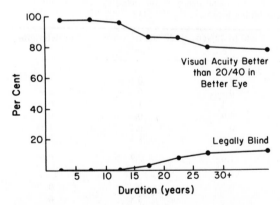

Figure 2 Percentage of insulin-taking subjects diagnosed to have diabetes before 30 years of age who participated in the WESDR baseline examination, with visual acuity of 20/40 or better, and of those with legal blindness, by duration of diabetes (reprinted with permission from Klein R, Klein BEK, Moss SE. Visual impairment in diabetes. *Ophthalmology* 1984; 91: 1–9)

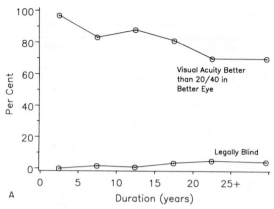

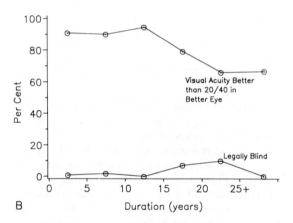

Figure 3 Percentage of subjects diagnosed to have diabetes after 29 years of age who participated in the WESDR baseline examination, with visual acuity of 20/40 or better, and of those with legal blindness, by duration of diabetes. (A) Taking insulin. (B) Not taking insulin

subjects in the WESDR population who were legally blind was highest in the older-onset groups. In the WESDR population, there were 41 older-onset persons taking insulin, 45 older-onset persons not taking insulin and 32 younger-onset persons who were legally blind. These data emphasize the need for ophthalmologic care for the large number of visually impaired, older-onset diabetic patients.

Few population-based prevalence data are available for comparison with data from the WESDR. The proportions of blindness reported in the WESDR are significantly higher than those reported in the 1976 National Health Interview Survey (NHIS) [4]. Visual impairment in that study was determined by the self-reported 'inability to read a newspaper', and the presence

Table 5 Percentage distribution of visual function by severity of retinopathy in the right eye of younger-onset diabetic subjects in the WESDR

Retinopathy status (right eye)	No.	Visual function				
		> 20/40	20/40 to 20/63	20/80 to 20/160	20/200 or worse	Not determined
No retinopathy (level 1)	337	96	2	1	0	1
Non-proliferative						
Early (levels 1.5–3)	309	96	3	1	0	0
Moderate to severe (levels 4–5)	161	94	4	2	0	0
Proliferative						
No DRS HRC* (levels 6–6.5)	117	72	9	4	15	0
DRS HRC						
level 7	35	57	11	9	23	0
Severe (level 8)	29	0	0	0	100	3
Not determined	8	0	0	0	100	0

*Diabetic Retinopathy Study high-risk characteristics for severe visual loss.
From reference 3, published with the permission of *Ophthalmology*.

and duration of diabetes was determined by self-reported physician's diagnosis of diabetes and the year of diagnosis. In a population-based study in Poole, England, Houston reported higher overall proportions of visual impairment (13%—20/40 or worse in the better eye) and legal blindness (1%), in non-insulin treated diabetic patients than in those treated with insulin, of whom 9% had visual impairment and 1% had severe visual impairment [16]. These acuities were 'corrected' only using a pinhole, and therefore might overestimate the degree of

impairment. On the basis of an earlier survey of registered blind people in England and Wales, Caird et al [12] reported that 2.8% of persons with diabetes were legally blind. Overall prevalence of blindness in the Danish population has been estimated by Nielsen to be between 0.3% and 0.5% [17]. Accurate population-based data on best corrected visual acuity in diabetic patients are needed to plan for future health care delivery. Longitudinal data are needed over time to assess the impact of new therapeutic and intervention strategies.

Table 6 Percentage distribution of visual function by severity of retinopathy in the right eye of older-onset diabetic subjects in the WESDR (1980–1982)

Retinopathy status (right eye)	No.	Visual function				
		> 20/40	20/40 to 20/63	20/80 to 20/160	20/200 or worse	Not determined
No retinopathy (level 1)	712	81	12	3	3	0
Non-proliferative						
Early (levels 1.5–3)	351	77	14	4	5	0
Moderate to severe (levels 4–5)	192	67	18	10	5	0
Proliferative						
No DRS HRC* (levels 6–6.5)	60	40	20	15	23	2
DRS HRC						
Level 7	16	37	25	19	19	0
Severe (level 8)	11	0	0	0	100	0
Not determined	28	0	7	7	86	0

*Diabetic Retinopathy Study high-risk characteristics for severe visual loss.
From reference 3, published with permission of *Ophthalmology*.

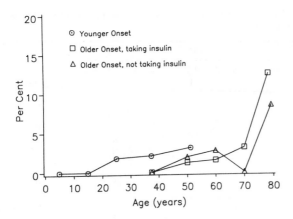

Figure 4 Four-year incidence of legal blindness (visual acuity 20/200 or worse in the better eye) in younger-onset patients taking insulin, older-onset patients taking insulin and older-onset patient not taking insulin, who participated in the WESDR

Incidence

Even fewer population-based data are available describing the incidence of visual impairment in diabetes [6, 18–21]. Reliable data are important for projecting needs for services and costs, assessing the impact of treatment, and defining etiologic relationships.

In the WESDR, the 4-year incidence of blindness was 1.5%, 3.2% and 2.7% in YO-I, OO-I and OO-NI groups, respectively [18]. On the basis of an estimated total of 113 new cases of blindness in 4 years among all diabetic patients in the study area (general population of 851 400), the annual incidence of blindness due to diabetes was calculated to be 3.3 per 100 000 population.

In the WESDR, the incidence of blindness increased with greater age at the baseline visit (Figure 4), increasing severity of diabetic retinopathy (Table 7) and poorer visual acuity at the baseline examination (Figure 5) in all three groups [18]. Increasing risk of blindness was also found with increasing durations of diabetes in both groups taking insulin (Table 8). In this study, progression of visual impairment, as measured by doubling of the visual angle (for example, changing from 20/20 to 20/40 or from 20/50 to 20/100), was associated with greater age at the time of the baseline examination, more severe retinopathy (Figure 6), and presence of macular edema in the three groups (Figure 7). It was also associated with longer duration of

diabetes, higher glycated hemoglobin levels, and presence of proteinuria in younger-onset and older-onset diabetic subjects taking insulin.

The 4-year incidence of legal blindness, as reported in the WESDR, is comparable to that reported by Caird et al [12]. Using data from the Radcliffe Infirmary in England, they estimated 5-year blindness rates of 2.4% and 2.0% in younger-onset and older-onset patients, respectively. The WESDR rates are higher than those reported by others using Model Reporting Area (MRA) data collected in 1970 [22]. On the basis of those data, annual incidence rates of blindness attributable at least in part to diabetes have been estimated to be 1.6–2.1 per 100 000 persons in the general population. Higher rates of blindness than those found in the WESDR have previously been reported by Nielsen [19, 20]. He reported a 1-year incidence rate of legal blindness (defined as a best corrected visual acuity of 20/200 or poorer in the better eye or visual angle of less than 20° in the better eye) of 3.7% in people with insulin dependent diabetes mellitus (IDDM) and 1.9% in people with non-insulin dependent diabetes mellitus (NIDDM) living on the Danish island of Falster. Dwyer et al [21] reported a lower rate in the population-based study of diabetic persons in Rochester, Minnesota, who had up to 20 years of follow-up. Among those who were not blind at the time of their diagnosis of diabetes, the cumulative incidence of subsequent bilateral blindness was 8.2%. Sjolie reported an annual incidence rate of blindness and/or death of 1% in younger-onset IDDM patients in Denmark [6].

Variations of reported incidence among populations may be due to differences in the time of the studies, composition of the populations, definitions of diabetes and blindness, measurement techniques to determine visual acuity, and availability of treatment regimens such as photocoagulation and other surgical and ocular interventions for retinopathy, cataracts and glaucoma.

CAUSES OF BLINDNESS AND VISUAL IMPAIRMENT

In the WESDR, diabetic retinopathy was the sole or contributing cause of visual acuity of 20/200 or worse vision in about 87% of eyes in younger-onset diabetic patients and 33% of eyes in older-onset patients [3]. The

Table 7 Four-year incidence of blindness in the right eye by retinopathy level at the baseline examination in the WESDR

| Baseline retinopathy level in the right eye* | Younger onset | | Older onset | | | |
| | No. | % | Taking insulin | | Not taking insulin | |
			No.	%	No.	%
1	307	0.3	178	4.5	343	3.2
1.5–2	166	0.6	65	3.1	65	4.6
3	119	2.5	67	10.4	33	6.1
4	133	4.5	102	12.7	33	24.2
5	3	0	4	0	0	–
6	96	6.2	31	6.5	2	–
7	21	23.8	4	0	1	–

*See reference 18 for definition of retinopathy levels. In brief, 1 = no retinopathy; 1.5–3 = early non-proliferative retinopathy; 4–5 = moderate to severe non-proliferative retinopathy; 6–7 = proliferative retinopathy.

lower rate of blindness attributable to retinopathy in the older-onset group was due to relatively higher frequencies of cataract, glaucoma and age-related macular degeneration in the older-onset patients. Houston reported that in Poole, England, retinopathy was the primary cause of visual disability in both insulin users and those not using insulin who were under 70 years of age; in those over 70 years of age, visual disability was primarily due to cataract [16].

The severity of retinopathy was also an important predictor of the 4-year incidence of visual loss in the YO-I, OO-I and OO-NI groups in the WESDR (Figure 6) [18]. It has been shown in the DRS that 25% of eyes with prolifer-

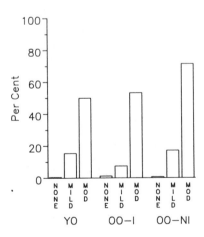

Figure 5 Four-year incidence of legal blindness in the WESDR by visual impairment status at the baseline examination (NONE, better than 20/40; MILD, 20/40 to 20/63; MOD, 20/80 to 20/160) in younger-onset patients taking insulin (YO), older-onset patients taking insulin (OO-I) and older-onset patients not taking insulin (OO-NI)

ative disease—characterized by new vessels at the optic disk, equalling or exceeding one-third of the disk area in extent; new vessels at the disk less than one-third of the disk area in extent, and preretinal or vitreous hemorrhage; and/or new vessels elsewhere associated with preretinal or vitreous hemorrhage—developed severe visual loss of 5/200 or worse over a 2-year period. The presence of macular edema was also positively associated with the prevalence and incidence of visual impairment in the WESDR (Figure 7) [3, 18]. In the presence of macular edema, older-onset WESDR participants were more likely to lose vision than were younger-onset WESDR participants with macular edema [18]. The ETDRS findings showed that 30% of eyes with clinically significant macular edema had deterioration of their visual acuity (manifested as doubling of the visual angle, for example 20/20 to 20/40 or 20/40 to 20/80) over a 3-year period [10].

OTHER FORMS OF VISUAL IMPAIRMENT

Although visual acuity is the usual definition of visual impairment, diabetic patients often develop other visual abnormalities. Before the development of retinopathy, disturbances in yellow–blue hue discrimination may be detected [23]. With the development of macular edema or ischemia, further deterioration in color vision is found [24]. This has important therapeutic significance for patients using test strips for either urine glucose testing [25] or home blood glucose monitoring [26], who must correctly interpret the test results.

Glare may be a problem for people with cataracts or blood in the vitreous, which causes

Table 8 Four-year incidence of blindness by duration of diabetes at the baseline examination in the WESDR

Baseline duration (yr)	Younger onset No. of participants (%)	Older onset	
		Taking insulin No. of participants (%)	Not taking insulin No. of participants (%)
0–4	157 (0)	78 (0)	204 (2.9)
5–9	232 (0)	83 (3.6)	151 (2.0)
10–14	162 (1.2)	78 (2.6)	54 (1.9)
15–19	117 (5.1)	106 (3.8)	54 (5.6)
20–24	73 (2.7)	75 (2.7)	27*(0*)
25–29	61 (4.9)	28 (10.7)	
30+	66 (0)	17 (5.9)	
$\rho^\dagger$	< 0.005	0.056	0.93

*Sample size and rate for duration of diabetes of 20 years or more.
†Based on a test for trend.
From reference 18, published with permission of *Ophthalmology*.

light to scatter [27]. This is particularly troublesome in brightly lit environments. Special polarizing filters in glasses are now available to minimize this problem.

Diabetic patients have reported numerous visual complaints after panretinal photocoagulation treatment [27]. These complaints include difficulty in adjusting to bright or dim lighting, trouble in distinguishing among dark colors, and problems judging distance and avoiding obstacles. Most of these disturbances were not related to the visual acuity after treatment.

PROGNOSIS

Visual impairment has been reported to be a significant predictor of mortality in the diabetic population. Berkow et al [28], in a review of a series of 180 blind diabetic patients who had received guide dogs, found that they lived for only 5.8 years, on the average, from the onset of blindness. In a prospective study of 709 patients taking insulin, diagnosed before 50 years of age and followed for 5–13 years, Davis et al [29] found that the 7-year survival rate was only 40% in those legally blind compared with 80% in those with no visual impairment in either eye at the baseline. Whereas visual impairment in the above studies was associated with severe diabetic retinopathy, a recent report by Podgor et al [30] described decreased survival in the presence of cataract in older-onset diabetic patients studied in the Framingham Eye Study. In the WESDR, after adjusting for age and sex, younger-onset patients who were legally blind at the baseline examination were 1.7 times more likely to die over a 6-year period than patients with no visual

impairment; for older-onset patients the rate ratio was 1.4 [31].

Ocular complications of diabetes are important predictors of poorer survival because of their strong association with risk factors for other systemic complications and with the factors that may themselves be the reason for death. These data suggest the need for close surveillance of all diabetic patients with ocular complications or visual impairment, because aggressive therapy for early renal disease, elevated blood pressure or cardiovascular disease may prolong life.

There is controversy over provision of renal dialysis for diabetic patients with end-stage renal disease [32, 33]. Blindness has been given as a reason for not offering dialysis to such patients; but Flynn recently demonstrated that motivated blind diabetic patients, after receiving training, were more successful than sighted diabetics in long-term maintenance of continuous ambulatory peritoneal dialysis [34].

PREVENTIVE STRATEGIES

As yet, there is no known medical therapeutic intervention that has been shown to prevent visual loss in persons with diabetes [35]. Although there is evidence suggestive of a relationship between control of blood pressure and blood glucose and progression of retinopathy, as yet there is no evidence from clinical trials of a beneficial effect from modifying these risk factors. It is hoped that more definitive therapeutic guidelines on the efficacy of tight metabolic control for preventing or reducing the progression of diabetic retinopathy will evolve

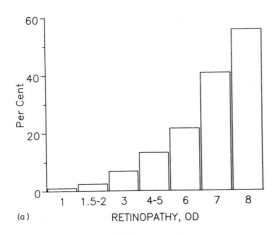

(a)

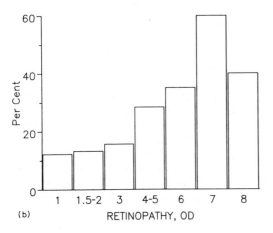

(b)

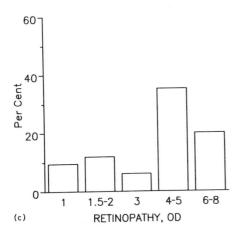

(c)

when data become available from two long-term, multicentered clinical trails—the Diabetes Control and Complications Trial [36] and the United Kingdom Prospective Diabetes Trial [37].

Findings from two other controlled clinical trials show that timely photocoagulation can reduce visual loss caused by diabetic retinopathy [9, 10]. The risk of severe visual impairment in eyes treated with panretinal photocoagulation for proliferative retinopathy was less than one-half that in untreated control eyes in the DRS [9]. In the ETDRS, after 36 months of follow-up, 12% of eyes with clinically significant macular edema assigned to immediate treatment had lost three or more lines of vision (for example, from 20/20 to 20/40 or 20/50 to 20/100) compared with 24% of eyes assigned to the control group [10].

Findings from the Diabetic Retinopathy Vitrectomy Study suggest that there is an advantage in earlier vitrectomy (within 3–6 months) in eyes with severe vitreous hemorrhage and decreased vision in younger-onset IDDM patients [38]. On the other hand, there is no advantage in early (less than 1 year) vitreous surgery for eyes of older-onset patients with decrease in vision due to vitreous hemorrhage.

On the basis of the findings from the DRS and ETDRS, several treatment recommendations have been made which, if followed, would be expected to lead to a decrease in the incidence of visual impairment due to diabetic retinopathy.

Recent studies suggest that several factors may limit physician and patient compliance with the recommendations from the DRS and

Figure 6 Four-year rate of doubling of the visual angle (for example, going from a visual acuity of 20/20 to 20/40, or from 20/40 to 20/80) by retinopathy severity level at the baseline examination (1, none; 1.5–2, retinal microaneurysms or blot hemorrhages only; 3, retinal microaneurysms and/or blot hemorrhages with hard exudate; 4–5, moderate to severe non-proliferative retinopathy consisting of retinal microaneurysms with cotton-wool spots and/or intraretinal microvascular abnormalities and/or venous beading and/or large blot hemorrhages; 6, proliferative retinopathy without DRS high-risk characteristics for severe visual loss; 7, proliferative retinopathy with DRS high-risk characteristics; 8, proliferative retinopathy which has caused severe loss of vision) in three groups (A, younger-onset patients; B, older-onset patients taking insulin; C, older-onset patients not taking insulin) who participated in the WESDR

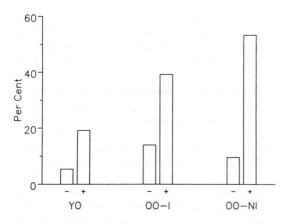

Figure 7 Four-year rate of doubling of the visual angle by presence (+) or absence (−) of macular edema by three groups: younger-onset group taking insulin (YO); older-onset group taking insulin (OO-I), and older-onset group not taking insulin (OO-NI), who participated in the WESDR

ETDRS [39]. First, retinopathy may go undetected: in the WESDR, only 33% of participants with retinopathy were aware of it [40]. Because diabetic retinopathy is usually asymptomatic, its detection by primary care physicians has required ophthalmoscopic examination. Without pupil dilation, trained examiners using direct ophthalmoscopy will miss 50% of cases of proliferative retinopathy [41]. Although 80% of primary-care physicians performed direct ophthalmoscopic examinations of their diabetic patients over a 12-month period, fewer than 1% dilated their patients' pupils before ophthalmoscopy [39]. Even under optimal conditions of examination through a dilated pupil, error rates of 74% for detection of retinopathy by internists and residents have been reported [42]. In addition, internists missed 52% of the diagnoses of proliferative disease, compared with general ophthalmologists, who missed 9%, and retinal specialists, who did not miss any. There are no data available on the ability of primary-care physicians and other non-ophthalmologists to detect clinically significant macular edema. For these reasons, the American Diabetes Association, the state of Kentucky, the American Academy of Ophthalmology and the Centers for Disease Control have developed a series of recommendations for eye care for diabetic patients [39]. All these programs suggest that it is important that the primary-care physician inform the patient at the time of diagnosis of diabetes that ocular

complications are associated with diabetes and may threaten sight, and that timely detection and treatment may reduce the risk of decreased vision. All diabetic patients 10–30 years old who have more than 5 years' duration of diabetes, and all diabetic patients diagnosed after 30 years of age, at the time of diagnosis of diabetes, should be referred to an eye specialist competent to detect retinopathy by examination through dilated pupils. All patients found to have reduced corrected visual acuity, elevated intraocular pressure or any other vision-threatening ocular abnormalities should be referred to an ophthalmologist with an interest in diabetic eye disease.

Unfortunately, a significant proportion of diabetic persons with vision-threatening eye disease have not been examined by an ophthalmologist [43]. In the WESDR, 34% of persons with either proliferative diabetic retinopathy with DRS high-risk characteristics for severe visual loss or clinically significant macular edema had not been seen by an ophthalmologist. The reasons for not having an ophthalmologic examination have been attributed to cost of examination, distance from an ophthalmologist, personal factors such as denial of a problem, dislike of bright lights and dilation, feelings that care by the primary-care physician or optometrist is adequate, or failure to be told by their doctor of the benefits or need for ophthalmologic care. This problem is exacerbated by living in rural areas where ophthalmologic care is not available [39]. In the USA, the Centers for Disease Control are currently evaluating various screening strategies designed to detect, refer and treat in a timely fashion patients with ocular complications associated with diabetes, so as to prevent visual loss. These programs involve education of both primary-care physicians and patients, and the use of trained non-ophthalmological examiners and/or evaluation of fundus photographs taken with a non-mydriatic camera. Data to demonstrate the efficacy of such programs are not yet available.

REHABILITATION

One of the more important, but often neglected, components of care for the diabetic person with visual impairment is rehabilitation. Visual impairment in diabetes may vary from minimal changes in color vision to total blindness, and often includes periods of rapid or slow progression with changes in vision due to recurrent vitreous hemorrhage and macular edema. Visually impaired diabetic patients on insulin therapy are confronted with the problems of identification of the type of insulin, determination of the amount of insulin in the vial, measurement of dose and location of injection sites. In addition, they are responsible for monitoring glucose levels using urine or blood test strips, daily foot care and other activities of daily living. Besides visual loss, many of these people are often quite ill with neuropathy, amputations, and renal and cardiovascular disease. They are often without adequate financial support. They face losing, or have lost, the ability to control their lives and have concerns about being burdensome to others. These problems usually lead to anxiety, guilt, anger, loss of self-esteem and difficulties in social adjustment.

In order to cope with these profound lifestyle changes, support systems are necessary, and often involve family members or friends and neighbors. However, in one study, only 51.2% of interviewed people with diabetes (none of whom was as yet legally blind) were found to have adequate support systems [44]. It is for these reasons that successful rehabilitation involves a team approach, consisting of social workers, psychologists, orientation and mobility instructors, and rehabilitation teachers, who are aware of the numerous, but specific, problems faced by the visually impaired person with diabetes. Depending on the degree of visual impairment, supportive rehabilitative services, including low-vision clinics, state vocational rehabilitation centers and schools for the blind, are available. Devices such as syringe magnifiers, dosage guides, needle guides, and vial and/or syringe holders may help improve insulin administration [7, 45]. In addition, the teaching of braille to the blind, although difficult in the tactilely impaired diabetic person, has been suggested in some cases. Helping the patient accept visual loss is probably the most important step in planning living arrangements and in developing coping strategies.

Acknowledgments

The authors are grateful to their collaborators, Barbara E.K. Klein, MD, MPH, Matthew D. Davis, MD, and David L. DeMets, PhD, and to Jean Espenshade, RN, PhD, and Polly Newcomb, PhD, who provided consultation and criticism.

The work was supported by grant EY 03083 (Dr R. Klein) from the National Eye Institute.

REFERENCES

1. Klein R, Klein BE. Vision disorders in diabetes. In Harris MI, Hamman RF (eds) Diabetes data compiled 1984. Washington, DC: US Government Printing Service, 1985: pp XIII, 1–36.
2. Palmberg PF. Diabetic retinopathy. Diabetes 1977; 26: 703–9.
3. Klein R, Klein BEK, Moss SE. Visual impairment in diabetes. Ophthalmology 1984; 91: 1–9.
4. Howie LJ, Drury TF. Current estimates from the Health Interview Survey: United States 1977. Vital Health Stat (10) 1978; no. 126.
5. Leibowitz HM, Krueger DE, Maunder LR et al. The Framingham Eye Study monograph. An ophthalmological and epidemiological study of cataract, glaucoma, diabetic retinopathy, macular degeneration and visual acuity in a general population of 2631 adults, 1973–1975. Surv Ophthalmol 1980; 24 (suppl.): 335–610.
6. Sjolie AK. Ocular complications in insulin treated diabetes mellitus. An epidemiological study. Acta Ophthalmol 1985; suppl. 172: 1–77.
7. Sorsby A. The incidence and causes of blindness in England and Wales 1948–1962. Reports on Public Health and Medical Subjects 114. London: HMSO, 1966.
8. Kahn HA, Hiller R. Blindness caused by diabetic retinopathy. Am J Ophthalmol 1974; 78: 58–67.
9. Diabetic Retinopathy Study Group. Photocoagulation treatment of proliferative diabetic retinopathy: clinical application of diabetic retinopathy study (DRS) findings (DRS Report 8). Ophthalmology 1981; 88: 583–600.
10. Early Treatment Diabetic Retinopathy Study Research Group. Photocoagulation for diabetic macular edema (Early Treatment Diabetic Retinopathy Study Report 1). Arch Ophthalmol 1985; 103: 1796–806.
11. Beetham WP. Visual prognosis of proliferating diabetic retinopathy. Br J Ophthalmol 1963; 47: 611–19.
12. Caird FI, Burditt AF, Draper GJ. Diabetic retinopathy: a further study of prognosis for vision. Diabetes 1968; 17: 121–3.
13. Aiello LM, Rand LI, Briones JC et al. Diabetic retinopathy in Joslin Clinic patients with adult onset diabetes. Ophthalmology 1981; 88: 619–23.
14. Klein R, Klein BEK, Moss SE et al. The Wisconsin

Epidemiologic Study of Diabetic Retinopathy. 2. Prevalence and risk of diabetic retinopathy when age at diagnosis is less than 30 years. Arch Ophthalmol 1984; 102: 520–6.

15. Klein R, Klein BEK, Moss SE et al. The Wisconsin Epidemiologic Study of Diabetic Retinopathy. 3. Prevalence and risk of diabetic retinopathy when age at diagnosis is 30 or more years. Arch Ophthalmol 1984; 102: 527–32.

16. Houston A. Retinopathy in the Poole area: an epidemiological inquiry. In Eschwège E (ed.) Advances in diabetes epidemiology. INSERM Symposium no. 22. Amsterdam: Elsevier, 1982: pp 199–206.

17. Nielsen NV. The prevalence and causes of impaired vision in diabetics. Acta Ophthalmol 1982; 60: 677–91.

18. Moss SE, Klein R, Klein BEK. The incidence of vision loss in a diabetic population. Ophthalmology 1988; 95: 1340–8.

19. Nielsen NV. Diabetic retinopathy. I. The cause of retinopathy in insulin treated diabetics. A one-year epidemiological cohort study of diabetes mellitus. The Island of Falster, Denmark. Acta Ophthalmol 1984; 62: 256–65.

20. Nielsen NV. Diabetic retinopathy. II. The cause of retinopathy in diabetics treated with oral hypoglycemic agents and diet regime alone. A one-year epidemiological cohort study of diabetes mellitus. The Island of Falster, Denmark. Acta Ophthalmol 1984; 62: 266–73.

21. Dwyer MS, Melton LJ III, Ballard DJ et al. Incidence of diabetic retinopathy and blindness: a population-based study in Rochester, Minnesota. Diabetes Care 1985; 8: 316–22.

22. Operational Research Department, National Society to Prevent Blindness. Vision problems in the US: a statistical analysis. New York: National Society to Prevent Blindness, 1980: pp 1–46.

23. Kinnear PR, Aspinall PA, Lakowski R. The diabetic eye and colour vision. Trans Ophthalmol Soc UK 1972; 92: 69–78.

24. Adams AJ, Zisman F, Ali E et al. Macular edema reduces B cone sensitivity in diabetics. Appl Optics 1987; 26: 1455–7.

25. Bresnick GH, Groo A, Palta M et al. Urinary glucose testing inaccuracies among diabetic patients. Effect of acquired color vision deficiency caused by diabetic retinopathy. Arch Ophthalmol 1984; 102: 1489–96.

26. Zisman F, Adams AJ, Linfoot J et al. Diabetic blood glucose monitoring: influence of color deficiencies (abstr). Invest Ophthalmol Vis Sci 1984; 25 (suppl.): 178.

27. Russell PW, Sekuler R, Fetenhour C. Visual function after panretinal photocoagulation: a survey. Diabetes Care 1985; 8: 57–63.

28. Berkow JW, Shugarman RG, Maumenee AE et al. A retrospective study of blind diabetic patients. JAMA 1965; 193: 867–70.

29. Davis MD, Hiller R, Magli YLM et al. Prognosis for life in patients with diabetes: relation to severity of retinopathy. Trans Am Ophthalmol Soc 1979; 77: 144–70.

30. Podgor MJ, Cassel GN, Kannel WB. Lens changes and survival in a population-based study. New Eng J Med 1985; 313: 1438–44.

31. Klein R, Moss SE, Klein BEK et al. The relation of ocular and systemic factors to survival in diabetes. Arch Intern Med 1989; 149: 266–72.

32. Medical Services Study Group of the Royal College of Physicians. Deaths from chronic renal failure under age 50. Br Med J 1981; 283: 283–6.

33. Audit in renal failure: the wrong target? Br Med J 1981; 283: 261–2.

34. Flynn CT. Why blind diabetics with renal failure should be offered treatment. Br Med J 1983; 287: 1177–8.

35. Klein R. Recent developments in the understanding and management of diabetic retinopathy. Med Clin North Am 1988; 72: 1415–37.

36. DCCT Research Group. The Diabetes Control and Complications Trial (DCCT). Design and methological considerations for the feasibility phase. Diabetes 1986; 35: 530–45.

37. Kohner EM, Aldington SJ, Nugent Z. Retinopathy at entry in the United Kingdom Prospective Diabetes Study (UKPDS) of maturity onset diabetes. Diabetes 1987; 36 (suppl. 1): 42A.

38. Diabetic Retinopathy Vitrectomy Study Research Group. Early vitrectomy for severe vitreous hemorrhage in diabetic retinopathy. Two-year results of a randomized trial. Diabetic Retinopathy Vitrectomy Study Report 2. Arch Ophthalmol 1985; 103: 1644–52.

39. Klein R, Moss SE, Klein BEK. New management concepts for timely diagnosis of diabetic retinopathy treatable by photocoagulation. Diabetes Care 1987; 10: 633–8.

40. Klein R, Klein BEK, Moss SE et al. The validity of a survey question to study diabetic retinopathy. Am J Epidemiol 1986; 124: 104–10.

41. Klein R, Klein BEK, Neider MW et al. Diabetic retinopathy as detected using ophthalmoscopy, a nonmydriatic camera, and a standard fundus camera. Ophthalmology 1985; 92: 485–91.

42. Sussman EJ, Tsiaras WG, Soper KA. Diagnosis of diabetic eye disease. JAMA 1982; 247: 3231–4.

43. Witkin SR, Klein R. Ophthalmologic care of persons with diabetes. JAMA 1984; 251: 2534–7.

44. Bluhm HP, Stone JB. Diabetic retinopathy patients: characteristics and rehabilitation implications. J Rehabil 1983; 49: 50–3.

45. Herget M. For visually impaired diabetics. Am J Nursing 1983; 6: 1557–60.

59
Diabetic Neuropathy

J.D. Ward

Royal Hallamshire Hospital, Sheffield, UK

Peripheral and autonomic nerves are significantly affected by the abnormal metabolism of diabetes mellitus, resulting in pathological change, functional disturbance and clinical morbidity. Unfortunately, in humans, it is not always possible to relate these three features accurately, and in trying to understand the basic mechanisms underlying 'diabetic neuropathy' it must be stressed that the bulk of our knowledge is based on work in experimental animals. The clinical features are varied and it is correct to refer to the *diabetic neuropathies*, whereas most of the animal work is reported as if only one 'clinical state' existed—indeed, detailed descriptions of the effects of nerve damage in animals are very limited. It may well be that each human clinical syndrome, while being related to a common aetiology, is finally caused by different factors. Only clinical observation will answer this question.

In this chapter the following major topics are reviewed:

(1) Histopathological changes observed in animals and humans,
(2) The biochemical pathways thought to be central to nerve damage—the sorbitol–myo-inositol–Na^+-K^+ATPase cycle, and the relationship to the enzyme aldose reductase,
(3) The role of microvascular changes in nerve disease,
(4) The physiological measurements that are available to assess nerve function and their relationship to natural history and clinical syndromes,
(5) A description of the clinical features of the peripheral neuropathies and their treatment —especially pain:
    So far it is somatic peripheral nerves that have been considered; however, they contain autonomic fibres and there is always an element of autonomic dysfunction in primarily somatic clinical syndromes,
(6) A review of autonomic function tests—both parasympathetic and sympathetic,
(7) A description of clinical autonomic neuropathy and its treatment,
(8) The distressing condition of impotence is also considered,
(9) Other topics include glycation of nerve proteins, autoimmune factors, mechanisms of pain, ischaemic resistance of diabetic nerve, and the abnormalities of blood flow related to neuropathy.

Attempts should be made to provide a definition of diabetic neuropathy—no easy task in view of the varied aetiological and clinical presentations. However, a standardized definition would enable more accurate assessment of natural history and therapeutic intervention.

International Textbook of Diabetes Mellitus. Edited by K.G.M.M. Alberti, R.A. DeFronzo, H. Keen and P. Zimmet
© 1992 John Wiley & Sons Ltd

HISTOPATHOLOGICAL CHANGE

Much of the reported pathological change in diabetic peripheral nerve is from animals— streptozotocin-induced diabetic rats or genetically diabetic Bio-Breeding (BB) rats. Although some changes seen in these animals are also reported in humans [1], great care must be exercised because other diabetic animals show quite different changes. The Chinese hamster, although having delayed conduction velocities, does not show much pathological change [2]; in diabetic dogs there are no changes in proximal nerves whereas segmental demyelination and axonal degeneration are present in the plantar nerves [3], suggesting a distal axonopathy as in humans, where many clinical effects are seen peripherally.

In human studies many morphological changes are observed and are often given different emphasis by different workers, suggesting that patient selection, age and site of biopsy may influence the exact type of lesion observed. Common lesions are axonal degeneration and loss, segmental demyelination and changes in Schwann cells, perineurial cells and endoneurial vessels [4]. There is likely to be a close functional relationship between Schwann cells, myelin and axons; hence segmental demyelination [5] and distal axonal atrophy [6] probably represent either an interrelated disease process or, if one is more prominent than the other, indicate differing primary insults.

As yet it is not possible, from human biopsy material, to correlate specific pathological features with clear-cut clinical syndromes. Indeed, there may be a very great discrepancy between histological change and clinical problems. Even in the absence of any clinical or investigative evidence of neuropathy, segmental demyelination and unmyelinated fibre degeneration with axonal sprouting is observed [7], indicating an active process despite clinical normality.

Although some changes have been described in the spinal cord, it is the peripheral nerves and, to a lesser extent, the nerve roots that are damaged. The more chronic sensorimotor neuropathy exhibits axonal degeneration and regeneration with axonal sprouts [8], while in acute, painful neuropathy small unmyelinated fibre loss is prominent [9]. Small myelinated and unmyelinated fibres are lost in severe neuropathy with marked loss of sensation [10]. Further support

for the dual presence of demyelination and axonal atrophy, but under separate influences, is supplied by the observation of segmental demyelination of fibres immediately proximal to distal axonal degeneration [11].

The major advantage of animal studies is that early in the diabetic state the evolution of structural change may be observed; these are well described by Sima et al [12]. At 3 months in the BB rat, large myelinated fibres show disorientation of neurofilaments, with bundles of neurofilaments in random orientation to the long axis of the axon. Severe axonal changes then progress from the periphery backwards— axonal atrophy and wallerian degeneration. Teased fibre preparations reveal myelin wrinkling and destruction of myelin in places, this spectrum suggesting early disorientation of the axonal cytoskeleton followed by axonal atrophy, degeneration and secondary demyelination. These features certainly bear striking similarities to some of the changes seen in human material from subjects with advanced neuropathy. Quantitative analysis at the same time shows a shift towards smaller-diameter fibres with atrophy of the endoneurial space. Moreover, fibre diameter is decreased over a given internodal length.

Paranodal swelling is also observed in the BB rat [13], and it is possible that this causes persistent nodal deformation and loss of strategic junctional complexes between terminal loops of myelin and the paranodal axolemma—'axoglial dysjunction' [14]—possibly leading to paranodal demyelination, resulting in delayed conduction velocities. It is these changes that appear to be prominent in human tissue as well [1]. Their possible relationship to biochemical mechanisms is discussed later, as are many histopathological features that suggest the role of microvessel disease in nerve damage.

Facts regarding changes in autonomic nerves are essentially descriptive and do little to clarify our understanding of the many abnormalities of function that occur in the autonomic nervous system. Loss of myelinated fibres in the vagus nerve, with enlargement and vacuolation of neurones, confirms severe derangement in subjects with advanced autonomic symptoms [15]. An inflammatory infiltrate has been observed in the ganglia, which is interesting in view of the suggested association between autonomic neuropathy and iritis [16]. For a list of other

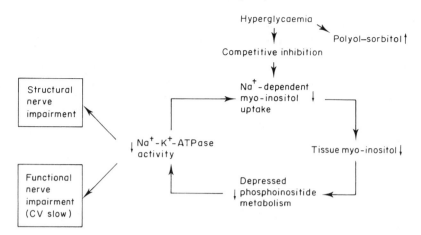

Figure 1 Theoretical link between hyperglycaemia and nerve dysfunction and damage, via sorbitol accumulation, myo-inositol depletion and N^+-K^+-ATPase activity

changes in tissues known to be involved in clinical autonomic syndromes, see reference 17.

BIOCHEMICAL MECHANISMS

Although there is reasonable evidence that in many instances the development of clinical neuropathy is related to the blood glucose level, the exact mechanisms leading to dysfunction or damage are not understood. A considerable amount of evidence, based on animal work, now supplies us with an acceptable theory linking hyperglycaemia, through sorbitol accumulation, myo-inositol depletion and Na^+-K^+-ATPase activity, with nerve dysfunction and damage [18].

Sorbitol accumulates in animal diabetic nerve in direct relationship to blood and nerve glucose. It is the reduction product of glucose through the action of the enzyme aldose reductase with further oxidation to fructose. Intimately related to this glucose-stimulated pathway is the cycle of events outlined in Figure 1. As described later, almost all of these abnormal events are prevented or reversed by control of blood glucose or inhibition of the enzyme aldose reductase. The use of therapeutic agents to block abnormal pathways that may have an important role in pathogenesis, independent of the blood glucose itself, obviously has great potential. As nerve metabolism is not dependent on the presence of insulin or on the actual level of glucose, the reduced energy production of diabetic peripheral nerve

which is attributable to reduced demand, must be mediated through other pathways [19]. Reduced Na^+-K^+-ATPase activity is the primary reason, in that it has been demonstrated that energy utilization in diabetic nerve is limited to the ouabain-inhibited respiratory fraction [20], an indicator of this activity.

The once-held view that sorbitol accumulation led to osmotic change as a cause of dysfunction and damage is unlikely to be correct, if only because of the relatively low concentrations of sorbitol (micromolar rather than millimolar) [21] and the fact that myo-inositol supplementation reverses the effects described in Figure 1 without any change in sorbitol concentration [22].

Impairment of nerve conduction velocity (CV) is a well-established feature of diabetic nerve (animal and human). Simple control of the blood glucose which results in reversal towards normal [23, 24] and such changes are probably related to fluid and electrolyte shifts resulting in a decreased capacity to transmit an applied electrical impulse. However, there are more logical explanations for such changes which are central to the whole modern view of 'metabolic derangement' in diabetic neuropathy. Aldose reductase inhibitors (ARI) administered to either humans or animals result in an improvement in CV [25], at the same time as they prevent depletion of nerve myo-inositol and reduction in Na^+-K^+-ATPase activity [26]. Myo-inositol supplementation also prevents these changes. The assumption, therefore, is that the abnormalities of function observed in all diabetic animals are intimately related to these abnormalities of myo-inositol and Na^+-K^+-ATPase. The use of cultured neuroblastoma cells indicates that intracellular sorbitol, as well as extracellular glucose, may inhibit sodium-dependent myo-inositol uptake [27]. The primary link seems more likely to be Na^+-K^+-ATPase, for myo-inositol feeding also produces improvement despite unchanged sorbitol concentrations, and myo-inositol depletion itself brings about reduced activity [28]. Greene et al have suggested that the pathway in Figure 1 becomes a self-perpetuating cycle that can be reversed only by normalization of blood glucose, dietary supplementation with myo-inositol or blockage of aldose reductase. Another important link may well be through reduced activity of protein kinase C, as this enzyme normalizes the decreased respiratory rate that has been associated with the decreased Na^+-K^+-ATPase activity of diabetic nerve [29]. In other tissues, protein kinase C stimulates Na^+-K^+-ATPase activity [30].

Returning to axoglial dysjunction, there may be an important link between structure, function and these metabolic abnormalities. In the BB rat such axoglial dysjunction is progressive and irreversible in longer-standing diabetes, whereas early reversal of hyperglycaemia prevents the abnormality [31]. Dysjunction improves together with paranodal swelling at the same time as there is improvement in CV and Na^+-K^+-ATPase activity, not only with normalization of blood glucose but also following myo-inositol supplementation or ARI administration [32]. The demonstration that changes do not reverse after longer periods of the diabetic state have important implications for earlier treatment in the human condition. Simple measurements of nerve fibre diameter and the presence of abnormal fibres in teased preparations were also much improved in streptozotocin-induced diabetic rats treated by continuous insulin infusion with an osmotic minipump to produce normoglycaemia [33].

Axonal Transport

Axonal transport of protein in nerve is of fundamental importance. In many toxic and metabolic neuropathies, changes in transport occur even before there are pathological changes in the fibres or clinical abnormality [34]. That such abnormalities are observed in diabetic animals indicates a toxic (endogenous or exogenous) effect of the disease. Transport may be quantitated by the measurement of endogenous proteins following pulse-labelling with radioactive precursors, estimation of the activity of endogenous transmitter enzymes or measurement of labelled proteins transported in a retrograde direction.

Accepting the evidence that many features of diabetic neuropathy are of a 'dying back' nature, then it is significant that there is altered transport in diabetic animals [35, 36]. Anterograde axonal transport provides vital tissue elements synthesized in the perikaryon to the distal axon; such elements comprise individual components differing in constituents and rate of transport. Retrograde transport returns protein constituents back to the head cell for re-use. Slow anterograde transport of axonal enzymes—choline acetyltransferase (CHAT)—and cytoskeletal components are undoubtedly deficient in animal diabetes [37, 38].

There is apparently a link between axonal transport and the myo-inositol pathway, in that the movement of CHAT in the streptozotocin-induced rat is reversed or prevented by administration of ARI agents or myo-inositol feeding of animals [35], although not all transported proteins are similarly affected. Fast anterograde protein transport is unchanged during administration of an ARI [39].

Nerve constriction experiments allow estimates of enzyme activity. In diabetic rats the axonally transported enzyme 6-phosphofructokinase does not accumulate on either side of a constriction; this is reversed by normalization of the blood glucose with insulin but not by an ARI [40]. On the other hand, the inhibition of fast axonal transport of protein, measured by injection of labelled H-leucine, is prevented by ARI, suggesting a further link with myo-inositol and sorbitol. As pressure palsies do occur in human diabetes, these may be prevented by glucose control or use of ARIs, although it is clear that not all aspects of nerve physiology and biochemistry are ameliorated by 'blocking agents'. It has been suggested that a classification of diabetic neuropathy might be based on abnormalities of axonal transport [41].

Other Possible Mechanisms

Numerous abnormalities of lipid chemistry have

been described in diabetic nerve in the last 30 years [42]; although such abnormalities undoubtedly contribute to abnormal function, they do not enhance our understanding of the mechanisms leading to nerve damage.

Similarly, glycation of nerve protein appears to represent a late manifestation of the disease. Long-term exposure of nerve myelin proteins to hyperglycaemia, in vivo and in vitro, leads to the formation of advanced glycation end-products and an alteration in myelin–macrophage interactions. This could serve as an initiating factor in segmental demyelination [43]. The potential role of glycation end-products is mentioned in the section dealing with treatment.

Nerve growth factor (NGF) may have a fundamental role [44, 45]. The retrograde transport of this factor is decreased in the ganglia of nerves known to develop a distal axonopathy, and the pattern of catecholamine fluorescence was found to be reduced in diabetic animal nerves and correlated with immunocytochemical staining for NGF.

Role of Aldose Reductase in Humans

Many of the abnormal pathways described above appear to be controlled by inhibition of the enzyme aldose reductase, although this does not apply to all aspects of axonal transport. Unfortunately, there are as yet few data from humans concerning the presence of these abnormal pathways or their relevance; the little that is available comes from patients with long-standing diabetes and advanced neuropathic syndromes, in contrast to the relatively 'clean' early studies in animals. In the extensive studies of Greene, Lattimer and Sima, in Ann Arbor and Winnipeg, their animal experimental results are supported by similar abnormalities in human tissue [12], although absolute concentrations of polyols are considerably below those of the BB rat. Essentially, sorbitol is increased and myo-inositol decreased. However, in the collection and analysis of human material there are likely to be differences due to variation in the metabolic state at the time of nerve biopsy, or even for some days before. Lack of exact matching of patients with regard to age, duration of diabetes and—more importantly—type of diabetes, make it inevitable that there will be some

variation in results from different centres. In a study of sural nerves biopsied before amputation of an ischaemic leg, concentrations of sorbitol and fructose were significantly higher in diabetic nerve compared with non-diabetic nerve, but concentrations of myo-inositol were not reduced [46] and neuropathy was not present. An earlier study also failed to demonstrate a relationship between polyol abnormalities and neuropathic severity [48]. The site of biopsy may be important, sural nerve being the only nerve available in humans. Returning to animal work, myo-inositol concentration was decreased soon after induction of diabetes and returned to normal after 2 months, and in this tissue sorbitol could not be detected in diabetic or non-diabetic animals [49].

It should be stressed that aldose reductase is a widely distributed enzyme; the more that it can be shown to have pathological relevance in other organs damaged in diabetes, the greater could be the therapeutic impact of its inhibition. The enzyme has now been purified from the testis of non-diabetic BB rats allowing the production of an antibody to it in rabbits, and hence precise tissue localization through immunological techniques [50]. In these animals the enzyme is present in retina and peripheral nerve; in the latter, it is found not only in the paranodal cytoplasm of the Schwann cells but also in the endothelial cells of endoneurial capillaries, suggesting a relationship between these biochemical abnormalities and the known microvascular changes seen in nerve. The classification of the types of aldose reductase is complex, there being three major forms, but they have been shown to be active in red cells, ocular tissue, muscle, brain and aorta [51]. Moreover, endothelial cells from human umbilical cord accumulate more intracellular sorbitol when exposed to high concentrations of glucose [52].

Red cell sorbitol could be used as a marker of the tissue activity of all these pathways. Concentrations in red cells certainly parallel changes in blood glucose [53], and they have been shown to return to non-diabetic levels under the influence of an ARI [54], although no improvement in neurological function was noted. Assuming that the duration of diabetes has no effect on the turnover of sorbitol in red cells, then this measurement may become an important part of the monitoring of long-term prospective treatment studies in diabetic complications.

Clinical Use of Aldose Reductase Inhibitors

As yet there is no convincing proof that the ARIs have any significant effect on established diabetic neuropathy; however, in all studies these agents (and there are at least five drugs actively under investigation) have been given to patients with nerves in a state of advanced damage, perhaps with the initiating biochemical pathways no longer relevant; early long-term prophylactic studies probably are necessary.

In a large number of diabetic subjects without neuropathy, administration of an ARI resulted in a significant improvement in CV—albeit rather small (0.70 m/s for motor nerves and 1.16 m/s for sensory nerves) [55]. A number of studies have been carried out in symptomatic neuropathy. In a double-blind, placebo-controlled crossover study there was improvement in only three measurements (pain, tendon reflexes and sural sensory potential amplitude), while clinical sensory testing seemed to deteriorate [56]. In a totally open-ended anecdotal study there was marked improvement in severe painful symptoms and CVs, which relapsed within days on withdrawal of the drug [57]. This study must be interpreted with great caution but it is a personal impression, reviewing studies of ARIs in established neuropathy, that there is a definite tendency for painful symptoms of relatively short duration to improve, perhaps supporting the view that early intervention (or prophylaxis) is more likely to be beneficial. Of importance in this context is a further study of 22 asymptomatic patients defined as having subclinical neuropathy, in which there was no improvement in either peripheral or autonomic function despite very adequate inhibition of red cell sorbitol by an ARI [58]. Many other trials are also reviewed in this paper [58].

The ARIs are seen by many as a method of treating or preventing a diabetic complication without regard to control of the blood glucose. Further care in interpretation must be exercised. No improvement in CV and symptoms is reported in one study over 4 weeks during which time the glycated haemoglobin was 11–12% [59]—but at what level of blood—nerve glucose concentration in humans is it no longer possible for these agents to exert their effect?

More encouraging results have now been reported by Sima and Greene [12], who carried out a large biochemical and morphological study in humans. Two sural nerve biopsies were performed 1 year apart. At entry to the study 27 subjects underwent biopsy to provide basal biochemical and morphological data, and 16 were biopsied 1 year later at a site on the sural nerve just proximal to that of the first biopsy. It was felt that these subjects were representative on clinical grounds. No significant changes on second biopsy were seen in the placebo group, whereas in the ARI-treated group there was a fourfold increase in regenerating myelinated nerve fibres and a 33% increase in the number of myelinated fibres per unit cross-sectional area of nerve. There was also evidence of 'repair' of certain myelinated fibre lesions described by these authors as characteristic of human diabetic neuropathy: e.g. axoglial dysjunction was decreased. Fibre regeneration was more evident in nerves that had shown lesser degrees of damage in the first biopsy, again indicating the need for early intervention in treating or preventing nerve damage in diabetes. Unfortunately, owing to the relatively small numbers of patients studied, it was not possible to relate structural repair to improvement in quantitative measures. This study underlines the need to improve electrophysiological measurement of the compound action potential amplitude, which is a direct measure of fibre number.

MICROVASCULAR DISEASE IN DIABETIC NERVE

Fagerberg was the first to describe changes in the microvessels in nerve, which were sclerosis and thickening of the walls [60]. Although microvessels are obviously diseased in retina and kidney, the role of such disease in neuropathy is less clear and has tended to be overshadowed by the attraction of the 'polyol explanation', a diffuse metabolic abnormality thought to be in keeping with the diffuse symmetrical nature of clinical diabetic neuropathy. However, clinical observation indicates that although there is usually a background neuropathy in most instances, there are many focal features that must be attributable to more local insults, the most likely being vascular. Moreover, electrophysiological studies indicate the patchy nature of involvement in function [61, 62] and, indeed, in 1929 Woltman and Wilder described 'patchy loss of myelin and fibres'

[63]. Although vessels have been shown to be abnormal (endothelial swelling and occlusion; basal lamina thickness) in a number of studies [61, 64, 65], no direct proof of a pathological effect of vessel disease was available until recently.

In diabetic rat sciatic nerve, endoneurial blood flow and oxygen tension are decreased [66]. Blood flow was measured using the hydrogen clearance technique, with platinum electrodes generating a current proportional to oxygen concentration. Blood flow was reduced by 33% with a similar decrease in oxygen tension, with an increase in vascular resistance suggesting a reduction in calibre or patency of vessels (or possibly increased blood viscosity). It is possible that there is a close relationship between biochemical abnormalities and ischaemia, and abnormal CVs and sorbitol accumulation were returned towards normal by administration of oxygen [67], although myo-inositol content was further decreased. In the BB diabetic rat, upon which much of the biochemical work has been carried out, vessel occlusion and endothelial swelling (identical to that seen in humans) has been demonstrated at an early stage in the life of the animal [68].

Non-diabetic rats kept hypoxic for 2 months developed abnormalities of electrophysiological function without the development of the abnormal biochemistry usually associated with diabetes [69]; studies with both diabetic and non-diabetic animals showed that some of the abnormalities could be prevented by maintaining animals in a high-oxygen environment [70]. More structural damage to sciatic nerve resulted from ligation of major arteries of supply in streptozotocin-induced diabetic rats than in normal rats [71]. In humans, clinical neuropathy develops in chronic obstructive airways disease [72]. All these facts encourage reinvestigation of the place of vessel disease in the aetiology of diabetic neuropathy.

More studies on human diabetic neuropathy are now available. In comparing 36 diabetic subjects with neuropathy, with 4 without neuropathy and 47 healthy subjects, there was a spatial distribution suggesting both diffuse and focal effects with regard to measures of fibre loss, demyelination and remyelination and the ratio of small to large fibre loss [73]. In an autopsy study, nerve roots and proximal-to-distal levels of lower limb nerves were compared in 8 controls and 15 diabetic neuropathic subjects. In the latter group fibre number and size, distribution and variability of density was again multifocal, more in keeping with a microvascular insult than with ischaemia [74].

Evidence continues to accumulate as to proliferation and thickening of endothelial cells and vessel walls in diabetic neuropathy [75]; however, more important is the direct demonstration of hypoxia (using a glass–platinum electrode technique similar to that described above) of sural nerve in vivo, in 15 diabetic patients with severe sensorimotor neuropathy, in whom significant vessel disease existed [76]. A totally unphysiological state was apparent, in that endoneurial oxygen partial pressure was 5 kPa, which was well below that of venous blood draining the foot and also lower than that in non-neuropathic subjects. In the diabetic subjects there was a reduction in endoneurial capillary density, thickening of capillary basement membrane and an increase in capillary diffusion distance [77]. In subdividing neuropathic subjects into those with severe or less severe neuropathy on clinical grounds, many of these vessel abnormalities were seen to be worse in the 'severe' group, and there were significant positive correlations between vascular indices and morphological abnormality such as fibre loss. This study indicates a point of vital importance with regard to the specific nature of small vessel disease: vessels were examined from skin and muscle biopsied at the same time as the sural nerve and none of the correlations with clinical or morphological severity was apparent; these vessels were very much less diseased. Thus, there is a specific neurochemical–vascular interaction occurring in nerve. Moreover, this observation precludes the extrapolation of muscle capillary abnormalities to the presence of microvascular disease in other tissues.

There would seem little doubt that vessel disease plays a part in human diabetic neuropathy. However, great care must be taken in the interpretation of reported studies. It has been pointed out by Sima that age has an effect on all small vessels, and indeed in one study [74] the controls were half the age of those with diabetes. It may be that there is some difference in pathological change in older diabetic subjects, or between those with type 1 or type 2 diabetes, suggesting that vessel changes do indeed become more important with age.

Resistance of Nerve to Ischaemia

Normally, occlusion of blood flow to a limb results in a rapid loss of any measurable conduction velocity or vibration perception threshold (VPT). In diabetes Steiness showed that this loss is greatly delayed and that VPT and CV are measurable for much longer periods [78]. This phenomenon may be demonstrated in animal diabetes [79] and other metabolic states [80], and may be attributable to the fact that diabetic nerve is usually relatively hypoxic and can withstand occlusion of its major blood supply for longer periods. It has been suggested that the known depression of Na^+-K^+-ATPase activity leads to Na^+ accumulation and K^+ loss, resulting in lowering of the resting potential [81]. Resistance of tail nerve action potentials to ischaemia in streptozotocin-induced diabetic rats is not affected by the administration of an ARI and may not be related to the polyol pathway [82]; its relationship to the level of blood glucose is a matter of debate. VPT measurement has demonstrated this resistance in 17 newly diagnosed subjects with non-insulin dependent diabetes mellitus; it persisted despite subsequent improvement in glucose control, again suggesting that it is unrelated to the metabolic pathways currently under investigation [83].

Haemorheological Abnormalities

There is no proof that abnormalities of platelets, coagulation or cellular deformability are a direct cause of vessel abnormality and nerve damage in diabetes. However, there is no doubt that there were many such abnormalities present in a wide range of diabetic subjects studied [84]. In the knowledge that small vessels in nerve are partly occluded and that platelet plugs have been observed in human [61] and animal [68] intraneural vessels, it seems likely that the microenvironment of flow must be restricted, with the addition of adverse effects on the endothelial cells themselves.

Summary

Diabetic peripheral nerve, resting as it does in a very abnormal metabolic environment, develops its own biochemical changes which seem to relate to dysfunction and a degree of morphological change. This state exists for years and yet only 20% of diabetic subjects develop a significant clinical problem. No doubt vascular factors become more important with age, but in humans, who may have a variety of clinical syndromes, other insults impinge on the already vulnerable nerve to produce more significant damage. While continuing with research into the fundamental (early) abnormalities in nerve, those treating patients should be looking for those features that may make one patient more likely to develop disease than another.

MEASUREMENT OF PERIPHERAL NERVE FUNCTION

In the clinical management of diabetic neuropathy it is not usually necessary to carry out physiological tests to determine the diagnosis or treatment. However, in any research study it is necessary to describe and classify the type of neuropathy accurately and this requires use of appropriate techniques. There is a growing need to carry out prospective studies into the natural history of nerve disease and the influence of various therapeutic regimens, making it essential to improve and standardize the techniques available. At present there is a wide variability in results, often with poor reproducibility. Moreover, the relationship of a measurement to the function and structure of the nerve is not always clear. Four types of measurement or assessment are considered below.

(1) Clinical assessment of symptoms and physical signs.
(2) Electrophysiological techniques.
(3) Measurement of vibration perception threshold.
(4) Measurement of thermal discrimination threshold.

Assessment of Symptoms and Signs

Such assessments are prone to inaccuracies but are essential, particularly in trials of symptomatic neuropathy. Studies of prophylaxis will almost certainly involve people without symptoms, but there is a need to identify symptoms if they eventually develop.

A standard list of questions is required regarding sensation or pain, with a score for each feature. The most complex of these, the neurological symptom score (NSS), allows a global assessment of all symptoms; although time-consuming to apply, it is the ideal [85], and does correlate with observed pathological changes within nerve. More detailed attempts have been made to 'stage' diabetic neuropathy [86], using a battery of clinical, electrophysiological and sensory functional tests. The following grading or staging system has been suggested by Dyck [87]:

Stage 0 (*no neuropathy*): no symptoms and fewer than two abnormalities of testing, including autonomic function.
Stage 1 (*asymptomatic neuropathy*): no symptoms but two or more abnormalities of functional testing.
Stage 2 (*symptomatic neuropathy*): symptoms of a 'lesser' degree along with two or more functional abnormalities.
Stage 3 (*disabling neuropathy*): 'disabling' symptoms and two or more functional abnormalities.

A simpler assessment of a specific symptom (e.g. pain, tingling, cramps) may be achieved by using the graphic linear pain score in which subjects mark their own assessment of symptom severity. This is a very effective method where serial measures are to be made.

A detailed comparison has been made of symptoms, signs and measures of electrical nerve conduction vibration and thermal testing [88]. Eighty-four patients had clinical neuropathy, 41 did not. Of those with neuropathy, 95% had abnormal CVs in two nerves, 82% abnormalities of vibration or thermal sensation, 80% abnormal NSS and 80% abnormal physical signs. Of those defined as having no neuropathy, 53% had no abnormalities at all, 15% CV abnormalities, 7% vibration and thermal abnormalities, 10% abnormal NSS and only 5% abnormal signs. Thus there seems to be a very reasonable correlation between accurate detailed clinical testing and physiological tests (although, clearly, there are patients who cross in both directions) and in long-term studies all these measures should be performed.

As with clinical symptoms, physical signs (reflexes, muscle strength, sensory deficit) may be listed and scored to produce a neurological disability score (NDS) [89]. However, reflexes may be present in the presence of severe pain, particularly if it is sudden in onset, and in the elderly there may well be reflex and sensory

change in the absence of any symptoms, again underlining the need to apply all measures.

An old method of sensory testing, with Frey's hairs, may well still have a place if the technique is performed carefully, for abnormal results are found in the fingers of subjects without symptoms [90]. Similarly, it is important to measure muscle strength [91].

Electrophysiological Measurements

Most electrophysiological measures are reliable and reproducible if performed with care by experienced personnel and with standardized temperature control of the limb. Measurements of nerve action potentials and somatosensory-evoked potentials (SEP) are used to assess sensory fibre function [92, 93]. Recordings of compound muscle action potentials, F-wave and distal latencies (coupled with needle electromyography) measure the function of motor axons. Much more sophisticated techniques are required for assessment of small myelinated fibres that carry autonomic stimuli [94]: amplitude and conduction velocities can be accurately quantitated. The latter tests are the most commonly and more easily performed, but the amplitude is the most meaningful parameter, being a function of the number and size of nerve fibres, i.e. the number of functioning axons. An early manifestation of axonal disease is the inability to carry repetitive impulses—hence the importance of developing techniques of evoked potentials, particularly evoked compound action potential amplitude, in studies of diabetic nerves in the early phase of disease [95]. A major drawback to interpretation of simple CVs is that they are dependent on so many factors—fibre size, myelination, nodal and internodal length, and fluid, glucose and electrolyte relationships at the time of measurement. Moreover CV only reflects myelinated fibres, a mere 25% of the fibre population. It is estimated that F-wave latencies are the most reproducible, with 2–3% variation, whereas the variation for CV is 4–7% and that for measurements of amplitude is 10–15% [96]. Thus each laboratory should supply its own range of results in normal subjects and groups of patients, with due regard to age.

There are many studies of simple CV in diabetic subjects without obvious neuropathy [97–99], greater abnormalities being seen in those with a longer duration of diabetes, and also in children [100–102]. Improvement in blood glucose control results in improved CV (motor more than sensory), an observation that has been confirmed on many occasiosn [24, 99] both in asymptomatic patients and in those with severe neuropathy. Impairment of all electrophysiological measures is more severe in the legs of those with diabetes than in the arms. Many patterns of electrophysiological abnormalities are described in differing clinical syndromes, confirming the existence of diffuse abnormalities of function with undoubted focal features— indeed, the multifocal pattern of abnormality must be considered in the design of clinical trials and in the assessment of aetiological hypotheses [96].

Measurement of the medial plantar sensory action potential (MPSAP) seems to be a useful and sensitive measure of large fibre function [103], as this action potential was undetectable in subjects in whom vibration and thermal thresholds were normal. Further measures to detect abnormalities at an early stage must be developed— e.g. measurement of the sural nerve sensory action potential [104] or of the Hoffman reflex from the soleus muscle [105].

Microneurography [92], although a test for studies of small number of patients in great detail, could allow measurement of extremely early change. Microelectrodes are inserted into a nerve and provide measures of sympathetic activity in C fibres, which are abnormal at an early stage and are not necessarily accompanied by other electrophysiological changes. This technique allows the indirect measure of CV in unmyelinated post-ganglionic C fibres by recording reflex latency following various stimuli.

Vibration Perception Threshold

The vibration perception threshold (VPT) provides a measure of large fibre function. In clinical practice a tuning fork is used, but quantitation requires an electrically driven vibrating stimulus in which the oscillations of the stylus are inversely related to the square root of the voltage supplied. The biothesiometer was developed by Steiness, who showed that VPT was significantly higher and more variable in diabetic than in normal subjects, was more abnormal in the foot than the hand, and was associated with loss of reflexes and sensory loss, although not with neurological symptoms or level of blood glucose [106]. Other

workers have subsequently demonstrated its use, correlating abnormality with CV [107] and thermal sensation [108], although in the latter study the relationship was not so marked, particularly in patients with acute painful neuropathy. Impaired VPT has been correlated with the presence of areas of high pressure in neuropathic feet and the risk of foot ulceration [109].

The vibrameter is a more recently developed instrument in which a spring-loaded system in the head of the device results in a constant pressure being applied, with much less likelihood of sideways movement of the stylus distorting the vibrating stimulus. It is important to control the pressure of the stylus head-piece [110]. The vibrameter head weight has a very significant effect on the index produced with this instrument. The biothesiometer is usually held by hand, and experienced operators do produce acceptably reproducible results. Care must be taken to apply the stylus in a symmetrical and vertical fashion and, as with any sensory testing, to allow the patient a period for adaptation and learning, so that apparent improvement is not due to 'practice'. However, this measurement has an inherent variation, more so in diabetic subjects and particularly in those with greater degrees of abnormality [111]. Age has a profound effect on responses, as shown in a survey of 519 subjects [112], again indicating the need for each group to establish its own normal range.

Thermal Discrimination Threshold

Relatively few studies of the thermal discrimination threshold (TDT) have been reported. It is a measure of small fibre function, and not surprisingly is always abnormal when measured in painful neuropathy [113]. A number of reliable instruments are now available [114] and it is important with this sensation to use a 'forced choice technique'. Two metal plates are held for one second consecutively against the site to be studied. The plates are electrically heated, water-cooled and installed in a spring-loaded handset, thus controlling the pressure of application. The plates are presented in a fixed order but can be changed so that either is neutral to or warmer than local skin temperature, and electrical switching between the plates is performed randomly as laid down by a predetermined table. The temperature difference between the plates is progressively reduced until the patient makes an error, and then increased until a correct response occurs and so on. The threshold is calculated as the mean of six such switches from 'hot' to 'cold'.

The best approach is to combine all measures including symptom scores into a semiautomated system in which the many results obtained are computerized; however, the system is expensive. This computer-assisted sensory examination [115] consists of stimulators, electromechanical translator, visual numerical display, computer and patient response keys. It is important that the computer controls the shape, magnitude and time of appearance of stimuli and subsequently their storage and analysis. Forced choice testing can therefore be applied to all measurements via the visual display.

A recent thorough comparison using such sophisticated equipment has been made of measurements of CV, VPT and TDT in diagnosing and staging diabetic neuropathy [116]. An exact definition of diabetic neuropathy is very difficult to achieve in view of the wide variations of nerve involvement: at one extreme there are asymptomatic subjects with slightly abnormal function tests; at the other there are those with severe clinical neuropathy (symptoms, signs) and grossly abnormal tests. Detailed knowledge of the relationships between abnormal function tests and clinical state would at least allow a 'staging' of the neuropathic state and a move towards reasonable standardization between different studies. In an analysis of 182 patients three detailed measures of symptoms and physical signs were made, together with tests of nerve conduction, VPT and TDT. The stricter the criteria for abnormality, the lower were the percentage found to be abnormal. Hence, one abnormality of nerve conduction from four measured nerves was found in 80%, but only in 21% was the abnormality present in all four nerves. Abnormalities of vibration were present in 44% and of thermal sensation in 35%. Abnormality of any two or more of the three clinical and three technical measures occurred in 64% of subjects. Although there was a reasonable correlation or association between various measures they were not nearly predictive enough to allow only one test to be used, hence the need to perform them all. This is well demonstrated in a study in which patients without any symptoms of neuropathy were compared with those with pain or a foot ulcer. Many discrepancies were demonstrated, although generally there was more evidence of small fibre damage in painful syndromes, and large fibre damage in those with foot ulcers [117]. This last study epitomizes all that has been written in this section. For meaningful prospective studies of diabetic neuropathy it is essential to carry out the following:

(1) Scoring of sensory symptoms
(2) Physical examination testing and scoring:
    sensation
    reflexes
    muscle strength
(3) Electrophysiology:
    CV on three nerves (two leg, one arm)
    Medial plantar sensory action potential
    Compound evoked action potential
    F-wave latency
(4) VPT
(5) TDT

Finally, it must be stressed that by performing all these measurements in a large population of diabetic subjects it is not necessarily possible to report on the incidence or prevalence of 'diabetic neuropathy', in that such a figure would depend entirely on the level of abnormality at which one chose to diagnose neuropathy: for example, if only nerve conduction abnormalities are considered, then 80% of subjects have neuropathy. Patients' subjective assessment of the magnitude of their problem and the physician's interest in neuropathy all profoundly affect such a figure. Should impotence be included as a neuropathic symptom, when vascular and psychological factors are known to play their part?

However, there is a need to produce a figure, as those in diabetic practice appreciate that neuropathic problems are common, and those in control of health care budgets need to be persuaded of the importance of such problems. On the basis of surveys in major diabetic clinics where the criteria for the diagnosis of neuropathy were strict, a reported prevalence of 13% in 1962 and 10.7% in 1985 would seem to be reasonable figures to quote [118, 119].

RELATIONSHIP OF NEUROPATHY TO BLOOD GLUCOSE CONTROL

As with the other complications of diabetes, the relationship between neuropathy and glycaemic control is difficult to ascertain. In many of the clinical syndromes described later there is a clear-cut relationship to hyperglycaemia at the time of presentation, but in many there are not, for example in chronic sensory neuropathy and diffuse motor neuropathy, particularly in older subjects. It is extremely difficult, if not impossible, to demonstrate a relationship between preexisting 'control' over many years and the presence of a clinical problem. The data documented by Pirart may underline the role of 'bad control' [120], although the diagnosis of neuropathy in such a large group of patients (4400) must have been rather haphazard. His reported incidence (19%) of neuropathy after 25 years is in keeping with the figures quoted above.

Over many decades numerous studies have been reported relating poor control to neuropathy and, in general, implicating high blood glucose levels [121, 122]. Improved functional assessment of nerve and better indices of control, such as glycated haemoglobin, reinforce this view, provided that it is agreed that abnormal function tests indicate nerve disease or a risk of neuropathy. As yet, none of our measurements have been shown to be predictive of future clinical disease.

It has already been mentioned that conduction velocities improve following reduction of blood glucose levels [123–125]. In a study of 36 subjects with a wide variety of clinical syndromes, glycated haemoglobin was significantly elevated compared with matched subjects without neuropathy [126]. There was also no association of neuropathy with HLA status. Similarly, meticulous control of blood glucose with insulin infusion pumps would appear to 'protect' individuals by improving electrophysiological function [127]. Other pump programmes have resulted in improvement of conduction velocities, but often sensory action potentials do not improve and these may be more meaningful indicators of structure and function [128].

Although children do not develop clinical neuropathic syndromes, impairment of nerve conduction does occur [129]. Indeed, there seems to be a relationship not only with glucose control but also with the M values as a measure of glycaemic excursions—widely fluctuating blood glucose levels may be more harmful than a steady state. Prospective studies should provide more useful information. In a 2.5-year follow-up of subjects between 16 and 19 years old, those

with less adequate glycaemic control had more deterioration in nerve function and in this group there was a greater incidence of retinopathy and microproteinuria [130]. Multivariate analysis suggested that, whereas there was a broad relationship between the development of all these complications and glycaemic control, it still existed in many individuals when control was discounted—other aetiological factors no doubt being involved. Conduction velocities do not always relate to other complications: in patients who did not produce C peptide, more retinopathy and microproteinuria was observed than in those who secreted C peptide, but nerve function was the same in both groups [131]. Such studies, while implicating blood glucose control to a certain extent, also stress the importance of regarding each complication as a separate aetiological issue. VPT has also been used as an indicator of healthier nerve function in relation to glucose control. This measure was significantly better after 2 years of 'improved control', as was glycated haemoglobin, compared with subjects on insulin who continued with their usual therapy [132]. In 80 young patients with insulin dependent diabetes mellitus (IDDM), VPT was undoubtedly better in those deemed to have better control, as was the state of the retina [133].

The level of blood glucose certainly seems to relate to the development of neuropathy, and particularly to the presence of abnormalities of functional tests, but clearly many other factors are involved in the progress to clinical disease.

CLINICAL FEATURES OF DIABETIC PERIPHERAL NEUROPATHIES

An attempt to classify the neuropathies is important for many reasons, including consideration of aetiology or the presence of different clinical syndromes indicating multiple factors in causation. The standard topographical classification was proposed by Bruyn and Garland [134]: they classified neuropathies as either *symmetrical*, predominantly sensory and distal polyneuropathy (diabetes pseudotabes; hyperalgesic type) or *asymmetrical*, predominantly motor and often proximal neuropathy (mononeuropathy; multiple mononeuropathy e.g. cranial neuropathy and diabetic amyotrophy; autonomic visceral neuropathy; radiculopathy).

Thomas suggested a simplification of this classification [42] into *symmetrical polyneuropathies* (sensory or sensorimotor neuropathies; acute or subacute motor neuropathy) and *focal and multifocal neuropathies* (cranial neuropathy; trunk and limb mononeuropathy; proximal motor neuropathy).

This chapter adopts the alternative approach of describing the clinical features presenting to the physician as a problem. There is considerable overlap in the mixture of features, although one usually predominates. Very often the clinical picture strongly suggests diffuse symmetrical involvement (metabolic effect) with a distinctly focal pattern superimposed (vascular effect). At all times it is important to consider causative factors in these individual syndromes. As clinical description is often a personal view of the author, the extensive bibliography involved in this clinical area is not individually quoted in this chapter, but all are listed in specific works [8, 17, 42]. It should be noted that in all the conditions described, a high percentage of subjects manifest abnormalities of autonomic function tests, although only a few have obvious clinical autonomic neuropathy. Impotence is common in all these syndromes. These tests and clinical features are considered separately later.

The following syndromes of peripheral diabetic neuropathies are described below:

(1) Chronic insidious sensory neuropathy
(2) Acute painful neuropathy
(3) Proximal motor neuropathy
(4) Diffuse symmetrical motor neuropathy
(5) The neuropathic foot
(6) Pressure neuropathies
(7) Focal vascular neuropathies
(8) Neuropathy present at diagnosis
(9) Treatment-induced neuropathy
(10) Hypoglycaemic neuropathy.

Chronic Insidious Sensory Neuropathy

Chronic insidious sensory neuropathy is by far the most common clinical problem of diabetic neuropathy. Symptoms vary from mildly irritating to extremely uncomfortable and painful. Typical symptoms consist of tingling, burning sensations, shooting or diffuse pains, muscle cramps and hypersensitivity of the skin to clothes and bedclothes. The legs are predominantly affected, but less severe symptoms may occur in

the hands, often with tingling and a numb sensation when touching fine objects. Symptoms are far worse at night, perhaps because they are then given more attention, or because the skin is warmed under the bedclothes. Allied to the painful sensations is a cold, numb sensation, which may encourage the patient to warm the feet directly in front of open heat, with disastrous results.

Reflexes are usually absent in the legs and patchy sensory loss is apparent, with impairment of vibration and position sense. Very occasionally the proprioceptive large fibres (or possibly the posterior columns) are severely affected and there is ataxia and a positive Romberg's sign; cerebrospinal fluid protein levels are typically elevated.

It is usual to find a considerable degree of muscle wasting and some weakness in this syndrome. Small muscles of hands and feet are badly affected, the latter leading to dropped metatarsal heads, loss of the arch of the foot and clawing of the toes. Such patients may well develop foot ulcers, although they are not at such great risk as those with the specific neuropathic foot. Proximal muscles such as the quadriceps are also wasted. It is interesting that very many older diabetic subjects without sensory symptoms or any muscle weakness will exhibit marked wasting on examination, attesting to the presence of a longstanding pathological process. This underlines the problem of whether to classify such an asymptomatic patient as having neuropathy.

Particularly high levels of blood glucose are not usually apparent in these patients—the onset is insidious; indeed, in many the control of blood glucose is fairly good.

Acute Painful Neuropathy

This syndrome is relatively rare but is a very distinct event, usually relating to poor metabolic control. There is sudden onset of very severe pains, mainly in the thighs but also in the lower limb, with profound muscle wasting and weakness, leading to depression and a state of 'diabetic cachexia', so great is the weight loss. Institution of insulin therapy (mandatory) results in considerable improvement in all symptoms and a gain in weight over a period of 6–12 months. Naturally, if therapy is started at a much earlier stage, extreme weight loss need not develop;

such patients often have considerable distention of veins when lying flat, indicating autonomic involvement. Reflexes are not always absent in such acute syndromes and sensory impairment is not marked. Clearly, metabolic factors are primarily involved here. The natural history of this condition, with almost guaranteed improvement [135], is in contrast to the chronic insidious sensory syndrome where most symptoms remain or worsen over a 5-year period [136].

Proximal Motor Neuropathy

Some features of proximal motor neuropathy are similar to those of acute painful neuropathy. However, the sudden onset of severe pain, at a time of poor metabolic control, is often confined to one thigh with extreme muscle wasting (amyotrophy of Garland). If muscle wasting is observed in the other thigh and lower leg, this suggests the presence of a focal neuropathy against a background of diffuse nerve damage. Nerve conduction studies support this view. Once again, control of blood glucose levels, usually with insulin, results in considerable improvement.

Diffuse Symmetrical Motor Neuropathy

Diffuse symmetrical motor neuropathy is being increasingly recognized and seems to be an overt manifestation of the common generalized muscle wasting. Profound muscle weakness and wasting of all muscle groups occurs over approximately 4 months while metabolic control is apparently good. In some cases weakness is so severe as to restrict the patient to a wheelchair existence. Muscle fasciculation is relatively common—indeed, it is not uncommon to see fasciculation in the first dorsal interosseous muscle in many diabetic subjects. These patients are older, mainly non-insulin dependent, and it is presumed that small vessel disease and, indeed, the effects of aging, play an important part in this syndrome. Sensory features are minor. Generally the outlook is poor, with only minimal return of power with physiotherapy. Occasionally, diffuse muscle involvement of this sort is seen in association with extreme hyperglycaemia, and recovery often results from control of blood glucose.

The Neuropathic Foot

It is important to regard the neuropathic foot as a distinct clinical entity, as it is an advanced form of pathological change involving peripheral and autonomic nerves, with arteriovenous shunting, vascular calcification and bone destruction. This subject is dealt with fully in Chapter 68.

Pressure Neuropathies

The diabetic nerve should be regarded as vulnerable to a number of insults, many as yet to be identified (it is known experimentally that nerves with segmental demyelination are sensitive to pressure and anoxia). Thus problems arise at vulnerable points, notably the peroneal nerve at the knee (foot drop) and the median nerve at the wrist (carpal tunnel syndrome). The latter is undoubtedly a feature in the diabetic clinic, where it may be dismissed as 'atypical arthritis', for the hand is often stiff with fixation of finger joints, or may be overlooked as an aspect of diabetic cheirarthropathy. Decompression of the median nerve beneath the flexor retinaculum improves symptoms although pain may return some years later, apparently more frequently in diabetic individuals than in non-diabetic persons.

The preponderance of neuropathic problems in the legs is assumed to be attributable to the increased vulnerability of the axon because of its length. Another possible cause, pressure on nerve roots at their exit in the spinal column, was not borne out by computed tomographic scanning of the lower spine, assessing nerve foramina and dimensions of the spinal canal in a selection of subjects with advanced lower limb neuropathy.

Focal Vascular Neuropathies

These are essentially the mononeuropathies and it seems very likely that they are due to focal vascular lesions. Lesions of nearly all the peripheral nerves have been described. With regard to the cranial nerves, palsies of nerves III and VII are the most common. At times of poor metabolic control, pain in the eye followed by paralysis of the globe is a typical picture. The sparing of pupillary constriction due to the peripheral situation of the nerve fibres of the iris is taken as evidence of a vascular lesion; and, indeed, sudden death in such a patient revealed vascular occlusion [137]. Intercostal nerve involvement leads to a 'bulge' or 'mass' developing at a costal margin on deep breathing, and a phrenic nerve lesion may be a cause of unexplained elevation of the diaphragm.

Neuropathy Present at Diagnosis of Diabetes

Occasionally a subject with longstanding undiagnosed diabetes will present with established neuropathy and other complications. However, an important observation is that 30% of peptide presenting with newly diagnosed diabetes are found to have 'neuropathic' symptoms on careful questioning and most of these (cramps, tingling, heaviness and weakness of legs) rapidly resolve with control of blood glucose levels. As this is a reversible situation, the reversible component should be elucidated at a relatively early stage in the disease. Are such subjects at risk of future neuropathy?

Treatment-induced Neuropathy

The condition known as 'insulin neuritis' has been recognized for years. It is usually an acute, painful sensory neuropathy, but generalized weakness may occur; it usually follows therapy with insulin but has been reported after diet and sulphonylurea treatment. A long period of hyperglycaemia before the event is usually documented, but no adequate explanation exists. It could be that in a subject with advanced nerve damage, the sudden fall in blood glucose concentration upsets a variety of adaptive changes of fluid balance within cells. Anterograde fast axonal transport (as shown by labelled methionine and fucose injected into ganglia) is decreased by 36% with acute lowering of blood glucose to hypoglycaemic levels in animals, an effect which could be abolished by producing a state of 'mild' hypoglycaemia for some days previously [138]. Sudden regeneration of axons, producing painful sprouts, has been suggested. The condition improves on continuation of glycaemic control.

Hypoglycaemic Neuropathy

Sensorimotor neuropathy of peripheral distribution with considerable atrophy of the small muscles of the hand has been described in association with insulinoma and insulin shock therapy [139]. Severe hypoglycaemia in animals results in loss of axons.

PAIN IN DIABETIC NEUROPATHY

Pain is a difficult sensation to quantitate and is profoundly influenced by individual personality. There is overlap of paraesthesia and pain. Many of the diabetic neuropathies are associated with pain, often local, and this occurs even when the predominant feature is motor [140]. In the neuropathic foot, pain sensation is so poor that trauma goes unnoticed, and yet such patients complain of painful tingling—the 'painful painless' foot. Painful sensory neuropathy is associated with involvement of small myelinated A delta and unmyelinated C fibres [141], these acting as nociceptive afferent pathways. Axonal degeneration and regeneration are manifested by sprouting of unmyelinated fibres [142], such sprouts also occurring in a neuroma and shown to have spontaneous activity as a source of pain. Injured nerves and axonal sprouts change from being impulse conductors to being impulse generators and a cause of pain [143]. These small unmyelinated fibres also have autonomic efferent activity which directly reduces the threshold stimulus of mechanoreceptors [144, 145]. Hyperglycaemia itself influences pain perception, for in non-diabetic subjects infusion of glucose to raise the blood glucose level results in a fall in pain threshold measurements [146] and, indeed, such pain thresholds are lower in diabetic subjects.

The known arteriovenous shunting that occurs in diabetic neuropathy [147] may also be a source of pain. Blood flow is increased in the legs of subjects with acute and chronic painful sensory neuropathy, with increase in skin temperature; such abnormalities were reversed when blood flow to the leg was occluded, with the intriguing observation that most subjects noted a relief of pain [148]. Many patients with the 'burning pain' type of symptom report relief by cooling their feet in cold water.

At all times in the assessment of pain in the diabetic leg, other causes should be considered, for example arteriosclerotic vascular disease, which may coexist anyway, and musculoskeletal diseases. Root pain from spinal cord disease such as lumbar disc lesion, cauda equina tumour or spinal stenosis, should not be overlooked. Proximal obstructive arterial disease apparently contributes little to nerve damage. Occasional clinical reports have suggested poor recovery from painful neuropathy in patients with ischaemia, and ligation of the blood supply to the sciatic nerve in diabetic rats results in more structural damage than in normal nerve [71].

In neuropathy (major vessel disease excluded)

there is an abnormal pattern of blood flow that is more marked in the 'neuropathic foot'. Arteriovenous shunting of blood occurs, as shown by the clinical observation of warm feet with visible bounding pulses in association with gross venous distension in the supine position —veins that do not collapse until the leg is elevated [149], oxygenated levels of blood from these veins [150] and Doppler ultrasonograms which suggest fast forward flow of blood [151] associated with increased volume of blood flow, as mentioned above. It is assumed that this abnormality is mainly due to autonomic dysfunction, aggravated by stiff, often calcified vessels [152]. There is some debate as to whether autonomic dysfunction is more common in subjects with neuropathic foot ulceration, perhaps relating to the fact that autonomic tests have been of systemic function rather than specifically in the legs. Using a technique in which activity of individual sweat glands is quantitated by counting active sweating points on a photograph of skin, subjects with ulceration show striking impairment of sweating as a test of local autonomic function [153]. In non-diabetic quadriplegic subjects with gross autonomic dysfunction, the Doppler sonogram and venous oxygenation are identical to those seen in the diabetic neuropathic foot [156].

TREATMENT OF PERIPHERAL NEUROPATHY

The most common clinical situation requiring treatment is that of pain or sensory disturbance. The muscle-wasting syndromes require physiotherapy and the diabetic foot needs a specialized approach, as described in Chapter 68. At all times, control of the blood glucose level is mandatory.

Diagnosis is usually straightforward but the possibility of spinal cord disease as a cause of symptoms must be considered, other peripheral neuropathies excluded and significant vascular disease excluded by assessment of the ankle pressure index (API) with Doppler ultrasound [147], although there will at times be a vascular ischaemic contribution to the pain. Earlier in this review the relationship of hyperglycaemia, clinical neuropathy and nerve function was established; effective glucose control will benefit many patients, even in those with longstanding resistant symptoms where continuous subcutaneous insulin infusion (CSII) may be necessary [155, 156]. Moreover, as the pain threshold falls when the blood glucose level is raised by glucose infusion in non-diabetic subjects, intensive efforts to produce normoglycaemia must be the main aim of therapy [146]. However, many older subjects may have significant symptoms in the presence of 'adequate' control.

The most effective sensory pain relief in diabetic neuropathy is achieved by the use of tricyclic drugs, for example imipramine, which has been established as effective in two double-blind trials [157, 158], although simple analgesics such as aspirin should be tried initially. Imipramine is administered usually at night, in doses of 50–150 mg, the benefits being related to blood levels of the drug; such benefits are often seen within the first week of therapy, suggesting a peripheral rather than central effect, i.e. not the effect on any associated depression. The benefits are probably achieved through modulation of receptor activity. If side-effects occur with this drug, other tricyclic drugs should be tried; enhanced benefit may result from the addition of a tranquillizer such as fluphenazine [159]. Diazepam or quinine may be particularly helpful for nocturnal muscle cramps. Over many years other sedative drugs (e.g. phenytoin and carbamazepine) have been variably reported as being of benefit and should be used if all else fails.

New Approaches to Therapy

Several recent reports are of great interest and their exact role in the future has yet to be decided (see below).

Aldose Reductase Inhibitors

Trials in progress of ARIs are yet to be reported, but it seems likely that these drugs may have to be administered at a much earlier stage in the natural history than hitherto, or even as prophylaxis.

Gangliosides

Gangliosides are complex sialoglycolipids found in high concentration in nervous tissue and are powerful initiators of dendritogenesis [160]. In animals, administration of mixed gangliosides results in improved peripheral nerve regeneration after injury [161], and improvement in nerve function in animals may be related to a reduction in slow axonal transport of acetyl-cholinesterase [162]. There are now a number of clinical trials that indicate improvement of electrophysiological nerve function in human diabetes, and some clinical improvement [163, 164]. In a study of 26 patients, although there was little improvement in functional tests, 4 patients showed improvement in compound motor action potentials in the common peroneal nerve, while no improvement was shown in the placebo-treated patients, suggesting a potential beneficial effect [165]. Here again, the suggestion is made that nerve damage is too far advanced to allow benefit from these theoretically effective agents.

Glycation of Nerve

Non-enzymatic glycation of nerve has now been described [166] (see Chapter 24). Glycation products derived from blood glucose and capable of crosslinking proteins accumulate on collagen, and extravasated low-density lipoprotein is covalently trapped in the subendothelial matrix of the arterial wall by these products, so that the plasma and matrix proteins become progressively resistant to physiological degradation. Prevention of this abnormality by aminoguanidine, an inhibitor of glycation, may lead to the demonstration of beneficial effects in peripheral nerve [167].

Gamma-linolenic Acid

Supplementation of the diet of diabetic subjects with γ-linolenic acid has been shown to improve conduction velocity [168], perhaps by restoring the normal concentration of long-chain essential fatty acids derived from linoleic acids. Further studies are required to establish whether this form of therapy will be effective.

Lignocaine Derivatives

Intravenous infusion of lignocaine, acting as a local anaesthetic, seems to have a beneficial effect on painful neuropathy, an effect which persists for a reasonable period after withdrawal of the infusion [169]. Mexiletine, a close structural analogue of lignocaine, when administered orally produced significant improvement in painful neuropathy in a randomized double-blind study [170].

Table 1 Approach to the treatment of painful neuropathy

1. Exclude other neuropathies and spinal cord disease
2. Improve blood glucose control as much as possible
3. Simple analgesics—aspirin, etc.
4. Tricyclic drugs (imipramine)
5. Tricyclic drugs plus fluphenazine
6. Lignocaine infusion—oral mexiletine
7. Other drugs:
   phenytoin
   carbamazepine
   gangliosides

The approach to the treatment of painful neuropathy is summarized in Table 1.

AUTONOMIC NEUROPATHY

Many diabetic subjects have demonstrable abnormalities of autonomic function without any evidence of clinical disease; there is a very extensive literature on this topic. Tests of autonomic function are assumed to be a measure of 'neurological' state and may be important methods of assessing therapy of diabetic complications. A review of these tests, their significance and correlation with other assessments of neurological function is therefore important. Troublesome clinical autonomic neuropathy, which presents with striking and intractable features, is fortunately a relatively rare event in practice.

Tests of Autonomic Function

Tests of autonomic function are essentially tests of the parasympathetic and sympathetic systems relating to cardiac and respiratory function. A large number of methods of stressing the autonomic system have been described and studied [171], ranging from immersing the face in cold water, through neck suction, to amyl nitrate inhalation. A series of tests are described below that are practical, meaningful and available for serial studies in patients. Although a clear-cut distinction between tests of the sympathetic and parasympathetic systems is often difficult, essentially the parasympathetic system is tested by measuring heart rate change during the Valsalva manoeuvre, deep breathing or on standing, and the sympathetic system by assessing blood pressure response to standing or sustained hand grip [172].

The electrocardiographic R–R interval shortens during inspiration and lengthens during expiration. The simplest and probably the best test methods are to measure the standard of the mean R–R during a period of quiet breathing [173], or to measure the difference between the maximum and minimum heart rates recorded over a period during deep breathing at six breaths per minute. A tendency of the heart rate to vary for other reasons during the test may be avoided by using vector analysis [174]. While attached to the electrocardiograph subjects must breathe at a standard rate and their position must not vary. If possible, smoking, coffee intake and known sympathomimetic and β-blocking drugs should be avoided before testing, and blood glucose control should be as stable as possible with strict avoidance of any tendency to hypoglycaemia [175]. With simple clinical control of the patient and standardization of the method, measurement of R–R variation provides an adequate measure of function and is abnormal at an early stage after the diagnosis of diabetes [176].

The *Valsalva manoeuvre* consists of forced expiration against a resistance which should be standardized (approximately 40 mm Hg), the force being maintained for 10–15 seconds. Tachycardia occurs during forced expiration secondary to decreased venous return, leading to a fall in cardiac output and baroreflex increase in vascular and cardiac sympathetic activity. Cessation of forced breathing is followed by increased cardiac output, leading to bradycardia secondary to an increase in cardiac parasympathetic activity. Quantitation of this test may be by relating a decrease in heart rate after the manoeuvre to the resting heart rate [177] or by calculation of the Valsalva ratio [178]—the maximum heart rate during the manoeuvre divided by the slowest rate thereafter. The lower limit of a normal ratio is accepted as 1:20 [179]. This ratio is not as sensitive as the R–R variation, being more related to overt clinical autonomic disease.

The heart rate response to standing is a simple test and correlates well with others [180]. In essence, all other methods of stressing cardiac function (which will be reflected by an autonomic compensation, leading to changes in heart rate and blood pressure) are useful as measures for serial assessment of neurological status, the simplest (e.g. hand grip responses) being the most effective if large numbers of patients are to be studied [179].

Plasma catecholamine responses allow a more sophisticated study of autonomic function, although perhaps not as adaptable to the investigation of large numbers of patients. Plasma noradrenaline reflects output from postganglionic sympathetic neuroeffector junctions. If these junctions are wide an increased leakage occurs into the circulation [181]. As in humans, plasma noradrenaline levels increase following stress, this may be used as a measure of sympathetic nervous activity in a fashion similar to that in the tests described above. Plasma [182] and arterial [183] noradrenaline are reduced in longstanding diabetes, although in poorly controlled subjects there is an exaggerated response to exercise [184]. Basal noradrenaline levels are lower in autonomic neuropathy, with a poor response to standing [185]. This hormone rises less after insulin administration in autonomic neuropathy with an increase in circulating renin [186].

In this complex field modifications to these basic tests are constantly being reported. Heart rate response to deep breathing, measured by comparing the longest R–R interval in expiration with the shortest in inspiration is simple [187] and this calculation may be made after forced breathing and standing [188]. Standing and hand grip seem superior to gradual head-up tilt as a test of vagal control [189]. The use of β-blocking agents may serve as a test in that blocking results in less R–R variation in diabetic subjects [190].

Pupillary function is easily accessible for evaluation since it reflects both parasympathetic and sympathetic activity. It is undoubtedly impaired in autonomic neuropathy [191]. Dilation is a function of the sympathetic system, and it is possible to study either system by the instillation of specific blocking agents [192]. The method of measurement requires a Polaroid camera, with a hood over the patient's head to achieve darkness [193]. Allowance for age must be made in any study. Using such techniques it seems that sympathetic fibre involvement precedes parasympathetic, suggesting that it may well be a sensitive early marker of neurological change.

Ventilatory reflexes can also be quantitated. Diabetic subjects exhibit impaired responses to hypoxia and hypercapnia, more so in those with autonomic neuropathy [194], and if a state of hyperoxic hypercapnia is induced the hypoxic drive to breathing is impaired in autonomic neuropathy [195] with a loss of ventilatory drive. During sleep, apnoea and breathing irregularities are common in those with abnormal cardiovascular reflexes and may partly explain the sudden death that can occur in subjects with severe neuropathy [196].

It does not appear that any one test of autonomic function will discriminate between minor variations in neurological states. There is a great need for careful standardization of method and production of normal values relating to age by each research group. Analysis of many published papers indicates that there is considerable overlap in degrees of abnormalities and a poor ability of many tests to provide adequate discrimination. Many subjects will show some abnormalities of these tests, and even children have been shown to have abnormality of R–R on standing [197]. For this reason it is important that a selection of tests are performed; economics and facilities will dictate what these will be. A reasonable 'package' would be R–R variation on shallow and deep breathing, heart rate and blood pressure response to standing and hand grip, the Valsalva manoeuvre, and pupillary responses, if possible. In an attempt to define one test it is apparent that the ratio between the mean R–R interval standing and the minimum during the first 5 beats on lying measures simple parasympathetic function, and the ratio between R–R maximum between beats 20 and 25 on standing and R–R minimum during 5 beats on lying assesses sympathetic function [198]. As with all diabetic complications, long-term natural history studies are required to assess the relevance of functional abnormalities of these tests. Twenty-three patients with impaired heart-rate response to deep breathing and blood-pressure response to rapid tilting appeared to develop symptoms of autonomic neuropathy during a period of 6 years [199]. In the future these indices will be used to assess the efficacy of therapeutic regimens. So far, varying reports of minor or no improvement have been received regarding the response of abnormal autonomic function tests in asymptomatic patients following improvement in blood glucose control, there being a trend to slight improvement. In clinically symptomatic patients, the Valsalva manoeuvre improved following CSII therapy, with further improvement in heart rate responses at 4 months, but these changes were not progressive [200]. Current interest in ARIs has resulted in many studies of autonomic function, again showing only marginal changes [201].

More local tests are required. There is still debate as to whether the abnormal blood flow of the neuropathic foot is related to autonomic dysfunction, this again depending on tests of central cardiac autonomic status [202–204]. However, if attention is paid to the abnormal limb itself, then gross impairment of sweating is apparent [153].

Relationship of Autonomic and Peripheral Neuropathy

In established autonomic neuropathy there will be distinct abnormalities of peripheral nerve function [205]. Similarly, in patients with peripheral neuropathy there are abnormalities of autonomic function tests. If both systems are tested in a group of diabetic patients some measurements correlate better than others. Conduction velocities in 35 patients did not correlate well with tests of autonomic function, whereas sural nerve sensory action potential was strongly associated. Distal motor nerve compound action potential and motor conduction velocity correlated with blood pressure fall as a measure of sympathetic function [206].

Clinical Features and Treatment of Autonomic Neuropathy

Once clinical autonomic neuropathy is established the patient often has evidence of other complications of diabetes. It is very unusual for any improvement to occur—indeed, in a 10-year study 71% of subjects were unchanged whereas 26% deteriorated [207]. Other studies have indicated a poor life expectancy once clinical disease is apparent [208]. All studies have indicated how patchy the disease may be, even within the same organ system. Not all features are necessarily present in each patient. The possible range of symptoms and signs in each system are described below.

Cardiac

Postural hypotension is rarely troublesome. Systolic pressure fall of greater than 30 mm Hg is taken as the abnormal point, but symptoms occur only with greater falls. Many subjects have no increase in plasma noradrenaline on standing, indicating vascular sympathetic damage [209]. However, there are many other complexly interrelated neurogenic, hormonal and metabolic factors involved, including vascular reactivity in response to insulin, dopamine receptors, antidiuretic hormone response to volume contraction and coexisting arteriosclerotic disease [201]. For severe symptoms a range of only partially effective treatments are available: elastic stockings, antigravity suits, mineralocorticoids, vasoconstrictors and atrial pacing [171]. Sensible advice against standing up too quickly and a drug such as fludrocortisone 0.1–0.2 mg daily usually helps.

Cardiac denervation. A fixed heart rate of approximately 90 beats per minute unresponsive to exercise or stress is the extreme end of the function tests described above [210], and may be the explanation for the sudden death seen in such patients and the occurrence of painless cardiac infarction. Diurnal electrocardiographic changes in QT interval are abolished in autonomic neuropathy, perhaps suggesting altered repolarization [211]. Ambulatory ECG monitoring in subjects without clinical heart disease but with autonomic neuropathy revealed ST depression more marked than that in non-neuropathic subjects [212], but arrhythmia was no more common in autonomic neuropathy although the mean hourly heart rate and minimum rate were much higher [213]. In a similar study, exercise produced abnormal ECG changes in diabetic subjects without a relationship to neuropathy [214]. Knowledge of this denervated state should lead to caution at times of stress, particularly at the induction of anaesthesia and during surgery.

Perhaps related to the poor sympathetic tone in the heart and peripheral vessels, there is now considerable evidence that cardiac function (assessed by many techniques) is impaired [215]. After exercise, heart rate and blood pressure increased less in those with autonomic neuropathy, and cardiac function (as assessed by radionuclide ventriculography) with regard to both left ventricular function and diastolic filling was defective [216].

Gastrointestinal

Gastric stasis (gastroparesis) and oesophageal immotility are well recognized and may give rise to troublesome symptoms in a few [217]. Measurements of gastric emptying are complex, being different for solid or liquid meals, and early or late emptying. Radioisotope methods measure oesophageal and gastric emptying of digestible solid, non-digestible solid and liquid meal components [218]. Recently, scintigraphic techniques have been developed and seem more simple and sensitive than other techniques, including intubation. Using such a technique, 58% of diabetic subjects had delayed gastric emptying of either the solid or liquid meal and there was a correlation with tests of autonomic function [219]. Symptomatic gastric retention and vomiting are all too obvious (although psychological factors have occasionally to be considered), but the fact that such a high percentage of randomly selected diabetic patients should be abnormal suggests that this may be a factor in erratic glucose control in some people. Manometry indicates absence of normal interdigestive motor cycles in the stomach [220], with antral hypermotility after ingestion of a solid meal. Pylorospasm may occur in subjects with clinical symptoms, and abnormal motility of the upper small gut is also demonstrable [221].

Metoclopramide results in improvement in gastric emptying and has proven clinical benefit [222], as does domperidone [223]. Cisapride in one-dose and long-term administration has proved to be effective in improving gastric emptying in diabetes by stimulating acetylcholine nerve endings [224]. Very rarely, if all else fails, gastroenterostomy may be necessary.

Diabetic diarrhoea is probably related to disordered small bowel motility, although not all those with abnormalities have diarrhoea [225]. Animal work suggests deficits of cholinergic and adrenergic innervation, microangiopathy and mucosal abnormalities [226]. That bacterial overgrowth must occur is suggested by the beneficial effects of tetracycline therapy [227]. After exclusion of other causes of diarrhoea (drugs, coeliac disease, colitis, tumour), therapy with codeine phosphate or loperamide should be tried before antibiotics.

Constipation may alternate with diarrhoea; little is known about its aetiology and treatment is very unrewarding. Megacolon has been reported [228]. External sphincter function is impaired and may lead to faecal incontinence, but functional tests seem to have little correlation with symptoms or therapeutic decision [229].

Excessive sweating after meals (gustatory sweating) may be an extremely unpleasant feature of autonomic neuropathy, occurring over the face and shoulders and often soaking the clothing [230]. Propantheline bromide relieves the sweating but often leads to intolerable dry mouth or constipation.

Bladder dysfunction is due to neuropathic changes in detrusor muscle afferent innervation [231], resulting in poor voiding, increased residual urine volume and, very occasionally, gross distention or total bladder paralysis. Pressure and reflex measurements are grossly abnormal and may be of diagnostic help on occasions [232]. Insidiously, the conscious sensation of bladder filling is lost and with efferent fibre loss (parasympathetic) the bladder fails to empty. Detailed urological assessment is important to exclude other causes of outflow obstruction. With an established problem a period of catheter drainage is warranted, followed by a regular drill of bladder emptying over 2–3 hours and prompt treatment of infection. Surgical resection of the bladder neck may be necessary but is followed by regrettable incidence of incontinence, destruction of the proximal sphincter leaving the patient dependent on the distal sphincter which itself may be neuropathic [233].

DIABETIC IMPOTENCE

Perhaps the most tragic complication of diabetes in human terms is impotence, afflicting approximately 40% of diabetic men [234]. The factors involved and resulting in failure of penile erection are neurological (peripheral and autonomic), vascular, hormonal and psychological. Treatment should be attempted only when all these factors have been assessed and the yardstick of success should not simply be regarded as 'return of erection'.

Assessment of the ability to achieve an erection helps to differentiate purely psychological influences. A number of devices are available and are usually used at night. Snap gauge fasteners measure maximal penile rigidity [235]. Nocturnal penile tumescence (NPT) records circumferential penile expansion and rigidity—a common phenomenon during sleep [236], the incidence of which reduces with age. Although many abnormalities of erectile ability have been described in diabetic men, more so in those with neuropathy, these measurements do not address

themselves to the fact that measured erection and rigidity may occur in a subject whose complaint is that the erection is not firm enough.

Electrophysiological measurements help to elucidate the extent of genital denervation and gross abnormalities will be more likely to occur in those with impotence. Basically, only the somatic innervation of the penile shaft may be assessed, and reduced conduction velocity is an early marker of neuropathy [237] and severely affected in proven impotence. Bulbocavernous reflex latency, a more invasive measurement, has proved to be an accurate measure and assists considerably in the exclusion of organic factors, gross abnormalities being present in organic impotence [238, 239].

Vascular factors are clearly also involved and may be easily evaluated by the use of Doppler ultrasound techniques [240]. In Lehman and Jacobs' study of diabetic impotence, 68% of men had evidence of vascular occlusion compared with only 26% with electrophysiological abnormalities. Arteriography with selective catheterization may be used, and infusion cavernosography has shown that there are venous leaks in organic impotence, whereas in the normal state there is no venous drainage during an erection [241].

The hormonal status in impotence is also abnormal. Plasma testosterone levels were low in 19% of the patients reported above [242] and, in a comparison of diabetic and non-diabetic impotence, serum free testosterone levels were reduced in the diabetic group together with an increase in urinary luteinizing hormone, findings that were not improved by meticulous control of the blood glucose [243].

In this complex field, psychological factors must play a large part. Even if such factors are not a primary cause, the onset of early awareness of slight inadequacy due to a physical cause could easily induce a serious but understandable psychological response. In these circumstances, early intervention, both organic and psychologically supportive, presumably would minimize this element. In assessing the role of different factors, 30% of subjects were thought to have psychological problems, although in only 19% of the total group were these regarded as important. In practice all factors are at work and the final end-point may be assessed by the visualization of erotic films by the patients, thus invoking the complexity of cerebral function. In fact, changes in penile diameter and penile pulse amplitude in response to 'sexual stimulation' failed to separate patients with organic disease from those with psychogenic symptoms. An erotic film resulted in less effective responses in diabetic subjects, not surprisingly least effective in those with autonomic dysfunction [244, 245].

As an obvious end-point of sexual achievement is present in the male, it is perhaps not surprising that 'sexual dysfunction' has been found to be no more common in diabetic women than in non-diabetic women [246]. Decreased libido is reported, with chronic tiredness and more evidence of emotional disturbance than in non-diabetic male spouses.

Treatment

In a condition where so many patients will not find a 'cure', considerable attention should be paid to psychological and clinical support of the patient in a constructive manner. Assessment will vary according to facilities available, but to ignore the problem—'it happens to diabetics' —is wrong. Not infrequently, totally diabetic marital or emotional problems are uncovered that can easily be solved. Where established organic impotence is beyond doubt, three lines of therapy are available:

(1) Coming to terms with an incurable situation. It may not present a major problem to a couple—but both partners must be assessed and considered. Other forms of physical comfort should be taught.
(2) Although no oral drug therapy is effective, direct injection of papaverine and phentolamine into the corpus cavernosum will induce satisfactory erections in a significant number of men [247, 248]. Priapism is a minor risk.
(3) Surgical implantation of a penile prosthesis —flexible or permanently rigid—is a technique to be offered only after detailed assessment and thought. Cultural factors influence the differing incidence of this treatment around the world. One study has shown that in the group selected most subjects were satisfied with the result [249]. Aids to erection based on the principle of suction applied to the penis, resulting in venous trapping, are available but have yet to be fully evaluated.

REFERENCES

1. Sima AAF, Nathaniel V, Bril V, McEwen TAJ, Greene DA. Histopathological heterogeneity of neuropathy in insulin-dependent and non-insulin dependent diabetes, and demonstration of axo-glial dysjunction in human diabetic neuropathy. J Clin Invest 1988; 81: 349–64.
2. Kennedy WR, Quick DC, Miyoshi T, Gerritsen GC. Peripheral neurology of the diabetic Chinese hamster. Diabetologia 1982; 33: 445.
3. Braund KG, Steiss JE. Distal neuropathy in spontaneous diabetes mellitus in the dog. Acta Neuropathol 1982; 57: 263.
4. Johnson PC, Coll SC, Cromey DW. Pathogenesis of diabetic neuropathy. Ann Neurol 1986; 19: 450–7.
5. Thomas PK, Lascelles RG. The pathology of diabetic neuropathy. Quart J Med 1966; 35: 489–509.
6. Yagihashi S, Matsumaja M. Ultrastructural pathology of peripheral nerves in patients with diabetic neuropathy. Tohoku J Exp Med 1979; 129: 357–66.
7. Malik R. Personal communication.
8. Thomas PK, Eliasson SG. Diabetic neuropathy. In Dyck PJ, Thomas PK, Lambert EH, Bunge R (eds) Peripheral neuropathy, vol. 2. Philadelphia: WB Saunders, 1984: pp 1773–810.
9. Archer A, Watkins PJ, Thomas PK, Sharma AK, Payan J. The natural history of acute painful neuropathy in diabetes mellitus. J Neurol Neurosurg Psychiat 1983; 46: 491.
10. Said G, Slama G, Selva J. Progressive centripetal degeneration of axons in small fibre type diabetic polyneuropathy. A clinical and pathological study. Brain 1983; 106: 791.
11. Sugimura K, Dyck PJ. Sural nerve myelin thickness and axis cylinder caliber in human diabetes. Neurology (NY) 1981; 31: 1087.
12. Sima AAF, Nathaniel V, Bril V, McEwen TAJ, Brown MB, Greene DA. Regeneration and repair of myelinated fibres in sural nerve biopsies from patients with diabetic neuropathy treated with an aldose reductase inhibitor. New Engl J Med 1988; 319: 548–55.
13. Sima AAF, Brismar T. Reversible diabetic nerve dysfunction: structural correlates to electrophysiological abnormalities. Ann Neurol 1985; 18: 21–9.
14. Sima AAF, Lattimer SA, Yagihashi S, Greene DA. Axo-glial dysjunction. A novel structural lesion that accounts for poorly reversible slowing of nerve conduction in the spontaneously diabetic Bio-breeding rat. J Clin Invest 1986; 77: 474–84.
15. Duchen LW, Anjorin A, Watkins PJ, Mackay JD. Pathology of autonomic neuropathy in diabetes. Ann Intern Med 1980; 92: 301.
16. Guy RJC, Richards F, Edmonds ME, Watkins

PJ. Diabetic autonomic neuropathy and iritis: an association suggesting an immunological cause. Br Med J 1984; 289: 343.

17. Dyck PJ. Pathology. In Dyck PJ, Thomas PK, Asbury AK, Winegrad AI, Porte D (eds) Diabetic neuropathy. Philadelphia: WB Saunders, 1987: pp 223–236.

18. Greene DA, Lattimer SA, Sima AAF. Sorbitol phosphorinositides and sodium potassium ATPase in the pathogenesis of diabetic complications. New Engl J Med 1987; 316: 599.

19. Greene DA, Winegrad AI. Effects of acute experimental diabetes on composite energy metabolism in peripheral nerve axons and Schwann cells. Diabetes 1981; 30: 967–74.

20. Greene DA, Lattimer SA. Impaired rat sciatic nerve sodium–potassium adenosine triphosphatase in acute streptozocin diabetes and its correction by dietary myo-inositol supplementation. J Clin Invest 1983; 72: 1058–63.

21. Clements RS. Diabetic neuropathy: new concepts of its aetiology. Diabetes 1979; 28: 604–11.

22. Greene DA, Lewis RA, Lattimer SA, Brown MJ. Selective effects of myo-inositol administration on sciatic and tibial motor nerve conduction parameters in the streptozocin-diabetic rat. Diabetes 1982; 31: 573–8.

23. Gregersen G. Variations in motor conduction velocity produced by acute changes of the metabolic state in diabetic patients. Diabetologia 1968; 4: 273–7.

24. Ward JD, Barnes CG, Fisher DJ, Jessop JD, Boher WR. Improvement in nerve conduction following treatment in newly diagnosed diabetics. Lancet 1971; i: 428–30.

25. Greene DA, Lattimer SA. Action of sorbinil in diabetic peripheral nerve. Relationship of polyol (sorbitol) pathway inhibition to a myo-inositol-mediated defect in sodium–potassium ATPase activity. Diabetes 1984; 33: 712–16.

26. Mayer JH, Tomlinson DR. The influence of aldose reductase inhibition and nerve myo-inositol on axonal transport and nerve conduction velocity in rats with experimental diabetes. J Physiol (London) 1983; 340: 25–6.

27. Yorek MA, Dunlap JA, Ginsberg BH. Myo-inositol metabolism in 41A3 neuroblastoma cells: effects of high glucose and sorbitol levels. J Neurochem 1987; 48: 53.

28. Simmons DA, Winegrad AI, Martin DB. Significance of tissue myo-inositol concentrations in metabolic regulation in nerve. Science 1982; 217: 848–51.

29. Greene DA, Lattimer SA. Protein kinase C agonists acutely normalize decreased ouabain-inhibitible respiration in diabetic rabbit nerve: implications for (Na, K)-ATPase regulation and diabetic complications. Diabetes 1986; 35: 242–5.

30. Hootman SR, Brown ME, Williams JA. Phorbol esters and A23187 regulate Na^+/K^+ pump activity in pancreatic acinar cells. Am J Physiol 1987; 252: G499–505.

31. Brismar T, Sima AAF, Greene DA. Reversible and irreversible nodal dysfunction in diabetic neuropathy. Ann Neurol 1987; 21: 504.

32. Greene DA, Chakrabarti S, Lattimer SA, Simma AAF. Role of sorbitol accumulation and myo-inositol depletion in paranodal swelling of large myelinated fibres in the insulin-deficient spontaneously diabetic bio-breeding rat. J Clin Invest 1987; 79: 1479.

33. McCallum KNC, Sharma AK, Blanchard DS, Stribling D, Mirrless DJ, Duguid IG, Thomas PK. The effect of continuous subcutaneous insulin infusion therapy on morphological and biochemical abnormalities of peripheral nerves in experimental diabetes. J Neurol Sci 1986; 74: 55.

34. Sidenius P, Jakobsen J. Axonal transport in human and experimental diabetes. In Dyck PJ, Thomas PK, Asbury AK, Winegrad AI, Porte D (eds) Diabetic neuropathy. Philadelphia: WB Saunders, 1987: pp 260–5.

35. Mayer JH, Tomlinson DR. Prevention of defects of axonal transport and nerve conduction velocity by oral administration of myo-inositol or an aldose reductase inhibitor in streptozotocin-diabetic rats. Diabetologia 1983; 25: 433–8.

36. Tomlinson DR, Mayer JH. Decreased axonal transport in diabetes mellitus—a possible contribution to the aetiology of diabetic neuropathy. J Auton Pharmacol 1984; 59–72.

37. Vitadello M, Filliatreau G, Dupont JL, Hassig R, Gorio A, Di Giamberadino L. Altered axonal transport of cytoskeletal protein in the mutant diabetic mouse. J Neurochem 1985; 45: 860–8.

38. Tomlinson DR, Sidenius P, Larsen JR. Slow component-a of axonal transport, nerve myo-inositol and aldose reductase inhibition in streptozotocin-diabetic rats. Diabetes 1986; 35: 398–402.

39. Whiteley SJ, Townsend J, Tomlinson DR, Willars GB. Fast anterograde axonal transport in wasted and non-wasted diabetic rats: effects of aldose reductase inhibition. Diabetes Res 1986; 3: 447.

40. Willars GB, Calcutt NA, Tomlinson DR. Reduced anterograde and retrograde accumulation of axonally transported phosphofructo-kinase in streptozotocin-diabetic rats: effects of insulin and the aldose reductase inhibitor 'Statil'. Diabetologia 1987; 30: 239.

41. Jakobsen J, Sidenius P, Braendgard H. A proposal for a classification of neuropathies

according to their axonal transport abnormalities. J Neurol Neurosurg Psychiat 1986; 49: 986.

42. Thomas PK, Ward JD. Diabetic neuropathy. In Keen H, Jarrett J (eds) Complications of diabetes. London: Edward Arnold, 1975: pp 151–77.

43. Vlassara H, Brownlee M, Cerami A. Accumulation of diabetic rat peripheral nerve myelin by macrophages increases with the presence of advanced glycosylation endproducts. J Exp Med 1984; 160: 197.

44. Schmidt RE, Modert CW, Yip HK, Johnson EM. Retrograde axonal transport of intravenously administered nerve growth factor in rats with streptozocin induced diabetes. Diabetes 1983; 37: 654.

45. Carson KA, Sar M, Hanker SJ. Immunocytochemical demonstration of nerve growth factor and histofluorescence of catecholaminergic nerves in salivary glands of diabetic mice. Histochem J 1982; 14: 35.

46. Hale PJ, Nattrass M, Silverman SH, Sennit C, Perkins CM, Uden A, Sundkvist G. Peripheral nerve concentrations of glucose, fructose, sorbitol and myo-inositol in diabetic and nondiabetic patients. Diabetologia 1987; 30: 464.

47. Reference deleted.

48. Dyck PJ, Sherman WR, Hallcher LM et al. Human diabetic endoneurial sorbitol, fructose and myo-inositol related to sural nerve morphometry. Ann Neurol 1980; 8: 590–6.

49. Llewelyn JG, Simpson CMF, Thomas PK. Changes in sorbitol, myo-inositol and lipid inositol in dorsal root and sympathetic ganglia from streptozotocin-diabetic rats. Diabetologia 1986; 29: 876.

50. Chakrabarti S, Sima AAF, Nakajima T, Yagishashi S, Greene DA. Aldose reductase in the BB rat: isolation, immunological identification and localization in the retina and peripheral nerve. Diabetologia 1987; 30: 244.

51. Srivastava SK, Ansari NH, Hair GA, Awasthi S, Das B. Activation of human erythrocyte, brain, aorta, muscle and ocular tissue aldose reductase. Metab Clin Exp 1986; 35: 114.

52. Koh MS, Misch KJ, Yuen CT, Rhodes EL. Accumulation of sorbitol in endothelial cells—a possible cause of diabetic microangiopathy. Diabetes Res 1986; 3: 217.

53. Vertommen J, Rillaerts E, Gysels M, De Leeuw I. Erythrocyte sorbitol content in diabetic patients: relation to metabolic control. Diabète Métab 1987; 13: 182.

54. Lehtinen JM, Hyvonen SK, Uusitupa M, Puhakainen E, Halonen T, Kilpelainen H. The effect of sorbinil treatment on red cell sorbitol levels and clinical and electrophysiological parameters of diabetic neuropathy. J Neurol 1986; 233: 174.

55. Judzewitsch RG, Jaspan JB, Polonsky KS et al. Aldose reductase inhibition improves nerve conduction velocity in diabetic patients. New Engl J Med 1983; 308: 119.

56. Young RJ, Ewing DJ, Clarke BF. A controlled trial of sorbinil, an aldose reductase inhibitor, in chronic painful diabetic neuropathy. Diabetes 1983; 32: 938.

57. Jaspan J, Herold K, Maselli R, Bartkus C. Treatment of severely painful diabetic neuropathy with an aldose reductase inhibitor: relief of pain and improved somatic and autonomic nerve function. Lancet 1983; ii: 758.

58. Martyn CN, Reid W, Young RJ, Ewing DJ, Clarke BF. Six month treatment with sorbinil in asymptomatic diabetic neuropathy: failure to improve abnormal nerve function. Diabetes 1987; 36: 987.

59. Lewin IG, O'Brien IAD, Morgan MH, Corrall RJM. Clinical and neurophysiological studies with the aldose reductase inhibitor, sorbinil, in symptomatic diabetic neuropathy. Diabetologia 1984; 26: 445.

60. Fagerberg SE. Studies on the pathogenesis of diabetic neuropathy. Acta Med Scand 1956; 156: 295.

61. Timperley WR, Boulton AJM, Davies-Jones GAB, Jarratt JA, Ward JD. Small vessel disease in progressive diabetic neuropathy associated with good metabolic control. J Clin Pathol 1985; 38: 1030–8.

62. Johnson PC, Doll SC, Cromey DW. Pathogenesis of diabetic neuropathy. Ann Neurol 1986; 19: 450–7.

63. Woltman HW, Wilder RM. Diabetes mellitus. Pathological changes in spinal cord and peripheral nerves. Arch Int Med 1929; 44: 577.

64. Williams E, Timperley WR, Ward JD, Duckworth T. Electron microscopical studies of vessels in diabetic peripheral neuropathy. J Clin Pathol 1980; 33: 462–70.

65. Powell HC, Rosoff J, Myers RR. Microangiopathy in human diabetic neuropathy. Acta Neuropathol (Berl) 1985; 68: 295–305.

66. Tuck RR, Schmelzer JD, Low PA. Endoneurial blood flow and oxygen tension in the sciatic nerves of rats with experimental diabetic neuropathy. Brain 1984; 107: 935.

67. Low PA, Tuck RR, Dyck PJ. Prevention of some electrophysiologic and biochemical abnormalities with oxygen supplementation in experimental diabetic neuropathy. Proc Natl Acad Sci USA 1984; 81: 6894.

68. Sima AAF, Thibert P. Proximal motor neuropathy in the BB-Wistar rat. Diabetes 1982; 31: 784.

69. Low PA, Schmelzer JD, Ward KK, Yao JK.

Experimental chronic hypoxic neuropathy: relevance to diabetic neuropathy. Am J Physiol 1986; 250: E94.

70. Low PA, Tuck RR, Takeuchi M. Nerve microenvironment in diabetic neuropathy. In Dyck PJ, Thomas PK, Asbury AK, Winegrad AI, Porte D (eds) Diabetic neuropathy. Philadelphia: WB Saunders, 1987: p 266.

71. Nukada H. Increased susceptibility to ischaemic damage in streptozocin-diabetic nerve. Diabetes 1986; 35: 1058.

72. Paramelle B, Vila A, Muller P. Fréquence des polyneuropathies dans les bronchopneumopathies chroniques obstructives. Presse Méd 1986; 15: 563.

73. Dyck PJ, Lais A, Karnes JL. Fibre loss is primary and multifocal in sural nerves in diabetic polyneuropathy. Ann Neurol 1986; 19: 425.

74. Dyck PJ, Karnes JL, O'Brien MS. The spatial distribution of fibre loss in diabetic polyneuropathy suggests ischaemia. Ann Neurol 1986; 19: 440.

75. Yasuda H, Dyck PJ. Abnormalities of endoneurial microvessels and sural nerve pathology in diabetic neuropathy. Neurology 1987; 37: 20.

76. Newrick PG, Wilson AJ, Ward JD. Sural nerve oxygen tension in diabetes. Br Med J 1986; 293: 1053.

77. Malik RA, Newrick PG, Sharma AK et al. Microangiopathy in human diabetic neuropathy: relationship between capillary abnormalities and the severity of neuropathy. Diabetologia 1987; 30: 538A.

78. Steiness IB. Influence of diabetic status on vibratory perception during ischaemia. Acta Med Scand 1961; 170: 319.

79. Seneviratne KN, Peiris OA. The effects of hypoxia on the excitability of the isolated peripheral nerves of the alloxan-diabetic rat. J Neurol Neurosurg Psychiat 1969; 32: 462.

80. Castaigne P, Cathala HP, Beaussart-Bolange L, Petrover M. Effect of ischaemia on peripheral nerve function in patients with chronic renal failure undergoing dialysis treatment. J Neurol Neurosurg Psychiat 1972; 35: 631.

81. Ritchie JM. A note on the mechanism of resistance to axonia and ischaemia in pathophysiological mammalian myelinated nerve. J Neurol Neurosurg Psychiat 1985; 48: 274.

82. Jaramillo J, Simard-Duquesne N, Dvornik D. Resistance of the diabetic rat nerve to ischaemic inactivation. Can J Physiol Pharmacol 1984; 63: 733.

83. Newrick PG, Boulton AJM, Ward JD. Nerve ischaemia resistance: an early abnormality in diabetes. Diabet Med 1987; 4: 517.

84. Greaves M, Preston FE. Haemostatic abnormalities in Diabetes. In Jarrètt J (ed.) Diabetes and heart disease. Amsterdam: Elsevier, 1984: pp 47–80.

85. Dyck PJ, Karnes JL, Daube J, O'Brien P, Service FJ. Clinical and neuropathologic criteria for the diagnosis and staging of diabetic polyneuropathy. Brain 1985; 108: 861.

86. Dyck PJ, Bushek W, Spring EM et al. The sensitivity and specificity of vibratory and cooling detection thresholds in the diagnosis of diabetic neuropathy. Diabetes Care 1987; 10: 432–40.

87. Dyck PJ. Detection, characterization, and staging of polyneuropathy assessed in diabetics. Muscle Nerve 1988; 11: 21.

88. Dyck PJ, Karnes J, O'Brien PC. Diagnosis, staging and classification of diabetic neuropathy and associations with other complications. In Dyck PJ, Thomas PK, Asbury AK, Winegrad AI, Porte D (eds) Diabetic neuropathy. Philadelphia: WB Saunders, 1987: pp 37–44.

89. Dyck PJ, Sherman WR, Hallcher LM et al. Human diabetic endoneurial sorbitol, fructose and myo-inositol related to sural nerve morphometry. Ann Neurol 1980; 8: 590.

90. Magelende R, McBride P, Mistretta CM. Light touch thresholds in diabetic patients. Diabetes Care 1982; 5: 311.

91. Aronson AE, Auger RG, Bastron JA et al. Clinical examination in neurology, 5th edn. Philadelphia: WB Saunders, 1981.

92. Cracco J, Castells S, Mark E. Spinal somatosensory evoked potentials in juvenile diabetes. Ann Neurol 1984; 15: 55.

93. Gupta PR, Dorfman LJ. Spinal somatosensory conduction in diabetes. Neurology 1981; 31: 841.

94. Fagius J. Microneurographic findings in diabetic polyneuropathy with special reference to sympathetic nerve activity. Diabetologia 1982; 23: 415.

95. Cruz MA. Spinal evoked potentials and single fibre EMG in diabetic neuropathy. Electromyogr Clin Neurophysiol 1986; 26: 499.

96. Daube JR. Electrophysiologic testing in diabetic neuropathy. In Dyck PJ, Thomas PK, Asbury AK, Winegrad AI, Porte D (eds) Diabetic neuropathy. Philadelphia: WB Saunders, 1987: pp 162–76.

97. Lawrence DE, Locke S. Motor nerve conduction velocity in diabetes. Arch Neurol 1961; 5: 483.

98. Mayer RF. Nerve conduction studies in man. Neurology 1963; 13: 1021.

99. Service FJ, Rizza RA, Daube JR, O'Brien PC, Dyck PJ. Near normoglycaemia improved nerve conduction and vibration sensation in diabetic neuropathy. Diabetologia 1985; 28: 722–7.

100. Eeg-Olofsson O, Petersen I. Childhood diabetic neuropathy: a clinical and neurophysiological study. Acta Paediatr Scand 1966; 55: 163.

101. Eng GD, Hung W, August GP, Smokvina MD.

Nerve conduction velocity determinations in juvenile diabetics: continuing study of 190 patients. Arch Phys Med Rehab 1976; 57: 1.

102. Gregersen G. Diabetic neuropathy: influence of age, sex, metabolic control and duration of diabetes on motor conduction velocity. Neurology 1967; 17: 972.

103. Levy DM, Abraham RR, Abraham RM. Small and large involvement in early diabetic neuropathy: A study with the medial plantar response and sensory thresholds. Diabetes Care 1987; 10: 441.

104. Abraham RR, Abraham RM, Wynn V. Autonomic and electrophysiological studies in patients with signs or symptoms of diabetic neuropathy. Electroencephalogr Clin Neurophysiol 1986; 63: 223.

105. Bertelsmann FW, Heimans JJ, Van Rooy JCGM, Visser SL. Comparison of Hoffman reflex with quantitative assessment of cutaneous sensation in diabetic neuropathy. Acta Neurol Scand 1986; 74: 121.

106. Steiness IB. Vibratory perception in normal subjects. A biothesiometer study. Acta Med Scand 1957; 158: 315–25.

107. Gregersen G. Vibratory perception threshold and motor conduction velocity in diabetics and non-diabetics. Acta Med Scand 1968; 183: 61–5.

108. Guy RJC, Clark PN, Watkins PJ. Evaluation of thermal and vibration sensation in diabetic neuropathy. Diabetologia 1985; 28: 131–7.

109. Edmonds ME, Blundell MP, Morris M, Thomas EM, Williamson M, Watkins PJ. The 'Combined Diabetic Foot Clinic'. A major development in diabetic foot care. Diabetologia 1982; 23: 468A.

110. Lowenthal LM, Hockaday TDR. Vibration sensory thresholds depend on pressure of applied stimulus. Diabetes Care 1987; 10: 100.

111. Bertelsmann FW, Heimans JJ, Van Rooy JCGM, Visser SL. Reproducibility of vibratory perception thresholds in patients with diabetic neuropathy. Diabetes Res 1986; 3: 463.

112. Bloom S, Till S, Sonksen P, Smith S. Use of a biothesiometer to measure individual vibration thresholds and their variation in 519 non-diabetic subjects. Br Med J 1984; 288: 1793.

113. Heimans JJ, Bertelsmann FW, Van Rooy JCGM. Large and small nerve fibre function in painful diabetic neuropathy. J Neurol Sci 1986; 74: 1.

114. Arezzo JC, Schaumburg HH, Laudadio C. Thermal sensitivity tester. Device for quantitative assessment of thermal sense in diabetic neuropathy. Diabetes 1986; 35: 590.

115. Dyck PJ, Karnes J, O'Brien PC. Detection thresholds of cutaneous sensation. In Dyck PJ, Thomas PK, Asbury AK, Winegrad AI, Porte D (eds) Diabetic neuropathy. Philadelphia: WB Saunders, 1987: pp 107–21.

116. Dyck PJ, Bushek W, Spring EM, Karnes JL, Litchy WJ, O'Brien PC, Service FJ. Vibratory and cooling detection thresholds compared with other tests in diagnosing and staging diabetic neuropathy. Diabetes Care 1987; 10: 432.

117. Young RJ, Zhou YQ, Rodriguez E. Variable relationship between peripheral somatic and autonomic neuropathy in patients with different syndromes of diabetic polyneuropathy. Diabetes 1986; 35: 192.

118. Fry IK, Hardwick C, Scott GW. Diabetic neuropathy: a survey and follow-up of sixty-six cases. Guys Hosp Rep 1962; 111: 113.

119. Boulton AJM, Knight G, Drury J, Ward JD. The prevalence of symptomatic diabetic neuropathy in an insulin-treated population. Diabetes Care 1985; 8: 125.

120. Pirart J. Diabetes mellitus and its degenerative complications. A prospective study of 4400 patients observed between 1947 and 1973. Diabetes Care 1978; 1: 168.

121. Brown MJ, Asbury AK. Diabetic neuropathy. Ann Neurol 1984; 15: 2.

122. Ward JD. Abnormal processes in the nerve. In Brownless M (ed.) Diabetes mellitus, vol 4. New York: Garland STPM Press, 1981: pp 87–113.

123. Mabin D, Darragon T, Manez JF. Influence of glycaemic control on peripheral nerve conduction in insulin-dependent diabetic subjects. Rev Electroencephalogr Neurophysiol Clin 1982; 12: 72.

124. Halar EM, Graf RJ, Halter JB. Diabetic neuropathy: a clinical, laboratory and electrodiagnostic study. Arch Phys Med Rehab 1982; 63: 298.

125. Agardh CD, Rosen I, Schersten B. Improvement of peripheral nerve function after institution of insulin treatment in diabetes mellitus. A case control study. Acta Med Scand 1983; 213: 282.

126. Boulton AJM, Worth RG, Drury J, Hardisty CA, Wolf E, Cudworth AG, Ward JD. Genetic and metabolic studies in diabetic neuropathy. Diabetologia 1984; 26: 15.

127. Dahl-Jorgensen K, Brinchman-Hansen O, Hanssen KF. Effect of near normoglycaemia for two years on progression of early diabetic retinopathy, nephropathy, and neuropathy: the Oslo Study. Br Med J 1986; 293: 1195.

128. Ehle AL, Raskin P. Increased nerve conduction in diabetics after a year of improved glucoregulation. J Neurol Sci 1986; 74: 191.

129. Commi G, Canal N, Lozza L. Peripheral nerve abnormalities in newly-diagnosed diabetic children. Acta Diab Lat 1986; 23: 69.

130. Young RJ, Macintyre CCA, Martyn CN et al. Progression of subclinical polyneuropathy in young patients with type I (insulin-dependent)

diabetes: association with glycaemic control and microangiopathy (microvascular complications). Diabetologia 1986; 29: 156.

131. Sjoberg S, Gunnarsson R, Gjotterberg M. Residual insulin production, glycaemic control and prevalence of microvascular lesions and polyneuropathy in long-term type I (insulin-dependent) diabetes mellitus. Diabetologia 1987; 30: 208.

132. Holman RR, Dornan TL, Mayon-White V et al. Prevention of deterioration of renal and sensory nerve function by more intensive management of insulin-dependent diabetic patients. A two-year randomised prospective study. Lancet 1983; i: 204.

133. Frighi V, Loughnane JW, Pozzilli P et al. Early signs of neuropathy and microangiopathy in young type I (insulin-dependent) diabetic patients: correlation with long-term metabolic control. Diabetologia 1987; 30: 521A.

134. Bruyn GW, Garland H. Neuropathies of endocrine origin. In Vinken PJ, Bruyn GW (eds) Handbook of clinical neurology, vol. 8. Amsterdam: North-Holland, 1970, p 29.

135. Archer AG, Watkins PJ, Thomas PK, Sharma AK, Payan J. The natural history of acute painful neuropathy in diabetes mellitus. J Neurol Neurosurg Psychiat 1983; 46: 491.

136. Boulton AJM, Armstrong WD, Scarpello JHB, Ward JD. The natural history of painful diabetic neuropathy—a 4-year study. Postgrad Med J 1983; 59: 556.

137. Asbury AK, Aldredge H, Hershberg R, Fisher CM. Oculomotor palsy in diabetes mellitus: a clinico-pathological study. Brain 1970; 93: 555.

138. Sidenius P, Jakobsen J. Anterograde fast component of axonal transport during insulin-induced hypoglycaemia in non-diabetic and diabetic rats. Diabetes 1987; 36: 853.

139. Jakobsen J, Sidenius P. Hypoglycaemic neuropathy. In Dyck PJ, Thomas PK, Asbury AK, Winegrad AI, Porte D (eds) Diabetic neuropathy. Philadelphia: WB Saunders, 1987: pp 94–9.

140. Boulton AJM, Ward JD. Diabetic neuropathies and pain. Clin Endocrinol Metab 1986; 15: 917–31.

141. Brown MJ, Martin JR, Asbury AK. Painful diabetic neuropathy: a morphometric study. Arch Neurol 1976; 33: 164–71.

142. Said G, Slama G, Selva J. Progressive centripetal degeneration of axons in small fibre diabetic polyneuropathy. Brain 1983; 106: 791–807.

143. Wall PD, Gutnick M. Properties of afferent impulses originating from a neuroma. Nature 1974; 248: 740–3.

144. Devor M. Nerve pathophysiology and the mechanism of pain in causalgia. J Autonom Nerv Syst 1983; 7: 371–84.

145. Akoev GN. Catecholamines, acetylcholine and excitability of mechanoreceptors. Prog Neurobiol 1980; 15: 269–94.

146. Morley GK, Mooradian AD, Levine AL, Morley JE. Mechanisms of pain in diabetic peripheral neuropathy: effect of glucose on pain perception in humans. Am J Med 1984; 77: 79–82.

147. Ward JD. The diabetic leg. Diabetologia 1982; 22: 141–7.

148. Archer AG, Roberts VC, Watkins PJ. Blood flow patterns in painful diabetic neuropathy. Diabetologia 1984; 27: 563.

149. Ward JD, Boulton AJM, Simms JM, Sandler DA, Knight G. Venous distension in the diabetic neuropathic foot. J Roy Soc Med 1983; 76: 1011.

150. Boulton AJM, Scarpello JHB, Ward JD. Venous oxygenation in the diabetic neuropathic foot: evidence of arteriovenous shunting? Diabetologia 1982; 22: 6.

151. Edmonds ME, Roberts VC, Watkins PJ. Blood flow in the diabetic neuropathic foot. Diabetologia 1982; 22: 9.

152. Edmonds ME, Morrison N, Laws JW, Watkins PJ. Medial arterial calcification and diabetic neuropathy. Br Med J 1982; 284: 928.

153. Ryder REJ, Kennedy RL, Newrick PG, Wilson RM, Ward JD, Hardisty CA. Severe autonomic denervation in the feet is an important component of diabetic neuropathic foot ulceration. Clin Sci 1988; 74 (suppl. 18): 12.

154. Van Den Hoogen F, Brawn LA, Sherriff S, Watson N, Ward JD. Arteriovenous shunting in quadriplegia. Paraplegia 1986; 24: 282.

155. Boulton AJM, Drury J, Clarke B, Ward JD. Continuous subcutaneous insulin infusion in the management of painful diabetic neuropathy. Diabetes Care 1982; 5: 386.

156. White NH, Waltman SR, Krupin T, Santiago JH. Reversal of neuropathic and gastrointestinal complications related to diabetes mellitus in adolescents with improved metabolic control. J Paediatr 1981; 99: 41–5.

157. Kvinesdal BB, Molin J, Froland A, Gram LF. Imipramine treatment of painful diabetic neuropathy. JAMA 1984; 251: 1727–30.

158. Young RJ, Clarke BF. Pain relief in diabetic neuropathy: the effectiveness of imipramine and related drugs. Diabet Med 1985; 2: 262–366.

159. Davis JL, Lewis SB, Gerich JE et al. Peripheral diabetic neuropathy treated with amitriptyline and fluphenazine. JAMA 1977; 238: 2291–2.

160. Gorio A, Carmignoto G, Ferrari G. Axon sprouting stimulated by gangliosides: a new model for elongation and sprouting. In Rapport MM, Gorio A (eds) Gangliosides in neurological and neuromuscular function, development and repair. New York: Raven Press, 1981: pp 175–95.

161. Kleinebeckel D. Acceleration of muscle re-innervation in rats by ganglioside treatment: an electromyographic study. Eur J Pharm 1982; 80: 243.

162. Marini P, Vitadello M, Bianchi R, Tribau C, Gorio A. Impaired axonal transport of acetylcholinesterase in the sciatic nerve of alloxan-diabetic rats: effect of ganglioside treatment. Diabetologia 1986; 29: 254.

163. Horowitz SH. Ganglioside therapy in diabetic neuropathy. Muscle Nerve 1986; 9: 531.

164. Crepaldi G, Fedele D, Tiengo A et al. Ganglioside treatment in diabetic peripheral neuropathy. Acta Diab Lat 1983; 20: 265.

165. Abraham RR, Abraham RM, Wynn V. The use of gangliosides in human diabetic neuropathy. Inserm 1984; 126: 575–84.

166. Vlassara H, Brownlee M, Cerami A. Excessive nonenzymatic glycosylation of peripheral and central nervous system myelin components in diabetic rats. Diabetes 1983; 37: 670.

167. Brownlee H, Vlassara A, Kooney P, Ulrich P, Cerami A. Inhibition of diabetes-induced arterial wall lipoprotein deposition and prevention of arterial wall collagen crosslinking by aminoguanidine. Diabetologia 1986; 29: 523A.

168. Jamal GA, Carmichael H, Weir AI. Gammalinolenic acid in diabetic neuropathy. Lancet 1986; i: 1098.

169. Kastrup J, Petersen P, Dejgard J, Hilsted J, Angelo HR. Treatment of chronic painful diabetic neuropathy with intravenous lidocaine infusion. Br Med J 1986; 292: 173.

170. Dejgard J, Petersen P, Kastrup J. Mexiletine for treatment of painful diabetic neuropathy. Lancet 1987; i: 911.

171. Pfeifer MA, Peterson H. Cardiovascular autonomic neuropathy. In Dyck PJ, Thomas PK, Asbury AK, Winegrad AI, Porte D (eds) Diabetic neuropathy. Philadelphia: WB Saunders, 1987: pp 122–33.

172. Young RJ, Ewing DJ, Clarke BF. Nerve function and metabolic control in teenage diabetics. Diabetes 1983; 32: 142.

173. Ewing DJ, Borsey DQ, Bellavere F, Clarke BF. Cardiac autonomic neuropathy in diabetes: comparison of measures of RR interval variation. Diabetologia 1981; 21: 18.

174. Weinberg CR, Pfeifer MA. An improved method for measuring heart rate variability: assessment of cardiac autonomic function. Biometrics 1984; 40: 855.

175. Mackey JD, Hayakawa H, Watkins PJ. Cardiovascular effects of insulin: plasma volume changes in diabetics. Diabetologia 1978; 15: 453.

176. Pfeifer MA, Weinberg CR, Cook DL et al. Autonomic neural dysfunction in recently diagnosed diabetic subjects. Diabetes Care 1984; 7: 447.

177. Bennett T, Farquhar IK, Hosking DJ, Hampton JR. Assessment of methods for estimating autonomic nervous control of the heart in patients with diabetes mellitus. Diabetes 1978; 27: 1167.

178. Ewing DJ, Campbell IW, Clarke BF. Assessment of cardiovascular effects in diabetic autonomic neuropathy and prognostic implications. Ann Intern Med 1980; 92: 308.

179. Ewing DJ. Cardiovascular reflexes and autonomic neuropathy. Clin Sci Molec Med 1978; 55: 321.

180. Ewing DJ, Campbell IW, Murray A, Neilson JM, Clarke BF. Immediate heart rate response to standing: simple test for autonomic neuropathy in diabetes. Br Med J 1978; 1: 145.

181. Cryer PE. Isotope derivative measurement of plasma norepinephrine and epinephrine in man. Diabetes 1976; 25: 1071.

182. Christensen NJ. Plasma catecholamines in long-term diabetics with and without neuropathy and in hypophysectomized patients. J Clin Invest 1972; 51: 779.

183. Neubauer B, Christensen NJ. Norepinephrine, epinephrine and dopamine contents of the cardiovascular system in long-term diabetics. Diabetes 1976; 25: 6.

184. Tamberlane W, Sherwin RS, Koivisto V, Hendler R, Genel M, Felig P. Normalization of the growth hormone and catecholamine response to exercise in juvenile-onset diabetic subjects treated with a portable insulin infusion pump. Diabetes 1979; 28: 785.

185. Caviezel F, Picotti GB, Margonato A et al. Plasma adrenaline and noradrenaline concentrations in diabetic patients with and without autonomic neuropathy at rest and during sympathetic stimulation. Diabetologia 1982; 23: 19.

186. Nakamaru M, Ogihara T, Higaki J. Plasma inactive renin in diabetic patients with neuropathy: a role for the sympathetic nervous system in the conversion in vivo of inactive renin. Acta Endocrinol 1983; 104: 216.

187. Smith SA. Reduced sinus arrhythmia in diabetic autonomic neuropathy: diagnostic value of an age-related normal range. Br Med J 1982; 285: 1599.

188. Weiling W, Van Brederode JF, De Rijk LG, Borst C, Dunning AJ. Reflex control of heart rate in normal subjects in relation to age: a data base for cardiac vagal neuropathy. Diabetologia 1982; 22: 163.

189. Weiling W, Borst C, Van Brederode JF, Van Dongen Torman MA, Van Montrans GA, Dunning AJ. Testing for autonomic neuropathy: heart rate changes after orthostatic manoeuvres and static muscle contractions. Clin Sci 1983; 64: 581.

190. Pfeifer MA, Cook D, Brodsky J et al. Quantitative evaluation of cardiac parasympathetic activity in normal and diabetic man. Diabetes 1982; 31: 339.

191. Smith SA, Smith SE. Reduced pupillary light reflexes in diabetic autonomic neuropathy. Diabetologia 1983; 24: 330.

192. Pfeifer MA, Cook D, Brodsky J et al. Quantitative evaluation of sympathetic and parasympathetic control of iris function. Diabetes Care 1982; 5: 518.

193. Smith SA, Dewhirst RR. A simple diagnostic test for pupillary abnormality in diabetic autonomic neuropathy. Diabet Med 1986; 3: 38.

194. Montserrat JM, Cochrane GM, Wolf C et al. Ventilatory control in diabetes mellitus. Eur J Respir Dis 1985; 67: 112.

195. Sobotka PA, Liss HP, Vinik AI. Impaired hypoxic ventilatory drive in diabetic patients with autoimmune neuropathy. J Clin Endocrinol Metab 1986; 62: 658.

196. Mondini S, Guilleminault C. Abnormal breathing patterns during sleep in diabetes. Ann Neurol 1985; 17: 391.

197. Mitchell EA, Wealthall SR, Elliott RB. Diabetic autonomic neuropathy in children: immediate heart-rate response to standing. Aust Paediatr J 1983; 19: 175.

198. Bellavere F, Cardone C, Ferri M, Guarini L, Piccoli A, Fedele D. Standing-to-lying heart rate variation. A new simple test in the diagnosis of diabetic autonomic neuropathy. Diabet Med 1987; 4: 41.

199. Sundkvist G, Lilja BO. Autonomic neuropathy in diabetes mellitus: a follow up study. Diabetes Care 1985; 8: 129.

200. Fedele D, Bellavere F, Cardone C et al. Improvement of cardiovascular autonomic reflexes after amelioration of metabolic control in insulin dependent diabetic subjects with severe autonomic neuropathy. Horm Metab Res 1985; 17: 410.

201. Hosking DJ. Autonomic neuropathy. In Alberti KGMM, Krall LP (eds) Diabetes annual 3. Amsterdam: Elsevier, 1987: pp 289–305.

202. Corbin DOC, Young RJ, Morrison DC, Hoskins P, McDicken WN, Housley E, Clarke BF. Blood flow in the foot, polyneuropathy and foot ulceration in diabetes mellitus. Diabetologia 1987; 30: 468.

203. Ahmed ME, Delbridge L, Le Quesne LP. The role of autonomic neuropathy in diabetic foot ulceration. J Neurol Neurosurg Psychiat 1986; 49: 1002.

204. Ahmed ME, Le Quesne PM. Quantitative sweat test in diabetics with neuropathic foot lesions. J Neurol Neurosurg Psychiat 1986; 49: 1059.

205. Ewing DJ, Burt AA, Williams IR, Campbell IW, Clarke BF. Peripheral motor nerve function in diabetic autonomic neuropathy. J Neurol Neurosurg Psychiat 1976; 39: 453–60.

206. Abraham RR, Abraham RM, Wynn V. Autonomic and electrophysiological studies in patients with signs or symptoms of diabetic neuropathy. Electroencephal Clin Neurophysiol 1986; 63: 223–30.

207. Ewing DJ, Martyn CN, Young RJ et al. The value of cardiovascular autonomic function tests: 10 years experience in diabetes. Diabetes Care 1985; 8: 491.

208. Ewing DJ, Campbell IW, Clarke BF. The natural history of diabetic autonomic neuropathy. Quart J Med 1980; 49: 95–108.

209. Hilsted J, Parving HH, Christensen NJ, Benn J, Galbo H. Haemodynamics in diabetic orthostatic hypotension. J Clin Invest 1981; 68: 1427.

210. Lloyd-Mostyn RN, Watkins PJ. Total cardiac denervation in diabetic autonomic neuropathy. Diabetes 1976; 25: 748.

211. Bexton RS, Vallin HO, Camm AJ. Diurnal variation of the QT interval—influence of the autonomic nervous system. Br Heart J 1986; 55: 253.

212. Hume L, Oakley GDG, Boulton AJM, Peach M, Hardisty CA, Ward JD. Ambulatory monitoring of the ST segment in diabetic men with and without peripheral neuropathy. Diabet Med 1986; 3: 545.

213. Hume L, Oakley GDG, Boulton AJM, Hardisty CA, Ward JD. Asymptomatic myocardial ischaemia in diabetes and its relationship to diabetic neuropathy: an exercise electrocardiography study in middle-aged diabetic men. Diabetes Care 1986; 9: 384.

214. Ewing DJ, Borsey DQ, Travis P, Bellauere F, Nielson JMM, Clarke BF. Abnormalities of ambulatory 24-hour heart rate in diabetes mellitus. Diabetes 1983; 32: 101.

215. Zola B, Kahn JK, Juni JE, Vinik AI. Abnormal cardiac function in diabetic patients with autonomic neuropathy in the absence of ischaemic heart disease. J Clin Endocrinol Metab 1986; 63: 208.

216. Kahn JK, Zola B, Juni JE, Vinik AI. Radionuclide assessment of left ventricular diastolic filling in diabetes mellitus with and without cardiac autonomic neuropathy. J Am Coll Cardiol 1986; 7: 1303.

217. Feldman M, Schiller LR. Disorders of gastrointestinal motility associated with diabetes mellitus. Ann Intern Med 1983; 98: 378.

218. Horowitz M, Collins PJ, Sherman DJC. Disorders of gastric emptying in humans and the use of radionuclide techniques. Arch Int Med 1985; 145: 1467–75.

219. Horowitz M, Harding PE, Maddox A et al. Gastric and oesophageal emptying in insulin-depen-

dent diabetes mellitus. J Gastroenterol Hepatol 1986; 1: 97–113.

220. Malagelda JR, Rees WDR, Mozzotta LJ, Go VLW. Gastric motor abnormalities in diabetic and postvagotomy gastroparesis: effect of metoclopramide and bethanechol. Gastroenterology 1980; 78: 286.

221. Mearin F, Camilleri M, Malagelda JR. Pyloric dysfunction in diabetes with recurrent nausea and vomiting. Gastroenterology 1986; 91(1): 268–71.

222. Ricci DA, Saltzman MB, Meyer C et al. Effect of metoclopramide in diabetic gastroparesis. J Clin Gastroenterol 1985; 7: 25.

223. Watts GF, Armitage M, Sinclair J et al. Treatment of diabetic gastroparesis with oral domperidone. Diabet Med 1985; 2: 491.

224. Horowitz M, Maddox A, Harding PE et al. The effects of a single dose and chronic administration of cisapride on gastric and oesophageal emptying in insulin dependent diabetes. Gastroenterology 1987; 92: 1899–907.

225. Camilleri M, Stanghellini V, Sheps SG, Malagelada JR. Gastrointestinal motility disturbances due to postganglionic sympathetic lesions (abstract). Clin Res 1984; 32: 489A.

226. DePonti F, Fealey RD, Malagelada J-R. Gastrointestinal syndromes due to diabetes mellitus. In Dyck PJ, Thomas PK, Asbury AK, Winegrad AI, Porte D (eds) Diabetic neuropathy. Philadelphia: WB Saunders, 1987: pp 155–61.

227. Malins JM, French JM. Diabetic diarrhoea. Quart J Med 1957; 26: 467.

228. Herr M, Pirovino M, Japp H, Buhler H, Schmid M. Diabetic gastroparesis and colonic distention tested with domperidone. Lancet 1980; ii: 1145.

229. Wald A, Tunuguntla AK. Anorectal sensorimotor dysfunction in fecal incontinence and diabetes mellitus. Modification with biofeedback therapy. New Engl J Med 1984; 310: 1282.

230. Pryor J, Parsons J, Goswamy R et al. In-vitro fertilisation for men with obstructive azoospermia. Lancet 1984; ii: 762.

231. Bradley WE. Diagnosis of urinary bladder dysfunction in diabetes mellitus. Ann Intern Med 1980; 92: 323.

232. Bhatia NN, Bradley WE, Haldeman S. Urodynamics: continuous monitoring. J Urol 1982; 128: 963.

233. Bhatia NN, Bradley WE, Haldeman S, Johnson B. Continuous ambulatory urodynamic monitoring. Br J Urol 1982; 54: 357.

234. McCulloch DK, Campbell IW, Wu FC, Prescott RJ, Clarke BF. The prevalence of diabetic impotence. Diabetologia 1980; 18: 279.

235. Ek A, Bradley WE, Drane RJ. Snap-gauge band: new concept in measuring penile rigidity. Urology 1983; 21: 63.

236. Bradley WE, Timm GW, Johnson B, Gallagher J. Continuous penile tumescence and rigidity monitoring in the evaluation of impotence. Urology 1985; 26: 4.

237. Lin JT, Bradley WE. Penile neuropathy in insulin-dependent diabetes mellitus. J Urol 1985; 133: 213.

238. Kaneko S, Bradley WE. Penile electrodiagnosis. Value of bulbocavernous reflex latency versus nerve conduction velocity of the dorsal nerve of the penis in diagnosis of diabetic impotence. J Urol (Baltimore) 1987; 137: 933.

239. Sarica Y, Karacan I. Bulbocavernous reflex to somatic and visceral nerve stimulation in normal subjects and in diabetics with erectile impotence. J Urol (Baltimore) 1987; 138: 55.

240. Lehman TP, Jacobs JA. Aetiology of diabetic impotence. J Urol 1983; 129: 291.

241. Wagner G, Green R. Impotence. New York: Plenum, 1981.

242. Murray FT, Wyss HU, Thomas RG, Spevack M, Glaros AG. Gonadal dysfunction in diabetic men with organic impotence. J Clin Endocrinol Metab 1987; 65: 127.

243. Bancroft J, Bell C. Simultaneous recording of penile diameter and penile arterial pulse during laboratory based erotic stimulation in normal subjects. J Psychosom Res 1985; 29: 303.

244. Bancroft J, Bell C, Ewing DJ et al. Assessment of erectile function in diabetic and non-diabetic impotence by simultaneous recording of penile diameter and penile arterial pulse. J Psychosom Res 1985; 29: 315.

245. Jensen SB. The natural history of sexual dysfunction in diabetic women: a 6 year follow up study. Acta Med Scand 1986; 219: 73.

246. Robinette MA, Moffat MJ. Intracorporal injection of papaverine and phentolamine in the management of impotence. Br J Urol 1986; 58: 692.

247. Sidi AA, Cameron JS, Duffy LM, Lange PH. Intracavernous drug-induced erections in the management of male erectile dysfunction: experience with 100 patients. J Urol (Baltimore) 1986; 135: 704.

248. Pfeifer M, Reenan A, Berger R, Best J. Penile prosthesis and quality of life. Diabetes 1983; 32: 77A.

249. Wiles PG. Successful non-invasive management of erectile impotence in diabetic men. Br Med J 1988; 296: 161–2.

60
Connective Tissue Disorders in Diabetes

Arlan L. Rosenbloom
University of Florida College of Medicine, Gainesville, Florida, USA

Connective tissue disorders in diabetes encompass the major long-term complications, which can be attributed to alteration in the quantity and quality of structural macromolecules of the extracellular matrix [1]. These alterations affect vascular basement membrane in the retina, kidney, heart and skeletal muscle, muscle fiber basement membrane (e.g. with cardiomyopathy) [2], nervous system basement membrane, lens capsule and crystallin, and trophoblastic basement membrane of the placenta in both gestational diabetes and overt diabetic pregnancies [3]. Other sections of this volume treat the connective tissue abnormalities in the major chronic complications and their biochemical basis (Chapters 55, 56, 59). This chapter reviews the abnormalities of interstitial connective tissue involving skeleton, joints, skin and periarticular tissues. Diabetic osteoarthropathy (also known as neuroarthropathy), which leads to the development of Charcot joints, is dealt with in Chapter 68. Gout and pseudogout (acute symptomatic chondrocalcinosis) appear to be related to diabetes only by chance or by the common bond of obesity and hyperlipidemia [4], and are not discussed further here, nor are skin problems that do not directly relate to the connective tissue abnormalities, including infection, dermatoses, lipodystrophies, cutaneous complications of treatment, and necrobiosis lipoidica diabeticorum; these have been reviewed recently [5].

This chapter discusses the following conditions: osteopenia in children and adults; hyperostosis; osteoarthritis; osteolysis; scleroderma diabeticorum; Dupuytren's disease; stiff hand syndrome of Lundbaek [6]; carpal tunnel syndrome; flexor tenosynovitis; adhesive capsulitis of the shoulder and shoulder–hand syndrome; and limited joint mobility (LJM). Among these abnormalities, LJM is unique in that it is common in childhood and adolescence, does not occur in the non-diabetic young population and is an important risk marker for other complications; a number of biochemical studies have been carried out on biopsy specimens of the associated thick, tight, waxy skin [7]. Furthermore, this condition needs to be delineated from the other joint disorders common in diabetes, to refine hypotheses about etiopathogenesis [8].

SKELETON

Osteopenia

Decreased bone mineral content is well recognized in both insulin dependent diabetes mellitus

International Textbook of Diabetes Mellitus. Edited by K.G.M.M. Alberti, R.A. DeFronzo, H. Keen and P. Zimmet

Table 1　Bone density in insulin dependent diabetes mellitus

Reference	Method	Population No./Ages (yr)	Controls No./Ages (yr)	Findings
12	PA	35/9–57	Previous studies	54% with BM loss > 10%, no sex difference
13	RG	107/4.5–18	Literature	41% males, 13% females with CT < 5th percentile
14	PA	196/6–26	124/6–26	29% males, 48% females with BM loss > 10%
15	PA	86/7–25 129/26–70	447/7–70	10% BM loss for group with 2× loss (14%) in young vs old (7%)
16	PA	34/7–18	Not specified	11.7% BM loss attributed to delayed bone age
17	RG	45/7–18	63/4–20	16% with CT > 2 SD below mean for age
18	PA	58/23–64	28/20–45	9.6% BM loss
19	PA/RG	78/8–25	Not specified	Decreased BM, CT
20	RG	206/7–20	Literature	85% below mean for age/sex; 22% below 2 SD — M 31%/F 12%

PA, photon absorptiometry; BM, bone mineral; RG, radiogrammetry; CT, cortical thickness.

(IDDM) and non-insulin dependent diabetes mellitus (NIDDM), although there is some controversy regarding this finding in NIDDM [9]. There is also controversy concerning the clinical significance of the osteopenia, i.e. whether there is an increased risk of skeletal fracture. The only population-based study, comprising 1000 persons with diabetes, failed to reveal an increased risk of fracture [10]. In NIDDM, increased weight appears to be associated with increased bone density, as is true in those without diabetes, and in one study this heavier group was far larger than the group with bone loss [11]; this admixture of patients might explain the difficulty in demonstrating a population risk [9].

Direct comparisons among various studies of bone integrity in diabetes is difficult. Various techniques have been used to demonstrate reduced bone mass including conventional radiographs, photon absorption densitometry, radiographic measurement of cortical width, resonance frequency of the ulna, total body neutron activation analysis, and x-ray microdensitometry. Controls in a number of reports are from previous studies or the literature, rather than concurrent and analyzed simultaneously. Finally, there are wide differences in age groups studied, as well as in diabetes types, and distinction is not always made between IDDM and NIDDM in a particular study, or between insulin use and other treatment.

Insulin Dependent Diabetes

Table 1 summarizes bone density studies by photon absorptiometry or radiogrammetry in IDDM patients. The photon absorption technique detects a transmission of radiation from a ^{125}I-crystal through the bones of the forearm. An analyzer determines bone width and mineral content, expressing bone density as grams of calcium per square centimetre of bone width. This method is precise and reproducible with a coefficient of variation of less than 4% at each site. Measurements correlate well with total body calcium and total skeletal weight estimates [12]. Hand radiogrammetry involves the measurement of cortical bone thickness and percentage cortical area at the midshaft of the second metacarpal bone on the left hand [13].

The original photon absorptiometry studies by Levin et al [12] included 35 IDDM patients of whom over half had osteopenia defined as greater than 10% bone mineral loss; there was no sex difference nor any difference in mean duration between those with more than 10% loss and those with less than 10% loss. Using the same technique in a much larger population of 190 patients aged 6–26 years compared with a control population matched for age and sex, Rosenbloom et al [14] found that 48% of girls and 29% of boys had more than 10% loss in bone density, and that this was much more severe in whites than in blacks. White females averaged 8.2% loss whereas white males averaged 4.7% loss and black females only 2% loss; there were not enough black males for analysis. Abnormalities seemed to be associated with the early stages of diabetes, particularly in the white females. During the first year of diabetes none of 8 white males but 10 out of 12 white females had a loss greater than 10%. When the groups were divided into those with duration of diabetes less than 5 years and those with duration greater than 5 years, most of the abnormality was seen in the first 5 years among white females. After 5 years, there was no sex difference in mean percentage bone mass change. The predominance of abnormality in white female youngsters with diabetes in this study is similar to the sex-specific and race-specific adult risk for bone loss.

The initial study of cortical thickness in 107 patients described a male preponderance (41% versus 13%) of abnormality defined as cortical thickness less than the fifth percentile of published controls, and in this study there was no effect of diabetes duration [13]. Later study in 45 patients found a somewhat lower overall abnormality of 16% with values greater than 2 SD below the mean for age, but no information was provided on sex differences [17]. The impression that these abnormalities were due to a failure to gain adequate endosteal bone rather than a loss of bone was derived from studies of Wiske et al [19], showing decreased cortical area with normal subperiosteal diameter among 78 patients aged 8–25 years. In the same group, radial midshaft determination by photon absorption correlated with the metacarpal cortical area. These authors also found a negative correlation between bone mass and duration of diabetes, in contrast to the studies describing either no effect of duration [13], improved bone mass with longer duration [12, 14] or a plateau after 3–5 years [15, 18]. Findings similar to those of Santiago et al [13] have been reported by Hough [20] among 206 patients aged 7–20 years, also using radiogrammetry: values less than 2 SD below the mean for reference standards were found in 31% of males and 12% of females. There was no relationship to duration of diabetes.

In addition to the differences in the influence of sex on the degree of bone abnormality, the racial difference noted by Rosenbloom et al [14] was not present in the study of Santiago et al [13]. Nielsen et al [16] correlated bone mineral loss with delayed sexual maturation, but this was not substantiated by Santiago et al [13] nor by Hough [20] in comparing osteopenic with non-osteopenic patients.

The mechanism of bone mineral loss remains unknown. In the reported studies where diabetes control has been examined, there has been no apparent effect of control measures at the time of study [14, 17, 18, 20], except in the report of McNair et al [15]. They found a strong correlation between bone mineral loss and fasting blood glucose concentration, glucosuria and insulin requirement, as well as declining C-peptide levels. They also suggested that the calcium loss was directly related to hyperglycemia and glucosuria, because urinary excretion of calcium and phosphorus correlated with these manifestations. Hough [20], however, was unable to demonstrate any great difference between osteopenic and non-osteopenic patients in terms of calcium or phosphate excretion, when these subjects were matched for age, size and diabetes control. Rosenbloom et al [14] found no correlation of bone mineral loss with serum concentrations of calcium, magnesium or alkaline phosphatase.

The bone mineral loss in young patients appears to be unrelated to type of diabetes. Ribs and vertebrae of 8 children and young adults dying with diabetes—4 secondary to cystic fibrosis and 2 owing to thalassemia major—had significant loss of bone mass, and this was true regardless of the etiology of the diabetes [21].

A wide variety of metabolic findings have been reported in association with osteopenia in IDDM, including increased alkaline phosphatase [17, 18, 20] and decreased levels of 1,25-dihydroxyvitamin D_3 and 25-hydroxyvitamin D_3 [17]. Hough [20] has done calcium loading studies that demonstrate intense intestinal hyperabsorption of calcium, absorptive hypercalciuria and phosphaturia, which (together with hypomagnesemia, hyperphosphatasemia and decreased circulating PTH) may form the basis of bone mass loss.

Non-insulin Dependent Diabetes

The original report of 101 NIDDM patients studied by photon absorption noted greater than 10% bone mass loss in 60%. Particularly noteworthy was that 80% of patients receiving oral hypoglycemic agents had osteopenia, compared with a not significantly different 57% for those on diet therapy alone, but highly significantly different from the 44% abnormal who were receiving insulin [12]. In this study, in contrast to IDDM patients in whom density improved with duration of diabetes, NIDDM patients showed no influence of diabetes duration on bone loss. Because of the presence of this finding at onset, its lack of relationship to control measures and to duration, and experimental evidence to suggest defective osteon formation, constitutional rather than metabolic factors were proposed as causative [12].

Quite different findings come from a study of

138 Belgian patients who had only a 20% rate of bone loss exceeding 10%. Most striking in this study was the presence of increased bone density in twice this proportion, with the greatest densities in those receiving oral hypoglycemic agents, who were also the heaviest patients [11]. Japanese investigators used microdensitometry of hand radiographs to examine 168 NIDDM patients and found bone mass clearly diminished in 26% and severely decreased in 12%. They noted that this densitometer pattern of osteopenia differed from that of typical osteoporosis in that the former showed less decrease in the relative width of the cortex but more marked decrease in the mean maximal density of the metacarpal bone. This indicated that the cortical bone width and volume in diabetes are relatively well preserved, whereas the mineral content is decreased compared with typical osteoporosis. They suggest that the preservation of volume may explain why there is no increased risk of fracture with this type of osteopenia. In contrast to the findings in IDDM, 25-hydroxyvitamin D_3 and 1,25-dihydroxyvitamin D_3 levels were not different among control subjects and those with NIDDM with or without osteopenia [22].

Hyperostosis

Hyperostosis may involve the spine as hyperostotic spondylosis (HS), the skull as hyperostosis frontalis interna, the pelvis as osteitis condensans ilii, the pelvic or other ligaments, or as large bony spurs at the heel or elbow [4, 23]. There may be a mild stiffness on arising in the morning, but spinal mobility is preserved and symptoms are usually absent. Heel and elbow pain can occur from calcaneal and olecranon spurs in about one-third of affected patients and dysphagia has been described in 16% of those with hyperostosis of the spine.

Whereas 2–4% of the general population may have hyperostotic changes, these changes are present in some 25% of the diabetes population. Of those with spine changes, 83% are male and 30% are obese. One-half of all patients with HS will have manifest or chemical diabetes. Obesity and diabetes appear to operate independently in the determination of this condition. Radiography reveals preservation of the disc spaces with hyperostosis seen as a line of calcification in the right anterolateral portion of the spine, typically in the thoracic region. Radiolucency is

seen between the deposited bone and the cortex of the underlying vertebral body. The principal differential diagnosis of HS is from ankylosing spondylitis, which occurs in a younger population and produces more serious problems, with morning stiffness and incapacitating loss of spinal movement. Radiographic differences are straightforward [23].

The etiology of hyperostosis in diabetes is not clear. It would be attractive to invoke growth hormone hypersecretion, in view of the similarity to acromegalic lesions, but growth hormone metabolism has been described as normal [23].

JOINTS

Osteoarthritis

Several studies have documented increased propensity for the development of osteoarthritis in diabetes, presumably reflecting the accelerated aging of cartilaginous tissue. A number of processes that have been described in vitro or with experimental diabetes, such as loss of glycosaminoglycans from articular cartilage, may be pertinent to the pathogenesis [23].

Osteolysis

Osteolysis of the fore foot is seen as a localized or generalized osteoporosis of the distal metatarsus and proximal phalanges. Pain is variable and there may be erythema over the joint, inevitably leading to a suspicion of cellulitis or osteomyelitis. The juxta-articular erosions may resemble those of rheumatoid arthritis and gout. The etiology of this lesion is unknown, and perfect reconstruction usually occurs spontaneously [23, 24].

SKIN AND PERIARTICULAR TISSUE

Scleroderma Diabeticorum

Fifty-four cases of scleroderma diabeticorum associated with longstanding IDDM as well as NIDDM have been summarized by Jelinek [25]. This condition occurs in middle-aged adults with a male preponderance (4:1) who have a longstanding history of poorly controlled diabetes and are obese. Ischemic heart disease, hypertension and retinopathy are common. There is thickening of the skin with a predilection for the posterior and lateral aspects of the neck and upper back, with induration extending to the face and anterior and posterior trunk and potentially involving most of the body. The condition has been described in whites, Orientals, and blacks. Prospective studies suggest that it may be more common than the number of reported cases suggests.

Hyperplasia of collagen is seen on histological examination, and one study has shown accumulation of glycogen in unmyelinated nerve fibers [26].

Dupuytren Disease

Dupuytren disease (DD) refers to subcutaneous fibrosis of the palmar aponeurotic space of the hands. In those without diabetes the process is sex-linked with a 6 : 1 male predominance, and occurs only in people of European origin. There has been argument in the literature about whether DD is more prevalent in persons with diabetes, but this question appears to be related to the failure to recognize milder expression in these patients. Not only does careful examination reveal that the true incidence approaches 40%, but, as with cardiovascular risk, the presence of diabetes abolishes the sex difference. However, women with diabetes tend to have knuckle pads, nodules and skin tethering without contraction. DD is also more radial in the hands of those with diabetes than in those without diabetes, affecting the third and fourth digits predominantly instead of the fourth and fifth. Characteristic lesions may precede the development of diabetes and are present in 16% of newly diagnosed older patients [27].

DD lesions causing sufficient contracture to be removed by surgery were found to contain higher contents of water, collagen and chondroitin sulfate, as well as increased proportions of soluble collagen and of reducible crosslinks, indicating synthesis of new collagen. The lesions also showed increased amounts of type III collagen and increased hydroxylation and glycosylation of reducible crosslinks, characteristics of granulation and scar tissues [28].

Peyronie disease, involving the penis, and Ledderhose disease, affecting the planter aponeurosis, are so rarely seen as to be difficult to relate to diabetes, although the impression is that they are more frequent with diabetes and have a similar pathogenesis to DD [23].

Stiff Hand Syndrome

This 'severe and sometimes incapacitating form of vascular disease of the hands' was described by Lundbaek in 1957, in 5 patients with long-standing IDDM [6]. The problem typically began with complaints of tingling or burning sensations in the hand, with increasing symptoms and the advent of pain aggravated by movement, leading in 2 patients to invalidism. The subcutaneous tissue of the fingers and palms was stiff and hard, and in 2 patients there were marked nail changes. There was no muscle atrophy. Radiographic study revealed calcification of the arteries of the hand in all 5 cases. Skin biopsy showed very few elastic fibers, but no other changes.

Carpal Tunnel Syndrome

Compression of the median nerve within the carpal tunnel at the wrist is the most common entrapment neuropathy, resulting in paresthesia of the thumb, index finger and little finger, with pain that is often worse at night. Diabetes is the most common associated disorder, accounting for 5–16% of cases [4].

In persons with diabetes, the disorder may not be due to nerve compression but a manifestation of diabetic neuropathy with decreased conduction velocity of both median and ulnar nerves with, in addition to typical thenar muscle atrophy, atrophy of the intrinsic and hypothenar muscles. The contractures involve the metacarpophalangeal and proximal interphalangeal joints of all fingers equally. The 23 patients with 'diabetic hand syndrome' described by Jung et al [29] included 6 who were not taking insulin. The average age of the 23 patients was 43 years and diabetes duration 17 years. These authors were impressed with the bilateral and symmetrical involvement of all distal and proximal interphalangeal and metacarpophalangeal joints and the involvement of the ulnar nerves, as indicators of the neuropathic etiology as opposed to an entrapment origin of this condition in their patients.

Flexor Tenosynovitis

Flexor tenosynovitis (FTS), also known as 'trigger finger' or stenosing tenovaginitis, can be congenital or hereditary in children, almost exclusively involving the thumb. In adults, it is estimated that one-third of multiple palmar FTS is due to diabetes, although the prevalence in those with diabetes is not known [4]. There is marked female predominance, predilection for the right hand, and preferential involvement of the thumb, middle and ring fingers. Fibrous tissue proliferates in the tendon sheath, particularly where the tendon is constricted in its passage through a fibrous ring or pulley or over a bony prominence, with swelling distal to this constriction and pain with movement of the enlarged segment through the narrowed ring. Palpable or audible crepitus may be present with movement; locking in flexion or extension occurs with impaction of the nodule proximal or distal to the thickened segment of tendon sheath [23].

Adhesive Capsulitis of the Shoulder and Shoulder–Hand Syndrome

Thickening of the joint capsule and its adherence to the head of the humerus results in marked reduction in the volume of the glenohumeral joint. In some cases this periarthritis may precede, accompany or follow diffuse swelling, coldness, erythema, tenderness and hyperhydrosis of the hand. Subsequently, swelling and vasomotor instability resolve, with the development of trophic skin changes and contractures. After weeks or months, the tenderness, swelling and vasomotor dysfunction completely resolve, with residual atrophic or dystrophic changes, finger contractures and occasionally frozen shoulder with atrophy of the shoulder girdle muscles. Osteoporosis of the bones of the hand and shoulder are seen. In addition to shoulder–hand syndrome, this has been referred to as reflex sympathetic dystrophy, causalgia, posttraumatic osteoporosis and Sudeck atrophy [4].

The above description of classic adhesive capsulitis and shoulder–hand syndrome appears to differ considerably from what is often seen with diabetes. In one large study, 11% of 800 patients with diabetes had frozen shoulder compared with 2.3% of 600 controls without diabetes [30]. Among 15 patients with frozen shoulder identified by the criteria of a history of pain for more than 3 months with over 50% loss of range of motion, in the absence of such causes as trauma, or myocardial infarction, minimal functional disability was noted, with the principal pain being relatively mild discomfort around the shoulder joint.

Prevalence of frozen shoulder was 45% among 29 individuals with finger joint stiffness, aged 23–65 years, with a duration of diabetes of 14–48 years. Ten of these people had Dupuytren's disease and 10 flexor tenosynovitis, in both situations considered not sufficient to account for the finger-joint limitation. Only 7% of subjects of similar age and diabetes duration without finger-joint limitation had frozen shoulder. In 10 out of the 13 with LJM and 1 out of the 2 controls, the frozen shoulder was bilateral, an uncommon circumstance in the spontaneous disease (5%). On radiographic examination, one patient was found to have periarticular calcification and no joint abnormalities were noted. Suspicion that finger contractures are attributable to more than the syndrome of LJM as described in young patients [7] arises from the findings of digital or radial artery calcification in 50% of those with finger-joint contraction, compared with 14% of controls, and of a fourfold increase in peripheral neuropathy in those with joint contracture. This study demonstrated important clinical, radiological and natural history differences from the isolated (not associated with diabetes) lesion, which would be expected in view of the histological findings in this condition (those of Dupuytren disease), in contrast to the inflammatory reaction (the synovial cell proliferation, collagen degeneration and infiltration by inflammatory cells) seen in the isolated syndrome [31].

Another study of 49 IDDM and 60 NIDDM patients, compared with 75 controls, found comparable frequencies of finger-joint contracture (50%) in both types of diabetes as opposed to 20% of controls; the contractures were all mild in the last group. Shoulder capsulitis was seen in 20% of IDDM patients, 18.3% of NIDDM patients and 5.3% of controls, applying criteria that were similar to, but somewhat less stringent than, those in the previous study. In this study, no correlation was observed between shoulder and finger-joint limitation [32]. In contrast to the study of Fisher et al [31], who eliminated half their original patient population on the basis of their joint contractures being obviously due to Dupuytren disease, osteoarthritis or flexor tenosynovitis, Pal et al [32] made no attempt to distinguish the causes of the finger-joint limitation.

Swedish investigators identified a subset of 60 diabetic patients with painful shoulder from a rehabilitative referral population. Their patients had difficulties in activities of daily living: in 25%, working capacity was affected and 42% also had restricted hip joint mobility. In contrast to the series of Fisher et al [31], this group had a rate of recovery comparable to that of the non-diabetic population, with 35% of the shoulders regaining normal mobility, 48% having clinical limitation and 17% having functional limitation over a median observation time of 29 months. IDDM was associated with worse prognosis. Nearly two-thirds of the group had associated hand syndromes [33].

Limited Joint Mobility

The initial observation of striking limitation of extension and flexion of the interphalangeal, metacarpophalangeal and wrist joints, in association with short stature, thick, tight, waxy skin, delayed sexual maturation and early microvascular complications, in 3 older teenagers with longstanding diabetes [34], was followed by the description of milder manifestations in 28% of 229 campers with diabetes aged 7–18 years [35]. Subsequent studies from Japan [36], Italy [37], Ireland [38], England [32, 39–41], Mexico [42], Ethiopia [43], Hungary [44] and from various populations in the US [45–54] have reported prevalences of 8–55% among IDDM patients, depending on the age of the population and the duration of diabetes, as well as the examination techniques; these studies are summarized in Table 2. Several reports have described LJM in NIDDM also, as summarized in Table 3: frequencies range from 25% to 76%, except for a single study which involved only patients not taking insulin [55].

There is no influence of sex or race on prevalence. In control pediatric populations, stiffness of the little fingers only was usually found in fewer than 2% (Table 2), whereas older populations may have as much as 20% involvement, probably related to occupation and aging (Table 3).

Changes begin in the metacarpophalangeal and proximal interphalangeal joints of the little finger and extend medially. The distal interphalangeal joint may also be involved, as may larger joints, most commonly wrist and elbow but also ankles and cervical and thoracolumbar

spine. The limitation is painless, unresponsive to physical therapy and non-disabling. Unrecognized cervical spine involvement can complicate endotracheal intubation [58].

Examination and Classification

The original method for demonstrating milder LJM was to have the patient place the hand on a flat surface palm down with the fingers fanned; the examiner would then determine contact with the plane surface by viewing at table level. Normally, the entire palmar surface of the fingers makes contact [59]. A simpler screening method is to have the patient attempt to approximate the palmar surfaces of the interphalangeal joints in the praying position with the fingers fanned. Whether this approximation is possible or not, the examiner extends the proximal and distal interphalangeal and metacarpal–phalangeal joints. In addition to finding these limited to less than 180° and 60° respectively, the examiner may find resistance to the permitted movement. Also noted will be thickening of the tissues surrounding the limited joints and inability to tent the skin, particularly over the dorsa of the fingers and hand. The examiner also attempts to extend the wrist maximally to at least 70° and the elbow to at least 180°. The ankle should flex maximally to at least 100°, the cervical spine lateral flexion should permit ear-to-shoulder juxtaposition and thoracolumbar spine lateral flexion should be at least 35° in young people [46].

This examination will reveal obvious LJM but, as noted, the clinical sensation of joint limitation without absolute reduction in maximum extension is quite subjective. Buithieu et al [60] compared metacarpal–phalangeal (MCP) and wrist maximal extension in 239 controls and 211 IDDM patients aged 9–30 years, and found a significant proportion of those without clinical LJM to have MCP and wrist limitation, defined as less than 2 standard deviations of the control mean. Those without apparent LJM (172) included 25% with MCP limitation and 13% with wrist limitation. Thus, earlier detection of LJM may be possible through objective measurement.

The staging of LJM has been useful in describing relationships of other findings to LJM and for patient follow-up. *No limitation* includes equivocal or unilateral findings. *Mild limitation* indicates involvement of one or two proximal

Table 2   Population-based studies of limited joint mobility (LJM) in IDDM (1975–86)

Reference	Age group (yr)	IDDM patients		Controls		Location
		No.	% LJM	No.	% LJM	
35	7–18	229	28	201	1	Florida
14	6–26	196	40	124	0	Florida
45	1–18	310	8	199	2	Chicago
36	3–18	68	30	92	1	Japan
46	1–28	309	30	–	–	Florida
37	?	210	9	–	–	Italy
38	5–57	115	36	90	3	Belfast
47	3–22	100	32	–	–	Boston
39	2–16	112	42	50	21	Nottingham
48	5–24	137	19	52	0	New Jersey
42	15–32	34	41	34	3	Mexico City
49	7–23	204	21	90	1	Florida
40	?	215	46	–	–	London
50	?	104	19	–	–	California
51	6–27	311	36	–	–	Florida
52	3–24	95	40	39	3	New York
43	14–62	110	44	300	2	Ethiopia
41	6–39	254	15	110	4	Bath
53	11–83	238	55	45	4	Boston
44	5–18	55	44	–	–	Hungary
54	7–25	375	33	–	–	California
32	18–82	49	49	75	20	Newcastle
60	3–30	211	19	239	0	Florida

interphalangeal (PIP) joints, one large joint, or only the MCP joints bilaterally. *Moderate limitation* refers to involvement of three or more PIP joints or one finger joint and one large joint bilaterally. *Severe limitation* refers to obvious hand deformity at rest or associated cervical spine involvement [46].

In describing 11 patients with severe LJM at the time that this problem was first being recognized, Benedetti and Noacco [61] used the term 'juvenile diabetic cheiroarthropathy', based on the Greek word for hand. This terminology would appear to be inadequate in view of the involvement of large joints as well, and with the absence of radiographic evidence for change

in the joint itself other than the periarticular thickening.

Natural History

Cross-sectional studies demonstrate that duration of diabetes is the most important variable in the appearance of LJM. However, when Rosenbloom et al [62] were able to determine the time of development of joint changes in 76 patients, they found that, although the age of onset of diabetes varied from infancy to adolescence, development of LJM occurred between the ages of 10 and 20 years in over 90%: in only 4 individuals was LJM detected before the age of 10 years. The 15 patients who had onset of

Table 3   Population-based studies of limited joint mobility (LJM) in NIDDM (1983–86)

Reference	Age group (yr)	NIDDM patients		Controls		Location
		No.	% LJM	No.	% LJM	
40	?	241	34	–	–	London
56	?	80	45	47	15	Montreal
43	28–79	190	25	300	2	Ethiopia
55	?	165	4	–	–	Italy
53	?	41	76	45	9	Boston
57	mean 55	168	47	100	26 M/9 F	Scotland
32	34–85	60	52	75	20	Newcastle

diabetes under 4 years of age developed their LJM at 11 to 16 years of age, indistinguishable from children with later-onset diabetes. When the population was evenly divided between those with onset under or over 7 years of age, a 2.5-year difference in the mean age of LJM onset was noted, despite a 6.3-year difference in the mean age of onset of diabetes, suggesting that age attained is much more important than duration of diabetes in the development of LJM. The interval between detection of mild LJM and progression to moderate or severe changes varies from 3 months to 4 years, with a mean of 2 years. After this period, progression (if any) is very slow. Many do not progress beyond mild changes.

In adult populations, about two-thirds of patients affected will have at least two fingers involved [38, 40]. One-half of young patients affected with more than 5 years' duration of diabetes will have moderate or severe limitation, defined as at least three interphalangeal joints or one finger joint and one large joint bilaterally. Approximately one-third of the affected group will have severe limitation, i.e. involvement of all the fingers and often of the cervical spine as well [61].

There is no relationship between LJM and diabetes control as measured by HbA_1 levels or clinical criteria in any of the controlled studies, but longitudinal data from diabetes onset have not been investigated. However, hepatomegaly has been noted in more severely affected patients [37, 59]. In one study, there was no correlation between loss of bone mineral content by photon absorptiometry and the presence or absence of LJM, which is to be expected in view of the different timing of these findings in the course of IDDM [14].

Effects on Growth

The original patients studied had growth failure [34, 61]. The subsequent population study demonstrated that more severe changes of LJM were associated with growth limitation, but that milder LJM was not [59]. A later study of individuals with more than 3 years' duration of diabetes, with onset before adolescence (thus permitting sufficient time for growth failure to occur), was more informative than previous cross-sectional studies; 142 such patients were assessed, including 31 with mild LJM and 43

with more severe changes. Of subjects without LJM, 68% were below the 50th percentile for height rather than the expected 50%, and most of this discrepancy was below the 25th percentile (38% versus expected 25%). Mild LJM resulted in four times the excess below the 25th percentile (72%), and moderate to severe limitation was not associated with significantly smaller stature (77% below the 25th percentile). The small proportion above the 75th percentile was similar for those without LJM (12%), and with mild or more severe LJM (both 10%) [62].

Differential Diagnosis

The differential diagnosis from other joint problems should be straightforward [7, 33]. Nevertheless, since our original description, numerous reports have referred to the various conditions listed in Table 4 as LJM, or have considered several of these conditions to be varying manifestations of the same process. LJM is easily distinguishable from Dupuytren disease, the only other condition involving the hand that is not associated with pain, by the absence of palmar fascial thickening and nodules in DD as well as the finger distribution. DD is not seen in young patients; in older patients, DD and LJM may be seen together [33, 40, 57]. All the other conditions are associated with pain and other characteristic findings, as noted in Table 4. Rheumatoid arthritis (RA) is not more frequent in diabetes, and patients with LJM do not meet the pain or inflammatory criteria for RA [7].

There have been several examples of diagnostic confusion in this area. The finding that LJM could precede the development of diabetes by 3 years in a teenage patient [63] has suggested an important constitutional component [23]. The patient described developed stiffness in the MCP and PIP joints and wrists more or less simultaneously, had thickening and contraction of flexor tendons in the palm, and progressive disability. Robertson et al [64] described a patient in her late 20s who had characteristic features of flexor tenosynovitis but was reported as 'juvenile diabetic cheiroarthropathy'. Three patients reported as having LJM appeared to have the diabetic hand syndrome, with additional features of shoulder–hand syndrome in one and flexor tenosynovitis in another [65].

The superimposition of other hand syndromes on LJM as patients age is not surprising [33].

Table 4 Differential diagnosis of joint syndromes involving the hand in diabetes

Condition	Usual fingers involved	Pain/ paresthesia	Muscle	Frequency	Other distinctive features
LJM	begins 5th, extends radially	No	Normal	50 + % of IDDM after 5 yr and puberty	Not disabling; associated with thick, tight, waxy skin
Dupuytren disease	3rd, 4th	No	Normal	Up to 40% over age 40 yr; 16% at diagnosis	Milder expression common in women; may precede diabetes
Flexor tenosynovitis	1st, 3rd, 4th	Yes	Normal	1/3 associated with diabetes	Marked female predominance; locking, disability
Carpal tunnel (diabetic hand)	All	Yes	Intrinsic, palmar atrophy	5–16% due to diabetes	Ulnar as well as median nerve involvement in diabetes
Stiff hand	All	Yes	Normal	Rare; IDDM > 20 yr	disability; calcified vessels; hard palmar skin, soft dorsal
Shoulder–hand (reflex dystrophy)	All	Yes	Atrophy	Shoulder limitation in 20% of older IDDM, NIDDM; reflex dystrophy unusual	Most bilateral; often associated with other hand syndromes

The presence of pain or paresthesia, neurologic findings, disability, finger locking, swelling, muscle atrophy, palmar skin or fascia thickening, or absence of greater involvement of the ring and little fingers could be indicators of additional problems. One would expect people with LJM to be at greater risk for other connective tissue proliferative problems and, perhaps, neuropathy.

Neuropathy

Kennedy et al [66] have noted prolonged nerve conduction velocity for the ulnar and median nerves in older patients with LJM, compared with those without LJM and comparable durations of diabetes. Also noted was decreased vibratory sense in both upper and lower extremities in the presence of LJM. Starkman et al [53] found that LJM was associated with a 4.3-fold relative risk of clinical neuropathy in IDDM.

Cardiac Function

Cardiac response to dynamic exercise in a group of otherwise healthy IDDM adolescents was compared with a non-diabetic control group by postexercise echocardiography. Abnormalities were found in the diabetic group in indicators of systolic function indicating subclinical cardiomyopathy. Twelve of the 25 patients had LJM. Five of the patients and one of the 26 controls had flat interventricular septal motion; all 5

IDDM patients with this abnormality had LJM [67].

Pulmonary Changes

Decreased elastic recoil at low lung volumes, with IDDM, was initially described in 11 young men who also demonstrated decreased pulmonary capacity [68]. The association of limited pulmonary capacity with LJM was first noted by Barta in a single patient [69]. A study of 12 adolescents and young adults with severe LJM who were matched for age, sex, height and duration of IDDM to 11 without LJM, found that LJM subjects had significantly less total lung capacity, thoracic gas volume, residual volume, forced vital capacity and forced expiratory volume (1 second). What could not be ascertained was whether these individuals had limited pulmonary compliance, decreased mobility of the chest wall, or both [70]. A subsequent report noted that 19% of IDDM patients had vital capacities more than 2 SD below those normal for age, but this was not associated with LJM [54]. In contrast, Madacsy et al [44] found that 24 patients with LJM had a significant decrease in total lung capacity, airway resistance and peak expiratory flow, compared with 26 without LJM.

Fibrous Disease of the Breast

Twelve women with breast lumps were identified

from among 88 with IDDM, aged 20–40 years, and 11 of these 12 were found to have LJM. The duration of their diabetes ranged from 8 years to 30 years, and all but one had retinopathy [71]. This would appear to be a significant association, but no data were provided about the prevalence of LJM in the rest of the population. The prevalence of breast lumps in this study (14%) is similar to that in non-diabetic populations.

Skin Changes

Thick, tight, waxy skin, most prominent over the dorsum of the hands and the forearms, was described in the initial patients and in about one-third of those with LJM described subsequently; this change was apparent only in those with moderate to severe LJM [34, 46, 59]. Siebold [48] examined primarily for skin changes by tenting, and found these to be more frequent than LJM but that LJM was present only in those who had skin changes (47 out of 137, of whom 26 had LJM). Similarly, a recent report noted that skin changes were present in 34% of patients without LJM, in 70% of those with mild LJM (involving only the fifth PIP joint) and in 100% of those with more severe limitation [54].

Ultrasound studies of 92 IDDM patients aged 20–38 years, with a wide range of disease durations, demonstrated that those with LJM had thicker skin than those without LJM, who in turn had thicker skin than those without diabetes [72]. Skin thickness assessed by ultrasound measurement was also noted to correlate with LJM in 80 measurements in a younger population [73].

Biopsy studies have shown thickening of the dermis and epidermis with accumulation of collagen and loss of skin appendages compared with control biopsies [50, 59].

The pathological features have been more carefully defined by Hanna et al [74]. They found clinical evidence of skin thickening in 22% of IDDM patients and 4% of controls. Full-thickness skin biopsy specimens from the forearm were analyzed in 9 patients with IDDM and thick skin, 4 patients with IDDM and clinically normal skin, 4 patients with progressive systemic sclerosis and 4 normal control subjects. They defined distinct differences from sclerodermatous and normal individuals: the IDDM patients with thick skin showed active fibroblasts and extensive collagen polymerization in the rough endoplasmic reticulum. Unlike scleroderma, in which there is bimodality of collagen fiber sizes, the thick skin of diabetes demonstrated predominance of large fibers, a finding that was also present in those with diabetes who did not have thick skin. Thus, the fibrosis in these two conditions appears basically different. Biochemical studies are discussed below.

Association with Microvascular Disease

The initial 7 patients with severe LJM involving fingers and large joints included 5 with clinically apparent retinopathy and/or proteinuria before the age of 18 years [59]. In a clinic population with diabetes duration of more than 4.5 years (the shortest duration at which microvascular complications were noted), 82 of 169 patients had LJM, of whom 41 also had microvascular complications, in contrast to only 10 of the 87 patients without LJM. Severity of LJM correlated directly with the frequency and severity of the microvascular disease. Life table analysis indicated an 83% risk for microvascular complications after 16 years of diabetes if joint limitation was present, but only a 25% risk in the absence of LJM. The combined risk of both groups was 42%, similar to rates reported by others. The differences between the LJM and non-LJM groups could not be accounted for by differences in patients' ages or durations of diabetes. The 4.5-fold greater likelihood of microvascular disease in the group with LJM in this population indicated that LJM identified a group exceptionally at risk for the development of early complications [46].

Benedetti and Noacco [37] reported that 8 of their 19 patients with LJM had clinical retinopathy, and this was exclusively in the group over 21 years of age (range 21–48 years) among whom only one individual did not have retinopathy. No data were provided on control populations. Among adult Irish patients with IDDM, retinopathy was present in 52.4% with LJM compared with only 12.3% without. Those with LJM and retinopathy had much longer durations of diabetes than those with LJM and no retinopathy. To assess whether the presence of LJM was a risk factor for the development of retinopathy, independent of duration of diabetes, two subgroups of 20 patients each, with and without LJM, were matched for duration. Retinopathy was much more common in the group with LJM (85% versus 40%), with a highly significant difference in the prevalence of proliferative retinopathy—70% in patients with LJM compared with 15% in patients with normal joint mobility [38].

A similar attempt was made to correct for duration of diabetes in a young population of 311 subjects aged 6–27 years undergoing fluorescein angiography to determine the prevalence of retinopathy. The relationship between LJM and retinopathy was highly significant ($P <$ 0.0001), and this was not due to the effect of duration on both complications: the interaction of LJM, retinopathy and duration was insignificant. The presence of LJM was predictive of associated retinopathy at the level of clinical recognition (more than 10 microaneurysms), with 43% of those with LJM and more than 4 years' disease duration having retinopathy compared with 15% having clinical retinopathy in this duration group without LJM [51]. Among the 45% of 110 Ethiopian patients with IDDM who had LJM, retinopathy was found to be twice as frequent as in those without LJM [43]. These findings of increased risk for microvascular disease attendant on the presence of LJM appear to be more difficult to substantiate in small groups of patients [42].

Among 150 Joslin Clinic patients under 40 years old, of whom 75 had LJM, the relative risk of retinopathy conferred by the presence of LJM was 3.7, and of preproliferative and proliferative retinopathy 4.2 [53]. Two-thirds of young patients with LJM reported from Hungary had preclinical retinopathy as opposed to one-third of those without LJM [44].

The largest survey reported, involving 375 persons aged 7–25 years, noted positive correlations between skin involvement, severity of joint limitation and diabetic retinopathy, although the latter was evaluated only through the undilated pupil [54].

Less impressive but significant correlation between LJM and microvascular disease is seen with NIDDM. This difference is particularly apparent in studies that involve both IDDM and NIDDM [40, 43, 56].

Biochemical Studies

Increased accumulation of dermal collagen which is relatively insoluble and resistant to enzymatic digestion, has been recognized as a characteristic of connective tissue aging in both IDDM and NIDDM [75]. In 2 out of 3 youngsters with multiple LJM and skin changes, Buckingham et al [50] described decreased acid solubility of skin collagen, suggesting increased crosslinkage; however, the 3 patients taken together did not have a significantly greater resistance of their collagen to digestion than did 7 non-diabetic controls, and no comparison was made to IDDM without LJM. In a subsequent study, skin biopsies from the lateral thigh of 23 patients with IDDM yielded 8 with less than 2.5% collagen extractable in 0.5 M acetic acid. Compared with the 15 with more than 2.5% acid-soluble collagen, there was no difference in age or mean duration of diabetes. However, the rates of retinopathy (50% versus 0%), LJM (63% versus 20%), skin changes (63% versus 20%), HbA_1 values greater than 12% (63% versus 27%) and decreased vital capacity (57% versus 0%) were all significantly different [75].

Skin collagen glycation is increased with diabetes but this does not correlate with LJM [76, 77] or microvascular complications [77]. This glycation correlates with HbA_1 level, and reflects the ketoamine link, an early step in the non-enzymatic browning reaction that leads to stable end-products. These stable end-products are fluorescent and thought to be responsible for increased crosslinking of collagen. Monnier et al [77] demonstrated that fluorescence of skin collagen (FSC) increased linearly with age, but that 95% of 41 IDDM patients had abnormal increases for age and that their FSC correlated with the presence of retinopathy, nephropathy and LJM.

The accumulation of stable end-products of the browning reaction, with increased crosslinking, dehydration and condensation of collagen, is quite distinct from the more hydrated and soluble collagen with increased reducible crosslinks in the thickened tissue of Dupuytren disease and shoulder capsulitis associated with diabetes [28, 31]. Thus, the suggestion that hypertrophied polyol pathway activity resulting in increased hydration of connective tissue, as in the connective tissue in Dupuytren disease, might also be associated with LJM appears unlikely [8].

Constitutional versus Metabolic Considerations

Attributing LJM and associated skin changes

to metabolic control is no easier than with the other long-term complications of diabetes. As with retinopathy, prepubertal duration is not as important as age attained in the appearance of LJM, suggesting the importance of other hormonal influences. No differences in HLA distribution between those with and without LJM have been described [66], and there is no difference in frequency of organ-specific autoimmunity [62].

A genetic component has been suggested by the observation of LJM in non-diabetic relatives of IDDM patients [39, 45]. Traisman et al [45] found a greater frequency of LJM among 106 non-diabetic siblings (9.4%) than among 310 probands (8.4%). In the oldest age group (15–18 years), however, 9% of siblings but 17% of patients had LJM. Data are not provided on duration of diabetes. The overall percentage for this patient population is lower than any other reported, except for that of the Italian investigators who used a handprint method for determining LJM, which would only pick up the more severe contractures [37]; Traisman et al [45] used techniques similar to those of Grgic et al [59]. Brice et al [39] found 42% of 112 IDDM patients aged 2–12 years to have LJM, with 78% of those with duration of diabetes of more than 7 years being affected; this is 3–4 times the prevalence reported by others for this largely preadolescent age group [61]. This diagnostic exuberance may explain their finding among 214 non-diabetic first-degree relatives, that 35% of the relatives of children with LJM were similarly affected, as were 13% of relatives of those children without LJM [39].

Rosenbloom and colleagues [49] examined 204 IDDM patients aged 7–23 years and 336 of their first-degree relatives. They also examined simplex and multiplex pedigrees with IDDM and normal controls. Only one of the non-diabetes-related normal controls had LJM; 3% of 225 non-diabetic parents were affected compare with 21% of the probands. Of the 108 non-diabetic siblings, only one had LJM. Three parents had adult-onset diabetes and had LJM. Of the non-diabetic relatives with joint limitation, none was related to a proband with LJM and all tested were negative for islet cell antibodies. Among 11 IDDM multiplex families with at least one member having joint limitation, the concordance rate for LJM was no greater than expected for age and duration of diabetes.

These authors concluded that the evidence for LJM being a metabolic consequence of diabetes included the virtual absence of limitation among first-degree relatives of probands, including probands with LJM, and that concordance for joint involvement was not increased in first-degree relatives with IDDM.

Further evidence for a metabolic explanation for LJM comes from its description in non-HLA associated, non-autoimmune IDDM, in 2 siblings with the syndrome of diabetes insipidus, diabetes mellitus and optic atrophy [78], as well as in 2 siblings with diabetes from infancy due to pancreatic hypoplasia [79].

As with other complications, the suggestion of a genetic component comes from the difficulty in identifying close correlation with control over the short term and the inability to recognize exceptional control in those individuals who do not develop LJM. The case previously noted in which purported LJM appeared years before clinical diabetes was clearly an erroneous classification of the joint problem [63]. However, LJM has been noted in a teenage sibling of a patient with IDDM who had mild impaired glucose tolerance, and 2 adolescents have been found to have LJM at the time of diagnosis of their diabetes [59, 62]. The latter circumstance does not preclude primary metabolic pathogenesis, as a substantial degree of hyperglycemia can be present for an extended time, particularly in an older child, before clinical symptoms appear.

Tissue culture studies provide the opportunity to examine genetically determined donor characteristics generations of cells removed from the donor metabolic milieu. The viability of cultured fibroblasts from 2 patients with severe LJM and growth failure was found to be completely normal for age, ruling against an inherent cellular defect in growth in these youngsters [80]. Seibold et al [48] studied 5 older patients with IDDM and 3 with NIDDM, all of whom had 'digital sclerosis'. They found that dermal fibroblasts produced less collagen and had less DNA replication but normal collagenase activity. However, there were only 3 controls, and they were substantially younger than all but 3 of the patients, a factor that would significantly alter the DNA replication and collagen synthesis results. Furthermore, there were no comparisons with age-matched people with diabetes who did not have 'digital sclerosis', because the purpose of this study was to demonstrate differences in vitro from systemic sclerosis, which these authors did. Systemic sclerosis is associated with increased collagen synthesis by fibroblasts in culture. The finding of decreased collagen production from cultured dermal fibroblasts from patients with diabetes is consistent with the decrease in collagen production in vivo by streptozotocin-induced diabetic rats [81]. These animals had specific decrease in collagen production in their bone and cartilage but normal non-collagen protein production. In contrast to the suggestion of a genetic component from the studies of Seibold et al [48], these studies in non-genetic diabetes, using fresh tissue, implicate a metabolic etiology.

The essential (apparently) metabolic derangement for the development of LJM and associated skin findings as well as other complications of diabetes that occur despite the type of diabetes (IDDM, NIDDM, secondary) must require a constitutional predilection, which is not specific. Monnier and colleagues [82] have suggested a means by which this constitutional factor may be expressed. They have found that the age-related collagen-linked fluorescence in skin biopsies from longstanding IDDM, reflecting advanced glycation end-products, was, as previously noted, greatly increased compared with controls. However, the rate of browning was not significantly different from normal in those without retinopathy but was 2.5 times greater in the presence of retinopathy. These findings suggested that there was a mechanism controlling the browning rate of collagen in those individuals who did not develop retinopathy.

An alternative metabolic pathway for keto-amine products could provide such a mechanism [83]. The oxidation of earlier glycosylation products to form relatively inert carboxymethyllysine rather than advanced glycosylation end products would reduce the ill effects of protein glycosylation. Differences in response to this process could explain different susceptibility to the development of complications. This raises the intriguing possibility of pharmacological intervention to prevent the development of long-term complications [84].

CONCLUSION

The abnormalities in bone, joints, skin and periarticular tissue described in this chapter cannot be attributed to a single pathogenic mechanism. Vascular insufficiency would appear to explain the stiff hand syndrome, and neuropathy the carpal tunnel syndrome as it appears in diabetes. As osteopenia is seen early in the course of diabetes and does not appear to worsen with duration, a basic metabolic abnormality concomitant with the development of hyperglycemia and unlikely to be related to other complications is probable. The lesions attributable to connective tissue proliferation, involving palmar fascia, the periarticular tissue, the tendon sheaths and the skin, may have the most relevance to the long-term disabling or fatal complications of diabetes in which connective tissue of basement membranes is abnormal.

Although the lesions of diabetes complications are frequently compared to those of aging, the skin and periarticular lesions (and perhaps the osteopenia) of diabetes either are unique or differ substantially from comparable lesions in non-diabetic individuals. This is true also for the complications of the retina, the heart, the kidneys and the peripheral nerves. Dupuytren disease has a different sex ratio and finger involvement in diabetes; adhesive capsulitis of the shoulder has a different natural history and histological picture in diabetes patients; and osteopenia does not appear to be associated with increased fracture risk as it is in those without diabetes.

LJM is the most intriguing of these lesions because of its early onset, the associated skin and lung changes, and the established relationship to retinopathy. The ready accessibility of skin for studies of thickness by non-invasive techniques and of biochemical and histologic changes by biopsy permits the testing of hypotheses regarding pathogenesis [82–84].

Acknowledgments

The author's work was supported by contracts with the Department of Health and Rehabilitative Services of the State of Florida for a Diabetes Research Education and Treatment Center, and a Regional Diabetes Program for Children (Children's Medical Services).

REFERENCES

1. Brownlee M, Cerami A. The biochemistry of the complications of diabetes mellitus. Ann Rev Biochem 1981; 50: 385–432.
2. Regan TJ, Lyons MM, Ahmed SS, Levinson GE, Oldewurtel HA, Ahmed MR, Haider B. Evidence for cardiomyopathy in familial diabetes mellitus. J Clin Invest 1977; 60: 885–9.
3. Luishner JRA, Tevaarwerk GJM, Clarson CL, Harding PGR, Chance GW, Haust MD. Analysis of the collagens of diabetic placental villi. Cell Molec Biol 1986; 32: 27–35.
4. Bland JH, Frymoyer JW, Newberg AH. Rheumatic syndromes in endocrine disease. Semin Arthr Rheum 1979; 9: 23–65.
5. Jelinek JE. The skin in diabetes. Philadelphia: Lea & Febiger, 1986.
6. Lundbaek K. Stiff hands in long-term diabetes. Acta Med Scand 1957; 158: 447–51.
7. Rosenbloom AL. Joint manifestations of diabetes in the young. In Serrano-Rios M, Lefèbvre PJ. (eds) Diabetes 1985. Amsterdam: Elsevier, 1986: pp 762–6.
8. Eaton RP. Aldose reductase inhibition and the diabetic syndrome of limited joint mobility: implications for altered collagen hydration. Metabolism 1986; 35 (suppl. 1): 119–21.
9. Hough FS. Alterations of bone and mineral metabolism in diabetes mellitus. Part I. An overview. S Afr Med J 1987; 72: 116–19.
10. Heath H, Melton LJ, Chic GP. Diabetes mellitus and risk of skeletal fracture. New Engl J Med 1980; 303: 567–70.
11. DeLeeuw I, Abs R. Bone mass and bone density in maturity-type diabetes measured by the ^{125}I photon-absorption technique. Diabetes 1977; 26: 1130–5.
12. Levin ME, Boisseau VC, Avioli LV. Effects of diabetes mellitus on bone mass in juvenile and adult-onset diabetes. New Engl J Med 1976; 294: 241–5.
13. Santiago JV, McAlister WH, Ratzan SK, Bussman Y, Haymond MW, Shackelford G, Weldon VY. Decreased cortical thickness and osteopenia in children with diabetes mellitus. J Clin Endocrinol Metab 1977; 45: 845–8.
14. Rosenbloom AL, Lezotte DC, Weber FT et al. Diminution of bone mass in childhood diabetes. Diabetes 1977; 26: 1052–5.
15. McNair P, Madsbad S, Christiansen C, Faber OK, Transbøl I, Binder C. Osteopenia in insulin-treated diabetes mellitus. Its relation to age at onset, sex and duration of disease. Diabetologia 1978; 15: 87–90.
16. Nielsen CT, Ibsen KK, Christiansen JS, Pieterson B, Uhrenholdt A. Diabetes mellitus, skeletal age and bone mineral content in children. Acta Endo-crinol 1978; suppl. 219: abstr. 58.
17. Frazer TE, White NH, Hough S et al. Alterations in circulating vitamin D metabolites in the young insulin-dependent diabetic. J Clin Endocrinol Metab 1981; 53: 1154–9.
18. McNair P, Christiansen MS, Madsbad S, Christiansen C, Transbøl I. Hypoparathyroidism in diabetes mellitus. Acta Endocrinol 1981; 96: 81–6.
19. Wiske PS, Wentworth SM, Norton JA, Epstein S, Johnston C. Evaluation of bone mass and growth in young diabetics. Metabolism 1982; 31: 848–54.
20. Hough FS. Alterations of bone and mineral metabolism in diabetes mellitus. Part II. Clinical studies in 206 patients with type I diabetes mellitus. S Afr Med J 1987; 72: 120–6.
21. Soejima D, Landing BH. Osteoporosis in juvenile-onset diabetes mellitus: morphometric and comparative studies. Pediatr Pathol 1986; 6: 289–99.
22. Ishide H, Seino Y, Matsukura S et al. Diabetic osteopenia and circulating levels of vitamin D metabolites in type 2 (noninsulin-dependent) diabetes. Metabolism 1985; 34: 797–801.
23. Crisp AJ, Heathcote JG. Connective tissue abnormalities in diabetes mellitus. J Roy Coll Phys (London) 1984; 18: 132–41.
24. Pastan RS, Cohen AS. The rheumatologic manifestations of diabetes mellitus. Med Clin North Am 1978; 62: 829–39.
25. Jelinek JE. Collagen disorders in which diabetes and cutaneous features coexist. In Jelinek JE (ed.) The skin in diabetes. Philadelphia: Lea & Febiger, 1986: pp 155–73.
26. Van De Staak WJBM, Bergers AMG. Ultrastructural abnormalities in the skin nerves of a patient with scleroderma adultorum (Buschke) and diabetes mellitus. Dermatologica 1975; 151: 223–7.
27. Noble J, Heathcote JG, Cohn H. Diabetes mellitus in the aetiology of Dupuytren's disease (DD). J Bone Joint Surg (Br) 1984; 66: 322–5.
28. Bazin S, LeLous M, Duance VC et al. Biochemistry and histology of the connective tissue of Dupuytren's disease lesions. Eur J Clin Invest 1980; 10: 9–16.
29. Jung Y, Hohmann TC, Gerneth JA et al. Diabetic hand syndrome. Metabolism 1971; 20: 1008–14.
30. Bridgeman JF. Periarthritis of the shoulder and diabetes mellitus. Ann Rheum Dis 1972; 312: 69–71.
31. Fisher L, Kurtz A, Shipley M. Association between cheiroarthropathy and frozen shoulder in patients with insulin-dependent diabetes mellitus. Br J Rheumatol 1986; 25: 1141–6.
32. Pal B, Andersen J, Dick WR, Griffiths ID. Limitation of joint mobility and shoulder capsulitis in insulin- and non-insulin-dependent diabetes mellitus. Br J Rheumatol 1986; 25: 147–51.
33. Morén-Hybbinette I, Moritz U, Schersten B. The clinical picture of the painful diabetic shoulder

—natural history, social consequences and analysis of concomitant hand syndrome. Acta Med Scand 1987; 221: 73–82.

34. Rosenbloom AL, Frias JL. Diabetes, short stature and joint stiffness—a new syndrome. Clin Res 1974; 22: 92A.

35. Grgic A, Rosenbloom AL, Weber FT, Giordano B. Joint contracture in childhood diabetes. New Engl J Med 1975; 292: 372.

36. Isshiki G, Osasa Y, Fujiwara Y, Izumi K, Kuno S, Okuno G. Joint contractures in childhood diabetes. In Mimura G, Kitagawa T, Hibi I. (eds) Childhood diabetes in Asia. Tokyo: Medical Journal Sha, 1979: pp 226–30.

37. Benedetti A, Noacco C. Hand changes in childhood onset diabetes. Pediat Adolesc Endocr 1981; 9: 149–55.

38. Kennedy L, Beacom R, Archer DB, Carson DJ, Campbell SL, Johnston PB, Maguire CJ. Limited joint mobility in Type I diabetes mellitus. Postgrad Med J 1982; 58: 481–4.

39. Brice JEH, Johnston DI, Noronha JL. Limited finger joint mobility in diabetes. Arch Dis Child 1982; 157: 879–80.

40. Lawson PM, Maneschi F, Kohner EM. The relationship of hand abnormalities to diabetes and diabetic retinopathy. Diabetes Care 1983; 6: 140–3.

41. Campbell RR, Hawkins SJ, Maddison PJ, Reckless JPD. Limited joint mobility in diabetes mellitus. Ann Rheum Dis 1985; 44: 93–7.

42. Garza-Elizondo MA, Diaz-Jouanen E, Franco-Casique JJ, Alarcon-Segovia D. Joint contractures and scleroderma-like skin changes in the hands of insulin-dependent juvenile diabetics. J Rheumatol 1983; 10: 797–800.

43. Mengistu M, Abdulkadir J. Limited finger joint mobility in insulin-dependent and non-insulin-dependent Ethiopian diabetics. Diabet Med 1985; 2: 387–9.

44. Madacsy L, Peja M, Korompay K, Biro B. Limited joint mobility in diabetic children: a risk factor of diabetic complications? Acta Paediatr Hungarica 1986; 27: 91–6.

45. Traisman H, Traisman ES, Marr TJ, Wise J. Joint contractures in patients with juvenile diabetes and their siblings. Diabetes Care 1978; 1: 360–1.

46. Rosenbloom AL, Silverstein JH, Lezotte DC, Richardson K, McCallum M. Limited joint mobility in childhood diabetes indicates increased risk for microvascular disease. New Engl J Med 1981; 305: 191–4.

47. Starkman H, Brink S. Limited joint mobility of the hand in type I diabetes mellitus. Diabetes Care 1982; 5: 534–6.

48. Seibold J. Digital sclerosis in children with insulin dependent diabetes mellitus. Arthritis Rheum 1982; 25: 1357–61.

49. Rosenbloom AL, Silverstein JH, Riley WJ, Maclaren NK. Limited joint mobility in childhood diabetes: family studies. Diabetes Care 1983; 6: 370–3.

50. Buckingham BA, Uitto J, Sandborg C et al. Scleroderma-like changes in insulin-dependent diabetes mellitus: clinical and biochemical studies. Diabetes Care 1984; 7: 163–9.

51. Rosenbloom AL, Malone JI, Yucha J, Van Cader TC. Limited joint mobility and diabetic retinopathy demonstrated by fluorescein angiography. Eur J Pediatr 1984; 141: 163–4.

52. Costello PB, Tambar PK, Green FA. The prevalence and possible prognostic importance of arthropathy in childhood diabetes. J Rheumatol 1984; 11: 62–5.

53. Starkman HS, Gleason RE, Rand LI, Miller DE, Soeldner JS. Limited joint mobility (LJM) of the hand in patients with diabetes mellitus: relation to chronic complications. Ann Rheum Dis 1986; 45: 130–5.

54. Buckingham B, Perejda AJ, Sandborg C, Kershnar AK, Uitto J. Skin, joint, and pulmonary changes in type I diabetes mellitus. Am J Dis Child 1986; 140: 420–3.

55. Rossi P, Fossaluzza V. Diabetic chieroarthropathy in adult non-insulin-dependent diabetes. Ann Rheum Dis 1985; 44: 141–2.

56. Fitzcharles MA, Duby S, Waddell RW, Banks E, Karsh J. Limitation of joint mobility (cheiroarthropathy) in adult non-insulin-dependent diabetic patients. Ann Rheum Dis 1984; 43: 251–7.

57. Larkin JG, Frier BM. Limited joint mobility and Dupuytren's contracture in diabetic, hypertensive, and normal populations. Br Med J 1986; 292: 1494.

58. Salzarulo HH, Taylor LA. Diabetic 'stiff joint syndrome' as a cause of difficult endotracheal intubation. Anesthesiology 1986; 64: 366–8.

59. Grgic A, Rosenbloom AL, Weber FT, Giordano B, Malone JI, Shuster JJ. Joint contracture—common manifestation of childhood diabetes mellitus. J Pediatr 1976; 8: 584–8.

60. Buithieu M, Rosenbloom AL, Conlon M, Thomas JL. Joint mobility and control in IDDM patients. Diabetes 1988; 37: 129A.

61. Benedetti A, Noacco C. Juvenile diabetic cheiroarthropathy. Acta Diabet Lat 1976; 13: 54–66.

62. Rosenbloom AL, Silverstein JH, Lezotte DC, Riley WJ, Maclaren NK. Limited joint mobility in diabetes mellitus in childhood: natural history and relationship to growth impairment. J Pediatr 1982; 101: 874–8.

63. Sherry DD, Rothstein RRL, Petty RE. Joint contractures preceding insulin-dependent diabetes

mellitus. Arthritis Rheum 1982; 25: 1362–4.

64. Robertson JR, Earnshaw PM, Campbell IW. Tenolysis in juvenile diabetic cheiroarthropathy. Br Med J 1979; 2: 971–2.

65. Eaton RP, Sibbett WL, Harsh A. The effect of an aldose reductase inhibiting agent on limited joint mobility in diabetic patients. JAMA 1985; 253: 1437–40.

66. Kennedy L, Richie C, Lyons TJ, Beacom R. Limited joint mobility in diabetes—some clinical and biochemical aspects. In Serrano-Rios M, Lefèbvre PJ (eds) Diabetes 1985. Amsterdam: Elsevier, 1986: pp 767–70.

67. Baum VC, Levitsky LL, Englander RM. Abnormal cardiac function after exercise in insulin-dependent diabetic children and adolescents. Diabetes Care 1987; 10: 319–23.

68. Schuyler MR, Niewoehner E, Inkley SR, Kohn R. Abnormal lung elasticity in juvenile diabetes mellitus. Am Rev Resp Dis 1976; 113: 37–41.

69. Barta L. Flexion contractures in a diabetic child (Rosenbloom syndrome). Eur J Pediatr 1980; 135: 101–2.

70. Schnapf BM, Banks R, Silverstein JH, Rosenbloom AL, Chesrown S, Loughlin G. Pulmonary function in insulin dependent diabetes mellitus with limited joint mobility. Am Rev Resp Dis 1984; 130: 930–2.

71. Soler NG, Khardori R. Fibrous disease of the breast, thyroiditis, and cheiroarthropathy in type I diabetes mellitus. Lancet 1984; i: 193–5.

72. Collier A, Matthews DM, Kellett HA, Clarke BF. Change in skin thickness associated with cheiroarthropathy in insulin dependent diabetes mellitus. Br Med J 1986; 292: 936.

73. Lieberman LS, Rosenbloom AL. Changes in growth and body composition related to control in children with diabetes. In Borms J, Hauspie R, Sand A, Susanne C, Hebbelinck M (eds) Human growth and development. New York: Plenum, 1984: pp 619–25.

74. Hanna W, Friesen D, Bombardier C, Gladman D, Hanna A. Pathologic features of diabetic thick skin. J Am Acad Dermatol 1987; 16: 546–53.

75. Kohn RR, Schnider SL. Glucosylation of human collagen. Diabetes 1982; 31 (suppl. 3): 47–51.

76. Perejda A, Buckingham B, Uitto J, Kaufman F, Sandborg C, Kershnar A. Correlation of increased collagen cross-linking with diabetic complications. Diabetes 1985; 34 (suppl. 1): 105A.

77. Monnier VM, Vishwanath V, Frank KE, Elmets CA, Dauchot P, Kohn RR. Relation between complications of type I diabetes mellitus and collagen-linked fluorescence. New Engl J Med 1986; 314: 403–8.

78. Fitzgerald GA, Greally JF, Drury MI. The syndrome of diabetes insipidus, diabetes mellitus and optic atrophy (DIDMOA) with diabetic cheiroarthropathy. Postgrad Med J 1978; 54: 815–17.

79. Winter WE, Maclaren NK, Riley WR, Toskes PP, Andres J, Rosenbloom A. Congenital pancreatic hypoplasia: a syndrome of exocrine and endocrine pancreatic insufficiency. J Pediatr 1986; 109: 465–8.

80. Rosenbloom AL, Rosenbloom EK. Insulin-dependent childhood diabetes: normal viability of cultured fibroblasts. Diabetes 1978; 27: 338–41.

81. Spanheimer RG, Umpierrez GE, Stumpf V. Decreased collagen production in diabetic rats. Diabetes 1988; 37: 371–6.

82. Monnier VM, Elmets CA, Frank KE, Vishwanath V, Yamashita T. Age-related normalization of the browning rate of collagen in diabetic subjects without retinopathy. J Clin Invest 1986; 78: 832–5.

83. Kennedy L, Lyons TJ. Non-enzymatic glycosylation. Br Med Bull 1989; 445: 174–90.

84. Brownlee M, Vlassara H, Klooney A, Ulrich P, Cerami A. Aminoguanidine prevents diabetes-induced arterial wall protein cross-linking. Science 1986; 232: 1629–32.

Macrovascular Disease

61

Cellular Mechanisms of Diabetic Large Vessel Disease

T. Ledet*, L. Heickendorff† and L.M. Rasmussen*

*Department of Pathology, University of Aarhus, and †Department of Clinical Chemistry, Kommunehospitalet, Aarhus, Denmark

For many years large vessel disease in diabetic patients has been an almost neglected area of research, but recently an increasing amount of information has emerged. Large vessel disease in diabetic individuals has been presented as a facet of classic atherosclerosis [1]. However, the challenge unfolded by the introduction of the concept of a specific diabetic macroangiopathy as a part of diabetic angiopathy should be recognized [2].

This chapter discusses the pathogenesis of large vessel disease in diabetic patients, chiefly in the context of current views regarding diabetic macroangiopathy and atherosclerosis in diabetes mellitus.

DIABETIC ANGIOPATHY—DIABETIC MACROANGIOPATHY

After the introduction of insulin treatment, it gradually became apparent that vascular damage is the greatest threat to patients with diabetes mellitus. In 1954, a hypothesis was put forward which considered the vascular changes expressed in the presence of one generalized specific vascular disease—an angiopathy—in individuals with long-term diabetes mellitus.

This nosological entity resulted from study of an unselected group of diabetic patients with a duration of diabetes of 15–25 years [3]. Nevertheless, a correlation between the duration of diabetes and large vessel disease was much more difficult to establish than that between duration and abnormalities in smaller vessels.

The concept of a specific generalized angiopathy is frequently misunderstood, but an analysis of the definition of diabetic retinopathy can be used to illustrate some of the most important aspects of the idea of a specific angiopathy in diabetic patients. Fundamentally, the word *specific* indicates the presence of an abnormality seen sooner or later, among *all* individuals with diabetes mellitus. Traditionally, diabetic retinopathy is considered to be a specific diabetic phenomenon. However, the individual lesions in the diabetic retina, apart from the microaneurysm, can be demonstrated in other diseases and not all patients with diabetes will develop retinopathy. Consequently, from a pedantic point of view, diabetic retinopathy is *not* a specific diabetic feature. Nevertheless, retinopathy must still be considered as a characteristic diabetic phenomenon as it is possible to diagnose diabetes mellitus by careful inspection of the background of the eye. It clearly appears

International Textbook of Diabetes Mellitus. Edited by K.G.M.M. Alberti, R.A. DeFronzo, H. Keen and P. Zimmet
© 1992 John Wiley & Sons Ltd

that the specificity of diabetic retinopathy is derived from the remarkable constellation of lesions in the retina. Thus, the term *specific angiopathy* implies a set of unique vessel changes and/or of constellations of abnormalities in the vessel wall seen in *most* patients with long-term diabetes mellitus.

The *generalization* of the vessel lesions is also a very important point in the hypothesis of a diabetic angiopathy. The various constellations of changes in the vessel wall may slowly pervade the total blood vessel system, giving rise to a variety of pictures in various organs.

Furthermore, the existence of a *causal* relationship between classic metabolic changes in diabetes mellitus and the development of vessel damage is an essential third requirement put forward in the hypothesis of a diabetic angiopathy.

In 1970, a landmark in research into diabetic angiopathy was the introduction of the term *diabetic macroangiopathy* [4]. This term was coined to indicate the presence of a non-atherosclerotic specific large vessel disease in diabetic patients. As a facet of diabetic angiopathy, diabetic macroangiopathy does not imply a set of abnormalities confined to certain territories in particular vessels as an early and severe type of atherosclerosis, but a variety of constellations, seen in the entire large blood vessel system.

Morphological Abnormalities

Atherosclerosis is commonly conceived as a disease involving the production of 'spotty' lesions of the intima as fatty streaks and fibrous plaques. In the opinion of most research workers, a disease pattern such as atherosclerosis is related to an alteration in lipoproteins or an abnormal passage of lipoprotein into the vessel wall.

Many reports of the prevalence and severity of artery disease in diabetic patients have emanated from studies carried out in the Tecumseh and Framingham communities in the USA, in civil servants in the Whitehall study in Britain, and in the World Health Organization multinational study. They all reported increased incidence of cardiac disease among diabetic subjects compared with non-diabetic subjects [5–8]. Consequently, information about the structural changes in the large vessel wall is of utmost importance. However, attempts to separate diabetic macroangiopathy from atherosclerosis on a morphological basis have been so infrequent that the amount of data available is rather limited; most studies have been designed to describe aspects of the lipid–atherosclerosis concept.

As early as 1937, abnormalities in the coronary arteries were analysed in histological sections obtained from 31 hearts from diabetic patients and 20 from non-diabetic patients [9]. No quantification was performed, but the author indicated the presence of a well-developed intimal thickening in the arteries of diabetic subjects. The next reasonable morphological investigation was published three decades later by Goodale et al [10]. In this analysis quantification was conducted on a carefully selected group of coronary arteries obtained from maturity onset diabetic patients and non-diabetic controls matched for age and sex. The thickness of the wall of the extramural arteries was found to be greater in samples from diabetic subjects compared with non-diabetic subjects. It was pointed out that lumen narrowing of the extramural arteries was not able to account for the frequency of myocardial infarction, although most of the diabetic patients were rather old.

In another investigation the thickness of the tunica media was shown to be significantly reduced in peripheral segments of the coronary arteries from type 2 diabetic patients compared with non-diabetic subjects [11]. This histomorphological study was performed on immersion-fixed hearts from 10 type 2 diabetic and 10 non-diabetic individuals, the thickness being determined by micrometer measurements. However, more recently a highly significant correlation between arterial wall thickness and duration of diabetes was observed in vivo in the common femoral artery [12]. The analysis was conducted on 19 young insulin-requiring diabetic patients and the measurements were made by a ultrasound technique. Unfortunately no information was available regarding wall thickness in non-diabetic subjects.

In a large, multinational study it became clear that the extent of raised lesions in the aorta and coronary arteries was higher in diabetic than in non-diabetic subjects. However, the evaluation was based on macroscopic inspection, and a difference in the detailed appearance cannot therefore be expected [13].

In a study of hearts from a large group of type 2 diabetic and non-diabetic subjects, the average number of coronary arteries with more than 75% narrowing was almost identical (2.5 versus 3.0) [14]. In this semiquantitative study all the non-diabetic individuals had suffered a fatal coronary event but matched the diabetic subjects with respect to age and sex. The diabetic patients with heart disease had more severe lumen narrowing than the diabetic patients without clinical heart disease. The degree of severe lumen reduction was observed to be the same in proximal as in distal segments from the group of diabetic subjects with coronary artery disease. Although no relationship between duration of diabetes and lumen size was demonstrated, the frequency of retinopathy was increased in the group of diabetic patients with heart disease compared with those diabetic individuals without heart disease. Data have been published from a recent important study of younger juvenile diabetic patients below the age when atherosclerosis usually develops [15]. In this investigation the extramural coronary arteries were subjected to the same semiquantitative analysis as above: the lumen size was decreased by 50% or more in about 50% of the length of the segments studied from diabetic patients, whereas severe lumen reduction was observed in only 1% of arteries from non-diabetic individuals.

A significant correlation between uniform narrowing of the femoral artery and duration of diabetes has been demonstrated in 47 insulin dependent diabetic patients who were analysed using angiography [16]. In another study recently published the internal diameter of the common femoral artery was also estimated in vivo in two groups of young type 1 diabetic patients using an ultrasound technique [17]. In the group of diabetic patients without any long-term complications the diastolic and systolic cross-sectional areas were the same as in a group of age-matched and sex-matched non-diabetic individuals. However, when the group of patients with severe late diabetic complications were analysed, the diastolic and systolic cross-sectional areas were found to be significantly reduced.

The frequency of diffuse coronary artery disease was found to be significantly higher in 185 subjects with predominantly type 2 diabetes compared with 185 age-matched and sex-matched non-diabetic subjects. The investigation was conducted as a combination of postmortem arteriography and histological analysis [18]. In another study the criteria for diffuse artery disease was based solely on evaluation of coronary arteriograms in vivo [19]. In this analysis no difference was observed, although the 37 type 1 and type 2 diabetic subjects were carefully matched for age, sex, blood pressure and hyperlipidaemia with 70 non-diabetic individuals.

The conclusion to be drawn from the data available at present is that the larger arteries from diabetic subjects develop thicker walls but at the same time thinner tunica media than those in non-diabetic individuals. The changes in the wall thickness appear to be correlated with the duration of diabetes. The arterial lumen is unchanged in young diabetic subjects without complications, but reduced in type 2 diabetic patients with heart disease and in young diabetic patients with severe long-term diabetic complications. The frequency of diffuse artery disease is increased among diabetic patients, and it is correlated with the duration of diabetes.

The composition of the arterial wall has been subjected to histological, histochemical and biochemical analysis. The extramural coronary arteries from 20 old diabetic patients (aged 50–70 years) and 20 non-diabetic individuals were given a semiquantitative histological and histochemical evaluation in our laboratory [20]. The arterial changes obtained from the diabetic patients were particularly prominent in the peripheral segments, as shown by accumulation of a PAS-positive material and deposition of calcium. Although no detailed analysis was performed, the amount of fat was also found to be increased. More recently we have expanded our investigations of the wall of the coronary arteries from individuals with type 2 diabetes [11]. Using a quantitative histochemical approach we have observed accumulation of material that was PAS positive but alcian blue negative (positive alcian blue indicates acid mucopolysaccarides) in tunica media from extramural coronary arteries obtained from type 2 diabetic individuals, together with an increase in the amount of connective tissue (Figures 1 and 2). It is important to emphasize that the results were also seen in areas devoid of atherosclerosis. Recently, quantitative immunohistochemical data were provided by study of aortas from a series of type 1 and type 2 diabetic patients. The results indi-

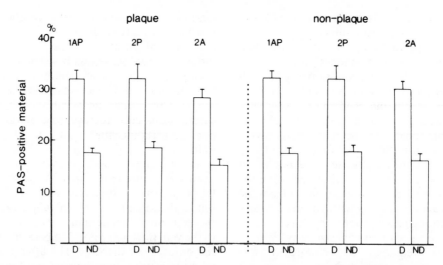

Figure 1 PAS-positive substance in tunica media from the extramural coronary arteries obtained from type 2 diabetic subjects. 1AP, average results from the first 3 cm of the anterior (A) and posterior (P) artery; 2A, peripheral segments of the anterior artery; 2P, peripheral segments of the posterior artery; D, diabetic cases; ND, non-diabetic cases

cate that part of the PAS-positive material seen in areas without atherosclerosis may correspond to fibronectin [21] (Figure 3). Moreover, we were able to demonstrate in the tunica media at the immunohistochemical level that the amount of such basement membrane components as type IV collagen and laminin were increased in the aorta [22]. An important clue is that the altera-

tions in the tunica media were found to be diffuse and unrelated to intimal lesions.

In 1949 arterial calcification was studied in 83 young diabetic subjects (aged 25–34 years), and a clear-cut relationship between calcification and duration of diabetes was demonstrated [23]. Ferrier [24] obtained in 1964 a series of data from low-voltage roentgenograms of the large

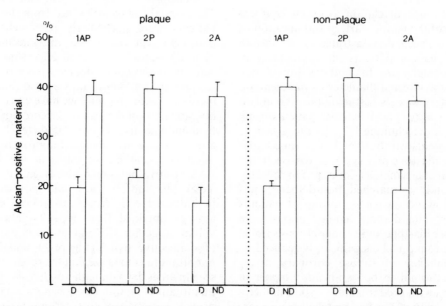

Figure 2 Histochemically measurable acid mucopolysaccharides (alcian blue positive material) in tunica media from extramural coronary arteries collected from type 2 diabetic individuals. D, diabetic cases; ND, non-diabetic cases

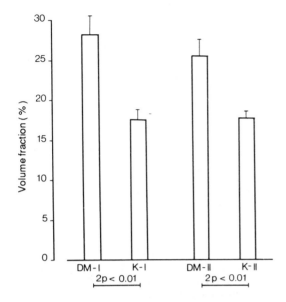

Figure 3 The areas of fibronectin in aortic tunica media from type 1 and type 2 diabetic subjects. Data ($\bar{x} \pm$ SEM) were obtained in areas without plaques. DM-I = type 1 diabetics, DM-II = type 2 diabetics, K-I and K-II = non-diabetics

vessels of amputated limbs from diabetic and non-diabetic individuals. A more pronounced medial calcification and luminal reduction of the metatarsal arteries was noticed among the diabetic subjects. Ferrier [24] and later Christensen [25] demonstrated that arterial linear calcification is a characteristic phenomenon in diabetes—quite different from the spotty lesions usually seen in severe atherosclerosis. An investigation published in 1971 described medial calcification as more extensive in the femoral artery and its ramifications among type 2 diabetic patients compared with non-diabetic subjects. Moreover, there was no difference in the amount of intimal calcification, but calcium deposition in the tunica media was statistically correlated with a decrease in glucose tolerance [26]. A strongly correlated relationship was recently demonstrated between linear medial calcification in the femoral artery and duration of diabetes in a group of 47 insulin dependent subjects in the age range 20–55 years [17].

It appears from analyses of the structure of the artery wall that a set of changes can be demonstrated in areas without the presence of classic atherosclerotic abnormalities. It is relevant to mention the accumulation of a PAS-positive substance, such connective tissue basement membrane components as fibronectin, type IV collagen and laminin, as well as the calcium deposition combined with a reduction in acid mucopolysaccharides. It is noteworthy that the peculiar PAS-positive but acid mucopolysaccharide-negative deposits in the small blood vessels are usually recognized as the histopathological indicator of diabetic microangiopathy [2, 27].

The functional consequences are unknown, although it has been calculated from measurements in vivo using an echocardiographic technique that aortic stiffness in both sexes is significantly increased in a group of young diabetic subjects compared with a group of healthy non-diabetic individuals [28]. Recent study of the biomechanical properties of aortic samples from type 1 diabetic subjects has demonstrated a marked reduction in the extensibility and an increase in the stiffness of the tissue [84]. It is noteworthy that the pronounced alterations of the diabetic aortic wall were found in areas with non-visible atherosclerosis and, furthermore, the changes could not be correlated to the grade of atherosclerosis in the thoracic aorta, indicating that the diabetic patient develops changes in the aorta independent of atherosclerosis. The diabetic patients showed no clinical manifestation of atherosclerosis or hypertension. The stiffness was clearly correlated with the duration of diabetes as well as with age, whereas there was no such age correlation in the healthy controls. Surprisingly, statistical analysis failed to reveal any correlation between stiffness and duration of diabetes in female patients. In a later study using an ultrasound technique, the stiffness of the femoral artery was demonstrated to be increased in diabetic individuals; this stiffness was also strongly correlated with duration of diabetes and with the arterial wall thickness [29].

Large Vessel Abnormalities in Experimental Diabetes

In order to obtain more information about the pathogenesis of diabetic large vessel disease, animals with experimental or spontaneous diabetes have been used. In 1949 Duff and McMillan published a series of surprising data which demonstrated that atherogenic diets given to alloxan-diabetic rabbits may well increase the plasma cholesterol [30], but the effect in developing large vessel abnormalities was less than that in non-diabetic rabbits. Several years later these interesting findings were confirmed by Kloeze and Abdellatif [31].

The effect of a cholesterol-rich diet on the development of large vessel abnormalities was studied for 4 months on alloxan-diabetic rabbits with and without the presence of cortisone [32]. Plaque formation in the diabetic rabbits was remarkably pronounced in the medium-sized coronary arteries, comprising mainly foam cells in the tunica intima. The body weight was identical in the two groups of rabbits, but the blood cholesterol levels were highest among the diabetic rabbits. Recently, morphological changes were analysed in aortas obtained from alloxan-diabetic rabbits fed a low-cholesterol diet for up to 40 weeks [33]; micrometer measurements demonstrated that the intima was significantly thicker in the diabetic group of rabbits. In addition, macroscopic quantification of the area of sudanophilic material on the surface of the aorta showed a significantly greater area in the diabetic than in the non-diabetic animals, and that the majority of lesions were small, raised plaques of collagen and smooth muscle cells.

Severe cardiovascular lesions have been demonstrated in diabetic rats fed a high-fat diet for 3–6 months [34–36]. Almost all studies dealt with diabetic rats with a high serum cholesterol level; in one study, however, advanced plaque composed of foam cells in the tunica media of large blood vessels was seen in diabetic rats which had serum cholesterol levels similar to those in the non-diabetic rats [34]. This investigation suggests the presence of an effect of diabetes independent of serum cholesterol. It has been demonstrated in our laboratory that the number of cells in the tunica media of the large coronary arteries is increased in rats with experimental diabetes of 9 months' duration [37]. Furthermore, it was observed that insulin treatment resulting in near-normal glucose metabolism suppressed the development of these changes.

The influence of diabetes and increased serum cholesterol has been analysed in a series of alloxan-diabetic squirrel monkeys [38]; the incidence of macroscopic lesions in the large vessels was found to be higher among the diabetic animals than among the controls. Another important study has demonstrated that monkeys with spontaneous diabetes on a normal diet develop larger plaques and more sudanophilia in the aorta than control animals [39]. The analyses were quantitative and the serum cholesterol was normal in both groups. Another noteworthy observation was the correlation between the incidence of aortic changes and the degree of abnormality of the intravenous glucose tolerance test.

The effect of experimental diabetes on the development of abnormalities in the large vessels is not easy to appraise. In most studies, high-fat diets or animals with high serum cholesterol levels have been used. However, some data clearly indicate that lesions can develop in the large vessels without a concomitant increase in the serum cholesterol level. These results suggest that a factor or factors in the diabetic metabolism may be of importance. The consequences of the changes in the vessel wall with experimental diabetes still remain to be elucidated. Two studies have been published assessing the biomechanical alterations after 30 and 95 days of diabetes; however, no influence on the biomechanical properties was detected [40, 41].

A hypothesis put forward in 1969 suggested that increased serum insulin levels induced by treatment may cause blood vessel damage in diabetic individuals [42]. The concept received support from a series of experiments with non-diabetic rats and chickens treated with large doses of insulin [43, 44]. These studies showed enhanced synthesis of cholesterol in the aortas. It has not been possible, however, to confirm these results using KK mice with increased levels of plasma insulin, or in diabetic rats treated with insulin [45, 46]; neither has it been possible to demonstrate an effect of insulin upon the transfer of cholesterol from plasma to the arterial wall [47]. The latter study was performed on 12 female rabbits, of which 6 were injected with 12 U zinc protamine insulin. All animals received radio-labelled cholesterol 22 hours before the aorta was removed for lipid estimation. Finally, our investigation [37] demonstrating a beneficial effect of insulin treatment on the development of lesions in large vessels from rats with experimental diabetes seriously undermines the insulin hypothesis.

Large Vessel Metabolism in Experimental Diabetes

It has been known for a long time that pronounced metabolic changes are found in vascular tissue of diabetic animals. In intima–media preparations of thoracic aorta from alloxan-diabetic rats and rabbits, the glucose uptake and the conversion of glucose to CO_2, glycogen, lipids and lactate is depressed (48–50). Glucose metabolism has also been shown to be impaired in Chinese hamsters with spontaneous diabetes [51].

A number of enzymes have been studied in the aortas of diabetic rabbits and rats. However, evaluation of enzymatic activity per se does not allow conclusions concerning activity in a given metabolic pathway: it is necessary to consider the enzymic activity in relationship to the flow of substrates and metabolites in the metabolic pathway before any conclusion can be drawn. It is difficult, therefore, to put into perspective the results published by Wolinsky et al [52, 53]. They found reduced activity of a number of hydro-lases in aortas from rats with experimental diabetes, but the substrates were not measured. On one occasion, however, a substrate for the acid cholesteryl-β-D-glucoside hydrolase (steryl-β-glucosidase) was found to be increased despite reduced enzymic activity. It has been shown that hexokinase activity is reduced in the aorta of diabetic rabbits, and similar results have been obtained in diabetic rats [54, 55]. The decreased glucose utilisation seen in aortic media–intima preparations from diabetic animals could be ascribed to impaired glucose phosphorylation, although it has not been possible to exclude a defect at the level of the phosphofructokinase reaction. Ågren and Arnquist [55] showed in 1981 that glucose-6-phosphate dehydrogenase and hydroxyacyl-CoA dehydrogenase were increased in an intima–media preparation from aorta of rats with diabetes of 2 weeks' duration. The same result was provided by a study on non-diabetic pigs with and without a high level of insulin antibodies [56]. However, the pigs with increased antibodies had pronounced glucose intolerance and increased plasma glucose although plasma insulin was elevated. Taking into consideration the data of Ågren and Arnquist [55], the results presented by Falholt et al [56] may well be ascribed to the diabetes-like condition rather than to the high insulin levels. Moreover, in the study of Ågren and Arnquist, insulin treatment normalised the changes observed in the enzymic activity [55]. It has been demonstrated in diabetic hamsters that injection of large amounts of insulin, resulting in

hyperinsulinaemia and hypoglycaemia, was able to normalise glucose metabolism in the aorta [51]. However, the long-term effects of abnor-malities of the various enzymes in the aorta of diabetic animals are not yet clear.

Recent studies have demonstrated that incu-bation of low-density lipoprotein (LDL) with glucose in vitro can result in glycation of lysine residues of LDL, with a resultant decrease in the binding of LDL to receptors on cultured human fibroblasts [57]. However, binding and degra-dation by normal fibroblasts of LDL obtained from 7 type 2 diabetic subjects and 10 non-diabetic subjects has been analysed [58]: the aver-age glucose value was 12.6 mmol/l in the diabetic group, but the results revealed no difference between diabetic and non-diabetic LDL. A sim-ilar result was found when LDL was bound and degraded by mouse peritoneal macrophages. A small but significant increase in cholesterylester synthesis and accumulation was seen in human monocyte-derived macrophages after incubation with LDL from type 1 diabetic patients [59] in whom the amount of non-enzymatic glycated LDL was higher than in the non-diabetic group. In a study performed recently on a few rabbits, it was demonstrated that, in the presence of antibodies against glycated LDL, the clearance rate of glycated LDL was greatly accelerated [60]; moreover, the uptake into the aorta of glycated LDL was considerably lower than that of native LDL. It appears from these studies that little if any effect on fibroblasts and macro-phages could be detected using non-enzymatic glycated LDL from type 1 and type 2 diabetic subjects. It appears that the presence of small amounts of antibodies against glycated LDL, which is to be expected in diabetic subjects, facilitates the degradation of glycated LDL and reduces the uptake into aorta. Consequently the importance of non-enzymatic glycated LDL in the development of lesions in the larger blood vessels in diabetic patients still remains to be elucidated.

TISSUE CULTURE AND LARGE VESSEL DISEASE: A MODEL IN VITRO

In recent years the use of tissue culture [61, 62] as a model of diabetic large vessel disease has provided important information for the under-standing of the pathogenesis of diabetic macro-angiopathy. The cells have mainly been derived

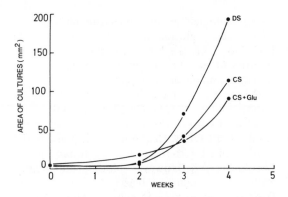

Figure 4 Effect of serum from type 1 diabetic and non-diabetic individuals with and without addition of glucose on growth of rabbit aortic smooth muscle cells in culture. DS, serum from diabetics; CS, serum from non-diabetics; CS + Glu, serum from non-diabetics with added glucose

from the tunica media or the tunica intima of various arteries. A popular culture system is based on repeated trypsin treatment of cells, but it is possible to grow cells in vitro without recourse to enzymes.

In our laboratory increased outgrowth and proliferation of rabbit arterial smooth muscle cells was seen after exposure to normolipaemic serum, either from juvenile diabetic individuals or from alloxan-diabetic rabbits [63, 64] (Figure 4). Similar results have been published using pooled sera from individuals with type 2 diabetes mellitus [65]. There have been several attempts to identify those components in diabetic serum responsible for the increased growth. Various concentrations of glucose added to serum from non-diabetic subjects were shown to have no effect [63, 65, 66]. A series of investigations using serum from type 1 diabetic males, ultrafiltration and dialysis indicated the presence of an active compound with a molecular weight between 3000 and 30 000 [64]. In a recent study, three serum samples taken from type 2 diabetic subjects were analysed, and it appeared that only a factor with a molecular weight below 3500 increased the growth of human arterial smooth muscle cells [67]; the factor was shown to be active after heating and not affected by lipid-dissolving agents.

In a study in vitro and in vivo the effect of endothelial denudation on growth of arterial smooth muscle cells was analysed. It became clear that the cell growth in intima–media preparations from rats with experimental diabetes

with poor or reasonable blood glucose control was identical [68]. It has been suggested that insulin may cause increased proliferation of cells in tissue culture. However, it was necessary for the cells to be starved for several days in the absence of serum before an insulin effect was shown, and only at rather high insulin levels (200–2500 μU/ml) [69–71]. In one study combining techniques in vitro and in vivo, insulin was found to reduce the incorporation of thymidine [68]. In our laboratory we have not been able to demonstrate an effect of insulin, and other groups have arrived at the same results [65, 72]. Finally, in serum from individuals with juvenile diabetes of recent onset, the growth promotion effect has been demonstrated although the concentration of serum insulin was 0–6 μU/ml [72].

Some years ago the increased serum growth hormone seen in diabetic subjects was suggested as one causal factor for the development of diabetic angiopathy [73]. Later, the frequency of small and large blood vessel disease was shown to be rather low among growth hormone-deficient dwarfs with a diabetic glucose metabolism [74]. In a series of studies we investigated the growth in tissue culture of arterial smooth muscle cells after addition of physiological amounts of human growth hormone (1 ng/ml), and found that the hormone increased growth significantly and that growth hormone anti-serum was able to normalise the growth effect of serum from diabetic subjects [75, 76]. Our results point to growth hormone as one possible factor in serum from diabetic individuals that may be responsible for the observed growth rate. It is therefore of considerable interest that Bettmann et al [77] have published data that show reduced proliferation of intimal smooth muscle cells after hypophysectomy in rats with vessel wall damage.

The effect of serum from diabetic subjects on the secretion of procollagen type I and type III was estimated in aortic smooth muscle cell cultures [78]; it became clear that serum from diabetic individuals enhanced type I collagen production. Fibronectin is a component of the basement membrane-like material obtained from aortic smooth muscle cells and also a component of other extracellular matrix material in the arterial wall. Data from the same tissue culture study demonstrated enhanced secretion of fibronectin in the presence of serum from diabetic subjects. High levels of glucose or ketones did not affect the production of collagen

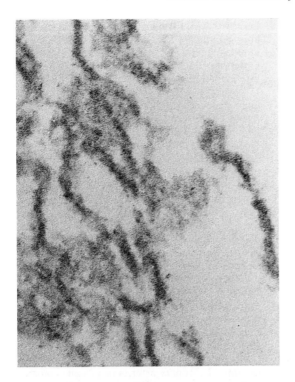

Figure 5 Electron micrograph of isolated basement membrane-like material obtained from cultured smooth muscle cells by a sonication–differential centrifugation procedure (× 60 000). Note absence of nuclei, cytoplasmic organelles, cell membranes, elastin and collagen fibres

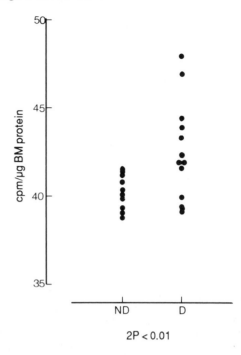

2P < 0.01

Figure 6 Effect of serum from type 1 diabetic patients on accumulation of basement membrane-like (BM) material. Cultures of smooth muscle cells from rabbit aortae were incubated with 0.5 μCi/ml ^{3}H-leucine and test sera. A significantly greater incorporation of leucine into BM is seen in cultures incubated with sera from diabetic persons (D; type 1) compared with sera from non-diabetic subjects (ND)

and fibronectin. Insulin (100 μU/ml), however, reduced secretion of collagens and fibronectin, whereas growth hormone (as did serum from diabetic subjects) augmented the elaboration of type I collagen and fibronectin.

In recent biochemical investigations the basement membrane-like material surrounding individual smooth muscle cells in the arterial wall has been isolated and to some extent characterized [79, 80] (Figure 5). Using serum from either type 1 or type 2 diabetic subjects, the accumulation of basement membrane-like material was found to be increased; this effect could not be ascribed to either reduced removal of the basement membrane-like material or the presence of high concentrations of glucose in the incubation medium [81] (Figure 6). It has not been possible to change the deposition rate of basement membrane-like material using various concentrations of insulin, ketones or glucagon [82]. However, human growth hormone (1 ng/ml) was able to enhance the accumulation of base-

ment membrane-like material isolated from cultures of aortic smooth muscle cells [83]. It could also be demonstrated, using radioactive sulphate, that the amount of glycosaminoglycans/acid mucopolysaccharides was reduced.

The data collected from these studies in vitro are compatible with the morphological observations of large amounts of PAS-positive material with reduced reaction for acid mucopolysaccharides in the extramural coronary arteries of subjects with type 2 diabetes. Moreover, our results in vitro suggest (but do not prove) that part of the development of diabetic macroangiopathy may be attributable to a factor or factors present in normolipaemic serum from diabetic individuals, and that the increased growth hormone level may be of some importance.

CONCLUSION

In this chapter we have compared and analysed published data related to the pathogenesis of large vessel disease in diabetic individuals. The prevailing opinion appears to be that diabetes mellitus accelerates the development of atherosclerosis. However, as an alternative, we have amassed data that point to the presence in diabetic subjects of a constellation of non-atherosclerotic large vessel abnormalities—a diabetic macroangiopathy. We now know that calcium deposition, accumulation of PAS-positive material, laminin, fibronectin, type IV collagen and connective tissue, as well as a lack of acid mucopolysaccharides, occur in the large vessel independent of the presence of atherosclerosis.

In our opinion, these facts emphasize that the concept of a specific diabetic macroangiopathy is a more fruitful working hypothesis than the usual theory of a relationship between atherosclerosis and diabetes mellitus. It is, of course, only one aspect of the pathogenesis of large vessel wall damage in diabetic subjects, but it provides a causal relationship (although the mechanism is still unknown) between such changes and the abnormal metabolism in subjects with diabetes mellitus.

REFERENCES

1. Ruderman NB, Haudenschild C. Diabetes as an atherogenic factor. Prog Cardiovasc Dis 1984; 26: 373–412.
2. Ledet T, Gøtzsche O, Heickendorff L. The pathology of diabetic cardiopathy: pathogenetic reflections. In Jarrett RJ (ed) Diabetes and heart disease. Amsterdam: Elsevier, 1984: pp 26–46.
3. Lundbaek K. Diabetic angiopathy—a specific vascular disease. Lancet 1954; i: 377–9.
4. Lundbaek K. Blood vessel disease. In Lundbaek K, Keen H (eds) Diabetes mellitus. Acta Diab Lat 1971; 8 (suppl. 1): 34.
5. Epstein FH, Ostrander LD, Johnson BC, Payne MV, Hayner NS, Keller JB, Francis T Jr. Epidemiological studies of cardiovascular disease in a total community—Tecumseh, Michigan. Ann Intern Med 1965; 62: 1170–87.
6. Kannel WB, McGee DL. Diabetes and glucose tolerance as risk factors for cardiovascular disease: the Framingham study. Diabetes Care 1979; 2: 920–6.
7. Reid DD, Brett GZ, Hamilton PJS, Jarrett RJ, Keen H, Rose R. Cardiorespiratory disease and diabetes among middle aged male civil servants. Lancet 1974; i: 469–73.
8. WHO multinational study of vascular disease in diabetics. Prevalence of small vessel and large vessel disease in diabetic patients from 14 centres. Diabetologia 1985; 28: 615–40.
9. Lefkovits AM. Coronary disease in diabetes mellitus. J Lab Clin Med 1937; 23: 354–7.
10. Goodale F, Daoud AS, Florentin R, Lee KT, Gittelsohn A. Chemicoanatomic studies of arteriosclerosis and thrombosis in diabetics. I: Coronary arterial wall thickness, thrombosis and myocardial infarcts in autopsied North Americans. Exp Molec Path 1962; 1: 353–63.
11. Dybdahl H, Ledet T. Diabetic macroangiopathy. Quantitative histopathological studies of the extramural coronary arteries from type 2 (non-insulin dependent) diabetic patients. Diabetologia 1987; 30: 882–6.
12. Christensen T, Neubauer B. Increased arterial wall stiffness and thickness in medium sized arteries in patients with insulin dependent diabetes mellitus. Acta Radiol Diagnosis 1988; 29: 299–302.
13. Robertson WB, Strong JP. Atherosclerosis in persons with hypertension and diabetes mellitus. Lab Invest 1968; 18: 78–91.
14. Waller BRF, Palumbo PJ, Roberts WC. Status of the coronary arteries at necropsy in diabetes mellitus with onset after age 30 years. Am J Med 1980; 69: 498–506.
15. Crall FV, Roberts WC. The extramural and intramural coronary arteries in juvenile diabetes mellitus. Am J Med 1978; 645: 221–30.
16. Neubauer B, Gundersen HJ. Calcifications, narrowing, and rugosities of the leg arteries in diabetic patients. Acta Radiol Diagnosis 1983; 24: 401–13.
17. Christensen T, Neubauer B. Internal diameter of common femoral artery in patients with insulin dependent diabetes mellitus. Acta Radiol Diagnosis 1988, 29: 423–5.
18. Vigorita VJ, Moore GW, Hutchins GM. Absence of correlation between coronary arterial atherosclerosis and severity or duration of diabetes of adult onset. Am J Cardiol 1980; 46: 535–42.
19. Dortimer AC, Shenoy PN, Shiroff RA, Leaman DM, Babb JD, Liedtke AJ, Zelis R. Diffuse coronary artery disease in diabetic patients. Fact or fiction? Circulation 1977; 57: 133–6.
20. Ledet T. Histological and histochemical changes in the coronary arteries of old diabetic patients. Diabetologia 1968; 4: 268–72.
21. Rasmussen LM, Heickendorff L. Accumulation of fibronectin in aortae from diabetic patients: a quantitative immunohistological and biochemical study. Lab Invest 1989; 61: 440–6.
22. Rasmussen LM, Heickendorff L, Ledet, T. Quantitative immunohistochemical studies of basement membrane components in the tunica media of aortas from diabetic patients. Submitted for publication.
23. Root HF. Diabetes and vascular disease in youth. Am J Med Sci 1949; 217: 545–53.

24. Ferrier TM. Radiologically demonstrable arterial calcifications in diabetes mellitus. Aust Ann Med 1964; 13: 222–8.

25. Christensen NJ. Muscle blood flow, measured by xenon[133] and vascular calcifications in diabetics. Acta Med Scand 1968; 183: 449–54.

26. Neubauer B. A quantitative study of peripheral arterial calcification and glucose tolerance in elderly diabetics and non-diabetics. Diabetologia 1971; 7: 409–28.

27. Ledet T. Diabetic cardiopathy. Quantitative histological studies of the heart from young juvenile diabetics. Acta Path Microbiol Scand (sect. A) 1975; 84: 421–8.

28. Thordarson H, Thorgeirsson G, Helgason T. Aortic stiffness in insulin dependent diabetics: an echocardiographic study. Diabet Med 1986; 3: 449–54.

29. Christensen T, Neubauer B. Arterial wall stiffness in insulin independent diabetes mellitus. Acta Radiol Diagnosis 1987; 28: 207–8.

30. Duff GL, McMillan GC. The effect of alloxan diabetes on experimental cholesterol atherosclerosis in the rabbit. J Exp Med 1949; 89: 611–30.

31. Kloeze J, Abdellatiff AMM. Effects of palm-kernel oil and sunflower seed oil on serum lipids and atherogenesis in alloxan diabetic rabbits. Atherosclerosis 1975; 22: 349–68.

32. Wellmann KF, Volk BWV. Experimental atherosclerosis in normal and subdiabetic rabbits. I. Short-term studies. Arch Path 1970; 90: 206–17.

33. Miller RA, Wilson RB. Atherosclerosis and myocardial ischemic lesions in alloxan-diabetic rabbits fed a low cholesterol diet. Arteriosclerosis 1984; 4: 586–91.

34. Still WJS, Martin JM, Gregor WH. The effect of alloxan diabetes on experimental atherosclerosis in the rat. Exp Molec Path 1964; 3: 141–7.

35. Wilson RB, Martin JM, Hartoft WS. Evaluation of the relative pathogenic roles of diabetes and serum cholesterol levels in the development of cardiovascular lesions in rats. Diabetes 1967; 16: 71–82.

36. Kalant N, Teitelbaum JI, Cooperberg AA, Harland WA. Dietary atherogenesis in alloxan diabetes. J Lab Clin Med 1964; 63: 147–57.

37. Baandrup U, Ledet T, Rasch R. Experimental diabetic cardiopathy preventable by insulin treatment. Lab Invest 1981; 45: 169–73.

38. Lehner NDM, Clarkson TB, Lofland HB. The effect of insulin deficiency, hypothyroidism, and hypertension on atherosclerosis in the Squirrel Monkey. Exp Molec Path 1971; 15: 230–44.

39. Howard CF Jr. Aortic atherosclerosis in normal and spontaneously diabetic *Macaca nigra*. Atherosclerosis 1979; 33: 479–93.

40. Andreassen TT, Oxlund H. Changes in collagen and elastin of the rat aorta induced by experimental diabetes and food restriction. Acta Endocrinol (Copenh) 1987; 115: 338–44.

41. Andreassen TT, Seyer-Hansen K, Oxlund H. Biomechanical changes in connective tissues induced by experimental diabetes. Acta Endocrinol (Copenh) 1981; 98: 432–6.

42. Stout RW, Vallance-Owen J. Insulin and atheroma. Lancet 1969; i: 1078–80.

43. Stout RW. Insulin stimulation of cholesterol synthesis by arterial tissue. Lancet 1969; ii: 467–8.

44. Stout RW. The effect of insulin on the incorporation of sodium $[1-^{14}C]$acetate into lipids of the rat aorta. Diabetologia 1971; 7: 367–72.

45. Chattopadhyay DP, Martin JM. Effect of insulin on the in vitro synthesis of sterol and fatty acid by aorta and liver from diabetic rats. J Atheroscler Res 1969; 10: 131–4.

46. Chobanian AV, Gerritsen GC, McCombs L, Brecher PI. Arterial lipid metabolism in diabetic animal models with reduced or elevated plasma insulin levels. In Schettler G, Weizel A (eds) Atherosclerosis III: Proceedings of the 3rd International Symposium. Berlin: Springer, 1974: pp 114–17.

47. Christensen S, Jensen J. Uptake of labelled cholesterol from plasma by aortic intima–media in control and insulin injected rabbits. J Atheroscler Res 1975; 5: 258–9.

48. Wertheimer HE, Bentor V. Influence of diabetes on carbohydrate metabolism of aortic tissue. Diabetes 1962; 11: 422–5.

49. Urrutia G, Beavan DW, Cahill GF. Metabolism of glucose-U-C[14] in rat aorta in vitro. Metabolism 1962; 11: 530–4.

50. Mulcahy PD, Winegrad AI. Effects of insulin and alloxan diabetes on glucose metabolism in rabbit aortic tissue. Am J Physiol 1962; 203: 1038–42.

51. Chobanian AV, Gerritsen GC, Brecher PI, McCombs L. Aortic glucose metabolism in the diabetic Chinese hamster. Diabetologia 1974; 10: 589–93.

52. Wolinsky H, Goldfischer S, Capron L, Capron F, Coltoff-Schiller B, Kasak L. Hydrolase activities in the rat aorta. I. Effects of diabetes mellitus and insulin treatment. Circ Res 1978; 42: 821–31.

53. Wolinsky H, Capron L, Goldfischer S, Capron F, Coltoff-Schiller B, Kasak LE. Hydrolase activities in the rat aorta. II. Effects of hypertension alone and in combination with diabetes mellitus. Circ Res 1978; 42: 831–9.

54. Yalcin S, Winegrad AI. Defect in glucose metabolism in aortic tissue from alloxan-diabetic rabbits. Am J Physiol 1964; 205: 1253–9.

55. Ågren A, Arnqvist H. Influence of diabetes on enzyme activities in rat aorta. Diabète Métab 1981; 7: 19–24.

56. Falholt K, Alberti KGMM, Heding LG. Aorta

and muscle metabolism in pigs with peripheral hyperinsulinaemia. Diabetologia 1985; 28: 32–7.

57. Gonen B, Jacobsen D, Farrar P, Schonfeld G. In vitro glycosylation of low density and high density lipoproteins. Diabetes 1981; 30: 875–8.

58. Kraemer FB, Chen YDI, Cheung RMC, Reaven GM. Are the binding and degradation of low density lipoprotein altered in type 2 (non-insulin dependent) diabetes mellitus? Diabetologia 1982; 23: 28–33.

59. Lyons TJ, Klein RL, Baynes JW, Stevenson HC, Lopes-Virella MS. Stimulation of cholesterylester synthesis in human monocyte derived macrophages by low-density lipoproteins from type 1 (insulin dependent) diabetic patients: the influence of non-enzymatic glycosylation of low-density lipoproteins. Diabetologia 1987; 30: 916–23.

60. Wiklund O, Witztum JL, Carew TE, Pittman RC, Elam RL, Steinberg D. Turnover and tissue sites of degradation of glucosylated low density lipoprotein in normal and immunized rabbits. J Lipid Res 1987; 28: 1098–109.

61. Fischer-Dzoga K, Jones K, Vesselinovitch D, Wissler RW. Ultrastructural and immunohistochemical studies of primary cultures of aortic medial cells. Exp Molec Path 1973; 18: 162–76.

62. Ross R. The smooth muscle cell. II. Growth of smooth muscle in culture and formation of elastic fibres. J Cell Biol 1971; 50: 172–86.

63. Ledet T, Fischer-Dzoga K, Wissler RW. Growth of rabbit aortic smooth muscle cell cultured in media containing diabetic and hyperlipemic serum. Diabetes 1976; 25: 207–15.

64. Ledet T. Growth of rabbit aortic smooth-muscle cells in serum patients with juvenile diabetes. Acta Path Microbiol Scand (sect. A) 1976; 84: 508–16.

65. Koschinsky T, Bunting CE, Schwippert B, Gries FA. Increased growth of human fibroblasts and arterial smooth muscle cells from diabetic patients related to diabetic serum factors and cell origin. Atherosclerosis 1979; 33: 245–52.

66. Turner IL, Bierman EL. Effects of glucose and sorbitol on proliferation of cultured human skin fibroblasts and arterial smooth muscle cells. Diabetes 1978; 27: 583–8.

67. Koschinsky T, Bunting CE, Rutter R, Gries FA. Sera from type 2 (non-insulin-dependent) diabetic and healthy subjects contain different amounts of a very low molecular weight growth peptide for vascular cells. Diabetologia 1985; 28: 223–8.

68. Capron L, Jarnet J, Kazandjian S, Housset E. Growth promoting effect of diabetics and insulin on arteries. An in vitro study of rat aorta. Diabetes 1986; 35: 973–8.

69. Stout RW, Bierman EL, Ross R. Effect of insulin on the proliferation of cultured primate arterial smooth muscle cell. Circ Res 1975; 36: 319–27.

70. Pheifle B, Ditschuneit HH. Ditschuneit H. Insulin as a cellular growth regulator of rat arterial smooth muscle cells in vitro. Horm Metab Res 1980; 12: 381–5.

71. King GL, Buzney SM, Kahn CR, Hetu N, Buchwald S, Macdonald SG, Rand LI. Different responsiveness to insulin of endothelial and support cells from micro and macrovessels. J Clin Invest 1983; 71: 974–9.

72. Ledet T. Growth hormone stimulating the growth of arterial medial cells in vitro. Absence of effect of insulin. Diabetes 1976; 25: 1011–17.

73. Lundbaek K, Christensen NJ, Jensen VA et al. Diabetes, diabetic angiopathy and growth hormone. Lancet 1970; ii: 131–3.

74. Merimee TJ, Fineberg ES, Hollander W. Vascular disease in the chronic HGH-deficient state. Diabetes 1973; 22: 813–19.

75. Ledet T. Diabetic macroangiopathy and growth hormone. Diabetes 1981; 30 (suppl.): 14–17.

76. Ledet T. Growth hormone antiserum suppresses the growth effect of diabetic serum. Studies on rabbit aortic medial cell cultures. Diabetes 1976; 26: 798–803.

77. Bettmann MA, Stemerman MB, Ransil BJ. The effect of hypophysectomy on experimental endothelial cell regrowth and intimal thickening in the rat. Circ Res 1981; 48: 907–12.

78. Ledet T, Vuust J. Arterial procollagen type I, type III, and fibronectin. Effects of diabetic serum, glucose, insulin, ketone, and growth hormone studied on rabbit aortic myomedial cell cultures. Diabetes 1980; 29: 964–70.

79. Heickendorff L, Ledet T. Arterial basement membrane-like material isolated and characterised from rabbit aortic myomedial cell-cultures. Biochem J 1983; 211: 397–404.

80. Heickendorff L, Ledet T. The carbohydrate components of arterial basement membrane-like material. Studies on rabbit aortic myomedial cell in culture. Biochem J 1983; 211: 735–41.

81. Rasmussen LM, Ledet T. Serum from diabetic patients enhances synthesis of arterial basement membrane-like material in cultured smooth muscle cells. Acta Path Microbiol Scand 1988; 96: 77–83.

82. Ledet T, Heickendorff L. Insulin, ketones, glucose and glucagon: effects on the arterial basement membrane in vitro. Acta Endocrinol (Copenh) 1987; 115: 139–43.

83. Ledet T, Heickendorff L. Growth hormone effect on accumulation of arterial basement membrane-like material studied on rabbit aortic myomedial cell cultures. Diabetologia 1985; 28: 922–7.

84. Oxlund H, Rasmussen LM, Andreassen TT, Heickendorff L. Increased aortic stiffness in patients with type 1 (insulin-dependent) diabetes mellitus. Diabetologia 1989; 32: 748–52.

62

Clotting Disorders in Diabetes

Donald E. McMillan

University of South Florida, Tampa, Florida, USA

The blood of vertebrates has sufficient properties in common for a number of useful general conclusions to be reached. Almost without exception, it contains cells that are equipped to carry oxygen to tissues and organs. Without exception it is able, when removed from its native environment, to turn from a fluid into a solid in a few minutes. As vertebrates have become larger, warmer and more active, the proportion of oxygen-bearing cells has risen and the cells have developed more efficient shapes and higher blood concentrations [1]. Coagulation, blood's property of changing from fluid to solid, has also become more complex, although its essential elements, coagulation-promoting cells [2] and fibrinogen [3], are present in all vertebrates. The coagulation-promoting cells, like the red blood cells, lose their cell nuclei and become much smaller as the evolutionary ladder is mounted, but always act on dissolved proteins to promote fibrinogen's ability to polymerize.

The coagulation process is a balance between groups of reactions, dominant most of the time, that keep the blood from coagulating, and an array of reactions that favor its coagulation when called into activity [4]. Coagulation may be necessitated by a small cut or venepuncture, or by a massive injury or extensive surgery. The process of response and balance between the two systems is affected by the extent of loss of vascular integrity.

PLASMA FIBRINOGEN

Our analysis starts with the plasma protein whose alteration is the final common denominator of the clotting process. Fibrinogen is a strikingly oblong, high molecular weight protein that is quite soluble in its native form [4]; however, when it is exposed to the enzymatic action of thrombin, it loses two areas that keep it from self-associating and comes out of solution, carrying platelets and erythrocytes with it.

Level and Turnover in Diabetes

The plasma level of fibrinogen is increased by the presence of diabetes [5–16]. Its inter-individual coefficient of variation is 18–20% and the average increase in diabetes is 22–30% (60–70 mg/dl), so that not all diabetics have an elevated fibrinogen level. The basis for the fibrinogen elevation has been investigated: not surprisingly, an increase in fibrinogen synthesis has been found, but a less anticipated finding is an *increased* rate of clearance of fibrinogen and

International Textbook of Diabetes Mellitus. Edited by K.G.M.M. Alberti, R.A. DeFronzo, H. Keen and P. Zimmet

shortening of its associated circulation half-life. Fibrinogen is produced by the hepatic parenchymal cells and has a half-life in the circulation of 2–4 days [17]. This contrasts with albumin, the major plasma protein produced by the liver, which has a half-life of 10–12 days [18]. The increased clearance rate means that synthesis is actually higher than suggested by the plasma level elevation. Two modifications in its metabolism are responsible: its synthesis is increased [19–21], as is the synthesis of its fellow acute phase reactants. The major acute phase protein, in both quantity and biologic role, is fibrinogen. It is present in plasma but not in serum, because it is consumed in the process of clot formation. Acute phase plasma protein synthesis rises in response to a wide variety of diseases and injuries [22] and is therefore not at all specific to diabetes. It has actually been reported that hyperglycemia can lower the fibrinogen level by accelerating plasma fibrinogen disappearance [21], but glucose intolerance without fasting hyperglycemia [13] is sufficient to raise fibrinogen levels.

Control of Acute Phase Protein Synthesis

Animal studies suggest that albumin is synthesized principally after meals whereas the acute phase proteins are made between meals. Glucose intolerance is associated with a disturbance of the glucagon/insulin ratio [23]. This changed hormonal influence on the liver can alter its pattern of protein synthesis [24–27]. The hormonal disturbance of diabetes favors interprandial over postprandial synthesis. Therefore in diabetes and conditions with altered protein intake or nitrogen balance, acute-phase proteins are high and plasma albumin is low.

Molecular Properties of Fibrinogen

Fibrinogen also differs from albumin in size: its molecular weight is 340 000 [4] whereas that of albumin is 65 000 [28]. Most importantly, fibrinogen, which is destined for use in forming a coagulum network, has a molecular structure that is much longer than it is wide; its hydrodynamic axial ratio is 20:1 [28], whereas albumin, an oncotic and carrier protein, has an axial ratio of 4.4:1 [28].

The difference in shape between fibrinogen and albumin affects two blood flow properties: it makes the plasma viscosity higher because fibrinogen, tumbling during flow, dissipates six times as much flow energy as albumin [28]; fibrinogen [29] and other very elongated macromolecules (e.g. dextran [30, 31] and polyvinylpyrrolidone [31]) increase the attraction between erythrocytes, causing them to aggregate, whereas albumin actually tends to reduce the tendency for erythrocytes to aggregate. The tendency for red cells to aggregate can be seen as very useful during the process of clotting. Aggregated red blood cells form a major part of the early clot. They are lost by being squeezed out as the fibrin network shrinks slowly under the influence of factor XIII [4] (see clot retraction, below). Not all erythrocytes are lost from the clot during its contraction; its dark red color is produced by those that remain.

Role of Fibrinogen in Blood Coagulation

Fibrinogen is designed to be irreversibly altered by the enzymatic action of thrombin [4]. Thrombin acts on two pairs of the three paired chains that form fibrinogen, to remove small segments that block its tendency to self-associate. The action of thrombin is not simultaneous on all four sites of each fibrinogen molecule, so that several intermediates are produced. The nonpolymerized intermediates can be measured together to estimate thrombin activity in the blood stream. Such a measurement results in a value often referred to as a fibrin degradation or split product level. However, the major products released by thrombin's enzymatic action are fibrinopeptide A from the two α chains and fibrinopeptide B from the two β chains [4]. Removal of one or both fibrinopeptide A chains allows a molecularly staggered (overlapping monomeric units) polymerization to begin, whereas loss of the fibrinopeptide B chains markedly reduces the negative charge that interferes with continuing polymerization.

The level of fibrinopeptide A has been studied in diabetes and tends to be elevated, especially when control is poor or vascular problems exist [32]. Its rise in the blood stream when hyperglycemia is induced is blocked by heparin, suggesting that thrombin generation is responsible [33]. This type of assay tends to be high in diabetes when advanced atherosclerosis is also present. Fibrinopeptide A level is also high in non-diabetics with advanced, clinically active

Table 1 Fibrinogen as a cardiovascular risk factor

Geographic area		Report year	Number of cases	Male/female	Study duration (yrs)	Number of events	Fibrinogen difference*	Conclusions v cholesterol/smoking
Framingham, US	[36]	1987	1499	662/837	14	369[1]	< 0.001 m 0.07 f	Fibr > smoking
Gothenburg, Sweden	[37]	1984	792	all m	14	189[1]	< 0.01	Fibr = cholest.
Gothenburg, Sweden	[38]	1987	789	all m	17	57[2]	< 0.01	Fibr > cholest.
Northwick Park, UK	[39]	1980	1510	all m	2–8	49[3]	< 0.01	Fibr > cholest.
Northwick Park, UK	[40]	1985	1274	all m	7–13	74[3]	< 0.01	Fibr > low class
Northwick Park, UK	[41]	1986	1511	all m	8–14	109[3]	0.02	Fibr > cholest.
Leigh, UK	[42]	1985	297	all m	7	40[1]	< 0.001	Fibr > cholest.
Cardiff, UK	[88]	1991	4860	all m	4	251[4]	< 0.001	Fibr., pl. visc. > chol.

[1]MI + stroke + deaths; [2]stroke only; [3]all deaths only; [4]all IHD.
*Comparison is of fibrinogen level in cardiovascular v. non-cardiovascular events.

atherosclerosis [34] and in death associated with intravascular thrombosis [35].

Fibrinogen Level and Artery Disease in Non-diabetics

Fibrinogen level measurement has been introduced into epidemiologic studies in recent years. English, Scandinavian and American groups (Table 1) interested in heart disease have found it to be an independent risk factor for coronary heart disease and stroke in the general population [36–42]. It is at least as effective as serum cholesterol in predicting future vascular events. In these studies fibrinogen level has been found to be higher in smokers. This latter observation can generate confusion. Fibrinogen is a predictor of future vascular events in non-smokers, but smoking is a poor predictor of future vascular events in normofibrinogenemic individuals. Cigarette smoking appears to stimulate a rise in fibrinogen level and cessation of smoking is associated with a slow fall in fibrinogen approaching 15 mg/dl [43]. Heredity plays a major part in determining an individual's fibrinogen level [44]. In many, but not all, of the cited studies, fibrinogen and cholesterol levels were nearly independent of each other. The collective observations suggest that some property of fibrinogen or its production is important in causing atherosclerosis or provoking occlusive thrombotic events. Continuing analysis and extension to other parameters in epidemiological studies should allow this important distinction to be made.

OTHER PLASMA COMPONENTS

Generation of Thrombin

Thrombin is generated from prothrombin by one of two procoagulant systems: the intrinsic system exists in the vascular space and the extrinsic system starts its procoagulant action in the extravascular space [4]. The result in either case is the enzymatic conversion of inactive prothrombin to fibrinogen-activating thrombin.

Uncontrolled intravascular or tissue blood coagulation is very undesirable and an impressive and complex array of procoagulant and anticoagulant protein molecules and reactions controlling thrombin and its formation have been identified. The discovery of this complex balancing system that controls the coagulation process has so far generated little information about diabetes or atherosclerosis. In two cardiovascular risk factor studies, procoagulant proteins other than fibrinogen were studied in an effort to examine whether the coagulation process was more widely involved. The levels of procoagulant proteins, factors VIIc and VIIIc, were higher in subjects with cardiovascular events in one study [39], whereas no difference in factor II–VII–X interaction (P & P method) or VIIIc could be found in the other, no matter what end-point was attempted [38]. The elevated factor VIIc level was found to be correlated with obesity and to rise following cessation of cigarette smoking by the group reporting its association with atherosclerosis [43]. Both factor VII and factor VIII levels have been reported to be elevated in diabetes [5, 12, 32].

Control of Thrombin Generation

In addition to the procoagulant intrinsic and extrinsic systems, an extensive number of similarly effective anticoagulants have been identified. Diabetes produces a large number of biochemical and metabolic changes. It should therefore come as no surprise that some unusual effects might be found in the procoagulation versus anticoagulation system when diabetes is present. Two examples linked to clotting prevention show the subtlety of interactions that can occur.

Dicoumarol was discovered more than 40 years ago after sweet clover was observed to cause bleeding in cattle. Its congeners now have a major role in chronic anticoagulant management. Their mechanism of action is competition with the quinone vitamin K, a cofactor in the formation of a unique carbon–carbon bond α to the γ carbon of glutamate in prothrombin, factor V, factor VII and factor IX [4]. The presence of this posttranslational modification, γ-carboxyglutamic acid, is necessary for the enzymatic actions of these procoagulants. Multiple sites are present in one area of each protein which bond with calcium ions to allow protein–protein non-covalent bonds to form and enzymatic action to take place. Without the γ-carboxyglutamic acid modification, the enzymatic activity necessary for coagulation does not occur. The coumarin anticoagulants act by blocking γ-carboxyglutamic acid formation.

Several years ago the development of paradoxic thrombosis in an individual receiving coumarin led to the discovery that an anticoagulant, protein C, shares this modification [4]. Protein C controls the activation of prothrombin by destroying activated factors V and VIII. The level of this anticoagulant protein has been measured in diabetes and found to be low [45]. As interference with γ-carboxyglutamate formation would also depress the levels of chemically similar procoagulant proteins, this finding supports the previously introduced concept that diabetes is a hypercoagulable state (see below).

Another anticoagulant protein affected in an unusual way by diabetes is antithrombin III [4]. This protein binds heparin non-covalently as a necessary feature of its irreversible binding reaction which inactivates thrombin. When antithrombin III is measured as a blood protein by an immunologic technique, it is found to be elevated in diabetes [46, 47]; however, when it is measured using its biologic activity it is found to be low [48]. The reason is linked to the effect of diabetes on heparin bioavailability. Heparin is also a cofactor in the perivascular–adipose tissue action of lipoprotein lipase. This reaction releases fatty acids from chylomicrons and very low-density lipoprotein molecules. Its activity is depressed in diabetes [48], apparently owing to reduced availability of heparin. The reduced activity of the supernormal antithrombin level may be a circulatory associate of tissue resistance to lipoprotein and chylomicron degradation. One possible explanation is that increased glycation of heparin binding sites blocks its interaction with its protein cofactor [49]. A similar interference has been proposed for a slowing in vitro of the action of plasmin on fibrin clots in diabetes [50]. Some caution in proposing that increased glycation is responsible for diabetic pathophysiologic aberrations is suggested by the level of glycation of fibrinogen, a plasma protein with a short half-life in diabetes (see above). Fibrinogen in diabetes has a degree of glycation only slightly different ($1.33 \, \text{mol/mol}$ versus $0.95 \, \text{mol/mol}$) from that of fibrinogen from non-diabetic subjects when it is purified and studied directly [51].

Fibrin Dissolution by Plasmin

The balance of procoagulants and anticoagulants continues after a vascular clot has formed. The trapped platelets release factors that favor proliferation of the clot while the circulation supplies anticoagulant proteins to keep it from spreading. The blood stream supplies an additional protein, plasmin, that is capable of releasing the carboxyl end of the fibrin (and fibrinogen) α chains, solubilizing the fibrin that formed the clot [4]. Plasmin is formed by enzymatic activation from the circulating protein, plasminogen. Either administered plasminogen activators, such as streptokinase, or an endothelially derived plasminogen activator act to split an arginine–valine bond to allow the plasminogen to alter its shape and become enzymatically active. Once activated, plasmin attacks both fibrinogen and fibrin, solubilizing the latter.

Plasminogen activator differs from the proteins that have already been discussed, in being formed by endothelial cells rather than by liver parenchymal cells. An early physiologic observation was the generation of clot-dissolving activity in local blood when a tourniquet is applied to a limb to stop the local circulation; this happens because endothelial plasminogen activator release is linked to this process. In many diabetic patients, limb flow stagnation-mediated release is impaired [52]. The impairment is not simply a result of poor diabetic control: the endothelium appears to have reduced plasminogen activator production in diabetes (see below). There is also evidence that obesity affects the control of blood levels of plasminogen activator by enhancing tissue release of an inhibitor of its activity [53]. Either reduced plasminogen activator release or increased plasminogen activator inhibitor release results in reduced effectiveness of the physiologic clot-dissolution system in diabetes.

von Willebrand Factor (vWF) in Diabetes

Another protein related to the coagulation system that is produced by the endothelium is the antihemophilic globulin component called either von Willebrand factor (vWF) or ristocetin cofactor [4]; the latter name is related to its measurement by platelet aggregation mediated by the antibiotic ristocetin. This factor also plays a part in platelet attachment to the subendothelium when endothelial cells are removed: it appears that endothelial cell production of plasminogen activator is impaired in diabetes whereas the production of vWF is increased [52–56]; the diabetic endothelium may be producing more of one protein and less of another. This is also true of the liver, where more fibrinogen and less albumin are produced, but in the case of the endothelial cells we have no sense yet of how such protein synthesis is controlled. There is other evidence of altered endothelial cell function in diabetes (see section on endothelial cells, below).

Protein Glycation and Clot Retraction in Diabetes

The β-chain amino-terminal valine is glycated in hemoglobin A_{1c}, but the more frequent chemical reaction is between glucose and lysine groups. In hemoglobin, the valine is so weakly basic that its positive charge is lost following glycation, thus affecting the physical properties of the hemoglobin molecule. There is normally so little reduction in basicity of lysine following glycation that protein charge is almost unaffected, but glycation causes a primary amine to become a secondary amine next to a double carbon bond, altering local chemical activity.

Proteins, including those in blood, when exposed to a supranormal glucose level undergo increased glycation in diabetes; alterations in behavior can occur, therefore, when lysine is glycated. Factor XIII, the clot retraction mediator, acts on fibrin to produce fibrin network contraction by crosslinking glutamine and lysine, especially near the C-terminal end of the α chain. Although potentially susceptible, the reaction is not known to be affected by the presence of diabetes.

A parallel reaction is thought to be responsible for erythrocyte removal when the red cells become too calcium-permeable. The same transglutamidase, known in the blood as factor XIII, is present on the red cell membrane inner surface and acts, when calcium is available, to crosslink the spectrin network present there to reduce the red cell's ability to stretch, allowing it to be phagocytized by macrophages. Preliminary evidence that the proportion of red cells that stretched poorly was high in diabetes [57] was combined with evidence that spectrin was even more vigorously glycated than hemoglobin to support interference by glycation [58]. This seemed particularly reasonable because of the 120-day circulatory lifetime of the erythrocyte (compare with the low degree of glycation of fibrinogen; see thrombin generation, above), but the completed red cell study failed to find any erythrocyte-stretching impairment in diabetes [59].

EXTRAVASCULAR EFFECTS OF HYPERGLYCEMIA

Collagen and Its Glycation in Diabetes

Collagen in extravascular areas activates platelet-mediated coagulation. The collagen group of connective tissue proteins also contains lysine and large amounts of another ketoamine acceptor, hydroxylysine. The lysine and hydroxylysine groups have a role in a number of posttranslational reactions that are responsible for the effectiveness of collagen as a connective tissue protein. Hydroxylysine is the site of enzymatically mediated transglycation: firstly galactose is added to the hydroxyl group on the carbon adjacent to the terminal amine, and then glucose is added to the galactose. This biochemical modification is very prominent in type IV collagen.

The amine groups of some of the lysines and hydroxylysines of the peptide chain take part in a reaction in which molecular oxygen, ferric iron and vitamin C have a role. The resulting aldehyde reacts with remaining amine groups to link chains of collagen together with covalent bonds. Transglycation of the sugars to hydroxylysine takes place after protein synthesis in fibroblasts and smooth muscle cells, and the oxidation of amine to aldehyde groups shortly afterward, but the crosslinking reaction is delayed until the time of extracellular collagen chain assembly. An interfering role for hyperglycemia has not yet been fully elucidated.

Extracellular collagen is a stimulator of platelet adhesion, aggregation and release reactions. Its modification by non-enzymatic attachment of glucose to lysines present in proteins could alter this relation. Collagen from diabetic patients has been found to have increased attachment of glucose and to be less soluble than non-diabetic collagen [60]. A small proportion of collagen can return to solution when connective tissue is finely divided; the fraction falls both with the age of the tissue and the age of the individual. The slow development of aldehyde–amine crosslinking accounts for some of the change. An even slower formation of interchain linkages by late modification of two keto-amine sites on adjacent peptide chains into an imidazole-containing chemical bridge [61] could play a part in the aging and diabetic processes.

There is little evidence yet how cell behavior is altered by the presence of excess intracellular glucose. The cataract model in hyperglycemia and hypergalactosemia suggests that broad interference with sulfur-mediated reduction reactions might be contributing to the desolubilization of lens protein.

CELLS AND COAGULATION IN DIABETES

Effects of Diabetes on Blood Platelets

Blood platelets are affected by the diabetic state. Interest in their potential role in the production of atherosclerosis by local release of a smooth muscle cell migration-promoting factor called platelet-derived growth factor has led to intensive studies in the last decade of platelet behavior in diabetes. An abnormality of platelet metabolism unique to diabetes has been documented and a pattern of interactions identified.

When platelet-rich plasma is exposed to an aggregation-promoting agent, the platelets coalesce, allowing more light to pass through the suspension. The change in light conductance has been used to measure degree of aggregation of blood platelets in disease. Platelet aggregation should be distinguished from two other platelet measurements—platelet adhesion and spontaneous platelet aggregation. The former is of direct physiologic consequence, as platelets are responsible for closing the hole in the antecubital vein produced when blood is drawn. The attachment of platelets to glass or another foreign surface is used to test this capacity, which has been found to be elevated in diabetes [5]. Spontaneous platelet aggregation in the circulation can be observed by indirect means and tends to be increased in poorly controlled type 1 in diabetics receiving insulin in management [62]. Either increased fatty acid levels or insulin–antibody complexes could be responsible.

Events in Platelet Aggregation

The aggregation reaction measures the predilection of platelets to adhere to each other. This process is promoted by substances that include epinephrine, collagen and adenosine diphosphate (ADP). Exposure to collagen at denuded vessel surfaces and the stress-related elevation of epinephrine are fairly obvious; the release by diabetic red blood cells of ADP is less obvious but has been reported to occur (see below). Normally, aggregation begins in such a way that mixing will restore the solution opacity to light if performed early enough but not after the reaction is well under way. Progression was thought to be due to a platelet shape change associated with the development of cytoplasmic projections, referred to as pseudopod formation, even though it has little resemblance to the process described by the same name in leukocytes. However, it has recently been shown that platelet aggregation will proceed to an irreversible state even when pseudopod formation is prevented by addition of a cationic amphophile such as chlorpromazine.

Blood β-Thromboglobulin

During its activation and aggregation, the platelet releases into its environment a number of substances that tend to favor blood coagulation. One of these, β-thromboglobulin, has been used to assess the spontaneous intravascular activation of platelets in diabetes.

Beta-thromboglobulin levels increase in the same situations that raise platelet aggregation —diabetes, aging and advanced atherosclerosis [32, 63, 64]. The major virtue of β-thromboglobulin measurement is its ease and reliability. The implication of a more procoagulant state with higher β-thromboglobulin levels is apparent.

Altered Platelet Size in Diabetes

A few reports of increased platelet size in diabetes should be mentioned because of the problems in data interpretation that they signal [65]. Platelets normally survive 9 days in the circulation, but this time is often shortened in diabetes [19]. The platelets gain density and lose volume during their circulating life just as erythrocytes do. It has been shown that young, large platelets are more metabolically active and more easily aggregated than old platelets. It is not known how early removal is accomplished in diabetes, but it seems likely that some of the changes described below could be attributable to the younger age of diabetic platelets.

Arachidonate Metabolism in Diabetic Platelets

One of the most intriguing aspects of platelet behavior in diabetes is the altered arachidonic acid metabolism found to be present except under ideal control [66]. The diabetic platelet stores at least normal amounts of arachidonate as membrane phospholipid glyceryl-2-arachidonate. The arachidonate is made available for chemical modification by being released by phospholipase A_2. Its turnover is high because diabetic platelets synthesize supranormal amounts of thromboxane [66–68], a substance that favors platelet aggregation [68]. Thromboxane may be added to increased vWF and fibrinogen blood levels on the list of factors present in diabetes that increase platelet aggregation. The diabetic platelets are already more capable of binding thromboxane [69] than normal platelets and they also interact more

with fibrinogen [70] and less with prostacyclin [71, 72] than normal platelets. A report of elevated calmodulin in diabetic platelets has not yet been integrated into this complicated picture [73].

Clotting and Endothelial Cells

Endothelial cell production of prostacyclin is impaired in diabetes, interfering with the resistance of each blood vessel to platelet adhesion [74]. In vitro, the exposure of cultured endothelial cells to high or medium glucose levels has been shown to affect even their DNA metabolism [75]. Cultured endothelial cells have also been shown to produce platelet-derived growth factor [76].

The endothelium is the barrier interfering with passage of plasma components into the extravascular space. Its cells have been cultured in vitro and studied, leading to a number of findings of interest. Most endothelial cells in the arterial system are elongated, with their long axis parallel to local blood flow. The cells in these areas show flattening of their cell nuclei as well, suggesting that they have adjusted to local flow. The responsiveness of endothelial cells to flow has been documented by experiments in vivo and in vitro. When a square segment of dog thoracic aorta was removed, turned at right angles to its original position and sewn back into the aortic wall, 2 weeks later all the cells had changed their direction of elongation to correspond to the flow pattern [77]. Endothelial cells in culture respond to the presence of stable overlying flow. A steady shear force of as little as 0.8 Pa is enough to force cultured endothelial cells to align with the flow pattern [78]. Intermittent or fluctuating force levels of the same magnitude do not produce cell alignment.

Erythrocytes and Blood Coagulation

Erythrocytes have a role in the coagulation process that has been identified already in this chapter. When the erythrocyte membrane is compromised and its contents released, its ADP acts to enhance platelet aggregation. Reduced erythrocyte deformability in diabetes has been proposed to cause increased platelet aggregation by this mechanism [79], although not all have found these erythrocyte changes [59].

CLINICAL CONSIDERATIONS

Diabetes as a Hypercoagulable State

Although diabetes can be considered to be a hypercoagulable state because of high blood fibrinogen and other procoagulant levels, increased platelet aggregation and impaired vascular resistance to coagulation, clinical case reports [80] are infrequent, and statistics on the frequency of clinically serious spontaneous intravascular coagulation in diabetes do not support this theory [81, 82]. Isolated cases do exist, but could easily represent the combination of established diabetes and unrecognized coagulation predisposition or toxin-producing infection.

As a number of therapeutic alternatives are available, the concept of a hypercoagulable state deserves careful appraisal. As stated above, factors identified as favorable to coagulation are known to be increased in diabetes and several factors controlling coagulation are reduced; however, the anticipated clinical consequence, disseminated intravascular coagulation, is uncommon. Parts of the system controlling the coagulation process are compromised but the overall system still seems to have the means to adjust and function normally. If some additional hereditary problem, such as the one that led to the discovery of protein C, is present, we may learn enough from studying future cases to recognize such diabetes-associated problems before they cause difficulty.

Diagnostic Implications in Diabetes

Some consideration should be given in diabetes management to the evaluation of the diabetic clotting state. At this time the most reasonable addition to our current periodic testing should be measurement of plasma fibrinogen level. The data supporting its value in predicting the development of cardiovascular problems in non-diabetics are impressive, and a longer-standing linkage between plasma fibrinogen and microvascular disease [7–11, 13–14] and an unfavorable prognosis [8] in diabetes already exists as well. Other measurements of the coagulation process do not appear to be justified simply by the presence of the diabetic state.

Current and Future Therapeutic Considerations

Measurement of plasma fibrinogen at least once during the course of diabetes implies that, if it is elevated, a plan likely to be beneficial should be made available to the patient concerned. Improved blood glucose control is obviously of value and its justification will be enhanced by the test, but some other possibilities should be considered as well. Probably one of the least risky is the administration of aspirin. Platelet thromboxane formation requires an attack on a carbon double bond by molecular oxygen mediated by the enzyme cyclooxygenase. This enzyme's activity is permanently disrupted by the transfer of the acetyl group from aspirin or another donor molecule: therefore, daily aspirin can control the biochemical abnormality of diabetic platelets. However, an effort to exploit this benefit in diabetic leg disease was unsuccessful, except in marginally reducing cerebrovascular events in stroke and symptomatic transient ischemia [83].

A similar cyclooxygenase pathway exists in endothelial cells, and acetylation also interferes with the favorable formation of prostacyclin, but reportedly at a somewhat higher blood level. For that reason it has been proposed that very modest doses of aspirin be used to alter platelet behavior without affecting endothelial cells. Another agent, ticlopidine, has been reported to interfere with the platelet reaction to ADP [84].

Lowering the plasma fibrinogen level would be a more direct approach. Several agents have been reported to lower fibrinogen; unfortunately, other effects that some of these agents (phenformin, clofibrate) have produced have led to their withdrawal from prescription availability. For several other drugs the evidence is insufficient. Studies failed to eliminate altered diabetic control as the basis for declining fibrinogen levels [21]. Despite these problems, there is a clear need for a safe agent that will lower fibrinogen levels by 20–40%. Agents with this potential have been developed in Europe [85, 86].

Fibrinogen can exert an adverse effect in diabetes, either through its known enhancement of coagulation rate or through its predilection to aggregate red blood cells. This is an important distinction in treatment because several agents have been reported to reduce red cell aggregation. Aspirin and other anionic amphophiles appear capable of enhancing erythrocyte charge, reducing aggregation propensity at the same time [87]. If red cell aggregation proves to be an important factor in the adverse role of fibrinogen, large but safe doses of such compounds may be helpful.

REFERENCES

1. Altman PL, Dittmer DS. Biology Data Book, vol. III, 2nd edn. Bethesda, Md: Federation of American Societies for Experimental Biology, 1974: pp 1849–53.
2. Maupin B: Blood platelets in man and animals, vol. 1. Oxford: Pergamon Press, 1969: pp 472–520.
3. Doolittle RF. The structure and evolution of vertebrate fibrinogen. Ann NY, Acad Sci 1983; 408: 13–27.
4. Bloom AL, Thomas DP. Hemostasis and thrombosis. Edinburgh: Churchill Livingstone, 1981.
5. Mayne EE, Bridges JM, Weaver JA. Platelet adhesiveness, plasma fibrinogen and factor VIII levels in diabetes mellitus. Diabetologia 1970; 6: 436.
6. Hart A, Cohen H, Thorp JM. Lipoprotein and fibrinogen studies in diabetes. Postgrad Med J 1971; 47: 435–9.
7. Van Haeringen NJ, Oosterhuis JA, Terpstra J, Glasius E. Erythrocyte aggregation in relation to diabetic retinopathy. Diabetologia 1973; 9: 20–4.
8. Jonsson A, Wales JK. Blood glycoprotein levels in diabetes mellitus. Diabetologia 1976; 12: 245–50.
9. Akazawa Y, Koide M, Yamadori E. Correlation between plasma fibrinogen level and vascular complications in diabetes mellitus. In Baba S, Goto Y, Fukui I (eds) Diabetes mellitus in Asia. Amsterdam: Excerpta Medica, 1976: pp 189–95.
10. De Silva SR, Shawe JEH, Patel H, Cudworth AG. Plasma fibrinogen in diabetes mellitus. Diabète Métab 1979; 5: 201–5.
11. Lowe GDO, Lowe JM, Drummond MM, et al. Blood viscosity in young male diabetics with and without retinopathy. Diabetologia 1980; 18: 359–63.
12. Tsianos EB, Stathakis NE. Soluble fibrin complexes and fibrinogen heterogeneity in diabetes mellitus. Thromb Haemost 1980; 44: 130–4.
13. McMillan DE. Physical Factors important in the development of atherosclerosis in diabetes. Diabetes 1981; 30: 97–104.
14. Cederholm-Williams SA, Dornan TL, Turner RC. The metabolism of fibrinogen and plasminogen related to diabetic retinopathy in man. Eur J Clin Invest 1981; 11: 133–8.
15. Sharma SC. Platelet adhesiveness, plasma fibrinogen and fibrinolytic activity in juvenile-onset and maturity-onset diabetes mellitus. J Clin Pathol 1981; 34: 501–3.
16. Van Oost BA, Veldhuyzen BFE, Van Houwelingen HC, Timmermans APM, Sixma JJ. Tests for

platelet changes, acute phase reactants, and serum lipids in diabetes mellitus and peripheral vascular disease. Thromb Haemost 1982; 48: 289–93.
17. McFarlane AS, Todd D, Cromwell S. Fibrinogen catabolism in humans. Clin Sci 1964; 26: 415–20.
18. Rothschild MA, Oratz M, Schreiber SS. Albumin synthesis. New Engl J Med 1972; 286: 748–57, 816–21.
19. Ferguson JC, MacKay N, Philip JAD, Sumner DJ. Determination of platelet and fibrinogen half-life with selenomethionine studies in normal and diabetic subjects. Clin Sci Molec Med 1975; 49: 115–20.
20. Bent-Hansen L, Deckert T. Metabolism of albumin and fibrinogen in type 1 insulin dependent diabetes mellitus. Diabetes Res 1988; 7: 159–64.
21. Jones RL, Jovanovic L, Forman S, Peterson CM. Time course of reversibility of accelerated fibrinogen disappearance in diabetes mellitus: association with intravascular volume shifts. Blood 1984; 63: 22–30.
22. Gordon AH. The acute phase plasma proteins. In Bianchi R, Mariani G, Mcfarlane AS (eds) Plasma protein turnover. Baltimore: Univ. Park Press, 1976: pp 381–94.
23. Unger RH. The milieu interieur and the islets of Langerhans. Diabetologia 1981; 20: 1–11.
24. Jeejeebhoy KN, Bruce-Robertson A, Ho J, Sodtke U. The comparative effects of nutritional and hormonal factors on the synthesis of albumin, fibrinogen and transferrin. Clin Symp 1973; 9: 217–47.
25. Miller LL, Griffin EE. Regulation of net biosynthesis of albumin, fibrinogen, alpha-1-acid glycoprotein, alpha-2- (acute phase) globulin and haptoglobin by direct action of hormones on the isolated perfused liver. In Litwack G (ed.) Biochemical actions of hormones. New York: Academic Press, 1975: pp 159–86.
26. Peavy DE, Taylor JM, Jefferson LS. Correlation of albumin production rates and albumin mRNA levels in livers of normal, diabetic and insulin treated diabetic rats. Proc Natl Acad Sci USA 1978; 75: 5879–83.
27. Koj A, Dubin A. On the hormonal modulation of acute-phase plasma protein synthesis in perfused rat liver. Acta Biochim Polon 1974; 21: 159–67.
28. Tanford C. Physical chemistry of macromolecules. New York: John Wiley, 1961: pp 394–6.
29. Rampling M, Sirs JA. The interactions of fibrinogen and dextrans with erythrocytes. J Physiol 1972; 223: 199–211.
30. Knox RJ, Nordt FJ, Seaman GV, Brooks DE. Rheology of erythrocyte suspensions: dextran-mediated aggregation of deformable and nondeformable erythrocytes. Biorheology 1977; 14: 75–84.

31. Sewchand LS, Canham PB. Modes of rouleaux formation of human red blood cells in polyvinyl-pyrrolidone and dextran solutions. Can J Physiol Pharmacol 1979; 57: 1213–22.

32. Rosove MH, Frank HJL, Harwig SSL. Plasma beta-thromboglobulin, platelet factor 4, fibrino-peptide A, and other hemostatic functions during improved short-term glycemic control in diabetes mellitus. Diabetes Care 1984; 7: 174–9.

33. Jones RL, Fibrinopeptide-A in diabetes mellitus. Diabetes 1985; 34: 836–43.

34. Serneri GGN, Gensini GF, Carnovali M, et al. Association between time of increased fibrino-peptide A levels in plasma and episodes of spontaneous angina: a controlled prospective study. Am Heart J 1987; 113: 672–8.

35. Meade TW, Howarth DJ, Stirling Y. Fibrinopeptide A and sudden coronary death. Lancet 1984; ii: 607–9.

36. Kannel WB, D'Agostino RB, Belanger AJ. Fibrinogen, cigarette smoking and risk of cardiovascular disease: insights from the Framingham Study. Am Heart J 1987; 113: 1006–10.

37. Wilhelmsen L, Svardsudd K, Korsan-Bengsten K, Larsson B, Welin L, Tibblin G. Fibrinogen as a risk factor for stroke and myocardial infarction. New Engl J Med 1984; 311: 501–5.

38. Welin L, Svardsudd K, Wilhelmsen L, Larsson B, Tibblin G. Analysis of risk factors for stroke in a cohort of men born in 1913. New Engl J Med 1987; 317: 521–6.

39. Meade TW, Chakrabarti R, Haines AP, North WRS, Stirling Y, Thompson SG. Haemostatic function and cardiovascular death: early results of a prospective study. Lancet 1980; i: 1050–4.

40. Markowe HLJ, Marmot MG, Shipley MJ. et al. Fibrinogen: a possible link between social class and coronary heart disease. Br Med J 1985; 291: 1312–14.

41. Meade TW, Mellows S, Brozovic M, et al. Haemostatic function and ischaemic heart disease: principal results of the Northwick Park Heart Study. Lancet 1986; ii: 533–7.

42. Stone MC, Thorp JM. Plasma fibrinogen a major coronary risk factor. J Roy Coll Gen Pract 1985; 35: 565–9.

43. Meade TW, Imeson J, Stirling Y. Effects of changes in smoking and other characteristics on clotting factors and the risk of ischaemic heart disease. Lancet 1987; ii: 986–8.

44. Hamsten A, Iselius L, De Faire U, Blomback M. Genetic and cultural inheritance of plasma fibrinogen concentration. Lancet 1987; ii: 988–90.

45. Vukovich TC, Schernthaner G. Decreased protein C levels in patients with insulin-dependent type I diabetes mellitus. Diabetes 1986; 35: 617–19.

46. Corbella E, Miragliotta G, Masperi R, Villa S, Bini A. Platelet aggregation and antithrombin III levels in diabetic children. Haemostasis 1979; 8: 30–7.

47. Matsuda T. Changes of antithrombin III. Alpha-2 macroglobulin, alpha-1-antitrypsin, C-1-inhibitor and alpha-S-plasmin inhibitor in arteriosclerotic diseases and diabetes mellitus. Rinsho Ketsueki 1978; 19: 947–54.

48. Lithell H, Krotkiewski M, Kiens B et al. Non-response of muscle capillary density and lipoprotein-lipase activity to regular training in diabetic patients. Diabetes Res 1985; 2: 17–21.

49. Brownlee M, Vlassara H, Cerami A. Inhibition of heparin-catalyzed human antithrombin III activity of nonenzymatic glycosylation. Diabetes 1984; 33: 532–5.

50. Brownlee M, Vlassara H, Cerami A. Nonenzymatic glycosylation reduces the susceptibility of fibrin to degradation by plasmin. Diabetes 1983; 32: 680–4.

51. Lutjens A, te Velde AA, van der Veen EA, van der Meer J. Glycosylation of human fibrinogen in vivo. Diabetologia 1985; 28: 87–9.

52. Almer LO, Pandolfi M, Aberg M. The plasminogen activator activity of arteries and veins in diabetes mellitus. Thromb Res 1975; 6: 177–82.

53. Vague P, Juhan-Vague I, Aillaud MF, Badier C, Viard R, Alessi MC, Collen D. Correlation between blood fibrinolytic activity, plasminogen activator inhibitor level, plasma insulin level and relative body weight in normal and obese subjects. Metabolism 1986; 35: 250–3.

54. Bensoussan D, Levy-Toledano S, Passa P, Caen J, Canivet J. Platelet hyperaggregation and increased plasma level of von Willebrand factor in diabetics with retinopathy. Diabetologia 1975; 11: 307–12.

55. Porta M, Peters AM, Cousins SA, Cagliero E, FitzPatrick ML, Kohner EM. A study of platelet-relevant parameters in patients with diabetic microangiopathy. Diabetologia 1983; 25: 21–5.

56. Davis TME, Moore JC, Turner RC. Plasma fibronectin, factor VIII-related antigen, and fibrinogen concentrations and diabetic retinopathy. Diabète Métab 1985; 11: 147–51.

57. Williamson JR, Kilo C, Sutera SP, Gardener RA, Boylan C, Chang KC. Shear induced deformation of red cells: decreased elongation and membrane rotation in diabetes. Horm Metab Res 1981; 11 (suppl.): 103–4.

58. McMillan DE, Brooks SM. Erythrocyte spectrin glucosylation in diabetes. Diabetes 1982; 31 (suppl. 3): 64–9.

59. Williamson JR, Gardner RA, Boylan CW et al. Microrheologic investigation of erythrocyte deformability in diabetes mellitus. Clin Hemorheol 1985; 5: 392.

60. Schnider SL, Kohn RR. Effects of age and diabetes mellitus on the solubility and nonenzymatic glucosylation of human skin collagen. J

Clin Invest 1981; 67: 1630–5.

61. Brownlee M, Vlassara H, Cerami A. Nonenzy-matic glycosylation and the pathogenesis of diabetic complications. Ann Intern Med 1984; 101: 527–37.

62. Davis JW, Hartman CR, Davis RF, Kyner JL, Lewis HD, Phillips PE. Platelet aggregate ratio in diabetes mellitus. Acta Haemat 1982; 67: 222–4.

63. Burrows AW, Chavin SI, Hockaday TDR. Plasma thromboglobulin concentrations in diabetes mellitus. Lancet 1978; i: 235–7.

64. Borsey DQ, Dawes J, Fraser DM, Prowse CV, Elton RA, Clarke BF. Plasma beta-thrombo-globulin in diabetes mellitus. Diabetologia 1980; 18: 353–7.

65. Eriksson U, Ewald U, Tuvemo T. Increased platelet volume in manifest diabetic rats. Uppsala J Med Sci 1983; 88: 17–23.

66. Mayfield RK, Halushka PV, Wohltmann HJ, Lopes-Virella M, Chambers JK, Loadholt CB, Colwell JA. Platelet function during continuous insulin infusion treatment in insulin-dependent diabetic patients. Diabetes 1985; 34: 1127–33.

67. Takahashi R, Morita I, Saito Y, Ito H, Murota S. Increased arachidonic acid incorporation into platelet phospholipids in type 2 (non-insulin-dependent) diabetes. Diabetologia 1984; 26: 134–7.

68. Halushka PV, Mayfield R, Wohltmann HJ et al. Increased platelet arachidonic acid metabolism in diabetes mellitus. Diabetes 1981; 30: 44–8.

69. Collier A, Tymkewycz P, Armstrong R, Young RJ, Jones RL, Clarke BF. Increased platelet thromboxane receptor sensitivity in diabetic patients with proliferative retinopathy. Diabetologia 1986; 29: 471–4.

70. DiMinno G, Silver MJ, Cerbone AM, Riccardi G, Rivellese A, Mancini M. Platelet fibrinogen binding in diabetes mellitus differences between binding to platelets from nonretinopathic and retinopathic diabetic patients. Diabetes 1986; 35: 182–5.

71. Betteridge DJ, El Tahir KEH, Reckless JPD, Williams KI. Platelets from diabetic subjects show diminished sensitivity to prostacyclin. Eur J Clin Invest 1982; 12: 395–8.

72. Akai T, Naka K, Akuda K, Takemura T, Fujii S. Decreased sensitivity of platelets to prostacyclin in patients with diabetes mellitus. Horm Metab Res 1983; 15: 523–6.

73. Paolisso G, Tirelli A, Coppola L, Verrazza L, Sgambato S, D'Onofrio F: Platelet calmodulin content in diabetic subjects and its relationship with diabetes-induced hyperaggregability. Diabetes Care 1986; 9: 549–50.

74. Johnson M, Harrison HE, Raftery AT, Elder JB. Vascular prostacyclin may be reduced in diabetes in man. Lancet 1979; i: 325–6.

75. Lorenzi M. Glucose toxicity for human endo-thelial cells in culture. Diabetes 1985; 34: 621–7.

76. Ross R. The pathogenesis of atherosclerosis—an update. New Engl J Med 1986; 314: 488–500.

77. Flaherty JT, Pierce JE, Ferrans VJ, Patel DJ, Tucker WK, Fry DL. Endothelial nuclear pat-terns in the canine arterial tree with particular reference to hemodynamic events. Circ Res 1972; 30: 23–33.

78. Dewey CF, Gimbrone MA, Bussolari SR, White GE, Davies PF. Response of vascular endo-thelium to unsteady fluid shear stress in vitro. Fluid dynamics as a localizing factor for athero-sclerosis. Schettler G (ed.) Berlin: Springer, 1983: pp 182–7.

79. Juhan I, Buonocore M, Jouve R, Vague P, Moulin JP, Vialettes B. Abnormalities of erythro-cyte deformability and platelet aggregation in insulin-dependent diabetics corrected by insulin in vivo and in vitro. Lancet 1982; i: 535–7.

80. Kwaan HC, Colwell JA, Suwanwela N. Dissemi-nated intravascular coagulation in diabetes mel-litus with reference to the role of increased plate-let aggregation. Diabetes 1972; 21: 108–13.

81. Jones EW, Mitchell JRA. Venous thrombosis in diabetes mellitus. Diabetologia 1983; 25: 502–5.

82. Kazmier FJ, Bowie EJW, O'Fallon WM, Zimmerman BR, Osmundson PJ, Palumbo PJ. A prospective study of peripheral occlusive arterial disease in diabetes. IV. Platelet and plasma func-tions. Mayo Clin Proc 1981; 56: 243–53.

83. Colwell JA, Bingham SF, Abraira C et al. Veterans Administration Cooperative study on antiplatelet agents in diabetic patients after amputation for gangrene. II. Effects of aspirin and dipyridamole on atherosclerotic vascular disease rates. Diabetes Care 1986; 9: 140–8.

84. Neumann V, Cove DH, Shapiro LM, George AJ, Kenny MW, Meakin M, Stuart J. Effect of ticlo-pidine on platelet function and blood rheology in diabetes mellitus. Clin Hemorheol 1983; 3: 13–21.

85. Roncucci R, Dehertogh R, Dormany JA et al. Effects of long-term treatment with suloctidil on blood viscosity erythrocyte deformability and total fibrinogen plasma levels in diabetic patients. Arzneim Forsch Drug Res 1979; 29: 682–4.

86. Lowe GDO, Morrice JJ, Forbes CD, Prentice CRM, Fulton AJ, Barbanel JC. Subcutaneous ancrod therapy in peripheral arterial disease improvement in blood viscosity and nutritional blood flow. Angiology 1979; 30: 594–9.

87. McMillan DE, Utterback NG, Wujeck JJ. Effects of anionic amphophiles on erythrocyte proper-ties. Ann NY Acad Sci 1983; 416: 633–41.

88. Yarnell JWG, Baker IA, Sweetnam PM et al. Fibrinogen, viscosity, and white cell count are major risk factors for ischemic heart disease. Cir-culation 1991; 83: 836–44.

63

Epidemiology of Macrovascular Disease and Hypertension in Diabetes Mellitus

R.J. Jarrett

United Medical and Dental Schools of Guy's and St Thomas's Hospitals, London, UK

There is a voluminous literature on the topic of diabetes and cardiovascular disease, including many reviews. However, for the modern reviewer most of this literature is redundant, principally because of the failure to distinguish between the two major varieties of diabetes—insulin dependent and non-insulin dependent. The impact of renal disease upon morbidity and mortality in insulin dependent diabetes mellitus (IDDM) is so enormous that it is imperative to consider cardiovascular disease—including hypertension—separately by type of diabetes. As far as possible this review does so, although for the first topic (atherosclerosis) the available literature does not allow a clear separation.

ATHEROSCLEROSIS

In the quarter-century following the introduction of insulin, there were numerous comparisons—chiefly from the USA—of the postmortem appearance of the coronary arteries in diabetic and non-diabetic subjects. The general observation was of more widespread and more severe coronary atherosclerosis in the diabetic subjects. The descriptions were, however, qualitative and said little or nothing about the possible effects of age at onset, type of diabetes or duration of diabetes. Some of these factors have only recently been investigated, either by postmortem examination or by angiographic techniques during life.

Waller et al [1] systematically re-examined the hearts of 229 diabetic subjects, whose age at onset was greater than 30 years, who had undergone autopsy at the Mayo Clinic between 1945 and 1975. Matched control patients were selected from patients with fatal coronary heart disease (CHD) from the same population. The authors attempted to answer three questions:

(1) Do the hearts of patients with diabetes and clinical CHD have more, less or similar amounts of coronary narrowing by atherosclerotic plaques than those of patients with CHD but no diabetes?

International Textbook of Diabetes Mellitus. Edited by K.G.M.M. Alberti, R.A. DeFronzo, H. Keen and P. Zimmet
© 1992 John Wiley & Sons Ltd

Table 1 Fatal cardiac events in diabetic and non-diabetic subjects with clinically evident CHD prior to death

Cause of death	Diabetic (%)	Non-diabetic (%)
Acute myocardial infarct	55	43
Sudden death	31	57
Congestive heart failure	14	0

Abstracted from Waller et al [1].

(2) Do the hearts of patients with diabetes and clinical CHD have more, less or similar amounts of coronary narrowing by atherosclerotic plaques than those of patients with diabetes but no clinical CHD?

(3) Among patients with onset of diabetes after 30 years of age, does the age at onset or the duration of diabetes correlate with the amount of coronary narrowing by atherosclerosis?

There were similar degrees of severe narrowing (more than 75%) by atherosclerotic plaques in the right, left anterior descending and left circumflex coronary arteries in each of the three groups of patients. The diabetic patients, however, had a significantly higher frequency of narrowing of the left main coronary artery, and within the diabetic group a higher frequency was found in those with a clinical history of CHD. When duration groups were constructed (1–5, 6–10, 11–25 and 26–40 years), no significant differences were observed for either degree of severe narrowing in the three major coronary arteries or the frequency of severe narrowing of the left main coronary artery. There were also no significant differences related to treatment of the diabetes.

An additional point of interest was a significantly different frequency in types of cardiac death between diabetic patients and controls (Table 1). These findings are in accord with several other reports.

Vigorita et al [2] performed a similar study, but used the technique of postmortem coronary angiography. Both the diabetic subjects and age-matched and sex-matched controls had undergone autopsy at the Johns Hopkins Hospital, Baltimore, between 1968 and 1978. Twenty-two per cent of all patients autopsied were studied, selection being predominantly 'the expectation of cardiac disease', and it can only be assumed

that selection was identical for diabetic and non-diabetic subjects. All abnormalities were graded according to severity. Compared with controls, diabetic subjects showed a significantly higher rate of coronary atherosclerosis and of infarcts. Within the diabetic group, there were no significant differences according to treatment (nil, diet, oral agents, insulin), nor was there a significant association with the duration of diabetes, even by univariate analysis.

In addition to these hospital-based studies, there are two population-based pathological studies. In the International Atherosclerosis Project [3], several diverse population groups were surveyed and standardised observations made upon the aorta and coronary arteries. According to the authors, 'With but few exceptions, mean extent of raised lesions ranks the geographic and ethnic groups in the order that would have been predicted from general knowledge of their relative economic status, standard of living, mortality from CHD, or other epidemiological variables which have long been known to be associated with atherosclerosis and its sequelae'. The severity of coronary atherosclerosis in the diabetic patients varied in parallel with the general severity in the population from which they were sampled, but the effect of diabetes was 'superimposed on any level of average severity of atherosclerosis'. The authors did not examine possible effects of the type of diabetes or of diabetes duration. In the Five Towns Study [4], standardised comparisons were made on postmortem material from Prague, Malmö, Tallinn, Yalta and Ryazan. The effect of diabetes was much greater in the coronary arteries than in the aorta. Even in non-hypertensive diabetic subjects, both raised and calcified lesions in the coronary arteries were more extensive than in the controls: indeed, the severity of coronary atherosclerosis in non-hypertensive diabetic subjects was similar to that in hypertensive non-diabetic subjects. The effect of duration was studied by comparing subjects who had been suffering from diabetes for less than or more than 10 years. Coronary atherosclerosis was more frequent in the latter group, but it appears that the comparison was not controlled for age at death or presence of hypertension.

Dortimer et al [5] compared the extent of coronary artery disease determined by coronary angiography in 37 living diabetic patients and 79 matched controls. Of the diabetic patients, only 7 were insulin treated. The controls were matched for age, sex and high or low risk factor status. In both groups the indication for angiography was chest pain; the severity of disease was assessed blind using a grading system. Of the diabetics, 43% had three-vessel disease compared with 25% of controls, a difference that escaped conventional statistical significance in these numbers ($0.1 > P > 0.05$). However, 68% of all vessels visualised in the diabetics were diseased compared with 46% in controls ($P < 0.005$). In addition, grade 3 or greater stenoses were significantly more frequent in the diabetic subjects.

Vigorito et al [6] performed a similar study in 34 diabetic subjects and 120 controls with CHD. In this study the controls were not individually matched, although on average they were similar in many respects to the diabetics. The major difference between the two groups was the significantly higher frequency of multiple vessel disease in the diabetic patients. By contrast, Verska and Walker [7] found no difference in severity of CHD as assessed by coronary angiography between 35 diabetic and 77 non-diabetic patients. These patients had, however, all been preselected as suitable for coronary bypass surgery, and so subjects with more extensive disease would have been excluded.

Weitzman et al [8] noted a substantially increased mortality rate, in diabetic and non-diabetic subjects alike, following a first myocardial infarct when the site of the infarct was anterior. There was some support in this study for a greater frequency of anterior infarcts in diabetic patients, thus contributing to the overall increase in mortality.

To summarise the above studies, it appears that at least in countries where atherosclerosis is common in the general population, coronary atherosclerosis is, on average, both more extensive and more severe in diabetic patients than in appropriately matched controls. There is insufficient evidence to distinguish between NIDDM and IDDM in this respect. At least in older (mainly NIDDM) diabetic patients, there is no good evidence of a positive association between duration and degree of coronary atherosclerosis.

There has been much less investigation of the cerebral and peripheral circulation. Chan et al [9], using non-invasive methods, compared the prevalence of carotid artery stenoses (50%

reduction or more) in 286 volunteer NIDDM subjects and 135 controls of similar age (mean 61 and 60 years, respectively); 7.3% of the diabetic subjects and 0.7% of controls had severe stenoses.

Strandness et al [10] compared a small group of diabetic patients (type not specified) with a group of controls, using non-invasive methods to study the peripheral circulation. The only notable difference was a greater prevalence of obstructive abnormalities in the arteries below the knee (anterior and posterior tibial and peroneal) in the diabetic patients, whose average age was 60 years. Elderly diabetic subjects also have an increased prevalence of medial calcification in peripheral arteries [11, 12], but this abnormality appears to have little or no correlation with atherosclerosis [13].

Kingsbury [14] studied 338 male, non-diabetic subjects referred to a surgical clinic specialising in peripheral vascular disease. Arteriography was performed in each subject and the degree of irregularity classified into three grades of severity. Oral glucose tolerance tests were also performed and it was found that, independent of age, both fasting and 2-hour blood glucose levels were related to the degree of irregularity. The mean ages of the men in the 'moderate' and 'extensive' disease categories were 59.2 years and 61.3 years respectively. It may be inferred from this study that men at increased risk of NIDDM (because of relative glucose intolerance) have more extensive peripheral arterial disease.

Mortality and Morbidity in IDDM

Coronary Heart Disease

Most of the published information on mortality in young-onset IDDM patients derives from cohort studies of the Joslin Clinic in Boston, Massachusetts [15, 16], the Steno Memorial Hospital in Copenhagen [17, 18] and (the only true population-based study) from Pittsburgh [19]. The latter study was able to compare black and white subjects and observed a higher relative mortality in the black population, with standardised mortality ratios (SMR) of 968 and 711, respectively. Each of the three cohort studies found renal disease to be the predominant cause of excess mortality, with cardiovascular causes becoming significant contributors above the age of 30 years. In the Pittsburgh study [19], SMRs for cardiovascular mortality were 1137 and 1591 for white males and females, respectively. No details were presented on the nature of the cardiovascular disease, presumably because the data were derived from death certificates. It is necessary at this point to remind the reader of the many problems in ascertaining the precise cause of death, particularly from death certificates. We do not know, for instance, how many 'sudden deaths' in diabetic patients may be related to autonomic neuropathy [20] rather than to coronary disease. In uraemic diabetic patients treated by dialysis, cardiovascular disease may apparently be the immediate cause of death, but nevertheless cannot be assumed to be identical, in terms of mechanisms involved, with that in non-uraemic diabetic patients.

Data from the Steno cohort demonstrate the much-diminished—although still significant—relative mortality risk in IDDM patients who remain free of proteinuria [18]. In the Joslin Clinic cohort the cumulative incidence of coronary heart disease mortality was also substantially lower in those who did not develop persistent proteinuria [16]. In neither study were lesser degrees of proteinuria (microalbuminuria) measured, and it is now known that this, too, is associated with a greater risk of clinical nephropathy and increased mortality [21, 22]. In the Steno study, the onset of proteinuria was followed by a substantially increased incidence of fatal and non-fatal coronary heart disease (Figure 1), and by average increases of serum cholesterol and blood pressure by comparison with matched, non-proteinuric controls [23]. Increases in blood pressure have also been demonstrated in microalbuminuric diabetic subjects [24, 25] (Table 2). It may be, therefore, that much (if not all) of the excess of coronary heart disease in IDDM can be attributed to the diabetic renal disorder.

Cerebrovascular Disease

There is no mortality or morbidity study of well-defined IDDM patients. In the Edinburgh prospective study [26], patients were separated into treatment categories, with 429 male and 505 female insulin-treated diabetic patients. Using death certificate data, cause-specific SMRs were calculated in comparison with the total population of Scotland. SMRs for cerebrovascular diseases were increased in the insulin-treated diabetic patients—166 for males and 135 for

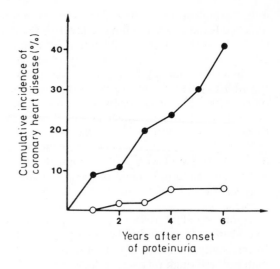

Figure 1 Cumulative incidence of coronary heart disease in IDDM subjects with (solid circles) and without (open circles) proteinuria. From reference 23, with permission

females—but in neither sex was the excess statistically significant.

A similar study in Warsaw [27] compared mortality rates in diabetic patients aged 30–68 years at diagnosis attending four clinics in Warsaw with those in the general population of Warsaw. Excess mortality from cerebrovascular disease was similar in men and women treated with insulin (SMR 162), but this difference was not statistically significant ($P > 0.05$), although numbers of deaths were few ($n = 13$). Fuller et al [28] analysed 1 181 357 death certificates from England and Wales for 1975 and 1976: of these, 3.7% mentioned diabetes. The certificates were specially coded for all mentioned underlying causes of death and a 'conditional proportional registration ratio' (CPRR) calculated for specific causes and by broad age groups. For the age group 15–45 years (at death)—and likely therefore to comprise predominantly IDDM subjects—the CPRRs for cerebrovascular disease were 162 and 240 for males and females, respectively. The CPRR for females was significantly increased ($P < 0.01$).

Thus, on the basis of a few studies, with obvious deficiencies, there is nevertheless some consensus that cerebrovascular mortality is increased in insulin-treated diabetic patients, although the excess is substantially less than that due to coronary heart disease.

Table 2 Comparison of blood pressure levels (mm Hg) in IDDM patients with and without increased urinary albumin excretion

	Albumin excretion rate (μg/min)			
	12.1–28.9	< 12.0	32.4–91.3	< 12.0
Systolic BP	119.0 ± 9.8	117.1 ± 9.5	135.5 ± 18.1*	117.9 ± 7.8
Diastolic BP	78.9 ± 8.5	76.4 ± 10.7	86.5 ± 8.9†	71.8 ± 7.2
Number of subjects	16	16	12	12

Values are means ± SD. BP, blood pressure in mm Hg.
* $P < 0.05$; † $P < 0.001$.
Abstracted from Wiseman et al [24].

Mortality and Morbidity in NIDDM

Coronary Heart Disease

Panzram recently reviewed reports from the years 1975 to 1985 on populations consisting predominantly or exclusively of patients with NIDDM [29]. These comprised studies from the USA, Europe and Japan. The ratio of observed to expected deaths from all causes ranged from 1.15 to 3.01, including both age-adjusted and age-specific data. For the latter, the ratios diminished with age at onset. Where ratios for CHD mortality were presented, they also tended to be higher than those for all-causes mortality. Where sex-specific data for CHD mortality were presented, some studies reported higher ratios in women [26, 30–32], whereas others found no difference [27, 33, 34]. The Japanese experience is of some interest: an excess mortality from CHD in diabetic patients appears to be of recent origin [35], from about 1970, and the proportion of cardiovascular deaths is lower than that obtaining in Europe and North America [33, 36] (Tables 3 and 4). By contrast, the proportion of deaths attributed to CHD in migrant Japanese

diabetics in Hawaii was almost identical to that in Europid diabetic patients on the island [37].

It has long been considered that the increased CHD risk associated with NIDDM is secondary to the diabetes, but there is now considerable evidence against this [38]. Thus a history of cardiovascular disease is more common in individuals who subsequently develop diabetes [39, 40] and the prevalence of CHD is already greater in patients at diagnosis, even when the diagnosis is made by population screening [41, 42]. Furthermore, an increased risk of CHD mortality has been demonstrated in subjects with glucose intolerance below that diagnostic of NIDDM [32, 43–45], where there is also an increased risk of developing NIDDM. Finally, if the increased risk of CHD were secondary to the diabetes, it would be expected that the risk would increase with duration (as it does for microvascular disease [46]). However, neither incidence [29, 47, 48] nor prevalence [49, 50] studies reveal such an association. In addition, two postmortem studies failed to find an association between the amount or degree of coronary artery wall disease and the duration of diabetes [1, 2].

Thus there is considerable circumstantial evidence to support the thesis that NIDDM and CHD are associated disorders and that an increased risk of CHD precedes the development

Table 3 Mortality in Japanese NIDDM patients, Osaka, 1962–81. Mean age at entry 50.5 years for men, 54.0 years for women

Cause of death	No. of deaths observed	No. of deaths expected	O/E ratio
All causes	201	137.2	1.46
Hypertensive heart disease	5	2.59	1.93
Ischaemic heart disease	21	9.08	2.31*
Cerebrovascular disease	33	28.61	1.15
Renal disease	24	2.03	11.82†

Abstracted from Sasaki et al [33].
* $P < 0.05$; † $P < 0.01$.

Table 4 Mortality in Japanese NIDDM patients, Tokyo; 3–7-year follow-up of patients seen 1976–80

Cause of death	No. of deaths observed	No. of deaths expected	O/E ratio
All causes	434	279.5	1.55
Ischaemic heart disease	64	27.1	2.36*
Cerebrovascular disease	59	60.4	0.97

Abstracted from Mihara et al [36].
* $P < 0.01$.

of significant hyperglycaemia. The genesis and expression of this risk is speculative and beyond the scope of this review, but it is worth noting that associations between levels of putative risk factors for both cardiovascular disease and diabetes (lipids, blood pressure, blood glucose and plasma insulin) have been demonstrated in children [51], i.e. long before the development of the clinical disorders.

Cerebrovascular Disease

Although the consensus is that cerebrovascular disease is more common in NIDDM, the reported dimension of the excess is less consistent than that for CHD. This may be in part because of methodological and nosological problems. Thus cerebrovascular disease or stroke comprises several disease entities which may be difficult to ascertain even in the clinical setting, let alone from the data available to epidemiologists. Some reports do attempt to distinguish between these entities but it is not possible to ascertain how successful they are. Data from death certificates are suspect when they rely on 'diabetes' and 'stroke' appearing on the same certificate, for it is merely an option for the certifier to mention diabetes when the stroke was the underlying cause of death. Furthermore, the certificate does not distinguish the type of diabetes. Data from cohorts of known diabetic subjects are more likely to be valid.

In the 20-year follow-up of the Framingham study population aged 45–75 years, the age-adjusted relative risks for 'brain infarct' were 2.7 and 3.8 for men and women respectively [30]. However, in a much larger population of 1010 primarily non-insulin dependent diabetic patients diagnosed between 1945 and 1969 in Rochester, Minnesota, the relative risks for a first stroke (undifferentiated) were 1.4 for both sexes and the difference was only significant in diabetic patients classified as hypertensive [52]. In this study, the ratio of ischaemic infarction to intracranial haemorrhage was greater in the diabetic cohort than in the general population (11 and 5 respectively).

A random sample of the population of two counties in eastern Finland was examined in 1972 and followed for 7 years [53]: 77 of 4034 men and 65 of 4334 women suffered a stroke or transient ischaemic attack. In multiple logistic analyses, diabetes (type not specified) was sig-

nificantly related in women to cerebral infarcts specifically and to all strokes, but was related in men to infarcts only.

In the UK a cohort of 5971 members of the British Diabetic Association recruited between 1965 and 1969 was followed for 11–14 years and cause-specific mortality ratios calculated by comparison with the general population of England and Wales [28]. In the older subjects (therefore predominantly with NIDDM), SMRs were 102 (males) and 175 (females) in the age range 45–64 years, and 145 (males) and 138 (females) for the age range 65 years and over. Only the latter SMR was significantly increased. In the Edinburgh study of known diabetic patients, coding of death certificates was done using International Classification of Disease (ICD) codes and a local system which eliminated most diagnoses of death ascribed to diabetes per se [26]. The results illustrate one of the problems of death certification data in this context. Thus, for diet-treated diabetics, SMRs for cerebrovascular disease deaths were 93 (males) and 136 (females) by ICD codes, and 121 (males) and 156 (females) by the local code. For subjects treated with oral agents the SMRs were 111 (males) and 170 (females) by ICD codes, and 166 (males) and 211 (females) by the local code.

In the prospective study of Hawaiian Japanese men [54], serum glucose level 1 hour after a glucose load was significantly related to the incidence (age-adjusted) of 'thromboembolic' stroke, fatal and non-fatal combined, but not to haemorrhagic stroke. By contrast, 9-year mortality rates from strokes were lower in glucose-intolerant men (known diabetic patients on specific medication or with 1-hour postload serum glucose levels of 225 mg/dl or above) than in normoglycaemic men [55]. Two studies in Japan showed no excess of deaths from cerebrovascular disease in NIDDM subjects compared with reference populations [33, 36] (Tables 3 and 4). By contrast, both studies reported excess mortality from CHD in the diabetic group. In the Whitehall study [43], the age-adjusted stroke mortality rate was significantly increased in men in the upper 5% of the blood glucose distribution—as with the CHD mortality rate.

In studies that differentiated between types of stroke, the association of NIDDM or elevated blood glucose was predominantly with non-haemorrhagic strokes [53, 54].

As the prevalence of strokes is not related to duration of NIDDM [56] and the incidence is higher in glucose-intolerant subjects [42, 53], the association of strokes and NIDDM evident in most of the populations studied may, as argued for CHD, not be one of cause and effect.

Peripheral Vascular Disease

As with cerebrovascular disease, there are considerable methodological problems in accurately identifying and classifying peripheral vascular disease. A history of intermittent claudication does not correlate well with modern methods of measuring the degree and distribution of arterial disease [57], and palpation of foot pulses is subject to considerable observer error [58]. Data on amputations may be reliable, but the decision to perform such surgery in a diabetic patient may be influenced by accompanying peripheral neuropathy.

Two prospective population studies provide data on intermittent claudication. In the 20-year follow-up of the Framingham population, the average age-adjusted incidence was 12.6 per 1000 for all diabetic men, 3.3 per 1000 for non-diabetic men, 8.4 per 1000 for all diabetic women and 1.3 per 1000 for non-diabetic women [30]. During the 5-year follow-up of men in the Israeli study [47], incidence rates were 2.2 times higher in previously diagnosed diabetic subjects and 2.3 times in newly diagnosed diabetic subjects. In both studies intermittent claudication was also more prevalent in subjects who subsequently became diabetic.

A Finnish study [59] compared 133 newly diagnosed diabetic patients aged 45-64 years with 144 randomly selected controls. Peripheral vascular disease was assessed by a history of intermittent claudication, absent foot pulses and an ankle–arm blood pressure ratio below 0.9. The prevalence of all three indicators was higher in diabetic patients of both sexes but the differ-

Table 5 Estimated amputation rates, USA, 1978 (rates per 10 000)

Age (years)	Non-diabetic	Diabetic	Type of amputation (%)		
			Toe	Foot	Leg
0–44	0.5	14.1	56.5	6.8	36.7
45–64	1.9	45.0	39.9	6.5	53.6
65+	9.9	101.4	24.4	3.2	72.4

Abstracted from Most and Sinnock [60].

Table 6 Self-reported absence of a lower extremity, USA, 1977 (rates per 1000)

Age group (years)	Diabetic	Non-diabetic
20–44	–	0.6
45–64	12.2	1.7
65+	23.2	3.5
20+	14.4	1.4

Data from 1977 Health Interview Survey, quoted by Palumbo and Melton [61].

ence reached conventional significance only for men with respect to absent pulses.

There are data on amputation rates from the USA that indicate much higher rates in diabetic patients, but they do not separate diabetes by type (Tables 5 and 6).

BLOOD PRESSURE AND HYPERTENSION

IDDM

Moss compared systolic blood pressures in 123 IDDM subjects aged 8–18 years and 889 controls all attending neighbouring summer camps [62]. Average levels—apparently age-adjusted —were 3–4 mm Hg higher in the diabetic subjects, but there was no adjustment for duration nor was there any measurement of urinary protein.

Kaas Ibsen et al [63] compared blood pressure levels in 151 diabetic children aged 2–19 years with those in a Danish reference population. Shortly after diagnosis, systolic blood pressure levels were similar, but diastolic (phase 4) levels were significantly lower in the diabetic children. After 5 years of diabetes, systolic levels remained similar in the two groups and significantly lower diastolic levels were confined to female diabetic subjects. Unfortunately, the blood pressures were measured in different positions—supine in the diabetic subjects and sitting in the reference population. Cruickshanks et al [64] measured blood pressure levels in 145 diabetic patients aged 9–16 years and compared them with 45 siblings of diabetics, not necessarily of the same diabetic probands. Systolic blood pressure on average was slightly and significantly higher in diabetic subjects of both sexes after age adjustment, but there was no significant difference in phase 4 diastolic levels. In girls, phase 5 diastolic level was higher in the diabetic patients. No adjustments were made for diabetes duration or for proteinuria.

Tarn and Drury [65] measured blood pressure levels in the families participating in the Barts–Windsor study. Measurements were made in 163 diabetic subjects aged 4–32 years, 232 non-diabetic siblings and 292 parents. Systolic pressures were not different overall nor in any 4-year age band, but phase 4 diastolic pressure was slightly and significantly higher (2.8 mm Hg) in diabetic males compared with their sibling group. There were no significant differences in diastolic pressure in the females whether phase 4 or 5 was used, nor in phase 5 in males. When mean blood pressure above the 90th centile for age and sex was considered, 17% of the diabetic subjects compared with 11% of the siblings exceeded this value. It may be relevant that 8 of 27 diabetic subjects (29%) in this category had increased albumin excretion, defined as a 24-hour urinary albumin excretion exceeding 12 μg/min or a random albumin concentration above 30 mg/dl. Furthermore, the respective parent groups of both diabetics and siblings with mean blood pressure levels above the 90th centile had significantly more individuals with borderline (blood pressure exceeding 140/90 mm Hg) or treated hypertension than the parents of the normotensive children.

The importance of albuminuria is illustrated by the case-control study of Wiseman et al [24] (see Table 2). Subjects were derived from a screening programme in the diabetic clinic in which overnight collections of urine were made for calculation of the albumin excretion rate (AER). All subjects were within 10% of ideal body weight, with negative Albustix tests for urinary protein, serum creatinine within the normal range and with no history of renal or urinary tract disease. Twenty-eight patients with AER above the normal range were identified and subdivided into two groups, termed 'low' and 'high' microalbuminuria respectively. They were individually matched for age, duration and gender with patients having an AER within the normal range. Four separate blood pressure readings were made in each subject by a single observer across the course of a day spent in a metabolic ward. Systolic and diastolic (phase 4) blood pressure levels showed no difference between the low microalbuminuria group and its control. However, both diastolic and systolic levels were significantly higher in the high micro-

Table 7 Rancho Bernardo study: mean blood pressure levels adjusted for age and obesity in white adults aged 50–79 years

Sex and diabetes status	No.	Mean blood pressure (mm Hg)	
		Systolic	Diastolic
Males			
Non-diabetic	1149	139.6	81.2
Diabetic:			
newly diagnosed	57	140.5	82.8
known	93	144.3	82.0
Females			
Non-diabetic	1453	135.4	79.8
Diabetic:			
newly diagnosed	41	136.3	79.1
known	53	142.9	82.4

Abstracted from Barrett-Connor et al [68].

albuminuria group. An association between degree of albuminuria and level of blood pressure in IDDM has been confirmed by other authors [25, 66, 67].

NIDDM

Many studies of blood pressure in NIDDM and reference populations do not control for degree of obesity, which is both related to blood pressure and tends to be greater in diabetic subjects. Similarly, studies that compare the prevalence of 'hypertension', including treatment in the definition, are subject to bias in that diabetic patients, being under regular medical supervision, have more opportunity to be subject to the diagnosis.

In a population study of subjects aged 50–79 years in California [68], mean blood pressure levels adjusted for age and body mass index (BMI) were lowest for non-diabetic subjects, intermediate for those with newly detected disease and highest for established diabetic subjects, but the differences were small and statistically significant only for women (Table 7).

In the Chicago Heart Association Detection Project in Industry study of 11 220 men and 8030 women aged 35–64 years, there were 377 male and 170 female known diabetic subjects [69]; it can be assumed that most were NIDDM. Blood pressure levels adjusted for age and relative weight did not differ significantly in the diabetic subjects of either sex. However, in subjects of both sexes with elevated blood glucose levels 1 hour after an oral glucose load, blood pressure levels were significantly raised even after adjustment for age and relative weight.

In the Bedford survey, blood pressure levels were compared between newly detected diabetic subjects, 'borderline diabetics' (roughly equivalent to 'impaired glucose tolerance') and a normoglycaemic reference population [70]. In men, mean systolic values adjusted for age and BMI were significantly higher in both hyperglycaemic groups, but diastolic values were higher only in the borderline diabetics. In women, only the adjusted systolic values were significantly higher in the hyperglycaemic groups.

The Whitehall study was confined to males working in the UK Civil Service [70]. All save known diabetic subjects had a blood glucose measurement 2 hours following a 50-g oral glucose load. Again, mean blood pressure levels were higher in borderline and newly detected diabetics; and, in multiple regression analysis, both systolic and diastolic blood pressure levels were significantly and independently related to the blood glucose level. In the diabetic patients participating in the study, average blood pressure levels were similar to those of the normoglycaemic controls, but it was not ascertained how representative these cases were, and they might, in any case, have been more accustomed to blood pressure measurement.

In the Framingham study [71], at the 12th examination, the prevalence of hypertension (systolic blood pressure over 160 mm Hg, diastolic blood pressure over 90 mm Hg) in diabetic subjects aged 50–79 years (presumably predominantly NIDDM) was higher than in non-diabetic subjects, and the difference was significant after adjustment for age and BMI. However, the dimensions of the difference after adjustment were not stated.

Associations between blood glucose (and plasma insulin)—both fasting and postload—with blood pressure, apparently independent of obesity, have been reported from several population surveys [51, 72–74]. A raised blood pressure may also be a weak predictor of subsequent diabetes, although this observation is potentially confounded by obesity [71, 75].

Thus, while glucose, insulin and blood pressure are demonstrably associated variables, and average blood pressure levels are higher in untreated persons with glucose intolerance both above and below the cut-off point for applying the label 'diabetic', we know virtually nothing about any subsequent effect of 'diabetes' upon blood pressure. However, when account is taken of potential confounding factors and diagnostic bias, it seems that hypertension is not a remarkable feature of NIDDM.

PROTEINURIA AND BLOOD PRESSURE IN NIDDM

Whereas the association of raised blood pressure and even modest degrees of proteinuria in IDDM is well established, the situation in NIDDM is confused. In the study of Fabre et al [76], diastolic hypertension was positively associated with 24-hour protein excretion, but blood pressure values were not adjusted for age or obesity.

In the Bedford study, significant positive correlations were obtained between systolic blood pressure and the logarithm of the albumin excretion rate in newly detected diabetic subjects [77]. A positive correlation of low degree was also noted in subjects with fasting hyperglycaemia, known diabetes and control subjects in a population aged 60–74 years in Denmark [78]. However, in another Danish study, in patients stratified by duration and urinary albumin concentration, there was no apparent association of the latter with blood pressure [79]. In a comparison of Europid and Asian Indian NIDDM patients, there was a significant association of blood pressure/hypertension with albumin/creatinine ratio in an early morning urine sample in the Indians, but not in the Europids [80].

The lack of consistency may in part be due to methodological differences, but an association of blood pressure and proteinuria appears to be less impressive in NIDDM than in IDDM.

CONCLUSION

It is clear that the relationships of cardiovascular disease and hypertension with diabetes differ between the two major varieties of diabetes. In IDDM the diabetes leads to a high rate of kidney disorder which in turn may cause hypertension and probably contributes to much of the excess of atherosclerosis and cardiovascular disease. In NIDDM the picture is less clear, but there is little direct evidence in favour of the view that hyperglycaemia is responsible for the increased risk of cardiovascular disease.

REFERENCES

1. Waller BF, Palumbo PJ, Lie T, Roberts WC. Status of the coronary arteries at necropsy in diabetes mellitus with onset after age 30 years. Am J Med 1980; 69: 498–506.
2. Vigorita VJ, Moore GW, Hutchins GM. Absence of correlation between coronary arterial atherosclerosis and severity or duration of diabetes mellitus of adult onset. Am J Cardiol 1980; 46: 535–42.
3. Robertson WB, Strong JP. Atherosclerosis in persons with hypertension and diabetes mellitus. Lab Invest 1968; 18: 538–51.
4. Zdanov VS, Vihert AM. Atherosclerosis and diabetes mellitus. Bull WHO 1976; 53: 547–53.
5. Dortimer AC, Shenoy PN, Shiroff RA, Leaman DM, Babb JD, Liedtke AJ, Zelis R. Diffuse coronary artery disease in diabetic patients. Fact or fiction? Circulation 1978; 57: 133–6.
6. Vigorito C, Betocchi S, Bonzani G, Guidice P, Miceli D, Piscione F, Condorelli M. Severity of coronary artery disease in patients with diabetes mellitus. Angiographic study of 34 diabetic and 120 nondiabetic patients. Am Heart J 1980; 100: 782–7.
7. Verska JJ, Walker WJ. Aorto-coronary by-pass in the diabetic patient. Am J Cardiol 1980; 35: 774–7.
8. Weitzman S, Wagner GS, Heiss G, Haney TL, Slome C. Myocardial infarction site and mortality in diabetes. Diabetes Care 1982; 5: 31–5.
9. Chan A, Beach KW, Martin DC, Strandness DE. Carotid artery disease in NIDDM diabetes. Diabetes Care 1983; 6: 562–9.
10. Strandness DE, Priest RE, Gibbons GE. Combined clinical and pathologic study of diabetic and non-diabetic peripheral arterial disease. Diabetes 1964; 13: 366–72.
11. Ferrier TM. Radiologically demonstrable arterial calcification in diabetes mellitus. Austr Ann Med 1964; 13: 222–8.
12. Neubauer B. Quantitative study of peripheral arterial calcification in elderly diabetics and non-diabetics. Diabetologia 1971; 7: 409–13.
13. Lindblom A. Arteriosclerosis and arterial thrombosis in the lower limbs. Acta Radiol 1950; 80 (suppl.): 38–48.
14. Kingsbury KJ. The relation between glucose tolerance and atherosclerotic vascular disease. Lancet 1966; ii: 1374–9.
15. Entmacher PS, Root HF, Marks HH. Longevity of diabetic patients in recent years. Diabetes 1964; 13: 373–7.
16. Krolewski AS, Kosinski EJ, Warram JH et al. Magnitude and determinants of coronary artery disease in juvenile-onset, insulin-dependent diabetes mellitus. Am J Cardiol 1987; 59: 750–5.
17. Andersen AR, Christiansen JS, Andersen JK, Kreiner S, Deckert T. Diabetic nephropathy in Type I (insulin-dependent) diabetes: an epidemiological study. Diabetologia 1983; 25: 496–501.
18. Borch-Johnsen K, Andersen PK, Deckert T. The effect of proteinuria on relative mortality in Type I (insulin-dependent) diabetes mellitus. Diabetologia 1985; 28: 590–6.
19. Dorman JS, LaPorte RE, Kuller LH et al. The Pittsburgh insulin-dependent diabetes mellitus (IDDM) morbidity and mortality study: mortality results. Diabetes 1984; 33: 271–6.
20. Page MMB, Watkins PJ. Cardiorespiratory arrest and diabetic autonomic neuropathy. Lancet 1978; i: 14–16.
21. Viberti GC, Hill RD, Jarrett RJ, Argyropoulos A, Mahmud U, Keen H. Microalbuminuria as a predictor of clinical nephropathy in insulin-dependent diabetes mellitus. Lancet 1982; i: 1340–2.
22. Mogensen CE, Christensen CK. Predicting diabetic nephropathy in insulin-dependent patients. New Engl J Med 1984; 311: 89–93.
23. Jensen T, Borch-Johnsen K, Kofoed-Enevoldsen A, Deckert T. Coronary heart disease in young Type I (insulin-dependent) diabetic patients with and without diabetic nephropathy: incidence and risk factors. Diabetologia 1987; 30: 144–8.
24. Wiseman M, Viberti G, Mackintosh D, Jarrett RJ, Keen H. Glycaemia, arterial pressure and micro-albuminuria in Type I (insulin-dependent) diabetes mellitus. Diabetologia 1984; 26: 401–5.
25. Mathiesen ER, Oxenboll B, Johansen K, Svendsen PA, Deckert T. Incipient nephropathy in Type I (insulin-dependent) diabetes. Diabetologia 1984; 26: 406–10.
26. Shenfield GM, Elton RA, Bhalla IP, Duncan LJP. Diabetic mortality in Edinburgh. Diabète Métab 1979; 5: 149–58.
27. Krolewski AS, Czyzyk A, Janeczko D, Kopczyński J. Mortality from cardiovascular diseases among diabetics. Diabetologia 1977; 13: 345–50.
28. Fuller JH, Elford J, Goldblatt P, Adelstein AM. Diabetes mortality: new light on an underestimated public health problem. Diabetologia 1983; 24: 336–41.
29. Panzram G. Mortality and survival in Type 2 (non-insulin-dependent) diabetes mellitus. Diabetologia 1987; 30: 123–31.
30. Kannel WB, McGee DL. Diabetes and glucose tolerance as risk factors for cardiovascular disease: the Framingham Study. Diabetes Care 1979; 2: 120–6.
31. Barrett-Connor E, Wingard DL. Sex differential in ischemic heart disease mortality in diabetics: a prospective population-based study. Am J Epidemiol 1983; 118: 489–96.

32. Jarrett RJ, McCartney P, Keen H. The Bedford Survey: ten-year mortality rates in newly diagnosed diabetics, borderline diabetics and normoglycaemic controls and risk indices for coronary heart disease in borderline diabetics. Diabetologia 1982; 22: 79–84.

33. Sasaki A, Uehara M, Horiuchi N, Hasagawa K. A long-term follow-up study of Japanese diabetic patients: mortality and causes of death. Diabetologia 1983; 25: 309–12.

34. Butler WJ, Ostrander LD, Carman WJ, Lamphiear DE. Mortality from coronary heart disease in the Tecumseh Study; long term effect of diabetes mellitus, glucose tolerance and other risk factors. Am J Epidemiol 1985; 121: 541–7.

35. Sasaki A, Kamado K, Horiuchi N. A changing pattern of causes of death in Japanese diabetics. Observations over fifteen years. J Chron Dis 1978; 31: 433–44.

36. Mihara T, Oohashi H, Hirata Y. Mortality of Japanese diabetics in a seven-year follow-up study. Diabetes Res Clin Pract 1986; 2: 139–44.

37. Kawate R, Miyanishi M, Yamakido M et al. Preliminary studies of the prevalence and mortality of diabetes mellitus in Japanese in Japan and on the island of Hawaii. Adv Metab Dis 1978; 9: 202–24.

38. Jarrett RJ. Type 2 (non-insulin-dependent) diabetes mellitus and coronary heart disease—chicken, egg or neither? Diabetologia 1984; 26: 99–102.

39. Ipsen J, Clark TW, Elsom KO, Roberts NJ. Diabetes and heart disease: periodic health examination programs. Am J Publ Health 1969; 59: 1595–611.

40. Wilson PWF, Anderson KM, Kannel WB. Epidemiology of diabetes mellitus in the elderly: the Framingham Study. Am J Med 1986; 80 (suppl. 5A): 3–9.

41. Keen H, Rose G, Pyke DA, Boyns DR, Chlouverakis C, Mistry S. Blood sugar and arterial disease. Lancet 1965; ii: 505–8.

42. Uusitupa M, Siitonen O, Aro A, Pyörälä K. Prevalence of coronary heart disease, left ventricular failure and hypertension in middle-aged, newly diagnosed Type 2 (non-insulin-dependent) diabetic subjects. Diabetologia 1985; 28: 22–7.

43. Fuller JH, Shipley MJ, Rose G, Jarrett RJ, Keen H. Mortality from coronary heart disease and stroke in relation to degree of glycaemia: the Whitehall Study. Br Med J 1983; 287: 867–70.

44. Pyörälä K, Savoleinen E, Kaukola S, Haapakoski J. High plasma insulin as coronary heart disease risk factor. In Eschwège E (ed.) Advances in diabetes epidemiology. INSERM Symposium 22. Amsterdam: Elsevier, 1982: pp 143–8.

45. Eschwège E, Richard JL, Thibult N, Ducimetière P, Warnet JM, Claude JR, Rosselin GE. Coronary heart disease mortality in relation with diabetes, blood glucose and plasma insulin levels: the Paris Prospective Study, ten years later. Horm Metab Res 1985 (suppl. 15): 41–6.

46. Jarrett RJ, Keen H. The WHO Multinational Study of Vascular Disease in Diabetes. 3. Microvascular disease. Diabetes Care 1979; 2: 196–201.

47. Herman JB, Medalie JH, Goldbourt U. Differences in cardiovascular morbidity and mortality between previously known and newly diagnosed adult diabetics. Diabetologia 1977; 13: 229–34.

48. Jarrett RJ, Shipley MJ. Mortality and associated risk factors in diabetics. Acta Endocrinol 1985; 110 (suppl. 272): 21–6.

49. Nielsen NV, Ditzel J. Prevalence of macro- and microvascular disease as related to glycosylated hemoglobin in Type I and II diabetic subjects: an epidemiological study in Denmark. Horm Metab Res 1985 (suppl. 15): 19–23.

50. Knuiman MW, Welborn TA, McCann VJ, Stanton KG, Constable IJ. Prevalence of diabetic complications in relation to risk factors. Diabetes 1986; 35: 1332–9.

51. Burke GL, Webber LS, Srinavasan SR, Radhakrishnamurty B, Freedman DS, Berenson GS. Fasting plasma glucose and insulin levels and their relationship to cardiovascular risk factors in children: Bogalusa Heart Study. Metabolism 1986; 35: 441–6.

52. Roehmholdt ME, Palumbo PJ, Whisnant JP, Elveback LR. Transient ischemic attack and stroke in a community-based diabetic cohort. Mayo Clin Proc 1983; 58: 56–8.

53. Salonen JT, Puska P, Tuomilehto J, Homan K. Relation of blood pressure, serum lipids, and smoking to the risk of cerebral stroke: a longitudinal study in Eastern Finland. Stroke 1982; 13: 327–33.

54. Kagan A, Popper JS, Rhoads GG, Yano K. Dietary and other risk factors for stroke in Hawaiian Japanese men. Stroke 1985; 16: 390–6.

55. Yano K, Kagan A, McGee D, Rhoads GG. Glucose intolerance and nine-year mortality in Japanese men in Hawaii. Am J Med 1982; 72: 71–80.

56. Welborn TA, Knuiman M, McCann V, Stanton K, Constable IJ. Clinical macrovascular disease in Caucasoid diabetic subjects: logistic regression analysis of risk variables. Diabetologia 1984; 27: 568–73.

57. Widmer LK, Greensher A, Kannel WB. Occlusion of peripheral arteries: a study of 6400 working subjects. Circulation 1964; 30: 836–52.

58. Meade TW, Gardner MJ, Cannon P, Richardson PC. Observer variability in recording the peripheral pulses. Br Heart J 1968; 30: 661–5.

59. Siiotenen O, Uusitupa M, Pyörälä K, Voutilainen

E, Länsimies E. Peripheral arterial disease and its relationship to cardiovascular risk factors and coronary heart disease in newly diagnosed non-insulin-dependent diabetes. Acta Med Scand 1986; 220: 205–12.

60. Most RS, Sinnock P. The epidemiology of lower extremity amputations in diabetic individuals. Diabetes Care 1983; 6: 87–91.

61. Palumbo PJ, Melton LJ. Peripheral vascular disease and diabetes. In Diabetes in America. NIH Publication no. 85-1468. 1985; pp XV 1–21.

62. Moss AJ. Blood pressure in children with diabetes mellitus. Pediatrics 1962; 30: 932–6.

63. Kaas Ibsen K, Rotne H, Hougaard P. Blood pressure in children with diabetes mellitus. Acta Paediatr Scand 1983; 72: 191–6.

64. Cruickshanks KJ, Orchard TJ, Becker DJ. The cardiovascular risk profile of adolescents with insulin dependent diabetes mellitus. Diabetes Care 1985; 8: 118–24.

65. Tarn AC, Drury PL. Blood pressure in children, adolescents and young adults, with Type I (insulin-dependent) diabetes. Diabetologia 1986; 29: 276–81.

66. Mogensen CE, Christensen CK. Predicting diabetic nephropathy in insulin-dependent patients. New Engl J Med 1984; 311: 89–93.

67. Parving HH, Hommel E, Mathiesen E et al. Prevalence of microalbuminuria, arterial hypertension, retinopathy and neuropathy in patients with insulin dependent diabetes. Br Med J 1988; 296: 156–60.

68. Barrett-Connor E, Criqui MH, Klauber MR, Holdbrook M. Diabetes and hypertension in a community of older adults. Am J Epidemiol 1981; 113; 276–84.

69. Pan W-H, Cedres LB, Liu K et al. Relationship of clinical diabetes and asymptomatic hyperglycemia to risk of coronary heart disease mortality in men and women. Am J Epidemiol 1986; 123: 504–16.

70. Jarrett RJ, Keen H, McCartney M, Fuller JH, Hamilton PJS, Reid DD, Rose G. Glucose toler-ance and blood pressure in two population samples: their relation to diabetes mellitus and hypertension. Int J Epidemiol 1978; 7: 15–24.

71. Wilson PWF, Anderson KM, Kannel WB. Epidemiology of diabetes mellitus in the elderly: the Framingham Study. Am J Med 1986; 80 (suppl. 5A): 3–9.

72. Florey C du V, Uppal S, Lowy C. Relation between blood pressure, weight, and plasma sugar and serum insulin levels in school children aged 9–12 years in Westland, Holland. Br Med J 1976; 1: 1368–71.

73. Persky V, Dyer A, Stamler J, Shekelle RB, Schoenberger J, Wannamaker J, Upton M. The relationship between post-load plasma glucose and blood pressure at different resting heart rates. J Chron Dis 1979; 32: 263–8.

74. Cederholm J, Wibell L. Glucose intolerance in middle-aged subjects—a cause of hypertension? Acta Med Scand 1985; 217: 363–71.

75. Medalie JH, Papier CM, Goldbourt U, Herman JB. Major factors in the development of diabetes mellitus in 10 000 men. Arch Int Med 1975; 135: 811–17.

76. Fabre J, Balant LP, Dayer DG, Fox HM, Vernet AT. The kidney in maturity onset diabetes mellitus: a clinical study of 510 patients. Kidney Int 1982; 21: 730–8.

77. Keen H, Chlouverakis C, Fuller JH, Jarrett RJ. The concomitants of raised blood sugar: studies in newly-detected hyperglycaemics. Guy's Hosp Rep 1969; 118: 247–54.

78. Damsgaard EM, Mogensen CE. Microalbuminuria in elderly hyperglycaemic patients and controls. Diabet Med 1986; 3: 430–5.

79. Mogensen CE. Microalbuminuria predicts clinical proteinuria and early mortality in maturity-onset diabetes. New Engl J Med 1984; 310: 356–60.

80. Allawi J, Rao PV, Gilbert R et al. Microalbuminuria in non-insulin-dependent diabetes: higher frequency in Indian compared with Europid patients. Br Med J 1988; 296: 462–4.

64

Metabolic Control and Macrovascular Disease

Matti Uusitupa*, Kalevi Pyörälä† and Markku Laakso†

*Department of Clinical Nutrition and †Department of Medicine, Kuopio University Hospital, Kuopio, Finland

Both insulin dependent diabetes mellitus (IDDM) and non-insulin dependent diabetes mellitus (NIDDM) are known to increase the risk of atherosclerotic vascular disease (ASVD), manifesting as coronary heart disease (CHD), cerebrovascular disease and peripheral vascular disease. So far, however, the underlying mechanisms for the accelerated atherogenesis in diabetes have remained poorly understood. Although diabetes may change cardiovascular risk factor levels in an atherogenic direction, population-based prospective studies have repeatedly shown that only a small proportion of the excess of ASVD in diabetes can be explained by the effects of diabetes on the levels of these risk factors [1–3]. Thus, the excessive occurrence of ASVD in diabetic patients must be mainly caused by diabetes itself or factors related to it (see Chapter 63). It is, however, important to notice that the major cardiovascular risk factors—elevated serum cholesterol, elevated blood pressure and smoking—have the same impact on the risk of ASVD in diabetic subjects as in non-diabetic subjects, i.e. the risk of ASVD increases similarly with increasing risk factor levels in diabetic and non-diabetic subjects, but at every level of a risk factor diabetic subjects have a marked excess of ASVD.

Diabetes may also lead to another form of macrovascular disease besides ASVD—medial sclerosis of large and medium-size arteries, especially in the lower limbs. The pathogenesis and clinical significance of medial sclerosis is still obscure, but it may have some role in the development of ischemic end-organ lesions in diabetes (see Chapter 61). This review of metabolic control and macrovascular disease does not deal with this specific type of macrovascular disease. Diabetic heart muscle disease is another diabetic complication that may contribute to the occurrence and prognosis of cardiac events in diabetic patients [1, 4, 5]. The particularly high occurrence of cardiac failure in diabetes, which is not fully explained by the high frequency of CHD or hypertension in diabetic patients, is apparently caused by diabetic heart muscle disease. This heart muscle disorder may also influence the precipitation of symptoms of CHD and have an adverse effect on the prognosis of diabetics in connection with an acute myocardial infarction. The possibility, therefore, exists that a part of the excess morbidity and mortality of diabetic

International Textbook of Diabetes Mellitus. Edited by K.G.M.M. Alberti, R.A. DeFronzo, H. Keen and P. Zimmet

patients ascribed to CHD may be explained by a direct effect of diabetes on the heart muscle.

There is increasing evidence that hyperglycemia is causally associated with the development of microangiopathic complications of diabetes [6, 7]. Because hyperglycemia is the most characteristic biochemical abnormality in diabetes, and because clinical and prospective epidemiological studies indicate that diabetes is associated with a markedly increased risk for ASVD, it is logical to consider the possibility that an abnormally high blood glucose level may have a role in enhanced atherogenesis in diabetic patients, either through its direct effects on the biology of the arterial wall or indirectly through mechanisms that become operative with the development of hyperglycemia.

HYPERGLYCEMIA AND ATHEROSCLEROTIC VASCULAR DISEASE

Mechanisms

Effect of Hyperglycemia on the Biology of the Arterial Wall

Endothelial cell injury has been considered to be an initial step in the pathogenesis of atherosclerosis [8]. High concentrations of glucose have been shown to inhibit the replication of cultured human endothelial cells [9]. It can be hypothesized, therefore, that an abnormally high blood glucose level may hamper the repair of endothelial lesions caused by various factors, thus favouring the penetration of atherogenic substances into subendothelial layers of the arterial wall. Increased cellular concentrations of glucose and sorbitol in hyperglycemic conditions have been shown to stimulate proliferation of human fibroblasts and smooth muscle cells, thus giving another hypothetical explanation of accelerated atherosclerosis in diabetes [10, 11].

Insulin may be one of the factors promoting atherogenesis through its effects on the cellular components and biochemical phenomena in the arterial wall [12, 13]. Impairment of the repair of endothelial damage under hyperglycemic conditions may allow insulin to come into contact with arterial smooth muscle cells, and their proliferation and migration may be stimulated thereby. Furthermore, insulin has been shown to stimulate synthesis of cholesterol in smooth muscle cells and of other lipids in the arterial wall. Thus the combination of hyperglycemia and hyperinsulinemia that is common in both types of diabetes and in impaired glucose tolerance may contribute to the development of atherosclerosis.

Hyperglycemia may also be involved in the development of atherosclerosis through accelerated glycation of various tissue proteins [11, 14–16]. The glycation of arterial wall collagen may alter the elasticity of the arterial wall and make it more susceptible to hemodynamic trauma, which may lead to endothelial injury and initiate the processes mentioned above.

Abnormalities of endothelial cell function leading to enhanced thrombogenesis have been observed in diabetes [11, 15, 17, 18]. The endothelial cells produce von Willebrand factor (vWF), which is a part of the factor VIII complex and a cofactor promoting platelet adhesion. Plasma levels of vWF are elevated in diabetics with ASVD and also in those free from clinical ASVD. Diabetes may also reduce prostacyclin synthesis by endothelial cells. Although the above abnormalities are not clearly related to the actual blood glucose level, they indicate the occurrence of disturbances in endothelial cell function in diabetes (see also Chapters 54, 62).

Monocytes, which, like tissue macrophages, may become transformed into lipid-laden foam cells, have a central role in the early stages of atherosclerosis [8]. The possibility exists that hyperglycemia or diabetes may alter the adherence of monocytes to arterial endothelium or the chemotaxis of monocytes, but at present there are no consistent data on such disturbances of monocyte function in diabetes [15].

Abnormalities of Serum Lipids and Lipoproteins in Relation to Hyperglycemia

Diabetes is associated with various abnormalities of serum lipids [2, 11, 15, 19–22]; because many of these abnormalities are related to metabolic control, they are briefly discussed here. In patients with IDDM adequately treated with insulin, levels of serum total cholesterol and low-density lipoprotein (LDL) cholesterol are quite normal, as are total and very low-density lipoprotein (VLDL) triglycerides, and high-density lipoprotein (HDL) cholesterol (which may protect against atherosclerosis) is frequently even elevated. However, in patients with IDDM who are in poor metabolic control and in patients with IDDM who have diabetic nephropathy, levels of serum total and LDL cholesterol, and of total and VLDL triglycerides, tend to be elevated whereas HDL cholesterol is lowered. In patients with NIDDM, levels of serum total and LDL cholesterol are either normal or slightly elevated, and serum total and VLDL triglycerides and VLDL cholesterol are commonly elevated; in contrast, HDL cholesterol is lower than normal. In addition, there are changes in the composition of lipoproteins, reflecting an increase in VLDL remnant production. Furthermore, synthesis of cholesterol-rich apolipoprotein E (apo-E) containing β-VLDL particles may be increased. Both VLDL remnants and β-VLDL particles have been suggested to be highly atherogenic through their stimulating effect on the formation of foam cells. Although these lipid abnormalities may reflect fundamental disturbances of lipid metabolism in NIDDM, some of them tend to be related to the degree of hyperglycemia, being most marked in poor glycemic control. Glycation of apolipoprotein B, the major apolipoprotein of LDL, may occur in diabetes to an extent that alters the catabolism of LDL [15, 16, 23, 24]. Other apolipoproteins also have been found to become glycated in the hyperglycemic diabetic patients [15, 16, 25]. Besides abnormalities in the levels and metabolism of lipoproteins and in the structure of apolipoproteins, alterations of fatty acid metabolism have been observed in diabetes [15]. An improvement in diabetic control enhances the conversion of linoleic acid to arachidonic acid, a precursor of prostanoids [26]. Thus, multiple abnormalities of lipid metabolism are associated with the glycemic control of diabetes and it is likely that these abnormalities contribute to enhanced atherogenesis in diabetic subjects.

Abnormalities of Hemostasis in Relation to Hyperglycemia

Several abnormalities of hemostasis occur in diabetes [2, 11, 15, 17, 18, 27]. Some of these abnormalities, associated with the function of endothelial cells, have already been mentioned. Hemostatic abnormalities may contribute to the precipitation of acute events of ASVD by accelerating thrombus formation, but they may also contribute more primarily to the atherosclerotic process per se. Increased adhesiveness and aggregation of platelets in vitro have been observed in diabetes and this may be of importance in the initiation of atherosclerotic lesions. The enhanced aggregation of platelets may be due to an increased synthesis of prostaglandins E_2 and F_2 and thromboxanes A_2 and B_2, and to a decreased production of prostacyclin which is an antiaggregating factor. Increased plasma levels of β-thromboglobulin and platelet factor 4, and decreased platelet survival have been reported in diabetics free from clinical ASVD, indicating indirectly that platelet aggregation and release reactions are increased in diabetes.

Information concerning the level of plasma fluid-phase clotting factors in diabetes is still conflicting, but increased plasma levels of factors V, VII and VIII have been observed in some studies. Elevated plasma fibrinogen concentration appears to be the most consistent finding among clotting factor abnormalities, and fibrinogen turnover has been found to be increased in diabetes. Furthermore, glycation of fibrinogen and antithrombin III has been suggested to lead to altered coagulation and a hypercoagulable state. Fibrinogen turnover and glycation tend to become normalized on control of hyperglycemia, unlike most other hemostatic abnormalities observed in diabetes.

There is some evidence that the fibrinolytic system may also be disturbed in diabetes, and production of plasminogen activator by the vein endothelium in response to venous occlusion has been reported to be decreased in IDDM and NIDDM. However, data concerning whole-blood fibrinolytic activity is contradictory, but several studies using euglobulin lysis time have shown a decreased fibrinolytic activity in diabetics as compared with non-diabetics. There is some evidence suggesting that both a decreased fibrinolytic activity [28] and an increased level of fibrinogen at baseline may predict increased cardiovascular morbidity and mortality in diabetic patients [29].

Blood Glucose and Hypertension

In epidemiological studies on non-diabetic subjects a positive relationship has been found between blood glucose and blood pressure levels over the whole range of measurement [30]. In addition, blood pressure levels and the prevalence of hypertension are higher in diabetic than in non-diabetic subjects (see Chapter 67). This is especially true with respect to patients with NIDDM and subjects with impaired glucose tolerance [1, 2, 31, 32]. In IDDM the appearance of elevated blood pressure is closely associated with the development of diabetic nephropathy, but a small elevation in blood pressure may occur in young patients with IDDM free from nephropathy [33]. One might argue therefore that the excess risk of ASVD in subjects with diabetes could be mediated through the elevated blood pressure. However, the excessive occurrence of ASVD is present also in normotensive diabetics and the risk of ASVD increases with increasing blood pressure levels in a similar manner in diabetic and non-diabetic subjects. Thus, it is unlikely that the relationship between blood glucose and blood pressure could be of central importance in explaining the susceptibility of diabetics for ASVD.

Hyperglycemia in Relation to ASVD in Non-Diabetic Subjects

The relationship between elevated blood glucose in an oral glucose tolerance test and ASVD in subjects without manifest diabetes was originally observed in two population studies, the Bedford Study [34] from the UK and the Tecumseh Study [35] from the USA, based on cross-sectional data. Subsequent follow-up of these two study populations demonstrated an association between blood glucose level and CHD mortality. In the Bedford Study, the 10-year CHD mortality was higher both in men and women with 'borderline' diabetes than in normoglycemic subjects of the same sex, the relative excess of CHD mortality associated with 'borderline' diabetes being more marked in women than in men [36]. In the 18-year follow-up of the Tecumseh Study population, blood glucose showed a positive association with CHD mortality in men but not in women [37]. In multivariate analysis, controlling for the effect of other risk factors, this association still remained statistically significant. In the Framingham Study based on the 16-year follow-up [38], the casual blood glucose level showed a non-linear, positive association with CHD incidence, with a marked increase in the incidence at blood glucose levels above 120 mg/dl. In the multivariate analyses of the Framingham Study

data, 'glucose intolerance' including also cases with previous diabetes, was found to be associated with the incidence of CHD independently of other risk factors [39]. In nine of the studies included in the International Collaborative Group report on asymptomatic hyperglycemia and CHD [40], the relationship between blood glucose level and CHD mortality was analyzed on the basis of postload blood glucose values. Cardiovascular and CHD mortality rates at the uppermost end of the blood glucose distribution curve (highest 2–10%) were twice as high or more than in lower blood glucose values in five of the nine studies. In multivariate analyses, however, with one single exception, blood glucose levels showed no predictive value with respect to cardiovascular or CHD death independent of other risk factors.

Follow-up results based on longer follow-up periods have been published from four studies included in the International Collaborative Group report. These are the Whitehall Study [41, 42], the Paris Prospective Study [43], the Helsinki Policemen Study [44], and the Chicago Heart Association Detection Project in Industry [45]. All four studies showed a non-linear relationship between fasting or postload blood glucose level and CHD mortality, with a marked increase in CHD mortality at the upper end of the distribution. The Whitehall Study [41, 42] and the Paris Prospective Study [43] showed that impaired glucose tolerance representing this upper end of the blood glucose distribution curve was associated with an excess of CHD deaths almost similar to that found in clinically manifest diabetes. After controlling for the effects of other risk factors, however, blood glucose variables did not show a significant independent relationship to CHD mortality in the Whitehall Study, the Paris Prospective Study and the Helsinki Policemen Study [41, 43, 44] (Figure 1). In the Chicago Heart Association Detection Project in Industry, asymptomatic hyperglycemia (1-hour postload plasma glucose ≥ 200 mg/dl) had, in univariate analyses adjusting for age, a significant association to 9-year CHD mortality both in men and women; after further adjustment for other risk factors, the excess risk associated with hyperglycemia persisted only in women [45].

Two other recent population-based studies have also shown an association between CHD mortality and blood glucose level. Barrett-

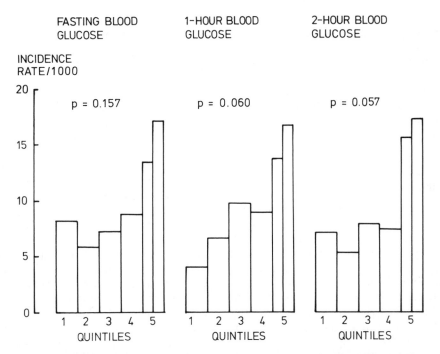

Figure 1 A non-linear association between the fasting, 1 and 2 hour blood glucose values after oral glucose load and the age-adjusted 9.5-year incidence of 'hard criteria' coronary heart disease (CHD death or non-fatal myocardial infarction) among 982 CHD-free Helsinki policemen. The top quintile for each blood glucose variable has been divided into two deciles. *P* values give the statistical significance for the overall association between blood glucose variables and CHD incidence based on likelihood statistics (reproduced from reference 44, with permission of the authors and *Acta Medica Scandinavica*)

Connor et al [46] reported that in the Rancho Bernardo Study this association was linear and independent of other risk factors in men, but in women only a non-significant, non-linear association was found on univariate analysis. In a 9-year follow-up of the cohort of Japanese ancestry living in Hawaii, asymptomatic hyperglycemia (1-hour postload serum glucose ⩾ 225 mg/dl) showed an independent association with CHD mortality [47]. In the Puerto Rico Heart Health Program population, however, casual blood glucose level was not related to CHD mortality [48].

Data concerning the association between fasting and postload blood glucose levels and cerebrovascular or peripheral vascular disease are scanty. In the Framingham Study population, casual blood glucose levels showed a curvilinear relationship to the incidence of atherothrombotic brain infarction, with a more marked increase in incidence at the upper end of the blood glucose distribution; however, previously diagnosed diabetics were included in the

analysis [39]. In the 10-year follow-up of the Whitehall Study population, the 2-hour postload blood glucose level exceeding 96 mg/dl was significantly predictive of stroke mortality independent of blood pressure and age [49]. In the Framingham Study a curvilinear relationship was also observed between casual blood glucose level and, peripheral vascular disease [39]; on the other hand, in the Israel Ischemic Heart Disease Study, the occurrence of peripheral vascular disease predicted the future development of diabetes, giving in a reverse way an indication that there is a relationship between impaired glucose tolerance and the presence of peripheral vascular disease [50].

To summarize, most of the published prospective studies on non-diabetic subjects indicate that there appears to be a positive non-linear association between the risk for ASVD and blood glucose level, with a sharp increase in cardiovascular and CHD mortality at 2-hour postload blood glucose levels from about 110 mg/dl to 200 mg/dl (6.1–11.1 mmol/l), i.e. at blood glucose levels much below those currently used for the diagnosis of diabetes. However, in multivariate analyses this association has not been independent of other risk factors in most of these studies, suggesting that the increased risk is mainly mediated through other factors associated with early disturbances of glucose metabolism, e.g. abnormalities in lipid and lipoprotein metabolism and elevated blood pressure.

Hyperglycemia in Relation to ASVD in Diabetic Subjects

Population-based prospective studies concerning the relationship between blood glucose level and ASVD suggest that, above a certain threshold level, hyperglycemia starts to enhance atherogenesis; this occurs either through its direct effects on the biology of the arterial wall or indirectly through other mechanisms associated closely with impaired glucose tolerance or early stages of diabetes, such as the appearance of abnormalities in lipid and lipoprotein metabolism or other disturbances discussed above. If hyperglycemia as such is causally associated with atherosclerosis, one would anticipate that among diabetic patients there would be a strong correlation between the degree of hyperglycemia and the extent of atherosclerosis or the occurrence of various manifestations of ASVD. The possibility exists, however, that a relatively small elevation of blood glucose level—below the current diagnostic criteria for the diagnosis of diabetes—may lead to enhanced atherogenesis (see above), and thus the relationship between blood glucose within the diabetic range and the occurrence of ASVD may become obscured. Elucidation of the possible relationship between the degree of hyperglycemia and the risk of ASVD in diabetes is extremely complex, for several reasons. First, characterization of the degree of hyperglycemia on the basis of a cross-sectional study or short-term assessment may not be relevant with respect to the average long-term hyperglycemia. Second, the duration of hyperglycemia exceeding a certain threshold level may be more important than the actual degree of hyperglycemia. Furthermore, if the duration of hyperglycemia is important, it may be impossible to separate the direct effect of hyperglycemia on the ASVD risk from the effects of other risk factors which become abnormal with the development of hyperglycemia. On the other hand, hyperglycemia may also become more severe with increasing duration of diabetes.

Degree of Hyperglycemia

Surprisingly few studies have attempted to elucidate the association between the degree of hyperglycemia and ASVD in diabetic patients. Most of them are, in addition, cross-sectional studies, and the assessment of glycemic control has usually been based on one single measurement of blood glucose or glycated HbA_1.

In the World Health Organization (WHO) Multinational Study of Vascular Disease in Diabetes [51], the relationship between fasting plasma glucose and the prevalence of different manifestations of ASVD was assessed in a pooled population of 3583 diabetic patients from nine different populations. Plasma glucose failed to show any association with the prevalence of major Q-wave electrocardiographic changes in the pooled population or in any of the nine populations. In our own study on 133 newly diagnosed middle-aged patients with NIDDM and 144 control subjects, fasting blood glucose levels measured at diagnosis were not related to the prevalence of CHD [52], nor was there any significant relationship between metabolic control and the appearance of CHD during the 5-year follow-up of these diabetic patients [53]. In analysis combining diabetic and non-diabetic subjects, diabetes itself had an independent association with the incidence of CHD [53]. In another cross-sectional study on 510 middle-aged patients with previously diagnosed NIDDM we did not observe any definite relationship between fasting blood glucose level and the prevalence of CHD [54]. Similarly, in a cross-sectional study carried out in Japan no relationship was found between blood glucose level and the occurrence of CHD in diabetic patients [55].

The prevalence of stroke in the WHO Multinational Study was almost twice as high in patients with plasma glucose levels over 250 mg/dl as in patients with levels below 150 mg/dl [51]. Furthermore, insulin-treated patients who had, on average, higher plasma glucose levels than those treated with diet only or with oral drugs, showed a prevalence of previous stroke twice that in diabetics receiving other types of treatment. However, in three other studies no significant relationship was found between the degree of hyperglycemia and the occurrence of cerebrovascular disease assessed on the basis of a history of previous stroke [54, 55] or by the occurrence of carotid artery occlusive disease diagnosed by oculo-plethysmography and phonoangiography [56].

Fasting plasma glucose in the WHO Multi-national Study was also higher in diabetics with leg artery disease (intermittent claudication, amputation) than in those without it [51]. The amputation frequency was roughly three times higher in patients with plasma glucose exceeding 250 mg/dl than in those with plasma glucose levels below 150 mg/dl. In some other studies, however, no significant relationship was observed between the occurrence of claudication and blood glucose level [53, 54].

The prevalence of diabetic complications in relation to different factors, including blood glucose and glycated hemoglobin levels, was examined in a cross-sectional study on 1084 Caucasoid diabetics—179 patients with IDDM and 905 patients with NIDDM—in rural Western Australia. In the first report from this study [57], in patients with IDDM the casual plasma glucose showed no definite relationship to the occurrence of ASVD. In contrast, in patients with NIDDM significant associations were found between plasma glucose level and CHD, and glycated hemaglobin level and peripheral vascular disease. In a later analysis combining both types of diabetics [58], macrovascular disease (defined as CHD, cerebrovascular disease or peripheral vascular disease) showed a significant association with diabetic control assessed by plasma glucose or glycated hemo-globin levels. This association was independent of age, plasma creatinine, systolic blood pressure, plasma cholesterol and HDL cholesterol level.

Duration of Hyperglycemia

The impact of duration of diabetes on the development of ASVD differs greatly in IDDM and in NIDDM; furthermore, various clinical manifestations of ASVD seem to have a different association with the duration of diabetes. In IDDM, which usually has its onset before the age of 30 years, ASVD can be considered as a late complication. In contrast, in NIDDM which is commonly preceded by a long period of impaired glucose tolerance or asymptomatic

hyperglycemia, ASVD and in particular CHD is a common finding at the diagnosis of the disease [1–3, 5, 53]. Furthermore, prospective studies of newly diagnosed and previously diagnosed patients with NIDDM have shown that the future risk of CHD in both groups of diabetics is almost equal [1–3]. These findings support the view, emphasized by Jarrett [59], that the dur-ation of NIDDM from its diagnosis is not clearly related to the risk of CHD. Duration of diabetes had no significant relationship to major Q-wave abnormalities in the ECG in the pooled data from the nine populations of the WHO study, although a weak but significant positive relation-ship was observed in diabetics in Tokyo and New Delhi [51]; nor did the duration of diabetes show any relationship to the prevalence of CHD in previously diagnosed patients with NIDDM in East Finland [54]. However, in the 5-year follow-up of patients with newly diagnosed NIDDM, the cumulative occurrence of CHD events gave some suggestion of a relationship between the duration of the disease and the risk of CHD [53]. A weak but significant relationship between the prevalence of macrovascular disease and the duration or age at onset of diabetes was reported in the study from Western Australia, including both types of diabetics. However, age was the most important time-related variable increasing the occurrence of macrovascular disease [58].

Autopsy and coronary angiographic studies give direct information about the severity of coronary atherosclerotic changes. Unfor-tunately, only a few studies, comprising mainly patients with NIDDM, have dealt with the severity of atherosclerosis in relation to the duration of diabetes. In a large autopsy study coordinated by the WHO, diabetics with more than 10 years' duration of the disease generally showed more extensive coronary atherosclerosis than those who had had diabetes for a shorter time [60, 61], but in two other studies no relationship was observed between the severity of atherosclerosis in coronary arteries and the duration of diabetes [62, 63]. In a coronary angiographic study on patients with sympto-matic coronary heart disease, the degree of coronary atherosclerosis was found to be similar in patients with impaired glucose tolerance and overt diabetes; this finding indirectly suggests the absence of a relationship between the extent of coronary atherosclerosis and duration of hyperglycemia [64]. In another coronary angiographic study on diabetic patients with symptomatic CHD, however, three-vessel disease appeared to be more common in patients with diabetes for 10 or more years than in those with a recent diagnosis of diabetes [65].

Although the occurrence of CHD seems to be only weakly related to the duration of diabetes, the occurrence of the two other major macrovascular complications—cerebrovascular disease and peripheral vascular disease—appears to be more consistently associated with a long duration of diabetes. In the WHO study the duration of diabetes was significantly longer in diabetics with previous stroke than in diabetics without stroke [51]. Similarly, an independent association between the duration of diabetes and the frequency of cerebrovascular disease was reported by Ishihara et al [55]. However, some other studies have failed to show an association between cerebrovascular disease and the duration of diabetes [54, 56]. In the WHO study the duration of diabetes was significantly longer in diabetics with 'leg vascular disease' (intermittent claudication or amputation) than in those without these manifestations of ASVD [51]. Several other studies have also shown that the duration of diabetes has a positive correlation with the occurrence of peripheral vascular disease [53, 57, 66–69].

Other Aspects Related to Hyperglycemia

On the basis of the Joslin Clinic's patient series, Krolewski et al [70] reported recently on the risk of premature CHD in a cohort of 292 patients with IDDM followed up for 20–40 years. CHD mortality was similarly increased in diabetics of both sexes, markedly exceeding that seen in non-diabetic subjects in the Framingham Study. CHD mortality was most increased in the diabetics with antecedent nephropathy, but the diabetics without nephropathy also showed a definitely increased CHD mortality compared with non-diabetic subjects from the Framingham Study population. Age at onset of IDDM did not contribute to the risk of premature CHD. The authors concluded that this finding is compatible with the hypothesis that the diabetic state acts mainly by accelerating progression of early atherosclerotic lesions that occur even in the absence of diabetes. Thus diabetes may act

as a promoter of atherosclerosis rather than as its initiator.

In accordance with the finding of Krolewski et al [70], Jensen et al [71], Winocour et al [72] and Borch-Johnsen and Kreiner [73] reported a striking increase in the occurrence of CHD in patients with IDDM who develop diabetic nephropathy, compared with those who remain free from nephropathy. The development of hypertension and the appearance of multiple lipid and lipoprotein abnormalities at early stages of diabetic nephropathy evidently contribute to this markedly increased risk of ASVD in patients with this diabetic complication, but other mechanisms may also be involved. Krolewski et al [70] suggested that diabetic nephropathy may act as a particularly powerful promoter of atherosclerosis and may influence mainly the progression of pre-existing atherosclerotic vascular lesions, but may have little or no effect on the initiation of the atherosclerotic process.

A recent study showed that a low glucose assimilation index, reflecting insulin insensitivity, was associated with death from vascular disease or with progression of atherosclerotic disease in an 18-year follow-up study of patients with IDDM [74].

Intervention Studies on the Relationship of Metabolic Control of Diabetes to ASVD

The purpose of the long-term treatment of diabetes is the prevention of late complications. There is increasing evidence from clinical trials concerning intensified insulin therapy in IDDM, that strict metabolic control may delay the appearance of microangiopathic complications [7]. However, with regard to the impact of the correction of hyperglycemia on the prevention of ASVD in diabetics, there is so far no direct proof supporting the view that strict metabolic control would delay or prevent the appearance of ASVD. The University Group Diabetes Program (UGDP) trial in the 1970s [75–80] raised concern about the possible contribution of different hypoglycemic drugs to the excessive cardiovascular mortality and morbidity in diabetic patients. This trial was designed to assess the efficacy of four different hypoglycemic drug treatments—tolbutamide, phenformin, standard-dose insulin, and variable-dose insulin—in the prevention of cardiovascular complications of NIDDM in comparison to placebo treatment. Increased cardiovascular mortality was observed in groups treated with tolbutamide and phenformin. These observations caused the discontinuation of the trial with these drugs, because of a suspicion of cardiovascular toxicity. The results of the UGDP trial subsequently have been the subject of criticism in many reviews, most recently by Fuller [81]. As indicated in that review, later studies carried out in patient groups with various degrees of glucose intolerance have not confirmed the increased cardiovascular morbidity and mortality associated with the use of oral antidiabetic agents. Despite its limitations, the UGDP trial so far remains the only long-term study attempting to resolve the effects of hypoglycemic agents on vascular complications in patients with NIDDM. The final results of this study concerning insulin therapy were published in 1982 [80]. The patients had been allocated to three groups: placebo (diet), standard dose of insulin and variable dose of insulin, each group consisting of about 200 patients with mild NIDDM. During the follow-up period, which in some cases was over 10 years, the best metabolic control was achieved by variable-dose insulin treatment. After 10 years the mean fasting blood glucose in the placebo group was 165 mg/dl, in the standard-dose insulin treatment group 174 mg/dl, and in the variable-dose insulin treatment group 120 mg/dl. All groups were, on average, in a reasonable state of metabolic control, compared with that seen in normal clinical practice. Despite the better control in the variable-dose insulin treatment group, no differences were found between the groups in cardiovascular mortality or morbidity.

Because the results of the UGDP trial remain controversial concerning the safety of oral antidiabetic drugs and the value of metabolic control in terms of prognosis in NIDDM, new large-scale studies attempting to resolve these controversies are needed. The UK Prospective Study now in progress may diminish uncertainty in this respect [82, 83]. The study includes patients with NIDDM who, after a 3-month introductory period on diet, are randomly allocated to diet therapy alone, sulfonylurea therapy (chlorpropamide or glibenclamide) or insulin therapy, with the exception of obese patients who are treated with metformin. The study design may give an opportunity to compare the different

treatment groups in terms of the effect of metabolic control on future ASVD, as after the first trial year patients on insulin or oral sulfonylurea drugs had a mean fasting plasma glucose level about 2.5 mmol/l (45 mg/dl) lower than that of patients on diet only. At this point in the trial the mean fasting plasma glucose levels were 6.8 mmol/l (122 mg/dl) in the insulin-treated group, 6.7 mmol/l (121 mg/dl) in the sulfonylurea-treated group and 9.3 mmol/l (167 mg/dl) in the diet-treated group.

The Diabetes Control and Complications Trial [84] is a multicenter, randomized clinical study in progress in the USA. It is designed to determine whether, in patients with IDDM, an intensive treatment regimen, accomplished with subcutaneous insulin infusion or multiple daily injections of insulin and aiming at maintaining blood glucose concentrations as close to normal as possible, will affect the appearance of early diabetic complications as compared with a regimen based on conventional insulin treatment. The results of a feasibility study for this trial indicated that the metabolic control achieved in the intensive treatment group during the first year was markedly better, in terms both of blood glucose profile and of glycated hemaglobin, than in the conventional insulin treatment group. At 12 months after entry the mean value for self-monitored seven-sample capillary blood glucose profile was 142 mg/dl in the experimental group and 232 mg/dl in the conventional treatment group. Although the primary aim of this trial is to investigate the importance of the maintenance of near-normoglycemia in the prevention of microangiopathic complications, it may also give valuable information concerning the relationship between the degree of hyperglycemia and the occurrence of ASVD.

Importance of Metabolic Control in the Prevention of ASVD in Diabetic Subjects

As indicated above, information from observational clinical and epidemiological studies concerning the relationship between metabolic control of diabetes and the occurrence of ASVD is scarce and difficult to interpret, and this applies even more to trial evidence—so far limited to one single trial, the UGDP trial. Pending more information from clinical and epidemiological studies and intervention trials in progress, the current assessment of the importance of the metabolic control of diabetes in the prevention of ASVD—including both primary and secondary prevention—has to be based on all available information as a whole, including results of studies on possible mechanisms by which hyperglycemia and associated metabolic and other disturbances may enhance atherogenesis and lead to clinical ASVD events.

An important finding emerging from clinical and epidemiological studies, which may be of central importance in consideration of the role of glycemic control in the prevention of ASVD in diabetic patients, is the apparent disparity in the glycemic 'threshold' above which the risks of microvascular disease and of ASVD begin to increase markedly. Information concerning the relationship of blood glucose levels and the risk of microvascular disease from several prospective studies uniformly support the hypothesis that a certain threshold of hyperglycemia is necessary before clinically significant diabetic microvascular disease occurs [6]. This threshold appears to approximate to a 2-hour blood glucose level of 200 mg/dl (11.1 mmol/l) in an oral glucose tolerance test or a fasting blood glucose level of 140 mg/dl (7.8 mmol/l). These blood glucose levels have, in fact, become the basis of the criteria recommended for the diagnosis of diabetes by the National Diabetes Data Group and the Expert Committee of the World Health Organization. Although the data from prospective studies concerning the relationship of blood glucose levels and the risk of ASVD are less uniform, interpreted in aggregate those data indicate that the glycemic threshold above which the risk of ASVD begins to increase sharply is at a much lower level than the threshold identified for microvascular disease. In terms of 2-hour blood glucose levels in an oral glucose tolerance test, the threshold above which the risk of ASVD begins to increase appears to be approximately 110 mg/dl (6.1 mmol/l). However, it should be taken into account that these observations concerning the threshold blood glucose levels are based on single measurements. An average blood glucose level over a diurnal blood glucose profile would be a better estimate of the degree of hyperglycemia.

Another point relevant in this context is the apparent disparity between the two main types of diabetes—IDDM and NIDDM—with respect to the extent of metabolic and other abnormalities associated with hyperglycemia. Although

it is an oversimplification, it may be argued that in IDDM, if normoglycemia or near-normoglycemia is achieved by careful insulin treatment, metabolic and other abnormalities concomitant with hyperglycemia will also become controlled. In NIDDM the situation appears to be different: in this type of diabetes a complex cluster of multiple metabolic and other abnormalities associated with hyperglycemia—including abnormalities in lipid and lipoprotein metabolism, elevation of blood pressure, hyperinsulinemia/insulin resistance and hemostatic abnormalities—emerges in the preclinical, often long-lasting phase of impaired glucose tolerance preceding the clinical diagnosis of NIDDM. On the other hand, in this type of diabetes some of the metabolic abnormalities, e.g. abnormalities in lipid and lipoprotein metabolism, are not always improved when hyperglycemia is corrected.

A third point relevant to the importance of metabolic control of diabetes in the prevention of ASVD in diabetic patients, is that made recently by the Joslin Clinic group of investigators [70]—the possibility that the diabetic state may act mainly as a promoter of the progression of already existing atherosclerotic lesions rather than as their initiator. In Western populations living in an 'atherogenic milieu', mainly determined by the typical diet and lifestyle of these populations, early atherosclerotic lesions in the coronary arteries of non-diabetic subjects have already begun to appear in men, on average, by the end of the second decade of life and in women about 10 years later [60]. There is a great interindividual variation in the appearance and progression of these lesions, but in middle age the majority of subjects in these populations already have clear-cut atherosclerotic lesions in the coronary arteries and in other parts of the arterial system, and in many subjects complicated stenosing lesions are present, setting the stage for subsequent clinical ASVD events. Seen against this background, IDDM which usually develops in childhood or young adult life would lead to an acceleration of the progression of atherosclerotic lesions in subjects who are otherwise prone to develop them. This would explain why patients with IDDM have an increased risk of premature ASVD, even in the absence of diabetic nephropathy which is accompanied with a particularly marked enhancement of the risk of ASVD through several mechanisms. Nevertheless, it should be noted that studies on the biology of the arterial wall have suggested mechanisms by which hyperglycemia could participate in the initial steps of the development of atherosclerotic lesions.

NIDDM usually becomes clinically manifest in middle age or later, at the time when a large proportion of subjects in Western countries, even without the additional effect of diabetes, already have advanced atherosclerotic lesions in their coronary and other arteries. As stated above, in this type of diabetes and in its precursor stage, impaired glucose tolerance, hyperglycemia is associated with a complex cluster of multiple metabolic and other abnormalities, which have a powerful capacity to enhance the progression of atherosclerotic arterial lesions and to precipitate clinical ASVD events. This may explain the puzzling finding that patients with newly diagnosed NIDDM have almost the same prevalence of CHD as patients with a longer duration of diagnosed NIDDM. The finding that the appearance of cerebrovascular disease and peripheral vascular disease are more clearly related to the duration of clinically diagnosed NIDDM than is the appearance of CHD, may be related to two issues: first, these manifestations of ASVD occur at a later age than CHD in non-diabetic subjects and thus there is a longer time span during which the accelerating effect of diabetes on their development may become evident; second, there may be dissimilarities between the relative importance of different factors accelerating the development of atherosclerotic lesions in the cerebral and peripheral arteries and in the coronary arteries.

The foregoing emphasizes the view that good metabolic control of a diabetic patient has to embrace more than merely the control of hyperglycemia in order to use all possible means of prevention of ASVD. With the aim of lowering serum cholesterol, the dietary recommendations to diabetics have been reconsidered [85, 86]; these guidelines are in accordance with the general guidelines for serum cholesterol lowering defined by the WHO Expert Committee on the Prevention of Coronary Heart Disease [87]. Thus, more emphasis is given in the diabetic diet on the reduction of dietary total and saturated fat, with replacement of saturated fat by unsaturated fat, as appropriate with respect to dietary fatty acid composition of the local food, reduction of dietary cholesterol to below 300 mg per day on average, and an increased intake of complex carbohydrate and fibre. Control of other major risk factors—elevated blood pressure and smoking—is also of great importance in a comprehensive approach to the prevention of ASVD in diabetic patients.

What, then, is the importance of correction of hyperglycemia in the prevention of ASVD in diabetic patients? Because hyperglycemia, both in IDDM and in NIDDM, is associated with several metabolic and physiologic abnormalities that enhance atherogenesis or may precipitate ASVD events, and as these abnormalities are (in part at least) reversible by the correction of hyperglycemia, there are good reasons to try to achieve a glycemic control which is as near normoglycemia as possible with respect to both primary and secondary prevention of ASVD. This goal is of central importance in the treatment of young patients with IDDM with respect also to the prevention of microvascular disease; the latter is, in turn, important with respect to the prevention of ASVD, because the appearance of diabetic nephropathy is associated with a marked increase in the occurrence of ASVD. With NIDDM the situation is different, because many patients already have clinical manifestations of ASVD at the time of diagnosis of diabetes. In patients with NIDDM, good control of hyperglycemia also tends to correct associated metabolic abnormalities to some extent; however, in this type of diabetes, which is usually associated with obesity, weight reduction and other measures assisting in the control of associated metabolic abnormalities are particularly important. As increased atherogenesis has already started to occur in the preclinical, usually undiagnosed, phase of NIDDM, one of the main goals of future research must be the development of better methods for the identification of those individuals who have the genetically determined trait for NIDDM and who thus are at increased risk of developing this type of diabetes and concomitant premature ASVD. Prevention of the advent of diabetes by avoidance of obesity (and possibly by other measures) and—if this is not successful—early correction of hyperglycemia and associated metabolic and other abnormalities, might then lead to improved prospects of prevention of ASVD in subjects who are at risk of NIDDM or are in its early stages.

REFERENCES

1. Pyörälä K, Laakso M. Macrovascular disease in diabetes mellitus. In Mann JI, Pyörälä K, Teuscher A (eds) Diabetes in epidemiological perspective. Edinburgh: Churchill Livingstone, 1983: pp 248–64.

2. Pyörälä K, Laakso M, Uusitupa M. Diabetes and atherosclerosis: an epidemiologic view. Diabetes Metab Rev 1987; 3: 463–524.

3. Jarrett RJ. The epidemiology of coronary heart disease and related factors in the context of diabetes mellitus and impaired glucose tolerance. In Jarrett RJ (ed.) Diabetes and heart disease. Amsterdam: Elsevier, 1984: pp 1–23.

4. Kannel WB, Hjortland M, Castelli WP. Role of diabetes in congestive heart failure. Am J Cardiol 1974; 34: 29–34.

5. Uusitupa M, Siitonen O, Aro A, Pyörälä K. Prevalence of coronary heart disease, left ventricular failure and hypertension in middle-aged, newly diagnosed type 2 (non-insulin-dependent) diabetic subjects. Diabetologia 1985; 28: 22–7.

6. Jarrett RJ. Microvascular disease in diabetes mellitus. In Mann JI, Pyörälä K, Teuscher A (eds) Diabetes in epidemiological perspective. Edinburgh: Churchill Livingstone, 1983: pp 248–64.

7. Hanssen KF, Dahl-Jørgensen K, Lauritzen T, Feld-Rasmussen B, Brinchmann-Hansen O, Deckert T. Diabetic control and microvascular complications: the near normoglycaemia experience. Diabetologia 1986; 29: 677–84.

8. Ross R. The pathogenesis of atherosclerosis—an update. New Engl J Med 1986; 314: 488–500.

9. Stout RW. Glucose inhibits replication of cultured human endothelial cells. Diabetologia 1982; 23: 436–9.

10. Turner JL, Bierman EL. Effects of glucose and sorbitol on proliferation of cultured human fibroblasts and arterial smooth muscle cells. Diabetes 1978; 27: 583–8.

11. Ganda OP. Pathogenesis of macrovascular disease including the influence of lipids. In Joslin's diabetes mellitus, 12th edn. Philadelphia: Lea & Febiger, 1985: pp 217–50.

12. Stout RW. The role of insulin in atherosclerosis in diabetics and non-diabetics. Diabetes 1983; 30 (suppl. 2): 54–7.

13. Stout RW. Insulin and atheroma—an update. Lancet 1987; i: 1077–9.

14. Kennedy L, Baynes JW. Non-enzymatic glucosylation and the chronic complications of diabetes: an overview. Diabetologia 1984; 26: 93–8.

15. Chait A, Bierman EL, Brunzell JD. Diabetic macroangiopathy. In Alberti KGMM, Krall LP (eds) Diabetes annual 1. Amsterdam: Elsevier, 1985: pp 323–48.

16. Peterson CM, Formby B. Glucosylated proteins. In Alberti KGMM, Krall LP (eds) Diabetes annual 2. Amsterdam: Elsevier, 1986: pp 137–55.

17. Colwell JA, Winocour PD, Lopes-Virella M, Halushka PV. New concepts about the pathogenesis of atherosclerosis in diabetes mellitus. Am J Med 1983; 75 (suppl. 58): 67–80.

18. Colwell J, Winocour PD, Halushka PV. Do platelets have anything to do with diabetic microangiopathic disease? Diabetes 1983; 32 (suppl. 2): 14–19.

19. Saudek CD, Eder HA. Lipid metabolism in diabetes mellitus. Am J Med 1979; 66: 843–53.

20. Goldberg RG. Lipid disorders in diabetes. Diabetes Care 1981; 4: 561–72.

21. Nikkilä EA. Plasma lipid and lipoprotein abnormalities in diabetes. In Jarrett RJ (ed.) Diabetes and heart disease. Amsterdam: Elsevier, 1984: pp 134–67.

22. Brunzell YD, Chait A, Bierman EL. Plasma lipoproteins in human diabetes mellitus. In Alberti KGMM, Krall LP (eds) Diabetes annual 1. Amsterdam: Elsevier, 1985: pp 463–89.

23. Witztum JL, Mahoney EM, Branks MJ, Fischer M, Elam R, Steinberg D. Nonenzymatic glucosylation of low-density lipoproteins alters its biological activity. Diabetes 1982; 31: 283–91.

24. Steinbrecher UP, Witztum JL. Glucosylation of low-density lipoproteins to an extent comparable to that seen in diabetes slows their catabolism. Diabetes 1984; 33: 130–4.

25. Curtiss LK, Witztum JL. Plasma apolipoproteins AI, AII, B, CI and E are glycosylated in hyperglycemic diabetic subjects. Diabetes 1985; 34: 452–61.

26. Tilvis RS, Helve E, Miettinen TM. Improvement of diabetic control by continuous subcutaneous insulin infusion therapy changes fatty acid composition of serum lipids and erythrocytes in Type 1 (insulin-dependent) diabetes. Diabetologia 1986; 29: 690–4.

27. Greaves M, Preston FE. Haemostatic abnormalities in diabetics. In Jarrett RJ (ed.) Diabetes and heart disease. Amsterdam: Elsevier, 1984: pp 45–80.

28. Meade TW, Chakrabarti R, Haines AP. Haemostatic function and cardiovascular deaths. Early results of the prospective study. Lancet 1980; i: 1050–4.

29. Schmechel H, Beikünfner P, Panzram G. Längsschnittuntersuchungen zur prognostischen Bedeutung des Plasmafibrinogens. Z Gesamte Inn Med 1984; 39: 453–7.

30. Jarrett RJ, Keen H, McCartney M, Fuller HJ, Hamilton PJS, Reid DD, Rose G. Glucose tolerance and blood pressure in two population samples: their relation to diabetes mellitus and hypertension. Int J Epidemiol 1978; 63: 54–64.

31. Drury PL. Diabetes and hypertension. Diabetologia 1983; 24: 1–9.

32. Christlieb AR. The hypertensions of diabetes. Diabetes Care 1982; 5: 50–8.

33. Tarn AC, Drury PL. Blood pressure in children, adolescents and young adults with Type 1 (insulin-dependent) diabetes. Diabetologia 1986; 29: 275–81.

34. Keen H, Rose G, Pyke DA, Boyns D, Chlouverakis C, Mistry S. Blood-sugar and arterial disease. Lancet 1965; ii: 505–8.

35. Ostrander LD, Francis T, Hayner NS, Kjelsberg MO, Epstein FH. The relationship of cardiovascular disease to hyperglycaemia. Ann Intern Med 1965; 62: 1188–98.

36. Jarrett RJ, McCartney P, Keen H, The Bedford Study: ten-year mortality rates in newly diagnosed diabetics, borderline diabetics and normoglycaemic controls and risk indices for coronary heart disease in borderline diabetics. Diabetologia 1982; 22: 79–84.

37. Butler WJ, Ostrander LD, Carman WJ, Lamphier DE. Mortality from coronary heart disease in the Tecumseh study. Long-term effect of diabetes mellitus, glucose tolerance and other risk factors. Am J Epidemiol 1985; 121: 541–47.

38. Framingham Study. An epidemiological investigation of cardiovascular disease (Section 26): some characteristics related to the incidence of cardiovascular disease and death—Framingham Study, 16-year follow-up. Washington, DC: US Government Printing Office, 1970.

39. Gordon T, Kannel WB. Predisposition to atherosclerosis in the head, heart and legs. The Framingham Study. JAMA 1972; 221: 661–6.

40. Stamler R, Stamler J (eds). Asymptomatic hyperglycaemia and coronary heart disease. A series of papers by the International Collaborative Group, based on studies on fifteen populations. J Chron Dis 1979; 32: 683–837.

41. Fuller JH, Shipley MJ, Rose G, Jarrett RJ, Keen H. Coronary-heart-disease and impaired glucose tolerance: the Whitehall Study. Lancet 1980; i: 1373–6.

42. Jarrett RJ, Shipley MJ. The Whitehall Study: comparative mortality rates and indices of risk in diabetics. Acta Endocrinol 1985; 110 (suppl. 272): 21–6.

43. Eschwège E, Ducimetière P, Thibult N, Richard JL, Claude JR, Rosselin GE. Coronary heart disease mortality in relation with diabetes, blood glucose and plasma insulin levels. The Paris prospective study, ten years later. Horm Metab Res (suppl. series) 1985; 15: 41–5.

44. Pyörälä K, Savolainen E, Kaukola S, Haapakoski J. Plasma insulin as coronary heart disease risk factor: relationship to other risk factors and predictive value during $9\frac{1}{2}$-year

45. Pan W-H, Cedres LB, Liu K et al. Relationship of clinical diabetes and asymptomatic hyperglycemia to risk of coronary heart disease mortality in men and women. Am J Epidemiol 1986; 123: 504–16.

46. Barrett-Connor E, Wingard DL, Criqui MH, Suarez L. Is borderline fasting hyperglycemia a risk factor for cardiovascular death? J Chron Dis 1984; 37: 773–9.

47. Yano K, Kagan A, McGee D, Rhoads GG. Glucose intolerance and nine-year mortality in Japanese men in Hawaii. Am J Med 1982; 72: 71–80.

48. Cruz-Vidal M, Garcia-Palmieri MR, Costas R, Sorlie PD, Havlik RJ. Abnormal blood glucose and coronary heart disease: the Puerto Rico Heart Health Program. Diabetes Care 1983; 6: 556–61.

49. Fuller JH, Shipley MJ, Rose G, Jarrett RJ, Keen H. Mortality from coronary heart disease and stroke in relation to degree of glycaemia: the Whitehall Study. Br Med J 1983; 287: 867–70.

50. Medalie JH, Papier CM, Goldbourt U, Herman JB. Major factors in the development of diabetes mellitus in 10 000 men. Arch Int Med 1975; 135: 811–17.

51. West KM, Ahuja MMS, Bennett PH et al. The role of circulating glucose and triglyceride concentrations and their interactions with other 'risk factors' as determinants of arterial disease in nine diabetic population samples from the WHO multinational study. Diabetes Care 1983; 6: 361–9.

52. Uusitupa M. Coronary heart disease and left ventricular performance in newly diagnosed non-insulin-dependent diabetics. Original Reports 6. Publications of the University of Kuopio, 1983.

53. Uusitupa MIJ, Niskanen LK, Siitonen O, Voutilainen E, Pyörälä K. 5-year incidence of atherosclerotic vascular disease in relation to general risk factors, insulin level and abnormalities in lipoprotein composition in non-insulin dependent diabetic and non-diabetic subjects. Circulation 1990; 82: 27–36.

54. Laakso M. Atherosclerotic vascular disease and its risk factors in non-insulin-dependent diabetics in East Finland. Original Reports 5. Publications of the University of Kuopio, 1986.

55. Ishihara M, Tukimura Y, Yamada T, Ohto K, Yoshizama K. Diabetic complications and their relationships to risk factors in a Japanese population. Diabetes Care 1984; 7: 533–8.

56. Kuebler TW, Bendick PJ, Fineberg SE, Markand ON, Norton JA Jr, Vinicor FN, Clark CMJ. Diabetes mellitus and cerebrovascular disease: prevalence of carotic artery occlusive disease and

follow-up of the Helsinki Policemen Study population. Acta Med Scand 1985; 701 (suppl.): 38–42.

associated risk factors in 482 adult diabetic patients. Diabetes Care 1983; 6: 274–8.

57. Welborn TA, Knuiman M, McCann V, Stanton K, Constable IJ. Clinical macrovascular disease in Caucasoid diabetic subjects: logistic regression analysis of risk variables. Diabetologia 1984; 27: 568–73.

58. Knuiman MW, Welborn TA, McCann VJ, Stanton KG, Constable IJ. Prevalence of diabetic complications in relation to risk factors. Diabetes 1986; 35: 1332–9.

59. Jarrett RJ. Type 2 (non-insulin-dependent) diabetes mellitus and coronary heart disease—chicken, egg or neither? Diabetologia 1984; 26: 99–102.

60. Kagan AR, Uemura K, Sternby NH et al. Atherosclerosis of the aorta and coronary arteries in five towns. Bull WHO 1976; 53: 485–638.

61. Zdanov VS, Vihert AM. Atherosclerosis and diabetes mellitus. Bull WHO 1976; 53: 547–53.

62. Waller BF, Palumbo PJ, Lie JT, Roberts WV. Status of the coronary arteries at necropsy in diabetes mellitus with onset after age 30 years. Analysis of 229 diabetic patients with and without clinical evidence of coronary heart disease and comparison to 183 control subjects. Am J Med 1980; 69: 498–506.

63. Vigorita VJ, Moore GW, Hutchins GM. Absence of correlation between coronary arterial atherosclerosis and severity or duration of diabetes mellitus of adult onset. Am J Cardiol 1980; 46: 535–42.

64. Hamby RI, Sherman L, Mehta J, Aintablian A. Reappraisal of the role of the diabetic state in coronary artery disease. Chest 1976; 70: 251–7.

65. Hamby RI, Sherman L. Duration and treatment of diabetes. Relationship to severity of coronary artery disease. NY State J Med 1979; 79: 1683–8.

66. Melton LJ, Macken KM, Palumbo PJ, Elveback LR. Incidence and prevalence of clinical peripheral vascular disease in a population-based cohort of diabetic patients. Diabetes Care 1980; 3: 650–4.

67. Janka HU, Standl E, Mehnert H. Peripheral vascular disease in diabetes mellitus and its relation to cardiovascular risk factors: screening with the Doppler ultrasonic technique. Diabetes Care 1980; 3: 207–13.

68. Beach KW, Strandness DE. Arteriosclerosis obliterans and associated risk factors in insulin-dependent and non-insulin-dependent diabetes. Diabetes 1980; 29: 882–8.

69. Paisey RB, Arredondo G, Villalobos A, Lozano O, Guevara L, Kelly S. Association of differing dietary, metabolic, and clinical risk factors with macrovascular complications of diabetes: a prevalence study of 503 Mexican type II diabetic subjects. I. Diabetes Care 1984; 7: 421–7.

70. Krolewski AS, Kosinski EJ, Warram JH et al. Magnitude and determinants of coronary artery disease in juvenile onset, insulin-dependent diabetes mellitus. Am J Cardiol 1987; 59: 750–5.

71. Jensen T, Borch-Johnsen K, Kofoed-Enevoldsen A, Deckert T. Coronary heart disease in young Type 1 (insulin-dependent) diabetic patients with and without diabetic nephropathy: incidence and risk factors. Diabetologia 1987; 30: 144–8.

72. Winocour PH, Durrington PN, Ishola M, Anderson DC, Cohen H. Influence of proteinuria on vascular disease, blood pressure, and lipoproteins in insulin dependent diabetes mellitus. Br Med J 1987; 294: 1648–50.

73. Borch-Johnsen K, Kreiner K. Proteinuria: value as predictor of cardiovascular mortality in insulin dependent diabetes mellitus. Br Med J 1987; 294: 1651–4.

74. Martin FIR, Hopper JL. The relationship of acute insulin sensitivity to the progression of vascular disease in long-term Type 1 (insulin-dependent) diabetic mellitus. Diabetologia 1987; 30: 149–53.

75. University Group Diabetes Program. A study of the effects of hypoglycemic agents on vascular complications in patients with adult-onset diabetes. I. Design, methods and baseline characteristics. Diabetes 1970; 19 (suppl. 2): 747–83.

76. University Group Diabetes Program. A study of the effects of hypoglycemic agents on vascular complications in patients with adult-onset diabetes. II. Mortality results. Diabetes 1970; 19 (suppl. 2): 785–830.

77. University Group Diabetes Program. Effects of hypoglycemic agents on vascular complications in patients with adult-onset diabetes. III. Clinical implications of UGDP results. JAMA 1971; 218: 1400–10.

78. University Group Diabetes Program. Effects of hypoglycemic agents on vascular complications in patients with adult-onset diabetes. IV. A preliminary report on phenformin results. JAMA 1971; 217: 777–84.

79. University Group Diabetes Program. Effects of hypoglycemic agents on vascular complications in patients with adult-onset diabetes. V. Evaluation of phenformin therapy. Diabetes 1975; 24 (suppl. 1): 65–184.

80. University Group Diabetes Program. Effects of hypoglycemic agents on vascular complications in patients with adult-onset diabetes. VIII. Evaluation of insulin therapy: final report. Diabetes 1982; 31 (suppl. 5): 1–81.

81. Fuller JH. Clinical trials in diabetes mellitus. In Mann JI, Pyörälä K, Teuscher A (eds) Diabetes in epidemiological perspective. Edinburgh: Churchill Livingstone, 1983: pp 265–90.

82. UK Prospective Study of Therapies of Maturity-

Onset Diabetes. I. Effect of diet, sulfonylurea, insulin or biguanide therapy on fasting plasma glucose and body weight over one year. Diabetologia 1983; 24: 404–11.

83. UK Prospective Study of Therapies of Maturity-Onset Diabetes. II. Reduction in HbA_{1c} with basal insulin supplement, sulfonylurea or biguanide therapy in maturity-onset diabetes. Diabetes 1985; 34: 793–8.

84. DCCT Research Group. Diabetes Control and Complications Trial (DCCT): results of feasibility study. Diabetes Care 1987; 10: 1–19.

85. World Health Organization Expert Committee on Diabetes Mellitus. Second report. Technical Report Series 646. Geneva: WHO, 1980.

86. American Diabetes Association. Nutritional recommendations and principles for individuals with diabetes mellitus: 1986. Diabetes Care 1987; 10: 126–32.

87. World Health Organization Expert Committee on the Prevention of Coronary Heart Disease. Technical Report Series 678. Geneva: WHO, 1982.

65

Clinical Features of Ischemic Heart Disease in Diabetes Mellitus

Ellison H. Wittels and Antonio M. Gotto
Department of Medicine, Baylor College of Medicine, Houston, Texas, USA

Macrovascular disease, seen as coronary artery disease (CAD), cerebrovascular disease or peripheral vascular disease, is the chief cause of death among people with diabetes mellitus. It is not entirely synonymous with atherosclerosis, although enhanced development of atherosclerosis would seem to be chiefly responsible for manifestations of macrovascular disease among diabetic patients.

Evidence of the particular susceptibility of the diabetic subject to atherosclerotic disease of the heart, legs and brain is extensive and incontestable [1, 2]. About three-quarters of deaths among North American diabetic patients are due to atherosclerotic disease, compared with about one-third of deaths in the general North American population [3, 4]. Diabetic death from atherosclerosis in fact bespeaks the success of diabetes treatment over this century. Between 1894 and 1915, in Joslin's series 64% of the patients died in diabetic coma [5]. Management advances—the introduction of insulin therapy in 1922, the development of oral hypoglycemic agents and improved diet strategies—have prolonged the lives of the majority of diabetic patients, thus increasing the incidence of long-term complications. For example, Kramer and Perlstein noted peripheral vascular disease in 58% of their diabetic patients seen between 1953 and 1956, compared with a 17% rate between 1921 and 1930 [6]. Currently, about 70% of patients with non-insulin dependent diabetes mellitus (NIDDM) in the USA are over age 55 years [7].

Coronary artery disease constitutes the greatest cardiovascular risk to diabetic patients and is therefore the major emphasis of this chapter. Twenty-year Framingham data reported by Kannel and McGee in 1979 showed the relative impact of diabetes to be greatest on intermittent claudication and congestive heart failure (Table 1), but CAD on an absolute scale to be the chief sequela [8]. The same report described diabetic men as having more than a 50% increased incidence of CAD events, and diabetic women as having a 200% increased incidence, compared with non-diabetic controls. Multiple other series support at least a twofold increase in CAD risk with diabetes [9–12]. The increased CAD risk may be related to dyslipidemia, although the

International Textbook of Diabetes Mellitus. Edited by K.G.M.M. Alberti, R.A. DeFronzo, H. Keen and P. Zimmet
© 1992 John Wiley & Sons Ltd

Table 1 Average annual age-adjusted incidence per 1000 specified cardiovascular events: 20 years' surveillance from Framingham*

	Men		Women	
	Diabetic	Non-diabetic	Diabetic	Non-diabetic
Cardiovascular disease	39.1	19.1	27.2	10.2
Cardiovascular disease death	17.4	8.5	17.0	3.6
Congestive heart failure	7.6	3.5	11.4	2.2
Intermittent claudication	12.6	3.3	8.4	1.3
Atherothrombotic brain infarction	4.7	1.9	6.2	1.7
Coronary heart disease	24.8	14.9	17.8	6.9

*Cohorts comprising men and women ages 45–74 years.
Reproduced from reference 8. [JAMA, 1979; 241: 2035–8] with permission. Copyright 1979, American Medical Association.

other risk factors common to diabetes—e.g. hypertension and obesity—may have major roles (see below).

Interestingly, however, although arterial wall changes in diabetic patients tend to be more severe than in non-diabetic controls with atherosclerosis (see below), the prevalence of artherosclerosis among diabetic patients varies considerably according to geography or ethnic origin fairly much in parallel with overall population differences in atherosclerosis frequency and severity. Such initial findings by the International Atherosclerosis Project [13], which examined some 23 000 sets of coronary arteries collected from 14 countries, have been supported by other studies, among them Japanese migration studies [14] and the World Health Organization (WHO) Multinational Study [15]. Thus, macrovascular disease would not seem to be as integral a part of the diabetic syndrome as microvascular disease, but diabetes does increase relative susceptibility to it [16].

ASYMPTOMATIC HYPERGLYCEMIA AND CAD RISK

Whether an excess risk of cardiovascular disease as is seen in frank diabetes extends to asymptomatic hyperglycemia is a question that has been much investigated and debated but not yet clearly answered. The Framingham Heart Study measured casual blood glucose values and reported a non-linear relation to CAD incidence at 16-year follow-up, with a marked increase in incidence at levels above 120 mg/dl [17]. Multivariate Framingham analyses have found an independent relation of glucose intolerance, a rubric in those analyses including diagnosed diabetes, and CAD incidence [18]. Both the Tecumseh and Bedford cross-sectional studies in

1965 reported higher age-adjusted postchallenge blood glucose levels among persons with CAD and/or other manifestations of atherosclerosis than among other members of the population in analyses excluding diagnosed diabetic subjects [19, 20]. By 1979, the International Collaborative Group saw the need for a comparative analysis and published the results of separate studies in 15 populations from 11 countries (representing about 40 000 subjects) [21], including reports from the Whitehall Study and the Chicago Heart Association Detection Project in Industry. Eleven of the studies had completed at least 4 years of follow-up; the other four were only cross-sectional. The group concluded that the results considered together did not indicate a consistent, strong, graded association [22].

Nearly all the International Collaborative Group studies found an increased prevalence of electrocardiographic abnormalities in the highest quintile, with an even stronger association seen in the upper 2.0–2.5% of glucose distribution in those studies with large enough numbers to allow analysis of this quantile. In most studies, however, the association did not prove to be independent on multivariate analysis. The subsequent full $7\frac{1}{2}$-year follow-up report from the Whitehall Study showed CAD mortality to be doubled above the 95th percentile ($\geqslant 96$ mg/dl) for 2-hour blood glucose levels, suggesting a threshold effect [23]. This finding prompted the Paris Prospective Study group to reanalyze their data, which did not support any independent relation between glucose and CAD in the collaborative publication. They reported a doubling threshold effect, but at a much higher 2-hour postload glucose level ($\geqslant 140$ mg/dl), enough to define impaired glucose tolerance [24].

The International Collaborative Group recognized many of its comparison's limitations, among them the differing protocols and methods of assessing glycemia. Only data on men were included because of the small number of numerator cases for women in the few studies that enrolled women. The possibility of incorrect classifications of subjects in terms of glycemia because of the use of glucose tolerance tests has been raised by several authors [25, 26]. One of these groups, Barrett-Connor et al [26], therefore assessed heart disease risk factors and death rates in 3625 non-diabetic men and women against fasting plasma glucose level because of the reduced intraindividual variability and smaller potential for misclassification of this parameter compared with postchallenge glucose level. At a 9-year follow-up, they reported a significant association of fasting glucose level with most risk factors; after adjustment for these factors, an independent and significant association of fasting glucose level (whether as a continuous or categorical variable) with all-cause, cardiovascular and ischemic heart disease mortality in men was found. The only significant association in women was with all-cause mortality at the highest glucose levels. The authors noted, however, that there were relatively few deaths among women, so that the different results in women may have reflected a lack of statistical power.

Other major studies that have appeared since the collaborative group analysis include a 10-year follow-up of the Bedford Survey [27], which found borderline postchallenge hyperglycemia to confer an excess risk of CAD death (but only in women), and an approximately 18-year follow-up in the Tecumseh Study [28], which showed excess CAD mortality after multivariate analysis among those with a high glucose score, the magnitude of the effect being less than among diagnosed diabetic patients. Twelve-year Gothenburg data in women showed no association between fasting blood glucose level and coronary end-points after the exclusion of diabetic subjects; the diabetic patients in this longitudinal population study had significantly increased rates of myocardial infarction (MI) and all-cause mortality [29]. The Chicago Heart Association Detection Project in Industry at 9-year follow-up of 11 220 men and 8030 women found CAD death to be associated not only with frank diabetes but also with asymptomatic hyperglycemia (1 hour postload), both associations greater for women in terms of relative risk

but greater for men in absolute risk. On multivariate analysis, the association with asymptomatic hyperglycemia was not independent for men but of borderline significance for women [30]. It is of interest that in this study's report in the International Collaborative Group publication, there had been no association of subdiabetic hyperglycemia with CAD mortality, even on univariate analysis. That report was made at 5-year follow-up and, as mentioned above, included data on men only. A small recent Finnish study found no association of fasting plasma glucose levels with coronary risk in any subgroup [31].

The question of asymptomatic hyperglycemia and CAD risk has been addressed in a number of the ongoing coronary risk studies among Japanese men. In one study a 1-hour postchallenge serum glucose level was recently found on multivariate analysis to be a significant predictor of CAD mortality in a large population at 12-year follow-up [32]. Among the Hawaiian Japanese men aged 45–70 years who constituted the population of the Honolulu Heart Program, it was found to be predictive of sudden cardiac death but not of non-fatal heart attack [33]; other predictors of cardiac death were blood pressure, cholesterol level, cigarette smoking, history of parental heart attack and electrocardiographic evidence of left ventricular hypertrophy or strain.

One Honolulu Heart Program analysis assessed the rates of CAD death and non-fatal MI at 12-year follow-up by postchallenge serum glucose level [34]. None of the men had a diagnosis of diabetes at entry. The authors found a consistent, graded increase in the adjusted relative risk of both CAD death and non-fatal MI, a trend that remained significant on multivariant analysis. The men who had a postchallenge glucose level between 157 mg/dl and 189 mg/dl (fourth quintile) had twice the age-adjusted risk of CAD death as those in the lowest quintile. No threshold effect was seen. Interestingly, however, postchallenge serum glucose levels did not independently correlate with autopsy-demonstrated coronary artery and aortic atherosclerosis in the Honolulu Heart Program [35].

PATHOLOGY

Diabetes affects the macrovascular and microvascular circulations and the myocardium.

Macrovascular disease in the form of CAD, cerebrovascular disease and peripheral vascular disease is the major cause of mortality among diabetic patients. The hallmark of macrovascular disease is the atherosclerotic plaque which is the same in diabetic and non-diabetic subjects [16, 36]. The Atherosclerosis Project demonstrated that the extent of raised lesions was greater in diabetic than in non-diabetic subjects [37]. Diabetic patients have an excess of atherosclerotic lesions with ulceration, thrombosis or hemorrhage [38].

Diabetic patients have been reported to have more atherosclerotic arterial wall changes [39]. They have also been reported to have more vessels involved: in one study 43% of diabetic subjects had three-vessel disease compared to 25% of non-diabetics [40]. Diabetic patients have been reported to have atherosclerotic changes that extend more peripherally [41, 42]. A statistically increased prevalence of left main coronary artery disease has also been reported in diabetic subjects (13%) compared to non-diabetic controls (6%) [43]. Not all studies have reported significant differences in the extent of atherosclerosis between diabetic and non-diabetic subjects [44, 45].

There is clinical and epidemiologic evidence to suggest that the increased risk of congestive heart failure among diabetics is not entirely attributable to accelerated atherosclerosis or increased rates of hypertension. The controversial 'diabetic cardiomyopathy' has been reviewed elsewhere [46]. The high incidence of bradycardia rhythms in diabetic patients has been thought to be secondary to the effects of microvascular disease on the cardiac conduction system.

Abnormalities of the small blood vessels, including microaneurysms of the coronary vessels, capillary membrane thickening, perivascular and interstitial fibrosis, scarring of adjacent tissues and myocytolysis, have been found within the heart [47]. These changes are similar to those observed in skeletal muscle, kidney, and the retina of patients with diabetes [48].

Proliferative lesions have been reported in all sizes of arterial branches and venules. In addition, arteriosclerosis-like lesions of small arteries and arterioles were 2–2.5 times more frequent among diabetic patients than non-diabetic [49]. The media of the intramural vessels

was observed to contain PAS-positive material. Although insulin dependent diabetes mellitus (IDDM) patients have not been shown to have endothelial cell proliferation, they do have an accumulation of PAS material in the intramural arteries [50].

DIABETES AND PROGRESSION OF ATHEROSCLEROSIS

Retinopathy, neuropathy and nephropathy in IDDM and NIDDM appear primarily related to the duration and severity of hyperglycemia, with age as a modulating factor. In contrast, macroangiopathy appears primarily related to attained age [51, 52]. Coronary atherosclerosis is more severe at all ages and occurs at a younger age in IDDM [53]. Alternatively, diabetic patients may already have underlying CAD when first diagnosed or may have an increased tendency for developing accelerated atherosclerotic heart disease [54]. It is also possible that an accelerated pace of atherogenesis is an early feature in the evolution of diabetes [55]. Finally, it has been proposed that individuals may develop diabetes who also possess the characteristics that predispose to CAD [56].

Sequential thallium scanning and exercise treadmill tests 1 and 2 years apart on asymptomatic middle-aged men showed that 77% of the diabetic subjects had abnormal results on retesting, while no control subject showed an abnormality [57]. The progression of atherosclerosis in adult diabetic patients may be independent of the progression of the diabetes. In NIDDM, there is considerable doubt whether the extent or severity of atherosclerosis is related to the duration or the severity of diabetes, the age of onset of the disease or the type of treatment [42, 44].

The effect of normalization of blood glucose concentrations on the prevention or delay of the rate of complications from coronary atherosclerosis has not been established. There is still significant controversy about the effect of diabetic control on the progression of coronary atherosclerosis [45]. However, the degree of control of the blood glucose did not affect the degree of coronary narrowing [43]. This contrasts sharply with the association between control of hyperglycemia and microvascular disease of the eyes and kidneys [50].

CAD IN DIABETIC FEMALES

Diabetic women have CAD mortality rates 3–4 times greater than non-diabetic women, while diabetic men experience a twofold excess in CAD mortality compared with non-diabetic men [30, 54, 58, 59]. In the Framingham Study, the relative increase in intermittent claudication, congestive heart failure and coronary heart disease attributable to diabetes was substantially greater for women than for men. Diabetes greatly reduces the relative protection that premenopausal females have from coronary disease [50]. Congestive heart failure is present to a greater extent in diabetic women than in diabetic men.

Borderline diabetes was associated with a greater mortality in women than in men. The Chicago Heart Association Detection Project in Industry found that women (but not men) with asymptomatic hyperglycemia had a significantly higher CAD death rate [30]. Interestingly, no increased incidence of angina pectoris, electrocardiographic changes indicative of ischemic disease, or stroke was observed in the Bedford population [60]. Women had a significantly increased incidence of MI and increased mortality 12 years after developing diabetes [59].

In children with IDDM, cardiovascular risk factors were reported to be more prevalent in girls than in boys. The increased risk found in adult diabetic females may relate in part to risk factors found in adolescence [61]. In the Framingham Study, female NIDDM subjects had higher serum cholesterol levels than their non-diabetic peers. Diabetic females have higher cholesterol and low-density lipoprotein (LDL) levels, higher blood pressure and more obesity than diabetic men. A low level of high-density lipoprotein (HDL) cholesterol in the presence of diabetes increases the risk of CAD in women relative to that in men. The risk is especially increased in diabetic women with superimposed obesity and low HDL cholesterol [62].

The presence of these risk factors does not explain the marked increase in cardiovascular mortality and morbidity in diabetic women [54, 58, 63]. Another explanation for the sex difference in CAD mortality among diabetic females is the more favorable survival rate in non-diabetic women compared with non-diabetic men [64].

TYPE 1 IDDM

Although cardiovascular mortality is relatively uncommon in young IDDM patients, it is increased when compared with that in non-diabetic young adults. In a group of diabetic patients, MI or atherosclerotic heart disease accounted for 2.5% of the deaths in individuals under 24 years old, 15% of deaths in those 25–34 years old and 39% of deaths in those 35–44 years old [65].

In a study of 9 patients with juvenile onset IDDM, significantly more atherosclerosis of the epicardial coronary arteries was found than in non-diabetic subjects of similar age and sex. Of the 9 patients, 6 had one or more of the four major arteries narrowed by more than 75%. Up to one-third of IDDM patients have symptoms of CAD by age 59 years and approximately one-third die by age 55 years [66].

Coronary artery disease is not an inevitable long-term complication of IDDM. In the study mentioned above, 3 of the 9 IDDM patients had no evidence of coronary atherosclerosis [67]. In another study, 73 juvenile onset IDDM patients were followed for a mean duration of 42.9 years. Major cardiac complications were found in 20% of the patients [68]. The presence of diabetes beginning at age 15 years or younger did not accurately predict the presence of clinical or anatomical CAD 20 years later. Several investigators have reported that juvenile IDDM patients with fewer episodes of ketoacidosis have less vascular disease subsequently [68, 69].

RISK FACTORS FOR CORONARY ARTERY DISEASE

The concept of risk factors evolved from prospective epidemiologic studies in the 1950s. The Framingham Study related personal characteristics to the subsequent occurrence of CAD. Risk factors may be directly causative, secondary manifestations of more basic underlying metabolic abnormalities, or early symptoms of disease. Risk factors for CAD have been identified based on their association with heart disease, prevalence in the general population, and data supporting their predictive value [70].

Hypertension, hypercholesterolemia and cigarette smoking are the three major modifiable risk factors for CAD. A low level of HDL cholesterol is also highly predictive of CAD. Male sex, type A personality, age over 40 years, obesity and a familial predisposition to pre-mature CAD are also predictors of coronary artery disease. Eventually, age itself becomes the strongest predictor of CAD, especially in an older population [51].

The prevalence of hypercholesterolemia, hypertension, low HDL cholesterol, hypertriglyceridemia and obesity is greater in diabetic than in non-diabetic subjects [54]. Smoking is more common in the non-diabetic population [71]. These features are present decades before the appearance of clinical evidence of diabetes [55]. The literature available indicates that the effect of risk factors on CAD is similar in both diabetic and non-diabetic populations [72]. Moreover, the increased risk of CAD in diabetic populations is not solely because of the increased prevalence of risk factors for CAD [54, 73]. Only part of the increased prevalence of CAD in diabetic patients can be explained by the high rate of risk factors in this group [55].

Cigarettes

Cigarette smoking is a risk factor for cardiovascular complications in both diabetic and non-diabetic people. Although the relative risk of smoking is comparable in both groups, the absolute risk contributed by smoking is greater in diabetic patients [71].

The Framingham Study reported that diabetic patients were less likely to smoke cigarettes than those without diabetes, although statistically significant differences were noted only for men [74]. Recently it has been shown that the prevalence of cigarette smoking is not different from the general population; diabetic subjects more than 50 years old were less likely to be smokers than the general population [75].

Hypertension

Approximately 2.5 million Americans are hypertensive and have either IDDM or NIDDM. Hypertension is twice as common among diabetic patients when compared with non-diabetic controls and commonly precedes the clinical onset of diabetes [76]. Greater age at examination, presence of proteinuria, larger body mass, male gender and longer duration of diabetes are associated with higher systolic blood pressure. The duration of diabetes has also been positively correlated with systolic blood pressure [77]. The

two conditions seem especially likely to be found together among the less socioeconomically advantaged. Individually, diabetes and hypertension are each more common among blacks than whites, with concurrent hypertension and diabetes occurring almost twice as frequently in blacks [78].

Hypertension occurs more frequently in NIDDM patients over 40–50 years old [36, 49]; and more frequently in diabetic males before age 50 years and in diabetic females after age 50 years [78]. Hypertension was detected in 21.9% of patients with the onset of diabetes before age 30 years, compared with 58% of patients diagnosed with diabetes after age 30 years [77]. Patients with IDDM have been reported to have higher systolic and diastolic blood pressures than their non-diabetic siblings [61]. While there is some controversy about the effect that treatment of glucose levels has on hypertension, it has been known for a number of years that the control of mild to moderate hypertension diminishes the rate of protein excretion and slows renal function deterioration [79].

There is a much higher mortality in diabetic patients compared with non-diabetic subjects with comparable degrees of hypertension [80]. Together, hypertension and diabetes accelerate the natural progression of atherosclerosis in all populations. In fact, the prevalence of atherosclerotic heart disease has not been reported to be significantly different between normotensive diabetic subjects and non-diabetic controls [76]. People with hypertension and diabetes consistently have more coronary artery atherosclerosis than people without hypertension or diabetes, regardless of age, sex, race or geographic location [37]. A patient with both diabetes and hypertension is twice as likely to develop CAD as a patient with hypertension alone [77, 81, 82].

Several explanations have been provided to explain the association between hypertension and diabetes. Higher rates of hypertension in diabetic populations could be due in part to detection bias, since hypertension is more likely to be discovered in those who are under medical care for other reasons. Diuretics or beta-blockers used to treat hypertension can increase blood glucose concentrations. Endocrinopathies including acromegaly and Cushing's disease cause both hypertension and carbohydrate intolerance, but are relatively uncommon.

Diabetes and hypertension may reflect an

underlying disorder that promotes both conditions. Extensive and diffuse proliferative lesions of the small blood vessels can progressively narrow the lumen, increase peripheral resistance to blood flow and account for the increased prevalence of hypertension among diabetic patients [76]. Insulin has been shown to increase renal reabsorption of sodium and increase sympathetic nervous system activity, which can increase blood pressure [83, 84].

Much of the increased association of diabetes and hypertension has been attributed to the association of hypertension and obesity, insulin resistance and hyperinsulinemia [85]. Adjustment for obesity reduced the association considerably, but a consistent association remained [86]. However, diabetic patients on 50 or more units of insulin per day had a lower prevalence of hypertension than other diabetic patients. This was attributed to suppression by adequate exogenous insulin of adrenocortical hormone secretion, which was postulated to be excessive and contributed to hypertension [76].

Obesity

In the Framingham Study, obesity was an independent risk factor for CAD. There is also significant association between the presence of obesity and diabetes. Approximately 70–80% of NIDDM patients are obese; 40–60% of markedly obese individuals will develop NIDDM [87]. In the Framingham Study, obesity occurred in 20.5% of diabetic men compared with 9.8% of non-diabetic men; and in 42.1% of diabetic women compared with 18.9% of non-diabetic women [54]. Among women, especially over age 50 years, the triad of obesity, diabetes and low HDL cholesterol was associated with a high risk of CAD [88]. The Veterans' Administration Normative Aging Study concluded that the effect of weight gain on fasting glucose levels was greatest in older men [89].

Other studies have documented a relationship between an excess quantity of body fat and an increased risk of CAD [90]. Excess abdominal fat has been associated with NIDDM, hypertension, hyperinsulinemia and CAD [91]. Body fat can be determined by body volume displacement or skinfold measurement. The waist/hip ratio (WHR) is used to determine the pattern of deposition of body fat. Excess abdominal fat is associated with an increased risk of CAD and

elevated plasma lipoproteins [92]. In women, the normal ratio is less than 0.8; in men the ratio is less than 1.0. An elevated WHR has been reported to correlate better with CAD risk than total body weight [93].

Obesity is associated with CAD risk factors including lack of exercise, hyperlipidemia, hypertension, low HDL levels [94] and diabetes. Obesity is associated with insulin resistance at the tissue level, increased insulin secretion and hyperinsulinemia. Hyperinsulinemia and its relationship to CAD is reviewed in this chapter. It is possible that obesity may be a marker for an underlying condition that makes the development of CAD and diabetes more likely to occur.

Hyperlipidemia

Hyperlipidemia has been found in approximately 50% of all diabetic patients [95]. The prevalence of hyperlipidemia in both IDDM and NIDDM may reflect the degree of glucose control [96]; this seems especially true of IDDM patients. However, no consistent or striking abnormalities have been consistently reported [97]. In diabetic patients, lipid levels reported to be abnormal include low HDL cholesterol, elevated very low-density lipoproteins (VLDL), elevated and abnormal LDL cholesterol and elevated triglycerides. In addition, there are often alterations in the composition of the apolipoproteins. Reduction of the apo-CII/apo-CIII ratio has been reported [36].

Cholesterol

Hypercholesterolemia is a major risk factor for CAD. In subhuman primates, diabetes causes increased susceptibility to atherosclerosis from hypercholesterolemia [86, 98]. Diabetic patients who develop atherosclerosis have been reported to have higher cholesterol levels than those who do not develop CAD. Framingham data showed the total plasma cholesterol concentration was elevated in diabetic women compared to non-diabetic women, but diabetic men who did or did not develop atherosclerotic cardiovascular disease had lower total serum cholesterol levels than non-diabetic men [86]. Low-density lipoprotein transports approximately 70% of the total plasma cholesterol. It is atherogenic. Patients with NIDDM are more likely to have raised LDL cholesterol levels than those with IDDM.

The level of LDL cholesterol varies according to glycemic control, tending to be increased in poorly controlled diabetic patients. Improved diabetic control results in decreased blood cholesterol which could reflect decreased VLDL synthesis which is catabolized to LDL. In NIDDM Pima Indians, the plasma cholesterol levels were higher among untreated diabetic subjects than among those treated with insulin. This reflected a generalized increase in hepatic lipid production and VLDL synthesis [99]. An increased LDL turnover in the adult onset diabetic patient has been demonstrated [100]. Increased LDL turnover could be important in the deposition of lipid-rich material in the arterial wall.

HMG-CoA reductase activity is insulin-dependent. Insulin deficiency results in depressed HMG-CoA reductase activity in hepatic microsomes in rats and mammalian cell cultures. Alternatively, it is possible that hyperinsulinism could stimulate hepatic cholesterol synthesis by its effect on HMG-CoA reductase [98].

Hyperglycemia can also impede the uptake of LDL. Hyperglycemia causes non-enzymatic glycation of LDL; LDL isolated from diabetic patients has had up to 5% of lysine residues glycated, which is 3–4 times higher than normal. It is possible that too much emphasis has been placed on the regulatory effect of non-enzymatic glycation of LDL as an important control mechanism of cholesterol homeostasis in diabetic patients. It is possible that the increased esterified/free cholesterol ratio is the more likely cause of effective regulation of cholesterogenesis in both NIDDM patients and non-diabetic subjects [101].

Glycated LDL binds poorly to LDL or apoprotein B/E receptors, but is readily bound and internalized by receptors present on macrophages or scavenger cells. Unlike the B/E receptor, the macrophage receptor is not subject to downregulation and an excessive accumulation of cholesteryl esters may occur. Lipid accumulation in these cells forms foam cells [36]. In addition, insulin deficiency may be associated with a diminished number of LDL receptors and thereby lead to decreased LDL binding. Changes in LDL receptors in poorly controlled diabetic patients has been reported [102].

A small, dense LDL particle has been linked to atherosclerosis [103, 104]. The LDL size is inversely related to plasma triglyceride and plasma insulin levels and directly related to a low HDL cholesterol level. The presence of small, dense LDL has been attributed to tissue insulin resistance [105]. Obese NIDDM patients as well as those with impaired glucose tolerance may be at increased risk for this subfraction of LDL.

Triglycerides

High VLDL and triglyceride levels are a hallmark of diabetes. The most common form of hyperlipidemia in NIDDM is elevation of VLDL triglycerides [95]. Whether hypertriglyceridemia is an independent risk factor for coronary atherosclerosis remains controversial. Several studies have found hypertriglyceridemia to be an independent risk factor for CAD [80], while others have reported that when HDL cholesterol levels were considered, hypertriglyceridemia was not an independent risk factor [88]. Both the Stockholm Prospective Study and the Uppsala Primary Prevention Study demonstrated a progressive association between hypertriglyceridemia and documented MI [106, 107]. In the Framingham Study, the triglyceride level was an independent risk factor for CAD only in women. There is evidence of an independent association between CAD and increased levels of triglyceride-rich VLDL remnants or intermediate density lipoprotein (IDL) [108].

Hypertriglyceridemia can be caused either by insulin deficiency or insulin excess. Patients with impaired glucose tolerance lose their normal tissue insulin sensitivity which leads to compensatory hyperinsulinism and stimulation of triglyceride synthesis and VLDL secretion by the liver. Among NIDDM patients there is an increased flux of unesterified fatty acids from adipose tissue to the liver, resulting in the stimulation of VLDL triglyceride synthesis and secretion.

Adipose tissue contains a hormone-sensitive lipase activated by epinephrine which releases free fatty acids. Insulin opposes this effect and exerts an antilipolytic action. The insulin-sensitive lipoprotein lipase breaks down chylomicrons and VLDL in the circulation at the endothelial cell. Insulin deficiency may produce profound hypertriglyceridemia due to a decrease in the activity of lipoprotein lipase [109]. Decreased levels of specific lipases participating in lipoprotein degradation have been documented in the aortic tissue of diabetic animals [110].

Type V is the only familial hyperlipidemia with a strong link to diabetes. In this genetic disorder, both chylomicrons and VLDL are increased. A relative deficiency of lipoprotein lipase exists and an oversynthesis of VLDL occurs. While poor control of blood glucose exacerbates hypertriglyceridemia, tight control does not eliminate it. When the hyperlipidemia is treated with diet and/or drugs, the lipoprotein pattern may shift from type V to type IV as the chylomicrons disappear. First-degree relatives may have either a type V or type IV pattern.

High-density Lipoprotein

In diabetic patients, as in the general population, HDL cholesterol values are strongly and inversely proportional to the incidence of CAD [111]. The level of HDL cholesterol is lower in diabetic men than in non-diabetic men, and statistically lower in diabetic women compared with non-diabetic women [62]; it is lower in NIDDM patients compared with those with IDDM [97]. The level of HDL cholesterol is lower in NIDDM patients treated with oral agents than in those treated with insulin. The subfraction most closely associated with vascular disease, HDL_2, also tends to be lower in NIDDM compared with IDDM patients. Overall, HDL cholesterol appears to be more strongly related to vascular disease in NIDDM patients than in IDDM patients [112, 113].

A close correlation between the levels of blood glucose and HDL cholesterol has been reported [114]. The difference in HDL metabolism appears to be related to differences in VLDL. Triglyceride-rich lipoprotein levels are usually inversely related to those of HDL cholesterol [115]. There is a tendency for higher triglyceride levels and therefore lower HDL cholesterol levels to occur in those with NIDDM compared with IDDM [116, 117]. The lower HDL cholesterol levels in NIDDM could be caused by obesity and insulin resistance leading to elevated serum triglyceride levels and low levels of serum HDL cholesterol [118].

The reported decrease in HDL and HDL cholesterol levels in diabetic compared with non-diabetic subjects disappeared when the glucose levels were normalized. However, in a study of 12 NIDDM patients, intensive insulin treatment controlled hyperglycemia and triglycerides but did not improve the abnormal HDL cholesterol

metabolism [117]. Therefore, other factors must be involved. While the level of apolipoprotein-A was the same in diabetic and non-diabetic subjects, there may be defective binding of cholesterol to apo-A in diabetic subjects [114].

THE ROLE OF DIABETES MELLITUS IN THE PATHOGENESIS OF ATHEROSCLEROSIS

The precise mechanism for the initiation and development of the atherosclerotic plaque is not completely understood. The 'response to injury hypothesis', with modifications, has been used to explain the development of the atherosclerotic plaque. Injury to the endothelium or endothelial cell dysfunction caused by hyperlipidemia, hyperglycemia, hypertension or cigarette smoking is widely held to be an essential event in the development of atherosclerosis. The relationship between atherosclerosis and coagulation has been extensively investigated. Physical disruption of the endothelial cell barrier exposes collagen and elastin fibers and initiates the process of platelet adherence and aggregation. Subsequent release of platelet derived growth factors and other growth factors, smooth muscle cell migration and proliferation, accumulation of extracellular glycosaminoglycans (GAG) matrix and accumulation of lipids ensue.

Recently, the important role of monocytes and macrophages in the formation of the atherosclerotic plaque has been recognized [119]. In hypercholesterolemic primates the monocyte is seen adhering to the endothelial cell and penetrating the endothelial barrier to enter the intima where it can become a lipid-accumulating macrophage or foam cell. After injury the endothelial barrier is normally restored and lesion formation subsides. However, if injury to the endothelium is continuous or repetitive or if endothelial regeneration is prevented, then the atherosclerotic plaque develops [120–122].

Hyperglycemia and Atherosclerosis

Diabetes can be associated with increased blood viscosity, abnormalities in platelet activation and function, enhanced production of growth factors, increased platelet aggregation, increased plasma fibrinogen levels and abnormalities in the composition of plasma lipids, all of which have been linked to the pathogenesis of atherosclerosis [123–125]. There is also interest in whether there is a genetically determined difference in the reaction of the vascular wall of diabetic subjects. This interest was spurred by reports of possible differences in response in the chlorpropamide alcohol flushing test, especially among those in whom flushing could be prevented by indomethacin [126].

In diabetic subjects, elevated plasma levels of von Willebrand factor (vWF), decreased prostacyclin release, decreased plasminogen activator and decreased lipoprotein lipase activity are evidence of endothelial cell damage and can potentiate atherosclerosis.

Hyperglycemia may be directly toxic to the endothelial cell wall. Both glucose and sorbitol stimulate arterial smooth muscle cell proliferation, considered essential for the development of the atherosclerotic plaque. Tissue hypoxia may be related to the atherosclerotic process. Hypoxia could stimulate activity of the polyol pathway in the diabetic patient, resulting in increased cell water content and further impairment of oxygenation of the arterial wall. In addition, hyperglycemia may reduce 2,3-diphosphoglycerate levels, further impairing tissue oxygen release [127]. Glycation of hemoglobin might also contribute to tissue hypoxia [128].

Glycation of LDL, collagen and other proteins can alter their degradation [129]. Glycated LDL cholesterol may be phagocytized by the macrophage and contribute to cholesteryl ester accumulation. Alternatively, altered glycated protein could cause autoantibody formation with an immune response and enhanced atherosclerosis. Hyperglycemia could affect vessel wall collagen directly or through non-enzymatic glycation.

Insulin

Higher fasting insulin levels or a greater insulin response to oral glucose has been reported in non-diabetic patients with proven atherosclerotic disease or at increased risk for CAD [130]. Several prospective studies of fasting and post-glucose insulin levels were correlated with the subsequent development of CAD. The Helsinki Policemen Study measured insulin levels fasting and at 1 hour and 2 hours following 60-g, 75-g or 90-g glucose challenges. After 5 years, this study showed that fatal and non-fatal MIs correlated with the highest 1-hour and 2-hour insulin levels [131]. The Paris Civil Servants Study was of adult men 43–54 years old who after fasting blood glucose and insulin measurement were given a 75-g glucose load; blood glucose and insulin levels were then measured again. Multivariate analysis showed that only the fasting insulin level correlated with the subsequent development of CAD [132, 133].

In diabetic subjects a relationship between insulin and atherosclerosis has been reported. In the Schwabing Study, endogenous insulin secretion, based on C-peptide concentration, was significantly higher than normal in NIDDM subjects with macrovascular disease and non-diabetic patients with CAD [134]. The Oxford Study of NIDDM patients demonstrated a correlation between fasting insulin concentrations and the appearance after 5 years of new electrocardiographic findings characteristic of CAD [135]. A higher insulin response to glucose has been demonstrated among diabetic patients with atherosclerosis compared with diabetic patients without atherosclerosis [136]. Those with mild glucose intolerance and NIDDM obese patients have higher insulin levels than non-diabetic controls [137].

Insulin levels in insulin-treated diabetic subjects are higher than in non-diabetic subjects, especially between meals and at night. In the diabetic patient receiving subcutaneous insulin, systemic levels are higher than the insulin level in the portal vein. Normally, insulin is secreted from the pancreas into the portal vein and then to the liver where 50% is degraded before it reaches the systemic circulation. Therefore, the level in the portal vein is higher than in the systemic circulation [138]. The Schwabing Study reported that either endogenous or exogenous hyperinsulinemia was increased in those with macrovascular disease [134].

Insulin has also been demonstrated to increase atherosclerotic lesions in experimental models and inhibit regression of diet-induced atherosclerosis. Selective insulin infusion into one of the femoral arteries of an alloxan-treated dog caused lipid accumulation and medial thickening compared to the opposite artery infused with saline [139]. Similarly, a group of chickens fed a normal diet plus insulin injections for 19 weeks developed lipid deposits in their arteries when compared to a control group fed a normal diet without insulin injections [140].

Several mechanisms may account for the atherogenic effect of insulin. The arterial wall is insulin sensitive. Insulin has been shown to stimulate cultured arterial smooth muscle cell proliferation in the primate and act as a growth factor. Elevated insulin levels are associated with several major cardiovascular risk factors including hyperlipidemia, obesity and hypertension. There is also interest not only in the insulin level but also in the role of insulin resistance as a primary cause of atherosclerosis [130].

Coagulation

The coagulation system appears to play a major role in both diabetic and non-diabetic subjects in the initiation and propagation (as well as in the complications) of atherosclerosis. While the effect of diabetes on CAD through an effect on thrombogenesis has been reported [141], there is still a residual effect of glucose intolerance after all the standard factors and fibrin are taken into account [142].

Among diabetic patients, increases in fibrinogen, factor VII and factor VIII have been reported [8, 142]. The glycoprotein manufactured by the endothelial cell, vWF, is a portion of the factor VIII complex. Von Willebrand factor can be measured in the blood either by ristocetin-induced platelet clumping or by immunologic techniques. Both methods have shown vWF levels to be elevated in diabetic subjects. Elevation of this factor appears to reflect endothelial cell damage.

Prostacyclin, a potent endogenous platelet antiaggregant and vasodilator, is manufactured in the endothelium from arachidonic acid. Several studies have demonstrated that its activity was reduced in diabetes [143]. Experimentally, better metabolic control with insulin has returned aortic or renal prostacyclin activity to normal [144]. Plasminogen activator converts plasminogen to plasmin which activates the fibrinolytic pathway. Decreased plasminogen activator activity has been reported in diabetic subjects [145].

Platelets

Altered platelet function has been observed in the majority of studies of diabetic humans and animals. Diabetic patients with or without vascular disease appear to have a greater rate of platelet production [146]. Platelet adhesiveness and aggregation contribute to the formation of the atherosclerotic plaque as well as acute thrombosis found with acute MI. Platelet adhesion and aggregation with subsequent release of platelet derived growth factor stimulate the proliferation of smooth muscle cells and contribute to the formation of the plaque.

Diabetic patients with or without vascular disease tend to have increased platelet adhesiveness and increased sensitivity to aggregating agents [146, 147]. Control of elevated glucose has not been reported to alter enhanced platelet reactivity [148]. Synthesis of thromboxane A_2, a potent vasoconstrictor and platelet aggregating agent, is elevated in diabetic patients with or without CAD as well as in patients with CAD without diabetes. A correlation has been reported between the plasma glucose level and arachidonic acid-stimulated thromboxane synthesis. These abnormalities may precede the development of clinically evident diabetes [149–151]. Most of the studies have been in vitro or animal models. Further studies will be needed to clarify platelet and clotting abnormalities which are directly related to diabetes or hyperglycemia and which are secondary to existing atherosclerosis and/or damage to the vascular endothelium.

Silent Ischemia

In 1962, researchers at the Joslin Clinic reported 42 of 100 diabetic patients with recent acute MI experienced no pain, versus only 6 non-diabetic patients [152]. Similarly, during 18 years of follow-up in the Framingham Study, 23% of all documented MIs were discovered only by routine follow-up electrocardiograms. Of these cases, 53% were classified as 'silent', while in the others histories of interim symptoms compatible with MI were reported [153]. Silent and less painful MI has been reported to occur more frequently in diabetic patients than in non-diabetics: in one analysis, 32–42% of diabetic patients had no chest pain compared with 6–15% of non-diabetic patients [154]. While this trend was seen at the 18-year follow-up it was not significant, possibly due to the low number of participants [153]. Interestingly, the 26-year follow-up Framingham data showed an increased incidence of silent infarction in diabetic men, but not in diabetic women [86].

Angina has also been reported to be an unreliable index of myocardial ischemia in diabetics with CAD. Nesto et al found a greater number of ischemic diabetic patients had painless ST-T changes on exercise testing compared to ischemic non-diabetic patients [155]. An increase in asymptomatic transient ST-T changes in all diabetic subjects compared to all non-diabetic subjects has also been reported [156].

Autonomic nervous system dysfunction has been suggested as a major cause of increased asymptomatic MI in diabetic patients [155–157]. Afferent fibers running through the cardiac sympathetic nervous system form the essential pathway for the transmission of cardiac pain. In a study of diabetic patients who died from painless MI, morphologic alterations of the nerves, including beaded thickening, hyperargentophilia, spindle shape, fragmentation and decreased number of fibers were found [158]. In addition, alteration of cardiac parasympathetic reflexes has been reported [157].

Other investigators have not found an increased rate of painless ischemia in diabetic patients [159–161]. The amount of pain medication used in the acute MI phase among hospitalized patients did not differ significantly between diabetic and non-diabetic subjects [159].

Silent ischemia may contribute to increased mortality by delaying diagnosis or making the diagnosis of previous infarction more difficult. Sudden death, common among patients with diabetic autonomic neuropathy, may be due to CAD producing arrhythmias or MI. With the high prevalence of CAD among diabetic patients, they should be closely monitored. Exercise testing and Holter monitoring are useful ways to assess the diabetic patient for ischemia.

Congestive Heart Failure

In the Framingham Study 18-year follow-up, diabetic men age 45–74 years had more than twice the frequency of heart failure compared with a non-diabetic cohort; diabetic women had a fivefold increase compared to non-diabetic women [147]. Even after other risk factors are accounted for, female diabetic patients were twice as vulnerable as males to congestive heart failure. In addition, diabetic patients with CAD develop cardiomyopathy more commonly than do non-diabetics with CAD [162]. The development of a diabetic cardiopathy may be related

to metabolic factors or microangiopathy [163].

A study of 49 untreated diabetic patients without evidence of clinical heart disease or hypertension demonstrated abnormalities of left ventricular function (compared with 32 control patients). These abnormalities included prolonged isovolumetric relaxation time, reduced E-F slope, and increased Weissler index (pre-ejection period/left ventricular ejection time) [163]. Studies on young CAD-asymptomatic diabetic patients support the existence of diabetic cardiomyopathy, but do not relate type, duration or severity of diabetes to the time of onset or degree of ventricular dysfunction [162]. The experiments of Baandrup et al in rats support these conclusions and emphasize the importance of careful insulin treatment in the prevention of diabetic cardiomyopathy [164].

Acute Myocardial Infarction

Rytter et al reported the prevalence of diabetes among acute MI patients as 9.7% versus 6.1% in an age-matched control group [165]. In Poland, Czyzk et al compared diabetic subjects to age-matched non-diabetic subjects and found the largest differences in mortality from MI to be in his youngest group (30–45 years) with the difference decreasing with age [161]. Meta-analysis shows diabetic patients have a statistically significant higher mortality from acute MI (31%) compared with non-diabetic subjects (19.5%) [166]. In contrast to the general population, the risk of MI is identical for diabetic men and women. However, diabetic women have a 40% greater mortality from MI than diabetic men [166].

Complications of Myocardial Infarction

Death from heart failure following acute MI is high among both diabetic and non-diabetic patients. In diabetic patients an increased incidence of postinfarction heart failure has been reported [167]; postinfarction mortality is especially high in obese diabetic women [168]. The increased incidence of left ventricular failure accompanying infarction in diabetic patients cannot be explained on the basis of enzymatically measured infarct size [169]. Stone et al suggest the factors responsible for the increased mortality may be related to underlying cardiomyopathy, acceleration of the atherosclerotic process, or an unidentified factor [170].

Mechanisms to explain the increased incidence of congestive heart failure in diabetic patients with acute MI include impaired reflex adaptation to hemodynamic stress from autonomic dysfunction, previous hypertension, small vessel CAD, an increased incidence of previously unrecognized infarction, underlying ventricular dysfunction or a combination of these factors. Diabetic patients may be prone to the development of excess extravascular lung water, even in the face of normal or mildly elevated left ventricular filling pressures. An alteration in capillary permeability associated with chronic diabetes, low plasma oncotic pressure from chronic disease, metabolic imbalance or vigorous resuscitation with crystalloids in the acute infarction phase could all increase extravascular fluid extravasation and heart failure [166].

The location of the infarction may also partly explain the increased incidence of heart failure and increased mortality in diabetic patients. Anterior wall MI frequently involves more heart muscle and is more disruptive to ventricular function than infarction in other areas of the heart. Diabetic subjects have been reported to have an increased frequency of anterior infarctions. Weitzman et al found the combination of diabetes and anterior infarct site to be associated with the highest mortality rate in their comparison of 60-day survival rates [171].

Cardiogenic shock is increased in diabetic compared with non-diabetic subjects [166, 172]. In a second series, approximately 26% of diabetic subjects had cardiogenic shock. The increased risk of cardiogenic shock may be secondary to the small vessel disease in diabetes. Rupture of the ventricular free wall, a complication of acute MI, has been found to occur 2.7 times more frequently in diabetic than in non-diabetic subjects. Female gender and hypertension which are relatively more common in diabetes have been independently linked to rupture of the myocardium [166].

Ketoacidosis occurring in association with acute MI is associated with a marked increase in mortality [173]. Normally, fatty acid oxidation provides most of the energy for the heart. When myocardial oxygen delivery falls, glucose becomes the main energy source for the ischemic heart muscle. Glucose use by the myocardium is enhanced by insulin. As in other acutely stressful conditions, there is an increased output of adrenal steroids and catecholamines which inhibit the action of insulin. The result can be impaired myocardial uptake of glucose. Insulin deficiency also increases lipolysis with subsequent increase in circulating free fatty acids and ketone bodies [174]. Free fatty acids may further exacerbate the metabolic imbalance by increasing myocardial oxygen demands, and have been associated with cardiac arrhythmias. However, the frequency of cardiac arrhythmias in patients with diabetes mellitus has been reported to be increased or unchanged compared to non-diabetic patients [166, 174].

TREATMENT OF ACUTE MI IN THE DIABETIC PATIENT

Some of the excess mortality among diabetic patients may be explicable on the basis of their higher frequency of hypertension, obesity or hyperlipidemia. A relationship between increased mortality from acute MI and preinfarction metabolic control has also been noted [165]. Poor metabolic control preceding acute MI could worsen the prognosis. Levels of HbA_{1c} correlated with prognosis, with a mortality rate (23%) much greater for those with normal HbA_{1c} values (less than 7.5%), compared with the mortality rate (33%) of those with borderline abnormal HbA_{1c} (7.5–8.5%), and compared with the mortality rate (63%) of those with clearly abnormal levels (greater than 8.5%). Cardiogenic shock was also a more common complication in acute MI among those with higher HbA_{1c} values.

There is uncertainty about the effect of treatment of diabetes on prognosis following acute MI. The intravenous infusion of insulin has been reported to markedly improve survival, especially in those who have been receiving oral hypoglycemic agents [174]. Others have reported that although the blood glucose concentration could be satisfactorily controlled between 100 mg/dl and 200 mg/dl in patients who were unable to eat, had cardiogenic shock or severe hyperglycemia, a decreased mortality could not be demonstrated [173].

Alternatively, complications from insulin therapy can lead to hypoglycemia with hyperepinephrinenemia, arrhythmia or extension of the infarction [72]. Oral hypoglycemic agents theoretically may be harmful at the time of acute

MI by increasing oxygen consumption through positive inotropic action. Insulin-treated NIDDM patients had a better prognosis than non-insulin-treated NIDDM patients [126]. Overall, no difference in mortality rates from acute infarction has been demonstrated between NIDDM and IDDM patients [175].

LONG-TERM SURVIVAL

Diabetes is an independent determinant of long-term mortality and reinfarction. Diabetic men surviving the acute phase of infarction have been shown to have a poorer long-term prognosis and a higher rate of reinfarction than non-diabetic men. The mortality rate was greater in diabetic patients compared to non-diabetic patients for 1–5 years after acute MI. The Gothenborg trial reported a 5-year mortality rate of 46% among diabetic men after acute MI, compared to a 27% mortality in non-diabetic men after acute MI [175, 176].

A high percentage of diabetic patients had angina pectoris after infarction which excluded them from taking a rate-limited exercise treadmill test [177]. Either diabetes contributes a unique characteristic that accounts for the poorer prognosis, or diabetic patients have accelerated atherosclerosis [178].

It is not clear what effect tight metabolic control has on short-term or long-term prognosis. The mortality rate has been reported to be highest in those requiring insulin for blood glucose control and least in those managed with diet alone. Causes of death included recurrent infarction, heart failure and arrhythmias [166]. A second study of survival when a cardiac event recurred revealed no difference between diabetic patients treated with insulin, diet, or oral agents [175]. Recently it has been reported that medications that cause β-blockade decrease mortality and reinfarction among diabetic patients following acute MI [179].

CORONARY ARTERY BYPASS SURGERY IN DIABETIC PATIENTS

For bypass surgery to be useful, the extramural vessels must support adequate distal flow. Discrepancies in the location, severity and diffuseness of coronary artery obstruction in diabetic patients remain. Angiographic studies to select patients suitable for bypass surgery might have excluded a large number of diabetic patients with diffuse inoperable disease. Alternatively, diabetic patients with more advanced disease might have been selected for study if there were a tendency to delay surgery on diabetic patients until later in their course.

Nevertheless, a substantial proportion of diabetic patients have been shown to be operable coronary disease. Small-caliber blood vessels less than 2 mm on arteriography should not be a specific contraindication to coronary bypass surgery among diabetic patients, in view of the probable underestimation of coronary artery diameter [180].

Results of Coronary Artery Bypass Surgery

There is increased morbidity and mortality in diabetic patients who have bypass surgery. Sternotomy complications, renal insufficiency and total hospital days are greater in NIDDM patients treated with oral hypoglycemics or diet and IDDM patients than in non-diabetic patients. Perioperative mortality was doubled in diabetic subjects: 9% versus 4% in non-diabetics. Other studies have also reported an increased perioperative mortality. A lower long-term survival rate has been reported in diabetic patients compared with non-diabetic patients after coronary bypass surgery [42, 44, 181]. Other investigators have found no difference in outcome [180]. The severity of diabetes was an important determinant of long-term survival [182]. Patients with NIDDM controlled by diet had a prognosis indistinguishable from non-diabetic patients, while diabetic patients receiving insulin had a poorer long-term prognosis. Another series found that IDDM patients had the same results from bypass surgery as NIDDM patients [180]. Graft flow rates play a significant role in the long-term outcome of coronary bypass surgery. The flow rates in coronary bypass grafts in diabetic subjects have been reported to be similar [44] or decreased compared to non-diabetic subjects [183]. The relief of angina pectoris after bypass surgery has been reported to be equal in diabetic and non-diabetic patients [55, 180, 181].

Diabetes is not a contraindication to coronary artery bypass grafting. Diabetes is a factor to be taken into account when evaluating a patient for coronary bypass grafting, but it should not disqualify a patient who would benefit from the surgery [180, 182].

CONCLUSION

As the population ages, the macrovascular complications of diabetes become more prevalent. Diabetic subjects, especially women, have increased morbidity and mortality from CAD. Diabetic patients have an increased incidence of risk factors which predispose to coronary atherosclerosis. In addition, hyperglycemia, hyperinsulinemia, increased platelet aggregation, altered coagulation and other metabolic changes all contribute to the atherosclerotic process.

There is still debate whether CAD is a direct result of hyperglycemia, insulin resistance or hyperinsulinemia. More information relating the presence of clinically apparent CAD and coronary atherosclerosis with duration, severity, therapy and degree of control will be necessary. Alternatively, individuals who develop diabetes may also possess the characteristics that predispose to CAD.

Congestive heart failure is more prevalent among diabetic patients, and the prognosis of diabetic patients with myocardial infarction is poorer than for non-diabetic patients. Coronary artery bypass surgery has increased mortality and morbidity in diabetic subjects, but is still indicated if the coronary anatomy makes the surgery technically impossible.

REFERENCES

1. Ganda OP. Pathogenesis of macrovascular disease including the influence of lipids. In Marble A, Krall LP, Bradley RF, Christlieb AR, Soeldner JS (eds) Joslin's Diabetes mellitus, 12th edn. Philadelphia: Lea & Febiger, 1985: pp. 217–50.

2. Jarrett R. Diabetes and the heart: coronary heart disease. Clin Endocrinol Metab 1977; 6: 389–402.

3. Steiner G. Atherosclerosis: the major complication of diabetes. Adv Exp Med Biol 1985; 189: 277–97.

4. Harris MI, Entmacher, PS. Mortality from diabetes: In National Diabetes Data Group (eds) Diabetes in America: diabetes data compiled 1984. NIH publ. no. 85–1468. Bethesda, MD: US Department of Health and Human Services, 1985: XXIX1–XXIX48.

5. Marble A. Late complications of diabetes: a continuing challenge. The Elliot P. Joslin Memorial Lecture of the German Diabetes Federation. Diabetologia 1976; 12: 193–9.

6. Kramer DW, Perlstein PK. Peripheral vascular complications in diabetes mellitus. Diabetes 1958; 7: 384–7. Citation derived from Santen RJ, Willis PW III, Fajans SS. Atherosclerosis in diabetes mellitus: correlations with serum lipid levels, adiposity, and serum insulin levels. Arch Int Med 1972; 130: 833–43.

7. National Diabetes Group, National Institute of Arthritis, Diabetes, and Digestive and Kidney Disease. National Institutes of Health data sheet on prevalence and incidence of diabetes in the United States, 1982. National Institutes of Health: Bethesda, 1982.

8. Kannel WB, McGee DL. Diabetes and cardiovascular disease: The Framingham Study. JAMA 1979; 241: 2035–8.

9. Kleinman JC, Donahue RP, Harris MI, Finucane FF, Madans JH, Brock DB. Mortality among diabetics in a national sample. Am J Epidemiol 1988; 128: 389–401.

10. Pyörälä K, Laakso M, Uusitupa M. Diabetes and atherosclerosis: an epidemiologic view. Diabetes Metab Rev 1987; 3: 463–524.

11. Pan W-H, Cedres LB, Liu K et al. Relationship of clinical diabetes and asymptomatic hyperglycemia to risk of coronary heart disease mortality in men and women. Am J Epidemiol 1986; 123: 504–16.

12. Heyden S, Heiss G, Bartel AG, Hames CG. Sex differences in coronary mortality among diabetics in Evans County, Georgia. J Chron Dis 1980; 33: 265–73.

13. Robertson WB, Strong JP. Atherosclerosis in persons with hypertension and diabetes mellitus. Lab Invest 1968; 18: 538–51.

14. Kawate R, Yamakido M, Nishimoto Y, Bennett PH, Harriman RF, Knowler W. Diabetes mellitus and its vascular complications in Japanese migrants on the Island of Hawaii. Diabetes Care 1979; 2: 161–70.

15. International Symposium on the Advances in Diabetes Epidemiology, 1982, Abbaye de Fontevraud, France. Advances in diabetes epidemiology. New York: Elsevier, 1982.

16. Keen H, Jarrett RJ, Fuller JH, McCartney P. Hyperglycemia and arterial disease. Diabetes 1981; 30 (suppl. 2): 49–53.

17. Framingham Study. An epidemiological investigation of cardiovascular disease. Section 26. Washington, DC: US Government Printing Office, 1970.

18. Gordon T, Kannel WB. Predisposition to atherosclerosis in the head, heart, and legs. The Framingham Study. JAMA 1972; 221: 661–6.

19. Ostrander LD Jr, Francis T Jr, Hayner NS, Kjelsberg MO, Epstein FH. The relationship of

cardiovascular disease to hyperglycemia. Ann Intern Med 1965; 62: 1188–98.

20. Keen H, Rose G, Pyke DA, Boyns D, Chlouverakis C, Mistry S. Blood-sugar and arterial disease. Lancet 1965; ii: 505–8.

21. Stamler R, Stamler J (eds). Asymptomatic hyperglycemia and coronary heart disease: a series of papers by the International Collaborative Group, based on studies in fifteen populations. J Chron Dis 1979; 32: 681–837.

22. International Collaborative Group. Joint discussion. International Collaborative Group. J Chron Dis 1979; 32: 829–37.

23. Fuller JH, Shipley MJ, Rose G, Jarrett RJ, Keen H. Coronary-heart-disease and impaired glucose tolerance: the Whitehall Study. Lancet 1980; ii: 1373–6.

24. Eschwege E, Ducimetiere P, Papoz L, Claude JR, Richard JL. Blood glucose and coronary heart disease (letter). Lancet 1980; ii: 472–3.

25. Pÿörälä K, Laakso M. Macrovascular disease in diabetes mellitus. In Mann JI, Pÿörälä K, Teuscher A (eds) Diabetes in epidemiological perspective. Edinburgh: Churchill Livingstone, 1983: pp 183–247.

26. Barrett-Connor E, Wingard DL, Criqui MH, Suarez L. Is borderline fasting hyperglycemia a risk factor for cardiovascular death? J Chron Dis 1984; 37: 773–9.

27. Jarrett RJ, McCartney P, Keen H. The Bedford Survey: ten year mortality rates in newly diagnosed diabetics, borderline diabetics and normoglycaemic controls and risk indices for coronary heart disease in borderline diabetics. Diabetologia 1982; 22: 79–84.

28. Butler WJ, Ostrander LD Jr, Carman WJ, Lamphiear DE. Mortality from coronary heart disease in the Tecumseh Study. Long-term effect of diabetes mellitus, glucose tolerance and other risk factors. Am J Epidemiol 1985; 121: 541–7.

29. Lapidus L, Bengtsson C, Blohmé G, Lindquist O, Nyström E. Blood glucose, glucose tolerance and manifest diabetes in relation to cardiovascular disease and death in women. A 12-year follow-up of participants in the population study of women in Gothenburg, Sweden. Acta Med Scand 1985; 218: 455–62.

30. Pan W-H, Cedres LB, Liu K et al. Relationship of clinical diabetes and asymptomatic hyperglycemia to risk of coronary heart disease mortality in men and women. Am J Epidemiol 1986; 123: 504–16.

31. Uusitupa MIJ, Niskanen LK, Siitonen O, Voutilainen E, Pÿörälä K. Five-year incidence of atherosclerotic vascular disease in relation to general risk factors, insulin level, and abnormalities in lipoprotein composition in non-insulin-

dependent diabetic and nondiabetic subjects. Circulation 1990; 82: 27–36.

32. Yano K, MacLean CJ, Reed DM et al. A comparison of the 12-year mortality and predictive factors of coronary heart disease among Japanese men in Japan and Hawaii. Am J Epidemiol 1988; 127: 476–87.

33. Kagan A, Yano K, Reed DM, MacLean CJ. Predictors of sudden cardiac death among Hawaiian-Japanese men. Am J Epidemiol 1989; 130: 268–77.

34. Donahue RP, Abbott RD, Reed DM, Yano K. Postchallenge glucose concentration and coronary heart disease in men of Japanese ancestry: Honolulu Heart Program. Diabetes 1987; 36: 689–92.

35. Reed DM, MacLean CJ, Hayashi T. Predictors of atherosclerosis in the Honolulu Heart Program. I. Biologic, dietary, and lifestyle characteristics. Am J Epidemiol 1987; 126: 214–25.

36. Steiner G. Atherosclerosis: the major complication of diabetes. Adv Exp Med Biol 1985; 189: 277–89.

37. Robertson WB, Strong JP. Atherosclerosis in persons with hypertension and diabetes mellitus. Lab Invest 1968; 18: 538–51.

38. Woolf N. Diabetes and atherosclerosis. Acta Diab Lat 1971; 8: 14–42.

39. Hamby RI, Sherman L. Duration and treatment of diabetes: relationship to severity of coronary artery disease. NY State J Med 1979; 79: 1683–8.

40. Dortimer A, Shenoy P, Shiroff R, Leaman D, Babb J, Liedtke A, Zelis R. Diffuse coronary artery disease in diabetic patients: fact or fiction? Circulation 1978; 57: 133–6.

41. Vigorita V, Moore G, Hutchins G. Absence of correlation between coronary arterial atherosclerosis and severity or duration of diabetes mellitus of adult onset. Am J Cardiol 1980; 46: 535–41.

42. Salomon NW, Page US, Okies JE, Stephens J, Krause AH, Bigelow JC. Diabetes mellitus and coronary artery bypass: short-term risk and long-term prognosis. J Thorac Cardiovasc Surg 1983; 85: 264–71.

43. Waller B, Palumbo P, Lie J, Roberts W. Status of the coronary arteries at necropsy in diabetes mellitus with onset after age 30 years: analysis of 229 diabetic patients with and without clinical evidence of coronary heart disease and comparison to 183 control subjects. Am J Med 1980; 69: 498–506.

44. Verska J, Walker W. Aortocoronary bypass in the diabetic patient. Am J Cardiol 1975; 35: 774–7.

45. Lemp G, VanderZwaag R, Hughes J et al. Association between the severity of diabetes mellitus

and coronary arterial atherosclerosis. Am J Cardiol 1987; 60: 1015–19.

46. Zonereich S. Diabetes and the heart. Springfield: Thomas, 1978.

47. Crall F, Roberts W. The extramural and intramural coronary arteries in juvenile diabetes mellitus—analysis of nine necropsy patients aged 19–38 years with onset of diabetes before age 15 years. Am J Med 1978; 64: 222–30.

48. Factor S, Okun E, Minase T. Capillary microaneurysms in the human diabetic heart. New Engl J Med 1980; 302: 384–8.

49. Blumenthal HT, Alex M, Goldenberg S. A study of lesions of the intramural coronary artery branches in diabetes mellitus. Arch Pathol 1960; 70: 27–40.

50. Kannel W, McGee D. Diabetes and glucose tolerance as risk factors for cardiovascular disease: the Framingham Study. Diabetes Care 1979; 2: 120–6.

51. Pirart J. Diabetes mellitus and its degenerative complications: a prospective study of 4400 patients observed between 1947 and 1973. Diabetes Care 1978; 1: 252–61.

52. Greene DA. Acute and chronic complications of diabetes mellitus in older patients. Am J Med 1986; 80 (suppl. 5A): 39–47.

53. Stout RW. Blood glucose and atherosclerosis. Atherosclerosis 1981; 1: 227–34.

54. Garcia M, McNamara P, Gordon T, Kannel W. Morbidity and mortality in diabetics in the Framingham population. Diabetes 1974; 23: 105–11.

55. Kannel W. Diabetic-atherogenic connection: a continuing puzzle. Cardiol 1987; 74: 333–4.

56. Jarrett RJ. Type 2 (non-insulin-dependent) diabetes mellitus and coronary heart disease—chicken, egg or neither? Diabetologia 1984; 26: 99–102.

57. Rubler S, Fisher V. The significance of repeated exercise testing with thallium-201 scanning in asymptomatic diabetic males. Clin Cardiol 1985; 8: 621–8.

58. Heyden S, Heiss G, Bartel AG, Hames CG. Sex differences in coronary mortality among diabetics in Evans County, Georgia. J Chron Dis 1979; 33: 265–73.

59. Lapidus L, Bengtsson C, Blohme G, Lindquist O, Nystrom E. Blood glucose, glucose tolerance and manifest diabetes in relation to cardiovascular disease and death in women: a 12-year follow-up of participants in the population study of women in Gothenburg, Sweden. Acta Med Scand 1985; 218: 455–62.

60. Jarrett R, McCartney P, Keen H. The Bedford Survey: ten year mortality rates in newly diagnosed diabetics, borderline diabetics and normoglycaemic controls and risk indices for coronary heart disease in borderline diabetics. Diabetologia 1982; 22: 79–84.

61. Cruickshanks K, Orchard T, Becker D. The cardiovascular risk profile of adolescents with insulin-dependent diabetes mellitus. Diabetes Care 1985; 8: 118–24.

62. Gordon T, Castelli WP, Hjortland MC, Kannel WB, Dawber TR. Diabetes, blood lipids, and the role of obesity in coronary heart disease risk for women: the Framingham Study. Ann Intern Med 1977; 87: 393–7.

63. Butler WJ, Ostrander LD Jr, Carman WJ, Lamphiear DE. Mortality from coronary heart disease in the Tecumseh study: long-term effect of diabetes mellitus, glucose tolerance and other risk factors. Am J Epidemiol 1985; 121: 541–7.

64. Barrett-Connor E, Cohn B, Wingard D, Edelstein S. Why is diabetes mellitus a stronger risk factor for fatal ischemic heart disease in women than in men? JAMA 1991; 265: 627–31.

65. Barrett-Connor E, Orchard T. Insulin-dependent diabetes mellitus and ischemic heart disease. Diabetes Care 1985; 8: 65–9.

66. van Hoeven KH, Factor SM. Diabetic heart disease: the clinical and pathological spectrum—Part I. Clin Cardiol 1989; 12: 600–4.

67. Crall FV Jr, Roberts WC. The extramural and intramural coronary arteries in juvenile diabetes mellitus: Analysis of nine necropsy patients aged 19 to 38 years with onset of diabetes before age 15 years. Am J Med 1978; 64: 221–30.

68. Paz-Guevara A, Hsu T, White P. Juvenile diabetes mellitus after forty years. Diabetes 1975; 24: 559–65.

69. Rot H, Barclay P. Diabetes of thirty-five years duration. JAMA 1956; 161: 801–6.

70. Kaplan N, Stamler J (eds). Prevention of coronary heart disease. Philadelphia: WB Saunders, 1983.

71. Mühlhauser I. Smoking and diabetes. Diabetic Med 1990; 7: 10–15.

72. Pyörälä K. Diabetes and coronary heart disease. Acta Endocrinol 1985; 110 (suppl. 272): 11–19.

73. Kannel W, McGee D. Diabetes and cardiovascular risk factors: the Framingham Study. Circulation 1979; 59: 8–13.

74. Brand FN, Abbott RD, Kannel WB. Diabetes, intermittent claudication, and risk of cardiovascular events: the Framingham Study. Diabetes 1989; 38: 504–9.

75. Jones RB, Hedley AJ. Prevalence of smoking in a diabetic population: the need for action. Diabet Med 1987; 4: 233–6.

76. Pell S, D'Alonzo CA. Some aspects of hypertension in diabetes mellitus. JAMA 1967; 202: 104–10.

77. Klein R, Klein B, Moss S, DeMets D. Blood

pressure and hypertension in diabetes. Am J Epidemiol 1985; 122: 75–88.

78. Working Group on Hypertension in Diabetes. Statement on hypertension in diabetes mellitus: final report. Arch Int Med 1987; 147: 830–41.

79. Parving HH, Andersen AR, Smidt UM, Svendsen PA. Early aggressive antihypertensive treatment reduces rate of decline in kidney function in diabetic nephropathy. Lancet 1983; i: 1175–9.

80. Ganda P. Pathogenesis of macrovascular disease in the human diabetic. Diabetes 1980; 29: 931–42.

81. Bild D, Teutsch SM. The control of hypertension in persons with diabetes: a public health approach. Publ Health Rep 1987; 102: 522–9.

82. Barrett-Connor E, Criqui MJ, Klauber MR, Holdbrook M. Diabetes and hypertension in a community of older adults. Am J Epidemiol 1981; 113: 276–83.

83. Weidmann P, Trost B. Pathogenesis and treatment of hypertension associated with diabetes. Horm Metab Res 1985; 15 (suppl.): 51–8.

84. Rowe JW, Young JB, Minaker KL, Stevens AL, Pallotta J, Landsberg L. Effect of insulin and glucose infusions on sympathetic nervous system activity in normal man. Diabetes 1981; 30: 219–25.

85. Ferrannini E, Buzzigoli G, Bonadonna R. Insulin resistance in essential hypertension. New Engl J Med 1987; 317: 350–7.

86. Kannel WB. Lipids, diabetes, and coronary heart disease: insights from the Framingham Study. Am Heart J 1985; 110: 1100–7.

87. Grundy S, Barnett J. Metabolic and health complications of obesity. Dis Mon 1990; 36: 669.

88. Gordon T, Castelli WP, Hjortland MC, Kannel WB, Dawber TR. Diabetes, blood lipids, and the role of obesity in coronary heart disease risk for women: the Framingham Study. Ann Intern Med 1977; 87: 393–7.

89. Borkan GA, Sparrow D, Wisniewski C, Vokonas P. Body weight and coronary heart disease risk: patterns of risk factor change associated with long-term weight change: the normative aging study. Am J Epidemiol 1986; 124: 410–18.

90. Barrett-Connor E. Obesity, atherosclerosis and coronary artery disease. Ann Intern Med 1985; 103 (suppl. 2): 1010–18.

91. Iverius PH, Brunzell J. Obesity and common genetic metabolic disorders. Ann Intern Med 1985; 103 (suppl. 2): 1050–1.

92. Despres JP, Moorjani S, Ferland M et al. Adipose tissue distribution and plasma lipoprotein levels in obese women: importance of intraabdominal fat. Arteriosclerosis 1989; 9: 203–9.

93. Bjorntorp P. Regional patterns of fatty distribution. Ann Intern Med 1985; 103 (suppl. 2): 994–5.

94. Brunzell JD. Obesity and coronary heart disease: a targeted approach. Arteriosclerosis 1984; 4: 180–2.

95. Winocour PH, Laker MF. Drug therapy for diabetic dyslipoproteinaemia: a practical approach. Diabet Med 1990; 7: 292–8.

96. Tzagournis M. Interaction of diabetes with hypertension and lipids: patients at high risk. Am J Med 1989; 86 (suppl. 1B): 50–4.

97. Schonfeld G. Diabetes, lipoproteins, and atherosclerosis. Metabolism 1985; 34: 45–50.

98. Frier BM, Sudek CD. Cholesterol metabolism in diabetes: the effect of insulin on the kinetics of plasma squalene. J Clin Endocrinol Metab 1979; 49: 824–8.

99. Bennion LJ, Grundy SM. Effects of diabetes mellitus on cholesterol metabolism in man. New Engl J Med 1977; 296: 1367–71.

100. Kissebah AH, Alfarsi S, Adams PW, Wynn V. The metabolic fate of plasma lipoproteins in normal subjects and in patients with insulin resistance and endogenous hypertriglyceridemia. Diabetologia 1976; 12: 501–9.

101. Owens D, Maher V, Collins P, Johnson A, Tomkin G. Cellular cholesterol regulation: a defect in the Type 2 (non-insulin-dependent) diabetic patient in poor metabolic control. Diabetologia 1990; 33: 93–9.

102. Lopes-Virella E, Sherer G, Wohltmann H. Diabetic lipoprotein deficient serum: its effect on low density lipoprotein uptake and degradation by fibroblasts. Metabolism 1985; 34: 1079–85.

103. Crouse JR, Parks JS, Schey HM, Kahl FR. Studies of low density lipoprotein molecular weight in human beings with coronary artery disease. J Lipid Res 1985; 26: 566–74.

104. Musliner T, Giotas C, Krauss R. Presence of multiple subpopulations of lipoproteins of intermediate density in normal subjects. Atherosclerosis 1986; 6: 79–87.

105. Barakat H, Carpenter J, McLendon V, Khazanie P, Leggett N, Heath J, Marks R. Influence of obesity, impaired glucose tolerance, and NIDDM and LDL structure and composition. Diabetes 1990; 39: 1527–32.

106. Aberg H, Lithell H, Selinus I, Hedstrand H. Serum triglycerides are a risk factor for myocardial infarction but not for angina pectoris. Result from a 10-year follow-up of Uppsala Primary Preventive Study. Atherosclerosis 1985; 54: 89–97.

107. Carlson LA, Bottiger LE. Risk factors for ischaemic heart disease in men and women. Acta Med Scand 1985; 218: 207–11.

108. Beigel Y, Gotto A. Lipoproteins in health and

disease: diagnosis and management. Cardiol Series 1986; 9: 1.

109. Reaven GM, Greenfield MS. Diabetic hypertriglyceridemia: evidence for three clinical syndrome. Diabetes 1981; 30 (suppl. 2): 66–75.

110. Wolinsky H, Goldfischer S, Capron L, Capron F. Hydrolase activities in the rat aorta. I. Effects of diabetes mellitus and insulin treatment. Circ Res 1978; 42: 821–31.

111. Masarei J, Kiiveri H, Stanton K. Risk factors for cardiovascular disease in a diabetic population. Pathol 1986; 18: 89–93.

112. Reckless JPD, Betteridge DJ, Wu P et al. High and low density lipoproteins and the prevalence of vascular disease in diabetes mellitus. Br Med J 1978; 1: 883–6.

113. Gordon T, Castelli WP, Hjortland MC et al. Diabetes, blood lipids and the role of obesity in coronary heart disease risk for women. The Framingham Study. Ann Intern Med 1977; 87: 393–7.

114. Lopes-Virella M, Stone P, Colwell J. Serum high density lipoprotein in diabetic patients. Diabetologia 1977; 13: 285–91.

115. Schaefer EJ, Anderson DW, Brewer Jr HB, Levy RI, Danner RN, Blackwelder WC. Plasma-triglycerides in regulation of HDL-cholesterol levels. Lancet 1978; ii: 391–3.

116. Laakso M, Pyörälä K, Sarlund H, Voutilainen E. Lipid and lipoprotein abnormalities associated with coronary heart disease in patients with insulin-dependent diabetes mellitus. Arteriosclerosis 1986; 6: 679–84.

117. Hollenbeck C, Chen Y, Greenfield M, Lardinois C, Reaven G. Reduced plasma high density lipoprotein-cholesterol concentrations need not increase when hyperglycemia is controlled with insulin in noninsulin-dependent diabetes mellitus. J Clin Endocrinol Metab 1986; 62: 605–8.

118. Garcia-Webb P, Bonser AM, Whiting D, Masarei JRL. Insulin resistance: a risk factor for coronary heart disease? Scand J Clin Lab Invest 1983; 43: 677–85.

119. Klagsbrun M, Edelman ER. Biological and biochemical properties of fibroblast growth factors: implications for the pathogenesis of atherosclerosis. Arteriosclerosis 1989; 9: 269–78.

120. Guyton JR. Lipid metabolism and atherogenesis. In Garson A Jr, Bricker JT, McNamara DG (eds) The science and practice of pediatric cardiology. Philadelphia: Lea & Febiger, 1990: pp 475–91.

121. Ross R. The pathogenesis of atherosclerosis: an update. New Engl J Med 1986; 314: 488–500.

122. Reidy M. A reassessment of endothelial injury and arterial lesion formation. Lab Invest 1985; 53: 513–20.

123. Colwell J, Winocour P, Lopes-Virella M, Halushka P. New concepts about the pathogenesis of atherosclerosis in diabetes mellitus. Am J Med 1983; 75: 67–80.

124. King G. Cell biology as an approach to the study of the vascular complications of diabetes. Metabolism 1985; 34 (suppl. 1): 17–24.

125. Turner JL, Bierman EL. Effects of glucose and sorbitol on proliferation of cultured human skin fibroblasts and arterial smooth-muscle cells. Diabetes 1978; 27: 583–8.

126. Barnett A, Pyke D. Chlorpropamide-alcohol flushing and large-vessel disease in non-insulin-dependent diabetes. Br Med J 1980: 261–2.

127. Ditzel J. Oxygen transport impairment in diabetes. Diabetes 1976; 25 (suppl. 2): 822–38.

128. Bunn HF, Gabbay KH, Gallop PM. The glycosylation of hemogloblin: relevance to diabetes mellitus. Science 1978; 200: 21–7.

129. Steiner G. Diabetes and atherosclerosis metabolic links. Drugs 1988; 36 (suppl. 3): 22–6.

130. Stout R. Insulin and atheroma. Diabetes Care 1990; 13: 631–54.

131. Pyörälä K. Relationship of glucose tolerance and plasma insulin to the incidence of coronary heart disease: results from two population studies in Finland. Diabetes Care 1974; 2: 131–41.

132. Ducimetiere P, Eschwege E, Papos L, Richard JL, Claude JR, Rosselin G. Relationship of plasma insulin levels to the incidence of myocardial infarction and coronary heart disease mortality in a middle-aged population. Diabetologia 1980; 19: 205–10.

133. Eschwège E, Richard JL, Thibault N, Ducimetière P, Warnet JM, Claude JR, Rosselin G. Coronary heart disease mortality in relation with diabetes, blood glucose and plasma insulin levels: the Paris Prospective Study, ten years later. Horm Metab Res Suppl 1985; 15: 41–6.

134. Standl E, Janka H. High serum insulin concentrations in relation to other cardiovascular risk factors in macrovascular disease of Type 2 diabetes. Horm Metab Res 1985; 15 (suppl.): 46–51.

135. Hillson R, Hockaday T, Mann J, Newton D. Hyperinsulinaemia is associated with development of electrocardiographic abnormalities in diabetics. Diabetes Res 1984; 1: 143–9.

136. Osonoi T, Onuma T, Kudo M, Tsutsui M, Ochiai S, Takebe K. Analyses of risk factors of ischemic heart disease in diabetics: multivariate analyses. Tohoku Exp Med 1983; 141 (suppl.): 517–21.

137. Stout R. Overview of the association between insulin and atherosclerosis. Metabolism 1985; 34 (suppl. 1): 7–12.

138. Horwitz DL, Starr JI, Mako ME, Blackard

WG, Rubenstein AH. Proinsulin, insulin, and C-peptide concentrations in human portal and peripheral blood. J Clin Invest 1975; 55: 1278–83.

139. Cruz AD Jr, Grande F, Hay L. Effect of intraarterial insulin on tissue cholesterol and fatty acids in alloxan-diabetic dogs. Circ Res 1961; 9: 39–43.

140. Stout R, Buchanan K, Vallance-Owen J. The relationship of arterial disease and glucagon metabolism in insulin-treated chickens. Atherosclerosis 1973; 18: 153–62.

141. Chakkabarti R, Meade T. Clotting factor platelet function and fibrinolytic activity in diabetics and in a comparison group. Diabetologia 1976; 12: 383.

142. Kannel W, D'Agostino R, Wilson P, Belanger A, Gagnon D. Diabetes, fibrinogen, and risk of cardiovascular disease: The Framingham experience. Am Heart J 1990; 115: 672–6.

143. Harrison H, Reece A, Johnson M. Decreased vascular prostacyclin in experimental diabetes. Life Sci 1978; 23: 251–6.

144. Harrison H, Reece A, Johnson M. Effect of insulin treatment on prostacyclin in experimental diabetes. Diabetologia 1980; 18: 65–8.

145. Almer L, Pandolfi M. Fibrinolysis and diabetic retinopathy. Diabetes 1976; 25 (suppl. 2): 807–10.

146. Colwell J, Winocour P, Lopes-Virella M, Halushka P. New concepts about the pathogenesis of atherosclerosis in diabetes mellitus. Am J Med 1983; 75 (suppl.): 67–76.

147. Gensini G, Abbate R, Favilla S, Neri S. Changes of platelet function and blood clotting in diabetes mellitus. Thromb Hemostasis 1979; 42: 983–90.

148. Jackson C, Greaves M, Boulton A, Ward J, Preston F. Near-normal glycaemic control does not correct abnormal platelet reactivity in diabetes mellitus. Clin Sci 1984; 67: 551–5.

149. Butkus A, Shirey E, Schumaher O. Thromboxane biosynthesis in platelets of diabetic and coronary artery disease patients. Artery 1982; 11: 238–51.

150. Halushka P, Rogers R, Loadholt C, Colwell J. Increased platelet thromboxane synthesis in diabetes mellitus. J Lab Clin Med 1981; 97: 87–96.

151. Halushka PV, Mayfield R, Colwell JA. Insulin and arachidonic acid metabolism in diabetes mellitus. Metabolism 1985; 34 (suppl. 1): 32–6.

152. Bradley RF, Schonfeld A. Diminished pain in diabetic patients with myocardial infarction. Geriatrics 1962; 17: 322–6.

153. Margolis JR, Kannel WB, Feinleib M, Dawber TR, McNamara PM. Clinical features of unrecognized myocardial infarction—silent and symptomatic. Eighteen year follow-up: the Framingham Study. Am J Cardiol 1973; 32: 1–5.

154. Nesto RW, Phillips RT. Asymptomatic myocardial ischemia in diabetic patients. Am J Med 1986; 80 (suppl. 4C): 40–6.

155. Nesto RW, Phillips RT, Kett KG, Hill T, Perper E, Young E, Leland OS Jr. Angina and exertional myocardial ischemia in diabetic and nondiabetic patients: assessment by exercise thallium scintigraphy. Ann Intern Med 1988; 108: 170–5.

156. Chiariello M, Indolfi C, Cotecchia MR, Sifola C, Romano M, Condorelli M. Asymptomatic transient ST changes during ambulatory ECG monitoring in diabetic patients. Am Heart J 1985; 110: 529–34.

157. Niakan E, Harati Y, Rolak L, Comstock J, Rokey R. Silent myocardial infarction and diabetic cardiovascular autonomic neuropathy. Arch Int Med 1986; 146: 2229–30.

158. Faerman I, Faccio E, Milei J, Nunez R, Jadzinsky M, Fox D, Rapaport M. Autonomic neuropathy and painless myocardial infarction in diabetic patients: histologic evidence of their relationship. Diabetes 1977; 26: 1147–58.

159. Christensen PD, Kofoed PE, Seyer-Hansen K. Painless myocardial infarction in diabetes mellitus: a myth? Danish Med Bull 1985; 32: 273–5.

160. Smith JW, Buckels LJ, Carlson K, Marcus FI. Clinical characteristics and results of noninvasive tests in 60 diabetic patients after acute myocardial infarction. Am J Med 1983; 75: 217–24.

161. Czyzk A, Krolweski AS, Szablowska S, Alot A, Kopczynski J. Clinical course of myocardial infarction among diabetic patients. Diabetes Care 1980; 3: 526–9.

162. Zarich SW, Nesto RW. Diabetic cardiomyopathy. Am Heart J 1989; 118: 1000–12.

163. Attali JR, Sachs RN, Valensi P et al. Asymptomatic diabetic cardiomyopathy: a noninvasive study. Diabetes Res Clin Pract 1988; 4: 183–90.

164. Baandrup U, Ledet T, Rasch R. Experimental diabetic cardiopathy preventable by insulin treatment. Lab Invest 1981; 45: 169–73.

165. Rytter L, Troelsen S, Beck-Nielsen H. Prevalence and mortality of acute myocardial infarction in patients with diabetes. Diabetes Care 1985; 8: 230–4.

166. Kereiakes DJ. Myocardial infarction in the diabetic patient. Clin Cardiol 1985; 8: 446–50.

167. Jaffe AS, Spadaro JJ, Schechtman K, Roberts R, Geltman EM, Sobel BE. Increased congestive heart failure after myocardial infarction of modest extent in patients with diabetes mellitus. Am Heart J 1984; 108: 31–7.

168. Tansey MJB, Opie LH, Kennelly BM. High mortality in obese women diabetics with acute myocardial infarction. Br Med J. 1977; 1: 1624–6.

169. Gwilt DJ, Petri M, Lewis PW, Nattrass M, Pentecost BL. Myocardial infarct size and mortality in diabetic patients. Br Heart J 1985; 54: 466–72.

170. Stone PH, Muller JE, Hartwell T et al. The effect of diabetes mellitus on prognosis serial left ventricular function after acute myocardial infarction: contribution of both coronary disease and diastolic left ventricular dysfunction to the adverse prognosis. J Am Coll Cardiol 1989; 14: 49–57.

171. Weitzman S, Wagner GS, Heiss G, Haney TL, Slome C. Myocardial infarction site and mortality in diabetes. Diabetes Care 1982; 5: 31–4.

172. Partamian JO, Bradley RF. Acute myocardial infarction in 258 cases of diabetes: immediate mortality and five-year survival. New Engl J Med 1965; 273: 458–61.

173. Husband DJ, Alberti KGMM, Julian DG. Methods for the control of diabetes after acute myocardial infarction. Diabetes Care 1985; 8: 261–7.

174. Clark RS, English M, McNeill GP, Newton RW. Effect of intravenous infusion of insulin in diabetics with acute myocardial infarction. Br Med J. 1985; 291: 303–5.

175. Ulvenstam G, Åberg A, Bergstrand R et al. Long-term prognosis after myocardial infarction in men with diabetes. Diabetes 1985; 34: 787–92.

176. Herlitz J, Malmberg K, Karlson BW, Ryden L, Hjalmarson A. Mortality and morbidity during a five-year follow-up of diabetics with myocardial infarction. Acta Med Scand 1988; 224: 31–8.

177. Smith JW, Buckels LJ, Carlson K, Marcus FI. Clinical characteristics and results of non-invasive test in 60 diabetic patients after acute myocardial infarction. Am J Med 1983; 75: 217–24.

178. Verska JJ, Walker WJ. Aortocoronary bypass in the diabetic patient. Am J Cardiol 1975; 35: 774–7.

179. Gundersen T, Kjekshus J. Timolol treatment after myocardial infarction in diabetic patients. Diabetes Care 1983; 6: 285–9.

180. Devineni R, McKenzie FN. Surgery for coronary artery disease in patients with diabetes mellitus. Can J Surg 1985; 28: 367–70.

181. Johnson WD, Pedraza PM, Kayser KL. Coronary artery surgery in diabetics: 261 consecutive patients followed four to seven years. Am Heart J 1982; 104: 823–7.

182. Lawrie GM, Morris GM Jr, Glaeser DH. Influence of diabetes mellitus on the results of coronary bypass surgery: follow-up of 212 diabetic patients ten to 15 years after surgery. JAMA 1986; 256: 2967–71.

183. Chychota NN, Gau GT, Pluth JR, Wallace RB, Danielson GK. Myocardial revascularization: comparison of operability and surgical results in diabetic and nondiabetic patients. J Thorac Cardiovasc Surg 1973; 65: 856–62.

66

Clinical Features and Treatment of Peripheral Vascular Disease in Diabetes Mellitus

Frank W. LoGerfo and Michael S. Rosenblatt
New England Deaconess Hospital, Boston, Massachusetts, USA

Optimum management of patients depends upon a clear understanding of the characteristics of occlusive vascular disease as it occurs in association with diabetes mellitus. In particular, there are some widespread misconceptions about vascular occlusive disease that can lead to inappropriate treatment. One of these is the idea that diabetic patients have a microvascular occlusive disease that impairs perfusion. This concept arose from an uncontrolled observational study demonstrating the presence of PAS-positive material in small vessels [1]. Subsequent controlled studies failed to demonstrate any small vessel occlusive disease associated with the diabetic state on the basis of histology [2] arterial casting [3] or vascular resistance [4]. Patients with diabetes mellitus do have a thickened muscle capillary basement membrane, but the capillaries are not narrowed [5]. The basement membrane thickening is associated with an albumin leak [6], but does not impair diffusion of oxygen [7]. Further details of this lesion are discussed in Chapter 54. However, the important point to remember is that there is no occlusive lesion in the microcirculation of patients with diabetes mellitus.

The pattern of macrovascular (atherosclerotic) occlusive disease in diabetes is somewhat altered (Figure 1). There is a predilection for atherosclerosis to occur in the tibial and peroneal arteries. However, this predilection is confined to the segment between the knee and ankle. The foot arteries in patients with diabetes are actually less involved with atherosclerosis when compared with non-diabetics [2, 3]. It is therefore incorrect to use the term 'small vessel disease' to describe any aspect of vascular occlusive disease in diabetic patients. The involvement of the tibial arteries is not a reflection of their size, as the smaller arteries in the foot are relatively spared. This is extremely important for clinical management because it is the basis for highly successful arterial reconstruction in diabetics [8].

In summary, there are two clinically import-

International Textbook of Diabetes Mellitus. Edited by K.G.M.M. Alberti, R.A. DeFronzo, H. Keen and P. Zimmet
© 1992 John Wiley & Sons Ltd

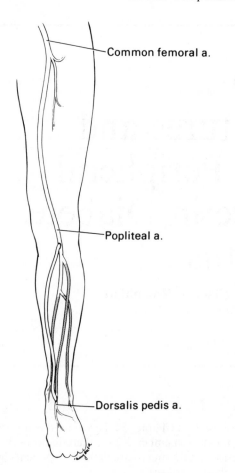

Figure 1 Distribution of infrapopliteal arterial disease (shaded area), with an example of a distal popliteal to dorsalis pedis artery bypass graft

ant characteristics of vascular disease in diabetes mellitus: first, there is no occlusive lesion in the microcirculation that might lead to inadequate perfusion or failure of an arterial graft; second, the tibial vessel occlusive disease often ends at the ankle, sparing the foot vessels. These circumstances allow for highly successful distal arterial reconstruction.

CLINICAL PRESENTATION AND EVALUATION OF THE SYMPTOMATIC PATIENT

The patient with a problem that may be related to disease of the peripheral arterial circulation should initially be evaluated in standard fashion with a thorough history and physical examination; a clinically based presumptive diagnosis

can then be made, which acts as a guide for possible further intervention. The second step involves the use of non-invasive tests that confirm or negate the presumptive diagnosis; these studies also help to quantitate the degree of arterial disease. A number of non-invasive tests have been developed that evaluate the arterial tree in an anatomic and functional fashion. The patient's measurements are then compared with reference measurements from a known population. The vascular surgeon then must determine whether the natural history of the disease and the severity with which it presents warrants intervention with either non-operative or operative alternatives, considering the risks and possible benefits afforded by the intervention [9].

The clinical presentation of diabetic patients with peripheral vascular disease is somewhat altered by the frequent presence of neuropathy. The details of neuropathy and its role in the development of foot lesions are discussed in Chapter 59. The important point to be made here is that diabetic patients often present with foot ulcers or small areas of gangrene when relatively mild ischemia is present. Because of the neuropathy, it is necessary to maintain a high arterial perfusing pressure to prevent ulceration at pressure points in the foot. When skin necrosis occurs, it should not be ascribed solely to neuropathy until the possibility of coexisting ischemia has been carefully evaluated.

A thorough physical examination is essential in the diabetic with lower extremity complaints. The peripheral pulses at all levels should be palpated. Although diabetics have a propensity toward atherosclerotic occlusion of the tibial arteries, it is not unusual to encounter atherosclerosis of the aorto-iliac region, as evidenced by diminished femoral pulses. In fact, in spite of the tibial vessel problem, the most common site of arterial occlusion in the diabetic (as in non-diabetics) is the superficial femoral artery [10] (Figure 2). Such patients have normal femoral pulses but no popliteal or distal pulses, and often they have both femoral and tibial artery occlusion. Patients who have only tibial vessel disease present with normal femoral and popliteal pulses but no foot pulses (dorsalis pedis or posterior tibial). In our experience, over 80% of these patients have diabetes mellitus [11]. For reasons to be described, examination of peripheral pulses is still the single most important step in the evaluation for ischemia.

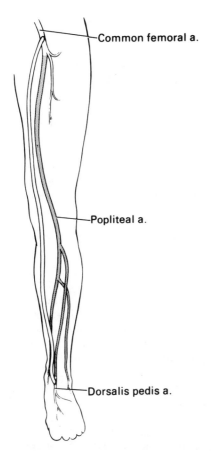

Common femoral a.

Popliteal a.

Dorsalis pedis a.

Figure 2 Distribution of superficial femoral artery disease with infrapopliteal arterial disease, with an example of a common femoral artery to dorsalis pedis artery bypass graft

The neurologic examination of the lower extremity is important in documenting the contribution of neuropathy to the pathogenesis of the patient's problem. Examination of the skin, especially careful visualization of all the areas between the toes, is essential in determining whether there is active infection. Evaluation of the tissue around an ulcer, looking for evidence of edema, capillary refill, pallor, dependent rubor and skin temperature, helps in assessing the degree of ischemia that is present, a rough gauge of the relative importance of arteriosclerosis in the presentation of an ulcer. Probing the base of an ulceration will give some indication as to the involvement of bony structures in the infectious and ischemic process. Plain radiographs of any lower extremity that has an ulcer or has a history of a healed ulcer but remains symptomatic should be undertaken as part of the initial evaluation. Careful examination of these films for evidence of bony involvement, either fracture or osteomyelitis, or evidence of deep soft tissue infection is required (see also Chapters 59 and 68).

A number of non-invasive techniques have been developed to measure arterial pressure in the lower extremity. Measurement of arterial pressures at different levels of the extremity, using a pneumatic cuff and a flow sensor, usually a Doppler ultrasound sensor, is the most commonly used technique [12]. After the cuff has been inflated at the proximal level, it is slowly deflated and the sensor over the distal vessel identifies the pressure at which flow resumes. This pressure is recorded for several points on the lower extremity, usually the high thigh, low thigh, calf and ankle.

A peculiar anatomic finding in diabetic patients is the presence of medial calcinosis of peripheral arteries. The artery is less compressible, and the indirect measurement of pressure within the vessel is artificially increased when compression is the basis of the measurement. Pressures in diabetic subjects are approximately 25 mmHg higher than those in non-diabetic subjects with similar intraluminal occlusive disease, down to the ankle level, so decisions based on these measurements must be adjusted appropriately [13]. An additional measurement of the toe blood pressure in diabetic patients has proved valuable, especially in patients with a foot lesion. Toe digital arteries are less likely to be calcified, so that occlusive pressure measurements more reliably reflect pressure within the digital artery. The measurement of the toe blood pressure in the diabetic compared with that in the non-diabetic patient reinforces the fact that diabetes does not cause 'small vessel disease' as both groups have the same pressures in the small vessels of the foot [14, 15].

When the tibial vessels are not compressible, other methods may be used to assess perfusing pressure. The most popular of these is pulse volume recording, a form of plethysmography. Plethysmography measures changes in volume over time. Cuffs are placed at segmental levels on the extremity, and the instrument records changes in the pressure of the cuff which reflect changes in the cuff volume, which in turn reflect momentary changes in limb volume [13]. These changes in limb volume have been correlated with direct intra-arterial pressure measurements, with good correlation over clinically relevant ranges [16]. The drawback of this technique is the absence of quantitative information in standardized form.

Examination of the Doppler waveform, specifically its phasic nature, is another test that can provide the experienced examiner with a qualitative view of the degree of stenosis [17]. Semi-quantitative information may be obtained by manipulation of ultrasound measurements, but usage of these ultrasound-derived analyses has not received wide acceptance. There is a paucity of other truly non-invasive techniques for quantitating flow. Semi-invasive techniques, including radioisotope flow studies, have been used to demonstrate physiologic significance of a vascular lesion, but these, too, have not achieved widespread acceptance.

Recently, the use of transcutaneous oxygen tension ($TcPo_2$) measurement in both health and occlusive disease has been used as a non-invasive measurement of limb perfusion [7, 18]. The patient with occlusive disease has significantly reduced $TcPo_2$ measurements compared with normals; this has been used to determine the possibility of ulcer healing and optimal amputation healing. In the diabetic with symptoms, $TcPo_2$ values are similar to those in non-diabetic individuals; similar findings are seen on comparing diabetics and non-diabetics without rest pain. However, diabetics with ulcers often have higher $TcPo_2$ levels than non-diabetics with ulceration, and sometimes ulcers or amputations fail to heal despite what would be an adequate level in a non-diabetic [7].

In summary, the most important step in evaluating ischemia in the diabetic foot is careful examination of pulses. When the pulses are absent, the value of non-invasive tests to confirm the diagnosis of ischemia is of limited value or accuracy. When a diabetic patient presents with a foot lesion and absent pulses, decisions are based primarily on clinical considerations.

For most patients presenting with claudication, the treatment program would include exercise, cessation of cigarette smoking, and possible pharmacologic interventions with medications such as pentoxifylline, a drug that theoretically decreases the stiffness of the red blood cell, thus allowing it to circulate more freely. In the case of the neurotrophic ulcer without underlying arterial occlusive disease, the treatment plan may center around local wound management and the use of special shoes to reduce the pressure on the insensate extremity. However, in the case of rest pain, ulceration or gangrene with absent pulses, surgical intervention is indicated to improve blood flow to the ischemic region. Factors important in this decision are the patient's general health, especially cardiac disease, the possibility of salvaging a functional limb, and the risk and benefit of any surgical procedure.

Once surgery has been selected, confirmation of the presumptive diagnosis with angiography must be considered. An accurate arteriogram of the entire lower extremity, including the foot vessels, is essential to successful arterial reconstruction in the diabetic.

ANGIOGRAPHY

Angiography in the diabetic patient carries an increased risk of precipitating renal insufficiency, and in some cases acute renal failure. At the same time, it is necessary to obtain high-quality arteriograms, including the foot arteries. Ionic iodide contrast compounds dissociate into an anion and cation with the anion acting as the iodinated radiopaque particle. With this dissociation into two ions, the contrast material is quite hypertonic. Several theories of nephrotoxicity are related to the hypertonicity of the contrast media [19, 20]. Experimental studies have demonstrated that infusion of hypertonic solutions causes a decrease in renal blood flow, which may be mediated by the renin–angiotensin system. Contrast medium itself may have a direct toxic effect on the renal cell. Differential degrees of renal injury were produced upon injection of a variety of contrast media of similar osmolarity, with the conclusion that contrast materials have nephrotoxic properties unrelated to their hypertonicity [21]. The hyperosmolarity of the media may cause a direct tubular injury, as evidenced by significant alteration in renal tubular sodium transport [22]. The hypertonicity may cause an abnormality in the viscosity of the blood, secondary to morphologic changes induced in red blood cells, thus causing microvascular obstruction within the kidney [23]. Several other theories relate to participation of urinary protein causing tubular obstruction [24], urate nephropathy secondary to uricosuric effect of contrast media [25], and the possible role of immunologic reactions with antibodies to contrast material inducing renal failure, either due to obstruction of tubules with antigen–antibody complexes or crossreactivity of antibody with renal cells [26].

In terms of predicting renal failure, the only factor that appears indisputably to be a risk factor is that of preangiographic renal insufficiency; if renal function is compromised to begin with, the patient runs a significantly higher risk of developing at least transient renal insufficiency; in some studies that risk is as high as 41% [27]. Conflicting reports in the literature as to the role of diabetes as an independent risk factor lead to uncertain conclusions: whereas some reports suggest no increase in renal insufficiency in diabetics [28–31], other studies demonstrate an increased risk for diabetics as a group [32–34]. The discrepancies between these studies may be explained by the findings of D'Elia et al [30] that the non-azotemic patients demonstrated a definite incidence of renal failure (2.5% of non-diabetics had creatinine change greater than 0.5 mg/dl, 2.0% of diabetics had the same creatinine change), but the azotemic group appeared to be at much higher risk for acute renal failure (20% of the non-diabetics had creatinine changes greater than 0.5 mg/dl, 38% of the diabetics with azotemia had the same degree of creatinine increase). There were no statistically significant differences between diabetic and non-diabetic patients when matched for degree of preangiogram azotemia. It is possible that the increased risk ascribed to diabetes may simply be that diabetics subjects tend to have a higher rate of preangiogram azotemia than the non-diabetic population.

Reports of pretreating patients with mannitol or furosemide, to increase renal blood flow and diuresis in an effort to limit the exposure of the kidney to recirculating contrast, have suggested some degree of protection [35–41]. A more common practice is hydration before, during and after the angiographic procedure, which has reportedly reduced the rate of measured renal dysfunction to near zero [28, 29, 42]. Although these data have been challenged [21], it seems likely that if adequate hydration can increase renal blood flow and reduce the exposure of the nephrons to a potentially toxic hypertonic dye, it should be performed in all patients who have no contraindication to hydration.

The absolute amount of dye (measured in grams of iodine) may play a part in the develop-

ment of acute renal insufficiency. Although there is no clear minimal amount of dye that is perfectly safe, it appears that a cut-off in the range of 80–90 g iodine represents the point where the risk of renal failure increases [32, 33]. The development of non-ionic contrast materials, which do not dissociate and therefore have lower osmolalities (at least in theory), should reduce the degree of renal failure attributable to hypertonic reactions [43–45].

The role of digital subtraction arteriography (DSA), a method for computer enhancement of images using lower volumes of contrast media, still remains somewhat controversial, especially in the imaging of the distal lower extremities. Although some reports [46–48] suggest that lower extremity calf vessels were seen better on occasion than those arteries seen by conventional techniques, it is not clear from these reports how many multiple projections and injections were required to visualize the calf and foot circulation. The quality of the standard arteriogram was questionable and the benefit thus gained by the DSA technique was a function of poor quality of the standard imaging techniques. Additionally, much of the benefit gained by the DSA study, i.e. better patient tolerance and lower theoretical total contrast load, may be offset by the decreased spatial resolution provided by DSA, especially when fine details of the arterial tree are necessary, as in arterial reconstruction of the distal lower extremity in the diabetic patient [49]. The tolerance issue might be dealt with by using the newer non-ionic media, although they may add considerably to the cost of the study. In light of the previous data presented, it might be best to limit the use of DSA to those patients with pre-existing renal disease.

In summary, postangiogram renal dysfunction appears to be a function of the ionic contrast material and occurs with greatest risk in the patient with pre-existing renal insufficiency. The total amount of dye seems to have a role, although renal failure has occurred with very low doses of contrast. Diabetes in and of itself may or may not be a risk factor, but clinically there is a higher incidence of pre-existing renal dysfunction in the diabetic population, so these patients are more at risk. Protection seems to be afforded by hydration, but it is not clear at present whether drug intervention is indicated. Non-ionic contrast agents should reduce the incidence of hypertonic renal injury, and DSA is

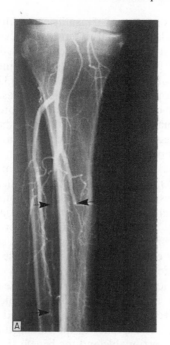
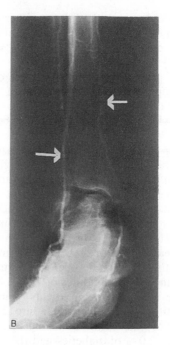
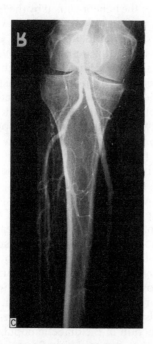
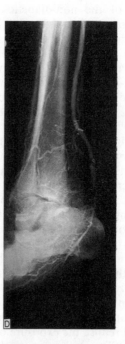

Figure 3 Arteriogram of a 74-year-old diabetic female with a non-healing ulcer on the plantar aspect of the right foot. (A) Popliteal artery trifurcation with demonstration of occlusions of the anterior tibial, posterior tibial and peroneal arteries distal to the trifurcation (dark arrows); (B) reconstitution of the anterior tibial and posterior tibial arteries at the ankle (white arrows); (C) postoperative angiogram demonstrating the popliteal artery with a proximal vein graft anastomosis at the level of the knee joint; (D) distal anastomosis of the vein graft to the posterior tibial artery at the level of the ankle, demonstrating the improved blood supply to the foot

useful in limiting the amount of contrast required in imaging patients with pre-existing renal insufficiency.

ARTERIAL RECONSTRUCTION

In general, arterial reconstruction in the diabetic patient is similar to that in the non-diabetic, with the exception of the lower extremity: here, the pattern of vascular disease and the associated problems of neuropathy and infection require some special attention. When a patient presents with evidence of infection, it is critically important to provide adequate drainage and antibiotic therapy as a first priority. Arterial assessment is performed as outlined above. If arteriography is necessary, it should be performed as soon as infection is under control, usually within 72 hours of admission.

Because of the pattern of atherosclerosis in diabetics, it is often necessary to perform arterial reconstruction to the distal tibial, peroneal or pedal arteries (Figure 3). Surprisingly, the results of vein bypass grafts to these distal vessels are now as good as—or better than—bypass grafts to the popliteal artery [50]. The widespread use of vein grafts *in situ* may in part be responsible for these improved results [51]. Not all would agree with this, and some report excellent results with reversed vein grafts as well [52]; however, there seems to be uniform agreement that prosthetic arterial grafts should not be used for arterial reconstruction to these distal vessels.

Minor amputation is frequently necessary before or after arterial reconstruction in the diabetic patient, usually as a consequence of deep ulceration or infection. However, in the presence of a normal restored circulation, these amputations will heal. As a consequence, the limb salvage rate on a modern vascular surgery service should be the same for diabetic and non-diabetic subjects [51, 53].

CONCLUSION

For the primary physician caring for diabetic patients with ischemic problems of the lower extremity, there are some guidelines that follow from the foregoing information:

(1) Ischemia should not be attributed to micro-vascular occlusive disease, a lesion that does not occur in the extremities of patients with diabetes mellitus.

(2) When there are absent pulses and a foot lesion, arteriography should be performed.

(3) Arteriography must include the arteries in the foot before the possibility of arterial reconstruction can be excluded.

(4) The results of distal arterial reconstruction in the diabetic patient should be as good as the results in non-diabetics.

If these guidelines are borne in mind, the incidence of limb loss due to the vascular complications of diabetes mellitus will be minimized.

REFERENCES

1. Goldenberg S, Alex M, Joshi RA, Blumenthal HT. Nonatheromatous peripheral vascular disease of the lower extremity in diabetes mellitus. Diabetes 1959; 8: 261–73.
2. Strandness DE, Priest RE, Gibbons GE. Combined clinical and pathologic study of diabetic and nondiabetic peripheral arterial disease. Diabetes 1964; 13: 366–72.
3. Conrad MC. Large and small artery occlusion in diabetics and nondiabetics with severe vascular disease. Circulation 1967; 36: 83–91.
4. Barner HB, Kaiser GC, Willman VL. Blood flow in the diabetic leg. Circulation 1979; 43: 391–4.
5. Siperstein MD, Unger RH, Madison LL. Studies of muscle capillary basement membranes in normal subjects, diabetic, and prediabetic patients. J Clin Invest 1968; 47: 1973–99.
6. Parving HH, Noer I, Deckert T et al. The effect of metabolic regulation on microvascular permeability to small and large molecules in short-term juvenile diabetics. Diabetologia 1976; 12: 161–6.
7. Wyss CR, Matsen FA, Simmons CW, Burgess EM. Transcutaneous oxygen tension measurements on limbs of diabetic and nondiabetic patients with peripheral vascular disease. Surgery 1984; 95: 339–45.
8. Auer, AI, Hurley JJ, Binnington HB, Nunnelee JD, Hershey FB. Distal tibial vein grafts for limb salvage. Arch Surg 1983; 118: 597–602.
9. Rutherford RB. In Rutherford RB (ed.) Vascular surgery, 2nd edn. Philadelphia: WB Saunders, 1984: p 1.
10. Gensler SW, Haimovici H, Hoffert P, Steinman C, Beneventano TC. Study of vascular lesions in diabetic, nondiabetic patients. Arch Surg 1965; 91: 617–22.
11. Sidawy AN, Menzoian JO, Cantelmo NL, LoGerfo FW. Effect of inflow and outflow sites

on the results of tibioperoneal vein grafts. Am J Surg 1986; 152: 211–14.

12. Allen JS, Terry HJK. The evaluation of an ultrasonic flow detector for assessment of peripheral vascular disease. Cardiovasc Res 1969; 3: 503.

13. Raines J. In Rutherford RB (ed.) Vascular surgery,. 2nd edn. Philadelphia: WB Saunders, 1984: pp 59–64.

14. Ramsey DE, Manke DA, Sumner DS. Toe blood pressure: a valuable adjunct to ankle pressure measurement for assessing peripheral arterial disease. J Cardiovasc Surg 1983; 24: 43–8.

15. Bone GE, Pomajzl MJ. Toe blood pressure by photoplethysmography: an index of healing in forefoot amputation. Surgery 1981; 5: 569–74.

16. Darling RC, Raines JK, Brener BJ, Austen WG. Quantitative segmental pulse volume recorder. A clinical tool. Surgery 1972; 72: 873–87.

17. Yao JS, Ricco J-B. In Rutherford RB (ed.) Vascular surgery, 2nd edn. Philadelphia: WB Saunders, 1984: p 85.

18. Franzeck UK, Talke P, Bernstein EF, Golbranson FL, Fronek A. Transcutaneous Po_2 measurements in health and peripheral arterial occlusive disease. Surgery 1982; 91: 156–63.

19. Malott JC, Fodor J. Advantages of non-ionic contrast media in vascular applications. Radiol Tech 1985; 56: 95–8.

20. Byrd L, Sherman RL. Radiocontrast-induced acute renal failure: a clinical and pathophysiologic review. Medicine 1979; 58: 270–9.

21. Talner LB, Rushman HN, Coel MN. The effect of renal artery injection of contrast material on urinary enzyme excretion. Invest Radiol 1972; 7: 311.

22. Ziegler TW, Ladens JH, Fanestil DD, Talner LB. Inhibition of active sodium transport by radiographic contrast media. Kidney Int 1975; 7: 68.

23. Schiantarelli P, Peroni F, Turone P, Rosati G. Effects of iodinated contrast media on erythrocytes. Invest Radiol 1973; 8: 199.

24. Rees E, Waugh WH. Factors in renal failure in multiple myeloma. Arch Int Med 1965; 116: 400.

25. Postelthwaite AE, Kelley WN. Uricosuric effect of radiocontrast agents. Ann Intern Med 1971; 74: 845.

26. Kleinknecht D, Delous J, Honberg JC. Acute renal failure after intravenous urography—detection of antibodies against contrast media. Clin Nephrol 1974; 2: 116.

27. Martin-Paredeero V, Dixon SM, Baker JD, Takiff H, Gomes AS, Busutill RW, Moore WS. Risk of renal failure after major angiography. Arch Surg 1 983; 118: 1417–20.

28. Eisenberg RL, Bank WO, Hedgock MW. Renal failure after major angiography can be avoided by hydration. AJR 1981; 136: 859–61.

29. Kuman R, Hull JD, Lathi S, Cohen AJ, Pletka

PF. Low incidence of renal failure after angiography. Arch Int Med 1981; 141: 1268–70.

30. D'Elia JA, Gleason RE, Alday M et al. Nephrotoxicity from angiographic contrast material. Am J Med 1982; 72: 719–25.

31. Cochran ST, Wong WS, Roe DJ. Predicting angiography-induced acute renal function impairment: clinical risk model. AJR 1983; 141: 1027–33.

32. Gomes AS, Baker JD, Martin-Paredero V, Dixon SM, Takiff H, Machleder HI, Moore WS. Acute renal dysfunction after major arteriography. AJR 1985; 145: 1249–53.

33. Lang EK, Foreman J, Schlegel JU, Leslie C, List A, McCormick P. The incidence of a contrast medium induced acute tubular necrosis following arteriography. Radiology 1981; 138: 203–6.

34. Alexander RD, Berkes SL, Abuelo JG. Contrast media-induced oliguric renal failure. Arch Int Med 1978; 138: 381–4.

35. Cruz C, Haicak H, Samhouri F, Smith RF, Eyler WR, Levin NW. Contrast media for angiography: effect on renal function. Radiology 1986; 158: 109–12.

36. Brown CB, Ogg CS, Cameron JS. High dose furosemide in acute renal failure: a controlled trial. Clin Nephrol 1981; 15: 90–6.

37. Becker JA. Prevention of radiocontrast induced acute renal failure with mannitol. Lancet 1980; i: 1147.

38. Old CW, Lehrner IM. Prevention of radiocontrast induced acute renal failure with mannitol. Lancet 1980; i: 885.

39. Barry KG, Cohen A, Knochel JP et al. Mannitol infusion. II. The prevention of acute functional renal failure during resection of an aneurysm of the abdominal aorta. New Engl J Med 1961; 264: 967–71.

40. Berman LB, Smith LL, Chisholm GD, Weston RE. Mannitol and renal function in cardiovascular surgery. Arch Surg 1964; 88: 239–45.

41. Eliahou HE. Mannitol therapy in oliguria of acute onset. Br Med J 1964; 1: 807–9.

42. Kerstein MD, Puyau FA. Value of periangiography hydration. Surgery 1984; 96: 919–22.

43. Bettman MA. Angiographic contrast agents: conventional and new media compared. AJR 1982; 139: 787–94.

44. Tornquist C, Almen T, Golman K, Hoftas S. Proteinuria following nephroangiography. VII. Comparison between ionic monomeric, monoacidic dimeric and nonionic contrast media in the dog. Acta Radiol (suppl.) 1980; 362: 49–52.

45. Gale ME, Robbins AH, Hamburger RJ, Widrick WC. Renal toxicity of contrast agents: iopamidol, iothalamate and diatrizoate. AJR 1984; 142: 333–5.

46. Dardik H, Miller N, Adler J et al. Primary and

adjunctive intra-arterial digital subtraction arteriography of the lower extremity. J Vasc Surg 1986; 3: 599–604.

47. Crummy AB, Strother CM, Sackett JF et al. Computerized fluoroscopy: digital subtraction for intravenous angiocardiography and arteriography. AJR 1980; 135: 1131–40.

48. Kaufman SL, Chang R, Kadir S, Mitchell SE, White RI. Intraarterial digital subtraction angiography in diagnostic arteriography. Radiology 1984; 151: 323–7.

49. Carmody RF, Yang PJ, Seeger JF, Capp MP. Digital subtraction angiography: update 1986. Invest Radiol 1986; 21: 899–905.

50. Cantelmo NL, Snow JR, Menzoian JO, LoGerfo FW. Successful vein bypass in patients with an ischemic limb and palpable popliteal pulse. Arch Surg 1986; 121: 217–20.

51. Hurley JJ, Auer AI, Hershey FB, Binnington HB, Woods JJ, Nunnelee JD, Milyard MK. Distal arterial reconstruction: patency and limb salvage in diabetics. J Vasc Surg 1987; 5: 796–800.

52. Taylor LM, Edwards JM, Phinney ES, Porter JM. Reversed vein bypass to infrapopliteal arteries. Modern results are superior to or equivalent to in-situ bypass for patency and for vein utilization. Ann Surg 1987; 205: 90–7.

53. Reichle FA, Rankin KP, Tyson RR, Finestone AJ, Shuman CR. Long-term results of femoro-infrapopliteal bypass in diabetic patients with severe ischemia of the lower extremity. Am J Surg 1979; 137: 653–6.

Other Complications

67

Arterial Hypertension in Diabetes Mellitus

Hans-Henrik Parving
Steno Memorial and Hvidöre Hospital, Copenhagen, Denmark

Arterial hypertension is a common problem in insulin dependent diabetes mellitus (IDDM) and non-insulin dependent diabetes mellitus (NIDDM) patients. Several clinical and population-based studies have demonstrated a higher prevalence of hypertension in IDDM and NIDDM patients compared with non-diabetic subjects [1–5]. Diabetic nephropathy is the main cause of hypertension in IDDM patients, whereas essential hypertension is dominant in NIDDM patients. Hypertension contributes to the major causes of morbidity and mortality in the diabetic population, i.e. macroangiopathy and microangiopathy [6–9]. This suggests that the hypertensive diabetic patient could benefit from more aggressive antihypertensive treatment initiated at a lower pressure level than generally recommended for the non-diabetic hypertensive patient. Another important issue concerns choice of antihypertensive treatment: should it be modified to take into account the concurrent diabetes?

This chapter reviews the aetiology, pathogenesis, clinical importance and treatment of arterial hypertension in diabetic patients.

CLASSIFICATION OF HYPERTENSION

All types of hypertension can occur in diabetic patients (Table 1) [2, 10, 11]. As previously mentioned, overt and incipient diabetic nephropathy are the main causes of hypertension in IDDM patients, whereas essential hypertension is most prevalent in NIDDM patients. Isolated systolic hypertension is frequently present in older diabetic patients. Supine hypertension with orthostatic hypotension occurs in some patients with longstanding diabetes complicated by severe autonomic neuropathy.

It might be expected that the endocrine causes of hypertension (and diabetes) would be more frequent in the hypertensive diabetic population. However, this question has not been looked at systematically, except in the case of phaeochromocytoma [12]. The higher frequency of renal artery stenosis in diabetes, mainly NIDDM [13], has not been confirmed [14]. The increased frequency of urinary tract infection in females with IDDM and NIDDM might be expected to lead to a higher prevalence of chronic interstitial nephropathy. Furthermore, obstructive nephropathy secondary to diabetic cystopathy is more prominent in longstanding diabetes [15].

International Textbook of Diabetes Mellitus. Edited by K.G.M.M. Alberti, R.A. DeFronzo, H. Keen and P. Zimmet

Table 1 Arterial hypertension in diabetes mellitus

IDDM	Hypertension of overt and incipient diabetic nephropathy
	Essential hypertension
	Isolated systolic hypertension
	Supine hypertension with orthostatic hypotension
NIDDM	Essential hypertension
	Isolated systolic hypertension
	Hypertension of diabetic nephropathy
	Supine hypertension with orthostatic hypotension
Endocrine causes	Thyrotoxicosis
	Myxoedema
	Cushing's syndrome
	Phaeochromocytoma
	Acromegaly
	Conn's syndrome
	Renovascular disease and other angiotensin II-dependent causes
	Synthetic oestrogen/ progestogen combinations
Other secondary causes	Other renal disease
	Coarctation
	Neurogenic causes

Modified from reference 11.

PATHOGENESIS OF HYPERTENSION IN DIABETES

The aetiology of essential hypertension remains unknown. Numerous concepts have been advanced to explain essential hypertension, as reviewed by Mendlowitz [16]. However, only areas where specific abnormalities have been demonstrated in diabetic patients are reviewed here. It should be mentioned that several studies have combined IDDM and NIDDM with and without complications (heterogeneous groups), which makes interpretation of the results difficult and sometimes impossible.

Incipient and Overt Diabetic Nephropathy

Incipient nephropathy is diagnosed clinically in IDDM patients if the following criteria are fulfilled: persistent microalbuminuria (urinary albumin excretion 20–200 μg/min or 30–300 mg per 24 hours); normal kidney function; sterile urine without ketonuria (below 2+); duration of diabetes 5 years or more; lack of frank hypertension (systolic blood pressure less than 160 mmHg, diastolic blood pressure less than

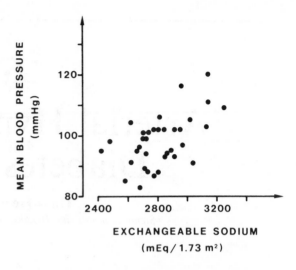

Figure 1 Exchangeable sodium versus mean blood pressure in 35 IDDM patients with elevated urinary albumin excretion (30–300 mg/24 hours, i.e. incipient diabetic nephropathy), $r = 0.54$, $P < 0.001$ (from reference 18, with permission)

105 mmHg); and no history of kidney or urinary tract disease [17]. Several studies have demonstrated elevated arterial blood pressure in this condition, as discussed later.

Recently, Feldt-Rasmussen et al [18] studied blood pressure, total exchangeable sodium, plasma and extracellular fluid volume, together with the renin–angiotensin–aldosterone system (RAAS) and catecholamines in IDDM patients with and without incipient nephropathy compared with non-diabetic controls. Exchangeable sodium was increased in IDDM patients but, more important, a correlation between mean arterial pressure and exchangeable sodium was demonstrated in patients suffering from incipient nephropathy ($n = 35$, $r = 0.54$, $P = <0.01$; see Figure 1). Extracellular fluid volume was elevated, whereas plasma volume was normal in IDDM patients with and without elevated urinary albumin excretion. The RAAS was normal, except for a significant reduction in angiotensin II in patients with incipient nephropathy. The plasma catecholamine concentrations were normal or slightly suppressed. We have confirmed these findings by demonstrating normal plasma volume, slightly evelated extracellular fluid volume and normal RAAS in IDDM patients with incipient nephropathy compared with non-diabetic controls [19].

Furthermore, plasma atrial natriuretic peptide concentrations were normal in incipient nephropathy.

Originally, the hypertension associated with diabetic nephropathy was regarded as a 'low renin–aldosterone hypertension', as reviewed by Christlieb [10]. However, this suggestion was based on findings in insulin-treated diabetic patients suffering from advanced nephropathy (serum creatinine 3.8 mg%) [20, 21]. In contrast, Björck et al [22] have demonstrated that the renin–angiotensin system is operative in IDDM patients with advanced nephropathy (serum creatinine 411 μmol/l). This suggests a role of the system in maintenance of hypertension, but sodium and fluid retention play the dominant part, as these patients nearly always suffer from oedema.

O'Hare et al [23] investigated the causes of hypertension in a heterogeneous group of diabetics (IDDM and NIDDM) with moderately advanced nephropathy, i.e. mean glomerular filtration rate (GFR) 49 ml/min. A significant correlation between blood pressure and exchangeable sodium ($r = 0.61$, $P < 0.01$) was demonstrated in nephropatic patients. Furthermore, the sodium–renin product was elevated in these patients, whereas plasma volume was unchanged. More recently, the pathophysiological importance of sodium/water retention and RAAS in hypertension has been investigated in the early stages of diabetic nephropathy in IDDM patients without oedema [18, 19]. Feldt-Rasmussen et al [18] found a 14% increase in exchangeable sodium in nephropathic patients (mean GFR 79 ml/min). Furthermore, a significant correlation between exchangeable sodium and blood pressure was observed in IDDM patients with and without nephropathy ($n = 70$, $r = 0.41$, $P < 0.01$). The RAAS was normal or slightly suppressed (angiotensin II) in nephropathy. Hommel et al [19] demonstrated enlargement of extracellular fluid volume (12%, $P < 0.01$) and normal plasma volume in IDDM patients with diabetic nephropathy (mean GFR 106 ml/min per 1.73 m^2). Furthermore, a significant correlation between mean arterial blood pressure and extracellular fluid volume was found in IDDM patients with and without nephropathy ($n = 79$, $r = 0.44$, $P < 0.001$). Finally, the RAAS was normal in nephropathic patients.

In conclusion, sodium and water retention

have a dominant role in initiation and maintenance of hypertension in incipient and overt diabetic nephropathy, whereas the contribution of the RAAS is smaller. However, it should be stressed that the RAAS seems to be inappropriately 'suppressed'. Finally, it should be recalled that there is no valid information with respect to the pathogenesis of hypertension in NIDDM patients suffering from diabetic nephropathy.

Hypertension Without Nephropathy

The great majority of NIDDM patients are obese. The association of obesity and hypertension is well recognized: several reports have demonstrated that approximately 50% of overweight subjects have high blood pressure [24]. Obesity and diabetes (NIDDM and IDDM) are both characterized by insulin resistance and hyperinsulinemia. The latter stimulates the sympathetic nervous system [25, 26], and several investigators have suggested that hyperinsulinemia and heightened sympathetic nervous system activity increase blood pressure by enhancing renal sodium reabsorption and by stimulating the heart and blood vessels, as reviewed by Landsberg [27]. Increased cardiovascular reactivity to plasma catecholamines has been demonstrated in normotensive and hypertensive diabetic patients [28, 29]. Normal plasma catecholamine levels have been reported, except in cases of autonomic neuropathy [28, 29].

DeFronzo [30] has studied the role of insulin on renal tubular sodium reabsorption and shown that there is significant sodium retention with physiological increments in plasma insulin concentration. Several studies have demonstrated that total exchangeable sodium is elevated by 5–10% in normotensive and hypertensive patients with NIDDM and IDDM [29, 31]. This rise can be reversed by diuretic therapy, which also reduces blood pressure [29]. Blood and plasma volumes are both normal in hypertensive NIDDM and IDDM patients [29, 31, 32]. Unfortunately, no information is available on extracellular fluid volume in non-nephropathic diabetic hypertension.

Plasma renin activity has been found to be normal or slightly reduced in hypertensive IDDM and NIDDM patients [20, 23, 31]. Plasma aldosterone concentration is within the normal range [20, 29, 31]. Improvement of metabolic control in a heterogeneous group of normotensive diabetic patients induces a significant reduction in plasma renin activity, plasma angiotensin II and plasma aldosterone, and a slight drop in blood pressure [33]. These findings document the need to define the degree of metabolic control when investigating the RAAS in diabetic patients. Several investigators have demonstrated elevated vascular reactivity to angiotensin II in normotensive and hypertensive diabetic patients [28, 29]. Furthermore, reduced distensibility of the microvascular bed (arteriolar hyalinosis) has been demonstrated in patients with longstanding IDDM and clinical microangiopathy [34, 35].

In conclusion, several factors contribute to the pathogenesis of hypertension in NIDDM and IDDM patients: these include obesity, hyperinsulinism, sodium retention, inappropriate suppression of the renin–angiotensin–aldosterone system, increased cardiovascular reactivity to catecholamines and angiotensin II, and increased resistance of the arteriolar system.

HYPERTENSION AND DIABETIC MICROANGIOPATHY

Incipient and Overt Nephropathy

Several studies have demonstrated elevated blood pressure in children and adult IDDM patients with incipient diabetic nephropathy compared with normoalbuminuric IDDM patients [36–38]. Recently, this observation was confirmed and extended in a cross-sectional study of 957 IDDM patients [39]. The patients were stratified into three groups: normoalbuminuric (< 30 mg per 24 hours), $n = 562$ (59%); microalbuminuric (31–299 mg per 24 hours), $n = 215$ (22%); and macroalbuminuric (> 300 mg per 24 hours), $n = 180$ (19%). The prevalence of arterial hypertension increased with enhanced albuminuria (normoalbuminuria, 19%; microalbuminuria, 30%; macroalbuminuria, 65%; $P < 0.01$). The prevalence of arterial hypertension rose in all three groups with increasing duration of diabetes (Figure 2). We have previously demonstrated a high prevalence (51%) of diastolic blood pressure elevation (above 95 mmHg) in young IDDM patients with diabetic nephropathy and normal serum creatinine [3]. Furthermore, we have demonstrated that the increase in arterial blood pressure to a

hypertensive level is an early feature of diabetic nephropathy [40]. Several studies have demonstrated that haemodynamic factors such as arterial hypertension and glomerular hypertension increase urinary albumin excretion and accelerate the development of glomerulopathy in diabetic animals [41]. More importantly, arterial hypertension accelerates the rate of decline in GFR in IDDM patients with nephropathy [42, 43]. Arterial blood pressure thus seems to have a complex relationship with diabetic nephropathy—nephropathy raising blood pressure, and blood pressure accelerating the course of nephropathy.

We have demonstrated a considerable reduction in urinary albumin excretion during acute blood pressure reduction in normotensive and hypertensive IDDM patients with incipient or overt diabetic nephropathy [17, 44]. Diminished urinary albumin excretion has also been demonstrated during long-term antihypertensive treatment with cardioselective β-blockers or angiotensin converting enzyme inhibition in normotensive IDDM patients with incipient nephropathy [45–47]. These findings suggest that reversible haemodynamic factors play an important part in the pathogenesis of microalbuminuria and macroalbuminuria. The simplest explanation of these findings may therefore be the correct one: a reduction of glomerular capillary hydraulic pressure induced by the reduction in systemic blood pressure.

In our prospective study, begun in 1976, the effect of early, aggressive antihypertensive treatment on kidney function in diabetic nephropathy was studied in 10 IDDM patients (mean age 29 years) [48, 49]. Figure 3 shows the average course of arterial blood pressure and kidney function in the 9 patients receiving long-term antihypertensive treatment (more than 6 years). Arterial blood pressure and albuminuria showed progressive increases during the control period ($P < 0.01$), whereas significant and fairly stable reductions occurred during the treatment period ($P < 0.01$). Antihypertensive treatment induced a progressive reduction in the rate of decline in GFR: 0.89 ml/min (before), 0.29 ml/min (during, 0–3 years) and 0.10 ml/min (during, 3–6 years) per month ($P < 0.01$). We have confirmed and extended the studies by Mogensen [42] and by Björck et al [50], and our own preliminary observations. The present and the two previous antihypertensive trials in diabetic nephropathy were

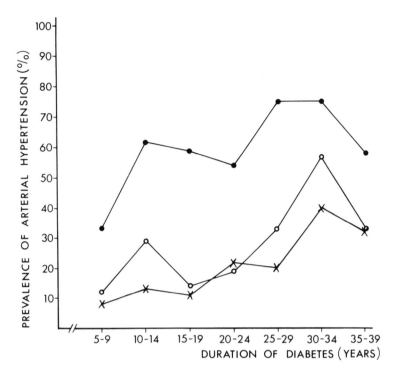

Figure 2 Prevalence of arterial hypertension in normoalbuminuric (crosses), microalbuminuric (open circles) and macro-albuminuric (solid circles) IDDM patients (from reference 39, with permission)

conducted as 'self-controlled' studies, in which each patient serves as his or her own control. This design was applied because it was considered unethical to run a parallel, untreated hypertensive group of patients with nephropathy, and because prognostic evaluations can be made from the slope of GFR, as discussed elsewhere [49].

In conclusion, effective antihypertensive treatment reduces albuminuria and postpones renal insufficiency in IDDM patients with nephropathy. Unfortunately, there is a complete lack of information on the effect of antihypertensive treatment in NIDDM patients with diabetic nephropathy.

Retinopathy

Several studies have suggested an association between elevated blood pressure and diabetic retinopathy [51, 52]. West et al [53] found no significant relationship between blood pressure and the frequency of retinopathy in NIDDM patients when systolic blood pressure was less than 170 mmHg, but above this level rates of

retinopathy were excessive, even in the non-proteinuric patients. Knowler et al [54] showed that the incidence of retinopathy (exudates) in NIDDM patients (Pima Indians) with systolic blood pressure of at least 145 mmHg was more than twice that of those with pressures less than 125 mmHg. This led the authors to suggest that control of blood pressure may reduce the incidence of retinal exudates in NIDDM patients. In a population-based study of IDDM patients, a higher diastolic blood pressure was found to contribute significantly to the severity of retinopathy [55]. Furthermore, carotid insufficiency or other causes of unilaterally and bilaterally reduced retinal blood flow (pressure), e.g. glaucoma, optic atrophy, myopia and extensive chorioretinal scarring, have been found to diminish the development of diabetic retinopathy, as reviewed by Rand et al [56]. These conditions all have in common a decreased retinal blood flow (pressure), as does panretinal photocoagulation, a treatment developed to mimic the antiretinopathic effects of these conditions.

Several investigators have demonstrated

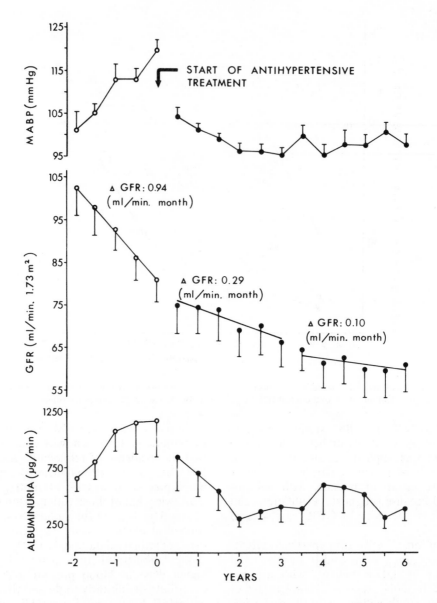

Figure 3 Average course of mean arterial blood pressure (MABP), glomerular filtration rate (GFR) and albuminuria before (open circles) and during (solid circles) long-term effective antihypertensive treatment of nine IDDM patients with nephropathy (from reference 49, with permission)

enhanced retinal blood flow in diabetics with little, if any, retinopathy [57, 58]. Atherton et al [59] showed that acutely induced hyperglycaemia enhances retinal blood flow in normal cats. The raised flow was due to an overriding of the normal autoregulatory response, i.e. the maintenance of constant blood flow despite wide variations in perfusion pressure. Sinclair et al [60] have demonstrated that autoregulation of retinal blood flow is impaired in simplex retinopathy and completely lost in proliferative retinopathy. In this context it should be mentioned that impaired autoregulation of blood flow has been demonstrated in many other tissues and organs (e.g. brain, skin and muscle) in longstanding diabetic patients, as reviewed by Parving et al [9]. The clinical significance of impaired autoregulation of blood flow is hypoperfusion during arterial hypotension (e.g. sleep) and hyperperfusion (capillary hypertension) during hypertensive episodes (e.g. stress and physical exertion). Osei et al [61] demonstrated abnormal retinal artery responses to stress in IDDM patients, and exercise induced a higher blood pressure response in IDDM patients who had had diabetes for some years [62]. Unfortunately, it must be stressed that no controlled study has been conducted to evaluate whether antihypertensive therapy may prevent the development or progression of diabetic retinopathy.

INVESTIGATION OF HYPERTENSION IN DIABETES

Measurements of blood pressure are generally carried out by using a mercury sphygmomanometer. A suitable cuff for adults should be 12–15 cm wide and 30–35 cm long; larger cuffs are needed for patients with fat arms, and smaller ones for children. Two or more blood pressure determinations in the supine or seated position (after at least 5 minutes rest) should be recorded, as well as the blood pressure after 2 minutes standing. Blood pressure should be taken at least once in both arms, and the arm with higher pressure subsequently used. The pressure at which the Korotkoff sounds are first heard is the systolic pressure. The diastolic pressure (phase V) is the pressure at which the sound disappears. Because most of the data concerning treatment have been related to phase V diastolic pressure, this should be used when deciding on the need for treatment. In patients whose initial diastolic blood pressure is in the range of 90–104 mmHg, further readings every 1 or 2 months over a period of 6 months should be obtained. Mild hypertension is confirmed if the diastolic blood pressure remains in the range 90–104 mmHg [63].

A medical history and complete physical examination for identifying any underlying cause of hypertension or for evidence of target organ damage (eyes, kidneys, heart, brain and peripheral vasculature) are essential. The following tests are recommended: haemoglobin, serum creatinine, potassium, total and high-density lipoprotein levels, complete urinalysis, electrocardiogram and ophthalmoscopic examination. As microalbuminuria is frequent in both IDDM and NIDDM, timed urine collections should be performed for determination of urinary albumin

excretion. In case of diabetic or non-diabetic kidney disease, GFR should be determined. In selected cases, such as those with severe hypertension or poor response to antihypertensive therapy, further investigations should be carried out, e.g. radioisotope renography, to exclude curable causes of hypertension.

ARTERIAL HYPERTENSION: DEFINITION AND THRESHOLD FOR INITIATING ANTIHYPERTENSIVE THERAPY

Normal adult blood pressure is arbitrarily defined as a systolic pressure equal to or below 140 mmHg together with a diastolic (phase V) pressure equal to or below 90 mmHg. Hypertension in adults is arbitrarily defined as a systolic pressure equal to or above 160 mmHg and/or diastolic pressure (phase V) equal to or above 95 mmHg. The term 'borderline hypertension' is used to denote blood pressure values between the normal and the hypertensive ranges as described above. The above-mentioned definitions are those produced by the World Health Organization Expert Committee on Hypertension [64]. According to the blood pressure level, hypertension is characterized as mild (diastolic pressure 90–104 mmHg), moderate (diastolic pressure 105–115 mmHg) or severe (diastolic pressure greater than 115 mmHg). Mild hypertension in adults is defined as a diastolic pressure (phase V) persistently between 90 mmHg and 104 mmHg (three to five readings over a period of 6 months) without obvious signs of left ventricular hypertrophy, or damage to the heart or other organs [63].

The beneficial effects of treating severe and moderate hypertension are well established. The evidence supporting the value of treating mild hypertension with antihypertensive drugs is not as clearly established as many believe [65]. However, most investigators recommend antihypertensive treatment if diastolic pressure is 100 mmHg or over [63–66].

Recently, the American Working Group on Hypertension in Diabetes suggested that diabetic patients with blood pressure of 140/90 mmHg or above (readings on two or more visits) should be considered for pharmacological treatment if a 3-month trial period of non-pharmacological treatment of mild hypertension is not effective in lowering blood pressure [67]. This recommendation is based on the additive impact on vascular disease of hypertension occurring in patients with diabetes mellitus. The Canadian Consensus Conference on Diabetes and Hypertension [68] proposed the following recommendations:

(1) Antihypertensive drug therapy should be initiated in diabetic patients with sustained diastolic blood pressure at or above 100 mmHg.

(2) Antihypertensive drug therapy should be initiated in patients whose sustained diastolic blood pressure is 90–99 mmHg and who have hypertensive target organ damage (left ventricular hypertrophy on electrocardiography, history or electrocardiographic evidence of myocardial infarction, history of intermittent claudication, serum creatinine level of 150 μmol/l or higher, or a creatinine clearance of 1 ml per second or less) *or* persistent proteinuria *or* proliferative diabetic retinopathy.

It is apparent that the two North American recommendations suggest that the blood pressure threshold for initiating antihypertensive drug therapy in diabetics should be lower than generally recommended in non-diabetics. However, there is an urgent need for well-designed, controlled studies to show whether antihypertensive therapy given for apparently mild hypertension among diabetics can reduce the excess morbidity and mortality from coronary heart disease, stroke, peripheral vascular disease and retinopathy. Finally, it should be recalled that approximately one-half the placebo-treated population at the end of 3 years' observation had a blood pressure below the criterion for entry, i.e. 95 mmHg, in the Australian National Blood Pressure Study [69].

TREATMENT

The goal of therapy should be not only to reduce morbidity and mortality but also to do so without adverse effects on the functional well-being of the patient. Unfortunately, it should be stressed that in diabetic patients there is a lack of well-designed trials comparing different antihypertensive drugs with respect to their efficacy, safety, side-effects and effects on quality of life; thus, no scientifically valid conclusion

can be drawn about an optimum drug regimen. Furthermore, diabetics are not a homogeneous group and no single regimen can be recommended for all. All classes of antihypertensive drugs have potential disadvantages, which may assume greater significance in certain groups of patients (Table 2). This section does not deal with the general side-effects of antihypertensive drugs but concentrates on those particularly relevant in diabetic patients: deterioration in glycaemic control and impaired recognition of hypoglycaemia. Furthermore, special attention should be paid to impotence and orthostatic hypotension, which frequently are present in the patient with longstanding diabetes. Finally, the choice of drug treatment will depend on the type of diabetes and the aetiology of the hypertension, e.g. nephropathic versus essential hypertension.

Non-pharmacological Therapy

Non-pharmacological treatment is particularly relevant for patients with mild hypertension and NIDDM. Approximately 85% of NIDDM patients are obese. Weight loss in these obese patients is of benefit in the treatment of both hypertension [70–72] and diabetes. Several studies have demonstrated that sodium and water retention is present in hypertensive IDDM and NIDDM patients with and without diabetic kidney disease, as discussed previously. Therefore, reduced sodium intake (approximately 80–100 mmol per day) should be recommended, even though no trials have been performed in diabetics. However, sodium restriction of the same magnitude reduces mean arterial blood pressure by an average of 7% in patients with essential hypertension [73]. Dodson et al [74] have demonstrated a beneficial effect on arterial hypertension in NIDDM patients treated with a high-fibre, low-fat and low-sodium diet for 3 months. Unfortunately, long-term compliance with these dietary recommendations is usually poor. Recently, moderate regular exercise has been demonstrated to reduce arterial blood pressure by 16/11 mmHg in untreated patients with essential hypertension [75]. Finally, hypertensive diabetic patients should avoid exogenous factors that may elevate blood pressure, e.g. excessive alcohol intake, smoking and non-steroidal anti-inflammatory drugs.

Table 2 Advantages and disadvantages of antihypertensive drugs in diabetic patients

Drug class	Advantages	Disadvantages
Diuretics	Reduction of excess body sodium and water	Deterioration in glycaemic control (NIDDM), may precipitate hyperosmolar coma, hyperlipidaemia, impotence
Potassium-sparing diuretics	Reduction of excess body sodium and water	Hyperkalaemia, impotence
Beta-adrenergic blockers	Postpones renal insufficiency in diabetic nephropathy, reduces microalbuminuria	Impaired recognition of hypoglycaemia, prolonged recovery from hypoglycaemia, pressor response to hypoglycaemia (IDDM and insulin-treated NIDDM), slight deterioration in glycaemic control (NIDDM)
Angiotensin-converting enzyme inhibitors	Postpones renal insufficiency in diabetic nephropathy, reduces micro- and macroalbuminuria, reduces excess body water	
Calcium entry blockers		Orthostatic hypotension (rare)
Arterial vasodilators		Sodium/water retention
Alpha-adrenergic blockers		Orthostatic hypotension, impotence, sodium/water retention
Centrally acting drugs		Orthostatic hypotension, impotence, sodium/water retention

Drug Treatment

Diuretics

Thiazide diuretics are effective in lowering blood pressure in hypertensive IDDM and NIDDM patients without nephropathy [29, 76, 77]. Thiazides normalize total body sodium and water in these patients [29]. Loop diuretics are frequently required to control sodium and fluid retention in patients with nephropathy.

It is well documented that thiazides bring about deterioration of glycaemic control in NIDDM patients, but it is important to remember that the degree of deterioration is dose related [77, 78]. Nowadays we tend to use lower doses of thiazide diuretics, and hence glycaemic deterioration may be less of a problem. The effect on metabolic control in IDDM patients is negligible or lacking. Several mechanisms contribute to the thiazide-induced hyperglycaemia: reduced insulin secretion (hypokalaemia), insulin resistance and a direct accelerating effect on hepatic glucose production, as reviewed by Struthers [78].

Thiazide diuretics increase blood levels of total and low-density lipoprotein (LDL) cholesterol and triglycerides, whereas high-density lipoprotein (HDL) cholesterol is unchanged [78, 79]. The clinical significance of such changes has not been adequately studied in diabetic patients.

The MRC study [80] clearly demonstrated that thiazides are associated with a significant incidence of impotence in non-diabetic patients, a problem likely to be more common in patients with longstanding diabetes. Relevant information on potassium-sparing diuretics is lacking in diabetes.

Beta-adrenergic Blockers

Beta-adrenergic blockers are some of the most commonly used first-line drugs in diabetics with essential hypertension [67, 68]; furthermore, they have a beneficial effect on kidney function in incipient and overt diabetic nephropathy [42, 45, 46, 48, 49].

The main hazards of β-adrenergic blockade in insulin-treated NIDDM and IDDM patients are impaired recognition of hypoglycaemia, delayed blood glucose recovery and pressor response to hypoglycaemia [67, 68, 78]. Careful instruction about this masking effect is of vital importance. Patients lacking hypoglycaemic warning symptoms should not be treated with β-blockers.

These adverse effects are less pronounced with the use of cardioselective β-adrenergic blockers [81]. However, the dose of the cardioselective blockers is crucial because cardiospecificity is a property that disappears when the dose of these drugs is increased. It should be stressed that the incidence of severe hypoglycaemic attacks does not seem to be elevated in IDDM patients receiving long-term β-blockade compared with a control group of IDDM patients [82].

The interaction between β-adrenergic blockers and glycaemic control in diabetes has been reviewed by Østman 883]. The overall deterioration in glycaemic control is small and most pronounced for the non-selective β-blockers.

It is well established that β-blockade increases plasma triglyceride levels and decreases HDL cholesterol in non-diabetic patients [78]. However, in the only study performed in diabetic patients no such effects were documented [84].

Angiotensin Converting Enzyme Inhibitors

Several studies have demonstrated that angiotensin converting enzyme (ACE) inhibition with captopril diminishes albuminuria [85, 86] and reduces the rate of decline in GFR in IDDM patients suffering from diabetic nephropathy [50]. Reduction in microalbuminuria during ACE inhibition with enalapril has also been reported in normotensive IDDM patients [47]. The beneficial effect of ACE inhibition in diabetic kidney disease is probably due to a reduction in glomerular capillary hydraulic pressure. This suggestion is supported by the results of micropuncture studies in normotensive streptozotocin-diabetic rats treated with ACE inhibition [87]: these studies showed that prevention of glomerular hypertension effectively protects against the subsequent development of glomerulopathy and proteinuria. Anderson et al [88] investigated the remnant kidney rat model and showed that glomerular hypertension was reduced by enalapril but not by a combination of thiazide, hydralazine and reserpine in spite of the same reduction in systemic blood pressure. Therefore, the authors concluded that unless glomerular capillary hydraulic pressure is reduced to near-normal values, control of systemic hypertension is insufficient to prevent progressive glomerular injury. In other words, not all antihypertensive drugs have the same ability to arrest progressive, renal disease.

Several small-scale studies have demonstrated that ACE inhibitors effectively reduce blood pressure in IDDM and NIDDM patients suffering from essential hypertension [89–91]. ACE inhibition influenced neither glycaemic control nor plasma lipids. Severe hyperkalaemia has not been reported in any of the above-mentioned studies, including those dealing with diabetic nephropathy.

Calcium Entry Blockers

The effect of calcium entry blockers on blood pressure, glycaemic control and plasma lipids has been evaluated in several short-term studies dealing with a limited number of NIDDM patients, as reviewed by Struthers [78], Ritchie and Atkinson [92] and Odigwe et al [93]. Most studies suggest that calcium entry blockers do not have a clinically significant effect on glycaemic control or plasma lipids. However, further long-term studies are required on the effect of calcium antagonists in the hypertensive diabetic patient.

Other Drugs

Passa [94] has reviewed the advantages, disadvantages and limitations of the various drugs used in diabetic patients (see also Table 2). Hydralazine combined with other antihypertensive drugs has been shown to be of value in slowing the progressive decline in GFR in diabetic nephropathy [49]. The main problems with α-adrenergic blockers and centrally acting drugs relate to orthostatic hypotension, high incidence of impotence and sodium/water retention.

SUGGESTIONS FOR ANTIHYPERTENSIVE DRUG TREATMENT

The choice of treatment is difficult, as there are no long-term comparative clinical trials of antihypertensive drugs in diabetic patients. The stepped-care approach to drug treatment should be applied. Valid scientific evidence (discussed previously) suggests that ACE inhibitors or cardioselective β-adrenergic blockers should be applied as a first step in IDDM and NIDDM patients with incipient and overt diabetic nephropathy. To control sodium and fluid retention, diuretics are nearly always required.

IDDM and insulin-treated NIDDM patients suffering from essential hypertension should probably be treated with diuretics, ACE inhibitors or calcium entry blockers as first-line drugs, with β-adrenergic blockers in the second or third line [68]. Beta-adrenergic blockers, ACE inhibitors or calcium entry blockers have been recommended as first-line drugs in NIDDM patients not receiving insulin [68]. Diuretics are regarded as a second or third choice in these patients.

REFERENCES

1. Pell S, D'Alonzo CA. Some aspects of hypertension in diabetes mellitus. JAMA 1967; 202: 104–10.
2. Christlieb AR. Diabetes and hypertensive vascular disease. Am J Cardiol. 1973; 32: 592–606.
3. Parving H-H, Andersen AR, Smidt UM, Oxenbøll B, Edsberg B, Sandahl Christiansen J. Diabetic nephropathy and arterial hypertension. Diabetologia 1983; 24: 10–12.
4. Klein R, Klein BEK, Moss SE, DeMets DL. Blood pressure and hypertension in diabetes. Am J Epidemiol 1985; 122: 75–89.
5. Panzram G. Mortality and survival in Type 2 (non-insulin-dependent) diabetes mellitus. Diabetologia 1987; 30: 123–31.
6. Kannel WB, Gordon T, Schwartz MJ. Systolic versus diastolic blood pressure and risk of coronary heart disease: the Framingham Study. Am J Cardiol 1971; 27: 335–46.
7. Kannel WB, Wolf PA, McGee DL, Dawber TR, McNamara P, Castelli WP. Systolic blood pressure, arterial rigidity and risk of stroke. The Framingham Study. JAMA 1981; 245: 1225–9.
8. Keen H. The prevalence of blindness in diabetics. J Roy Coll Phys 1972; 7: 53–60.
9. Parving H-H, Viberti GC, Keen H, Christiansen JS, Lassen NA. Hemodynamic factors in the genesis of diabetic microangiopathy. Metabolism 1983; 32: 943–9.
10. Christlieb AR. The hypertensions of diabetes. Diabetes Care 1982; 5: 50–8.
11. Drury PL. Diabetes and arterial hypertension. Diabetologia 1983; 24: 1–9.
12. Freedman P, Moulton R, Rosenheim ML, Spencer AG, Willoughby DA. Phaeochromocytoma, diabetes and glycosuria. Quart J Med 1958; 27: 307–21.
13. Shapiro AP, Perez-Stable E, Monsos SE. Co-existence of renal arterial hypertension and diabetes mellitus. JAMA 1965; 192: 813–16.
14. Munichoodappa C, D'Elia JA, Libertino JA, Gleason RE, Christlieb AR. Renal artery stenosis in hypertensive diabetics. J Urol 1978; 121: 555–8.
15. Frimodt-Møller C. Diabetic cystopathy. II: Relationship to some late-diabetic manifestations. Dan Med Bull 1976; 23: 279–86.
16. Mendlowitz M. Some theories of hypertension: fact and fancy. Hypertension 1979; 1: 435–41.
17. Hommel E, Mathiesen ER, Edsberg B, Bahnsen M, Parving H-H. Acute reduction of arterial blood pressure reduces urinary albumin excretion in Type 1 (insulin-dependent) diabetic patients with incipient nephropathy. Diabetologia 1986; 29: 211–15.
18. Feldt-Rasmussen B, Mathiesen ER, Deckert T, Giese J, Christensen NJ, Bent-Hansen L, Nielsen MD. Central role for sodium in the pathogenesis of blood pressure changes independent of angiotensin, aldosterone and catecholamines in insulin-dependent diabetes mellitus. Diabetologia 1987; 30: 610–17.
19. Hommel E, Mathiesen ER, Giese J, Nielsen MD, Schütten HJ, Parving H-H. On the pathogenesis of arterial blood pressure elevation in insulin-dependent diabetic patients with incipient and overt nephropathy. Scand J Clin Lab Invest 1989; 49: 537–44.
20. Christlieb AR, Kaldany A, D'Elia JA. Plasma renin activity and hypertension in diabetes mellitus. Diabetes 1976; 25: 969–74.
21. Christleib AR, Kaldany A, D'Elia JA, Williams GH. Aldosterone responsiveness in patients with diabetes mellitus. Diabetes 1978; 27: 732–7.
22. Björck S, Dalin K, Herlitz H, Larsson O, Aurell M. Renin secretion in advanced diabetic nephropathy. Scand J Urol Nephrol 1984; 79: 53–7.
23. O'Hare JA, Ferriss JB, Brady D, Twormey B, O'Sullivan DJ. Exchangeable sodium and renin in hypertensive diabetic patients with and without nephropathy. Hypertension 1985; 7 (suppl. II): 43–8.
24. Berchtold P, Jorgens V, Finke C, Berger M. Epidemiology of obesity and hypertension. Int J Obesity 1981; 5 (suppl. 1): 1–7.
25. Landsberg L, Young JB. Insulin-mediated glucose metabolism in the relationship between dietary intake and sympathetic nervous system activity. Int J Obesity 1985; 9 (suppl. 2): 63–8.
26. Rose JW, Young JB, Minaker KL, Stevens AL, Pallota J, Landsberg L. Effect of insulin and glucose infusions on sympathetic nervous system activity in normal man. Diabetes 1981; 30: 219–25.
27. Landsberg L. Diet, obesity and hypertension: an hypothesis involving insulin, the sympathetic nervous system, and adaptive thermogenesis. Quart J Med 1986; 236: 1081–90.
28. Christlieb AR. Vascular reactivity to angiotensin II and to norepinephrine in diabetic subjects. Diabetes 1976; 25: 268–74.
29. Weidmann P, Beretta-Piccoli C, Keusch G et al. Sodium–volume factor, cardiovascular reactivity

and hypotensive mechanism of diuretic therapy in mild hypertension associated with diabetes mellitus. Am J Med 1979; 67: 779–84.

30. DeFronzo RA. The effect of insulin on renal sodium metabolism. A review with clinical implications. Diabetologia 1981; 21: 165–71.

31. De Châlet R, Weidmann P, Flammer J, Ziegler WH, Beretta-Piccoli E, Veller W, Reubi FC. Sodium, renin, aldosterone, catecholamines and blood pressure in diabetes mellitus. Kidney Int 1977; 12: 412–21.

32. Parving H-H, Rasmussen SM. Transcapillary escape rate of albumin and plasma volume in short and long-term juvenile diabetics. Scand J Clin Lab Invest 1973; 32: 81–6.

33. O'Hare JA, Ferriss JB, Tworney BM, Gonggrijp H, O'Sullivan DJ. Changes in blood pressure, body fluid volumes, circulating angiotensin II and aldosterone with improved diabetic control. Clin Sci 1982; 63: 415–18.

34. Faris I, Agerskov K, Henriksen D, Lassen NA, Parving H-H. Decreased distensibility of a passive vascular bed in diabetes mellitus: an indicator of microangiopathy. Diabetologia 1982; 23: 411–14.

35. Kastrup J, Lassen NA, Parving H-H. Diabetic microangiopathy, a factor enhancing the functional significance of peripheral occlusive arteriosclerotic disease. Clin Physiol 1984; 4: 367–9.

36. Mathiesen ER, Oxenbøll B, Johansen K, Svendsen PA, Deckert T. Incipient nephropathy in Type 1 (insulin-dependent) diabetes. Diabetologia 1984; 26: 406–10.

37. Wisemann M, Viberti GC, Mackintosh D, Jarrett RJ, Keen H. Glycaemia, arterial blood pressure and microalbuminuria in Type 1 (insulin-dependent) diabetes mellitus. Diabetologia 1984; 26: 401–6.

38. Mathiesen ER, Saurbrey N, Hommel E, Parving H-H. Prevalence of microalbuminuria in children with Type 1 (insulin-dependent) diabetes mellitus. Diabetologia 1986; 29: 640–3.

39. Parving H-H, Hommel E, Mathiesen E, Skøtt P, Edsberg B, Bahnsen M, Lauritzen M, Mongaard P, Lauritzen E. Prevalence of microalbuminuria, arterial hypertension, retinopathy and neuropathy in patients with insulin dependent diabetes. Br Med J 1988; 296: 156–160.

40. Parving H-H, Smidt UM, Friisberg B, Bonnevie-Nielsen V, Andersen AR. A prospective study of glomerular filtration rate and arterial blood pressure in insulin-dependent diabetics with diabetic nephropathy. Diabetologia 1981; 20: 457–61.

41. Hostetter TH, Rennke HG, Brenner BM. The case for intrarenal hypertension in the initiation and progression of diabetic and other glomerulopathies. Am J Med 1982; 72: 375–80.

42. Mogensen CE. Long-term antihypertensive treat-ment inhibiting progression of diabetic nephropathy. Br Med J 1982; 285: 685–8.

43. Hasslacher C, Stech W, Wahl P, Ritz E. Blood pressure and metabolic control as risk factors for nephropathy in Type 1 (insulin-dependent) diabetes. Diabetologia 1985; 28: 6–11.

44. Parving H-H, Kastrup J, Smidt UM, Andersen AR, Feldt-Rasmussen B, Christiansen JS. Impaired autoregulation of glomerular filtration rate in Type 1 (insulin-dependent) diabetic patients with nephropathy. Diabetologia 1984; 27: 547–52.

45. Christensen CK, Mogensen CE. Effect of antihypertensive treatment of progression of incipient diabetic nephropathy. Hypertension 1985; 7: 9–13.

46. Friedman PJ, Dunn PJ, Jury DR. Metoprolol and albumin excretion in diabetes. Lancet 1986; ii: 43.

47. Marre M, Leblanc H, Suarez L, Guyenne T-T, Menard J, Passa P. Converting enzyme inhibition and kidney function in normotensive diabetic patients with persistent microalbuminuria. Br Med J 1987; 294: 1448–52.

48. Parving H-H, Andersen AR, Smidt UM, Svendsen PA. Early aggressive antihypertensive treatment reduces rate of decline in kidney function in diabetic nephropathy. Lancet 1983; i: 1175–9.

49. Parving H-H, Andersen AR, Smidt UM, Hommel E, Mathiesen ER, Svendsen PA. Effect of antihypertensive treatment on kidney function in diabetic nephropathy. Br Med J 1987; 294: 1443–7.

50. Björck S, Nyberg G, Mulec H, Granerus G, Herlitz H, Aurell M. Beneficial effects of angiotensin converting enzyme inhibition on renal function in patients with diabetic nephropathy. Br Med J 1986; 293: 471–4.

51. Kornerup T. Blood pressure and diabetic retinopathy. Acta Ophthalmol (Copenh) 1957; 35: 163–74.

52. Ishihara M, Yukimura Y, Aizawa T, Yamada T, Ohto K, Yoshizawa K. High blood pressure as risk factor in diabetic retinopathy development in NIDDM patients. Diabetes Care 1987; 10: 20–5.

53. West KM, Erdreich LJ, Stober JA. A detailed study of risk factors for retinopathy and nephropathy in diabetes. Diabetes 1980; 29: 501–8.

54. Knowler WC, Bennett PA, Ballintine EJ. Increased incidence of retinopathy in diabetics with elevated blood pressure. New Engl J Med 1980; 302: 645–50.

55. Klein R, Klein BEK, Moss SE. A population-based study of diabetic retinopathy in insulin-using patients diagnosed before 30 years of age. Diabetes Care 1985; 8: 71–6.

56. Rand LI, Kroleweski AS, Aiello LM, Warram

JA, Baker RS, Maki T. Multiple factors in the prediction of risk of proliferative diabetic retinopathy. New Engl J Med 1985; 313: 1433–8.

57. Kohner EM. The problems of retinal blood flow in diabetes. Diabetes 1976; 25 (suppl. 2): 839–44.

58. Soeldner JS, Christacopoulos PD, Gleason RE. Mean retinal circulation time as determined by fluorescein angiopathy in normal prediabetic and chemical-diabetic subjects. Diabetes 1976; 25 (suppl. 2): 903–8.

59. Atherton A, Hill DW, Keen H, Young S, Edwards EJ. The effect of acute hyperglycaemia on the retinal circulation of the normal cat. Diabetologia 1980; 18: 233–7.

60. Sinclair SH, Graunwald JE, Riva C, Braunstein SN, Nichols CW, Schwartz S. Retinal vascular autoregulation in diabetes mellitus. Ophthalmology 1982; 89: 748–50.

61. Osei K, Fields PG, Cataland S, Graig EL, George JM, O'Dorisio TH. Abnormal retinal artery responses to stress in patients with type 1 diabetes. Am J Med 1985; 78: 595–601.

62. Karlefors T. Exercise test in male diabetics. Acta Med Scand 1966; 180 (suppl 449) 449.

63. Memorandum from the WHO/ISH. 1986 guidelines for the treatment of mild hypertension. Hypertension 1986; 8: 957–61.

64. WHO. Arterial hypertension. Report of a WHO Expert Committee on Hypertension. Technical Report Series 628. Geneva: WHO, 1979.

65. Freis ED. Should mild hypertension be treated? New Engl J Med 1982; 307: 306–9.

66. Editorial. Treatment of hypertension: the 1985 results. Lancet 1985; ii: 645–7.

67. Working Group on Hypertension in Diabetes. Statement on hypertension in diabetes mellitus. Arch Int Med 1987; 147: 830–42.

68. Wilson TW, Parving H-H, Larochelle P, Zinman B, Dawson KG. Specificity of hypertension therapy in diabetes. In Hamet P (ed) Report of the third consensus conference on hypertension and diabetes in Canada. Montreal: Canadian Hypertension Society, 1988, 17–27.

69. Management Committee of the Australian Therapeutic Trial in Mild Hypertension. Untreated mild hypertension. Lancet 1982; i: 185–91.

70. Chiang BN, Pereman LV, Epstein FN. Overweight and hypertension. A review. Circulation 1969; 39: 403–21.

71. Heyden S. The working man's diet. II: effect of weight reduction in obese patients with hypertension, diabetes, hyperuricaemia and hyperlipidaemia. Nutr Metab 1978; 22: 141–59.

72. MacMahon SW, MacDonald GJ, Bernstein L, Andrews G, Blacket RB. Comparison of weight reduction with metoprolol in treatment of hypertension in young overweight patients. Lancet 1985; i: 1233–6.

73. MacGregor GA, Markandu ND, Best FE, Elder DM, Carn JM, Sagnella GA, Squires M. Double-blind randomized cross-over trial of moderate sodium restriction in essential hypertension. Lancet 1982; i: 351–4.

74. Dodson PM, Pacy PJ, Bal P, Kubicki AJ, Fletcher RF, Taylor KG. A controlled trial of a high fibre, low fat and low sodium diet for mild hypertension in Type 2 (non-insulin-dependent) diabetic patients. Diabetologia 1984; 27: 522–6.

75. Nelson L, Jennings GL, Ester MD, Korner PI. Effect on changing levels of physical activity on blood-pressure and haemodynamics in essential hypertension. Lancet 1986; ii: 473–6.

76. Pacy PJ, Dodson PM, Kubicki AJ, Fletcher RF, Taylor KG. Comparison of the hypotensive and metabolic effects of bendrofluazide therapy and high fibre, low fat, low salt diet in diabetic subjects with mild hypertension. J Hypertens 1984; 2: 215–20.

77. Dornhorst A, Powell SH, Pensky J. Aggravation by propranolol of hyperglycaemic effect of hydrochlorothiazide in Type II diabetics without alteration of insulin secretion. Lancet 1985; i: 123–6.

78. Struthers AD. The choice of antihypertensive therapy in the diabetic patient. Postgrad Med J 1985; 61: 563–9.

79. Grimm RH, Leon AS, Huinnhake PB, Lenz K, Hannon P, Blackburn H. Effects of thiazide diuretics on plasma lipids and lipoproteins in mildly hypertensive patients: a controlled trial. Ann Intern Med 1981; 94: 7–11.

80. Report of the Medical Research Council Working Party on Mild to Moderate Hypertension. Adverse reactions to bendrofluazide and propranolol for the treatment of mild hypertension. Lancet 1981; ii: 539–43.

81. Lager I, Blohmé G, Smith U. Effect of cardioselective and non-selective beta-blockade on the hypoglycaemic response in insulin-dependent diabetics. Lancet 1979; i: 458–62.

82. Barnett AH, Leslie D, Watkins PJ. Can insulin-treated diabetics be given beta-adrenergic blocking agents? Br Med J 1980; 280: 976–8.

83. Østman J. Beta-adrenergic blockade and diabetes mellitus. A review. Acta Med Scand 1983; 672: 69–77.

84. Benfield GFA, Hunter KR. Oxprenolol, methyldopa and lipids in diabetes mellitus. Br J Clin Pharmacol 1982; 13: 219–22.

85. Taguma Y, Kitamoto Y, Futaki G et al. Effect of captopril on heavy proteinuria in azotemic diabetics. New Engl J Med 1985; 313: 1617–20.

86. Hommel E, Parving H-H, Mathiesen ER, Edsberg B, Nielsen MD, Giese J. Effect of captopril on kidney function in insulin-dependent diabetic

patients with nephropathy. Br Med J 1986; 293: 467–70.

87. Zatz R, Dunn BR, Meyer TW, Andersen S, Rennke HG, Brenner BM. Prevention of diabetic glomerulopathy by pharmacological amelioration of glomerular capillary hypertension. J Clin Invest 1986; 77: 1925–30.

88. Anderson S, Rennke HG, Brenner BM. Therapeutic advantage of converting enzyme inhibitors in arresting progressive renal disease associated with systemic hypertension in the rat. J Clin Invest 1986; 77: 1993–2000.

89. Matthews DM, Wathen CG, Bell D, Collier A, Muir AL, Clarke BF. The effect of captopril on blood pressure and glucose tolerance in hypertensive non-insulin-dependent diabetics. Postgrad Med J 1986; 62 (suppl. 1): 73–5.

90. Gambaro G. Captopril in the treatment of hypertension in Type 1 and Type 2 diabetic patients. J Hypertens 1985; 3 (suppl. 2): 149–51.

91. Passa P, LeBlanc H, Marre M. Effects of enalapril in insulin-dependent diabetic subjects with mild to moderate uncomplicated hypertension. Diabetes Care 1987; 10: 200–4.

92. Ritchie CM, Atkinson AB. Towards better management of the diabetic patient with raised blood pressure. Diabet Med 1986; 3: 301–5.

93. Odigwe CO, McCulloch AJ, Williams DO, Tunbridge WMG. A trial of the calcium antagonist nisoldipine in hypertensive non-insulin-dependent diabetic patients. Diabet Med 1986; 3: 463–7.

94. Passa P. Le traitement de l'hypertension artérielle chez les diabètiques. Diabète Métab 1980; 6: 287–98.

68

The Diabetic Foot

M.E. Edmonds and P.J. Watkins

King's College Hospital, London, UK

One of the most destructive complications of diabetes is the loss of a limb. In a recent review of hospital admissions in 1981, for the population of East Anglia in the UK, diabetic patients with peripheral circulatory disorders represented the largest proportion of admissions (and daily-occupied beds) [1]. In the USA 50–70% of all non-traumatic amputations occur in diabetic patients [2], and this totals between 20 000 and 32 000 amputations annually [3]. The economic cost of the diabetic foot is enormous: hospital costs exceeded $200 million in the USA for the year 1980 [4].

Ulceration of the diabetic foot is due to trauma in the presence of neuropathy or ischaemia. Once the skin has been broken, superadded infection causes further problems. The underlying pathology, the nature and course of the disease and its management are quite distinct in neuropathic and ischaemic feet. Neuropathy results in a warm, numb, dry and usually painless foot in which the pulses are palpable. It leads to three main complications: the neuropathic ulcer, the neuropathic (Charcot) joint and neuropathic oedema; ulcer healing, with or without limited surgery, is the rule. In contrast, the ischaemic foot is cold and the pulses are absent. It is complicated by rest pain, ulceration from localised pressure necrosis and gangrene. Results of conservative treatment are less satisfactory than for neuropathic lesions, and vascular reconstruction and angioplasty have a definite role.

NEUROPATHIC FOOT

Pathophysiology

The presence of neuropathy is a prerequisite for the development of the highly characteristic lesions when the circulation is intact. At the very least, the small nerve fibres are damaged, causing diminished thermal and pain sensation [5, 6] and sympathetic denervation, leading to an increased peripheral circulation [7–9] and diminished or absent sweating. Loss of other sensory modalities is usually demonstrable as well and the feet are sometimes anaesthetic, but occasionally a dissociated sensory loss is observed with intact large-fibre modalities (vibration perception and light touch) [6]. The neuropathy that develops in leprosy has many similar features, and lesions in the feet are almost identical.

The severity of the sensory loss in the neuropathic ulcerated foot varies considerably, and ranges from mild impairment to complete loss of both thermal perception (small fibres) and vibration perception (large fibres) in about half the patients [10]. Boulton et al [11] suggested that vibration perception in these patients always

International Textbook of Diabetes Mellitus. Edited by K.G.M.M. Alberti, R.A. DeFronzo, H. Keen and P. Zimmet
© 1992 John Wiley & Sons Ltd

exceeds 30 volts when assessed using a biothesio-meter, and this test may be a useful method for ascertaining feet at risk of ulceration.

Autonomic (small-fibre) denervation is also an essential component of the neuropathic foot lesions. Our patients with neuropathic ulcers all have evidence of cardiac vagal denervation (reduced heart-rate variability) [12], but of greater relevance is the evidence for peripheral sympathetic denervation [13]. Its consequences are an increased blood flow, increased rigidity of the arterial wall with evidence of medial calcification, and diminished sweating.

The arterial wall in diabetic neuropathic patients is abnormally stiff. This increased stiffness has been inferred from raised systolic ankle pressures, shortened transit times of the pulse wave form, and an increase of the elastic modulus [8]. The pressure index (the ratio of the ankle systolic pressure to the brachial systolic pressure) is sometimes considerably higher (over 1.2) than normal (1.0–1.2); even in ischaemic patients, in whom it should be less than 1.0, this ratio may exceed 1.3–2.0 in patients with rigid, incompressible arteries.

The cause of arterial stiffening is at least in part due to medial calcification (Mönckeberg's sclerosis) which is a feature of severe diabetic neuropathy [14]. Vascular calcification has been observed commonly (78–90%) in patients with neuropathic (Charcot) joints [15], and also occurs on the operated side after sympathectomy [16]. Sympathetic denervation may be responsible for medial degeneration, and we speculate that this is followed by calcification. Peripheral blood flow may nevertheless be normal or raised even when extensive calcification is present.

Sympathetic denervation of peripheral vessels also causes a substantial increase of peripheral blood flow. The neuropathic foot has long been described as excessively hot with bounding pulses [17]. The normal triphasic Doppler sonograms are altered showing patterns characteristic of high diastolic flow (Figure 1), and there is ample evidence for arteriovenous shunting as well [7, 8]. Plethysmographic measurement of blood flow in the great toe shows that it is on average five times normal [9]. The changes are described in detail in Chapter 59.

Vascular responses in the neuropathic foot are also abnormal [18]. Apart from a limitation of maximal blood flow in response to heating, there is a marked diminution of vasoconstriction in the dependent foot—93% reduction in capillary flow in normal subjects compared with 85% reduction in neuropathy subjects [9]. The failure to vasoconstrict contributes to the excessive blood flow when upright, and to the oedema which to a greater or lesser extent often develops in severe neuropathy. Increased capillary permeability in long-term diabetes must also contribute to this problem.

The presence of substantial arteriovenous shunting might in theory jeopardise capillary nutritional blood flow. New methods of examination show that this is not the case. Measurement of capillary blood flow by laser Doppler flowmetry shows, overall, a higher flow than normal and this is further confirmed by direct visualisation of capillary blood flow velocity using television microscopy [19].

Sympathetic denervation of richly innervated capillaries also causes increased uptake by bone of technetium methylene diphosphonate, giving very striking isotopic scans of bones that appear normal on conventional radiography [20]. It is likely that this causes a resorption of bone leading to osteopenia, as it does in other situations such as paraplegia. We have

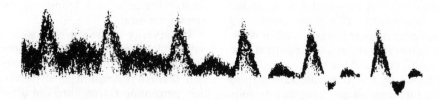

Figure 1 Doppler ultrasonogram from the posterior tibial of a young female patient with painful neuropathy. On the left the pattern is that of typical neuropathy, showing the normal upward deflection of forward flow followed by a continuous forward flow throughout diastole with complete loss of the expected reverse flow. After sympathetic stimulation by coughing the appearance of the sonogram becomes normal on the right, showing a typical triphasic pattern with deflection of forward flow followed by reversed and later again forward flow in diastole (A.G. Archer, unpublished observation)

found some evidence of cortical bone thinning in the feet and hands of severely neuropathic diabetic patients [21]. This might predispose to the extensive bony destruction which occurs in Charcot neuroarthropathy, and this is discussed below.

Uncontrolled inflammatory responses may occur in the neuropathic foot. There are several clinical features that suggest this possibility: thus, the very rapid development of cellulitis which may spread within hours, the inappropriate amounts of callus which form at the sites of minor metatarsal fractures and the astonishingly destructive effects of salicyclic acid in corn plasters all suggest that failure to control inflammation could contribute to the pathology of the diabetic foot.

Sweating

Diminished sweating is a feature of sympathetic denervation in the neuropathic foot. New, sophisticated methods of assessing sweating have led to renewed interest in this field [22]; it is now possible to assess peripheral (preganglionic and postganglionic) sympathetic function, postganglionic function by the axon reflex using iontophoresis with acetylcholine or by the thermoregulatory smear test and by direct stimulation of sweat glands with pilocarpine, or by recording the sympathetic discharge as a galvanic skin response.

The most common sweating deficit occurs in the feet in the classic 'stocking' distribution. It is associated with other autonomic defects, although the cardiovascular abnormalities tend to develop first [23]. It is responsible for the dry, cracked skin characteristic of the neuropathic foot and which serves as a portal of entry for infection. Although sweating is absent in the majority of ulcerated feet, it is retained in about one-quarter of these patients, and an even greater proportion of those with Charcot arthropathy [23]. The role of sweating loss in the genesis of diabetic foot lesions may need reappraisal.

Pressure and Deformity

The presence of excessive pressure is a prerequisite for the development of a neuropathic ulcer. Foot ulcers are unusual unless the vertical pressure exceeds $10 \, \text{kg/cm}^2$ [24]. Elevated foot pressures are more likely to be present when the foot is deformed. The presence of neuropathy, even in its very earliest form with relatively mild sensory defects, may itself predispose to elevated foot pressures [24]. Patients with foot ulcers tend to be heavier than others, although weight does not itself necessarily cause high foot pressure. Although these vertical forces are obviously important, shear forces must also be instrumental in damaging the neuropathic foot, and the sites of healed ulcers have been shown to correspond to the sites of maximal shear forces. However, little is known regarding the magnitude of shear forces, and this remains an important, relatively unexplored area of research.

Deformities of the feet are more likely to be associated with abnormal pressures. Abnormalities are congenital or acquired as a result of neuropathy. Congenital abnormalities may be more common, although this has not been systematically investigated. Neuropathy may cause weakness of the small muscles of the foot with clawing of the toes and prominence of the metatarsal heads, and this may be one reason for reduced toe loading in neuropathic patients. Some patients have congenitally clawed toes, and the distinction from those with a neuropathic basis may be impossible by that stage of foot ulceration. Other deformities that predispose to abnormal pressures include hallux rigidus, hammer toes and bunions [25]. The most severe abnormalities are those of the Charcot neuroarthropathic foot: they are very liable to ulceration, especially when there is a 'rocker-bottom' sole (see below).

Oedema

The presence of foot oedema may not only underlie the development of foot ulcers when the shoes become too tight, but also (in theory at least) could impede healing of established ulcers. Oedema is common in elderly patients, but in diabetic patients there are additional reasons for its occurrence, either from neuropathy or less commonly from fluid retention or nephrotic syndrome in patients with diabetic nephropathy.

Oedema is a complication of severe diabetic neuropathy. It has long been recognised and was observed in 35 of 125 patients with neuropathy described by Martin [26]. It is therefore not a rare phenomenon, although severe intractable oedema resulting from neuropathy is exceptional. This form of oedema probably results from the major haemodynamic abnormalities associated with neuropathy. Thus, the high blood flow, vasodilatation and arteriovenous shunting resulting from sympathetic denervation lead to abnormal venous pooling. Oedema probably occurs because of loss of the venivasomotor reflex, which normally occurs on standing and results in an increase in precapillary resistance: the inability of the foot to compensate for the rise in venous pressure would thus predispose to oedema formation. Relief of oedema by administration of the sympathomimetic agent ephedrine [27] lends further strength to the argument that sympathetic failure is the cause of the oedema, and is discussed in greater detail below.

Complications of the Neuropathic Foot

Neuropathic Ulcer

Pathogenesis. Neuropathic ulcers result from noxious stimuli (unperceived by the patient because of loss of pain and sensation) which cause mechanical, thermal and chemical injuries. Direct mechanical injuries result from treading on nails and other sharp objects. However, the most frequent cause of ulceration brought about by mechanical factors is the neglected callosity. This results from excess friction on the tips of the toes and from high vertical and shear forces under the plantar surface of the metatarsal heads on walking.

The repetitive mechanical forces of gait eventually result in callosity formation, inflammatory autolysis and subkeratotic haematomas [28, 29]. The callosities are painless and are neglected by the patient. Tissue necrosis occurs below the plaque of callus and results in a small cavity filled with serous fluid. This eventually breaks through to the surface with ulcer formation.

Thermal injuries cause direct trauma and damage to the epithelium. This often results from bathing the feet in excessively hot water, the injudicious use of hot-water bottles, from resting the feet too close to a fire or radiator, or from walking barefoot on hot sand during holidays in warm climates.

Chemical trauma can result from the use of keratolytic agents. They often contain salicylic acid which causes ulceration in the diabetic foot. When corn cures are applied, callus tissue is softened and macerated and provides a point of entry for bacteria. Corn cures destroy non-keratinized cells in the subcutaneous tissues; the result is ulceration and sepsis. We recently reported 7 patients who developed foot ulceration and sepsis after application of corn cures [30]; 4 patients had such extensive tissue necrosis that they needed forefoot surgery.

When the epithelium is damaged in the skin of the diabetic foot, infection can supervene, caused by organisms from the surrounding skin which are usually *Staphylococcus aureus* or streptococci. Cellulitis can develop, with abscess formation and tracking of pus to infect underlying tendons and bones and to cause septic arthritis. Occasionally, both staphylococci and streptococci are present together and these can combine to produce a rampant cellulitis that extends rapidly through the foot, producing marked necrosis within only a few hours. Enzymes from these bacteria are angiotoxic and cause thrombosis of vessels in situ. If both vessels are thrombosed in a toe, then it becomes necrotic and gangrenous and this is probably the basis of 'diabetic' gangrene in which tissue necrosis is seen only a few centimetres away from a bounding dorsalis pedis pulse. Anaerobic organisms flourish in deep-seated infections.

Severe sepsis in the diabetic foot is often associated with gas in the soft tissues. Subcutaneous gas may be detected by direct palpation of the foot and the diagnosis is confirmed by the appearance of gas in the soft tissue on the radiograph. Although clostridial organisms have previously been held responsible for this presentation, non-clostridial organisms are more frequently the offending pathogens. These include *Bacteroides*, *Escherichia* and anaerobic streptococci.

Both aerobic and anaerobic organisms can spread rapidly to the blood stream and occasionally result in life-threatening bacteraemias [31].

Fungal infections also occur but usually do not cause systemic upset. However, infections of toenails (tinea unguium) and interdigital spaces (tinea pedis) by such fungi as *Trichophyton* and *Candida albicans* can serve as portals of entry for bacteria.

Management. This falls into three parts: removal of callus, eradication of infection and reduction of weight-bearing forces.

The callus that surrounds the ulcer must be removed by expert chiropody. Excess keratin should be pared away with a scalpel blade to expose the floor of the ulcer and allow efficient drainage of the lesion and re-epithelialisation from the edges of the ulcer.

A bacterial swab should be taken from the floor of the ulcer after the callus has been removed. A superficial ulcer may be treated in the outpatient department and oral antibiotics prescribed, according to the organism isolated, until the ulcer has healed. The patient should be instructed to dress the ulcer daily. A simple, non-adhesive dressing should be applied, after cleaning the ulcer and surrounding tissue with an antiseptic.

If cellulitis is present the limb is threatened and hospital admission should be arranged as a matter of urgency. The limb should be rested and, after blood cultures have been taken, intravenous antibiotics administered. Suitable antibiotics are benzylpenicillin (2 mega units 6-hourly) plus flucloxacillin (500 mg 6-hourly) plus metronidazole (1 g per rectum 8-hourly). This antibiotic regimen may need revision after the results of bacterial cultures are available. If gram-negative organisms have been isolated, gentamicin or a cephalosporin may be indicated.

In the neuropathic foot, it is important that all necrotic tissue be removed and abscess cavities drained surgically. If gangrene has developed in a digit, a ray amputation to remove that toe and part of its associated metatarsal is necessary and is usually very successful [25].

Reduction of weight-bearing forces is necessary, both in the acute stages and also in the long-term management. In the presence of sepsis, bed rest is ideal and will obviously remove the weight-bearing forces to promote healing. Proper care should be taken of the heels, and foam wedges used to protect the heels from pressure in bed. If such measures are not taken, the risk of ulceration is high. However, bed rest is not always possible. In the short term, a plaster cast that conforms to all the contours of the foot (a 'total contact' plaster) can be applied to 'unload' the ulcer and reduce shear forces [2]. In the long term, redistribution of weight-bearing forces can be achieved by special footwear which is fashioned from casts of the patient's foot. Insoles made of closed-cell polyethylene foams such as Plastazote have energy-absorbing properties. These can be heated and

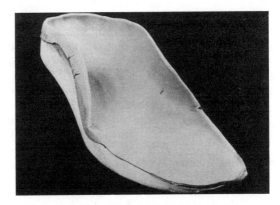

Figure 2 Moulded Plastazote insole

moulded to the shape of the foot to cushion the foot and to spread the weight-bearing forces evenly on the sole (Figure 2). When subjected to wear and tear, Plastazote insoles can lose their resilience and it is now possible to use more durable materials such as Poron. Indeed, composite insoles are often made with an upper layer of polyethylene foam for total contact and a lower layer of microcellular rubber for resilience (Figure 3). When there has been previous ulceration, a rigid weight-distributing cradle is required, as well as cushioning, to relieve weight from high-pressure areas and to transfer it to other less vulnerable areas. Recently, Plastazote cradles have been manufactured often with 'windows' cut out (and filled in with cushioning material such as Neoprene) for weight relief under high-pressure areas [32].

Moulded insoles must be accommodated in extra-depth shoes. When the foot is not deformed, shoes fashioned from commercial

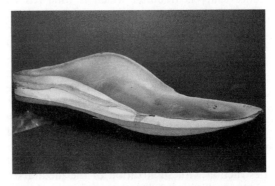

Figure 3 Composite insole with upper layer of polyethylene foam for total contact and a lower layer of microcellular rubber for resilience

lasts and available 'off the shelf' can be used. If the patient has a foot deformity with healed trophic ulcers, it is necessary to make individual lasts from casts of the patient's foot. In either case, the heels must be low, and slipping is prevented by using laces; the forefoot should be broad and square and the uppers of high-quality leather which will adapt to toe pressure. When pressure points are not adequately relieved by cushioned insoles it is necessary to modify the soles of the shoe. When the ulcer is under the plantar surface of the great toe, a rigid rocker sole allows the shoe to rock like a seesaw on a pivot under the centre of the shoe, minimising contact between the forefoot and floor during gait. If the ulcer is under the metatarsal heads, a metatarsal bar placed just proximal to the heads can reapportion weight-bearing forces along the shafts.

Neuropathic Joint (Charcot Joint)

Pathogenesis. The most frequent location of the neuropathic joint is the tarsal–metatarsal region, followed by the metatarsophalangeal joints and then the ankle of subtalar joints [33]. The initial presentation is often a hot, swollen foot which can be uncomfortable in up to one-third of cases and is often misdiagnosed as cellulitis or gout. The precipitating event is usually a minor traumatic episode such as tripping. If the patient presents within a few days radiographs are often normal, although isotope bone scans may be grossly abnormal [34, 35] with localised areas of high uptake representing excessive osteoblastic activity and heralding eventual radiological abnormalities. A common early radiological abnormality is fracture, which is followed by osteolysis, bony fragmentation and finally joint subluxation and disorganisation. In addition to fracture, erosions, periosteal new bone formation and sclerosis are also prominent bony findings in the development of the Charcot joint. Sclerosis is usually associated with lucency in the heads of the metatarsals, the final appearance being similar to the Freiberg's infraction lesion associated with osteonecrosis of the epiphysis of the metatarsal head. These initial bony abnormalities eventually lead to secondary joint destruction with subluxation of the metatarsophalangeal joints, dislocation of the tarsal, subtalar and ankle joints, fragmentation of bone and soft-tissue calcification [36, 37].

The process of destruction takes place over a few months only and leads to two classic deformities: the rocker-bottom deformity, in which there is displacement and subluxation of the tarsus downwards, and the medial convexity, which results from displacement of the talonavicular joint or from tarsometatarsal dislocation. If these deformities are not accommodated in properly fitting footwear, ulceration at vulnerable pressure points often develops.

The development of Charcot osteoarthropathy depends on both peripheral autonomic and somatic defects. It is suggested that the evolution is as follows. Sympathetic denervation of arterioles causes an increase of blood flow which in turn causes rarefaction of bone, making it prone to damage even after minor trauma. Bone formation and structure are closely linked with vascular changes. Large venules containing rapid linear velocities of blood flow cause resorption of bone spicules [38]. In animals, the site of maximum bone-calcium loss after paraplegia corresponds to areas of maximum blood flow, which may lead to increased resorption of bone [39]. Recent histological studies of Charcot joints have shown marked increase in vascularity with vessel dilatation and trabecular resorption by large numbers of osteoclasts [40]. Thus, increased bony blood flow can lead to bony resorption and susceptibility to fracture (see above). Loss of sensation from somatic neuropathy permits abnormal mechanical stresses to occur, normally prevented by pain. Relatively minor trauma can then cause major destructive changes in susceptible bone.

Management. It is essential to make the diagnosis early, before extreme joint destruction has taken place. The initial presentation of unilateral warmth and swelling in a neuropathic foot after an episode of minor trauma is suggestive of a developing Charcot joint.

There is no definite treatment that halts the progression of the disease, but immobilisation may help. Treatment comprises rest (ideally bed rest), or the avoidance of weight-bearing by the use of crutches until the oedema and local warmth have resolved. Alternatively, the foot can be put in a well-moulded non-walking plaster cast. Immobilisation is continued until bony repair is complete, usually a period of 2–3 months. Indomethacin may be useful in painful cases. In long-term management, special shoes and insoles should be fitted to accommodate deformity and prevent ulceration, which is the major hazard of the deformed foot. Although the eventual deformity may be substantial, walking is not often affected and patients usually retain full mobility.

Neuropathic Oedema

Pathogenesis. This has been discussed earlier in this chapter.

Management. The use of a sympathomimetic agent, by stimulating vasoconstriction, might be expected to reduce this form of oedema and, indeed, ephedrine has a rapid and substantial effect on relieving neuropathic oedema [27]. It results in a rapid decrease of weight, a reduction in peripheral diastolic flow and an increase in sodium excretion, all associated with rapid diminution of oedema over a few days. The effect of ephedrine is possibly complex, and as well as its peripheral effects, it may have central effects on the control of salt and water homeostasis. The usual dosage of ephedrine is 15–30 mg thrice daily, although it may be necessary to increase this to 60 mg thrice daily.

In the reported study of the use of ephedrine in neuropathic oedema, all patients had prolonged diastolic flow as shown by Doppler sonography of the foot pulse before ephedrine. Immediately after the introduction of the drug there was a return to the normal triphasic pattern, with a considerable reduction of diastolic flow. These peripheral effects of ephedrine may have been augmented by its inotropic effect on the myocardium, with a rise in cardiac output.

Sympathomimetic agents have been noted previously to reduce aldosterone secretion [41] and this may account for the efficacy of ephedrine. It has a direct pressor activity on afferent glomerular vessels [42], thus increasing wall tension. The rise in transmural pressure gradient leads to a reduction in renin and aldosterone secretion [43]. Alternatively, ephedrine may reduce aldosterone secretion by acting directly on the adrenal cortex where aldosterone secretion is held under maximal tonic suppression by dopamine [44]. Dopaminergic pathways may be deficient in autonomic neuropathy, allowing aldosterone secretion to continue unchecked, with resultant sodium retention. Ephedrine

releases dopamine from nerve terminals and this may explain its mechanism of action. Furthermore, dopamine is known to increase sodium excretion by a direct action on tubular transport [45].

Side-effects of ephedrine were notably absent in this study despite the relatively high dosage taken by one patient (60 mg thrice daily). Blood pressure was observed closely, both in the supine and standing positions, in view of previous reports of hypertension in the recumbent position. However, there was no significant change in the supine systolic or diastolic pressure after the introduction of ephedrine. Similarly, the mean systolic and diastolic blood pressure on standing was little altered and, indeed, it is well known that no improvement results when treating patients with postural hypotension.

ISCHAEMIC FOOT

Pathophysiology

The main factor responsible for a reduction in blood supply to the foot is atherosclerosis of the large vessels of the leg. In the diabetic patient such atherosclerosis is often multisegmental, bilateral and distal, involving tibial and peroneal vessels [46]. Occlusion can be particularly extensive in foot vessels of the diabetic patient. Conversely, involvement of the aortoiliac vessels is twice as common in non-diabetic as in diabetic subjects. The predilection of atherosclerosis in diabetes for the vessels below the knee is unexplained.

The actual histopathology of the large vessel wall is similar to that in non-diabetic patients with atherosclerosis. Fatty deposits occur in plaques within the intima. The plaques are most commonly localised at bifurcations, on the posterior walls of arteries and where the arteries are compressed by muscle fascia, as in the adductor canal [47].

In the diabetic ischaemic foot, obstructive disease is common in the metatarsal arteries [48] and this reduces communication in and between the plantar and dorsal arterial arches. The digital arteries are thus converted into 'end arteries' [49]. Many bacteria can elaborate angiotoxic substances which cause a septic thrombosis. Advancing infection can thus obliterate digital arteries and the tissue perfused by that artery then becomes necrotic, followed by rapid advancement of sepsis through the foot.

So-called 'small vessel disease' involving capillaries and arterioles has been thought to contribute substantially to impaired circulation in the feet. However, the significance of obliterative lesions of arterioles and capillaries with endothelial proliferation and basement membrane thickening is not known, and their role, if any, in the development of ischaemic foot lesions remains to be elucidated [50]. Although there is little evidence of an occlusive microvascular disease, functional abnormalities of the capillaries, such as increased leaking of albumin from the capillaries to the interstitium, may be important [51]. However, previous emphasis on small vessel disease in the diabetic foot has led to therapeutic nihilism and inappropriate care, especially if it is thought to be responsible for the ischaemic lesions.

The concomitant presence of neuropathy in the ischaemic foot obviously predisposes to minor trauma, which can lead to ulceration. However, the presence of neuropathy is not a prerequisite, and, indeed, in non-diabetic patients with these lesions sensation (thermal and vibration) is often intact. We have found a distinctive pattern of sensory impairment in ischaemic diabetic feet, with early involvement of the larger nerve fibres (vibration perception) when thermal (small-fibre) sensation is still intact [52]; this presents a different pattern from that seen in the classic neuropathic lesions described above, in which small (thermal) fibres are affected first. Some ischaemic diabetic patients are free from neuropathy, and in others it is very advanced.

Investigation of the Ischaemic Limb

The non-invasive techniques used to evaluate the peripheral circulation include measurements of systolic pressures at ankle and toe levels, the examination of blood velocity waveforms obtained by Doppler ultrasound [53], pulse volume recordings [54] and the measurement of transcutaneous Po_2 [55].

Ankle systolic pressure can be measured using a 12-cm cuff and a Doppler probe placed over the pedal vessels. When the ankle systolic pressure is divided by the brachial systolic pressure, the pressure index is derived; in normal subjects

this is usually greater than 1.1. Between 5% and 10% of diabetic patients have stiff, non-compressible peripheral vessels causing an artificially elevated systolic pressure, and a pressure index greater than 1.5 [56]. The most likely cause for this is calcification in the medial arterial wall. Nevertheless, recent studies have shown that the pressure index can be a useful guide to healing: 87% of ulcers in feet with a pressure index greater than 0.6 healed, compared with 40% with a pressure index less than 0.6 ($P < 0.05$, chi-squared test) [57]. Absolute toe pressures can provide a further method for deciding the likelihood of success of healing of an ulcer or of a minor amputation [58]. Healing is doubtful if the toe pressure is below 30 mm Hg.

The Doppler waveform becomes abnormal distal to an obstructing lesion, with loss of the normal rapid systolic upstroke and a loss of diastolic flow. With diminishing flow, the waveform becomes flattened before it finally disappears. Several methods of signal analysis have been proposed to quantify the changes in flow waveform and provide an index of severity of arterial disease [53].

Plethysmographic techniques may be useful in the diabetic leg. The pulse volume recorder is a quantitative segmental plethysmograph that can assess variations in arterial volume in a specific limb segment [59]. The technique is less affected by the rigidity of calf vessels and may have more prognostic significance regarding the healing of minor amputations than the measurement of the pressure index.

The measurement of transcutaneous Po_2 has been used to evaluate tissue perfusion in the ischaemic leg. A recent study, measuring differences between limb and trunk transcutaneous Po_2, has demonstrated that regional oximetry may be superior to Doppler pressures in assessing the adequacy of local limb perfusion [55].

Ulceration and Gangrene of the Ischaemic Limb

Pathogenesis

Tissue necrosis in the ischaemic limb is usually associated with minor trauma, often complicated by infection. The trauma may be caused by direct pressure from tight shoes or socks, thermal or chemical injuries and injudicious cutting of the nails. When external pressures on localised areas of skin exceed capillary pressure, tissue necrosis follows. Initial incidents are often trivial and lead to trivial injuries. However, they are frequently neglected and rapidly lead to ulceration. Ulcers present as areas of necrosis, often surrounded by a rim of erythema. In contrast to the neuropathic foot, callus tissue is usually absent. Furthermore, ulceration in the ischaemic foot is often painful, although this varies from patient to patient according to the coexistence of a peripheral neuropathy. In the ischaemic foot, the most frequent sites of ulceration are the great toe, medial surface of the head of the first metatarsal, the lateral surface of the fifth metatarsal and the heel. These are often complicated by secondary infection with aerobic and anaerobic organisms. Ultimately, gangrene occurs: the patient notices marked pain in an infected toe, which becomes discoloured and finally black.

Medical Treatment

Medical management is indicated if the ulcer is small and shallow and is of recent onset (within the previous month). Furthermore, it is the mainstay of treatment for those patients in whom reconstructive surgery is technically not feasible, or impossible because of widespread cardiovascular or cerebrovascular disease. It is important to eradicate infection with prompt and specific antibiotic therapy. The organisms do not differ from those in the neuropathic foot, and mainly comprise staphylococci and streptococci, although in deep-seated ulcers anaerobes and gram-negative bacteria may be isolated. Often these patients have pedal oedema which predisposes to ulceration [60]. In one series, cardiac failure accounted for two-thirds of oedematous feet, and this necessitated diuretic treatment, with care to avoid dehydration [25].

Made-to-measure footwear should be prescribed to accommodate deformity in the foot. Regular chiropody should be performed to remove necrotic tissue from the ulcers, and in the case of subungual ulcers, to cut back the nail to allow drainage of pus from the ulcer. Ischaemic ulcers are often painful and pain relief is an important part of conservative treatment. Smoking should be banned, obesity treated and optimal control of the diabetes obtained. With such conservative treatment, up to 70% of ischaemic ulcers can be healed [57].

Surgical Treatment

The possible options for surgical treatment are arterial reconstruction, angioplasty, sympathectomy and finally amputation.

Arterial reconstruction. The indications for arterial reconstruction are intractable rest pain, ulceration that has not responded to medical treatment, and necrotic toes which require amputation in order to save the limb and also an increase in arterial inflow to make the procedure successful. Although the non-invasive Doppler investigations help to locate the site of arterial disease, arteriography is needed to assess whether arterial reconstruction is possible.

When aortoiliac disease is suspected from a weak femoral pulse and a damped femoral Doppler sonogram, percutaneous transfemoral arteriography should be performed. In the presence of a good femoral pulse and no clinical signs of proximal disease, direct femoral arteriography should be performed. This method is useful for the demonstration of superficial femoral artery, popliteal and distal tibial and peroneal occlusions. The branches of the popliteal artery may be better seen by passing a catheter from the common femoral artery through the superficial femoral artery to the popliteal artery. A bolus of dye can then be injected to demonstrate the distal leg and foot vessels [61]. Regardless of the type of arteriography, the minimum of contrast dye should be injected and the patient should be kept well hydrated to prevent renal shutdown.

The most striking arteriographic finding is one of stenotic and occlusive lesions of the branches of the popliteal artery. The popliteal and superficial femoral arteries may show some atherosclerotic plaques and the iliac artery and aorta may be relatively unaffected. If a stenosis of the aorta or iliac arteries is present, then aortoiliac or aortofemoral reconstruction should be performed. If the block is in the femoral artery, then a reversed saphenous vein graft acting as bypass from the common femoral to the popliteal artery is frequently carried out; this has resulted in high rates of limb salvage, even in elderly diabetic patients [62].

However, there is a predilection to stenosis in the branches of the popliteal artery, and it is now possible to perform femoral artery to distal tibial or peroneal artery bypass using reversed saphenous vein grafts [63]. Recently, methods of using the saphenous vein in situ have been developed, thus preserving the vasa vasorum and minimizing endothelial injury [64]. A limb salvage rate of 74% at 2 years was obtained in a group of 26 patients (88% diabetic) who presented with threatened limbs and in whom bypass procedures to the distal vessel were carried out [65].

Angioplasty. Angioplasty is a recently developed technique which uses intraluminal balloons to dilate stenosis in obstructed arteries. Lower-extremity vessel dilations are usually performed with a double-lumen catheter, the inner lumen allowing direct percutaneous insertion of the dilating catheter over a guide wire [66]. The procedure is performed under local anaesthetic, and has been used to dilate stenoses in the iliac, femoral and popliteal arteries. The lesions most suitable for angioplasty are focal stenoses less than 4 cm long and occlusions shorter than 10 cm.

At present iliac artery angioplasties have a greater success rate than femoral and popliteal dilations. The 2-year patency rate for dilation of iliac artery stenoses ranges from 87% to 100% [67], compared with aortofemoral bypass graft patency rates of 96% in 2 years. In the femoral artery, patency rates after angioplasty vary from 72% to 84%, compared with patency of 90% with femoral popliteal bypass. Experience with popliteal artery dilation is very limited, with 50% remaining patent after 2 years [68]. The relative roles of angioplasty and surgery are undergoing reassessment. They may well be complementary measures: for example, an iliac artery stenosis should be dilated before a femoral artery occlusion is treated by a saphenous vein bypass. At present, angioplasty is particularly useful for patients unable to undergo major arterial reconstruction.

Sympathectomy. Lumbar sympathectomy may have a specific role in the relief of ischaemic rest pain in a foot that is neither rapidly deteriorating nor improving. In a recent controlled prospective trial, neurolytic chemical block was somewhat more successful than placebo injection in relieving pain, although there was no improvement in haemodynamic blood flow measurements [69]. The explanation for this probably lies in the destruction of afferent pain fibres which are not functionally part of the sympathetic trunk but which travel with the sympathetic fibres, leaving the trunk in the rami communicantes and relaying in the dorsal root ganglia.

Amputation. Amputation of a digit or a ray may be necessary because of severe tissue lesions in the ischaemic foot. However, it rarely succeeds unless the foot is also revascularised by arterial reconstruction or angioplasty. Below-knee amputation is indicated for rampant infection, extensive tissue destruction or intractable rest pain in a limb in which reconstruction has not been possible or has failed.

THE FOOT IN DIABETIC NEPHROPATHY

Foot ulcer, sepsis and gangrene resulting from peripheral vascular disease, neuropathy, or both together, are common in patients with diabetic nephropathy and renal failure. These problems and their management are, in general, similar to those in diabetes uncomplicated by renal disease. The most striking difference in nephropathy patients is the presence of extensive digital arterial calcification, which occurs both in feet and hands [70, 71]. Digital gangrene of toes and fingers occurs predominantly in those with calcified vessels and is almost specific for patients with diabetic renal failure: it can occur in any of these patients, whether on dialysis or receiving transplantation. Of 80 patients with diabetic nephropathy who received a renal transplant, 11 developed digital gangrene; all had severe digital calcification. The pathophysiological changes that precipitate digital gangrene are not clearly understood.

ORGANISATION OF DIABETIC FOOT CARE: THE DIABETIC FOOT CLINIC

It is vital that there is close liaison between chiropodist, shoe-fitter, physician and surgeon in the care of the diabetic foot; since 1981, diabetic foot problems (including those with diabetic nephropathy) have been treated within a special Diabetic Foot Clinic at King's College Hospital [25]. It has provided intensive chiropody, close surveillance, prompt treatment of foot infection and a footwear service by the attending shoe-fitter. Essential aspects of management are specially constructed shoes, intensive chiropody and precise antibiotic therapy.

Over a 3-year period, 148 patients with neuropathic ulcers and 91 patients with predominantly ischaemic ulcers were treated in the Foot Clinic, where healing was achieved in 204 out of 238 (86%) neuropathic ulcers and 107 out of 148 (72%) ischaemic ulcers. Healing time was 10.3 ± 10.2 weeks (mean $\pm$ SD) in neuropathic ulcers and 14.0 ± 11.4 weeks in ischaemic ulcers. Patients attended for chiropody every 3.5 ± 1.0 weeks during healing and 7.4 ± 1.5 weeks after healing to prevent reaccumulation of callus in the neuropathic foot, as well as for meticulous care of the nails in both neuropathic and ischaemic feet. Recurrence of ulceration was reduced by special footwear. In patients who accepted and wore special footwear, the relapse rate was 26% compared with 83% in patients who continued to wear their own shoes against advice.

The effect of the Foot Clinic on the number of major amputations and minor operations (which comprised drainage operations and 'ray' amputations) was assessed by comparing the number of such procedures in both neuropathic and ischaemic patients from the Diabetic Clinic for 2 years before the establishment of the Foot Clinic with the number of procedures performed for the 3 years after. In the 2 years before the clinic was established, there were 11 and 12 major amputations yearly. This was reduced during the following 3 years to 7, 7 and 5 amputations, respectively. Similarly, the number of minor operations was reduced from yearly figures of 27 and 29 for the 2 years before the establishment of clinic, to 16, 21 and 15 per year for the 3 years following.

Prevention

The ultimate treatment is, of course, prevention, and this therapeutic approach must be through education of the patient in foot care and regular examination of the feet by the physician.

It has been shown that patients who develop foot lesions have significantly less knowledge of diabetes, including foot care [72]. Moreover, Assal et al have shown clearly that education reduces the number of major amputations in a diabetic clinic population [73].

Routine examination of the feet in diabetic patients is an important part of management in order to identify those at risk of ulceration, and to prevent its occurrence.

Foot Deformities

These are simple to discover, and constitute the greatest threat to the diabetic foot. Early advice on footwear (see above) is probably the most effective preventive measure that can be taken.

Callus Formation

Callus forms readily in diabetic neuropathy; active and regular treatment by a chiropodist will prevent ulceration. Skin cracks should also be sought.

Pulses

Absence of both dorsalis pedis and posterior tibial pulses, sometimes associated with bruits over the femoral arteries, should alert the physician to the presence of peripheral vascular disease and the need for special investigations and treatment. The use of simple Doppler equipment greatly facilitates this examination: assessment of the pressure index (ratio of ankle systolic pressure to brachial systolic pressure) is very simple, indicating ischaemia if it is below 1 (with a poor prognosis if it is below 0.6).

Neuropathy

Ankle (and knee) jerks should be examined, although absence of ankle jerks is so common that it gives only limited information regarding the severity of neuropathy.

Quantitative evaluation of sensory neuropathy is valuable and most readily undertaken by use of a biothesiometer [5] to assess the vibration perception threshold. Foot ulcers do not usually occur unless the reading is greater than 30 volts, and this vlaue may indicate feet at risk.

Evaluation of thermal sensation, pain awareness and sweating are all of importance but the equipment for these tests is complex and available only in specialist centres.

Autonomic function tests are desirable but not essential: it is unusual for foot ulcers to develop unless autonomic neuropathy is present.

CONCLUSION

Ulceration of the non-ischaemic diabetic foot depends on the presence of neuropathy, and is especially likely to occur in areas of the foot where high pressure (often associated with foot deformities) leads to the development of excessive callus which eventually breaks down and ulcerates.

Damage to small nerve fibres is the essential element of the neuropathy, causing loss of thermal and pain sensation, and sympathetic defects leading to diminished sweating and grossly altered haemodynamics. The arteries in the feet of these patients are rigid, and blood flow greatly increased both in skin and bones, causing both oedema and osteopenia; nutritive capillary flow remains unimpaired. Ulceration in ischaemic feet results from pressure necrosis. The presence of neuropathy is not essential but, when present, renders the foot vulnerable to minimal trauma. The main reduction in blood supply to the foot is related to atherosclerosis of the large vessels of the leg which, in the diabetic patient, is often multisegmental, bilateral and distal, involving tibial and peroneal vessels.

The feet of diabetic patients must be carefully examined for the presence of deformities, callus formation, evidence of ischaemia and neuropathy in order to institute effective measures.

Optimum care of the diabetic foot is provided in a diabetic foot clinic where the skills of chiropodist, shoe-fitter and nurse receive full support from physician and surgeon. Many lesions of the diabetic foot are avoidable and thus patient education is of immense importance.

REFERENCES

1. Williams DRR. Hospital admission of diabetic patients: information from hospital activity analysis. Diabet Med 1985; 2: 27–32.
2. Brand PW. The diabetic foot. In Ellenberg M, Rifken H (eds) Diabetes mellitus. New York: Medical Examination Publishing, 1983: pp 829–49.
3. West KM. The epidemiology of diabetes and its vascular lesions. New York: Elsevier, 1978.
4. Kozak GO, Rowbotham JL. Diabetic foot disease: a major problem. In Kozak GP, Hoar SC, Rowbotham JL et al (eds) Management of diabetic foot problems. Philadelphia: WB Saunders, 1984: pp 1–8.
5. Guy RJG, Clark CA, Malcolm PN, Watkins PJ. Evaluation of thermal and vibration sensation in diabetic neuropathy. Diabetologia 1985; 28: 131–7.
6. Jamal GA, Weir AI, Hansen S, Ballantyne JP. An improved automated method for the measurement of thermal thresholds in patients with peripheral neuropathy. J Neurol Neurosurg Psychiat 1985; 48: 361–6.
7. Scarpello JH, Martin TR, Ward JD. Ultrasound measurements of pulse wave velocity in the peripheral arteries of diabetic subjects. Clin Sci 1980; 58: 53–7.
8. Edmonds ME, Roberts VC, Watkins PJ. Blood flow in the diabetic neuropathic foot. Diabetologia 1982; 22: 9–15.
9. Archer AG, Roberts VC, Watkins PJ. Blood flow patterns in painful diabetic neuropathy. Diabetologia 1984; 27: 563–7.
10. Said B, Slama G, Selva J. Progressive centripetal degeneration of axons in small fibre type diabetic polyneuropathy. A clinical and pathological study. Brain 1983; 106: 791–807.
11. Boulton AJM, Kubrusly DM, Bowker JH. Impaired vibratory perception and diabetic foot ulceration. Diabet Med 1986; 3: 335–7.
12. Edmonds ME, Nicolaides KH, Watkins PJ. Autonomic neuropathy in diabetic foot ulceration. Diabet Med 1986; 3: 56–9.
13. Watkins PJ, Edmonds ME. Sympathetic nerve failure in diabetes. Diabetologia 1983; 25: 73–7.
14. Edmonds ME, Morrison N, Laws JW, Watkins PJ. Medial arterial calcification and diabetic neuropathy. Br Med J 1982; 284: 928–30.
15. Sinha S, Munichoodappa CS, Kozak GP. Neuroarthropathy (Charcot joints) in diabetes mellitus. Medicine (Baltimore) 1972; 51: 191–210.
16. Goebel FD, Fuesse HS. Mönckeberg's sclerosis after sympathetic denervation in diabetic and non-diabetic subjects. Diabetologia 1983; 24: 347–50.
17. Pryce TD. On diabetic neuritis with a clinical and pathological description of three cases of diabetic pseudo-tabes. Brain 1893; 16: 416–524.
18. Tooke JE. The microcirculation in diabetes. Diabet Med 1987; 4: 189–96.
19. Flynn MD, Tooke JE, Watkins PJ. Abnormal capillary blood flow in the diabetic neuropathic foot, assessed by direct television microscopy. Diabet Med 1986; 3: 587A.
20. Edmonds ME, Clarke MD, Newton S, Barrett JJ, Watkins PJ. Increased uptake of bone radiopharmaceutical in diabetic neuropathy. Quart J Med 1985; 57: 843–55.
21. Cundy TF, Edmonds ME, Watkins PJ. Osteopaenia and metatarsal fractures in diabetic neuropathy. Diabet Med 1985; 2: 461–4.
22. Low PA, Fealy RD. Sudomotor neuropathy. In Dyck PJ, Thomas PK, Asbury AK, Winegrad AI, Porte D (eds) Diabetic neuropathy. Philadelphia: WB Saunders, 1987: pp 140–5.
23. Ahmed ME, LeQuesne PM. Quantitative sweat test in diabetics with neuropathic foot lesions. J Neurol Neurosurg Psychiat 1986; 49: 1059–62.
24. Boulton AJM, Betts RP, Franks CI, Newrick

PG, Ward JD, Duckworth T. Abnormalities of foot pressure in early diabetic neuropathy. Diabet Med 1987; 4: 225–8.

25. Edmonds ME, Blundell MP, Morris HE, Thomas EM, Cotton LT, Watkins PJ. Improved survival of the diabetic foot; the role of a specialised foot clinic. Quart J Med 1986; 232: 763–71.

26. Martin MM. Diabetic neuropathy. Brain 1953; 76: 594–624.

27. Edmonds ME, Archer AG, Watkins PJ. Ephedrine: a new treatment for diabetic neuropathic oedema. Lancet 1983; i: 54–5.

28. Edmonds ME. The diabetic foot. Med Internat 1985; 13: 551–3.

29. Delbridge L, Ctercteko G, Fowler C, Reeve TS, LeQuesne LP. The aetiology of diabetic neuropathic foot ulceration. Br J Surg 1985; 72: 1–6.

30. Edmonds ME, Foster A. 'Corn cures can damage your feet'. An important lesson for diabetic patients. Diabet Med 1986; 3: 564A.

31. Sapico FL, Bessman AN, Canawati HN. Bacteraemia in diabetic patients with infected lower extremities. Diabetes Care 1982; 5: 101–4.

32. Tovey FI. Establishing a diabetic shoe service. Pract Diabetes 1985; 2: 5–8.

33. Sinha S, Frykberg RG, Kozak GP. Neuroarthropathy in the diabetic foot. In Kozak GP (ed.) Clinical diabetes mellitus. Philadelphia: WB Saunders, 1983: pp 415–25.

34. Eymontt MJ, Alavi A, Dalinka MK, Kyle GC. Bone scintigraphy in diabetic osteoarthropathy. Radiology 1981; 140: 475–7.

35. Park H-M, Wheat LJ, Siddiqui AR. Scintigraphic evaluation of diabetic osteomyelitis: concise communication. J Nucl Med 1982; 23: 569–73.

36. Gondos B. Roentgen observations in diabetic osteopathy. Radiology 1968; 91: 6–13.

37. Kraft E, Spyropoulos E, Finby N. Neurogenic disorders of the foot in diabetes mellitus. AJR 1975; 124: 17–24.

38. McClugage SG, McCuskey RS. Relationship of the microvascular system to bone resorption and growth in situ. Microvasc Res 1973; 6: 132–4.

39. Verhas M, Martinello Y, Mone M et al. Demineralisation and pathological physiology of the skeleton in paraplegic rats. Calcif Tissue Int 1980; 30: 83–90.

40. Brower AC, Allman RM. Pathogenesis of the neurotrophic joint; neurotraumatic vs neurovascular. Radiology 1981; 139: 349–54.

41. Greenough WB, Sonnenblick EH, Januszewicz V et al. Correction of hyperaldosteronism and of massive fluid retention of unknown cause by sympathomimetic agents. Am J Med 1962; 33: 603–14.

42. Weiner N. Norepinephrine, epinephrine and the sympathomimetic amines. In Goodman LS, Gilman A (eds) The pharmacological basis of therapeutics, 6th edn. New York: Macmillan, 1980: pp 138–75.

43. Davis JO, Freeman RH. Mechanisms regulating renin release. Physiol Rev 1976; 56: 1–56.

44. Carey RM, Thorner MO, Ortt EM. Effects of metoclopramide and bromocriptine on renin–angiotensin–aldosterone system in man. J Clin Invest 1979; 63: 727–35.

45. Goldberg LI, Weder AB. Connections between endogenous dopamine, dopamine receptors and sodium excretion: evidence and hypothesis. In Turner P, Shand E (eds) Recent advances in clinical pharmacology 2. Edinburgh: Churchill Livingstone, 1980: pp 149–66.

46. Strandness DE Jr, Priest RE, Gibbons GE. Combined clinical and pathologic study of diabetic and non-diabetic peripheral arterial disease. Diabetes 1964; 13: 366–72.

47. Wheelock FC, Gibbons GW, Marble A. Surgery in diabetes. In Marble A, Krall LP, Bradley RF, Christlieb AR, Soeldner JS (eds) Joslin's Diabetes mellitus. Philadelphia: Lea & Febiger, 1985: pp 712–31.

48. Ferrier TM. Radiologically demonstrable arterial calcification in diabetes mellitus. Austr Ann Med 1967; 13: 222–6.

49. O'Neal LW. Surgical pathology of the foot and clinicopathologic correlations. In Levin ME, O'Neal LW (eds) The diabetic foot. St Louis: CV Mosby, 1983: pp 162–200.

50. Logerfo FW, Coffman JE. Vascular and microvascular disease of the foot in diabetes. New Engl J Med 1984; 311: 1615–19.

51. Parving HH, Rasmussen SM. Transcapillary escape rate of albumin and plasma volume in short and long term juvenile diabetics. Scand J Clin Lab Invest 1973; 32: 81–7.

52. Das A, Flynn MF, Goss D, Foster A, Watkins PJ. Abnormal peripheral nerve function in the diabetic ischaemic limb. Diabet Med 1987; 4: 378.

53. Levin ME, O'Neal LW. Peripheral vascular disease. In Ellenberg M, Rifkin H (eds) Diabetes mellitus: theory and practice, 3rd edn. New York: Medical Examination Publishing, 1983: pp 803–28.

54. Darling RC, Raines JK, Brenner BJ, Austen WG. Quantitative segmental pulse and volume recorder: a clinical tool. Surgery 1972; 72: 873–87.

55. Hauser CJ, Klein ST, Mehringer CM, Appel P, Shoemaker WC. Assessment of perfusion in the diabetic foot by regional transcutaneous oximetry. Diabetes 1984; 33: 527–31.

56. Raines JK, Darling RC, Beth et al. Vascular laboratory criteria for the management of peripheral vascular disease of the lower extremities. Surgery 1976; 79: 21–9.

57. Edmonds ME, Gilbey S, Walters HW et al.

Improved survival of the diabetic ischaemic foot. Diabet Med 1985; 2: 506A.

58. Barnes RW, Thornhell B, Nix L, Rittgers SE, Turley G. Prediction of amputation wound healing. Roles of Doppler ultrasound and digit photoplethysmography. Arch Surg 1981; 116: 80.

59. Gibbons GW, Campbell DR. Non-invasive diagnostic studies. In Kozak GP, Hoar CS, Rowbotham JL et al (eds) Management of diabetic foot problems. Philadelphia: WB Saunders, 1984: pp 91–6.

60. Lithner F, Tornblom N. Gangrene localised to the lower limbs in diabetics. Acta Med Scand 1980; 208: 315–20.

61. Staple TW. Radiography of the diabetic foot. In Levin ME, O'Neal LW (eds) The diabetic foot. St Louis: CV Mosby, 1983: pp 201–31.

62. Reinhold RB, Gibbons GW, Wheelock FC, Hoar CS. Femoral popliteal bypass in elderly diabetic patients. Am J Surg 1979; 137: 549–55.

63. Reichle FA, Rankin KP, Tyson RR. Long term results of femoro-infrapopliteal bypass in diabetic patients with severe ischaemia of the lower extremity. Am J Surg 1979; 137: 653–6.

64. Leather RP, Shah DM, Karmody AM. Infrapopliteal bypass for limb salvage: increased patency and utilization of the saphenous vein used in situ. Surgery 1981; 90: 1000–8.

65. Samson RH, Gupta SK, Scher LA et al. Treatment of limb-threatening ischaemia despite a palpable popliteal pulse. J Surg Res 1982; 32: 535–9.

66. Greenfield AJ. Femoral, popliteal and tibial arteries: percutaneous transluminal angioplasty. AJR 1980; 135: 927–35.

67. Nieman HL, Brabdt TD, Greenberg M. Percutaneous transluminal angioplasty: an angiographer's viewpoint. Arch Surg 1981; 116: 821–8.

68. Sprayregen S, Sniderman KW, Sos TA et al. Popliteal artery branches: percutaneous transluminal angioplasty. AJR 1980; 135: 945–50.

69. Cotton LT, Cross FW. Lumbar sympathectomy for arterial disease. Br J Surg 1985; 72: 678–83.

70. Grenfell A, Watkins PJ. Clinical diabetic nephropathy: natural history and complications. Clin Endocrinol Metab 1986; 15: 783–805.

71. Gonzalez-Carrillo M, Moloney A, Bewick M et al. Renal transplantation in diabetic nephropathy. Br Med J 1982; 285: 1713–16.

72. Delbridge L, Appleberg M, Reeve TS. Factors associated with the development of foot lesions in the diabetic. Surgery 1983; 93: 78–82.

73. Assal J-P, Gfeller R, Ekoe J-M. Patient education in diabetes. In Bostrum H, Ljungstedt N (eds) Recent trends in diabetes research. Stockholm: Almqvist & Wiksell, 1981: pp 276–90.

69

The Prevention and Screening of Diabetic Complications

M. McGill and D.K. Yue

Royal Prince Alfred Hospital, Camperdown, NSW, Australia

Complications of diabetes remain a serious cause of morbidity and mortality despite modern advances in the management of this disease. Once complications are present in a clinically severe form they cannot readily be reversed, even by meticulous diabetic control. The precise stage at which diabetic complications become irreversible is not known; the multicentre Diabetes Control and Complications Trial (DCCT) currently in progress should provide valuable information in this regard [1]. Three previous studies have shown that diabetic retinopathy of moderate severity does not improve significantly, despite periods of tight diabetic control ranging from 8 months to 2 years [2–4]: in fact, quite unexpectedly there was transient deterioration in retinopathy when diabetic control was improved. There is a similar irreversibility of advanced diabetic nephropathy [5, 6]. Clinicians witness too often the inexorable decline of renal function once a patient has developed persistent proteinuria and a plasma creatinine greater than 200 μmol/l. The persistence of numbness and pain and the recurrence of foot ulceration in patients with diabetic neuropathy further attest to our inability to reverse severe diabetic complications.

Clearly, it would be a major advance if treatment strategies could be developed to prevent the occurrence of diabetic complications. However, as prevention of complications cannot be realized with our current state of knowledge, attention has turned to their early detection. This is necessary because, by the time symptoms are volunteered by patients, complications may already be well advanced. This notion of screening for diabetic complications is based on the premise that therapy is available and, indeed, is more effective if the complications can be treated early in their natural history. It is possible that, if complications can be detected early, maintenance of normoglycaemia or other therapeutic interventions will be more effective in preventing their deterioration. These assumptions are valid to different extents for the various complications of diabetes.

In this chapter we first discuss the general principles of preventing diabetic complications and the value of screening. Factors specific to each complication are then discussed, and a table summarizes our recommendations for screening procedures to be used in clinical practice.

International Textbook of Diabetes Mellitus. Edited by K.G.M.M. Alberti, R.A. DeFronzo, H. Keen and P. Zimmet
© 1992 John Wiley & Sons Ltd

PRIMARY PREVENTION VERSUS SECONDARY PREVENTION

Attempts to prevent a diabetic complication can be implemented before any evidence of this complication is detectable (primary prevention), or when it is already present (secondary prevention), aiming to slow the deterioration of this complication. This distinction of primary versus secondary prevention is arbitrary as it depends on the sensitivity of the techniques used in the detection of the complication. For example, the decision about whether a patient has diabetic retinopathy would depend on whether clinical examination with direct ophthalmoscopy, retinal photography or fluorescein angiography was used in its detection.

It could reasonably be expected that any preventive measure is likely to be more effective in primary than in secondary prevention. On the other hand, any method of primary prevention would need to be implemented for a longer period before its efficacy became clinically obvious and could be proven statistically. This is particularly relevant in the case of diabetic complications, which generally occur in clinically severe forms only after about 10 years of diabetes.

A further observation which adds to the complexity of the problem is that many diabetic patients have the disease for many years without developing significant complications, whereas others are affected by severe complications after shorter periods of relatively mild diabetes. These factors make it exceedingly difficult to prove scientifically that a particular therapeutic modality is useful in the primary prevention of diabetic complications.

Even if the efficacy of a primary preventive measure could be validated, the measure would be applied for many years to many patients, some of whom would not develop severe complications in any case. As such, its use could only be justified if the measure had few side-effects and did not seriously impair the patient's quality of life.

Some of these difficulties with primary prevention can be lessened by concentrating on secondary prevention. In this situation, it would take less time to prove the efficacy of a preventive measure, and any side-effects of treatment could be more readily accepted on a risk–benefit basis. Of course, secondary prevention faces the problem that the diabetic complications may already be in an irreversible phase.

Methods of Preventing Diabetic Complications

From the considerations outlined above, it can readily be understood that not many therapeutic manoeuvres have been shown to be unequivocally effective in preventing diabetic complications. Strategies can be broadly divided into those aiming at achievement of normoglycaemia and those aiming to act independently of blood glucose control.

Maintenance of near-normoglycaemia is usually achieved with a regimen of multiple daily insulin injections or continuous subcutaneous insulin infusions. Results from already completed studies of 1–2 years' duration, and preliminary data from the DCCT, have established that good diabetic control with glycated haemoglobin levels close to the normal range can, indeed, be achieved in patients randomly assigned to such intensive insulin treatment [1–4]. However, this degree of good diabetic control is achieved at the price of increased frequency and severity of hypoglycaemic episodes, occurring approximately three times more frequently than in conventionally treated patients [1]. The patients participating in these trials were selected for their compliance and ability to comprehend treatment regimens. In an unselected diabetic population not under the rigorous supervision of a clinical trial, the degree of diabetic control achieved would be considerably worse and the risk of hypoglycaemia even greater. It is clear, therefore, that there remains a need for alternative methods of preventing or modifying diabetic complications.

From the pharmacological point of view, the aldose reductase inhibitors have been investigated intensively as a possible means of reversing or preventing a wide range of diabetic complications [7, 8]. The results thus far have been disappointing and inconclusive, and it is not known if this is because they have been used too late in patients whose complications are too advanced. Treatment of hypertension has been shown to be effective in retarding the development of diabetic nephropathy and vascular disease [9, 10], but the best antihypertensive regimen for diabetic patients remains controversial. The angiotensin converting enzyme (ACE) inhibitors may have a special role in this regard, as some preliminary reports suggest that they act specifically to preserve renal function in diabetic patients [11, 12]. Many other methods of modifying diabetic complications have been advocated and are discussed in individual sections.

Is Treatment More Effective if Implemented Early?

There is no doubt that laser photocoagulation cannot help patients who are already blind from the results of diabetic retinopathy, and there would also be no argument that intensive foot-care education or treatment of diabetic neuropathy cannot restore limbs already lost due to amputation. In the case of diabetic nephropathy, treatment of blood pressure cannot be expected to reverse renal failure in a patient requiring transplantation or dialysis.

Leaving aside these extreme examples, there are also reasonable data to support the philosophy that early detection and treatment of diabetic complications are, indeed, worthwhile goals. This is best established in the case of diabetic retinopathy, where large prospective studies have established the level of visual acuity below which laser treatment becomes less effective [13, 14]. There is also evidence that treatment of hypertension can retard the progression of diabetic nephropathy in patients with moderate renal impairment [9, 10]. Implementation of foot-care education in high-risk patients can reduce the need for further hospitalization and amputation [15].

What is less certain is whether this policy of early treatment to produce better results is also applicable to patients at even earlier stages. For example, these would include patients with minimal background retinopathy with no immediate threat to vision, patients with subtle electrophysiological changes of nerve function but no overt diabetic neuropathy, and patients with early evidence of diabetic nephropathy in the form of microalbuminuria. The answers to these questions will have an important bearing on our commitment to screening and early treatment, and will require further systematic studies.

Methods of Screening for Diabetic Complications

The methods used for the screening of diabetic complications should be appropriate for the resources and treatment available. For example, it would not be rational to use the valuable time of an ophthalmologist or physician to screen for macular oedema as an early warning of diabetic maculopathy unless there was the facility for laser treatment of detected cases.

DIABETIC RETINOPATHY

Prevention

There are no conclusive data to prove that any treatment is effective in the primary or secondary prevention of diabetic retinopathy. Although the report by Job et al appeared to support the value of good diabetic control in this regard, there was poor adherence of patients to their assigned treatment regimens and, by modern standards, relatively imprecise assessment of diabetic retinopathy [16]. More recent studies have shown that the maintenance of near-normoglycaemia for approximately 1 year did not significantly improve existing diabetic retinopathy [2–4]. In fact, there was some deterioration due to the increased appearance of soft exudates. As soft exudates are signs of retinal infarction there was considerable concern that their emergence might herald the development of proliferative retinopathy. Fortunately, this has not eventuated in these studies and by 2 years the retinopathy was no worse in patients undergoing intensive insulin treatment. These carefully conducted studies were performed on relatively small numbers of patients and the results were not conclusive, but they certainly did not give great encouragement for the rapid reversal of diabetic retinopathy. The precise benefit of tight glycaemic control on the primary and secondary prevention of diabetic retinopathy awaits the results of the much larger DCCT study [1]. In experimental studies, good diabetic control with insulin has been reported to normalize the early permeability changes of the retinal vessels demonstrable by vitreous fluorophotometry, but the clinical relevance of this observation is unproven [17].

The efficacy of other pharmacological treatments in the prevention of diabetic retinopathy is disappointing, even though they may have a sound theoretical basis. Aspirin has been tried as a method of normalizing the increased platelet aggregation and adhesion in diabetes, but its effect on retinopathy is small [18]. Although the pericytes of retinal vessels contain aldose reductase, clinical usage of aldose reductase inhibitors does not appear to have a dramatic benefit on retinopathy [18]. Other factors such as cessation of smoking and treatment of hypertension are non-specific and have not been formally tested in prospective clinical trials [18].

Early Treatment

There is good evidence that laser photocoagulation is more effective if given before significant visual loss has taken place [13, 14]. In patients with proliferative retinopathy, laser treatment can induce regression of neovascularization before the occurrence of vitreous haemorrhage. Its greater efficacy in treating diabetic maculopathy when the visual acuity is better than 6/24 is also well established. Furthermore, with early treatment fewer laser burns are required, resulting in less damage to the peripheral field of vision. More recently, the report of the Early Treatment Diabetic Retinopathy Study suggests that patients with the earliest form of diabetic maculopathy, manifested only by macular oedema with minimal or no visual loss, may benefit from prophylactic laser treatment [19]. Whether such aggressive preventive treatment will stand the test of time remains to be seen.

Screening for Diabetic Retinopathy

Screening for diabetic retinopathy is particularly important as many patients feel that they could not have retinopathy unless vision is impaired.

Visual Acuity

Every diabetic patient should have pinhole (corrected) visual acuity checked at approximately yearly intervals. This is particularly important for the detection of diabetic maculopathy, where a gradual decline in vision is an important warning sign even if examination of the fundi does not reveal any obvious abnormality. Visual loss due to bleeding in proliferative retinopathy is usually more dramatic in onset and is rapidly reported by the patient; here, visual acuity testing will only confirm the obvious. It is important to note that, although testing of visual acuity is essential, it is an inadequate screening procedure by itself. Diabetic

maculopathy should be detected before impairment of vision has occurred, and severe proliferative retinopathy may be present with perfectly normal vision until the occurrence of a catastrophic haemorrhage.

In a large diabetic clinic the testing of visual acuity is often left to the most junior staff and passed from one individual to the other. This practice should be discouraged, as inconsistency and inexperience in testing preclude the information being used in a meaningful way. To overcome this problem at our Diabetes Centre, we have a nurse with expertise in diabetic eye disease who coordinates the annual screening of retinopathy.

Examination of the Optic Fundus

This is the most important and cost-effective step in screening for diabetic retinopathy. It should be performed with pupils adequately dilated with sympathomimetic drops, the effects of which can be readily reversed to allow patients to resume driving within a short period. The risk of precipitating acute glaucoma is very small and should not deter routine dilatation of pupils for examination. A good-quality direct ophthalmoscope is a perfectly satisfactory tool for the screening of diabetic retinopathy. Although an indirect ophthalmoscope gives a wider field of vision and is better in patients with cataracts, it is not essential for the screening of diabetic retinopathy.

For the purpose of screening, the most important skill to be acquired by the examiner is the ability to distinguish a normal fundus from an abnormal one. This is not difficult, as microaneurysms, haemorrhages and exudates are readily visible and, with practice, the presence of new vessels can also be recognized. More subtle clinical skills, such as the ability to detect macular oedema and to distinguish soft from hard exudates, are not essential for the purposes of screening. In fact, with the exception of gross cystic changes, macular oedema cannot be detected readily by direct ophthalmoscopy. The choice of person to perform the screening depends on the clinical situation. In the private office, clinicians need to assess their own ability to detect retinopathy, and if they are not confident then referral is essential. In a large diabetic clinic, logistics and available resources become the determining factors. In many centres the availability of ophthalmologists is limited and their time would be better spent on the treatment and detailed assessment of patients with diabetic retinopathy rather than on screening. In this situation, screening can safely be performed by physicians provided that they are experienced in the examination of diabetic fundi. In our Diabetes Centre with approximately 1500 patients, screening is performed by physicians: over a 12-month period the false negative rate (determined by random referral of patients to ophthalmologists for assessment) was about 14%. Most of the retinopathy missed was mild and only 2 patients subsequently required laser treatment. If a patient is found to have normal vision and a normal fundus on examination, the probability of significant retinopathy requiring treatment being missed is small. Generally speaking, once diabetic retinopathy is detected the patient should be referred for more detailed assessment by ophthalmologists or specially trained physicians.

Retinal Colour Photography

In recent years there have been major advances in the standardization of retinal colour photography for the purpose of quantitating diabetic retinopathy [20]; this has arisen from the requirement of clinical trials to have a reproducible and objective assessment of diabetic retinopathy. This technique is sensitive but laborious to perform and not required for the routine screening of diabetic retinopathy. Photographs that cover less extensive fields are often used for the purpose of clinical records; they can also be taken with a non-mydriatic camera. For screening purposes, these photographs are not superior to direct examination of the fundi by an experienced observer.

Fluorescein Angiography

Occasional examples can be cited where direct examination and visual acuity reveal little abnormality of the fundus and yet fluorescein angiography demonstrates lesions requiring laser treatment. Nevertheless, in most clinical situations fluorescein angiography is not required for the screening of diabetic retinopathy. Its main use is in localizing areas of non-perfusion, assessing the state of capillary beds around the macula and identifying small areas

of new vessels in patients with clinically obvious retinopathy.

Who Should be Screened and How Often?

There is no strict rule about screening. Young patients with IDDM of abrupt onset should be screened routinely from 5 years after the onset of diabetes. Before this time, they rarely develop diabetic retinopathy requiring treatment. Up to 20% of patients with NIDDM (presumably because of its more insidious onset) have some retinopathy at their first presentation and they should be routinely screened even at this early stage [21]. In patients with normal visual acuity and fundal appearance, screening should be repeated at approximately yearly intervals. Patients are unlikely to develop severe retinopathy requiring treatment within this period.

DIABETIC NEPHROPATHY

Prevention

The aetiology of diabetic nephropathy is poorly understood and there are no conclusive data to prove that any intervention is effective in preventing its occurrence. Cross-sectional studies and clinical experience point to a relationship between poor glycaemic control and diabetic nephropathy. It is logical to assume that maintenance of good glycaemic control early in the course of the disease should prevent diabetic nephropathy, but it is not known what degree of control is necessary and how early this must be implemented. In patients with established diabetic nephropathy manifested by proteinuria and elevated levels of plasma creatinine, renal function deteriorates at a rate characteristic of that patient and is little influenced by diabetic control [6].

In recent years it has been suggested that the high glomerular filtration rate (GFR) found in many patients with IDDM may play a part in the pathogenesis of diabetic nephropathy [22, 23]. If this hypothesis is correct, then measures that lower the GFR may paradoxically protect the kidney in the long term. Restriction of dietary protein may be one such method of modulating the GFR [23–26]. It is known that a protein load can increase the GFR whereas protein restriction has the opposite effect. Strict protein restriction (20 g per day) used in the symptomatic treatment of end-stage renal failure is unpalatable and requires essential amino acid supplementation; compliance of the patient with this diet is doubtful. Moderate protein restriction to approximately 0.6 g/kg body weight is better tolerated by patients and is more suitable for long-term clinical trials in the prevention of diabetic nephropathy. In short-term studies, modest protein restriction of this degree can decrease the GFR, lower the filtration fraction and reduce proteinuria and microalbuminuria: these are indications that modest protein restriction may also prevent the development of clinical diabetic nephropathy; however, this remains unproven at this stage.

Early Treatment of Diabetic Nephropathy

Because of our inability to modify advanced diabetic nephropathy, increasing attempts are being made to identify earlier stages of nephropathy by the measurement of albumin excretion rate. Patients who have increased albumin excretion but not overt proteinuria are said to have 'microalbuminuria' and are at high risk of developing subsequent overt proteinuria [27–29]. There is considerable interest in whether this early phase of diabetic nephropathy can be reversed or halted. Results are not conclusive, but it appears that in patients who receive the intensive insulin treatment regimen, microalbuminuria can be reversed after 1–2 years of good diabetic control [30]. Whether this can be translated into long-term success in the prevention of overt diabetic nephropathy is not known at present.

Perhaps the most important aspect in the prevention and early treatment of diabetic nephropathy is control of hypertension [31] (see also Chapter 67). Its role in retarding the deterioration of renal function in patients with established nephropathy has been documented. In patients with microalbuminuria the treatment of hypertension may be equally important. As a group, patients with microalbuminuria have mildly elevated blood pressure, although not to a level that would normally be considered to require treatment. This degree of mild hypertension (e.g. 135/90 mmHg) has been termed 'microhypertension' and its presence may be the factor perpetuating further damage to the glomerular structures in diabetes. Treatment of microhypertension, together with meticulous control of diabetes, may be what is required in the long term to prevent overt diabetic nephropathy. There is little information about which is the best antihypertensive regimen for patients with overt or incipient diabetic nephropathy. Recently, there is some evidence that the ACE inhibitors may have a protective action on the diabetic kidney above and beyond their antihypertensive effect [11, 12]. This interesting possibility is the subject of several studies in progress at the moment.

Screening for Diabetic Nephropathy

Detection of Proteinuria by Test Strips

On a clinical level, this is the single most important test in the screening for diabetic nephropathy. It is easily done and any reading of 2 + or above almost invariably means the presence of diabetic nephropathy. When 2 + of proteinuria is detected, further tests such as measurement of the creatinine clearance and quantitative estimation of daily protein excretion should be carried out. Testing for proteinuria with test strips is an integral part of any screening procedure. The presence of proteinuria is the single most important determinant of overall prognosis and indicates that hypertension must be treated vigorously.

Measurement of Plasma Creatinine and its Clearance

Plasma creatinine measurement by itself is not a sensitive indicator of early diabetic nephropathy. Its performance is less cost-effective than the detection of proteinuria with test strips in identifying high-risk patients, particularly when dealing with a large number of patients. Similarly, although the measurement of creatinine clearance is a good clinical test of renal function, it is not suitable for screening purposes. Generally speaking, measurement of plasma creatinine and its clearance should be reserved for the quantitative rather than the qualitative assessment of renal impairment.

Detection of Microalbuminuria

Detection of microalbuminuria can identify patients at risk of developing overt diabetic nephropathy so that their microhypertension and hyperfiltration can be treated. Although there is evidence that this concept is worth pursuing, it is still an experimental approach with unproven long-term benefit. Apart from Mögensen's work, there are few data on the relevance of microalbuminuria in NIDDM patients [28]. At this stage, whether an institute should undertake the task of screening for microalbuminuria will depend on its patient population, resources and research interest. As microalbuminuria is a predictor of long-term kidney disease, its measurement will be meaningful only for those patients with a reasonable life expectancy.

There is no unanimous agreement about the optimal method of collecting urine for the measurement of albumin excretion. Mögensen et al advocated the collection of urine over an accurately timed period of several hours with the patient at rest and under supervision [22]. This has an advantage over 24-hour urine samples, in that the completeness of collection and the exercise activity of the patient can be adequately controlled. The collection of overnight urine or samples taken at random has also been used successfully [27, 32, 33]. Obviously, each laboratory must standardize its own procedure of urine collection for the purpose of measuring albumin excretion rate. When microalbuminuria is detected, it should be confirmed by another collection as there can be considerable fluctuations in its early stages [31]. In older NIDDM patients, other causes of increased albumin excretion, such as cardiac failure, renal calculi and infection, should be excluded.

Who Should be Screened and How Often?

The detection of proteinuria by test strips is cheap and should be performed at approximately yearly intervals. This is an undervalued procedure which not only doctors, but all health professionals including nurses, should be encouraged to perform. As with diabetic retinopathy, IDDM patients are unlikely to have significant proteinuria until after 5 years of diabetes, but patients with NIDDM may already be at risk at the time of diagnosis. Indication for screening for microalbuminuria has already been discussed.

DIABETIC NEUROPATHY AND FOOT PROBLEMS

Prevention

Prevention of neuropathy and its associated foot problems is obviously desirable; but, again, no method has yet been proved scientifically to be effective (see Chapter 68). A correlation between hyperglycaemia and electrophysiological abnormalities has been shown in a number of studies [34, 35]. Tightening of metabolic control can also improve nerve conduction and reduce neuropathic pain by raising the pain threshold [36]. However, the relationship between these acute changes and the prevention of neuropathy in the longer term is equivocal. Most workers believe that good diabetic control early in the course of diabetes will minimize the risk of diabetic neuropathy.

Many aldose reductase inhibitors are being tested extensively in clinical trials but have not been proved to be effective in the prevention of diabetic neuropathy. In a study of diabetic patients with no symptoms of neuropathy, and in laboratory animals with diabetes, it has been shown that these agents can improve nerve conduction [37, 38]. Dramatic responses have also been reported in some patients with symptomatic neuropathy, but placebo effects were not excluded [39]. In more controlled studies on patients with severe clinical neuropathy, the benefits of aldose reductase inhibitors have not been dramatic and are certainly not proved beyond doubt [40]. Attempts to give these agents at an earlier stage of neuropathy are thwarted by toxicity, making a large-scale, long-term primary trial difficult to justify. Other pharmacological and nutritional approaches, such as myo-inositol supplementation and vitamin treatment, have also been advocated for the prevention and early treatment of neuropathy, but have not been shown to be effective.

Thirty per cent of newly diagnosed diabetic patients, if questioned specifically, will be found to have some neuropathic symptoms. For the most part these symptoms resolve with treatment of the hyperglycaemia. It has been postulated that this subset of patients with early and reversible neuropathic symptoms may be particularly at risk for the subsequent development of significant neuropathy [41]. As such, they may be suitable for testing various strategies of early treatment and prevention, but this hypothesis remains to be tested.

Until specific measures to prevent neuropathy are available, screening and education of patients with clinical neuropathy and those at high risk of developing foot problems must remain the cornerstone of treatment.

Screening for Neuropathy and Foot Problems

Neurological Assessment

The most common method used for the screening and detection of peripheral neuropathy is clinical neurological assessment (see Chapter 59). However, this is time-consuming, subjective and has large interexaminer variations, especially in the testing of sensation. Qualitative data collected on a patient cannot be easily compared serially to document any deterioration. For the purpose of screening it is necessary to streamline the procedure of assessment. This should include enquiry about the presence of numbness or pain in both feet, and testing for ankle jerks. Generally, patients with well-preserved ankle jerks are unlikely to have neuropathy of sufficient severity to cause ulceration. Even if neuropathic pain is present in these individuals, it is likely to respond to control of hyperglycaemia.

Neurophysiological Testing

Motor and sensory nerve conduction velocities are often abnormal in subclinical or clinical neuropathy [34, 35]. However, they do not always correlate well with the clinical status of the peripheral nerves and do not differentiate between early manifestations of neuropathy and transient abnormalities of nerve conduction at the time of poor diabetic control. Neurophysiological testing requires expensive equipment and expertly trained individuals. It is not practical or necessary in the screening of diabetic patients for neuropathy and foot problems.

Semiquantitative Measurement of Sensation

From the considerations outlined above, it is clear that simpler and more objective means of screening and documenting nerve function are necessary. In part, this need can be fulfilled by measurement of the vibration perception threshold (VPT) using a biothesiometer [42]. This is an inexpensive instrument which is electrically driven; it can be used to determine the vibratory sensory perception by applying it to a standard position, such as the undersurface of the great toe, and increasing the amplitude until a response is given by the patient. The biothesiometer provides a quantitative measurement of the large-fibre function of the peripheral nerves. Although the reading increases with age and each institute must determine its own normal range, generally a reading greater than 30 V indicates increased risk of developing foot ulceration. It is relatively cheap and can be used after minimal training for rapid screening of patients to select those most at risk. The results of the VPT can be affected by the pressure that is applied at the contact point, and a newer machine that standardizes this variable is available [43]. However, for screening purposes in a busy diabetic clinic or private consulting room, the ordinary biothesiometer appears to be adequate.

In some patients, damage of small nerve fibres that control temperature and pain sensation may predate large-fibre damage. An efficient and reproducible method of measuring temperature sensation is required. This is available in the form of a temperature discriminator in which patients are asked to indicate the smallest temperature difference that they can detect. Apart from selecting patients already at risk, serial measurements of this nature would also help to identify patients whose condition is deteriorating.

Screening of Patients at High Risk of Developing Foot Problems

Once neuropathy is advanced, there is little evidence to show that the neuropathy can be reversed or that the progression of the damage can be slowed. However, the morbidity from peripheral neuropathy can be reduced by identifying those patients most at risk of developing foot ulceration and providing them with intensive foot-care education. Hospitalization from diabetic foot disease is an all-too-common occurrence, leading to high emotional and economic costs for all involved.

Historically, it has often been accepted by health professionals that foot disease is an inevitable consequence of diabetes. There is now good evidence to show that this pessimism is not necessary [44] (see Chapter 68).

Screening is also necessary because the conventional wisdom, that detailed foot-care advice is essential for all diabetic individuals, is not practical. One reason for this is that the education may not have been delivered at the most effective time. Is it appropriate to advise 15-year-old patients with IDDM of recent onset not to go barefoot, when it is highly likely that they will continue to do so and not face any immediate problem? It is, perhaps, better to reserve these life-style restrictions for the time when patients have demonstrable early neuropathy and enter a high-risk phase. A streamlined, efficient and effective system of identifying these patients at risk needs to be developed. A simple checklist can be used to screen all diabetic patients and allocate them into either a low-risk or a high-risk group. Patients who are categorized into a low-risk group present no real problem; it would be sufficient to offer them some simple, common-sense guidelines, such as advice to wear comfortable shoes. Patients, categorized into a high-risk group require intensive foot-care education and management.

Some characteristics of the high-risk foot that should be included in the checklist are listed below.

(1) The presence of an ulcer: this is frequently missed, by both patients and health professionals, owing to lack of attention to the feet.
(2) A past history of ulcer: without intervention, the causal factors of the original ulcer will lead to further problems. Disappointingly, it is all too common to see ulcers recur.
(3) Abnormal sensation: impairment of the pain sensation allows mechanical, chemical and thermal damage to occur without the diabetic patient's knowledge. A biothesiometer reading greater than 30 is indicative of impaired sensation and is a convenient method of replacing the time-consuming sensory testing.
(4) Absent ankle jerks: this is a physical sign which is relatively objective and easy to elicit. When ankle jerks are unequivocally present, the patient generally is not at high risk of developing neuropathic ulcers.
(5) Biomechanical problems of the foot: muscle wasting and claw toes are indicative of subtle motor neuropathy which also increases the formation of corns and calluses—areas susceptible to ulceration.
(6) Dry, cracked skin: decreased sweating attributable to coexisting autonomic dysfunction leads to dry, cracked skin, which predisposes to infection.
(7) The presence of other complications: peripheral vascular disease further increases the problem due to neuropathy.
(8) Patients with impaired vision: this applies especially to the elderly, who cannot see and manage their feet properly.

Once these high-risk patients have been identified, a programme of intensive education should be undertaken. As stated earlier, these people require instruction beyond the customary 'you need to be careful about your feet'. In addition to theoretical knowledge they will often need practical demonstrations on how to dry between their toes, how to inspect the bottom of their feet and how to cut their nails. With increasing recognition of the importance of diabetic foot disease, many clinics now have a combined diabetic foot service which includes the expertise of podiatrists, physicians, orthotists, specialist nurses and surgeons (orthopaedic and vascular). The resources of these individuals are often stretched to the utmost. This problem can be partially overcome by training a diabetes nurse specialist to have clinical expertise in diabetes foot care beyond the theoretical knowledge now possessed by most educators. The diabetes nurse specialist can play an important part by implementing an effective screening program to identify the high-risk patients, providing the necessary intensive foot-care education and referring them to the appropriate member of the foot-care team. This would permit more efficient use of the podiatrists' and doctors' time.

AUTONOMIC NEUROPATHY

Prevention

Currently, the results from any measures that may lead to the prevention of autonomic neuropathy are disappointing. Tightening of glycaemic control confers no major benefit in improving or reversing symptoms of established disease. Some early autonomic dysfunction detected by sophisticated electrophysiological testing can be reversed by insulin infusion, but the long-term benefit remains unproven [45, 46]. Studies of the effect of aldose reductase inhibitors on autonomic neuropathy are few and findings have been inconsistent, with little (if any) improvement in cardiovascular tests [45, 46]. Ewing et al state 'the possible role of aldose reductase inhibitors may . . . lie more in primary prevention of diabetic neuropathy.' [46].

Screening for Autonomic Neuropathy

The case for routine screening of diabetic complications is weakest in relation to autonomic neuropathy. The tests available are either insensitive, non-specific or require expensive equipment. Moreover, when autonomic neuropathy is detected, little or no specific treatment is available. Autonomic neuropathy tests are usually requested to determine whether impotence in a patient is due to autonomic neuropathy. In this context, testing of autonomic neuropathy is further hampered by its patchy distribution, and testing the cardiovascular reflexes may not accurately reflect the erectile function of the penis. In practice, patients who do not have peripheral neuropathy rarely have significant autonomic involvement. Patients with unequivocal autonomic dysfunction, however, do have a bad prognosis.

A number of tests are used in the screening of autonomic neuropathy, most of which depend on testing the variability of heart rate or blood pressure during various manoeuvres [45, 46]. No single test is entirely satisfactory. We use three tests when screening our patients: these are (a) variation of heart rate during the Valsalva manoeuvre: this is performed by asking the patient to blow into a syringe connected to a manometer and maintain the pressure at 40 mmHg; (b) variation of heart rate during respiration: this is performed by asking the patient to inspire and expire deeply for 12 cycles within 1 minute; and (c) postural change in blood pressure. These tests are simple and can be done at the bedside, but an experienced person must be involved in the testing to ensure accurate results. In our clinic we arbitrarily designate those patients with two or more abnormal tests as having autonomic neuropathy, and they can proceed to more detailed autonomic tests if the clinical situation is appropriate.

MACROVASCULAR DISEASE

The prevention of macrovascular disease in diabetic patients by the treatment of hyperlipidaemia and hypertension has been dealt with elsewhere in this book. Although there are no specific data confirming the efficacy of such treatment in diabetes, it is generally accepted as an important preventive measure. With the increasing trend toward treating even minor elevations in serum lipid and blood pressure, larger numbers of diabetic patients are considered to require therapeutic intervention. This will certainly make the already intrusive regimen of low-fat, low-protein and low-salt diet, regular medications and repetitive glucose monitoring even more cumbersome.

Perhaps of even greater importance is the need to help diabetic patients give up smoking, a notoriously difficult objective. In a recent survey of diabetic patients, smokers were found to have a better knowledge of the general dangers of smoking than non-smokers [47]. They were, however, quite ignorant of the potential of smoking to aggravate diabetic complications. Clearly, it is not sufficient to provide patients with general information alone and it may be necessary to emphasize the interaction between smoking and diabetic complications. In another study it was found that immediately upon diagnosis of diabetes, patients were more reluctant to join an antismoking programme conducted by a nurse practitioner than if they were approached 2 months later [48]. Perhaps patients already experience too much stress and too many changes in life-style when diabetes is first discovered. The better personal rapport with the nurse practitioner after 2 months of treatment may also be an important factor. Although antismoking counselling is undoubtedly time-consuming, its importance is such that further evaluation of the optimal strategy in advising patients to give up smoking must be explored.

Careful physical examination of the peripheral pulses is as valuable as the more sophisticated investigations in the screening for peripheral vascular disease in diabetes. Although Doppler examination is often used, it is potentially misleading due to the hardening of the arteries that occurs in diabetes.

PSYCHOLOGICAL ASPECTS OF SCREENING FOR DIABETIC COMPLICATIONS

The psychological impact of screening for diabetic complications should not be underestimated, but there is a dearth of information in this regard. Many health professionals feel uncomfortable discussing diabetic complications with patients and either avoid the issue or resort to scare tactics. One consequence of either approach may be entrenched denial, making screening and early treatment of diabetic complications difficult. Alternatively, repeated warnings that diabetic complications are imminent and that screening is essential may generate enormous and unnecessary anxiety. A question that must be asked is whether screening increases or allays anxieties. Our experience during screening is that IDDM patients are more aware of the possible complications, and can be either very relieved or nervous that 'something is being done'. The older NIDDM patients often feel that their disease is mild and they are just having 'routine tests', which does not affect their stress levels.

A particularly difficult case is that of a child with diabetes. Children are unlikely to develop significant diabetic complications that will require treatment before puberty. There is no clear consensus about whether they should have routine assessment for diabetic complications to assure the family that the child is complication-free and to encourage the habit of screening, or whether they should be spared the unnecessary anxiety at this stage.

In addition to these dilemmas, better guidelines must be developed by appropriate research on how best to counsel patients if early complications (when no treatment is deemed to be necessary) or severe complications (when no improvement is considered to be likely) have been detected.

CONVENIENCE FOR PATIENTS: A ONE-VISIT SCREENING PACKAGE

Traditionally, the comprehensive screening for diabetic complications requires a patient to attend doctors and laboratories on more than one occasion. This is inconvenient and means that many patients omit one or more important screening procedures. To overcome this problem, we have developed a convenient service

Table 1 Screening for diabetic complications: a 3-hour package

Complications	Recommended measurements
Retinopathy	1. Corrected visual acuity
	2. Direct ophthalmoscopy with pupils dilated
Nephropathy	3. Test-strip detection of proteinuria
	4. Measurement of microalbuminuria or proteinuria by a 2.5-hour urine collection when 350 ml of water is drunk after an initial rest period of 30 minutes
	5. Measurement of blood pressure
Neuropathy and problems	6. Enquiry about neuropathic foot symptoms
	7. Testing of ankle reflexes
	8. Examination of feet for high-risk features
	9. Recording of biothesiometer result
Peripheral vascular disease	10. Enquiry about claudication
	11. Examination of foot pulses
Autonomic neuropathy (optional)	12. Postural change in blood pressure
	13. Heart rate variation in response to deep breathing
	14. Heart rate variation during Valsalva manoeuvre

which can screen for all major diabetic complications in a 3-hour visit. Details of the procedures are shown in Table 1. The duration chosen is sufficient for an accurately timed collection of urine, to measure microalbuminuria and total protein excretion. While this is proceeding, other complications are assessed by an assembled team of one doctor, two nurses and a podiatrist. With proper organization, many patients can be screened in the same session to improve its cost-effectiveness. Results are sent to referring doctors with recommendations for treatment if required. Both patients and doctors have found this to be a convenient service. In addition, it is an excellent forum for the collection of data and for teaching.

REFERENCES

1. DCCT Research Group. Diabetes Control and Complication Trial (DCCT): results of feasibility study. Diabetes Care 1987; 10: 1–19.
2. Dahl-Jørgensen K, Brinchmann-Hansen D, Hanssen KF et al. Rapid tightening of blood glucose control leads to transient deterioration of

retinopathy in insulin dependent diabetes mellitus: the Oslo Study. Br Med J 1985; 290: 8–15.

3. Kroc Collaborative Study Group. Blood glucose control and the evaluation of diabetic retinopathy and albuminuria: a preliminary multicenter trial. New Engl J Med 1984; 311: 365–72.

4. Lauritzen T, Larsen HW, Frost-Larsen K et al. The Steno study group: effect of 1 year of near-normal blood glucose levels on retinopathy in insulin-dependent diabetes. Lancet 1983; i: 200–4.

5. Viberti GC, Bilous RW, Mackintosh D et al. Long term correction of hyperglycaemia and progression of renal failure in insulin dependent diabetes. Br Med J 1983; 286: 598–602.

6. Jones RH, Hayakawa H, Mackay JD et al. Progression of diabetic nephropathy. Lancet 1979; i: 1105–6.

7. Cogan DG. Aldose reductase and complications of diabetes. Ann Intern Med 1984; 101: 82–91.

8. Greene DA, Lattimer S, Ulbrecht J et al. Glucose-induced alterations in nerve metabolism: current perspective on the pathogenesis of diabetic neuropathy and future directions for research and therapy. Diabetes Care 1985; 8: 290–9.

9. Mögensen CE. Long-term anti-hypertensive treatment inhibiting progression of diabetic nephropathy. Br Med J 1982; 285: 685–8.

10. Parving H-H, Andersen AR, Smidt UM et al. Early aggressive antihypertensive treatment reduces rate of decline in kidney function in diabetic nephropathy. Lancet 1983; i: 1175–8.

11. Bjorck S, Nyberg G, Mulec H et al. Beneficial effects of angiotension converting enzyme inhibition on renal function in patients with diabetic nephropathy. Br Med J 1986; 293: 471–4.

12. Hommel E, Parving HH, Mathiesen E et al. Effect of Captopril on kidney function in insulin-dependent diabetes patients with nephropathy. Br Med J 1986; 293: 467–70.

13. Diabetic Retinopathy Study Research Group. Photocoagulation treatment of proliferative diabetic retinopathy. Clinical application of diabetic retinopathy study (DRS) findings. DRS report no. 8. Ophthalmology 1981; 88: 583–600.

14. British Multicentre Study Group. Photocoagulation for diabetic maculopathy: a randomized controlled clinical trial using the xenon arc. Diabetes 1983; 32: 1010–16.

15. Assal JP, Gfeller R, Ekol JM. Patient education in diabetes. In Bostrum H, Ljungstedt N (eds) Recent trends in diabetes research. Stockholm: Almqvist & Wiksell, 1981: pp 276–90.

16. Job D, Eschwega E, Guyot C et al. Effect of multiple daily insulin injection on the course of diabetic retinopathy. Diabetes 1976; 25: 463–7.

17. Cunha-Vaz JG, Fonseca JR, Abreu JR et al. Follow-up study by vitreous fluorophotometry of early retinal involvement in diabetes. Am J Ophthalmol 1978; 86: 467–73.

18. Kohner EM, Sharp PS. Diabetic retinopathy. In Alberti KGMM, Krall LP (eds) Diabetes annual 3. Amsterdam: Elsevier, 1987: pp 252–88.

19. Early Treatment of Diabetic Retinopathy Study Research Group. Photocoagulation for diabetic macular oedema. Arch Ophthalmol 1985; 103: 1796–806.

20. Klein BE, Davis MD, Segal P et al. Diabetic retinopathy: assessment of severity and progression. Ophthalmology 1984; 91: 10–17.

21. Owens DR, Jones D, Shannon AG et al. Retinopathy in newly presenting NIDDM patients. Diabetes 1987; 36 (suppl. 1): 416A.

22. Mögensen CE. Early glomerular hyperfiltration in insulin-dependent diabetics and late nephropathy. Scand J Clin Lab Invest 1986; 201–6.

23. Viberti GC, Wiseman MJ. The kidney in diabetes: significance of the early abnormalities. Clin Endocrinol Metab 1986; 15: 753–82.

24. Cohen DC, Dodds RH, Viberti GC. Reduction of microalbuminuria and glomerular filtration rate by dietary protein restriction in type I insulin dependent diabetic patients: an effect independent of blood glucose control and arterial pressure changes. Diabetologia 1986; 29: 528A.

25. Bending JJ, Dodds R, Keen H et al. Lowering protein intake and the progression of diabetic renal failure. Diabetologia 1986; 29: 516A.

26. Kupin WL, Cortes P, Dumler F et al. Effect on renal function of a change from high to moderate protein intake in type I diabetic patients. Diabetes 1987; 36: 73–9.

27. Viberti GC, Jarrett RJ, Mahmud U et al. Microalbuminuria as a predictor of clinical nephropathy in insulin-dependent diabetes mellitus. Lancet 1982; i: 1430–2.

28. Mögensen CE. Microalbuminuria predicts clinical proteinuria and early mortality in maturity onset diabetes. New Engl J Med 1984; 310: 356–60

29. Mathieson ER, Oxenball K, Johansen PA et al. Incipient nephropathy in type I (insulin-dependent) diabetes. Diabetologia 1984; 26: 406–10.

30. Feldt-Rasmussen B, Mathiesen E, Deckert T. Effect of two years of strict metabolic control on the progression of incipient nephropathy in insulin-dependent diabetes. Lancet 1986; ii: 1300–4.

31. Mögensen CE. Early diabetic renal involvement and nephropathy. Can treatment modalities be predicted from identification of risk factors. In Alberti KGMM, Krall LP (eds) Diabetes annual 3. Amsterdam: Elsevier, 1987: pp 306–24.

32. Cowell CT, Rogers S, Silink M. First morning urinary albumin concentration is a good predictor of 24 hour urinary albumin excretion in children

with type I (insulin-dependent) diabetes. Diabetologia 1986; 29: 97–9.

33. Viberti GC, Jarrett RT, Mahmud U et al. Microalbuminuria as a predictor of clinical nephropathy in insulin-dependent diabetes mellitus. Lancet 1982; i: 1430–2.

34. Ward JC, Baarnes CG, Fisher DJ et al. Improvement in nerve conduction following treatment in newly diagnosed diabetics. Lancet 1971; i: 428–30.

35. Graf RJ, Halter JB, Pfeifer MA et al. Glycemic control and nerve conduction abnormalities in non-insulin dependent diabetic subjects. Ann Intern Med 1981; 94: 307–11.

36. Morley GK, Mooradian AD, Levine AS et al. Mechanism of pain in diabetic peripheral neuropathy. Effect of glucose and pain threshold in humans. Am J Med 1984; 77: 79–82.

37. Judzewitsch RG, Jaspan J, Polonsky KS et al. Aldose reductase inhibition improves nerve conduction in diabetic patients. New Engl J Med 1983; 308: 119–25.

38. Yue DK, Hanwell M, Satchell P et al. The effect of aldose reductase inhibition on motor nerve conduction velocity in diabetic rat. Diabetes 1982; 31: 789–94.

39. Jaspan J, Maselli R, Herold K et al. Treatment of severely painful diabetic neuropathy with an aldose reductase inhibitor; relief of pain and improved somatic and autonomic nerve function. Lancet 1983; ii: 758–63.

40. Young RJ, Ewing DJ, Clark BF. A controlled trial of Sorbinil, an aldose reductase inhibitor, in chronic painful diabetic neuropathy. Diabetes 1983; 32: 928–42.

41. Ward JD. Diabetic neuropathies. In Belfiore F, Molinetti GM, Williamson JR (eds) Vascular and neurological complications of diabetes mellitus. Karger: Basel, 1987: 146–59.

42. Boulton AJM, Ward JD. Diabetic neuropathies and pain. Clin Endocrinol Metab. 1986; 15: 916–31.

43. Lowenthal LM, Hockaday TDR. Vibration sensory thresholds depend on pressure of applied stimulus. Diabetes Care 1987; 10: 100–2.

44. Edmonds ME. The diabetic foot: pathophysiology and treatment. Clin Endocrinol Metab 1986; 10: 910.

45. Ewing DJ, Clark BF. Autonomic neuropathy: its diagnosis and prognosis. Clin Endocrinol Metab 1986; 15: 855–88.

46. Ewing DJ, Clarke BF. Diabetic autonomic neuropathy: present insights and future prospects. Diabetes Care 1986; 9: 648–65.

47. Fowler P, Hoskins P, McGill M, Dutton S, Yue DK, Turtle JR. Anti-smoking programme for patients: the agony and the ecstasy. Diabetic Med 1989; 6: 698–702.

48. McGill M, Yue DK. Diabetic complication assessment service: a new concept. Diabetes Care 1989; 12: 8.

49. Nelson R, Pettitt D, Carraher M, Baird R, Knowler W. Effect of proteinuria on mortality in NIDDM. Diabetes 1988; 37: 1499–504.

50. Zeller K, Whittaker M, Sullivan L, Raskin P, Jacobsen H. Effect of restricting dietary protein on the progression of renal failure in patients with insulin-dependent diabetes mellitus. N Engl J Med 1991; 324: 78–84.

Diabetes and Public Health

70

Screening for Diabetes and Other Categories of Glucose Intolerance

Gary Dowse*, Paul Zimmet* and K.G.M.M. Alberti†

*International Diabetes Institute, Caulfield, Australia, and †Department of Medicine, University of Newcastle upon Tyne, UK

The need for and methods of screening for diabetes mellitus and related disorders of abnormal glucose tolerance have caused confusion and conflict for several decades. Contributing to this has been: (a) the lack of standardized diagnostic criteria; (b) inadequate understanding of the natural history of glucose intolerance; (c) failure to include control populations in evaluation; (d) lack of appropriate cost–benefit analysis; and (e) naïve enthusiasm for unsubstantiated therapeutic interventions.

Following the establishment of compatible and internationally accepted classifications and diagnostic criteria by the National Diabetes Data Group (NDDG) [1] and the World Health Organization (WHO) [2, 3], it was hoped that research workers might be able to answer many of the questions that remained concerning screening for the diabetes syndrome. Unfortunately, to date most of the questions remained unresolved.

This chapter focuses on screening directed toward detecting presymptomatic stages of the major forms of the diabetes syndrome, namely insulin dependent diabetes mellitus (IDDM), non-insulin dependent diabetes mellitus (NIDDM), impaired glucose tolerance (IGT) and gestational diabetes mellitus (GDM). Malnutrition related diabetes mellitus (MRDM), the epidemiology of which is still poorly understood, is not considered here. Discussion of screening for specific complications can be found elsewhere in this book.

It is pertinent first to consider recognized definitions of screening; its potential scope within both the population and the health services; and those attributes of disease, screening test and health system thought to be desirable for successful screening programs. Methods of evaluating screening services are discussed in general terms, before considering the historical development of screening as applied to diabetes detection, together with some reflections on limitations in our current knowledge of the relative prognostic value of glucose intolerance with normal basal glucose levels versus fasting hyperglycemia and raised glycated protein levels. Following this, various methods of

International Textbook of Diabetes Mellitus. Edited by K.G.M.M. Alberti, R.A. DeFronzo, H. Keen and P. Zimmet
© 1992 John Wiley & Sons Ltd

screening are considered, and finally the potential application of screening to different categories of the diabetes syndrome is discussed.

DEFINITION AND RATIONALE FOR SCREENING

'Screening' was defined by the US Commission on Chronic Illness [4] as 'the presumptive identification of unrecognized disease or defect by the application of tests, examinations or other procedures which can be applied rapidly. Screening tests sort out apparently well persons who probably have a disease from those who probably do not'. The Commission further stated that 'a screening test is not intended to be diagnostic', and specified that persons with conditions detected by screening exercises should be referred to their physician for definitive diagnosis and treatment if appropriate.

Thus defined, screening is implicitly a tool for use in the prevention of onset of disease or complications of disease. Screening can be considered as a means of 'primary' prevention of resultant diseases such as coronary heart disease and stroke through identifying individuals with modifiable risk factors such as cigarette smoking or hypercholesterolemia. By analogy, screening to detect IGT (considered here as a 'risk factor' for onset of diabetes) and obesity could also be considered as primary preventive measures for NIDDM.

More conventionally, however, screening fulfils a 'secondary' preventive function through detection of presymptomatic disease, and intervention is directed towards preventing the development of complications. In some instances, treatment may lead to disease *cure* (e.g. tuberculosis discovered on screening radiograph), but in the context of chronic non-communicable diseases such as hypertension and diabetes, disease *control* is the aim, with a resultant reduction in associated morbidity and mortality.

SCOPE OF SCREENING

Screening may take place on a number of levels with varying implications for health sector costs. In the past, screening for diabetes has commonly taken place in tents or caravans situated in diverse locations such as municipal parks and suburban shopping centres. In such 'mass' or 'community' screening programs, whole populations are subjected to simple and quick tests. Mass screening exercises are often conducted by lay groups such as diabetes associations and, given their usual random occurrence, are 'mass' only in a desultory fashion. This type of screening is probably more effective at fund-raising and creating community awareness than in positively influencing disease in screenees [5].

Alternatively, such programs may be sponsored by government health authorities. In these cases, coverage of the population is more complete, goals are more likely to have been clearly defined, and program planning more considered (although often not matched by results). At present, however, there are no non-infectious diseases for which mass indiscriminate screening of whole communities is likely to offer overall benefit.

For chronic diseases, 'selective', 'discriminate' or 'high risk' screening offers the most attractive and cost-effective approach [6, 7]. This, too, can be considered on two levels. First, there are organized and usually government-sponsored programs where a serious attempt is made to cover all of the target group. These programs require a captive population, either through the responsible authorities visiting a common gathering point of the target screenees, or by requiring individuals to visit special facilities. In the first case, the best examples are routine screenings of school students carried out in some countries for conditions such as deafness or poor vision, and Mantoux or Heaf tuberculin testing to determine the requirement for BCG innoculation. As examples of the latter case, immigrants are required to have a chest x-ray for tuberculosis detection before entrance to some countries, and commercial pilots are required to undertake electrocardiographic examination before licence endorsement.

Secondly, and more commonly, selective screening is conducted on an opportunistic 'case-finding' basis by physicians or other health workers in subgroups of the population considered to be at high risk of the disease in question, at the time of a visit, usually for some unrelated matter. This is the situation in which most diabetes and cardiovascular disease (CVD) screening is undertaken in both developed and underdeveloped countries.

The extent to which such screening is institutionalized and standardized varies considerably both within and between countries. Factors determining the extent of screening activities in any particular country include the degree of economic development, the nature of the disease burden, the structure of—and resources available to—the primary health care network, and the extent of community, political and physician interest in disease prevention activities.

'Multiphasic' screening, whereby a number conditions may be screened for at one time, perhaps at regular intervals, has been considered a more cost-effective manner of screening [6, 7], and diabetes has been a component of such programs in the past [8]. Multiphasic screening is commonly performed in hospital practice, particularly in older patients, when a range of hematological, biochemical and microbiological investigations are routinely and rather indiscriminately carried out at the time of admission. The extent of multiphasic screening within any community probably bears a positive relation to wealth, and an inverse relation to health status [7].

The diabetes screening literature is replete with epidemiological studies, the principal aims of which are to describe the prevalence and distribution of glucose intolerance, and to a greater or lesser extent, to investigate etiological factors and natural history. Although these studies often attempt to arrive at their prevalence estimate by application of 'screening tests' [9, 10] or may compare the characteristics (in terms of sensitivity, specificity and predictive value) of various procedures in relation to their 'gold standard' definition [9–11], they should be seen primarily as descriptive epidemiologic studies. Their consideration as studies of screening, or even as 'screening programs' [10, 12] may in part be responsible for the lack of evaluated projects conceived and conducted as screening programs, and incorporating specific interventions.

Recommendations for screening for a range of conditions, such as diabetes, hypercholesterolemia, and breast and cervical cancer, have been made periodically by review bodies and as commentaries in leading medical journals, but considerable controversy surrounds many of the issues involved [13–19]. Even if recommendations were unanimous, however, there will always remain variation in the enthusiasm with which, firstly, doctors and other health workers offer the suggested screening service, and secondly, the target population takes advantage of services offered [20].

It has been a common observation in developed countries that those who tend to ask for and accept screening (the 'worried well') are often those who least need it. Individuals from the lower socioeconomic groups, where rates of chronic diseases are higher, are less likely to be screened [7]. To counter this trend, awareness must be improved and resources made available in appropriate areas. A goal of complete uptake (even in clearly defined high-risk groups) seems unrealistically Utopian for most societies without some form of rigid institutionalism. Given the lack of convincing evidence for cost-effectiveness of screening programs, it seems unlikely at this stage that governments will warmly embrace such major structural change to health services.

DESIRABLE CHARACTERISTICS FOR SCREENING PROGRAMS

Important principles that need to be considered before the establishment of screening programs were succinctly proposed by Wilson and Jungner [21] in 1968. Their points are presented in modified fashion under the three major headings of disease characteristics, test characteristics, and program and health system characteristics, in Table 1.

Consideration of current knowledge concerning glucose intolerance and screening for diabetes indicates clearly that these criteria are not readily satisfied. Shortcomings are alluded to more specifically in subsequent sections.

Assessment of Screening Tests

The *repeatability* or *reliability* (the amount of agreement when a test is repeated or reassessed) of a screening test is not only an important determinant of its validity (the degree to which a test correctly classifies people with respect to the condition of interest), but it also influences the level at which referral for further testing is desirable. For tests with poor repeatability, lower thresholds will be required to ensure that the same individuals are detected than for tests with greater repeatability. A lack of repeatability is more important for screening tests (where subject misclassification has undesirable consequences) than for tests used in epidemiological surveys, where misclassification of individuals does not unduly influence estimates of disease

Table 1 Desirable characteristics for disease screening programs

Disease characteristics

1. The disease should be an *important* health problem — This could be considered in terms of prevalence, severity (attributable morbidity and mortality), and economic and social cost to the community
2. The natural history of the condition should be adequately understood, particularly the rate and determinants of progression from inapparent to symptomatic disease
3. There should be a detectable preclinical phase to the condition
4. A safe and accessible form of treatment must be available
5. There should be clear indications of when, how and in whom to use the treatment—it should necessarily improve the course and prognosis of the condition in detected presymptomatic individuals

Test characteristics

6. The test should be safe and acceptable to screenees
7. It should detect presymptomatic disease with appropriate validity (sensitivity and specificity) and repeatability, and the assessment of the usefulness of a screening test should include consideration of these indices

Program and health system characteristics

8. Facilities and staff for follow-up of positive screenees for definitive diagnostic testing and subsequent treatment must be available
9. Costs of screening, subsequent diagnostic testing and resultant treatment should be acceptable in comparison with costs which would have been incurred in the absence of the program, and/or in the face of alternative uses
10. Screening should be a continuing process, implying the need for at least some systematic integration into health care services and training of appropriate personnel. Moreover, the program must reach its target population

frequency, on the assumption that the variation in measurements is random and will average out [22].

Although laboratory methods are available for measuring blood glucose accurately and precisely [23], there is still considerable random biological variation in any individual's blood glucose results, even under the standardized conditions of an oral glucose tolerance test (OGTT) [8, 24]; this has important implications for misclassification rates, particularly in subjects whose levels fall close to cut-off values. It should be noted, however, that a test can be highly repeatable but still have poor validity (as reflected by sensitivity and specificity).

The *sensitivity* of a screening test refers to its ability to identify correctly subjects with the disease or condition of interest [6, 7]. A test with 80% sensitivity will correctly detect 8 out of 10 diseased individuals—those not identified are called 'false negatives' (Table 2). These people gain little from a screening test and may be indirectly harmed if, for instance, they subsequently ignore the development of symptoms because of the false reassurance of a negative test. A lack of sensitivity may have disastrous consequences for conditions such as phenylketonuria, where a missed diagnosis may lead to irreparable brain damage. False-negative screenees in diabetes screening programs are less likely to come to great harm. In screening for gestational diabetes, however, it has been argued that tests with greater sensitivity are required than those employed in non-pregnant subjects—this implies a lowering of the values accepted as indicating a positive test [25–27].

Specificity is the ability of a screening test to identify correctly 'normal' individuals [6, 7]. A test that misclassifies 1 out of 10 well persons as having the disease has a 90% specificity (Table 2). The misclassifed subject is a 'false positive' and suffers through the inconvenience, expense and anxiety of undergoing unnecessary further diagnostic tests.

An ideal screening test should be both highly sensitive and specific, but unfortunately a compromise must usually be reached, as sensitivity and specificity have an inverse relationship—increasing specificity will result in more false-negative screenees and a lack of sensitivity (Figure 1). A lack of specificity (with corresponding increased sensitivity) will result in increased costs to a screening service, because of the need for false-positive screenees to undergo further diagnostic tests. Highly specific screening tests are desirable in situations where definitive diagnositic tests may be expensive, dangerous or unpleasant, and when a lack of sensitivity is not critical (such as for diseases with long preclinical phases where the consequences of a false-negative screen for prognosis are unlikely to be grave). Glucose intolerance fits into the latter category—a more specific test will result in relatively more false-negative screenees, but delayed diagnosis may not be critical for long-term prognosis, although this remains conjectural.

Predictive value (PV) is a useful indicator in assessing the cost-effectiveness of a screening

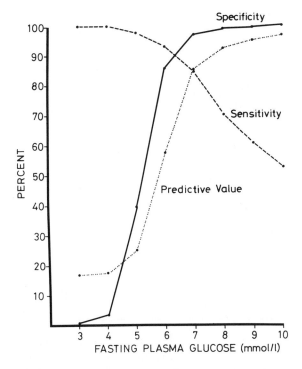

Figure 1 The relationship of sensitivity, specificity and predictive value at different levels of fasting plasma glucose as a screening test for undetected or untreated NIDDM in Micronesian Nauruans aged 20–74 years (NIDDM defined as plasma glucose value 11.1 mmol/l or above, 2 hours following a 75-g OGTT)

program [7]. The PV of a positive test is the proportion of test positives who are proven to have the condition following definitive testing. For instance, if 100 of 1000 tested individuals have a positive screen, but only 25 are confirmed to have the condition, then the PV of the test is 25%. Conversely, the PV of a negative test is the proportion of those with a negative test who truly do not have the disease (Table 2). Predictive value is very prevalence dependent; it can be improved by applying the test in subgroups with higher prevalence. This relationship is illustrated in Figure 2. It can be seen that, at any screening cut-off level, the PV of fasting plasma glucose testing for detection of NIDDM (defined by the 2-hour glucose value alone) is greater in the higher-prevalence population.

High-risk screening takes advantage of the relationship between PV and prevalence: not only is expense spared by excluding the majority of the population from screening in the first place, but fewer unnecessary follow-up diagnostic tests are undertaken because of the higher predictive value of the screening test which arises implicitly through screening in higher-prevalence subgroups. For abnormalities of glucose tolerance these include older age groups, the overweight, those with a family history, women with a history of GDM, and certain ethnic groups with high prevalence. The latter include Asian Indians in immigrant communities [28], Micronesian and Polynesian Pacific Island populations [29], and aborigines of Australia [30] and the Americas [31].

A further point concerning screening for glucose intolerance in high-prevalence populations is that the sensitivity of screening tests is also improved [9, 32]. For categoric ('yes/no') conditions such as cancer, the sensitivity and specificity of screening tests are unrelated to disease prevalence. However, for a continuously distributed parameter such as plasma glucose and where diagnostic thresholds are fixed, a screening test will have higher sensitivity in populations where the glucose distribution is shifted to the right, or where the distribution is bimodal [9]. This increased sensitivity has also been attributed to more severe hyperglycemia in diabetics of high-prevalence populations relative to diabetics in low-prevalence populations [9]. The phenomenon can be appreciated from Figure 3 where the behaviour of fasting plasma glucose levels as a screening test for NIDDM in different populations is plotted. At any cut-off level the sensitivity of the test is greatest in the high-prevalence population. The relationship is somewhat more complicated, however, as indicated by the lower sensitivities in the intermediate-prevalence population. As also demonstrated in Table 3, it would appear that innate differences in glucose metabolism between populations may influence the performance characteristics of a particular screening test.

EVALUATION OF SCREENING PROGRAMS

Many disease screening programs have been instituted in the past without proper evaluation either before their establishment or during their operation [33]. Both screening procedures and programs for diabetes have generally been poorly evaluated. Fortunately, there is now

Table 2   Method of determining screening test characteristics in relation to true disease status (all numbers are hypothetical)

	True disease status		
	Positive	Negative	Total
Screening test status			
Positive	a (40)	b (100)	$a + b$ (140)
Negative	c (10)	d (900)	$c + d$ (910)
Total	$a + c$ (50)	$b + d$ (1000)	$a + b + c + d$ (1050)

Prevalence	$=$	$\dfrac{a + c}{a + b + c + d}$	$=$	$\dfrac{50}{1050}$	$=$ 4.8%
Sensitivity	$=$	$\dfrac{a}{a + c}$	$=$	$\dfrac{40}{50}$	$=$ 80.0%
Specificity	$=$	$\dfrac{d}{b + d}$	$=$	$\dfrac{900}{1000}$	$=$ 90.0%
Predictive value (+ve test)	$=$	$\dfrac{a}{a + b}$	$=$	$\dfrac{40}{140}$	$=$ 28.6%
Predictive value (−ve test)	$=$	$\dfrac{d}{c + d}$	$=$	$\dfrac{900}{910}$	$=$ 98.9%

recognition of the need for proper evaluation [13, 34].

Costs and Benefits

Evaluation must rest finally with some form of cost–benefit analysis where attempt is made to rationalize the costs and benefits that accrue to three diverse elements: screened individuals, the health services and the community at large. The major points requiring consideration are summarized in Table 4. At the level of individuals, costs may include the following: financial loss due to travel, time off work, and further medical consultation and diagnostic testing; the pain and discomfort of procedures undergone; and the unnecessary anxiety caused to false-positive screenees. Benefits include the earlier diagnosis of disease with resulting improved health and longevity, and the reassurance of good health in correctly identified, disease-free individuals.

For health services, costs that need to be considered are the direct and indirect costs associated with staff and resources (test materials, facilities, etc.) involved in the screening program, and the ensuing costs of further consultations, diagnostic investigations and treatment (which might in some cases be unwarranted). On the beneficial side, intervention in the early stages of disease

might lead to monetary savings on more expensive treatment, hospitalization and rehabilitation services. Although they carried out an incomplete cost–benefit analysis, Genuth et al. [35] calculated that expenses accrued over 6 years to a mass screening program in Cleveland in the USA could be offset if 4.2% of 8400 previously undetected diabetics were spared 1 week of hospitalization which they might have required if diagnosis was left until the appearance of symptoms. However, even if their figures for the direct and indirect costs of the program were correct, and although the possibility of such savings on hospitalization seems superficially to be eminently plausible, evaluation based on numerous assumptions is always questionable.

For the community, the costs of a screening program can be considered mainly in terms of the opportunity cost of scarce resources (money, personnel and facilities) diverted from other potential uses, either within the health context (such as primary prevention) or outside it (social welfare, education, and so on). Benefits of the screening program to the community might conversely follow from overall savings on health expenditure which can be put to other uses, and as described in the literature of diabetes screening, a much-vaunted role in increasing public awareness and education [8]. It is likely, however, that there are much more efficient methods

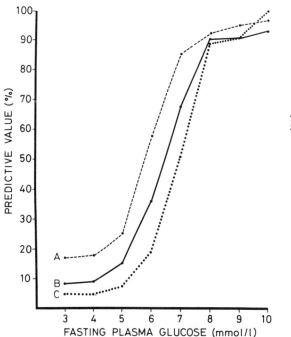

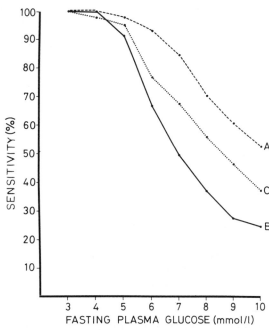

Figure 2 Predictive value of different levels of fasting plasma glucose as a screening test for undetected or untreated NIDDM in adults aged 20–74 years in three populations with varying disease prevalence (NIDDM defined as plasma glucose value 11.1 mmol/l or above 2 hours following a 75-g OGTT). A, Micronesian Nauruans (prevalence 17.1%); B, Fijian Indians (prevalence 8.7%); C, Fijian Melanesians (urban) (prevalence 5.1%)

Figure 3 Sensitivity of different levels of fasting plasma glucose as a screening test for undetected or untreated NIDDM in adults aged 20–74 years in three populations with varying disease prevalence (NIDDM defined as plasma glucose value 11.1 mmol/l or above, 2 hours following a 75-g OGTT). A, Micronesian Nauruans (prevalence 17.1%); B, Fijian Indians (prevalence 8.7%); C, Fijian Melanesians (urban) (prevalence 5.1%)

of educating the public about diabetes than through screening programs.

Measures and Pitfalls

Important indices that need to be considered in evaluation of screening programs include the following *process* measures—the proportion of the target population who actually receive screening, the prevalence of disease detected in screenees, total expenditure on the program, the cost per screenee and case detected, and the predictive value of a positive test.

Additionally, important measures of *outcome* must be reckoned with. In the first instance, the frequency of complications such as proteinuria, retinopathy, hypertension and ischemic heart disease, already present at the time of diagnosis, can be compared in screen-detected and symptom-detected cases. Subsequently, measures of morbidity (number of hospitalizations, days

off work, frequency of development of particular complications and mortality) can be determined and compared with a reference group.

It is important to consider, however, potential biases that act to exaggerate the efficacy of screening [7]. Firstly, it is possible that those cases detected by screening represent the milder end of the disease spectrum with better prognoses (more severe cases present earlier in their course with symptoms) and might not normally have high complication rates anyway. This is known as *length bias*. *Lead-time bias* operates where screen-detected cases appear to take longer to develop complications, and survive longer, than do symptom-detected cases: in reality this may be a false impression due to the fact that their diagnosis has effectively been brought forward in time.

Comparisons might also be biased by inclusion amongst screen-detected groups of a

Table 3 Characteristics of fasting plasma glucose measurement as a screening test for NIDDM in various Pacific Island populations (see footnote for criteria)

Population	Number	Prevalence of undetected NIDDM* (%)	Sensitivity (%)	Specificity (%)	Predictive value (%)	
					Positive test	Negative test
Fijian Melanesians						
Rural	466	1.3	50.0	99.6	60.0	99.3
Urban	838	5.1	55.8	99.2	80.0	97.6
Western Samoans (Polynesian)						
Rural	714	2.2	87.5	99.9	93.3	99.7
Urban	701	6.6	69.6	99.4	88.9	97.9
Fijian Indians	1211	8.7	39.0	99.5	87.2	94.5
Nauruans (Micronesian)						
20–44 years	959	8.3	71.3	99.2	89.1	97.4
45–74 years	318	43.7	75.5	95.0	92.1	83.3

Fasting plasma glucose value of 7.8 mmol/l or above constitutes a positive screening test. For purposes of illustration, NIDDM is defined as a plasma glucose value of 11.1 mmol/l or over 2 hours following a 75-g OGTT.
* Limited to all adults aged 20–74 years with both fasting and 2-hour specimens, and not on hypoglycemic medications (includes some previously diagnosed but untreated cases).

number of misclassified individuals, or those who may under normal circumstances (that is, without medical intervention) have reverted to normal glucose tolerance. This phenomenon is known as *pseudodisease* [7]. It is unclear how often this may occur amongst those whose glucose levels fall within the NIDDM range, but the high frequency of 'reversion' to normal tolerance in individuals originally classified as having IGT is well documented [36].

A fourth factor that may bias evaluation of diabetes screening programs is *prognostic selection*, whereby those who are willing to attend screening services are likely to be more health conscious and amenable to undergoing treatment and changing life-style than are those not interested enough to undergo screening in the first place [7].

Methods of Evaluation

Comparison of clinical characteristics and outcome measures between screen-detected and symptom-detected cases is a common method of evaluation (often used for cancer screening programs), but is subject to the four sources of bias described above. The extent of such biases is difficult to determine, however, and little can be done to account for them beyond being aware of their potential influence, if this form of evaluation is undertaken.

Another less than satisfactory approach is to compare outcome measures before and after the start of screening activities. It may be difficult to discount the influence of temporal changes in disease patterns, although the incorporation of a control population into the 'before and after'

Table 4 Costs and benefits associated with disease screening programs

Level	Costs	Benefits
Individuals	Financial: travel, loss of earnings, medical consultation, diagnostic tests, treatment Other: pain and discomfort of procedures, anxiety	Improved health outcome Reassurance of health Potentially improved earning capacity
Health services	Direct and indirect costs of staff and resources allocated to screening Further diagnostic investigations and treatment	Potential savings on treatment and rehabilitation services needed if disease had not been detected early
Community	Opportunity cost of resources diverted from other potential uses to screening program	Potential benefit of savings on overall health expenditure diverted to other uses Public awareness and education

design may allow a reasonable assessment of the influence of secular trends. The use of a 'before and after' comparison (with or without a control group) requires that appropriate measures of disease outcome have been collected in the past, and, in order to optimize the chance of drawing conclusions, that the newly introduced screening service is implemented widely [7, 37]. Case-control techniques have been utilized successfully in studies of cancer screening programs [7], but are likely to be very difficult to apply to evaluation of diabetes screening.

Experimental methods will ultimately give the most objective answer to questions concerning the efficacy of screening services. Unfortunately, logistic and ethical considerations preclude the use of randomized controlled trials. It would be most difficult to randomize asymptomatic individuals to screening versus non-screening groups, and it would be equally impractical and perhaps unethical to screen individuals for glucose intolerance but act on the result in only half of the screenees. Thus, it would appear that the most satisfactory method of assessing diabetes screening programs will be by comparing outcome measures between control or reference communities and a demonstration 'screening' community. The problems of ensuring comparability of such areas will need to be considered, but the method is the most likely to provide acceptable evidence for the impact of diabetes screening services.

The need for proper evaluation of diabetes screening programs has long been recognized. A meeting of experts held in Atlanta, USA, in 1979 [13] formally recommended that screening in non-pregnant populations should be conducted only in the context of well-designed research projects, some of which might specifically attempt to evaluate the effectiveness of screening. To date, apart from studies that have assessed the validity of alternative screening tests [9, 11], no properly controlled evaluated studies of diabetes screening programs have been reported. There is, therefore, no convincing evidence for the efficacy of screening asymptomatic non-pregnant persons for glucose intolerance.

HISTORY OF SCREENING
FOR DIABETES

Early attempts to detect diabetes by screening were based on tests for glycosuria performed in World War I military recruits and life insurance applicants (see review by West [8]). After World War II, screening programs in the USA began to be instituted on a mass basis in a number of states, apparently following the lead of the American Diabetes Association, and often involving contributions from both government and lay groups [8, 35].

Screening for diabetes has not been so warmly embraced outside the USA. Surveys in places such as Birmingham, UK [38], Busselton, Australia [20] and Bergen, Norway [39] were primarily epidemiological studies which also attempted to answer questions about community screening programs. A mass screening project in Ferrara, Italy was recently reported to have favourably influenced the rate of progression of IGT to clinical diabetes, and to have led to a reduction in the incidence of NIDDM in this community [40]; however, there are many potential biases in this study, and the optimistic conclusions of the authors seem unwarranted.

One of the better-documented and better-evaluated programs was that conducted during the 1960s and 1970s in Cleveland, USA, on over 600 000 persons, and based on a screening blood glucose test 2 hours following a 75-g glucose load [34, 35, 41]. Eventually, this mass screening program was downgraded to a more discriminating program wherein community detection for gestational diabetes was initiated, and further screening was performed only on request, particularly in subjects over the age of 40 years [41]. The reasons for the change largely reflected the lack of specificity and poor predictive value of the screening test [35, 41], with consequent worries concerning incorrect disease labelling in false-positive screenees [34], and the recognition that not enough was known about either the natural history of lesser degrees of glucose intolerance or the effectiveness and safety of treatment in this group [34, 41].

A consensus conference in Atlanta, USA, in 1978 recommended that evidence available at that time did not support the need for either community *or* high-risk (except in pregnancy) screening programs for detection of states of asymptomatic glucose intolerance [13]. Their conclusions were drawn against the background of (a) availability of more objective assessment of diabetes screening programs [41]; (b) a growing interest by epidemiologists in the study of diabetes [8]; and (c) results of the University Group Diabetes Project (UGDP) which suggested that treatment of asymptomatic NIDDM with oral hypoglycemic agents did not favourably influence disease end-points [42]. Notwithstanding dissenting voices [43], the view of the Atlanta Workshop has largely prevailed since that time [14, 19, 44, 45], although some continue to advocate screening high-risk individuals, such as those with a family history of diabetes, and the obese [3, 43]. Surprising statements such as 'Diabetes mellitus is so rampant in the United States that the clinician should screen everyone for it routinely . . .' [46] still appear in major textbooks.

Recently, the American Diabetes Association released a position statement [100] which appears to legitimize community and physician screening programs for NIDDM, although the statement did recommend that measurement of blood glucose should only be performed in subjects with demonstrated risk factors. As subsequently pointed out by Nathan and Singer [101], this liberalization of the 'official' attitude to screening seems unfounded, as there is little new evidence to challenge the previous consensus view that screening for NIDDM is inappropriate [13, 14, 19, 44, 45].

Despite calls for more research into the effectiveness of diabetes screening programs [13, 43], little new work has appeared recently. A report from New South Wales, Australia, looked at the results of mass detection exercises in that state based on random blood glucose measurement ascertained with portable reflectance meters, and found the test to be insensitive and surprisingly non-specific, and that a high proportion of positive screenees did not seek follow-up testing [5].

LIMITATIONS IN SCREENING FOR GLUCOSE INTOLERANCE—WHEN IS IT DIABETES?

There is no doubt that IDDM is a life-threatening disease, and that symptomatic NIDDM patients require therapy. There remains some doubt, however, whether asymptomatic individuals who have normal levels of fasting blood glucose, but who demonstrate abnormalities of glucose tolerance in response to glucose loads, will benefit from treatment [43, 47].

The current criteria for diagnosis of IGT and diabetes [1–3] are largely based on studies showing an excess of complications in those who fall into certain ranges of glucose intolerance, defined by the 2-hour postload glucose level [48–50]. However, it can be argued that particularly in the IGT range, the results are inconclusive [47, 51]. A number of longitudinal studies have documented the variable natural history of the IGT category: over a 6-year period, around one-third of Nauruans with IGT progress to NIDDM, one-third remain glucose intolerant, and one-third revert to normal glucose tolerance [36]. This 'instability' is even more marked (for both IGT and NIDDM, so defined) if glucose tolerance tests are performed more closely together in time [24, 52, 102, 103]. It is therefore essential for clinical diagnosis that before an asymptomatic individual is labelled as diabetic, at least one repeat test value should be in the diabetic range [3].

Unfortunately, longitudinal studies that have demonstrated a gradation in mortality and coronary heart disease incidence with increasing levels of glucose intolerance have been based on single initial glucose tolerance tests. The potential for misclassification of an individual's real glucose tolerance status (acceptable for epidemiological studies where the aim is prevalence estimation) [3] will therefore weaken the ability of these studies to show differences between groups. It remains possible that elevations of risk seen in individuals with 'IGT' may be spurious due to the presence of a number of misclassified 'diabetics'.

Of more concern, however, is the notion that diabetic glucose intolerance per se (in the diabetic range based on 2-hour postload values, but with normal fasting glucose levels) may not really be diabetes [8]. It may be a stage in the evolution of diabetes; however, at present it is not particularly clear from published studies to what extent morbidity and mortality attributed to individuals classified as NIDDM on the basis of glucose tolerance testing can be divided between those with fasting hyperglycemia (which should be most of those prone to continuous hyperglycemia on a day-to-day basis) on the one hand, and those who show elevated 2-hour levels only when subjected to the unnatural stress of a glucose tolerance test, on the other. It has been cogently argued that diabetes might best be defined in terms of sustained elevations of basal glucose levels, as reflected in levels of glycated proteins [47].

The late Kelly West remained unconvinced that mild states of glucose intolerance had major adverse implications for health [8]. Data from a longitudinal study conducted in the Micronesian Nauruan population, who have one of the highest incidence rates of NIDDM yet recorded [36], support this view. Nauruans with high 2-hour plasma glucose concentrations, but normal fasting glycemia, suffer microvascular complication rates (microalbuminuria and retinopathy) more compatible with rates seen in individuals with IGT than in diabetics who have fasting hyperglycemia [104]. Furthermore, over a 6-year follow-up period (1982–87), both mortality and hospital admission rates in a group of 68 Nauruans with normal fasting but diabetic 2-hour postload glucose levels were similar to rates in those with normal and impaired glucose tolerance (Table 5). The differences were independent of treatment instituted on the basis of the baseline glucose values. These and other data suggest that fasting hyperglycemia may most effectively distinguish those at risk of adverse outcomes [104]. Individuals with glucose intolerance in the diabetic range, but with normal fasting glycemia, in fact appear to have more in common with the IGT category.

It does not yet appear sufficiently clear that a glucose tolerance test should be required to define 'diabetes'. In clinical practice very few cases of diabetes are diagnosed on the basis of an OGTT, whereas OGTTs are the corner-stone of most modern epidemiological studies of NIDDM. This has led to a curious imbalance between diabetes defined clinically versus that defined epidemiologically. Reanalysis of existing data sets along the lines of those performed in Nauruans, should help to clarify the importance of abnormal tolerance with normal fasting values. Longitudinal population studies with baseline data on both glycated proteins and glucose tolerance related to subsequent development of complications and mortality are keenly awaited. The implication for diabetes screening is that if the argument of Duncan and Heiss [47] is valid, it may not be worth screening for glucose intolerance, and measures of either fasting glucose levels or glycated proteins may be more appropriate—and certainly simpler.

It is likely, however, that the situation is much more complicated. The sustained elevated level

Table 5 Six-year mortality and three-year hospital admission data for Micronesian Nauruans with varying degrees of glucose intolerance and fasting glycemia (limited to subjects with baseline values available for fasting plasma glucose and for plasma glucose 2 hours following a 75-g OGTT)

	Diabetic		Impaired glucose tolerance ($7.8 \leqslant 2PG < 11.1$ mmol/l, FPG < 7.8 mmol/l)	Normal glucose tolerance ($2PG \geqslant 7.8$ mmol/l, FPG < 7.8 mmol/l)
	Fasting hyperglycemia (FPG $\geqslant 7.8$ mmol/l)	Fasting normoglycemia ($2PG \geqslant 11.1$ mmol/l, FPG < 7.8 mmol/l)		
Number studied	307	68	280	884
Mortality (1982–87)				
Percentage	24.8	7.4	6.4	3.5
95% CI	20.0–29.6	1.2–13.6	3.5–9.3	2.3–4.7
Hospital admissions (1982–84)				
Percentage with at least one admission	45.0	29.4	28.2	23.8
95% CI	39.4–50.6	18.6–40.2	22.9–33.5	22.4–25.2

FPG, fasting plasma glucose; 2PG, plasma glucose 2 hours following 75-g OGTT; CI, confidence interval.

of insulin seen in many subjects with IGT (and NIDDM), before decompensation [53], may in itself be an important risk factor for cardiovascular disease, independent of glucose levels [54]. Following decompensation, with a fall in insulin levels and a rise in glucose levels, the latter might become the important risk factor. Hence, even if diabetes is not defined 'correctly', screening to detect asymptomatic hyperinsulinemic glucose intolerance might still be of value, provided that treatment is shown to influence prognosis favourably in those so detected.

METHODS AVAILABLE FOR DIABETES SCREENING

Diabetes is currently defined either by classic symptomatology and clearly elevated fasting or casual blood glucose levels, or by the demonstration of abnormal glucose levels during a standardized OGTT [1–3]. Assessment of screening tests for presymptomatic disease must therefore be made against this latter standard, notwithstanding reservations concerning the OGTT as discussed above. In a special class are immunological and genetic screening tests that may be used to identify individuals at increased risk for development of IDMM; their potential is judged in relation to their success in predicting disease onset.

Methods are considered here from the point of view of their usefulness solely as diagnostic screening tools, irrespective of their application in the clinical and self-monitoring context, and notwithstanding questions concerning the utility of screening itself.

Urine Glucose Testing

There is no place for urine testing as a screening tool where there is a means available (including reflectance meters) to measure blood glucose. Urine testing has neither acceptable sensitivity nor specificity [8, 23, 52]. Its use can be advocated only where blood testing is either not available, or is particularly expensive. Even in the latter situation, however, costs involved in confirmatory testing in positive screenees (depending on the level accepted as positive) may eventually outweigh savings due to initial use of urine tests. The renal threshold for glucose varies with age (higher), sex (lower in men), pregnancy (lower) and ethnic group, as well as demonstrating wide

variability between individuals [8, 23]. Hence the validity of urinary glucose as a standard screening test is highly questionable. Furthermore, sensitivity and specificity will vary depending on the level of glycosuria deemed significant, the state of hydration of subjects and the type of test strips used.

Its sensitivity has been shown to rise from 16.7% for fasting values to 72.7% for 2-hour postload values, with corresponding falls in specificity from 97.9% to 77.4% and predictive value (positive test) from 33.3% to 22.2%, using current diagnostic criteria in a British population [52]. In comparison with other potential screening tests such as fasting blood glucose, 2-hour blood glucose and glycohemoglobin, these figures are unappealing [8, 52].

Some research [49] and public health-oriented [40] screening programs have in the past employed glycosuria as the initial screen in a multistage process. Such a method cannot be recommended, for a number of reasons. Firstly, the prevalence of glucose intolerance will be underestimated because of the insensitivity of the first test. Secondly, if descriptive epidemiology and exploration of etiological hypotheses are to be pursued, then cases detected through such a multistage procedure are unlikely to be typical, leading to biased results. Thirdly, if the principal aims relate to public health, and are presumably based on the belief that treating detected cases will improve their prognosis, then there seems little point in using an instrument acknowledged to be inferior.

The utility of testing urine with multitest strips as a screening tool during hospital admissions, primary health care contacts and at general practitioner visits can also be questioned, unless there are specific indications for assessing other parameters such as hematuria and proteinuria. If one is really interested in screening for diabetes, then more sensitive and specific methods are indicated. However, where symptoms of diabetes are present, a positive urine test will be strongly supportive of the diagnosis.

Glycated Proteins

Tests for glycohemoglobin and its subfractions and, to a lesser extent, other glycated proteins such as glycated albumin and fructosamine, are generally accepted as useful guides to control of blood glucose over variable preceding periods of weeks to months. However, initial enthusiasm for their usefulness as diagnostic and screening tools has waned in most [11, 23, 55] but not all [47, 52] quarters.

Glycohemoglobin testing has been shown to have superior sensitivity and specificity to casual blood glucose measurement in detecting NIDDM [56], although these authors noted that glucose determination was cheaper, simpler and quicker. However, studies have shown that glycohemoglobin is inferior to fasting blood glucose as a screening test for detecting both NIDDM and the combined group of IGT and NIDDM [11, 56]. Furthermore, combinations of glycohemoglobin and fasting plasma glucose measurements have not been found to improve predictive value relative to fasting plasma glucose alone [11].

Glycohemoglobin measurement is also less effective when compared against 2-hour postload glucose as a single screening test. With equivalent sensitivity of 90%, Forrest et al [52] found that a screening 2-hour postload glucose test had 93.3% specificity and 47.9% predictive value for NIDDM confirmed in a second full OGTT (WHO criteria), as against 64.5% and 9.5%, respectively, for the screening glycohemoglobin. However, the latter's specificity was higher (85.3%), but still with a low predictive value of 14%, at the same level of sensitivity, when compared against 'probable' NIDDM as determined from the screening 2-hour glucose value [52]. This difference apparently reflects the larger intraindividual coefficient of variation for the 2-hour blood glucose level, compared with glycohemoglobin.

Considerable but variable (perhaps related to methods) overlap has been observed in the glycohemoglobin distributions of subjects with normal, impaired and diabetic glucose tolerance, respectively [11, 52, 57, 105], which further emphasizes the inadequacies of glycohemoglobin measurement as a screening test for diabetes.

Serum fructosamine testing, largely because of its cheapness and ease of determination, was initially proposed as a potentially useful tool for diabetes screening [58], but this early enthusiasm has not been vindicated in population screening exercises [59, 60]. The evidence suggests that the method has inappropriate sensitivity and predictic value for detection of glucose intolerance [55, 59, 60, 105]. Serial serum fructosamine

measurements have been suggested as a potential method for detecting onset of GDM during the third trimester [55], but the utility of this technique awaits evaluation.

The conclusion must be, therefore, that with diabetes defined in terms of the glucose tolerance test, measurements of glycated proteins do not yet offer sufficient ability to discriminate between subjects with normal and abnormal glucose tolerance. However, as has been discussed earlier, the validity of the OGTT for diagnosis of 'real' diabetes [8, 47, 57, 104] has been questioned. Until data on the relative prognostic value of glycated proteins and mild abnormalities of glucose tolerance are available, an open mind must be kept on the usefulness of glycated protein measurement as a screening and diagnostic test [47, 57].

Blood Glucose and the OGTT

The various forms of abnormal glucose tolerance are defined in terms of raised blood glucose levels; with the diagnostic level depending on the nature of the specimen (venous or capillary whole blood, or plasma) and whether the blood is collected randomly (in relation to eating habit and time of day), in a fasting state, or at specified intervals following a standard glucose load [1–3]. It is hardly surprising, therefore, that blood glucose levels are currently the best means of detecting states of glucose intolerance.

The choice of biochemical methods and instruments used in the assay of glucose is discussed elsewhere in this book. It is worth emphasizing, however, that provided there is proper attention to detail, even portable reflectance meters give results with considerable accuracy and precision [23], although use of these meters by inadequately trained personnel and under non-standardized conditions (e.g. abnormal heat and humidity) may lead to spurious results [5].

Random (or casual) blood glucose testing has been shown, at equivalent levels of sensitivity, to have inferior specificity to both glycohemoglobin and fasting blood glucose measurement in detecting diabetes amongst a group selected in such a way as to include individuals at the higher end of the glucose distribution [56]. Depending on the cut-off level, casual blood glucose testing will always lead to a substantial number of misclassified individuals. The choice of high levels will improve specificity and predictive value of a positive test, but at the cost of a large number of false-negative subjects. Setting lower levels will improve sensitivity but lead to very poor specificity and predictive value, with increased costs related to the extra confirmatory tests required in false-positive subjects. Random plasma glucose testing has also been found to substantially under-estimate the prevalence of NIDDM (as determined using a 75-g OGTT) in a study of Micronesian Nauruans [106], indicating the disadvantages of using random glucose values in epidemiological studies.

Fasting whole blood (or plasma) glucose measurement has superior discriminatory power for diabetes when compared with measurement of glycated proteins such as glycohemoglobin [11, 56] and fructosamine [60]. The margin varies depending on the method by which subjects are chosen. With cut-off points set at equivalent levels of sensitivity, fasting glucose is more specific and has higher predictive value than glycohemoglobin [56].

Both the NDDG [1] and WHO [2, 3] recommend 75 g of glucose (or equivalent dissolved in water for the OGTT in adults, and diagnostic criteria are based on this load. There seems little sense in the continued use of 50-g, 100-g or other loads, except perhaps for particular research purposes. For diagnosis of GDM, however, the NDDG and the American Diabetes Association continue to recommend the complicated O'Sullivan criteria, based on a 50-g screening glucose load, followed by a diagnostic 100-g 3-hour OGTT [1, 26, 27, 61]. The WHO has made life easier for the rest of the world by retaining the 75-g load [3]. It is hoped that when further data become available concerning the prognostic significance of GDM and IGT in pregnancy, as defined by the WHO, the way will be clear for a single international standard for GDM.

Unfortunately, the NDDG and WHO guidelines were not sufficiently dogmatic in emphasizing that 75 g of glucose referred to 75 g of *anhydrous* glucose. The result has been that 75 g of glucose *monohydrate* (equivalent to 68 g of anhydrous glucose) has been used widely both in epidemiological studies and in clinical practice [104]. In effect, there are now two 'standard' 75-g loads and it does not seem that either can claim ascendancy.

Although surveys and screening programs have in the past used timed *postprandial* glucose

estimates based on both 'standard' and non-standard test meals [8, 62], there is nothing to recommend the method over the standardized OGTT. Certainly, a high postprandial blood glucose level, at an appropriate time interval, should be specific for diabetes, but questions will remain about sensitivity. Moreover, an oral glucose drink, whether a proprietary or 'homemade' product, is considerably quicker, easier and cheaper to prepare than a 'gourmet' meal.

Comparisons of differently timed blood collections taken during an OGTT, whether using NDDG or WHO criteria, show that fasting glucose has strikingly inferior sensitivity to both 2-hour [9, 11, 32] and 1-hour [9, 11, 63] postload glucose levels for diagnosis of diabetes. The 1-hour glucose value (NDDG criteria) has poorer specificity, however, than either fasting or 2-hour glucose levels [9].

In a study comprising both high-prevalence Mexican-Americans and moderate-prevalence Anglo-Americans, 2-hour postload blood glucose measurement was found to be the optimal single test for classifying diabetes according to both NDDG criteria, where it had specificity of over 99% and sensitivity of over 93%, and WHO criteria, with specificity of 100% (by definition), and sensitivity of over 90% [9].

Harris et al [63], comparing the NDDG and WHO criteria, found that the 2-hour postload glucose had a sensitivity of 97% using either system, and concluded that the WHO criteria provided a simpler, inclusive classification scheme. They recommended that in situations where multiple venepunctures were undesirable (such as epidemiological surveys and large screening programs) the 2-hour glucose level very satisfactorily classified individuals as having diabetes, IGT or neither. The WHO Study Group [3] also recommended that the 2-hour value alone was sufficient in these circumstances, noting that it was more robust against non-fasting subjects.

It should be emphasized again that, for clinical diagnosis, glucose tolerance tests are usually unnecessary [3]. For screening asymptomatic individuals to detect glucose intolerance, whether in the IGT or diabetes range, however, the inescapable conclusion is that casual and fasting blood specimens, and glycated proteins, are inadequate and that an OGTT is required.

It has been observed (Figure 3 and Table 3) that fasting glucose has greater sensitivity in populations with higher prevalence of diabetes [9, 28], related to differences in the distribution of glucose values between populations [9]. Thus, in high-prevalence groups (certain ethnic groups and the elderly being most appropriate), fasting glucose measurement may be deemed sufficiently sensitive to suit local screening requirements, when balanced against the extra cost and inconvenience associated with the OGTT. Where more sensitivity is necessary, a screening OGTT with 2-hour glucose will be favoured.

Unfortunately, the OGTT has poor intra-individual repeatability, particularly in the IGT range [24, 52, 102, 103], and clinicians should therefore seek further supportive blood glucose results from asymptomatic positive screenees before a final diagnosis is made. Moreover, as discussed previously, the lingering suspicion that individuals with glucose intolerance but normal fasting glucose and glycated protein levels may not in essence be 'diabetic', needs to be addressed by researchers [47, 57, 104].

TO SCREEN OR NOT TO SCREEN?

Insulin Dependent Diabetes Mellitus

First-degree relatives who are either HLA identical or HLA haploidentical to a proband with IDDM have an increased risk of developing the disease [64]. Furthermore, a high proportion of family members developing diabetes carry islet cell antibodies (ICA) for months to years before onset of disease, and overt decompensation may be heralded by a diminished acute insulin response during intravenous glucose tolerance tests [65, 66], and also by IGT as indicated by an OGTT [67]. On the basis of such evidence there has been optimism that it might one day be possible to prevent progress to overt diabetes in individuals found to harbour these immunological, genetic and biochemical markers [44, 66, 68, 69].

The problem of the efficacy of screening for IDDM is much simpler than that posed for NIDDM, in that IDDM is an all-or-none phenomenon, and that untreated it is incompatible with life. For NIDDM, GDM and IGT, the important question is whether disease endpoints can be altered favourably by early detection and treatment—that is, does screening have

a useful secondary preventive function? For IDDM, we need 'simply' to know if the disease can be prevented from occurring (primary prevention) in positive screenees and, even if the ultimate onset of the disease cannot be prevented, whether early identification and education of the 'at risk' will lead to significant savings (in human and economic terms) on morbidity and early mortality associated with disease onset.

First-degree relatives are an easily identified 'at risk' group, and their numbers can be readily reduced to a 'very high risk' group by HLA typing, ICA testing and glucose tolerance tests. If, however, onset of disease in this high-risk group cannot be prevented, then their identification through a series of increasingly invasive tests cannot be justified [70, 71]. Less intrusive education of family members in general concerning their increased risk, the identification of early symptoms and the importance of not delaying medical attention in the event that such symptoms arise, is likely to be both considerably more cost-effective and humane than specific prediction of risk in individuals.

Notwithstanding the arguments above, the vast majority of cases of IDDM are sporadic in origin [72], and hence even if primary prevention of onset in screen-detected susceptibles from IDDM families were possible, most cases in the community will continue to present symptomatically. Population-based screening of children for ICA and even for susceptibility genes has been seriously suggested by some [69]; at present, this would appear to be both expensive and unrealistic [70].

The last decade has provided exciting insights into the etiopathogenesis and early natural history of IDDM, and the possibility of prevention. However, this remains only a distant possibility. Not until properly conducted experimental trials have demonstrated successfully that the incidence of IDDM can be significantly reduced in screen-detected susceptibles from IDDM families will it be reasonable to *consider* the place of screening for IDDM [107, 108]. Even if primary prevention in high-risk individuals does become tenable in the years to come, it is difficult to foresee that screening could ever be applied beyond the confines of first-degree relatives of those suffering from IDDM. Hopes for prevention of the bulk of IDDM cases appear to lie with environmental modification [73].

Non-insulin Dependent Diabetes Mellitus

There are, at the time of writing, no appropriately conducted studies demonstrating that detection and treatment of those with asymptomatic NIDDM leads to significant reduction in morbidity and mortality. The only positive supportive data appear to result from an incompletely reported Italian study which has compared symptom-detected diabetics and screen-detected subjects with IGT who subsequently progressed to diabetes. This study found that there were no significant differences in rates of retinopathy, cataract, neuropathy or hyperlipidemia, but that there was a significant excess of macrovascular disease in a symptom-detected group [40]. It appears, however, that the symptom group may have had worse disease (29% required insulin versus 4.8% in the screened subjects). The comparison is also subject to important biases, as discussed earlier in the chapter, and many crucial methodological details of the study, such as whether investigators were aware of the group to which subjects belonged when they assessed complications, were not discussed.

On the negative side, the controversial University Group Diabetes Project (UGDP) results provide compelling evidence (in the face of no convincing contrary data) that pharmacological treatment does not influence the course of chronic microvascular and macrovascular complications of NIDDM [42, 74, 75]. This study compared two insulin treatment regimens, two oral hypoglycemic agents and a placebo agent in individuals with asymptomatic diabetes of less than one year's duration. This group is likely to be similar to those detected by screening, and particularly by a high-risk screening strategy. There were no significant reductions for drug compared with placebo treatment for total or cardiovascular mortality, rates of retinopathy and blindness, proteinuria, or peripheral vascular disease, over a follow-up period of up to $14\frac{1}{2}$ years and despite good control of fasting blood glucose in one of the insulin treatment groups [75]. Oral hypoglycemic agents were withdrawn during the trial because of apparent adverse effects on cardiovascular and total mortality [42, 74, 75]. Each of the five treatment groups received dietary advice, and the study does not assess whether this alone may influence complication rates.

There are a number of short-term experimental studies that have shown improvements in glucose tolerance and insulin resistance in subjects with NIDDM in response to strict dietary and life-style change [76, 77]. Intensive insulin therapy has also been shown to reverse metabolic abnormalities in NIDDM [78]. However, the duration of these effects and the implications for long-term complications remain unknown.

West [43], reviewing experimental and other evidence for the value of early diabetes detection, felt that screening programs would be more effective than education alone in reducing the number of undiscovered asymptomatic cases, and in decreasing the proportion of cases presenting late with gangrene and ketoacidosis. This seems a rather insubstantial argument on which to recommend screening and it is, indeed, likely that effectively run and appropriately directed media campaigns will be a more cost-effective means of educating the wider community about diabetes.

Currently, the best evidence available for evaluating the potential usefulness of screening asymptomatic individuals for NIDDM is the UGDP study. The failure to show a beneficial effect (and the possibility of a harmful effect) of treatment in a group of individuals likely to be similar to those detected by screening asymptomatic adults for NIDDM, cannot be ignored [44]. Screening cannot be justified without firm evidence that treatment improves prognosis in such cases. Until contrary data appear, it would seem unwise to recommend either mass or high-risk screening strategies for NIDDM, except, perhaps, in a few remarkable high-prevalence populations. Certainly, the recently released American Diabetes Association position statement condoning high-risk community screening for NIDDM in the US population seems ill-advised [100, 101], as does an Australian recommendation to screen for NIDDM (and IGT) by periodic OGTTs in adults [109]. Even the Atlanta Workshop's earlier statement that blood glucose screening might 'be justified as one of several components in programs to detect and control the risk factors associated with cardiovascular diseases' [13] seems unwarranted. At present, it would seem better advice that attention be concentrated on factors for which there is more evidence that intervention may be of value— such as cigarette smoking, hypertension and hyperlipidemia [79].

Impaired Glucose Tolerance

Subjects with IGT have been shown in a number of studies to be at high risk of progressing to NIDDM, although the majority will not progress during follow-up periods of at least 10 years [36, 80]. The factors that best predict progression from IGT to NIDDM appear to be fasting and 2-hour blood glucose levels, decreased insulin response, and obesity [36, 53, 80, 81, 104], but at present the ability to identify successfully those *individuals* who will progress to NIDDM has not been demonstrated.

There is conflicting evidence as to the effectiveness of therapeutic intervention in IGT. Neither the Bedford [81] nor the Whitehall [80] studies showed that treatment with oral hypoglycemic agents (tolbutamide and phenformin, respectively) or diet lessened the rate of deterioration to NIDDM over 5-year or 10-year periods. A follow-up study of women with postgestational IGT as defined by an intravenous glucose tolerance test also failed to note a significant effect of treatment with oral hypoglycemic agents. Stowers et al. [82] did not find any difference in subsequent rates of glucose intolerance in women treated with either diet or diet plus chlorpropamide. Their study did not include a control group, so the effectiveness of dietary advice cannot be ascertained.

Sartor et al. [62], however, found significant reductions in diabetes incidence from IGT in groups treated with either diet alone, or with combination diet and tolbutamide, compared with a non-treated group. In contrast to the UGDP study [42, 74, 75], the drug treatment group did not experience increased cardiovascular or total mortality. These workers concluded that progression from IGT to NIDDM could be prevented by treatment with diet and sulfonylureas (at adequate doses) and advocated the development of screening procedures for identification of those with IGT, followed by active treatment [62].

Unfortunately, for a number of reasons—including the manner in which IGT was defined, and the fact that the non-treatment group had worse baseline glucose tolerance and more frequently family histories of diabetes than the treatment groups—this study is inconclusive. Certainly, if analysed on the basis of the original treatment groups, there does not appear to be any advantage of tolbutamide treatment over diet alone in reducing diabetes incidence or mortality [62].

More compelling, perhaps, are the results of Cederholm [110], who found that a combination of dietary advice and encouragement of physical activity resulted in significant improvements in glucose tolerance, blood pressure, body mass index, total cholesterol and triglycerides over a period of 6 months in a randomized controlled study of Swedish subjects with IGT. However, longer-term follow-up information on outcome in these subjects is not available, and a possible bias was introduced as the treatment and control groups were studied over unequal periods (6 versus 10 months, respectively) [110].

Regrettably, no new data have appeared that can clarify the contradictions posed by these studies. Until convincing evidence of efficacious therapeutic interventions is forthcoming, there are no grounds for recommendation of screening activities directed specifically at detection of IGT [14, 44].

Gestational Diabetes Mellitus

This discussion is limited to the merits of detection of previously unrecognized abnormal glucose tolerance during pregnancy. Unfortunately, despite recommendations by a number of review groups [13, 26, 27], the last decade has produced surprisingly little informative new research relating screening, diagnostic criteria and therapeutic interventions to perinatal and maternal outcomes.

Despite the acceptance of (almost) standardized criteria for glucose intolerance in non-pregnant women [1–3], considerable confusion remains over standards for GDM. The WHO Study Group advocates the same criteria irrespective of pregnancy [3], whereas the NDDG [1] and American Diabetes Association (ADA) [26, 27] continue to recommend 50-g oral glucose screening tests and diagnostic criteria that have their basis in those originally proposed by O'Sullivan and Mahan in 1964 [61]. These criteria were developed statistically (mean glucose level plus 2 standard deviations) but were subsequently shown to be associated with maternal and perinatal outcome [83], at a time when the general level of obstetric and perinatal care was inferior to current standards [44]. However, particularly in North America, the O'Sullivan criteria have become so entrenched that there has been a blinkered approach to fresh research into screening and diagnostic standards for GDM [111]. Curiously, some workers and review groups have recognized the need for proper evaluation of programs in relation to outcomes, but at the same time recommended widespread introduction of screening and therapeutic intervention on the basis of often uncontrolled and ill-substantiated findings [26, 27, 84].

West [43] considered that there was insufficient evidence that glucose intolerance in the absence of fasting hyperglycemia was an independent risk factor for complications in pregnancy. This view has been supported by studies using the relatively low fasting values of the O'Sullivan or similar criteria [85–87], and more recently, the higher fasting cut-off value (7.8 mmol/l in plasma) of the WHO criteria [88].

Li et al. [88] compared the WHO and NDDG criteria in women at risk of developing GDM and found that 51% of women with GDM by NDDG standards had normal glucose tolerance according to WHO criteria. Moreover, there were no major differences in perinatal outcome between treatment and control groups in women who were either normal or IGT by WHO standards. This is an important finding, and if verified should lead to more widespread acceptance of the simpler WHO criteria for GDM. These results also support the assertion that fasting hyperglycemia may be more important in determining adverse outcomes of pregnancy than glucose intolerance alone [43].

In contrast, Pettitt et al [89], using WHO criteria but based only on the 2-hour postload glucose level, concluded that screening for and recognition of IGT in pregnancy was worthwhile in the highly NIDDM-susceptible Pima Indian population. They found trends for increasing rates of perinatal mortality, macrosomia and toxemia—but not for congenital malformations or prematurity—with increasing glucose intolerance. Examination of their data, however, shows that with the exception of macrosomia, the evidence for significantly higher rates in women with impaired glucose tolerance is not convincing. Indeed, the 2-hour level of 11.1 mmol/l seems to distinguish most clearly the group at risk of serious complications. A more recent paper from the same workers confirms this [90]. There were no significant differences in rates for any perinatal or maternal complications between women with

IGT in pregnancy and normal glucose tolerance (WHO criteria). A higher rate of Caesarean sections in women with IGT may reflect obstetric practice more than necessity. Again, an obvious elevation in complication rates occurred only at 2-hour glucose levels above 11.1 mmol/l.

It has been shown that the offspring of known diabetic mothers suffer high rates of obesity and diabetes in later life, and much of this effect has been attributed to the abnormal intrauterine environment [91, 92]. GDM and even IGT in pregnancy may convey similar risk at glucose levels that may not be of immediate danger to the mother or baby [90].

This raises the question of the level of 'complication' attributed to glucose intolerance during pregnancy that is deemed sufficiently serious to warrant attempts at detection and control of maternal glucose. Is it worth (in economic and human terms) screening and treating perhaps hundreds of women with mild glucose intolerance to prevent a few offspring from developing NIDDM perhaps 50 years later? In the more immediate scenario, there are doubts whether even macrosomia in its own right is a sufficient justification [88, 93].

Braveman et al [93] suggested that complication rates associated with GDM may have been overestimated as a result of a selective underreporting of the presence of GDM in uncomplicated deliveries. There is also reasonable evidence that IGT in pregnancy has complication rates similar to those of women with normal glucose tolerance [88–90]. Moreover, the efficacy of, and relative indications for, insulin versus dietary intervention in GDM remain unclear [94–97]. In this climate, recommendation of routine screening for GDM by glucose tolerance tests seems rash [98].

The 1985 International Workshop-Conference on Gestational Diabetes recommended that *all* pregnant women should undergo 50-g oral glucose screening tests between the 24th and 28th week of pregnancy. Although not clearly stated, by implication they intended that diagnostic 100-g OGTTs should be reserved for positive screenees and those at particular risk for GDM [27]. The 1985 WHO Study Group advocated screening for GDM, but elaborated neither on the method to be used, nor the degree of coverage intended in the pregnant population [3].

The American recommendations for continued use of the O'Sullivan criteria seem irksome [111] and are rarely followed elsewhere. There is now some documentation that a single plasma glucose test performed 2 hours after a 75-g glucose load and interpreted by WHO criteria adequately identifies women at risk of complicated pregnancies [88–90]. Furthermore, if evidence can be presented that complication rates in those with normal fasting values but 'diabetic' (11.1 mmol/l or over) 2-hour postload values by WHO criteria are not greatly dissimilar from rates in control groups, then the Utopian quest for routine screening OGTTs may be discarded. A more pragmatic, less expensive and (it is hoped) more valid and frequently used recommendation for routine screening during pregnancy, based on fasting glucose levels alone, might be possible.

That the issue is a complex one is undoubted. However, unless screening and treatment regimens for GDM are established now on the basis of properly controlled and evaluated studies, physicians and pregnant women may bear the cost and discomfort of unnecessary procedures and treatment for many years to come.

CONCLUSIONS

Many physicians nurture the hope that IDDM and NIDDM may be preventable. There are grounds for belief that primary prevention of many cases of NIDDM may be achievable through promoting a generally healthy life-style [70, 99]. Enthusiasts even foresee the day when primary prevention of IDDM might be possible through environmental modification [73]—but in the meantime, hopes rest on preventing the small proportion of cases that occur in high-risk family members detected by immunogenetic screening [66, 68, 70]. However, therapeutic intervention has not yet proved successful, and on humane grounds routine screening of first-degree relatives of IDDM probands cannot be advocated.

It is known that most communities harbour a considerable number of adults with asymptomatic glucose intolerance. The concept of 'screening for diabetes' was born for the salvation of these individuals. The expectations have not, however, been fulfilled: to date there is no sound evidence that detection and treatment of asymptomatic glucose intolerance results in improved longevity or quality of life. Whether screening in 'high-risk' individuals is a legitimate activity remains unproven and cannot be recommended as routine [13]. It is likely that funds might be better spent on education campaigns relating to symptoms of diabetes and healthy life-style promotion than on diabetes screening programs. There are definite grounds for advocating some form of screening for GDM, but the evidence for routine glucose tolerance testing is not as convincing as many think it to be.

There is considerable need for well-planned and properly evaluated controlled trials of outcomes in screened and unscreened populations. Studies should continue to ask whether any form of screening for glucose intolerance is appropriate in the general or high-risk population, and to clarify the nature of the screening test most appropriate to pregnancy. The questions are important and have long remained unanswered. The studies may be difficult, unglamorous and time-consuming, but are essential. Widespread recommendation of screening procedures and interventions not proven to be efficacious should no longer be tolerated.

REFERENCES

1. National Diabetes Data Group. Classification and diagnosis of diabetes mellitus and other categories of glucose intolerance. Diabetes 1979; 28: 1039–57.
2. World Health Organization Expert Committee on Diabetes Mellitus. Second Report. Technical Report Series 646. Geneva: WHO, 1980.
3. Diabetes Mellitus: Report of a WHO Study Group. Technical Report Series 727. Geneva: WHO, 1985.
4. Commission on Chronic Illness. Chronic illness in the United States: prevention of chronic illness, vol, 1. Cambridge, Mass: Harvard University Press, 1957.
5. Moses RG, Colagiuri S, Shannon AG. Effectiveness of mass screening for diabetes mellitus using random blood glucose measurements. Med J Aust 1985; 143: 544–6.
6. Whitby LG. Screening for disease: definitions and criteria. Lancet 1974; ii: 819–21.
7. Morrison AS. Screening in chronic disease. Monographs in epidemiology and biostatistics, vol. 7. New York: Oxford University Press, 1985.
8. West KM. Epidemiology of diabetes and its vascular lesions. New York: Elsevier, 1978.
9. Haffner SM, Rosenthal M, Hazuda HP, Stern MP, Franco LJ. Evaluation of three potential

screening tests for diabetes mellitus in a biethnic population. Diabetes Care 1984; 7: 347–53.

10. Hoskins PL, Handelsman DJ, Hannelly T, Silink M, Yue DK, Turtle JR. Glycosylated hemoglobin as an index of the prevalence and severity of diabetes in biethnic Fiji. Diabetes Res Clin Pract 1987; 3: 257–67.

11. Modan M, Halkin H, Karasik A, Lusky A. Effectiveness of glycosylated hemoglobin, fasting plasma glucose, and a single post load plasma glucose level in population screening for glucose intolerance. Am J Epidemiol 1984; 119: 431–44.

12. Stern E, Blau J, Rusecki Y, Rafaelovsky M, Cohen MP. Prevalence of diabetes in Israel: epidemiologic survey. Diabetes 1988; 37: 297–302.

13. Herron CA. Screening in diabetes mellitus: report of the Atlanta Workshop. Diabetes Care 1979; 2: 357–62.

14. Editorial. Screening for carbohydrate intolerance. Lancet 1980; i: 1174–5.

15. McNeil JJ. Cholesterol: action or caution? Med J Aust 1988; 148: 1–3.

16. Editorial. Screening for breast cancer. Lancet 1985; i: 851–2.

17. Canadian Task Force on Cervical Cancer Screening Programs. Cervical cancer screening programs. Summary of the 1982 Canadian Task Force report. Can Med Assoc J 1982; 127: 581–9.

18. Canadian Task Force on the Periodic Health Examination. The periodic health examination. Can Med Assoc J 1979; 121: 1193–254.

19. Frame PS. A critical review of adult health maintenance: part 4. Prevention of metabolic, behavioural, and miscellaneous conditions. J Fam Pract 1986; 23: 29–39.

20. Welborn TA, Cullen KJ, Balazs N. Diabetes detection in mass health examinations. Three-year experience from Busselton. Med J Aust 1972; 2: 133–7.

21. Wilson JMG, Jungner G. Principles and practice of screening for disease. Geneva: WHO, 1968.

22. Rose G, Keen H, Jarrett J. Epidemiologic methods in diabetic macrovascular disease. Diabetes Care 1979; 2: 91–7.

23. Alberti KGMM. Tools for the diagnosis of diabetes. In Krall LP (ed.) World book of diabetes in practice, vol 2. Amsterdam: Elsevier, 1986: pp 16–20.

24. Riccardi G, Vaccaro O, Rivellese A, Pignalosa S, Tutino L, Mancini M. Reproducibility of the new diagnostic criteria for impaired glucose tolerance. Am J Epidemiol 1985; 121: 422–9.

25. Merkatz IR, Duchon MA, Yamashita TS, Houser HB. A pilot community-based screening program for gestational diabetes. Diabetes Care 1980; 3: 453–7.

26. American Diabetes Association Workshop-Conference on Gestational Diabetes. Summary and recommendations. Diabetes Care 1980; 3: 499–501.

27. American Diabetes Association. Summary and recommendations of the 2nd International Workshop-Conference on Gestational Diabetes Mellitus. Diabetes 1985; 34 (suppl. 2): 123–6.

28. Taylor R, Zimmet P. Migrant studies in diabetes epidemiology. In Mann JI, Pyorala K, Teuscher A (eds) Diabetes in epidemiological perspective. Edinburgh: Churchill Livingstone, 1983: pp. 58–77.

29. Zimmet P. Type 2 (non-insulin-dependent) diabetes—an epidemiological overview. Diabetologia 1982; 22: 399–411.

30. Cameron WI, Moffitt P, Williams DRR. Diabetes mellitus in the Australian Aborigines of Bourke, New South Wales. Diabetes Res Clin Pract 1986; 2: 307–14.

31. Knowler WC, Bennett PH, Hamman RF, Miller M. Diabetes incidence and prevalence in Pima Indians: a 19-fold greater incidence than in Rochester, Minnesota. Am J Epidemiol 1978; 108: 497–504.

32. Taylor R, Zimmet P. Limitation of fasting plasma glucose for the diagnosis of diabetes mellitus. Diabetes Care 1981; 4: 556–8.

33. Holland WW. Screening for disease. Taking stock. Lancet 1974; ii: 1494–7.

34. Houser HB, Mackay W, Verma N, Genuth S. A three-year controlled follow-up study of persons identified in a mass screening program for diabetes. Diabetes 1977; 26: 619–27.

35. Genuth SM, Houser HB, Carter JR, Merkatz I, Price JW, Schumacher OP, Wieland RG. Community screening for diabetes by blood glucose measurement. Results of a five-year experience. Diabetes 1976; 25: 1110–17.

36. King H, Zimmet P, Raper LR, Balkau B. The natural history of impaired glucose tolerance in the Micronesian population of Nauru: a six-year follow-up study. Diabetologia 1984; 26: 39–43.

37. Barker DJP, Rose G. Epidemiology in medical practice, 3rd edn. Edinburgh: Churchill Livingstone, 1984.

38. Birmingham Diabetes Survey Working Party. Five-year follow-up report on the Birmingham diabetes survey of 1962. Br Med J 1970; 3: 301–5.

39. Aspevik E, Jorde R, Raeder S. The diabetes survey in Bergen, Norway, 1956. Acta Med Scand 1974; 196: 161–9.

40. Morsiani M, Beretta P, Pareschi PL, Manservigi, D, Bottoni L. Long-term results in preventive medicine for type II diabetes. Acta Diab Lat 1985; 22: 191–202.

41. Genuth SM, Houser HB, Carter JR, Merkatz

IR, Price JW, Schumacher OP, Wieland RG. Observations on the value of mass indiscriminate screening for diabetes mellitus based on a five-year follow-up. Diabetes 1978; 27: 377–83.

42. University Group Diabetes Program. A study of the effects of hypoglycemic agents on vascular complications in patients with adult-onset diabetes. VI. Supplementary report on non fatal events in patients treated with tolbutamide. Diabetes 1976; 25: 1129–53.

43. West KM. Commentary. Community screening programs for diabetes? Diabetes Care 1979; 2: 381–4.

44. Bennett PH, Knowler WC. Early detection and intervention in diabetes mellitus: is it effective? J Chron Dis 1984; 37: 653–66.

45. Larkins RG. To screen or not to screen—the diabetic dilemma. Med J Aust 1985; 143: 537.

46. Seltzer HS. Diagnosis of diabetes. In Ellenberg M, Rifkin H (eds) Diabetes mellitus: theory and practice, 3rd edn. New York: Medical Examination Publishing Co., 1983: pp 441.

47. Duncan BB, Heiss G. Nonezymatic glycosylation of proteins—a new tool for assessment of cumulative hyperglycaemia in epidemiological studies, past and future. Am J Epidemiol 1984; 120: 169–89.

48. Fuller JH, McCartney P, Jarrett RJ, Keen H, Rose G, Shipley MJ, Hamilton PJS. Hyperglycemia and coronary heart disease: the Whitehall Study. J Chron Dis 1979; 32: 721–8.

49. Jarrett RJ, McCartney P, Keen H. The Bedford survey: ten year mortality rates in newly diagnosed diabetics, borderline diabetic and normoglycaemic controls and risk indices for coronary heart disease in borderline diabetics. Diabetologia 1982; 22: 79–84.

50. Jarrett RJ. Do we need IGT? Diabet Med 1987; 4: 544–5.

51. Stamler R, Stamler J, eds. Asymptomatic hyperglycemia and coronary heart disease. J Chron Dis 1979; 32: 683–837.

52. Forrest RD, Jackson CA, Yudkin JS. The glycohaemoglobin assay as a screening test for diabetes mellitus: the Islington diabetes survey. Diabet Med 1987; 4: 254–9.

53. Sicree RA, Zimmet PZ, King HOM, Coventry JS. Plasma insulin response among Nauruans. Prediction of deterioration in glucose tolerance over 6 yr. Diabetes 1987; 36: 179–86.

54. Ducimetière P, Eschwège E, Papoz L, Richard JL, Claude JR, Rosselin G. Relationship of plasma insulin levels to the incidence of myocardial infarction and coronary heart disease mortality in a middle-aged population. Diabetologia 1980; 19: 205–10.

55. Ashby JP, Frier BM. Is serum fructosamine a clinically useful test? Diabet Med 1988; 5: 118–21.

56. Ferrell RE, Hanis CL, Aguilar L, Tulloch B, Garcia C, Schull WJ. Glycosylated hemoglobin determination from capillary blood samples. Utility in an epidemiologic survey of diabetes. Am J Epidemiol 1984; 119: 159–66.

57. Verrillo A, de Teresa A, Golia R, Nunziata V. The relationship between glycosylated haemoglobin levels and various degrees of glucose intolerance. Diabetologia 1983; 24: 391–3.

58. Baker JR, O'Connor JP, Metcalf PA, Lawson MR, Johnson RN. Clinical usefulness of estimation of serum fructosamine concentration as a screening test for diabetes mellitus. Br Med J 1983; 287: 863–7.

59. Baker J, Metcalf P, Scragg R. Fructosamine concentrations in general population of Kawerau. Diabetes Care 1988; 11: 239–45.

60. Swai ABM, Harrison K, Chuwa LM, Makene W, McLarty D, Alberti KGMM. Screening for diabetes: does measurement of serum fructosamine help? Diabet Med 1988; 5: 648–52.

61. O'Sullivan JB, Mahan CM. Criteria for the oral glucose tolerance test in pregnancy. Diabetes 1964; 13: 278–85.

62. Sartor G, Schersten B, Carlstrom S, Melander A, Norden A, Persson G. Ten-year follow-up of subjects with impaired glucose tolerance. Prevention of diabetes by tolbutamide and diet regulation. Diabetes 1980; 29: 41–9.

63. Harris MI, Hadden WC, Knowler WC, Bennett PH. International criteria for the diagnosis of diabetes and impaired glucose tolerance. Diabetes Care 1985; 8: 562–7.

64. Walker A, Cudworth AG. Type 1 (insulin-dependent) diabetic multiplex families. Mode of genetic transmission. Diabetes 1980; 29: 1036–9.

65. Srikanta S, Ganda OP, Eisenbarth GS, Soeldner JS. Islet cell antibodies and beta-cell function in monozygotic triplets and twins initially discordant for type I diabetes mellitus. New Engl J Med 1983; 308: 322–5.

66. Srikanta S, Ganda OP, Rabizadeh A, Soeldner JS, Eisenbarth GS. First-degree relatives of patients with type I diabetes mellitus. Islet-cell antibodies and abnormal insulin secretion. New Engl J Med 1985; 313: 461–4.

67. Rosenbloom AL, Hunt SS, Rosenbloom EK, MacLaren NK. Ten-year prognosis of impaired glucose tolerance in siblings of patients with insulin-dependent diabetes. Diabetes 1982; 31: 385–7.

68. Stiller CR, Dupre J, Gent M et al. Effects of cyclosporine immunosuppression in insulin-dependent diabetes mellitus of recent onset. Science 1984; 223: 1362–7.

69. Jarett L, Soeldner JS, Lernmark A, Rizza RA,

Santiago J. Panel discussion 1: diagnosis, classification, and value of screening for diabetes mellitus. Clin Chem 1986; 32: B30–6.

70. Tuomilehto J, Wolf E. Primary prevention of diabetes mellitus. Diabetes Care 1987; 10: 238–48.

71. Bell DSH, Acton RT, Barger BO, Vanichanan C, Clements RS. Futility of predicting onset of type 1 diabetes mellitus. Diabetes Care 1987; 10: 788–9.

72. Bennett PH. Changing concepts of the epidemiology of insulin-dependent diabetes. Diabetes Care 1985; 8 (suppl. 1): 29–33.

73. Diabetes Epidemiology Research International. Preventing insulin dependent diabetes mellitus: the environmental challenge. Br Med J 1987; 295: 479–81.

74. University Group Diabetes Program. Effects of hypoglycemic agents on vascular complications in patients with adult-onset diabetes. III. Clinical implications of UGDP results. JAMA 1971; 218: 1400–10.

75. University Group Diabetes Program. Effects of hypoglycemic agents on vascular complications in patients with adult-onset diabetes. VIII. Evaluation of insulin therapy: final report. Diabetes 1982; 31 (suppl. 5): 1–81.

76. Savage PJ, Bennion LJ, Flock EV et al. Diet-induced improvement of abnormalities in insulin and glucagon secretion and in insulin receptor binding in diabetes mellitus. J Clin Endocrinol Metab 1979; 48: 999–1007.

77. O'Dea K. Marked improvement in carbohydrate and lipid metabolism in diabetic Australian Aborigines after temporary reversion to traditional lifestyle. Diabetes 1984; 33: 596–603.

78. Scarlett JA, Gray RS, Griffin J, Olefky JM, Kolterman OG. Insulin treatment reverses the insulin resistance of type II diabetes mellitus. Diabetes Care 1982; 5: 353–63.

79. Puska P, Tuomilehto J, Salonen J et al. The North Karelia project. Evaluation of a comprehensive community programme for control of cardiovascular diseases in North Karelia, Finland 1972–1977. Copenhagen: WHO/EURO, 1981.

80. Jarrett RJ, Keen H, Fuller JH, McCartney M. Worsening to diabetes in men with impaired glucose tolerance ('borderline diabetes'). Diabetologia 1979; 16: 25–30.

81. Keen H, Jarrett RJ, McCartney P. The ten-year follow-up of the Bedford study (1962–1972): glucose tolerance and diabetes. Diabetologia 1982; 22: 73–8.

82. Stowers JM, Sutherland HW, Kerridge DF. Long-range implications for the mother. The Aberdeen experience. Diabetes 1985; 34 (suppl. 2): 106–10.

83. O'Sullivan JB. Establishing criteria for gestational diabetes. Diabetes Care 1980; 3: 437–9.

84. Beard RW, Gillmer MDG, Oakley NW, Gunn PJ. Screening for gestational diabetes. Diabetes Care 1980; 3: 468–71.

85. Little RR, McKenzie EM, Shyken JM, Winkelmann SE, Ramsey LM, Madsen RW, Goldstein DE. Lack of relationship between glucose tolerance and complications of pregnancy in nondiabetic women. Diabetes Care 1990; 13: 483–7.

86. Mestman JH. Outcome of diabetes screening in pregnancy and perinatal morbidity in infants of mothers with mild impairment in glucose tolerance. Diabetes Care 1980; 3: 447–52.

87. Gabbe SG. Effects of identifying a high risk population. Diabetes Care 1980; 3: 486–8.

88. Li DFH, Wong VCW, O'Hoy KMKY, Yeung CY, Ma HK. Is treatment needed for mild impairment of glucose tolerance in pregnancy? A randomized controlled trial. Br J Obstet Gynaecol 1987; 94: 851–4.

89. Pettitt DJ, Knowler WC, Baird HR, Bennett PH. Gestational diabetes: infant and maternal complications of pregnancy in relation to third-trimester glucose tolerance in the Pima Indians. Diabetes Care 1980; 3: 458–64.

90. Pettitt DJ, Bennett PH, Knowler WC, Baird HR, Aleck KA. Gestational diabetes mellitus and impaired glucose tolerance during pregnancy. Long term effects on obesity and glucose tolerance in the offspring. Diabetes 1985; 34 (suppl. 2): 119–22.

91. Pettitt DJ, Aleck KA, Baird HR, Carraher MJ, Bennett PH, Knowler WC. Congenital susceptibility to NIDDM. Role of intrauterine environment. Diabetes 1988; 37: 622–8.

92. Freinkel N, Metzger BE, Phelps RL, Dooley SL, Ogata ES, Radvany RM, Belton A. Gestational diabetes mellitus. Heterogeneity of maternal age, weight, insulin secretion, HLA antigens, and islet cell antibodies and the impact of maternal metabolism on pancreatic B-cell and somatic development in the offspring. Diabetes 1985; 34 (suppl. 2): 1–7.

93. Braveman P, Showstack J, Browner W, Selby J, Teutsch S, Sepe S. Evaluating outcomes of pregnancy in diabetic women. Epidemiologic considerations and recommended indicators. Diabetes Care 1988; 11: 281–7.

94. Beard RW, Hoet JJ. Is gestational diabetes a clinical entity? Diabetologia 1982; 23: 307–12.

95. Persson B, Stangenberg M, Hansson U, Nordlander E. Gestational diabetes mellitus (GDM). Comparative evaluation of two treatment regimens, diet versus insulin and diet. Diabetes 1985: 34 (suppl. 2): 101–5.

96. Kalkhoff RK. Therapeutic results of insulin

therapy in gestational diabetes mellitus. Diabetes 1985; 34 (suppl. 2): 97–100.

97. Widness JA, Cowett RM, Coustan DR, Carpenter MW, Oh W. Neonatal morbidities in infants of mothers with glucose intolerance in pregnancy. Diabetes 1985; 34 (suppl. 2): 61–5.

98. Jarrett RJ. Reflections on gestational diabetes mellitus. Lancet 1981; ii: 1220–2.

99. Zimmet P. Primary prevention of diabetes mellitus. Diabetes Care 1988; 11: 258–62.

100. American Diabetes Association. Position statement: screening for diabetes. Diabetes Care 1989; 12: 588–90.

101. Nathan DM, Singer DE. Screening for diabetes (letter). Diabetes Care 1990; 13: 542–3.

102. Yudkin JS, Alberti KGMM, McLarty DG, Swai ABM. Impaired glucose tolerance: is it a risk factor for diabetes or a diagnostic ragbag? Br Med J 1990; 301: 397–402.

103. Swai ABM, McLarty DG, Kitange HM, Kilima PM, Masuki G, Mtinangi BI, Chuwa L, Alberti KGMM. Study in Tanzania of impaired glucose tolerance: methodological myth? Diabetes 1991; 40: 516–20.

104. Dowse GK, Zimmet PZ. The prevalence and incidence of non-insulin-dependent diabetes mellitus. In Alberti KGMM, Mazze R (eds) Frontiers of diabetes research: current trends in non-insulin-dependent diabetes mellitus. Amsterdam: Elsevier, 1989: pp 37–59.

105. Guillausseau PJ, Charles MA, Paolaggi F et al. Comparison of HbA_1 and fructosamine in diagnosis of glucose-tolerance abnormalities. Diabetes Care 1990; 13: 898–900.

106. Finch CF, Dowse GK, Collins VR, Zimmet PZ. Quantifying the extent to which random plasma glucose underestimates diabetes prevalence in the Nauruan population. Diabetes Res Clin Pract 1990; 10: 177–82.

107. Lipton R, LaPorte RE, Becker DJ, Dorman JS, Orchard TJ, Atchison J, Drash AL. Cyclosporin therapy for prevention and cure of IDDM: epidemiological perspective of benefits and risks. Diabetes Care 1990; 13: 776–84.

108. American Diabetes Association. Position statement: prevention of type I diabetes mellitus. Diabetes 1990; 39: 1151–2.

109. Couch MHA (ed). Health assessment for adults. Sydney: CCH Australia, 1989.

110. Cederholm J. Short-term treatment of glucose intolerance in middle-aged subjects by diet, exercise and sulfonylurea. Upsala J Med Sci 1985; 90: 229–242.

111. Naylor CD. Diagnosing gestational diabetes mellitus: is the gold standard valid? Diabetes Care 1989; 12: 565–72.

71a

Organization of Care: The Diabetic Clinic—A Center of Knowledge

U. Rosenqvist

Stockholm County Council Teaching Center for Diabetes, Karolinska Hospital, Stockholm, Sweden

The goal of the diabetic clinic is the health and well-being of diabetic patients.

The main point made in this chapter is that the diabetic clinic has an important function as a center of knowledge. The implications of this for the design and operation of the clinic are set forth.

TWO FORMS OF KNOWLEDGE

There are two distinct forms of knowledge. One is knowledge that can be formulated and written down—'propositional knowledge'. The other kind of knowledge is aptly called 'tacit knowledge': this is knowledge that we cannot put down on paper. Such knowledge becomes visible only in its practical application, in the actions we take. Tacit knowledge is what makes it possible for us to distinguish a face in the crowd, to realize that a person is ill by the mere sight of him, to feel a patient's nervousness 'in the air', to know how to utilize a team in an efficient way, etc.

There are well-established methods for the monitoring and accumulation of propositional knowledge, and such knowledge can be rapidly transferred through various kinds of media. It is vital that the diabetic clinic utilizes existing propositional knowledge and builds new knowledge of this type through a regular inflow of information from external sources and by generating new information through regular reviews of the clinic's own operations. Modern textbooks should be made available and used, and the team should also be enabled to make searches, using tools such as the *Index Medicus* and the *Science Citation Index*. In the future it is to be hoped that different sources of information will be available on compact discs in the clinic. Holding regular seminars for literature review is another tested way to stimulate knowledge exchange and growth within the team.

In this context it is also worth remembering that we enlarge our knowledge when we have an opportunity to reflect on previous experience and knowledge. People find it easiest to learn things that they perceive a need for; this holds true both for patients and staff. The team leader or teacher therefore has to adopt the role of acting as a guide and adviser, rather than simply handing down quantities of facts.

International Textbook of Diabetes Mellitus. Edited by K.G.M.M. Alberti, R.A. DeFronzo, H. Keen and P. Zimmet

Tacit knowledge, on the other hand, can only be acquired by observing and participating in practice. Crafts are learned by apprenticeship; provision should therefore be made for the same kind of practical training for the diabetic clinic staff. Single-way screens and videotaping can be used for such purposes and can constitute a tool for reviewing one's own practice. An interview with a patient, for example, can be greatly improved by recording it and then listening to the tape with another member of the staff. Breaks in the communication between patient and staff will become apparent, and staff members can learn to avoid them. Another routine that might help to improve practical application is to induce the team to reflect regularly on the question of how they behave in dealing with 'difficult' patients. The Balint group is a model for improving professional care, especially with regard to the handling of psychosocial problems [1].

This short review will, it is hoped, have delineated these two types of knowledge and have indicated that they call for different learning strategies.

THE SERVICE MANAGEMENT CONCEPT

Now that we have stated the central role of knowledge in the diabetic clinic, how should we organize the clinic and staff it, and how should the patient be involved, in order to enhance the quality of care?

The diabetic clinic and its functions can well be organized in terms of the 'service management' concept [2]. This concept focuses on the encounter between patient and staff as the critical moment of service delivery (Figure 1). Support for the encounter is derived from knowledge, experience, attitudes, support routines and a proper organization. At the moment of encounter the efficiency of the whole diabetic clinic is tested. The concept also emphasizes the active role of the patient as the 'customer' of the service system. From the service management concept, it follows that the development of the diabetic clinic services should take its point of departure from a critical analysis of what is essential to make the encounter as productive as possible. What knowledge is needed, what back-up does the staff need and which support routines can be used?

Three areas of the clinic's work can be distin-

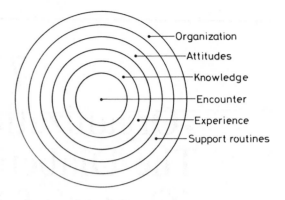

Figure 1 The encounter between individual patients and staff members is central to the diabetic clinic activities. The outcome of the encounter is supported by appropriate knowledge, previous experiences, the right attitudes, proper support routines and organization of the diabetic clinic

guished: the 'front stage', where patients and staff meet, the 'back stage' (or back room) where support is generated for the staff, and a third stage outside the clinic where the patients live their own lives. The third stage is the one towards which the clinic's activity must be geared. In order to live a full life, the patients need basic education about their disease, and must acquire essential skills and the ability to cope with everyday life, which may involve irregular hours and odd activities.

THE ENCOUNTER

Modern teaching theory tells us that we should not just transmit knowledge but, rather, encourage the students to ask for information in order that the knowledge may be integrated with their basic concepts and affect their behaviour. The staff member's task is to acquaint patients with the extent of the knowledge available and involve them in a frank dialogue to elucidate the patients' areas of interest.

As the diabetic condition and its treatment affect all areas of patients' lives, the matter of involving the patient in a frank discussion is of immense importance. The measures taken to achieve good metabolic control can never be considered in isolation from the patient's experience of quality of life. Thus patients' self-knowledge, their preferred way of living, their fears and joys in life, their previous experiences of the disease and of encounters with the health care system, their way of defining their health status, etc., are constituents of the dialogue, as well as the staff member's knowledge about the condition and its treatment.

To engage in a dialogue that allows the patient a more active role, and that permits broader and deeper areas of the patient's life and personality to surface, is often difficult for the staff member. Special training is therefore needed in therapeutic attitudes and interview techniques [3–5]. Support routines are also needed that can help staff members develop this new professional skill.

ORGANIZATION

From an organizational point of view, patient education with the above content will have to take time and will require a good rapport between patient and staff in order for a true dialogue to be established. In order to promote this climate, the staff will need special training in interviewing methods. For example, video sessions make it possible for the staff to find flaws in their teaching technique. Teaching skills can be improved by systematic training [3]. Initially the 'interview' teaching approach will be more time-consuming, but it should lead to a better-informed patient capable of acting on the basis of integrated knowledge, rather than simply being compliant. Brochures, books, computer and video programs, etc., may then be used to *supplement* the individual teaching and to enhance the patient's interest in acquiring more knowledge. The ever-present learning situation should be encouraged by patients sharing experiences with each other and with staff, etc. Lectures for both patients and staff, as practised at the International Diabetes Centre in Minneapolis, is one way of emphasizing the learning role of everyone involved.

Because of the nature of tacit knowledge acquisition, it would be preferable if the patient initially could work only with a few team members so that tacit knowledge is retained and fully shared between patient and staff members. The patient's often-voiced quest for continuity of care most certainly stems from the fact that a relatively long time is needed to acquire tacit knowledge, in comparison with propositional knowledge.

The pedagogic situation has been described at some length so that we may examine what implications it will have on the organization and staffing of the diabetic clinic. First, it follows that every team member—even those recruited as specialists, dietitians or nurses—must acquire sufficient basic knowledge from other members for each of them to be able to respond to the patient's questions, even if they touch on a field outside their own professional sphere. Special arrangements should therefore be made for individual members to share their knowledge and experiences with the rest of the team. One way to strengthen the team members' overall knowledge would be to rotate the student teaching assignments so that team members are obliged to penetrate different knowledge areas and integrate them with their own knowledge base. The patient, of course, must also be able to integrate different areas of knowledge, and all of the staff should attain at least the same level in areas above and beyond their special field.

Preferably, the team should encompass the following specialists: a diabetologist; a registered nurse with special diabetes training; a dietitian; a chiropodist; a psychologist; and a social worker. In addition, there should be at least one person able to review and audit the records of the diabetes service. The roles of the different team members should be clarified within the team.

Team building and the development of each staff member, both with regard to the diabetes service and individual personalities, should be done in a systematic way [4]. Similarly, the replacement of team members should be planned in advance. It is necessary to achieve only a slow turnover of staff, in order to retain and enhance the knowledge 'pool' within the team. Managers should make every effort to have all members stay for a long period; unplanned staff replacements can be detrimental to quality care.

SUPPORT ROUTINES

The 'back stage' of the clinic should be organized to reduce the load on the staff at the moment of patient encounter. This would imply that records should be typed, filed and readily available. A separate *diabetes register* can be of great help for an audit if the records are kept together with those of non-diabetic patients. All encounters with the patient should be recorded in a *single document*. 'One body, one mind and one record' can simplify the exchange of information between staff members. The record should also have a *checklist* in order to provide a rapid review of such items as frequency of eye examinations, goals for treatment agreed upon, etc. In fact, the checklist can be developed for easy extraction of data that can later be used for annual audits. The *audit* is another backstage support routine that can help the staff pose questions and reflect on their performance. What should be looked for in the audit should therefore be developed within the team and preferably also with input from the patients. The central issue will be to find answers to the question, 'How can the quality of care be improved?'

The diabetes register can also provide mailing addresses for newsletters to the patients.

REGULAR MEETINGS

The staff need to discuss problems and exchange experience in order to increase their knowledge. Open, free dialogue in regular meetings should be encouraged. Time should be reserved not only for a 'technical' discussion about the work, but also for discussions on attitudes and ethical issues and for reflection on the group process. Minutes should be kept and decisions concerning individual patients should be noted in their records.

The amount of time that should be set aside for this kind of meeting cannot be specified. In our experience it is better to meet every week, even if only for 30 minutes, than to have long and perhaps tiring meetings at monthly intervals.

SELF-HELP GROUPS

Patient self-help groups can be a great support to patients in coping with their disease and with the medical care system [6]. It has been observed, though, that too strong an input by the staff may smother the initiative of the self-help group. The staff can therefore help to set up groups, for example of parents of diabetic children, but should then let the group live its own life.

CONCLUSION

The quality of diabetes care in the diabetic clinic depends on knowledge both of a propositional and of a tacit nature. The encounter between individual patients and staff members is the critical moment of service delivery. This encounter should be the point of departure for an analysis of what is critical in order to generate high-quality service.

Patient teaching should not be merely a handing-out of information, but should help patients ask for what they specifically need. This can be achieved through a true dialogue between staff and patient.

The staff members need back-up from those 'back stage' for their encounters with patients. Support routines and a regular forum for the exchange of knowledge, experience and time for reflection are vital for the development of knowledge among the staff.

High-quality diabetes care in the diabetic clinic is founded on knowledge and resources but, first and foremost, it depends on human interaction. Staff development is therefore an essential task of the management of the diabetic clinic.

Development of quality care has to be a continuous process of reviewing, reflection and adjustment.

REFERENCES

1. Balint M. The doctor, his patient and the illness. New York International 1972.
2. Normann R. Service management. Stockholm: Liber, 1987.
3. Cook S, Cohen RM. Evaluating a workshop for improving diabetes patient education programs: is it really successful? Diabet Educ 1986; 12: 48–50.
4. Mazze RS, ed. Professional education in diabetes. Proceedings of the Diabetes Research and Training Centers Conference. Washington DC: US Dept of Health and Human Services Public Health Service NIH, 1980.
5. Assal J-P, Berger M, Gay N, Canivet J, eds. Diabetes education. How to improve patient education. International Congress Series 624. Amsterdam: Excerpta Medica, 1983.
6. Chesler M. Self-help groups as intervenors in patient–provider conflict in health care. University of Michigan, Ann Arbor, MI: Center for Research on Social Organization, 1987, no. 342, March.

71b

Organisation of Care: The Diabetes Care Centre— A Focus for More Effective Diabetes Treatment and Prevention

J.J. Bending* and H. Keen†

* District General Hospital, Eastbourne, UK, and † Guy's Hospital, London, UK

The advent of insulin injection therapy in the treatment of diabetes in the 1920s was the major impetus to the creation and rapid proliferation of diabetic clinics in many countries. The distribution of insulin solution and the means for its injection was hardly less important than the need to instruct the patient in injection technique, correct dosage measurement, the basis of timing and balancing dietary carbohydrate against insulin action, the recognition and correction of hypoglycaemia—indeed, the whole spectrum of diabetes knowledge and understanding that has become so familiar today. In addition, private doctors took on the responsibility for the insulin treatment of individual diabetic patients, although the acquisition of special skills and experience for optimum management was sometimes a problem. With the increasing recognition of the prevalence and importance of non-insulin dependent diabetes mellitus (NIDDM) and the organised treatment and monitoring of people with this disease, NIDDM patients progressively came to dominate diabetic clinics numerically. Many aspects of the treatment of these patients were also considered to be appropriate to management by practitioners at primary health care level; from this has grown the notion of shared care, where the use of community and hospital health care resources are most rationally adapted and blended to meet the varying needs of individual patients.

As the possibilities for improving health care for people with diabetes have evolved, the limitations of the traditional hospital-based clinic to meet modern expectations for providing adequate diabetes care have become apparent [1]. Typically, the hospital diabetes clinics have,

International Textbook of Diabetes Mellitus. Edited by K.G.M.M. Alberti, R.A. DeFronzo, H. Keen and P. Zimmet
© 1992 John Wiley & Sons Ltd

over the last few decades, found themselves coping with increasing numbers of patients expected to wait for long periods in crowded waiting rooms for brief consultations with a changing succession of doctors, sometimes of junior status with limited interest or experience in diabetes. This has become inefficient in terms of optimal health outcomes, and unacceptable to the recipients as an approach to the management of a life-long disorder. The crowded hospital outpatient clinic is an unsuitable setting for the provision of adequate diabetes education and is inadequate for the systematic and careful screening for, and management of, the long-term complications of the disease.

It is against this background that the diabetes care centre has emerged as a necessary and effective modern solution for the provision of diabetes care. The seeds of this evolution go back to individual endeavours such as the centre established in East Berlin nearly four decades ago [1], and paralleled by independent development initiatives in places as far apart as Britain [1], New Zealand [2] and Canada [3]. In the UK, from this perception of needs, the concept of the district diabetes centre has evolved, constituting a new 'centre of gravity' for the organisation of diabetes care on a district-wide basis, positioned between hospital and community services with the goal of integrating both into effective and locally appropriate schemes for the care of the diabetic patient [4]. The District Diabetes Centre initiative is developing a pivotal role in what we believe could become a 'New Deal for Diabetes' [5].

COMMUNITY DIABETES CARE WORLD WIDE

Several models for diabetes care in the community have been implemented world wide and these have been reviewed recently [6]. Initiatives have come out of a number of countries, ranging from Sweden, India (Kashmir) and China to the USA, Yugoslavia (Croatia) and the USSR. The Swedish model has defined several potential barriers to the implementation of community diabetes care programmes, including lack of knowledge about diabetes, lack of coordination within public health agencies, lack of guidelines for care, and lack of contact with hospital-based specialists [7]. Attempts have been made to overcome these barriers systematically by developing

care on the basis of locally defined evaluations of experience and need rather than imposing a rigid programme from above [6]. The conclusion from this is clearly that not only do needs for diabetes care require to be addressed individually on a national, regional and district level, but that the diabetes care programme has to be fashioned, especially at the local level, by the staff, patients and carers who are to be the final users of the programme.

Thus the selection of a diabetes care programme will depend on local conditions and traditions and will vary widely. The range of options extends from the facilities available in industrialised countries like Sweden, with highly developed health care systems, functioning primary health care centres and well-trained physicians and nurses, to those in developing nations where local health care may be dependent on community workers (e.g. schoolteachers) with relatively little medical training [6]. The emphasis in all these models is on the need for elaborating a clear statement of feasible aims and goals which call for close and well-functioning cooperation between different agencies and levels of care with the Diabetes Care Centre and supplying the focus for the integration of locally structured resources.

THE DIABETES CARE CENTRE

The functioning of the diabetes care centre is geared ideally to provide a forum for diabetes care that differs totally in its atmosphere and operation from the traditional diabetic clinic and its limitations. The centre offers patients access throughout the week to the trained team of doctors, nurses, dietitians and chiropodists. It has the potential to transform the approach to diabetes both in the patients and in those who care for them, offering the space, facilities, skills and (especially) greater time to provide for the broad range of needs of diabetic people.

In the UK, the prospect of a diabetes centre in every health district is a real aspiration. There are doubters [8], but this goal is sponsored by the British Diabetic Association who enthusiastically support this development [4]. The first centres in the UK developed from very diverse origins, but the improved quality of organisation and care provided by these centres has been universally and enthusiastically endorsed by both carers and recipients of care generally [4]. Where the old-style clinic remains alongside a centre, it is able to assume a principal role in 'problem finding'. In this situation, the main function of the diabetes centre becomes 'problem solving' [5].

The Role of the Diabetes Care Centre

The emphasis of the diabetes care centre is very much that of health promotion—directed to the image of the healthy diabetic person rather than the sick patient. It lends itself to the provision of diabetes care and education, including dietetic instruction (e.g. 'hands on' in the diet demonstration kitchen, as well as in theory), which may be conveyed to the diabetic clientèle (and family members, etc., when appropriate) both individually and in groups. As well as providing a suitable venue for the instruction of people with diabetes and their relatives, the centre provides a natural focal centre for the planned teaching and training of medical, nursing and other staff. A 'home base' for the diabetes care team, the centre can also offer a major resource as a point of contact and information for general practitioner and community nursing services.

The diabetes care centre lends itself to regular and systematic screening for detection and prevention of diabetic complications. It forms a suitable meeting place for supportive activities of many types, young diabetic groups, parents' groups, diabetes slimming groups, local branch Diabetic Associations, and so on.

The diabetes centre can also tackle the major problem of the 'lost patients'—people with diagnosed diabetes who have broken clinical contact and are receiving little, if any, diabetic care from either hospital or community. These diabetic patients are particularly at risk; in some UK communities they may constitute as many as one-half of those with diabetes [9–11]. They often first come to the attention of the hospital or family practitioner when some potentially preventable disaster such as visual loss or gangrene threatens or has occurred. A computerised district diabetes register, based in the diabetes centre, compiled with the collaboration of community and hospital agencies, can form a central record of those at risk and greatly facilitate the targeting of the provision of diabetes care and the effective screening for complications such as retinopathy in this most vulnerable group.

Table 1 General principles for the function of a district diabetes centre

---

Coordination of community and hospital diabetes services: integration of primary, secondary and tertiary levels of care

Development of overall district plan for diabetes care (approx 250 000 population)

Training of personnel in providing diabetes health care skills

Regular patient review for routine care and anticipatory screening

Education resource centre for patients and their families (individually and in groups)

Centre for monitoring and audit of quality and effectiveness of diabetes care

Venue for joint specialised clinics—obstetric, ophthalmologic, foot-care, renal and vascular, depending on local expertise and facilities

Opportunity for organisation and conduct of basic research and clinical trials

Meeting place for professional and client groups

Base for regular meetings of diabetic groups (e.g. branches of national Diabetic Association)

Centre for organising local awareness compaigns, public education, etc.

The Structure of the Diabetes Centre

The form that the diabetes care centre takes will obviously depend in large part on the economic and cultural status of the society and upon its medical care structure. However, a number of generally applicable principles can be listed, to be met in a way most appropriate to local conditions (Table 1).

Diabetes Centre Design

Accommodation for the diabetes centre should ideally be dedicated for the provision of diabetes care; the design must, however, be adaptable to meet particular local needs and resources [5]. Centres will differ in urban and rural communities, and in industrial and developing societies.

An example of an idealised, diagrammatic, functional plan is shown in Figure 1. Usually within reach of (and sometimes even on the premises of) a general hospital, to facilitate access to specialised personnel and services, the

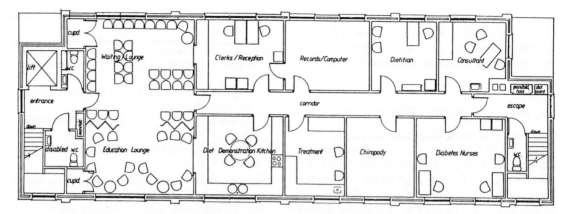

Figure 1   Idealised, functional plan for a diabetes care centre

centre must also look outwards into the community and its health agencies. It must strive to be seen by them as a readily accessible resource. Both its structure and its functional organisation should accommodate visits by appointment, casual 'drop-in' visits, regular clinical review for routine and anticipatory treatment, and systematic teaching.

The Diabetes Care Centre Team

The centre brings together health-care staff from both hospital and community and aims to provide as much as possible of the variety of skills necessary for effective and sustained provision of diabetes care. The team is ideally led by a physician with a special interest and training in diabetes. It should include diabetes specialist nurses, dietitians, chiropodists and administrative/organisational staff. Other support staff may comprise junior medical staff in training, social workers, educationalists and other visiting staff with ophthalmic, renal, obstetric or orthopaedic skills—who may take part in joint sessions.

Diabetes Specialist Nurses

One of the most important developments in the provision of satisfactory and effective care for people with diabetes has been the emergence in many countries of the diabetes specialist nurse. As part of a general expansion of the role of the nurse in health care, this development recognises the important contribution in sustained education and support for people with diabetes which the overextended doctor is often unable to

supply. The role of the diabetes specialist nurse has been recognised in the St Vincent Declaration initiative described below. It includes much of the essential infrastructure of modern diabetes care. In particular, it greatly enhances the involvement, comprehension and motivation of diabetic patients themselves in the process of diabetes care, an essential component in the successful application of modern knowledge. The boundaries of the nurse's role have not yet been fully defined and set, but what has emerged is the urgent need for programmes of advanced nurse training. This should encompass not only the clinical techniques of diabetes care but also the deeper understanding of the emotional and social implications of long-term disorders like diabetes. Such courses have already been developed and are increasing in number as their effectiveness is recognised. The rapid expansion of this cadre of trained personnel is a clear recognition of this cost-efficient and effective means of improving the expectation of health and life for people with diabetes.

Diabetes specialist nurses frequently are responsible for the day-to-day running of the diabetes care centre, and provide the backbone to much of its activities. This dedicated group of professionals possess the skills, inclination and time to provide the close and prolonged engagement with the patient that is necessary to deliver sustained education, motivation and technical instruction. This strategy has proved very effective, both professionally and economically [12]. The traditional role of the doctor as chief provider of care, with the patient as its passive recipient and the nurse as an ill-defined intermediary, has been superseded by this more effective new relationship. Health-care professionals now try to adopt an advisory and supportive role by enabling the patient to become a main agent in securing the necessary level of care.

DIABETES INTEGRATED CARE AND THE DIABETES CARE CENTRE

The trend to 'dehospitalise' as much as possible of the routines of diabetes care has laid more emphasis on the community-based family practitioners, community nurses and other health aides. Such initiatives in primary care settings in the UK have recently been reviewed [13]. In the UK, the concept of community-based miniclinics was first described by Thorn and Russell in the early 1970s. These clinics were run by interested local practitioners in collaboration with the local hospital-based diabetes specialist [14]. More than ten years ago Hill described a similar shared-care scheme in Poole [15]. Local refresher courses for community-based medical staff were organised. Communication was much facilitated by a cooperation booklet, which was carried by the patient and which linked the hospital and community components of that patient's individually designed care plan. It made clear who takes specific responsibilities in such a scheme of regular care. In another approach, an itinerant clinical assistant or diabetes specialist arranged a round of collaborative visits to interested general practitioners to review patients [16] with diabetes or set up a network of diabetes nurse specialists to care for these patients in the practice [17].

These initiatives have produced promising evaluations [13], but the longer-term outcomes of the major efforts put into these schemes has been relatively disappointing [18–19]. The failure to influence patterns of diabetes care more widely has not been due to lack of goodwill nor to any lack of realisation of the importance of coordinating the agencies for diabetes care. The deficiency has, in our view, been the absence of an established diabetes centre, of the type we describe, to maintain and develop these pioneering initiatives. There is a clear need to organise, implement and monitor long-term policies for diabetes on a district-wide basis; the concept of the district diabetes centre has emerged from this perception of need. The importance of continuity of care along these lines has recently been highlighted in the UK by the mushrooming of many small-scale 'health promotion' clinics in general practice. Although in principle this increase in care available for patients with diabetes is to be welcomed, it is essential that a high quality of care is provided. This can be achieved by the creation of clinical guidelines, regularly reviewed and updated, and opportunities for training to meet the desirable clinical structure and function [20]. The diabetes care centre should play a constructive and valuable part in this expanded provision of care of diabetic patients: it can set standards, provide training and information and ensure continuous review and updating of practice.

DIABETES CARE ORGANISATION VERSUS HEALTH SERVICE REORGANISATION

A series of goals aimed at improving health care and research for people with diabetes in Europe was agreed between the lay and professional Diabetes Associations and their respective Government Health Departments at a meeting in St Vincent, Italy in 1989. The St Vincent Declaration [21] calls for measures to attain a sustained improvement in health and a life approaching normal expectation in quality and quantity. Health service organisation and reorganisation must make real provision for the care structures that have evolved, and some recent patterns appear to move away from this need [20]. Health services world wide, faced by burgeoning costs, will be increasingly exposed to downward pressures relating to short-term costs. The long-term advantages of diabetes care in a personal, clinical and (for governments) economic sense—the leg not amputated, the eye not blind, the stroke not suffered—make the evaluation of initiatives in diabetes care such as the district diabetes centre vital. To those enthusiasts who were the pioneers, those developing and providing these advances and, above all, the clients who are the recipients of these improvements in care provided, the benefits are already clear.

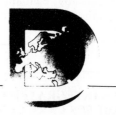

DIABETES MELLITUS IN EUROPE:
A PROBLEM AT ALL AGES IN ALL COUNTRIES.
A Model for Prevention and Self Care
SAINT VINCENT (ITALY), 10-12 OCTOBER 1989

A Meeting Organized by WHO and IDF in Europe

Diabetes Care and Research in Europe
The Saint Vincent Declaration

Representatives of Government Health Departments and patients organisations from all European countries met with diabetes experts under the aegis of the Regional Offices of the World Health Organisation and the International Diabetes Federation in St. Vincent, Italy on October 10–12, 1989. They unanimously agreed upon the following recommendations and urged that they should be presented in all countries throughout Europe for implementation.

Diabetes mellitus is a major and growing European health problem, a problem at all ages and in all countries. It causes prolonged ill-health and early death. It threatens at least ten million European citizens.

It is within the power of national Governments and Health Departments to create conditions in which a major reduction in this heavy burden of disease and death can be achieved. Countries should give formal recognition to the diabetes problem and deploy resources for its solution. Plans for the prevention, identification and treatment of diabetes and particularly its complications – blindness, renal failure, gangrene and amputation, aggravated coronary heart disease and stroke – should be formulated at local, national and European regional levels. Investment now will earn great dividends in reduction of human misery and in massive savings of human and material resources.

General goals and five-year targets listed below can be achieved by the organised activities of the medical services in active partnership with diabetic citizens, their families, friends and workmates and their organisations; in the management of their own diabetes and the education for it; in the planning, provision and quality audit of health care; in national, regional and international organisations for disseminating information about health maintenance; in promoting and applying research.

General goals for people – children and adults – with diabetes
● Sustained improvement in health experience and a life approaching normal expectation in quality and quantity.
● Prevention and cure of diabetes and of its complications by intensifying research effort.

Source: Diabetic Medicine 1990; 70: 360. Reproduced by permission of IDF/WHO European Region and John Wiley & Sons Ltd.

Five-year targets

Elaborate, initiate and evaluate comprehensive programmes for detection and control of diabetes and of its complications with self-care and community support as major components.

Raise awareness in the population and among health care professionals of the present opportunities and the future needs for prevention of the complications of diabetes and of diabetes itself.

Organise training and teaching in diabetes management and care for people of all ages with diabetes, for their families, friends and working associates and for the health care team.

Ensure that care for children with diabetes is provided by individuals and teams specialised both in the management of diabetes and of children, and that families with a diabetic child get the necessary social, economic and emotional support.

Reinforce existing centres of excellence in diabetes care, education and research. Create new centres where the need and potential exist.

Promote independence, equity and self-sufficiency for all people with diabetes – children, adolescents, those in the working years of life and the elderly.

Remove hindrances to the fullest possible integration of the diabetic citizen into society.

Implement effective measures for the prevention of costly complications
- Reduce new blindness due to diabetes by one third or more.
- Reduce numbers of people entering end-stage diabetic renal failure by at least one third.
- Reduce by one half the rate of limb amputations for diabetic gangrene.
- Cut morbidity and mortality from coronary heart disease in the diabetic by vigorous programmes of risk factor reduction.
- Achieve pregnancy outcome in the diabetic woman that approximates that of the non-diabetic woman.

Establish monitoring and control systems using state of the art information technology for quality assurance of diabetes health care provision and for laboratory and technical procedures in diabetes diagnosis, treatment and self-management.

Promote European and international collaboration in programmes of diabetes research and development through national, regional and WHO agencies and in active partnership with diabetes patients organisations.

Take urgent action in the spirit of the WHO programme, "Health for All" to establish joint machinery between WHO and IDF, European Region, to initiate, accelerate and facilitate the implementation of these recommendations.

At the conclusion of the St. Vincent meeting, all those attending formally pledged themselves to strong and decisive action in seeking implementation of the recommendations on their return home.

REFERENCES

1. Ling P, Lovesay JM, Mayon-White VA, Thomson J, Knight AH. The diabetic clinic dinosaur is dying: will diabetic day units evolve? Diabet Med 1985; 2: 163–5.
2. Beavan DW, Scott RS, Helm AM et al. IDF Bull 1983; 28: 5.
3. Hunt JA. Twenty-five years of a diabetes education centre. Diabet Med 1990; 7: 400–6.
4. Day JL, Spathis GS (eds). District Diabetes Centres in the United Kingdom. A report on workshop held by the Diabetes Education Study Group on behalf of the British Diabetic Association. Diabet Med 1988; 5: 372–80.
5. Bending J, Keen H. A new deal for diabetes. J Roy Coll Phys Lond 1989; 23: 251–4.
6. Rosenqvist U, Luft R. Diabetes care in the community. In Alberti KGMM, Krall LP (eds) Diabetes annual 4. Amsterdam: Elsevier, 1988: pp 162–78.
7. Carlson A, Rosenqvist U. Control program implementation. On the importance of staff involvement. Scand J Primary Health Care 1988; suppl. 1: 105–12.
8. Daggett P. Diabetes centres: an important development or another gimmick? (editorial). Diabet Med 1988; 5: 723.
9. Yudkin JS, Boucher BJ, Schopelin KE, Harris BT, Claff HR, Whyte NJD. The quality of diabetic care in a London health district. J Epidemiol Commun Health 1980; 34: 277–80.
10. Moor JM, Gadsby R. Non insulin-dependent diabetes in general practice 1. Practitioner 1984; 228: 675–9.
11. Mellor JG, Samantha A, Blandford RL, Burden AC. Questionnaire survey of diabetic care in general practice in Leicestershire. Health Trends 1985; 17: 61–3.
12. Nabarro JDN. The diabetes specialist nurse. Diabetes Newsline (British Diabetic Association) July 1985; 7–8.
13. Wood J. A review of diabetes care initiatives in primary care settings. Health Trends 1990; 39–43.
14. Thorn PA, Russell RG. Diabetic clinics today and tomorrow; mini-clinics in general practice. Br Med J 1973; 2: 534–6.
15. Hill RD. Community care service for diabetics in the Poole area. Br Med J 1976; 2: 1137–9.
16. Baksi AK, Brand J, Nicholas M et al. Non-consultant peripheral clinics: a new approach to diabetic care. Health Trends 1984; 16: 38–40.
17. Mallows C, Nicholas MK, Beable AE, Waterfield MR, Baksi AK. An evaluation of nurse specialist diabetic clinics. Pract Diabetes 1990; 7: 21–3.
18. Hayes TM, Harries J. Randomised controlled trial of routine hospital clinic care versus routine general practice care for type II diabetics. Br Med J 1984; 289: 728–30.
19. Day JL, Humphreys H, Alban-Davies H. Problems of comprehensive shared diabetics care. Br Med J 1987; 294: 1590–2.
20. Keen H. Bending J. Diabetes care and the White Paper—will it work for patients? J Roy Coll Phys Lond 1989; 23: 210–11.
21. International Diabetes Federation. Diabetes care and research in Europe: the Saint Vincent Declaration. Diabet Med 1990; 7: 360.

71c
Organisation of Care: Problems in Developing Countries—India

A. Ramachandran and M. Viswanathan

Diabetes Research Centre, Madras, India

India is the second most populous country in the world, accounting for 15% of the world's population [1]. The population in India has grown from 273 million in 1931 to 685 million in 1982 [2] and 746 million in 1984, as estimated by the Population Reference Bureau of Washington [3]. The increase in the growth rate has been mostly due to the dramatic decline in the crude death rate, from 38 per 1000 population in the 1920s to 19 in the 1960s and 12.5 in 1981 [2].

Diabetes mellitus is a universal disease and affects populations all over the world. Hence the large population of India poses a major challenge, as the number of diabetic patients would be very high even with a low prevalence rate. This is particularly true because a large number of individuals could have undetected diabetes.

According to the statistics currently available, the prevalence of diabetes is low in many developing countries. However, half the population in most of these countries is under 20 years old [4]. The average life expectancy has improved considerably in India over the years, and similar trends are seen in other developing nations. We must, therefore, anticipate that when infectious diseases come under better control, there will be a tremendous increase in the number of people with diabetes.

PREVALENCE OF DIABETES IN INDIA: THE MAGNITUDE OF THE PROBLEM

It is well known that the prevalence of diabetes varies in different geographical regions. In his epidemiological studies, West has reported that the prevalence of diabetes is low in countries where a high-carbohydrate diet is consumed [5], which includes India. Most earlier studies also have shown a low prevalence of diabetes in India [6]. A large, multicentric study in 1979 by the Indian Council of Medical Research (ICMR) reported that the overall prevalence of diabetes (in subjects over 15 years old) was 1.8%, with a higher rate in urban (2.1%) than rural (1.5%) areas [6]. Over the years, a spate of papers have appeared in the literature showing a high prevalence of diabetes in the migrant Indian populations living outside India in places such as South Africa, Fiji, Trinidad, Singapore [7] and the UK [8]. One of the interesting findings was that the rural–urban difference seen among

International Textbook of Diabetes Mellitus. Edited by K.G.M.M. Alberti, R.A. DeFronzo, H. Keen and P. Zimmet

other ethnic groups was conspicuously absent among Indians in Fiji [7]. A recent survey of known diabetic patients in Southall, London, showed higher rates of diabetes among Asians compared with whites [8].

The high prevalence of diabetes among Indians living abroad compared with other ethnic groups (Europeans, blacks, Chinese or Malays) is not only surprising but also interesting. There are no clinically identifiable factors among Indians, different from the others in the population, that could have caused their higher rates of diabetes. For example, there was no difference in the prevalence of obesity between Indians and whites in the Southall population [8]. A high prevalence of diabetes among the migrant Indian populations probably indicates that Indians as a race have a higher susceptibility to develop diabetes. As long as these people remain in India the conditions are not optimal to bring out their carbohydrate intolerance; this may be because of poverty, low energy intake, low fat intake and low prevalence of obesity [9, 10]. Settlement in more affluent societies abroad makes a dramatic change in life-style, and this could be responsible for unmasking diabetes. This is supported by the high degree of familial aggregation among Indians with diabetes [11, 12]. A comparative study between Indians and Europeans showed that a positive family history was present more often among Indians [12]. A high prevalence of diabetes among offspring in families where one or both parents are diabetic has been noted [13, 14]. These findings suggest that hereditary factors have a significant role in the aetiopatho-genesis of diabetes among Indians. Obesity is considered to be the most important environmental factor in the pathogenesis of diabetes. The lack of obesity in most of the diabetic patients implies that hereditary factors are probably more important in the Indian patients. Consanguineous marriages are common in Indian communities: this is a result of a high proportion of marriages arranged by parents for their children; they prefer to choose brides and bridegrooms from their own caste. Many wealthy families prefer marriages among their own relatives so that the wealth does not go out of their families. Consanguinity may therefore be one of the reasons for the high degree of familial aggregation in diabetes among Indians.

There are new data emerging that the prevalence of diabetes in India is not low, as hitherto believed, especially among the affluent. A recent survey of known diabetic patients in Darya Ganj [15] showed a high prevalence of diabetes, comparable to that of Indians in Southall. Even with a conservative estimate of 2%, there are about 14 million people with diabetes requiring medical attention, and by rough estimates, an equal number may have diabetes not yet detected. Thus, this huge population with diabetes is a formidable challenge to the health authorities, especially with the limited resources available in India.

The other major problem is the high prevalence of NIDDM among the young. The high prevalence of maturity-onset diabetes in the young (MODY) has been reported, not only from India [16] but also among Indians in South Africa [17]. In the original description by Tattersall, it was reported that MODY patients are less prone to vascular complications [18]. However, subsequent studies in Indian MODY patients showed that although macrovascular complications are infrequent, the specific micro-vascular complications are equally common in MODY as in classic NIDDM [19, 20]. The higher proportion of NIDDM in the young increases the clinical load of the physicians, especially when most hospitals are understaffed.

The next major challenge is the existence of malnutrition related diabetes mellitus (MRDM). Although diabetes is more common among the affluent societies of the developed nations, it is disquieting to note that diabetes does not spare the malnourished in the developing countries. The occurrence of MRDM is widely recognised, and the World Health Organization has included it in the major classification of diabetes [21]. A detailed description of MRDM is given in Chapter 8. The practical problems in the management of MRDM are multiple. A majority of MRDM patients come from very low socio-economic groups and cannot afford even the bare necessities of life. The cost of treatment is high, as they require large doses of insulin, and need hospitalisation frequently for acute illnesses. Earlier it was believed that as MRDM was a secondary form of diabetes, such patients were not prone to the specific vascular complications of diabetes. However, recent studies have shown that MRDM patients do develop complications similar to those of NIDDM [22–24]. Thus it is clear that the management of MRDM constitutes another formidable task in India.

MALDISTRIBUTION OF PHYSICIANS IN THE POPULATION

India is predominantly an agricultural nation. The vast majority of cultivators are small farmers in the villages; about 80% of the total population live in rural areas. The total turnover of medical graduates is approximately 12 500 every year from the 110 medical colleges in our country. The statistics brought out by the Directorate General of Health of the Government of India show that there are 615 531 institutionally qualified medical persons in India [25]. This should give a physician to population ratio of 1 : 1100. Unfortunately, this is not the case: almost 75% of the medical partitioners work in urban areas catering for the needs of only 20% of the country's population, and barely 25% of the medical practitioners serve the overwhelming 80% of the rural population. This formidable mismatch in the distribution of physicians and population makes hardly one doctor available for 20 000 people in the rural areas [26].

LITERACY

The literacy rate in India as a whole is still very low, although it has improved from 29% in 1971 to 36% in 1981 [25]. The literacy rate is particularly poor among women, being only 25% in 1981 [25].

Public awareness about diabetes is essential for early diagnosis and treatment. Moreover, the success of treatment of any chronic metabolic disorder such as diabetes depends on constant motivation, encouragement and interaction with medical and paramedical personnel. The essential component leading to the success of such a system is a reasonable level of literacy in the population. Thus, it is understandable that the present low level of literacy in the Indian population is a formidable challenge, especially in the rural areas. Added to this is the problem of the use of different languages in different states in the Republic of India. Although a large proportion of the population speak the national language, Hindi, more than 20 regional languages are spoken in the Indian subcontinent [27]. This

obviously interferes with the effective implementation of health care delivery programmes.

Shortage of trained personnel for teaching lay people regarding diabetes is yet another problem [28]. In many developed nations, there are regular training programmes for nurses and other paramedical staff regarding diabetes education. A new cadre of 'patient educators' has been developed and funds are made available for diabetes education programmes. There have been a number of reports about the impact of education on the management of diabetes [29]. It is true that well-organised education programmes can achieve results even in developing countries. Our own studies have shown the effectiveness of organised education programmes in spite of differences in literacy and language [30]. However, such programmes are available only in very few institutions in India. Therefore millions of diabetic patients are not exposed to any kind of formal education at all.

DIFFICULTIES IN COMMUNICATION AND TRANSPORT

As mentioned earlier, most Indian people live in villages; such villages have inadequate electricity supplies, telephone connections and transport facilities. There is little doubt that these inadequacies are major impediments to health care. Emergencies in diabetes can be fatal if not attended to promptly. Moreover, successful treatment of patients with diabetes depends on regular contact with or visit to the caring physician. Earlier reports have shown that insulin dependent diabetes mellitus (IDDM) is rare in India [31–33]. In an analysis of diabetic patients with age of onset below 30 years, only 22% were found to have IDDM [34], so that acute emergencies are less likely. There are thousands of villages in India where people have to walk or travel by bullock cart for miles to obtain even simple medical aid. At present, we are not sure whether there are IDDM patients in the remote villages of India who die before receiving any type of medical attention.

A more challenging problem is the scarcity in rural areas of laboratory facilities, which are essential for the proper care of diabetic patients. In India, facilities for even ordinary clinical and biochemical investigations are available only in large towns and cities. Thus patients in villages have to travel long distances for any sort of laboratory test. In towns, the institutions run by the government have laboratories that offer services free of cost to the poor. However, most of these laboratories are overcrowded and overloaded. Hence, many seek the services of private laboratories; but these are expensive and usually cannot be afforded by the average citizen.

RELIGIOUS BELIEFS AND TABOOS

Although a majority of the population are Hindus, there are many other religious groups in India such as Muslims, Sikhs, Christians, etc. Even among the Hindus, there are subclasses which vary in different areas of the country. Being an ancient country with an ancient social order, there are many religious customs and rituals that have been practised for hundreds of years. Scientific and technological progress has not changed the life-style and habits of the vast majority of people, especially in the rural areas. Moreover, there are many ancient systems of medicine practised in India, such as Ayurveda, homeopathy, Siddha, Unani, etc. Most of these native systems have been practised by generations of certain families and by people belonging to a particular caste. The faith of the common man in these systems of native medicine is unflinching. As diabetes is a chronic disorder without cure, it is no wonder that people, especially the uneducated, seek all other possible methods of treatment, although such treatment may not help them in any way.

Another major handicap is the infrequency with which women consult physicians. This is particularly true of Muslim women, who practise the custom of wearing 'pardha' ('purdah') which prohibits them being seen by men. Many authors have implicated this taboo as one of the possible causes of reports of the low prevalence of diabetes among women in India, compared with men.

Remedies for diabetes prescribed by native medical men include neem tree leaves, bitter gourd juice, honey, etc. Some quacks have made fortunes selling wooden tumblers made from a particular tree, claiming that cold water kept in the tumbler for a few hours has an antidiabetic action. One of the very strong misconceptions about food is that a diabetic should avoid rice. In India the food is mainly cereal-based and people, especially in South India, consume rice and preparations made from rice as their staple

food [35]; a cereal-based diet is comparatively cheap. The misconceptions are shared by people throughout India and thus interfere with the proper implementation of diabetes care in Indian societies.

LIMITED RESOURCES

From the above description it is evident that there are many major problems and challenges in diabetes health care in India. Above all, the resources to meet these challenges are very limited. Among the Asian countries, India has limited financial resources: the gross national product (GNP) per capita (1982) in India was 260 US dollars compared with $300 in China, $320 in Sri Lanka, $580 in Indonesia and $5980 in Singapore [36].

There are no systems of health insurance comparable to those existing in the developed Western countries. All the general hospitals run by the governments in different states offer treatment free of cost to the low-income groups. However, the medical attention given in many of these hospitals is far from satisfactory as they are overcrowded. Moreover, most of the funds are spent on problems with higher priorities, such as family planning, leprosy, tuberculosis and other infectious diseases. Thus, except for a few large teaching hospitals, most hospitals do not have facilities to look after metabolic diseases. Diabetic clinics offering specialised health care are very few in India.

India's position today is unique in that it shares all the health and economic problems of developing countries, and at the same time the incidence of diabetes, atherosclerosis and ischaemic heart disease is not very low. In the years to come, with the control of communicable diseases and a simultaneous increase in the average life expectancy, the population in this country will be facing major chronic health problems. This is especially true of diabetes, in the light of the findings that Indians as a race have been shown to have a high genetic susceptibility to diabetes.

Thus new strategies are imperative for the health care delivery system in India. A comprehensive approach is necessary for planning and implementing prevention and control programmes for non-communicable diseases, including diabetes, with common underlying risk factors [37]. This necessitates an integrated programme for primary diabetes care with a new public health strategy, generation of a reliable database, development of personnel for diabetes health care, and appropriate laboratory technology.

REFERENCES

1. Nortman DL. Population and family planning programmes, 12th edn. A Population Council Fact Book. New York: Population Council, 1985: p 56.
2. Ministry of Health and Family Welfare. Year book 1982–83. Family welfare programme in India. New Delhi: Government of India, 1984: p 1.
3. UNICEF. An analysis of the situation of children in India, New Delhi: UNICEF Regional Office for South Central Asia, 1984: pp 1–107.
4. Miller L. The scope of diabetes mellitus in developing countries: diabetes at the grass roots. IDF Bull 1983; 28: 17.
5. West KM. Epidemiology of diabetes mellitus and its vascular lesions. New York: Elsevier, 1978.
6. Ahuja MMS. Epidemiological studies on diabetes mellitus in India. In Ahuja MMS (ed.) Epidemiology of diabetes in developing countries. New Delhi: Interprint, 1979: pp 29–38.
7. Taylor R, Zimmet P. Epidemiology of diabetes: migrant studies. In Mann JI, Pyorala K, Teuscher A (eds). Diabetes in epidemiological perspective. New York: Churchill Livingstone, 1983: pp 58–77.
8. Mather HM, Keen H. The Southall Diabetes Survey: prevalence of diabetes in Asians and Europeans. Br Med J 1985; 291: 1081–4.
9. Mohan V, Ramachandran A, Viswanathan M. Tropical diabetes. In Alberti KGMM, Krall LP (eds) Diabetes annual 2. Amsterdam: Elsevier, 1986: pp 30–8.
10. Ramachandran A, Gallaghar F, Mohan V et al. Comparative study of clinical pattern of diabetes from two referral centres for diabetes in the USA and India. J Diab Assoc Ind 1986; 26: 83–8.
11. Viswanathan M, Ramachandran A, Mohan V, Snehalatha C. Familial aggregation in diabetes mellitus. An analysis of 4000 cases. J Diab Assoc Ind 1977; 17: 9–13.
12. Mohan V, Sharp PS, Aber VR, Mather HM, Kohner EM. Family histories of Asian and European non-insulin dependent diabetic patients. Pract Diabetes 1986; 3: 254–6.
13. Viswanathan M, Mohan V, Snehalatha C, Ramachandran A. High prevalence of Type 2 (non-insulin dependent) diabetes among offspring of conjugal Type 2 diabetic parents in India. Diabetologia 1986; 28: 907–10.
14. Ramachandran A, Mohan V, Snehalatha C, Viswanathan M. Prevalence of non-insulin

15. Verma NPS, Mehta SP, Madhu S, Mather HM, Keen H. Prevalence of known diabetes in an urban Indian environment: the Darya Ganj diabetes survey. Br Med J 1986; 293: 423.
16. Mohan V, Ramachandran A, Snehalatha C, Mohan R, Bharani G, Viswanathan M. High prevalence of maturity onset diabetes of the young among Indians. Diabetes Care 1985; 8: 371–4.
17. Asmal AC, Dayal B, Jialal I, Leary WP, Omar MAK, Pillay NL, Thandaroyen FT. Non-insulin dependent diabetes mellitus with young age at onset in Blacks and Indians. S Afr Med J 1981; 60: 93–6.
18. Tattersall RB, Fajans SS. A difference between the inheritance of classical juvenile onset and maturity onset diabetes of young people. Diabetes 1975; 24: 44–53.
19. Ramachandran A, Snehalatha C, Mohan V, Viswanathan M. Vascular complications in Asian Indian non-insulin dependent diabetic patients. J Med Assoc Thai 1987; 70 (suppl. 2): 180–4.
20. Fajans SS. Heterogeneity between various families with non-insulin dependent diabetes of the MODY type. In Kobberling J, Tattersall RB (eds) Genetics of diabetes mellitus. London: Academic Press, 1982: p 251.
21. WHO Study Group on Diabetes Mellitus. Technical Report Series 727. Geneva: WHO, 1985.
22. Mohan R, Rajendran B, Mohan V, Ramachandran A, Viswanathan M. Retinopathy in tropical pancreatic diabetes. Arch Ophthalmol 1985; 103: 1487–9.
23. Ramachandran A, Mohan V, Kumaravel TS, Velmurugendran CU, Snehalatha C, Chinnikrishnudu M, Viswanathan M. Peripheral neuropathy in tropical pancreatic diabetes. Acta Diab Lat 1986; 23: 135–40.
24. Ramachandran A, Mohan V, Snehalatha C, Usha Rani KS, Shanmughasundaram S, Sivarajan N, Viswanathan M. Left ventricular dysfunction in fibrocalcific pancreatic diabetes. Acta Diab Lat 1987; 24: 81–4.
25. Choudhuri SK. Demographic trends in India and the tasks ahead (editorial). J Ind Med Assoc 1986; 84: 169–71.
26. Lalitha Rao. Presidential address of the Indian Medical Association—1985. J Ind Med Assoc 1985; 83: 87–90.
27. Ramachandran A, Mohan V, Shobana R, Viswanathan M. Challenges in patient education in India. IDF Bull 1985; 30: 18.
28. Saxl ER. Lay people's involvement in diabetes education in developing countries. IDF Bull 1983; 28: 18–19.
29. Beggan MP, Cregan D, Drurry MI. Assessment

of the outcome of an educational programme of diabetes self care. Diabetologia 1982; 23: 246–51.

30. Shobana R, Indira P, Ramachandran A, Mohan V, Premila L, Viswanathan M. Effectiveness of patient education in a multilingual multiliterate population. J Med Assoc Thai 1987; 70 (suppl. 2): 219–22.

31. Patel JC, Dhirwani MK, Kadekar SG. Analysis of 5481 subjects with diabetes mellitus. In Patel JC, Talwalkar NG (eds) Diabetes mellitus in the tropics. Bombay: Diabetic Association of India, 1966: p 94.

32. Guptha OP. The study of juvenile diabetes in Ahmedabad. J Assoc Phys Ind 1964; 12: 89–93.

33. Krishnaswami CV, Chandra P. The significance of certain epidemiological variants in the genesis of juvenile insulin dependent diabetes. The need for a global programme of cooperation. Tohuku J Exp Med 1983; 141 (suppl.): 161–70.

34. Ramachandran A, Mohan V, Snehalatha C et al. Clinical features of diabetes in the young as seen at a diabetes centre in South India. Diabetes Res Clin Pract 1988; 4: 117–25.

35. Viswanathan M, Ramachandran A, Mohan V, Snehalatha C. High carbohydrate, high fibre diet in diabetes. J Diab Assoc Ind 1981; 21 (suppl. 1): 90–6.

36. Thandanand S, Vannasaeng S, Nitiyanant W, Vichayanarat A. Diabetes in developing countries in 1985: present situation in Asia. Bull Deliv Health Care Diabetes Dev Countr 1986; 7: 3–8.

37. Bajaj JS, Madan R. Integrated program for primary diabetes care: special emphasis on developing countries. IDF Bull 1986; 31: 95–9.

71d

Organization of Care: Problems in Developing Countries—Malaysia

B.A.K. Khalid

Faculty of Medicine, Universiti Kebangsaan Malaysia, Kuala Lumpur, Malaysia

Malaysia is a developing country situated in South-East Asia: it consists of peninsular, or West Malaysia, and East Malaysia which is made up of the two Borneo states of Sabah and Sarawak. West Malaysia, with a population of about 13 million people, is more developed than East Malaysia, which has a population of about 3 million people only. Malaysia was under British colonial rule until 1957 when it gained independence, but the British rule has left its legacy of good roads, railways, schools and hospitals, and the judicial, police and administrative systems.

The country is rich in natural and mineral resources: it is the world's largest producer of tin, natural rubber, palm oil, tropical hardwoods and pepper; petroleum and natural gas have, however, become the largest export earner in the last decade. Like many other developing countries in the region, Malaysia is also rapidly becoming industrialized; it is now a major exporter of silicon chips and microelectronic components, and has started to produce its own motor car. Herein lies one major problem of providing health care, including diabetic care,

to the population: industrialization has brought about rapid expansion of towns and cities, with consequent strain on the existing health services.

ORGANIZATION OF HEALTH CARE

Malaysia has a well-organized and planned health care system, part of which it inherited from the British colonial administration. The health care system is aimed at providing 'health for all', so that even the remotest villages are served with basic health and medical care. The bottom of the pyramid for providing health care therefore is the village health clinic, usually staffed by specially trained village nurses. The next level is the rural health centre, where there are more nurses, a medical assistant who has had 4 years of basic medical training, and a doctor who visits the centre once or twice weekly and in emergencies. The next level of health care is the district hospital, where there is at least one doctor, assisted by medical assistants and trained nurses and technologists. These district hospitals are usually situated in the smaller

International Textbook of Diabetes Mellitus. Edited by K.G.M.M. Alberti, R.A. DeFronzo, H. Keen and P. Zimmet

towns. The larger towns have larger district hospitals which may be staffed by a physician, a surgeon, an obstetrician and gynaecologist and supporting resident medical officers. The district hospitals then refer patients to the general hospitals, which are found in each capital city or town of each of the 13 states of Malaysia. Difficult cases from the general hospitals are referred to the Kuala Lumpur General Hospital, which is the national reference hospital and teaching hospital for the National University of Malaysia. The standard of health and medical care for each illness, including diabetes, increases with the level of sophistication of the health service offered at each tier.

Health Services for Diabetes Care

Diabetes care includes diagnosis of diabetes, managing the disease once diagnosed, monitoring of diabetes control, detection of diabetic complications and managing the complications. At the village health clinic, the village nurse is trained to recognize diabetes, and screens for it by urine testing for reducing substances using Benedict's solution. Ketone testing is not usually available, but testing for urinary proteins is done using sulphosalicylic acid. The patient is usually referred to the nearest rural health centre, where the medical assistant or visiting doctor may confirm the 'diagnosis' by repeating Benedict's test on fresh urine specimens and sending the blood sample to the district hospital for glucose testing. If the patient is not too ill, then treatment with sulphonylurea and/or metformin is given. There are no facilities for blood glucose measurements at the rural centre. If the patient is ill, with secondary infection, or is obviously acidotic or comatose, or has not responded to the medications as shown by persistent sugar in the urine, then he or she will be referred to the nearest district hospital with physician and inpatient care available. At the district hospital, tests for levels of blood glucose, urea and electrolytes, blood cultures, blood gases, electrocardiographic and radiographic tests are usually available. Patients may be stabilized at the district hospital, or if their condition deteriorates, they may be transferred to the state general hospital at the state capital. At most state general hospitals, modern medical care is available for management of diabetes and its complications. However, facilities for measurement of

haemoglobin A_{1c}, fructosamine, islet cell antibodies and C-peptide are not available. These sophisticated tests are only available at the General Hospital in Kuala Lumpur. Similarly, fluorescein angiography and laser photocoagulation therapy are only available at the General Hospital in Kuala Lumpur and at a few new private hospitals mushrooming in Kuala Lumpur and the bigger towns. Dialysis for diabetes is still very limited and confined to the general hospitals only.

PROBLEMS IN ORGANIZATION OF DIABETIC CARE

Like other developing countries, Malaysia has its fair share of problems in maintaining and improving the above health organization for the care of diabetes and other diseases. These problems can be categorized as follows.

Financial Resources

One major problem is the lack of financial resources. Every developing country needs to finance development in that country, and development projects that bring in financial returns are usually favoured, such as oil refineries and industrial estates. Service-oriented projects such as development of health care are usually not a top priority. The national economy had been badly affected by the recent drop in primary commodity prices, including the price of petroleum oil. Funds for health and diabetes care were therefore sparse. There was a lack of funds for the purchase of new equipment and diagnostic reagents. Even blood test strips for glucose monitoring are very hard to come by, and are not available at rural health centres. Malaysia is also a tropical country where infectious diseases such as hepatitis, gastroenteritis, dengue, leptospirosis, typhus, malaria and tuberculosis are still endemic. Priority in the allocation of funds for provision of health care is therefore given to these diseases, rather than to diabetes.

Technical Expertise

For proper diabetes care, there is a need for a team of experts, including diabetic education nurses, dietitians, physicians and biochemists to perform laboratory tests or develop new ones such as HbA_{1c} assays. As in other developing countries, there is a grave shortage of such 'technical experts' for diabetes care, because (a) very few are suitably trained; (b) the dietitians, nurses and doctors are needed to provide health care for other illnesses as well—there is no room for specialization; (c) those who are well trained are sometimes underutilized in terms of their expertise in diabetes care, but are made to perform routine nursing, laboratory work or general medical duties; (d) a significant number of trained experts refused to return to Malaysia from where they were trained, e.g. in Britain or Australia; and (e) experts may emigrate to these Western countries when they cannot tolerate the local working conditions. This last 'brain drain' problem is common to developing countries, with no easy solution in sight. One major problem and cause for migration is job dissatisfaction, due to lack of instruments, inadequate staffing with consequent overwork, and lack of opportunity for career development by improving expertise in diabetic care and opportunity for diabetes research.

Maldistribution of Resources and Expertise

Malaysia is one of the rapidly developing countries in Asia, with massive programmes for rural development and industrialization. As mentioned above, the oil wealth and rapid industrialization have also brought about many problems, including health care for diabetes.

The large towns and cities are rapidly expanding. There is a higher standard of living in the urban areas; expectations are high, for education, amenities and health care. The medical services and technology in the general hospitals tend to be of a high standard, compared with those in rural areas. There are many private hospitals, providing high-class medical care, available for large fees. Many in the urban areas can afford this 'high-technology' type of health and diabetic care. However, rapid development has caused large rural-to-urban migration, with consequent large, poor, urban squatter populations and gross overcrowding of the government-financed general hospitals.

The rural areas have lower standards of living, with areas of abject poverty. The population may be large in some areas, for example in the rice-growing districts; however, in many parts of Malaysia, the population in the rural areas may be small and scattered, hence the need for village health clinics. As stated earlier, the technology for diagnosis and management of diabetes in the clinics and health centres is extremely limited, to Benedict's solution testing of urine only. Many cases of diabetes, or diabetes in pregnancy, may have been undetected, underdiagnosed and untreated.

Problems of Diagnosis of Diabetes and its Complications

The diagnosis of diabetes entails the measurement of blood glucose, whether done fasting, randomly or during a glucose tolerance test. Obviously, this is a major problem in the rural districts. It is not possible to provide a glucose analyser and a trained technologist to every rural health centre: blood samples, or the patient, will have to be sent to the nearest district hospital to confirm the diagnosis. In some areas this is not a major problem, but in the sparsely populated rural areas, this may mean a trek or boat ride lasting 2–3 days. Similarly, management and diagnosis of complications of diabetes, such as nephropathy, retinopathy and pulmonary tuberculosis, would entail sending the patient to the district hospital or general hospital.

Problems of Planning

The organization of medical services for diabetes care has been hampered not only by lack of finance, experts and equipment, by remote villages and overcrowded city hospitals, but also by the lack of hard data on the prevalence of diabetes in rural and urban populations, as well as in the various major racial groups of Malaysia. Health planners need such information to help plan future health services. If it can be shown that the prevalence of diabetes in the major races of Malaysia is as high as that in Fiji or Nauru, surely the government will take more heed of the problem? If it can be shown that the prevalence of diabetes is related to urbanization and improved socioeconomic status, then perhaps the government will realize that rapid development may mean more funds for diabetic health care. The government has realized that diabetes and cardiovascular disease may be major health problems and has supported a major nationwide study to assess the extent of the problem. Results are not yet available for public perusal, but the government has now directed that public awareness and education about these diseases should be enhanced.

SUMMARY

Malaysia has a well-organized health care system which is directed towards 'health care for all by the year 2000'. Health care is made available to the most remote areas, with a system of referral to high-technology hospitals if need be. The health services for diabetes care are available to the population, although high-technology and expert services are confined to the state general hospitals and a few district hospitals. Problems in organization of diabetes care occur because of several factors, including lack of financial resources, lack of expertise and maldistribution of resources and expertise. There is also a profound lack of data on the prevalence of diabetes and its complications; thus, because the extent and severity of the problem is not known, diabetes does not have priority in national health planning.

71e

Organisation of Care:
Problems in Developing
Countries—Tanzania

D.G. McLarty

Muhimbili Medical Centre, Dar es Salaam, Tanzania

A doctor working in Zaïre, one of Tanzania's neighbouring countries, has expressed the following view on diabetes care in that country [1]:

> Zaïre cannot afford to treat degenerative diseases like diabetes or heart failure. If you start treatment for 100 new patients this year they will survive, and next year there will be those patients and another 100 new patients and so on each year. So no hospital can afford to treat them free and insulin for a day costs 10 pence. A school teacher earns 40 pence a day on which to feed and clothe his wife and family.

Should diabetic patients, therefore, in poor countries like Zaïre and Tanzania be abandoned to the vagaries of the natural history of the disease or, in the case of insulin dependent diabetes mellitus (IDDM) patients, almost certain death?

Most Third World countries, including Tanzania, have experienced an unprecedented drop in living standards over the past 4–5 years. There has been a deterioration in all human welfare indicators such as childhood malnutrition, educational standards and functioning health centres [2]. Can Tanzania, therefore,

direct resources to the care of the chronic sick when the basic needs of the majority remain unmet? Many would agree with the doctor quoted above and consider that any attempt to establish an effective national network of care for diabetic patients, and for all with chronic diseases, is at present totally unrealistic.

In spite of all the problems, however, we in Tanzania believe that something can be done. Diabetic patients should not be left to die in a world with enormous resources of wealth and knowledge. A first, faltering step has therefore been taken towards the integration of diabetic care into the primary health-care system, and in the pursuit of a more effective union betweeen tertiary and primary care.

MEDICAL SERVICES IN TANZANIA

The Country

The United Republic of Tanzania was formed by the union of Tanganyika (mainland Tanzania) and Zanzibar. It lies on the eastern side of the African continent just south of the equator. Mainland Tanzania is surrounded by Kenya and

International Textbook of Diabetes Mellitus. Edited by K.G.M.M. Alberti, R.A. DeFronzo, H. Keen and P. Zimmet
© 1992 John Wiley & Sons Ltd

Table 1 Tanzania: some health and socioeconomic statistics

Area of Tanzania (km^2)	945 000
Total population (millions)	22.5
Population density (persons/km^2)	25.3
Crude birth rate	49 per 1000
Crude death rate	14 per 1000
Population growth rate (%)	3.5
Rural population (%)	85
Urban population (%)	15
Infant mortality rate	115 per 1000
Adult literacy rate (%)	85
Life expectancy at age 1 (years)	60
Life expectancy at birth (years)	55
Income per capita per annum (US $)	300
Government expenditure on health (% total budget 1987/88)	3.6
Health expenditure per capita per annum (US $, 1989/90 budget)	2.0
Population within 5 km walking distance from a health facility (%)	73

From reference 3, with permission.

Table 2 Health personnel development in Tanzania

	1961	1969	1971	1973	1980*
MCH aides/village midwives	400	545	650	780	2500
Health auxiliaries	150	180	230	325	800
Nurse/midwife A	388	683	838	934	1960
Nurse/midwife B	984	1619	2110	2690	4100
Rural medical aides	380	462	544	621	2800
Medical assistants	200	249	289	335	1200
Assistant medical officers	32	103	115	140	300
Doctors					
Tanzanian	12	90	155	231	700
Foreign	413	355	324	302	130
Total	2959	4286	5280	6328	14490

* Target figures.

Uganda to the north, Rwanda, Burundi and Zaïre to the west, Malawi and Zambia to the southwest, Mozambique to the south and the Indian Ocean to the east. Some facts about the country, including health statistics, are shown in Table 1 [3].

Structure of Health Services

Since independence, the delivery of health care to the rural areas of the country has been a government priority. As physicians are expensive to train, emphasis has been placed on the training of other cadres of health-care workers such as medical assistants and rural medical aides.

The development of health personnel in Tanzania since independence in 1961 until 1980 is shown in Table 2 [4]. Table 3 [5] shows the number of existing health facilities, with targets for the year 2000. In view of the current serious economic situation, it is uncertain whether these targets can be met. Emphasis, however, will continue to be placed on the development of primary health-care services, and it is within the context of existing primary health-care facilities in two districts of Tanzania that a programme has been started for the care of patients with diabetes and other chronic diseases.

Some reasons why attention should be paid to the care of patients with diabetes and other chronic diseases in developing countries are listed below.

(1) The denial of basic care to the diabetic patient is, we believe, similar to the denial of food to the hungry; 'for even hunger and thirst are diseases, . . . and if they lasted long, would kill us' [6].

(2) Life expectancy in most developing countries is increasing. The number of people reaching the age of increased susceptibility to these problems is therefore growing.

(3) Many developing countries have recorded marked increases in non-infectious diseases related, possibly, to changing life-styles, urbanisation, smoking, etc. These changes are occurring at a time when the great burden of infectious diseases remains. Preventive measures must be introduced if epidemics of coronary heart disease [7], diabetes [8] and tobacco-associated neoplasms [9] are not to follow. Education leading to increased awareness of problems such as diabetes among patients and public can, for example, lead to a reduction of chronic disability and death and the saving of resources.

PROGNOSIS FOR DIABETIC PATIENTS IN TANZANIA

Only one study on the natural history of diabetes in Africa has been reported, from Harare, Zimbabwe [10]. In 1977, 107 diabetic patients were admitted to the Harare General Hospital; 9 (8.4%) died before discharge. Six years later 93 of the 98 surviving patients were traced: of these, 38 (41%) had died, 21% within 1 year of discharge. Twenty-five (50%) of the 50 men in the series were heavy drinkers, and 32 of the 98

Table 3 Existing and projected health facilities in relation to administrative units

Administrative level	No. of units	Type of facility	No. of facilities in 1981	Projected, year 2000
Village	8300	Village health post	233	5300
Wards	1963	Dispensary	2600	
Division	360	Health centre	239	
District	104	District hospital	81	104
Regions	20	Regional hospital	17	20
Zone	5	Consultant hospital	4	5

patients (32%) had diabetes secondary to pancreatic or hepatic disease. Treatment with insulin was required by 84 patients (85.7%); in this series, therefore, most patients were classified as IDDM.

In June 1981 a diabetic register was opened at Muhimbili Medical Centre, Dar es Salaam. This hospital sees most African patients diagnosed as diabetic in the city. By 31 May 1987, 1250 patients had been registered. After a minimum follow-up period of 22 months, 205 (16.4%) of the 1250 patients were known to have died, 126 (61.5%) in hospital and 79 (38.5%) in the community. At least a further 71 were likely to have died [11].

Among those patients in whom the cause of death was known, diabetic ketoacidosis accounted for 50% of the deaths in patients with diabetes requiring insulin. Cardiovascular and renal diseases accounted for 24% of the deaths in patients with diabetes not requiring insulin (Table 4). In all patients, infections accounted for 30.3% of deaths where the cause was known. Infection also contributed to many of the deaths

due to diabetic ketoacidosis. If the causes of death at home were known and the fate of patients lost to follow-up, acute metabolic complications and infections would account for the majority of deaths. Most diabetic patients in Dar es Salaam therefore die from preventable causes, and this in the country's major city where diabetic services are available. In most parts of the country prognosis must be considerably worse. The need for improved diabetic care is obvious.

PROBLEMS AND SUGGESTED SOLUTIONS IN THE ORGANIZATION OF DIABETIC CARE

Problem 1: Lack of Resources—Financial and Material

At the National Level

Tanzania is one of the world's poorest countries. Its economy, like its political system, is based on a centrally planned socialist model. Education and health services have, up to now, been pro-

Table 4 Causes of death of 126 diabetic patients known to have died in hospital in Dar es Salaam, Tanzania

	Type of diabetes		
	Requiring insulin	Not requiring insulin	Uncertain
No (%) dying of:			
Diabetic coma (ketoacidotic, hyperosmolar)	19 (50)	1 (2)	
Hypoglycaemia	2 (5)	1 (2)	3 (12)
Infection:			
of extremities (including gangrene and septicaemia)	3 (8)	12 (19)	7 (28)
tuberculosis and other chest infections	6 (16)	2 (3)	5 (20)
diarrhoeal diseases	3 (8)	1 (1)	
Cardiovascular and renal diseases		15 (24)	1 (4)
Liver disease	1 (3)	5 (8)	3 (12)
Cancer		10 (16)	1 (4)
Miscellaneous		5 (8)	1 (4)
Unknown	4 (11)	11 (18)	4 (16)
Total	38 (100)	63 (100)	25 (100)

From reference 11, with permission.

vided free, although the worsening economic situation has raised questions as to how much longer this can be sustained.

The amount of money allocated for the health and social welfare services is insufficient to maintain the current health infrastructure. Per capita expenditure on health is approximately US $2.0 per person per annum. It is unlikely that the amount available for health care will increase in the foreseeable future: if diabetic care is to be improved, additional resources have to be found.

Possible sources of additional funding include:

(1) Non-governmental organisations within and outside Tanzania. The Lion's Club of Dar es Salaam has, for example, been one valuable source of financial help. To most people in the north, diabetes is an unknown problem in developing countries, and yet it is much more common than leprosy, for which at least two relief associations exist in the UK. People are moved by the mutilating injuries of leprosy; yet diabetes, because of the increased effect of infection, can be a more destructive and disabling disease.

(2) Increased effectiveness of self-help groups such as the Tanzania Diabetes Association. Diabetes associations are still in their infancy in most developing countries, and members have yet to appreciate the potential of cooperative action in seeking to further their welfare. The strong mutual concern that exists within the African extended family should provide a solid foundation for the future effectiveness of diabetic associations. If supplies of essential drugs and equipment were available, many members of the association would be willing to contribute a token fee, which, in turn, could go towards the welfare of the poorest patients.

(3) The development of links between diabetic associations in developing countries and those in developed countries should be encouraged. The Tanzania Diabetes Association has appreciated financial and material help from the British Diabetic Association. Links could even be encouraged between members of diabetic associations at an individual level.

At the Personal Level

Most diabetic patients are poor. Many live in villages which may be 4 or more hours' walk from the nearest bus stop. A journey to Dar es Salaam four times a year to collect insulin may consume a peasant farmer's entire annual income. Other patients live far from the main centres, and access for them to centralised resources is impossible. Most patients in such areas live and die without the diagnosis of diabetes ever having been made.

A possible solution is for tertiary levels of care to be brought into the community. However, before this can be done, and services planned, more information has to be obtained about the prevalence of diabetes in the community.

Problem 2: How Common is Diabetes in the Community?

Little is known about the prevalence of diabetes in most sub-Saharan countries. A number of studies indicate prevalence rates varying from 0–6% [12–13]. Using the World Health Organization (WHO) criteria for the diagnosis of diabetes, a prevalence of 0.5–1.3% has been found in people aged 15 years and over in a number of different African communities in Tanzania [14]. Most of these cases are of NIDDM, and most, in the rural areas, are asymptomatic. The mild and asymptomatic nature of many cases may be one reason why diabetes was rarely diagnosed in the past. It is possible that diet, exercise and low body weight prevent the emergence of symptoms, but if such patients are exposed to a different life-style the disease may become clinically evident. On the other hand, patients with undiagnosed IDDM are unlikely to be encountered in community surveys unless large numbers of adults and children are studied over a long period. There is strong evidence in Tanzania that the reason why IDDM was considered rare was due to the fact that most cases remained undiagnosed. Failure to diagnose diabetes may occur even when patients do present to government health services. In one series of 35 patients with diabetic ketoacidosis admitted to Muhimbili Medical Centre, 8 (22.9%) remained undiagnosed even after admission to the medical wards [15]. Awareness of diabetes, therefore, both among health workers and among the general public is limited. Although most patients present with classic symptoms, we have found in Dar es Salaam that only 10% attributed their symp-

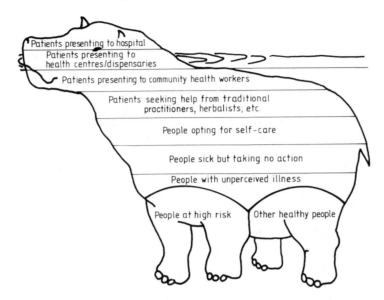

Labels within figure:
Patients presenting to hospital
Patients presenting to health centres/dispensaries
Patients presenting to community health workers
Patients seeking help from traditional practitioners, herbalists, etc.
People opting for self-care
People sick but taking no action
People with unperceived illness
People at high risk
Other healthy people

Figure 1 Like the hippo, most ill-health remains under the surface, unrecorded and unreported (redrawn from reference 16, with permission)

toms to diabetes, and 65% attended a health unit at least three times before the diagnosis of diabetes was made.

The risk of basing impressions of the frequency of any disease on hospital statistics is shown in Figure 1 [16]. The frequency of any problem must be based on careful community-based studies. There is, to date, no published evidence indicating an increase in the frequency of diabetes in Tanzania greater than might be expected from increases due to increased utilization of health services, increased population at risk, etc.

Problem 3: Lack of Recognition of Interdependence of Primary and Tertiary Health Care

Primary health care is often falsely viewed as an alternative to hospital-based health care. It may exist autonomously in the delivery of immunisation and maternal and child health-care programmes, but, in the care of the chronic sick, cooperation is essential between all levels of health care.

Successful follow-up and care of patients with chronic diseases such as diabetes will require, at the *primary care level*:

(1) a system of primary health care with adequate communications, available transport and adequate supervision;

(2) a team of informed primary health-care workers;
(3) a system of referral to and from the primary health-care unit;
(4) supplies of essential drugs, and some provision for the small number of patients who have need for drugs outside the essential drug programme.

Requirements at the *tertiary care level* are:

(1) a system of referral to the primary health-care worker;
(2) an appreciation of what can be done by the primary health-care workers, and readiness to instruct, supervise and encourage them;
(3) identification of those diseases amenable to chronic care in rural areas;
(4) realism about drugs;
(5) sympathy for the patients so that their return to the clinic does not involve them in undue hardship.

Plans in Tanzania for Community-based Care of the Chronic Sick, Including Diabetic Patients

As stated earlier, the Government of Tanzania has a declared priority for primary health care. Pilot projects have been started in two districts in Tanzania, which seek to incorporate the care of patients with diabetes and other chronic diseases into the existing primary health-care system. Seminars have been held in both districts, at which village health workers, rural medical aides and medical assistants have been trained in (a) recognition of the cardinal features of the main non-infectious diseases, including diabetes; (b) criteria for identification of loss of control and complications; (c) criteria for referral to the second and third tiers of the health-care system; and (d) relevant preventive measures. The evaluation of this programme will take some time, and its introduction on a national level many years; it is, however, a first step.

Problem 4: Problems Related to Personnel

Most developing countries, including Tanzania, face problems with respect to personnel. These can be summarised as manpower, motivation and the magnetism of cities.

Manpower

Tanzania has one doctor for every 56 000 people, and each year the country's one medical school produces approximately 40 graduates. It has been government policy, as stated previously, to concentrate on the training of other cadres of health-care workers such as medical assistants and rural medical aides, as training costs are less, as well as expectations. The doctor/person ratio given above is therefore misleading, as there are many other health-care workers. Experience has shown that a motivated nurse or medical assistant may be worth several poorly motivated medical graduates, and, for the foreseeable future, the provision of basic health services in the community must be dependent on cadres other than that of medical graduates.

Unfortunately many medical assistants have ceased to see their vocation as an end in itself and view themselves as ill-trained doctors. 'Must we continue to be assistants for the rest of our lives?' they ask. Such feelings, if frustrated, can lead to loss of interest and motivation.

Motivation of Health-care Workers

The main cause of lack of motivation is probably low levels of pay. The past few years have seen a significant reduction in the value of health workers' monthly income. A government salary is barely sufficient to meet survival needs for more than 1 or 2 weeks out of 4. The situation in most sub-Saharan countries is now such that if ways are not found of improving conditions of service, programmes seeking to improve the organisation of care for the chronic sick are unlikely to succeed. For effective care of the diabetic patient at both tertiary and primary care levels, those caring for them must, at least, be partially freed from anxieties concerning their own survival. For the village health worker, support and encouragement should come from the community. Such support varies from one community to another; often it is inadequate. National diabetes associations could act as a source of support and encouragement for health workers involved in diabetic care.

The Magnetism of Cities

In most developing countries, doctors prefer to live and work in cities. The reasons are clear. This phenomenon, however, must be recognised by all who seek to establish community-based health care for diabetic patients living in rural areas. The solution to this problem lies, as indicated above, in adequate provision for health-care workers. Governments often cannot provide this, and alternative solutions must be found.

Problem 5: Use of Alternative Health-care Facilities

In the organisation of care for diabetic patients, the use by patients of alternative health-care facilities should be recognised. Orthodox or Western-type health services provide only a small proportion of the total health care in Tanzania. In Dar es Salaam, approximately 35% of all new diabetic patients have first sought traditional treatment. In one study the mean duration of treatment in those who sought traditional treatment was 27 weeks, while the mean duration of symptoms for all patients was 16 weeks. Attempts have been made in a number of countries to incorporate the contribution of traditional healers into the primary health-care system. Results have been variable, but generally the union is fraught with difficulties. The fact that the symptoms of diabetes may resolve spontaneously adds to the problem of assessing claims for traditional medicines. Nevertheless, such claims are worthy of attention and further investigation.

Problem 6: Compliance

The problem of compliance is frequently mentioned in discussions on the care of diabetic patients in Tanzania and other African countries. Corrigan, for example, working in Mwanza, Tanzania, has reported that only 177 (40.6%) of 436 patients seen over an 8-year period continued to attend the diabetic clinic [17]. Health workers often speak of the patients' 'failure' to comply, whereas this 'failure' may be due to the most understandable reasons: the patient may, for example, be unable to afford travel expenses to the clinic. Other reasons for lack of compliance include disappointment and inability to accept the concept of a disease for which there is no permanent cure, as well as reasons already referred to, such as the use of alternative health-care systems. Death is another major reason for 'default'.

The problem of compliance highlights the need for effective communication between tertiary and primary health-care workers. Alternatively, if there is no community-based health-care system, those who care for diabetic patients at the tertiary level in towns must have a nurse or other health worker who is able to follow patients in their homes. Diabetic associations may assist these patients who find it difficult to attend for economic reasons.

REFERENCES

1. Masters D. Pray that the vision will not grow dim. Medical Bulletin of Baptist Doctors Missionary Fellowship 1985; 118: 7–11.
2. Brittain V. Living standards in Third World fall. Guardian Weekly 1987; 137: 8.
3. Kavishe FP. Proposal for a 5-year national programme on the prevention and control of iodine-deficiency disorders in Tanzania. Report no. 1095. Dar es Salaam: Tanzania Food and Nutrition Centre, 1987.
4. Chagula WK, Tarimo E. Meeting basic health needs in Tanzania. In Newell KW (ed.) Health by the People. Geneva: World Health Organization, 1975: p 161.
5. Guidelines for the implementation of the primary health care programme in Tanzania. Dar es Salaam: Ministry of Health and Social Welfare, 1983.
6. Donne J. In Simpson EM (ed.) Sermons on the Psalms and Gospels. Berkeley: University of California Press, 1963: p 35.
7. Dodu SRA. Coronary heart disease in developing countries: the threat can be averted. WHO Chronicle 1984; 38: 3–7.
8. Taylor R, Thoma K. Mortality patterns in the modernized Pacific Island nation of Nauru. Am J Publ Health 1985; 75: 149–55.
9. Scrimgeour EM, Jolley D. Trends in tobacco consumption and incidences of associated neoplasms in Papua New Guinea. Br Med J 1983; 266: 1414–16.
10. Castle WM, Wicks AC. A follow-up of 93 newly diagnosed African diabetics for 6 years. Diabetologia 1980; 18: 121–3.
11. McLarty DG, Kinabo L, Swai ABM. Diabetes in tropical Africa: a prospective study, 1981–7. II. Course and prognosis. Br Med J 1990; 300: 1107–10.
12. Teuscher T, Balliod P, Rosman JB, Teuscher A. Absence of diabetes in a rural West African population with a high carbohydrate/cassava diet. Lancet 1987; i: 765–8.
13. McLarty D. Diabetes in Africa. In Krall LP (ed.) World book of diabetes in practice. Amsterdam: Elsevier, 1985: pp 218–28.
14. McLarty DG, Swai ABM, Kitange HM et al. Prevalence of diabetes and impaired glucose tolerance in rural Tanzania. Lancet 1989; i: 871–5.
15. Rwiza HT, Swai ABM, McLarty DG. Failure to diagnose diabetic ketoacidosis in Tanzania. Diabet Med 1986; 3: 181–3.
16. Nordberg EM. The true disease pattern in East Africa, Part 1. E Afr Med J 1983; 60: 446–52.

71f
Organization of Care: Diabetes Community Programs as Part of Primary Health Care in the Community

Jaakko Tuomilehto

Department of Epidemiology, National Public Health Institute, Helsinki, Finland

During the 10–15 years in which it has been realized that properly organized and delivered diabetes control programs are necessary [1, 2], it is a paradox that in spite of great advances in our knowledge concerning diabetes mellitus and recent technological developments, organized health care for prevention and control of diabetes in most parts of the world has fallen behind. Although several studies have documented some improvements [3–5], control of diabetes, defined as the application of existing knowledge and technology to reduce diabetes-related mortality and morbidity, remains a major challenge. The magnitude and severity of this problem has been recognized and more systematic approaches to improve the care of diabetic patients, mainly through individual patient education and nutritional counselling, have been designed and implemented [1, 2, 5–8].

Control of diabetes in the community must be distinguished from control in individual patients. Community and individual efforts are, of course, independent and complementary. The development of community control programs was previously hampered by a lack of consensus on the objectives and strategies of diabetes management [2]. It has also been realized that the creation of sophisticated health services, including highly qualified personnel with predominantly curative approaches, to give excellent support to a few diabetic patients rather than helping the total population of diabetics in the community, has not produced a generally satisfactory result.

International Textbook of Diabetes Mellitus. Edited by K.G.M.M. Alberti, R.A. DeFronzo, H. Keen and P. Zimmet

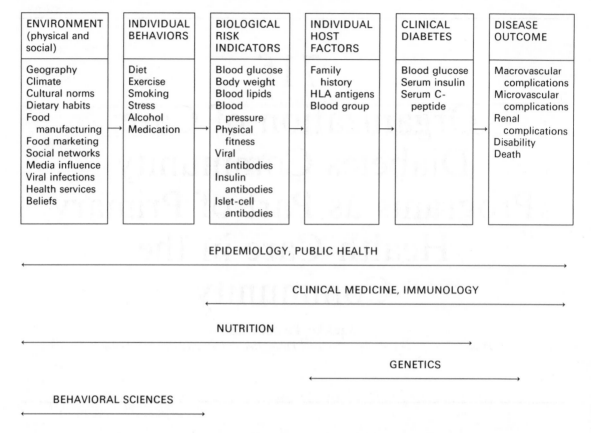

Figure 1 Sequence of factors leading to diabetes. The major disciplines and their scope, needed for research related to community-based prevention and control programs, are also shown

DIABETES AND OTHER NON-COMMUNICABLE DISEASES

Research into the etiology of diseases has largely relied on an approach according to category, which means that each disease has been considered separately. This approach has proved to be useful in defining the etiology, treatment and potential for prevention of infectious diseases, genetic disorders and some relatively rare non-communicable diseases (NCD), but it has not solved the problem of the major NCDs which now account for more than two-thirds of mortality and severe morbidity. Typically, these major NCDs (such as cancer, cardiovascular disease and diabetes) have a multifactorial etiology, involving several environmental factors that interact with each other and with certain host factors, i.e. genetic susceptibility (Figure 1). That several NCDs have common etiologic

factors has been shown in many studies [9–14], and this fact forms the scientific basis for the 'integrated approach' for prevention and control of NCD [15].

The environmental factors associated with the onset of disease do not seem to be very different for specific NCDs: they include cigarette smoking, high saturated fat intake, a low ratio of polyunsaturated to saturated fats in the diet, low fiber intake, high salt intake, low vitamin A, C and E intake, lack of physical activity, etc. Furthermore, these factors are also important for the successful resolution and the prevention of severe complications related to NCDs. Therefore, not only does the prevention of these diseases have a common basis, but the treatment of these NCDs also has much in common, especially with regard to non-pharmacologic therapeutic approaches that are always aimed at reducing the levels of causal factors of diseases.

Pharmacologic treatment, in contrast, typically aims at controlling only the symptoms of the particular disease or blocking its natural history with actions that may sometimes even precipitate another disease, e.g. some forms of antihypertensive drug therapy may have a diabetogenic effect.

Epstein and Holland [16] recently stated that the case for an integrated approach to controlling NCD does not only stand or fall with the hypothesis of linked common causes; irrespective of other considerations, the integration of community health programs to prevent NCD might be more effective and efficient in that it makes better use of available resources, both in terms of personnel and money. Furthermore, existing programs aiming at the control of only one disease may influence individuals to adopt healthier life-styles in other ways as well, and integration can be achieved simply by managerial unification of a set of preventive activities.

Although diabetes may sometimes be directly associated with inconvenient and even serious health problems, per se, it is not usually the main cause of death [17]. However, diabetes is a major factor contributing—usually directly—to increased mortality and morbidity, especially in cardiovascular diseases. In diabetic patients other known risk factors (smoking, hypertension, hypercholesterolemia) play as important a part as in non-diabetic subjects. Therefore, it is not wise (and probably not even justifiable) to start a community program for diabetes only without integrating it with interventions aimed at the more general prevention of cardiovascular diseases.

INTERVENTION STRATEGIES

In the development and implementation of a community control program, a full community assessment is essential. Community analysis should provide as comprehensive an understanding as possible of the situation at the start of the program; it should provide a basis for selecting priorities and appropriate methods of intervention; it should also indicate how continuous follow-up can be carried out through the program and thereby help to determine the course of the activities. As the most important intervention methods in diabetes control programs are health education of the public, patient education and organization of health primary

care, community analysis should be designed in such a way that these control issues are satisfactorily covered. The review of existing data from earlier studies, statistics and other sources is invaluable.

Epidemiological knowledge about diabetes and its complications in the target population provides the essential basis for the program: prevalence, incidence, mortality and their distribution within and between different population groups; the factors influencing the natural course of diabetes, and their prevalence [6]. It is also important to understand the social and cultural features of the population and the country. Information about health behaviour related to diabetes and its risk factors, about factors in the community influencing these behaviour complexes, and about community leadership and social interaction, are essential for program development and implementation.

Much of the success of any community program depends on the support of the population. For this reason information on how people and their official representatives see the problems and how they feel about the possibilities of solving them, should be part of the community analysis. Because the program would also depend heavily on their cooperation, the knowledge, attitudes and therapeutic practices of the health personnel should be surveyed too. The main objectives of a program are usually set by the perceived health needs of the community.

There is much evidence of the feasibility and effectiveness of primary and secondary prevention of major non-communicable diseases. Primary prevention has been defined as all measures designed to reduce the incidence of a disease in a population by reducing its onset. Secondary prevention includes all measures designed to reduce the prevalence of a disease in a population, by shortening its course and duration [18]. Both types of prevention are necessary to achieve effective control of major NCDs, including non-insulin dependent diabetes mellitus (NIDDM), in the community. Knowledge about the natural history of the disease, effective intervention methods, occurrence of the disease and the quality of the existing health care system will dictate the priorities between different types of intervention used in the health program. Ideally, primary prevention should take precedence, because intervention after the clinical stages of a disease have been reached will have

Ideal situation	Priority of the activities of community health programs	Current situation in diabetes care
Primary prevention of disease	Stage 1	Treatment of diabetic patients
Treatment of cases with a disease	Stage 2	Treatment of complications due to diabetes
Prevention of complications due to a disease	Stage 3	Prevention of complications due to diabetes
Treatment of complications due to a disease	Stage 4	Primary prevention of diabetes

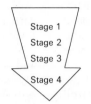

Figure 2 Priority order of different intervention strategies in community health programs, with special reference to diabetes care

only a limited impact on the mass epidemic of NIDDM and other major NCDs experienced in developed countries and in many developing countries today. Unfortunately, we cannot claim that such a priority setting actually obtains with regard to diabetes care (Figure 2).

In the development of methods for modern community health programs, diabetes-related activities might even serve as a model for more general NCD prevention and control in some countries. Diabetes care has several important components that can be effectively incorporated into primary health care services. These include the following, at the very least:

(1) health education of the public;
(2) guided patient self-care;
(3) continuous education of patients;
(4) training of health personnel and lay workers;
(5) community participation;
(6) organizing and maintenance of primary diabetes health care supported by specialist consultations;
(7) attempts to improve the environment;
(8) social support;
(9) development of diabetes registers or other relevant information systems.

NEED FOR PRACTICAL DEMONSTRATION PROGRAMS FOR PREVENTION AND CONTROL OF DIABETES

Community demonstration programs for diabetes control are a key step in putting the current knowledge of proven effective prevention and control strategies into practice in the community (Figure 3). The prerequisite for a demonstration program is an adequate level of health services in the community. Such a program can only be fully justified when it is implemented within the existing health care system and social structure of the community. In countries where the health care system is heterogeneous it has become obvious that lack of coordination among various resources and providers of care has contributed to inadequate prevention and primary care; this has also led to an ineffective use of resources.

It is important that community demonstration programs adopt a problem-oriented planning process where problems and resources are first identified. This means that some level of community analysis will be carried out. Unfortunately, the database needed for a comprehensive community diagnosis concerning diabetes is completely, or almost completely, lacking in most communities. It is, therefore, often the historical situation that will determine the objectives and resources available; e.g. the fact that the prevalence of NIDDM is extremely high in the USA among some Indian tribes [19–21] and in Australia among the aboriginals, or that in Finland the incidence of IDDM is the highest in the world [22], or that the population of the island republic of Nauru has developed a major diabetes epidemic during the past 50 years [23].

It must be borne in mind that community demonstration programs are not planned, in the experimental sense, to test a formal hypothesis about the causal effects of risk modification. Rather, they test the feasibility and effects of complex yet practical interventions based on available knowledge. They should also be planned in such a way that they could be applied elsewhere, if successful. The great advantage of community demonstration programs is that

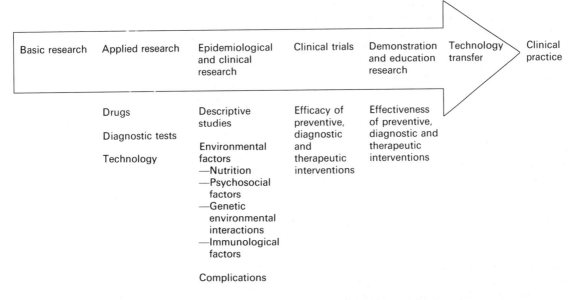

Basic research	Applied research	Epidemiological and clinical research	Clinical trials	Demonstration and education research	Technology transfer	Clinical practice
	Drugs	Descriptive studies	Efficacy of preventive, diagnostic and therapeutic interventions	Effectiveness of preventive, diagnostic and therapeutic interventions		
	Diagnostic tests					
	Technology	Environmental factors				
		—Nutrition				
		—Psychosocial factors				
		—Genetic environmental interactions				
		—Immunological factors				
		Complications				

Figure 3 Spectrum of medical research in diabetes leading to clinical practice applications

their findings are valid in real-life circumstances. It is clear that when such programs are carefully designed, their effectiveness and impact can be assessed.

Figure 1 presents a schematic model of stages in the natural course of diabetes, highlighting major factors or elements that have a role during this course, and tracing the progress of the disease from environmental and behavioral origins through a pathophysiological process to the clinical manifestations of diabetes. The genetic susceptibility of individuals is the major modifying factor in pathophysiological reactions to environmental exposure.

Community demonstration programs should apply medical and epidemiological knowledge simultaneously to identify health problems. This knowledge should also be used to set priorities in selecting objectives for such health programs. Another principle of community demonstration programs is that they use knowledge from social and behavioral sciences to design the actual program content. This implies an interdisciplinary approach in the planning, implementation and the evaluation of the program. Many of these principles can be seen in existing diabetes control activities [1, 5]. However, these principles have not been applied in a systematic way in community programs for diabetes, but mainly for clinical management of individual diabetic patients [24–26].

DESIGN OF COMMUNITY DEMONSTRATION PROGRAMS FOR PREVENTION AND CONTROL OF NCD

Several components of the design of community demonstration programs in non-communicable diseases have to be considered to strengthen the causal inference that the program itself is responsible for changes observed during the program evaluation period. Blackburn [27] stated that at the very least the following issues require careful attention a priori.

Control. Experimental community health intervention has to be compared in reference populations that are similar in size and structure, but which should have separate trade and communication borders.

Repetition. Program activities must be introduced in stages in the intervention communities. Staged introduction has not only practical managerial implications, but it amounts to a repetition of the experiment and generally strengthens the inference with each repetition, if the changes noted are in one direction.

Sensitive trend assessments. Cross-sectional, retrospective and prospective measurements of mortality, morbidity, levels of known risk factors, and social and behavioral indicators are used to characterize community risk and disease trends. Cohort analyses of those originally surveyed provide sensitive indicators of individual change. A number of other measurements, e.g. those of anthropological observations, medical care, community events, perceived health, personnel experiences, etc. are important to complete the trend data.

Dose–effect measurement. The design of community demonstration programs allows for a wide range of exposures to different intervention strategies, from those maximally exposed in the intensive intervention communities to those minimally exposed in the reference communities. A graded response strengthens the inference.

Maximal intervention. A consistent series of activities using multiple strategies should continue at an intensive level for 5–10 years, providing a systematically planned intervention for prevention and control of diabetes by methods that are postulated to be synergistically effective.

Linkage. Links are established (a) between components of the intervention program and its mass campaigns, (b) short-term behavior changes and their risk factor sequelae, and (c) between population risk factor trends and disease trends.

Pooling. Pooling of results in several intervention communities within and between different health intervention programs, compared with those of several reference communities, reduces variability and increases the power to detect trends. If this were not done, it might be difficult to separate the effects of the program from changes occurring spontaneously in the community.

Design limitations. There are many limitations in research related to demonstration programs. It is usually not feasible to apply randomized assignment of multiple study units, i.e. entire communities, for several reasons. The characteristics to be dealt with in complete matching are possibly far more numerous than the analytical units involved. The nature of community health programs precludes the experimental control of too many variables. It is not always certain whether the items chosen to be monitored in the program are the best to reflect changes. Reliabil-

Table 1 Principles of community demonstration programs for diabetes control to be taken into consideration

1.	These programs serve as a link translating current knowledge of proven effective intervention measures into health care practice
2.	Objectives and methodologies to address the problems must be clearly defined
3.	They should not be planned only to test etiological hypotheses
4.	They should apply medical/epidemiological knowlege to identify problems, and should also use social/behavioral knowledge to design the actual intervention measures
5.	Prerequisites are: adequate level of health care commitment of the local health authorities to support the program community analysis at baseline identification of problems to be solved during the program
6.	Programs should be first tested in 'pilot' areas
7.	Results (e.g. feasibility, effectiveness, costs, etc.) must be evaluated

ity of many interesting issues like the effects of socioeconomic factors associated with diet, exercise, smoking and drinking habits, etc., is often unknown.

The Main Components of a Demonstration Program

The practical framework of a diabetes control program consists of three components: (a) planning, (b) implementation of the intervention program, and (c) evaluation. Although these usually occur sequentially in time, in many cases they operate simultaneously as the program proceeds. Table 1 summarizes the main issues that form the principles of community demonstration programs.

Planning

The major elements in program planning are (a) the identification of the problem; (b) definition of objectives; (c) establishment of the program organization; and (d) the preparatory steps.

Identification of the problem in each community is carried out by means of the 'community analysis' (community diagnosis) which should provide a comprehensive understanding of the situation at the start of the program. Data on risk factors and modifying factors contributing to the existence of the problem should be assessed by various means, sometimes by rapid

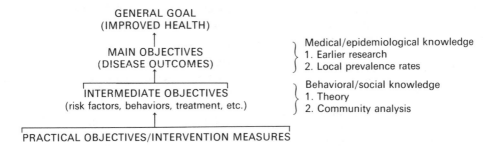

Figure 4 Establishment of the hierarchy of objectives in a community-based health program

surveys. Expert opinions are often very useful for review in planning seminars [28].

The intermediate objectives are those requiring the expenditure of resources. They are designed on the basis of the available medical and epidemiological knowledge of methods of influencing the health problems identified. The practical objectives and actual intervention measures should then be based on careful community analysis and on understanding of the main determinants of the intermediate objectives (Figure 4). Usually the historic development of each community health program dictates the program organization which has to be integrated into the existing health care and community structure. During the preparatory steps, various organizational and coordination aspects of the program can be evaluated and adjusted accordingly.

Implementation

The goal is to implement the program activities systematically according to its objectives and principles. Within the overall framework of the program, its actual implementation can be sufficiently flexible to adjust in response to the local opportunities. Integrating the program into the social organization of the community is necessary in order to ensure community participation and availability of various community resources, especially those outside the health sector [29]. The practical activities of the program have to be carried out mainly by the community. However, expert advice and consultations by others are needed to support the community's efforts.

The program activities have to be simple and practical in order to facilitate enactment in the entire community. Simple basic services for the largest possible proportion of the population are preferred to highly sophisticated services for a few people. Integration of several intervention measures will mean better use of the existing resources and avoid duplication of activities. To identify and mobilize all community resources, it is necessary to work closely with both official agencies and voluntary organizations.

The following groups of program activities need to be considered and developed:

(1) media-related and general educational activities;
(2) training of local health personnel and other active groups;
(3) organization of health services—primary health care, specialized supportive services, etc.;
(4) community activities for the modification of the environment;
(5) information services for monitoring the development of the program, and for providing feedback.

Many of these above-mentioned groups of activities have been used in diabetes care, but not very extensively in the framework of a community-based program [1, 3–5, 7, 26, 28]. Experience from existing diabetes care projects can provide useful information for the community analysis which is an essential step in the planning of integrated NCD prevention programs.

Evaluation

Any preventive or therapeutic action and its outcome must be continually evaluated to justify the program's continuation [29–31]. Therefore, an evaluation component is needed for any efficient diabetes prevention and control program in order to carry out the following strategic actions:

(1) add to the knowledge of disease etiology;

(2) evaluate the feasibility and effects of primary, secondary and tertiary prevention activities;

(3) evaluate the effectiveness of secondary prevention activities;

(4) devise and test new intervention strategies for disease prevention.

Evaluation can be divided into two components: (a) internal or formative evaluation, and (b) external or summative evaluation. The evaluation of community programs for diabetes control must be distinguished from the more research-oriented clinical trials or those narrower interests that focus on one aspect of the intervention, such as diabetes patient education.

Internal evaluation is carried out during the program to provide rapid feedback to the program workers, management and public. Data is mainly used to develop the program further. It is also used to assess the adequacy of the program and provide information for the review of progress during the intervention.

The main aim of external evaluation is to assess the overall feasibility, efficiency, effects, impact and other results of the program over a given time. External evaluation is used to assess whether the main objectives have been attained, and to what extent. It can also be used to identify which were the major factors contributing to the results, positive or negative. An expert group in some way external to the daily community activities is usually responsible for external evaluation. For national health policy the assessment of cost-effectiveness of the program is of great interest and significance, but it is usually very difficult to carry out [32, 33].

ADVANTAGES OF USING DIABETES AS A MODEL FOR INTEGRATION WITH OTHER NCD

Public Awareness of the Problem

It is well known that the public is aware of diabetes as a chronic, life-long disorder. A large body of data about the management of diabetes and about the beneficial effects of treatment on diabetic patients has been accumulated. Therefore, relatively little community education is needed to make people aware of diabetes as a health problem. What people and decision makers usually do not know is the magnitude of the diabetes problem in their own communities.

Existing Media-related and General Educational Activities

The strongest support for an integrated approach in prevention and control of major NCDs comes from the fact that these diseases have common causal factors, and that many recommendations for treatment include similar instruction for different diseases. This is a great advantage for health education. Numerous mass media activities on diabetes, especially those related to symptoms, diet, treatment and prevention of complications, are regularly seen in many countries [34]. Thus, we have a number of media experts who could also provide assistance for more comprehensive educational activities related to other NCDs [35]. Health education concerning diabetes has a longer tradition than that relating to cancer or cardiovascular diseases in many countries [36]. However, little attention has been paid so far to the primary prevention of diabetes.

Diabetes Patient Education

Diabetes education has become an essential part of any modern diabetes control program. The philosophy of self-care and health education for an improved long-term quality of life is probably nowhere better illustrated than when using self-management of diabetes as a model [3, 4, 25, 26].

Training of Health Personnel and Other Active Groups

Diabetes has been a major area for the continuous training of personnel in many medical and paramedical groups. This training has usually had clearly defined goals and aimed at providing practical skills for the participants [4, 5, 7, 28, 37–40]. This is why it is an excellent model for integration with other NCDs [41]. Furthermore, not only specialist doctors but also various other groups, including lay people in the community, have taken part in training concerning diabetes. Such training has traditionally stressed the importance of a multidisciplinary approach, which is one of the key strategies in the integrated prevention and control of NCDs [14, 16, 41, 42].

Organization of Health Services

Because diabetes is a disease usually of long

duration, it is natural that health services for diabetes are fairly well organized in most developed countries. They are, in fact, sometimes too specialized and lack the strong support of primary health care which is the essential requirement for any community health program. The comprehensive use of voluntary organizations and other non-medical community resources is well known in diabetes care. Because treatment for diabetes is usually long-term, the services developed provide a good model for other NCDs as well. These activities include not only models for clinical services, but also educational programs for families and community lay people [29, 34, 39, 42, 43].

Modification of Environment

Traditionally, diabetes has been a disease with a visible impact on our environment. Food production, manufacturing and marketing have accepted the needs of diabetic citizens. The role of community organizations and active individuals in this development must be appreciated by all those who are dealing with diabetes care. The success of this development has confirmed that the modification of the environment is feasible. Moreover, these achievements not only are important for a small group of diabetic patients in the community, but the trend to produce healthier alternatives for the daily diet of the whole population has greatly benefited from the lead given by those interested in diabetes care. Recently, it has been realized that dietary guidelines for diabetes are, in fact, almost the same as those for prevention of cardiovascular diseases or cancer. On the topic of population-based strategies of disease control, Rose [44] has said, 'Once a social norm of behaviour has become accepted and once the supply industries have adapted themselves to the new pattern, then the maintenance of that situation no longer requires effort from individuals. The health education phase aimed at changing individuals is, we hope a temporary necessity . . .'. This may be somewhat idealistic, but it underlines the importance and potential of environmental modification for health.

Information Systems for Management and Feedback

Until recently, information systems for diabetes care have not been very impressive when compared with those developed for cancer or cardiovascular diseases. The lack of systematic databases and international standardization in diabetes may reflect the earlier opinion of many experts that the diabetes problem could be solved by clinical and laboratory research alone, without public health involvement. Unfortunately, we now know that diabetes is rapidly increasing in most populations in the world [19–23, 45–48]. Because there has not been a systematic collection of data on possible causes of this increasing trend, we can only guess the reasons behind it.

Yet diabetes is one of the disorders that easily can be defined for epidemiological purposes, much more easily than, for instance, ischemic heart disease, arthritis or some forms of cancer. It is surprising that the international classification of diabetes in its present form was developed only in the late 1970s [2, 45, 49]. The present development, however, seems to be rather promising, as a number of epidemiological surveillance programs have been initiated or are being planned in various countries [22, 46, 49].

MAJOR CONSTRAINTS

The main constraints do not lie in the theoretical aspects of this issue of integrated prevention and control of diabetes, but concern more practical decisions and capabilities of working for a common goal. First of all, we are now faced with a historic decision which we could postpone with ease, using such commonly accepted excuses as 'We do not know enough', 'There is no final proof', 'Are you sure this action does not carry any risks?', etc.

Another constraint is that the resources will never be adequate to do all that needs to be done. However, many successful public health programs may eventually even bring about cost reduction and lessen the burden to the community. The old adage is that prevention is better than cure (or at least less expensive than treatment). The program for the integrated prevention and control of major NCDs could, in theory, save even more expense than a program designed for one disease only. In practice, however, such 'savings' may be difficult to identify because of the complex way in which the health care systems are developing and because demands are usually much greater than the resources available.

REFERENCES

1. Luft R, Lindmark C, Andersson B, Bergström I, Larsson Y, Ljunggren H. Underlag till vard-program för diabetes. Socialstyrelsens vard-programnämnd 1977.
2. WHO Expert Committee on Diabetes Mellitus. WHO Technical Report Series 646. Geneva: World Health Organization, 1980.
3. Wibell L, Walinder O. Success and failure in patient education in diabetes. Skandia International Symposia: Recent trends in diabetes research. Stockholm: Almqvist & Wiksell, 1981.
4. Mazzuca SA, Moorman NH, Wheeler ML et al. The Diabetes Education Study: a controlled trial of the effects of diabetes patient education. Diabetes Care 1986; 9: 1–10.
5. Leichter SB, Allweiss P. National consensus standards for diabetic patient education programs: a first step in solving an important puzzle. Arch Int Med 1984; 144: 1137–8.
6. Herman WH, Sinnock P, Brenner E et al. An epidemiologic model for diabetes mellitus: incidence, prevalence and mortality. Diabetes Care 1988; 7: 367.
7. Beaven DW, Scott RS. The organization of diabetes care. In Krall LP, Alberti KGMM (eds) World book of diabetes in practice, vol. 2. Amsterdam: Elsevier, 1986: pp 284–7.
8. Litonjua Augusto D. Asia—special area problems and solutions. In Krall LP, Alberti KGMM (eds) World book of diabetes in practice, vol. 2. Amsterdam: Elsevier, 1986: pp 239–42.
9. Hinkle LE Jr, Wolff HG. Ecologic investigations of the relationship between illness, life experience and the social environment. Ann Intern Med 1958; 49: 1373–88.
10. Epstein FH, Francis T Jr, Hayner NS, et al. Prevalence of chronic diseases and distribution of selected physiologic variables in a total community, Tecumseh, Michigan. Am J Epidemiol 1965; 81: 307–22.
11. Abrahamson JH, Gofin J, Peritz E, Hopp C, Epstein LM. Clustering of chronic disorders—a community study of coprevalence in Jerusalem. J Chronic Dis 1982; 35: 221–30.
12. Manton KG, Patrick CH, Stallard E. Mortality model based on delays in progression of chronic diseases: alternative to cause elimination model. Publ Health Rep 1980;95: 580–5.
13. Fries FJ. Aging, natural death, and the compression of morbidity. New Engl J Med 1980; 303: 130–5.
14. Grabauskas V, Tuomilehto J. Integration of diabetes control with that of other non-communicable diseases. In Tuomilehto J, Zimmet P, King H, Pressley M, (eds) Diabetes mellitus. Primary health care prevention and control. International Diabetes Federation. Singapore: International Press, 1982: pp 51–60.
15. Glasunov IS, Grabauskas V, Holland WW, Epstein FH. An integrated programme for the prevention and control of noncommunicable diseases. A Kaunas report. J Chron Dis 1983; 36: 419–26.
16. Epstein FH Holland W. Prevention of chronic diseases in the community—one-disease versus multiple-disease strategies. Int J Epidemiol 1983; 12: 135–7.
17. Fuller JH, Elford J, Goldblatt P, Adelstein AM. Diabetes mortality: new light on an underestimated public health problem. Diabetologia 1984; 24: 336–41.
18. Hogarth J. Glossary of health care. Public health in Europe 5, Copenhagen: WHO Regional Office for Europe, 1975: p 302.
19. Knowler WC, Bennett PH, Hamman RF, Miller M. Diabetes incidence and prevalence in Pima Indians, a 19-fold greater incidence than in Rochester, Minnesota. Am J Epidemiol 1978; 108: 497–505.
20. Gardner LI, Stern MP, Haffner SM, et al. Prevalence of diabetes in Mexican Americans: relationship to percent of gene pool derived from native American sources. Diabetes 1984; 33: 86–92.
21. Brosseau JD, Eelkema RC, Crawford AC, Abe TA. Diabetes among the three affiliated tribes: correlation with degree of Indian inheritance. Am J Publ Health 1979; 69: 1277–8.
22. Rewers M, LaPorte RE, King H, Tuomilehto J. Trends in the prevalence and incidence of diabetes: insulin-dependent diabetes mellitus in childhood. World Health Stat Q 1988; 41: 179–89.
23. Zimmet P, Taft P, Guinea A, Guthrie W, Thoma K. The high prevalence of diabetes mellitus on a Central Pacific island. Diabetologia 1977; 13: 111–15.
24. Stern MP, Pugh JA, Gaskill SP, Hazuda HP. Knowledge, attitudes, and behavior related to obesity and dieting in Mexican Americans and Anglos: the San Antonio heart study. Am J Epidemiol 1982; 115: 917–28.
25. Rosenthal MM. Resistance to change: the case of the Swedish Diabetes Primary Care Program. In Luft R, Rosenqvist U (eds) Diabetes care as a model for primary health care (in press).
26. Vinicor F, Cohen SJ, Mazzuca SA et al. Diabeds: a randomized trial of the effect of physician and/or patient education on diabetes patient outcomes. J Chron Dis 1987; 40: 345–56.
27. Blackburn H. Research and demonstration pro-

jects in community cardiovascular disease prevention. J Publ Health Pol 1983; 4: 398–421.

28. Smith CK, Taylor TR, Gordon MJ, WAMI Family Medicine Collaborative Research Group. Community based studies of diabetes control: program development and preliminary analysis. J Fam Pract 1982; 14: 459–67.

29. Tuomilehto J, Neittaanmäki L, Salonen JT, Puska P, Nissinen A. Community involvement in developing comprehensive cardiovascular control programs. A case study in North Karelia, Finland. Yearbook Pop Res Finland 1983; 21: 75–98.

30. Cook T, Campbell D. Quasi-experimentation. Design and analysis issues for field settings. Chicago: Rand McNally, 1979.

31. World Health Organization. Development of indicators for monitoring progress towards health for all by the year 2000. Geneva WHO, 1981.

32. Jönsson B. Diabetes: the cost of illness and the cost of control. Acta Med Scand 1983; Suppl. 671: 19–27.

33. Entmacher PS, Sinnock P, Bostic E, Harris MI. Economic impact of diabetes. In National Diabetes Data Group: Diabetes in America. NIH Publication no. 85–1468. Bethesda, Md: 1985: pp XXXII-1-13.

34. Tupling H, Webb K, Harris G, Sulway M, eds. You've got to get through the outside layer. A handbook for health educators, using diabetes as a Model. Sydney: Diabetes Education & Assessment Programme of Royal North Shore Hospital of Sydney and Northern Metropolitan Health Region of the Health Commission of New South Wales, 1981.

35. Davidson PO, Davidson SM. Behavioral medicine: changing health lifestyles. New York: Brunner Mazel, 1980.

36. Elliott PJ. The prevention of diabetes mellitus. JAMA 1921; 76: 79–84.

37. Beaven DW, Dodge JS, Kilpatrick JA, Spears GFS. Education and diabetes: attitudes, opinions and needs of New Zealand doctors. NZ Med J 1975; 81: 95–100.

38. Mazzuca SA. Diabetes patient education: the state-of-the-art. Patient Educ Newslett 1983; 6: 1–3.

39. National Commission on Diabetes. Diabetes education for health professionals, patients and the public. Part 5, vol. III, Reports of Committees, Subcommittees and Workgroups. DHEW Publication no. NIH 76–1031. Washington, DC: US Government Printing Office, 1976.

40. Weinberger M, Cohen SJ, Mazzuca SA. The role of physicians' knowledge and attitudes in effective diabetes management. Soc Sci Med 1984; 19: 965–70.

41. Mazzuca SA. Does patient education in chronic disease have therapeutic value? J Chron Dis 1982; 35: 521–9.

42. Miller J, Grover PL. Guidelines for making health education work. Publ Health Rep 1976; 91: 248–53.

43. Puska P, Nissinen A, Salonen JT et al. The community-based strategy to prevent coronary heart disease: conclusions from the ten years of the North Karelia project. Ann Rev Publ Health 1985; 6: 147–93.

44. Rose G. Sick individuals and sick populations. Int J Epidemiol 1985; 14: 32–8.

45. WHO Study Group. Diabetes mellitus. Technical Report Series 727. Geneva: WHO, 1985.

46. Dahlqvist G, Gustavsson KH, Holmgren G et al. The incidence of diabetes mellitus in Swedish children 0–14 years of age. A prospective study 1977–1980. Acta Pediatr Scand 1982; 71: 7–14.

47. National Diabetes Data Group: Diabetes in America: diabetes data compiled 1984. NIH Publication no. 85–1468. Washington, DC: US Government Printing Office, 1985.

48. Åkerblom HK, Reunanen A. The epidemiology of insulin-dependent diabetes mellitus (IDDM) in Finland and in Northern Europe. Diabetes Care 1985; 8 (suppl. 1): 10–16.

49. National Diabetes Data Group: Classification and diagnosis of diabetes mellitus and other categories of glucose intolerance. Diabetes 1979; 28: 1039–57.

72

Diabetic Life Problems: Insurance, Driving, Employment

Leo P. Krall

Joslin Diabetes Center, Boston, Massachusetts, USA

Here, this late in the book, are issues that can be disturbing and disruptive in the life of the person with diabetes. Although all of the preceding topics are important for those with diabetes and their physicians, they may not appear as important to the person trying to earn a living as such mundane problems as 'How can I get insurance?', or 'Can I make a living without my car?', or 'Can I get a decent job?'

The natural mantra of the medical profession is to assure patients that if they take proper care of themselves, they can live a perfectly 'normal' life, which is not completely true. In a survey of a dozen diabetes texts published in the last 10 years, only three had any mention of these topics: book A discussed them in 20 pages out of 1090; book B had 30 pages out of 950, and book C had 12 pages out of 380 to discuss, even remotely, these problems so vital to the patient. These matters are usually left to the diabetes associations and lay groups to pursue.

In the USA alone, the lowest estimate of the total impact of diabetes is at least US $14 billion annually [1]. This may not, however, mean as much to individuals as the fact that they may not be able to protect their families with adequate life-insurance or cannot find suitable employment because of antidiabetes bias. The late Dr Elliott P. Joslin stated in his earliest text (1916) that 'the way persons with diabetes live and their ability to make a living have much to do with the success of their treatment' [2]. Three topics of importance for the diabetic life, discussed in this chapter in order of available information, are the basics of insurance, the right to drive an automobile, and employment with or without discrimination.

INSURANCE

Life-insurance, or 'assurance' in some countries, is, in its simplest form, an annual gamble between the insured and the insurer (i.e. the company). In the case of *term* (renewable each year) life-insurance, the company estimates the odds according to actuarial figures (life tables) and says: 'We bet you will live at least another year'. The insured says: 'I'll bet I do not'. At the end of the year, the company says 'You lose. Do

International Textbook of Diabetes Mellitus. Edited by K.G.M.M. Alberti, R.A. DeFronzo, H. Keen and P. Zimmet
© 1992 John Wiley & Sons Ltd

you want to try another year? It will cost you more'. Usually the insured is happy to agree. In *ordinary* life-insurance, the betting is life-long. People (including diabetic patients) have been living longer, but the life tables do not always reflect this very rapidly. The best policies are those where entire employment groups are insured. A problem here is that if the insured wish to leave their job, does the insurance go with them?

The improved life expectancy has led to a liberalized approach. At present, diabetes classification states that impaired glucose tolerance and gestational diabetes are separate entities and not necessarily considered to be stages of diabetes, as is true for 'potential' and 'previous' glucose tolerance abnormalities. Increasingly, diabetic patients may obtain protection at standard rates [3]. In spite of this, many still are considered as substandard, paying much higher premiums when policies are available. Insulin dependent diabetes mellitus (IDDM) is still associated with the highest risks; life-insurance companies claim that excess mortality is highest among those whose diabetes began at a very young age and that better mortality data come from older age groups with non-insulin dependent diabetes mellitus (NIDDM). Mortality tended to increase with duration of diabetes, but in all categories there was a tenfold impact on mortality if proteinuria was found at the time of examination for insurance, whereas obesity caused only a modest increase in mortality rates [3].

Petrides et al agree that evaluation of diabetic patients for insurance has changed because of better diabetes therapy: they set out the German experience that age of the patient at time of diagnosis, the type of treatment, the state of metabolism and patient compliance help to determine the risk for life-insurance [4]. The German Diabetes Association has energetically pushed for better insurance for its members. In almost every country, the same factors used to evaluate life-insurance for diabetic patients are also considerations in health insurance. Of course, each country differs: for example, the socialized European nations have provision for all diseases equally. In Denmark, all life-insurance companies are regulated, meaning they are not permitted to compete for policies (K. Borch-Johnsen, personal communication). An official board makes decisions on all such policies and decides substandard risks individually. These cannot be appealed, meaning that patients and physicians must depend on this board. Prior to the setting up of this board, premiums were based on diabetes type and age at diagnosis, and patients were divided into subgroups depending on degree of 'regulation' of diabetes control: the best regulated had the lowest premium rates; those with complications were often declined. However, the groups were not always clearly defined, or were difficult to evaluate. Steno Hospital studies [5] showed early proteinuria to be the leading cause of excess mortality. At present, rates are lowest for subjects with NIDDM. Those with persisting proteinuria exceeding 0.5 g per 24 hours are declined insurance, but 'occasional proteinuria' does not influence these rates. If there is proliferative retinopathy without proteinuria, the policy is deferred for 2 years. If after that time there is still no proteinuria, insurance is provided at the standard diabetes rate. However, if proteinuria persists, the policy is refused. Age at diagnosis is important because the premiums decrease with increased age at diagnosis. Somewhat similar regulations have been adopted in Norway and Sweden.

A classic study by Goodkin and Wolloch [6] concerning a 20-year follow-up of insured diabetic patients showed that:

(1) mortality declines progressively with increasing age at time of diagnosis;
(2) mortality increases with increased duration of the disease until the 15th year of disease, after which it flattens out;
(3) mortality rates are much higher with the same duration of the disease in IDDM than in NIDDM subjects;
(4) the age at onset of diabetes is the most significant factor in mortality, with the highest rates of onset of diabetes at age 14 years and under;
(5) a group of patients with poor metabolic control shows 2.5 times the mortality of the relatively well-regulated group;
(6) those people treated with diet alone, or diet and medication, show a much lower mortality rate than those with IDDM;
(7) the overweight diabetic shows a higher mortality than does the standard or underweight diabetic;
(8) the presence of albuminuria is an extremely unfavorable prognostic sign.

A questionnaire [7] was sent to 33 European member organizations of the International Diabetes Federation in 18 countries; answers were received from 19 organizations in these countries. In answer to the question 'Are insulin-requiring diabetics accepted for life-insurance?' 6 answered 'yes', while others stated 'almost never' or 'possibly' depending on duration, lack of complications, disability, etc.; 3 replied 'no, none available'. As to 'Are insulin-requiring diabetics charged a higher premium than non-diabetics?', 10 answered 'yes', 5 'no', 1 'some-times'. The amount of excess premium was 'vari-able', 'depends on health', '0–100%'. 'Were oral agent-treated patients accepted?'—14 'yes', 3 'treated individually'.

In summary, with better actuarial statistics, insurance companies are taking a more enlight-ened view regarding the issuing of life-insurance to groups previously considered substandard, but many people still encounter difficulty or much higher rates for coverage if they have diabetes.

A partial answer may be the effectiveness of increasingly aggressive diabetes associations seeking insurance for their members in group plans. Members of the American Diabetes Asso-ciation (ADA), for example, can find group term life-insurance with coverage up to US $66 000, depending on certain criteria, for ages 5–59 years (with certain limitations).

As for the future, Entmacher and Bale [8] conclude that unless intervention occurs, with new and more effective treatment, there may not be more dramatic increases in life expectancy among diabetics in the foreseeable future—but who knows the future?

Some things can be done: (a) even better data should be developed, proving that better-treated diabetic patients survive for longer; (b) diabetes organizations must be both vigilant and more aggressive in demanding equitable treatment for their members; (c) those who are in diabetes-prone categories should get the insurance they require, as early as possible; (d) those with diabetes should look for positions that include group insurance, or join groups that might get them more favorable consideration.

DRIVING

The right to be able to drive an automobile is not only one of the most cherished tribal rights of adulthood, but increasingly a necessity in modern life. However, it is important to remem-ber that in most of the world, driving is generally a privilege rather than a right.

In the USA, regulation is mostly left to the individual states, which means that regulations vary greatly. At present, all 50 states permit those with diabetes to drive, although some require a physician's statement that the applicant is in good health, that the diabetes is adequately 'controlled' and that the applicant does not suffer such reactions as might threaten judgment or consciousness. Krosnick [9] listed hypogly-cemia, poor judgment, poor or blurred vision, defective reflexes or impaired sensation to the feet as well as retinopathy as the main reasons why New Jersey, for example, requires a diabetic driver cited for a motor violation or accident to complete a form, and the driver's physician to submit an exhaustive report expressing whether or not diabetes would interfere with highway safety. This is then reviewed by a medical advis-ory panel who make recommendations to the director of the Division of Motor Vehicles.

Unquestionably, motor vehicle accidents are a leading cause of death in much of the world. Long ago a study [10] showed that drivers with diabetes and also those with other chronic conditions averaged more than twice as many accidents per million miles of driving as did drivers with no known conditions, although more recent studies seem to differ from this evaluation. A very recent one [11] concluded that many drivers with diabetes do, indeed, have more accidents than non-diabetic drivers, but the risks were smaller than those in previous studies and did not warrant restrictions on driv-ing privileges. Furthermore, many people with diabetes do not make this known on their license applications, as shown in a UK report [12], which stated that, of 250 patients with IDDM, 41.8% had not mentioned this on their license applications. There is also increased use of high-powered boats, snowmobiles and other powered vehicles, with almost no regulation.

In the European survey previously mentioned [7] to which there were 19 responders, the ques-tion 'Must you mention diabetes in applying for a driving license?' received the answer 'yes' for a personal license in 13 countries and for an occupational license in 16. The question 'Is there a distinction in application forms by therapy?' received 14 'yes' answers, 3 'no', and 4 responses stated that special examinations by a diabetologist or eye physician were required. The German Democratic Republic had the most stringent regulations: everyone, not only diabetic patients, must have examinations that may include blood and urine glucose testing. The question whether occupational driving licenses are issued to diabetic patients using insulin elicited the following responses: for taxicabs, 4 'yes', 13 'no'; for buses, 2 'yes', 15 'no'; for trucks, 3 'yes', 3 'yes, if the license preceded the diabetes', 11 'no'.

Some rules were strange. One nation did not permit insulin-using diabetic patients to drive a taxi or bus, but truck driving was permitted. In another, no bus driving was allowed but both taxi and truck driving were permitted. All allowed driving by those taking oral hypoglycemic agents, although this is under review in several nations. One nation did not permit sulfonylurea agents but biguanides were satisfactory. There is a tremendous difference in regulations in countries adjacent to each other and, indeed, the coming of the European Economic Community (EEC) in 1992 should permit the International Diabetes Federation to encourage the standardization of regulations in this area.

Petrides et al [4] have commented that in the Federal Republic of Germany there were no rigid legal guidelines for granting or revocation of drivers' licenses for diabetic patients, the decision resting with a physician experienced in diabetes. Furthermore, in Germany all patients are supposed to carry 'diabetic passes' that contain all pertinent findings concerning health care.

Even a tropical paradise such as New Caledonia (J. Henri, personal communication), about 1800 km east of New Zealand, with a population of about 150 000, has problems as there are estimated to be 15 500 persons with diabetes (10%). Long-distance driving ability is determined by the Medical Commission of the Highway Code. Ordinarily a driving license is granted there for a lifetime, but diabetes patients must declare the condition to obtain the first driver's license. With NIDDM, the medical examination will determine the duration of the driving permit, which is renewable with further medical examinations. Persons with IDDM may not drive a truck weighing more than 3500 kg or a car with more than nine seats including that of the driver. However, if a license has been obtained before the onset of diabetes, the patient can continue to drive a private car without declaring the condition and the license is permanent, but a medical examination is required in case of a serious traffic offense.

Songer et al [13] reported a case-control study, examining motor vehicle accident experiences of 158 IDDM patients and 158 non-diabetic siblings. They found that the overall accident risk of those with diabetes and the control subjects did not differ significantly but, for some reason, female diabetic drivers showed an increased risk for motor vehicle accidents (about 5 times higher than in the female control subjects). Hypoglycemia-related accidents were evident on a cumulative basis but did not appear to explain the accident difference in women. This excess risk compared with female non-diabetics is difficult to explain.

US Interstate Commerce

Although individual US states permit trucks (lorries) to be driven *within* the state, in some cases—such as Texas and California—distances are enormous. Interstate truck driving is not permitted to persons using insulin. On 3 November 1987 the Federal Highway Administration (FHA), Department of Transportation (USA) reaffirmed its previous ruling that 'the weight of medical evidence supported prohibiting insulin-using diabetics from driving commercial motor vehicles in interstate commerce' [14]. It is to be noted that the Federal Railroad Administration has no prohibition for operating locomotives if a physician qualifies an engineer (train driver). Under pressure from petitioners, FHA is now reviewing this rule. Perhaps it is thought that those driving trucks within state boundaries are more likely to make shorter trips, are nearer their homes, or at least stop for meals and are not likely to be driving long-distance vehicles or to be driving through the night, with longer hours, infrequent stops and irregular meals. On the other hand, the ADA has recommended certain criteria and procedures for evaluating insulin-requiring diabetics requesting a waiver, and feels that such persons should be given driving permission if there is no other disqualifying disease [15]. The ADA has stated its policy: 'Any person, whether insulin-dependent or non-insulin-dependent, should be eligible for any driver's or pilot's license for which he or she is individually qualified'; in other words, people should be considered as individuals rather than as a class of persons.

For its part, the FHA has stated that longer driving fatigue increases the probability of an accident, especially in insulin dependent persons, and further estimates that the likelihood of accident due to hypoglycemic reactions would be 1.5–3 times greater if IDDM drivers were to drive interstate.

The Department of Transportation has proposed establishing minimal testing and licensing standards, to be implemented by the states for commercial, bus and truck drivers. There are about 5.5 million drivers who would have to obtain such a license by April 1992; this has not been resolved.

This type of effort is, of course, not limited to the USA. A subcommittee of Diabetes Australia set out recommendations to modify the regulations in Australia, citing many inequities [16]: for example, in some Australian states, even those drivers taking oral agents are not allowed to transport goods in heavy trucks. The goal is to develop a system that would consider individual cases; those satisfactorily treated with diet and/or oral agents would be reviewed annually; diabetic patients using insulin would be subject to a more inclusive annual medical report that would include listing of any insulin reactions in the previous year.

Cockram et al [17] cited a case in which an insulin-treated driver of a heavy goods vehicle (HGV) had his license revoked although he had been treated since 1967 with insulin, with an excellent record and no evidence of diabetes complications. He had two minor hypoglycemic reactions during the 1970s while asleep. In 1977 he had a road traffic accident with no other vehicles involved; his blood glucose level was within normal range. His license was then reviewed in 1979 and revoked in 1982 although he had driven nearly 1 000 000 km miles with no diabetes-involved accidents. The case went to the High Court on an important point of law, and the driver then retained his license on the basis that he did not 'suffer from a disease or disability likely to cause the driving by him . . . to be a source of danger to the public'. In this strict legal context, the word 'likely' is taken to mean more than a bare possibility—it could happen—but less than a probability. In the UK there is no general statutory restriction banning diabetic patients from driving either ordinary

vehicles or HGVs. In another case, the High Court established that 'it would be wrong to refuse renewal of HGV licences on the grounds that . . . it could not be said that an insulin-taking diabetic would not suffer hypoglycaemia in the future'. The question to ask is whether diabetes renders a subject a likely source of danger to the public while driving.

In January 1983 a European directive by the member states of the EEC required that HGV licenses should not be granted to insulin dependent first-time applicants after 1 January 1983. Lasche [18] comments that persons driving with diabetes do have accidents, preventable or not, and cites a number of these, pointing out that in his state (Florida), 33 325 drivers had to submit medical reports during the past 30 years due to questionable ability to drive a motor vehicle safely: of these, 1798 or 5.4% required a report because of diabetes and this number has remained constant throughout these 30 years. He notes that in the UK, diabetes, whether with insulin or not, is designated as a 'prospective disability', with the issuing of a full driving license restricted to a maximum of 3 years, with the possibility of renewal. Cockram et al [17] also cite a study [19] concerning an outpatient diabetes clinic population, which revealed that 49% of the men and 19% of the women had experienced hypoglycemia while driving and fewer than half of these had carbohydrate available, indicating that many patients with diabetes either are insufficiently educated in the prevention of hypoglycemic reactions, or ignore what they have learned.

It is also pertinent to point out that in this increasingly litigious world, there are increased risks of lawsuits filed regardless of legal virtue. If a physician treating a patient with either oral agents or insulin, although properly informing the patient of the potential dangers of hypoglycemia, fails to document this on the office chart, he or she might be accused of inadequately treating the patient. There have been several lawsuits based on the fact that a patient had a motor vehicle accident and allegedly had not been warned of these dangers. With an increasing number of lawyers involved in suing for real or imaginary reasons, the necessity for adequate patient information, well documented, must not be overlooked. One of the stranger cases is one recently filed, in which a commercial truck driver using insulin went to a completely strange physician, to whom he did not reveal his diabetes history. The physician, finding nothing abnormal, signed the license application form. Some days later, the driver was found dead in his truck alongside the road in another state—cause of death not known. The estate of the deceased sued the physician for signing the application for the license even though the former patient allegedly lied to him! This was ultimately rejected by the courts, but not before much mental anguish to the physician involved.

EMPLOYMENT

Little is found in the medical literature concerning the problems of employment of those with diabetes. Most of the reports are found in health-care professional or lay literature, as developed by the various diabetes associations. Yet of all the problems faced by all of us, except for maintenance of good health, the prospect of being unable to earn a livelihood is one of the most threatening aspects of any chronic disease.

Anyone who cannot qualify for proper employment or who is suboptimally employed will suffer drastic changes in life-style, as well as in psychological state. The young diabetic patient entering the job market today continues to have problems, although the situation has improved slightly because of federal and state legislation of the past 10 years in many countries. Older persons with diabetes are more likely to be working, because many of them had been employed when their diabetes became apparent, and they either had established good work records or have kept their condition secret. The problem is not whether a person is truly disabled, but whether others, including present or future employers, consider him or her to be handicapped.

Previous National Health Interview Surveys (NHIS) some years ago estimated that less than two-fifths (36.9%) of all diabetic patients 20 years of age and older were in the labor force. As in the general population, participation in the world of work differs with age, sex, race, education, health status and many other factors: men with diabetes are almost twice as likely as women with diabetes to participate in the work force; black diabetic patients have lower employment rates than do white diabetic patients; those with little education have much lower rates than those with more years of training, while patients with limitations due to their diabetes or its complications are less likely to work than those without such limitations. The question here is how much of this lack of work is due to real inability, perceived inability, or prejudice?

These difficulties, of course, are not limited to the USA. In the previously cited European survey [7], the 19 responders to the question 'Are any jobs closed to diabetics or difficult for them to get?' gave 13 'yes' answers, 1 'no' and 5 'sometimes'. The jobs that were closed were termed 'dangerous', although this was not defined. In the study, the civil service, the armed services, aviation, police, security, transport, working at heights, hard physical labor, night work, locomotive driving, the fire brigade, and using heavy machinery were included in the list of 'closed' jobs.

The question 'Must those with insulin-requiring diabetes leave their jobs when this develops and they already are employed?' received the answers 'yes' (10), 'no' (4) and 'sometimes' (5). As might be expected, the 'yes' and 'sometimes' groups included aviation, army, navy, bus drivers, mining, police, security and heavy transport.

'Must they leave their jobs if they develop diabetes using oral hypoglycemic agents?': 'yes', 0; 'no', 14; 'sometimes', 5.

There may be veiled difficulties of employment in some occupations for diabetic employees. This implies that, in the face of official non-discrimination policies, there can be an amazing amount of discrimination. Diabetic applicants felt that they were assigned inappropriate shifts, irregular hours and hard physical work. Again, many became the first unemployed in periods of higher levels of job unavailability, and found it difficult to get jobs in competition with non-diabetic applicants, although they were equally well qualified.

A fairly comprehensive recent study [20] examined 158 IDDM individuals and compared them with 158 matched non-diabetic siblings in a case-controlled design to evaluate the effect of diabetes on employability. Overall, the IDDM patients reported more job refusals (56% versus 42%). They were also less likely to be employed at the time (55% versus 73%). Results suggested that hiring practices may still be discriminatory but that, once hired, the employment experiences of both groups appeared to be similar, provided that no diabetes complications developed.

With regard to education leading to jobs, diabetic patients often were not encouraged to seek education in medical and nursing schools (and, the author has been informed, were actually discouraged from doing so), allegedly because of irregular hours and training for strenuous jobs. In China, for example, some persons with diabetes finishing the 12th grade are discouraged from seeking advanced education, such as college, because of the misplaced fear that their life-span would be too short. It is said that sometimes physicians deliberately avoid diagnosing diabetes in these youngsters until after they have been in college long enough to have tenure.

The problem of employment guidelines is difficult. Both employers and their insurance companies prefer as few problems as possible. Employers are afraid of insulin reactions, about which they know very little, and fear injuries, damage to expensive machinery or worse. One can scarcely blame those diabetic patients who do not advertise their condition during job interviews, because they sense that many times there will be covert, if not overt, prejudice. There have been many attempts at job counseling for diabetics, some of which are impractical. One such states that the job to be sought should fit the mental and physical ability of the diabetic individual, training should be complete, the diabetic metabolism should be 'well balanced', hypoglycemia avoided, etc.; no one states just how this ideal state should be achieved. Almost all of this advice includes a list of proscribed careers and occupations allegedly *not* for diabetic patients, especially those requiring insulin; yet (except for many aviation-related jobs and the military) some workers with diabetes are successfully doing each of these. The answer is that those with diabetes or other chronic conditions should be judged on an individual basis, rather than as a group.

Another problem is that mass testing for many conditions, including diabetes, requires low-cost procedures that are capable of being performed by relatively unskilled people and that are cost-effective as well, considering the numbers involved with licenses for driving, as well as certain employment opportunities. Although this may be possible in a completely socialized medical system, it is much less feasible in some other countries, especially when medical authorities are not always in agreement as to what the criteria could or should be. This situation can best be resolved by associations of diabetic patients and their well-wishers educating both patients and organizations [21]. This is necessary because, as shown in this chapter, different sections of the same government have different regulations: for example, US Department of Defense directives not only prohibit those with diabetes from joining the military, but previously stated that 'diabetes mellitus in both natural parents is disqualifying' [22]; this latter provision was rescinded in 1990 [23].

Disability?

Is a person with diabetes a disabled person or not? Many, if not most, diabetic patients believe they are perfectly normal and not disabled in the absence of complications; yet most of the protective laws come under the heading of 'disabled persons'. To obtain the protection of these laws they must assume disability, but this label already compromises them. Legally, the diabetic patient cannot have it both ways.

Another advance in recent years was the passage of the Federal Rehabilitation Act of 1973 by the Congress of the United States (Title 5) [24] entitling all qualified 'handicapped' persons to equal job opportunities and treatment. Whether the patient or the physician considers the patient to be handicapped does not matter, as the regulations consider diabetes to be a handicap, and the law requires employers to hire qualified diabetics and promote them on the same basis as non-diabetic people. The qualifications for the particular job must be the sole consideration in hiring. Section 101 states that each state rehabilitation agency must try to hire qualified handicapped people and promote those who are qualified. Section 501 does the same for all the departments in the executive branch of the federal government. Section 503 covers those with federal contracts for more than $2500 per year (about 50% of the businesses and industries in the USA). Section 504 covers schools, colleges, hospitals and health and social agencies receiving federal monies.

Many states and local governments have laws similar to the Federal Rehabilitation Act and in some states they apply to all businesses. The effect of these laws and more recent clarifications shift the focus to job placement rather than employability, depending on whether or not an individual can perform a specific job; if so, in theory he or she must be hired (although this often does not occur in practice). The original provisions were limited in 1984 by a Supreme Court ruling defining the recipients of federal funds as restricted to a specific department of an organization rather than the entire organization. This was corrected in a 1988 law.

In fact, the United Nations through its constituent health body, the World Health Organization, recognized these problems and named 1983–92 the Decade of Disabled Persons. At a meeting convened in August 1987 to review implementation of actions concerning disabled persons, appropriate resolutions were passed.

With regard to the prohibition against those with IDDM from driving large trucks between states, some suggestions have been made that drivers should carry complete testing outfits in their cabs; blood glucose levels should be maintained between 60 mg/dl and 140 mg/dl when fasting and 140–200 mg/dl at other times, to be tested within 1 hour of driving and every 4 hours while driving [25]. These suggestions, of course, refer to an ideal situation, but from the viewpoint of the regulatory authorities and the industry appear to be impractical, making it simpler not to permit IDDM patients to drive, unjust though this may be. The ADA has set up a network of attorneys in many states who agree to represent or help people with diabetes to find adequate counsel if they are the victims of discrimination.

There have been some notable victories in the fight against discrimination. The state of California used to follow the federal regulations against insulin-using truck drivers driving trucks interstate. A recent California Court of Appeals decision ruled that the state should be willing to grant exceptions to truckers whose diabetic control was such that they presented no danger on the highway [26]. There have also been notable reversals of discriminating rules. A building repairman was hired and in his application he made no secret of his insulin dependent diabetes. The physical examination showed considerable glycosuria. He was denied employment as 'out of control'. A medical review board upheld the decision, as did the state Civil Service Commission, insisting that 'good control' was a requirement for the position. Several years later, the case came before the Circuit Court of Appeals. The Court ruled that the city could not make good control a condition of employment but rather job restriction had to be connected directly to either 'business necessity or safe performance'. The Court did not state that the man's diabetes was in *good* control but only that *lack of control* was not in itself a valid job restriction. Furthermore, the Court stated that if a person has a handicap but is qualified to do a job, it is up to the employer to prove that the medical restrictions for denial of employment make sense. This was an important shift in the burden of proof [27]. The courts are gradually determining that a person with a medical condition must be shown to be incapable of doing the job, rather than being barred from a job because of potential problems that may never occur.

The Aviation Industry and Diabetes

With the enormous increase in the number of airline passengers and the many new airlines and planes, many airports are inundated with the volume of traffic. The spate of recent accidents reminds us that the 'friendly skies' are becoming crowded. Although flying on scheduled flights is more than 30 times safer than traveling by car on highways, the number of 'near mid-airs' (the term pilots use when two planes come dangerously close in the air) has increased. Those reported in the USA alone were 311 in 1982, 475 in 1983, 589 in 1984, 777 in 1985 and 812 in 1986, and the numbers continue to increase [28]. It is obvious that pilot and aircrew health is increasingly under survey.

There have been accidents, admittedly rare, where the health of the pilot was presumed to be the cause. One of these two decades ago killed 80 passengers [29]. The Civil Aeronautics Board (CAB) blamed the pilot's heart failure: this charter pilot had a history of heart disease for 18 years and of diabetes for $3\frac{1}{2}$ years, which the CAB stated could remain undetected during the FAA examination, claiming that the pilot deliberately falsified his license application. Concerning diabetes, the Federal Aviation Administration (FAA) explicitly states that diabetics requiring any medication for control, oral or otherwise, are disqualified [30], and the *Guide for Aviation Medical Examiners* [31], paragraph 21-K, states that the finding of glycosuria or proteinuria at the time of examination is cause for deferral by the examiner. Although diabetes requiring hypoglycemic drugs for control is disqualifying, a past history of such medication may not be disqualifying: a history of diabetes itself is not disqualifying but a period of control of at least 90 days by diet alone is required.

Age-specific license denial rates for airline pilots increase with age, with the highest rate being at age interval 55–59 years. The overall highest rates for denial, according to condition, are for (a) cardiovascular, (b) neuropsychiatric and (c) miscellaneous conditions; the latter includes endocrine diseases (most often diabetes). Paragraph 21-N, part B of the *Guide for Aviation Medical Examiners* states, 'A blood glucose determination is not a routine part of the FAA medical examination for any class of medical certification. However, the examination includes routine urinalysis' [31].

The ADA has in the past expressed the opinion that a 'person intimately concerned with the safe operation of aircraft should not be an individual with diabetes requiring insulin or oral hypoglycemic agents for control'. Since then, because of improvements in treatment and monitoring of diabetes and new, more effective, testing, the ADA policy on drivers' and pilots' licenses adopted by the Board of Directors in October 1985 states, 'Any person with diabetes, whether insulin-dependent or non-insulin-dependent, should be eligible for any driver's or pilot's license for which he or she is individually qualified'.

A first-class medical certificate is required for airline transport pilots. It is valid for 6 months, and renewal requires another history and physical examination. With the improvement in techniques of diabetes monitoring and treatment, the gradual age increase of the pilot population and widespread use of oral hypoglycemic agents and their acceptance in many areas of employment, more than 100 pilots have been given waivers and permitted to fly (J.N. Fisher, personal communication). At the time of writing (March 1991), no other national licensing body is known to have permitted this. There have been efforts in this respect for conditions other than diabetes: if, for example, a pilot has a bypass in one leg permitting normal blood flow and function, is he not capable of flying? To some extent this has been allowed, as is the medical certification of a pilot with surgically treated coronary disease [32].

Several years ago the FAA asked the American Medical Association to review the medical standards for civilian pilots and to recommend new or revised standards for all fields of medicine. The FAA charge stated, 'the report must consider pertinent advances in the field of medicine since 1959, and determine what changes in FAA medical standards, if any, are warranted, and the rationale for such changes', with final standards to be developed by the FAA. There was a total of 77 physicians covering all areas of medicine, with 5 in the endocrinology/diabetes section. This massive undertaking culminated in a report to the FAA [33], which suggested the granting of waivers to carefully monitored pilots using oral hypoglycemic agents. The report continued to recommend that persons taking insulin should be denied certification at this time, but recommended the removal of the 'absolute prohibition against certifying persons taking oral hypoglycemic agents'. However, it also gave very strict guidelines concerning what appear to be trial approvals rather than 'blanket' waivers. The arguments against permission for the use of insulin accepted that pilots were usually very responsible people, very technically educated and motivated; nevertheless, the climate of medicolegal risk prevailed at this time. The committee also presented data defining reasonable control to avoid reactions, etc. Although this outcome may be a disappointment to those who insist that diabetic patients are capable of doing any job, it must be remembered that even the pleas for equal access to any job 'for which he or she is individually qualified' contain a warning that the FAA and other such agencies should make decisions on what constitutes qualification.

Other Airline Personnel

The health regulations concerning cabin attendants are determined by individual airlines concerned with the safety of their passengers. Recently, several of these attendants were discharged from their flight duties, although some were given other employment not involving flying.

The functions of these employees include service in all its aspects, public relations, maintaining control of the passenger areas and, most important, assisting passengers in cases of emergency. They are, as a group, well trained and disciplined with a strong sense of responsibility.

D.S. was 25 years old with an exemplary work record for $3\frac{1}{2}$ years when she had a classic onset of diabetes in 1980. She required insulin and undertook an intensive course of diabetes education, carefully regulating her diabetes with an average dose of 20 units of NPH and 5–8 units of regular insulin daily. Her blood glucose levels were in a satisfactory range and the glycolated hemoglobin normal after her initial period of regulation. She suffered no hypoglycemic reactions and was under constant medical surveillance. When she was discharged, her union sued to retain her job. The position of the airline was that she might have a reaction during an emergency when she should be helping passengers evacuate a plane. Statistics were developed showing that the chances of this type of situation in a wrecked plane where there were survivors were infinitesimal. An intelligent, alert, well-educated and motivated young person with a strong job incentive and access to nourishment need never have a significant reaction. Her union believed that she should be judged as an individual and not as part of a class. Reactions, which are largely preventable, should be dealt with by the same discipline as other infractions of airline regulations. She was reinstated, and this has now happened to several other cabin attendants with different airlines. They are evaluated as individuals and given a certain time period to prove that they can handle the job. This is *not* a 'blanket' ruling, but each person is judged individually. These reinstated attendants proved their ability and demonstrated a willingness to accept the disciplines of diabetes and still perform their duties.

Since this chapter was first drafted, because of petitions from various interested organizations the FAA has convened an advisory panel to determine whether diabetic air traffic controllers can continue to perform their duties while using insulin. There were relatively few individuals with diabetes among the (approximately) 20 000 US controllers; they had been carrying out their duties (with insulin waivers) with no known or proven mishap. In response to an ATCS union petition, the FAA is trying to determine whether, using modern up-to-date testing devices and proper education, these controllers can be adequately monitored, preserving their employment functions while still ensuring complete air traffic safety. Because of advances in diabetes management there are increasing pressures for greater flexibility in employment of diabetic individuals. The ADA has presented a new petition [34] to the Federal Agency to reconsider the rulings that now prohibit interstate truck drivers and airline pilots from becoming licensed. It will be some time before these matters are resolved.

The small steps of the past have become more definite in the direction of employment equality for those with diabetes to be able to work effectively at many, or even most, jobs.

In summary, those with diabetes must handle their medical condition so well that there is no doubt of their ability to function. There must be a willingness of physicians, and especially diabetes associations, not only to educate but to bring proper pressures to bear on employers and legislators, to prevent and avoid discrimination in all fields of endeavor. However, the burden of proof starts with the diabetic patients themselves. In short, in keeping with the philosophy that people should not be denied anything because something untoward might occur, those with diabetes should be viewed as innocent, unless proved guilty.

REFERENCES

1. Entmacher PS, Pomeroy S, Bostic E, Harris MI. Impact of diabetes. In Diabetes in America. NIH Publication 85-1468, 1985: p 11.
2. Joslin EP. Diabetes mellitus. Philadelphia: Lea & Febiger, 1916.
3. Krall LP, Entmacher PS, Drury TF. Life cycle in diabetes: socioeconomic aspects. In Marble A, Krall LP, Bradley RF, Christlieb AR, Soeldner JS (eds) Joslin's Diabetes mellitus, 12th edn. Philadelphia: Lea & Febiger, 1985: pp 907–36.
4. Petrides P, Weiss L, Loffler G, Wieland PH. Die Zuckerkrankheit. Munich: Urban & Schwartsenberg, 1983: pp 97–101.
5. Borch-Johnsen K, Andersen PD, Deckert T. The effect of proteinuria on relative mortality in Type 1 (insulin-dependent) diabetes mellitus. Diabetologia 1985; 28: 590–6.
6. Goodkin G, Wolloch LB. A long-term study of insured and declined diabetics. Trans Assoc Life Ins Med Directors 1968; LXI: 211–36.
7. Social rights of diabetic patients in Europe. Alvsjo: Swedish Diabetic Association, 1986: pp 4–30.
8. Entmacher PS, Bale GS. Insurability and life expectancy of diabetics. In Rifkin H, Raskin P (eds) Diabetes mellitus, vol. 5. Bowie, Md: Robert J. Brady, 1981: pp 341–5.
9. Krosnick A. Yes, you can get a driver's license. Diabetes Forecast 1982; 35: 16.

10. Waller JA. Chronic medical conditions and traffic safety. Review of the California experience. New Engl J Med 1965; 273: 1413.

11. Hansotia P, Broste SK. The effect of epilepsy or diabetes mellitus on the risk of automobile accidents. New Engl J Med 1991; 324: 22.

12. Frier BM, Matthews, DM, Steel JM, Duncan LJP. Driving and insulin-dependent diabetes. Lancet 1980; i: 1232.

13. Songer TJ, LaPorte RE, Dorman JS, Orchard TJ, Cruickshanks KJ, Becker DJ, Drash AL. Motor vehicle accidents and IDDM. Diabetes Care 1988; 11: 701–7.

14. Federal Register 1990; 55: 40128–41037.

15. Federal Register, Part IV, Department of Transportation, Federal Highway Administration, 49 CFR part 391. Qualification of drivers; Diabetes; proposed rule, 5 October 1990.

16. Diabetes and Driving. Diabetes Conquest 1984 (winter); 11–13.

17. Cockram CS, Dutton T, Sonksen PH. Driving and diabetes: a summary of the current medical and legal position based upon a recent heavy goods vehicle (HGV) case. Diabet Med 1986; 3: 137–40.

18. Lasche EM. The diabetic driver (editorial). Diabetes Care 1985; 8: 189–91.

19. Clarke B, Ward JB, Enoch BA. Hypoglycaemia in insulin-dependent diabetic drivers. Br Med J 1980; 281: 586.

20. Songer TJ, LaPorte RE, Dorman JS, Orchard TJ, Becker DJ, Drash AL. Employment spectrum of IDDM. Diabetes Care 1989; 12: 615–22.

21. Whitehouse FW. How to deal with barriers to employment. Diabetes News 1990; 9: 38–41.

22. Fisher JN. Diabetics need not apply (editorial). Diabetes Care 1989; 12: 659–60.

23. Kussman MJ, Clement SC. Change in army policy (letter). Diabetes Care 1990; 13: 903.

24. Friedman GJ. Employability of the diabetic. In Rifkin H, Raskin P (eds) Diabetes mellitus, vol. 4. Bowie: Robert J. Brady, 1981: pp 335–40.

25. Ratner RE, Whitehouse FW. Motor vehicles, hypoglycemia and diabetic drivers. Diabetes Care 1989; 12: 217–22.

26. Thiesen C. Your employment rights. Diabetes Self-Management 1988; Jan/Feb: 26–30.

27. Zagoria RB. The tides are turning. Diabetes Forecast 1986; 39: 22–6.

28. Magnuson E. Be careful out there. Time, 12 January 1987: 24–32.

29. Pilot hid heart flaw . . . 80 died. Boston Globe, 4 April 1987.

30. Dark SJ. Characteristics of medically disqualified airline pilots. Report no. FAA-AM-83.5. Washington: Federal Aviation Administration Office of Aviation Medicine, 1983.

31. Guide for aviation medical examiners. Washington: Federal Aviation Administration, 1981.

32. Sands MJ Jr. Aviation medical certification after coronary artery surgery. New Engl J Med 1982; 307: 52.

33. Engelberg AL, Gibbons HL, Doege TC. A review of the medical standards for civilian airmen. Synopsis of a two-year study (special communication). JAMA 1986; 255: 1589–99.

34. Petition for Rulemaking and for Other Agency Action of the American Diabetes Association, before the Department of Transportation. Federal Aviation Administration, 14 CFR part 67, 21 February 1991.

73

The Economics of Diabetes Care

Thomas J. Songer

Department of Epidemiology, University of Pittsburgh, USA

Over the last 20 years, expenditure on medical care has risen extensively throughout the world [1, 2]. Health care expenditures have risen much faster than the cost increases reported in other sectors of the economy. One consequence of these large increases is that individuals with chronic disease face an increasing financial burden because of their long-term medical care needs and a changing reimbursement strategy among third party payers. Diabetes mellitus, as described in this book, is currently a leading cause of premature morbidity and mortality in the general population, and is also probably a major factor in the economic costs of living for individuals with diabetes.

It is important to know the economic costs in diabetes care for several reasons. Appropriate knowledge of the expenditure related to diabetes can assist governments and health care organizations in allocating scarce resources, attracting additional resources and managing available assets to control the health and socioeconomic burdens of diabetes. Comparison of the distribution of costs in different countries can provide information about the advantages or disadvantages of different health care practices, reimbursement mechanisms and utilization patterns between the countries. Finally, knowledge of the

costs incurred by individuals with diabetes can help clinicians and educators to provide useful advice to their patients about controlling and reducing the burdens of diabetes on an individual level.

In general, there are two economic practices that can be used to assist in diabetes planning and policy; descriptive studies of the cost of diabetes, and evaluativeness studies of the cost–benefit, cost–utility or cost-effectiveness of diabetes interventions. Studies of the economic costs of diabetes show the amount of resources that are used or lost due to diabetes. Estimates of the cost of diabetes can provide information to help guide priorities for the allocation of research funds, hospitals, physicians, treatment programs, etc. to diabetes care. Such studies can also provide baseline data for evaluating subsequent policy, reimbursement, health care practice or technological changes.

Cost–benefit, cost–utility or cost-effectiveness studies differ substantially from cost of illness studies. They consider the costs of a diabetes program or treatment relative to the benefits obtained. Comparisons with an alternative program or treatment are often made in an attempt to guide the direction of future resources and therapies. One current example is the evaluation

International Textbook of Diabetes Mellitus. Edited by K.G.M.M. Alberti, R.A. DeFronzo, H. Keen and P. Zimmet

of diabetes education programs for determining the appropriate setting and method of education for the diabetes patient.

Economic studies can thus be of major value in the diabetes field. This review examines the status of the economic analyses for diabetes mellitus. The first section describes the methodologies used in the classic studies of the cost of illness, and those used in estimating the previous costs of diabetes. Next, the estimated overall expenditures in diabetes mellitus and its components are reviewed, followed by a discussion on the use of cost–benefit and cost-effectiveness analysis in diabetes.

METHODOLOGY IN THE ESTIMATION OF THE COST OF DIABETES MELLITUS

General Methods of Estimating the Cost of Illness

The costs of illness are usually subdivided into two categories: the direct and indirect costs of disease. Direct economic costs of disease include the expenditure for medical care and treatment of the illness (hospital care, physician services, nursing-home care, drugs and other medical needs). These direct costs are often easily measured by surveys and studies. Indirect economic costs include the societal costs of morbidity, disability and premature mortality. These nonmedical costs of disease are not easily measured or calculated. A third category, the psychosocial costs of illness, is often mentioned as another dimension in the cost of illness, but usually is not included because of the difficulty in measuring these costs. Discussions on measuring the direct, indirect and psychosocial costs of illness are detailed elsewhere [3–7].

Much debate surrounds the valuation of the indirect costs of illness. There are two general methodologies used to estimate indirect costs: the human capital approach, and the 'willingness to pay' approach [34]. In the human capital approach, individuals are regarded as producing output in their lifetime that can be valued as equal to each individual's earnings during that time. Indirect expenses, then, are seen as the earnings, present and future, lost to that individual and his or her employer as a result of the illness.

The main criticism of the human capital approach is that it values life in terms of the earnings of the individual. Changes in life-style due to disease are expressed by changes in the earnings of the individual. Thus, the human capital approach may economically undervalue some segments of society relative to others (e.g. women, the young and the elderly) because people are valued by their baseline earnings. To answer this criticism, the 'willingness to pay' approach was proposed. In this approach, life and life-style changes are valued as equal to the amount that the individuals are willing to spend to reduce their risk of death or illness [8, 9]. This methodology, however, has been very difficult to implement and has been used in very few cost-of-illness studies. The human capital approach has been the only methodology used in the cost-of-diabetes studies.

Designs Applied in Estimating the Cost of Diabetes

Internationally, there are few studies on the cost of diabetes. The majority of studies have been conducted in the USA. Although many developing countries may not have the population-based and diabetes-specific data needed to complete a cost-of-diabetes study, many nations do have the necessary data or the capacity to generate it. These data generally include information on (a) the utilization of health services (hospital and physician care, medications, etc.) in the diabetes population or a sample thereof, (b) the cost of health services, (c) the number of persons with diabetes who are unable to work due to disability, (d) the number of persons working and the average earnings of workers in the general population, (e) mortality in the diabetes population and life expectancy in the general population, and (f) the prevalence or incidence of diabetes.

Table 1 lists the designs used for estimating the cost of diabetes, overall, or the components of diabetes care in previous studies. There have been three primary study designs used to estimate the costs of diabetes, each distinguished by the type of data used to determine a cost estimate. These designs include estimates from diagnostic category data, estimates from the experiences or responses of diabetic individuals, and estimates projected from previous cost studies. All are based on the human capital method of valuing life.

Table 1 Past and potential methodologies in cost of diabetes studies

Type of study	Benefits	Limitations
Aggregate estimates of costs from general population surveys and statistics	Has been the primary source of the cost of diabetes information Easy and inexpensive to complete, if data are available Has been the only source of data used for estimating the indirect costs of diabetes due to mortality and morbidity	Use of aggregated data neglects the characteristics of subgroups Data often are not available Uses primary diagnosis data only; costs when diabetes is a secondary diagnosis are not known Uses underlying cause of death data only; costs for diabetes as a contributing cause of death are not known Fails to separate IDDM costs from NIDDM costs Uses data for severely disabled diabetics only; neglects the costs of less severe forms of disability Per-capita costs are difficult to derive
Cost projections from previous estimates of the cost of diabetes	Relatively quick, easy and inexpensive to conduct	Assumes that the changes in costs of diabetes are equal to the changes in inflation rates and prevalence rates Error rate is higher since based on previous estimates
Individual estimates of costs from general population data of the NMCES, NMCUES	Availability of data on individuals with diabetes permits the evaluation of costs within the subgroups Gives more precision to the estimates since it is based on individual expenditures Has been used to provide data on the direct costs of diabetes	Has not been used to assess the indirect costs of diabetes Fails to separate IDDM costs from NIDDM costs Not easy and very expensive to complete
Individual estimates of costs from diabetes population registries	Provides more precise estimates of the cost of diabetes since (a) looking at the cost of the individual, (b) can distinguish cost of IDDM, (c) can look at subgroup characteristics, and (d) are representative of the diabetes population Many diabetes registries currently exist	An underutilized source of data for the cost of diabetes, has been used for data on the cost of diabetes care, therapies, etc. No registries for NIDDM exist Registries are expensive to establish
Individual estimates of costs from non-population-based diabetes groups	Have been used to estimate the cost of diabetes care, therapies, procedures, etc. Very simple to complete Good source of hypothesis-generating data	Usually not representative of the diabetes population Do not provide data that will adequately describe the cost of diabetes

Aggregate Estimates from General Population Data

The majority of the economic cost data in diabetes have been based on national health, health care, disability and mortality statistics. National statistics often are broken down by diagnostic categories based on the International Classification of Diseases (ICD) codes. In general, data are attributed to the diabetes mellitus category only when diabetes is listed as the primary diagnosis or reason for a health-care visit, disability or cause of death.

Previous studies have used two general computational methods to determine the direct costs of disease from diagnostic category data: the 'top down' and 'bottom up' approaches. Details on the calculation procedures for these methods are provided elsewhere [10]. Indirect costs have been calculated in a fairly standard manner in the literature. Procedures for estimating indirect costs are provided by Rice [3].

The diagnostic category data design has been widely used to estimate the costs of diabetes because the data have been easily available and it is a relatively inexpensive study to conduct. However, serious limitations are present in the design that may underestimate the true costs of diabetes. Estimates based exclusively on figures where diabetes is the primary diagnosis, cause of death or reason for disability miss the health care costs incurred by diabetic individuals where diabetes is a secondary or tertiary factor. Diabetes mellitus, biologically, is a leading cause of blindness, renal failure, heart disease and lower-limb amputations. Cardiovascular disease is the major cause of death for most diabetic patients [11]. The critical point is that often individuals with complications associated with diabetes (e.g. heart disease) do not have diabetes listed as the primary diagnosis upon hospitalization [12] or as the underlying cause of death [11, 13]; some account should be taken of the costs incurred by these individuals. Furthermore, as chronic diseases such as heart disease occur frequently in the general population, analyses using control groups of non-diabetic individuals are needed to separate the excess morbidity costs related to diabetes from those costs that would be expected to occur normally.

Another limitation of this design is that costs related to insulin dependent diabetes mellitus (IDDM) or non-insulin dependent diabetes mellitus (NIDDM) may not be estimated accurately. The ICD diagnostic category for diabetes considers only the general definition of diabetes: subgroups of diabetes, such as IDDM and NIDDM, are not entirely distinguishable in diagnostic category data. In addition, it is not possible to determine the economic impact of diabetes from the perspective of the individual with diabetes, or of the family.

Cost Projections from Previous Estimates

Diabetes cost estimates have also been predicted from the results of previous cost studies. In this study design, cost estimates determined in a previous study and changes in the health care utilization and mortality rates associated with diabetes, as well as the change in prevalence and inflation rates, were utilized to forecast the economic costs of diabetes. The advantage of this design is that it is even more easy and inexpensive to conduct. However, major limitations

concerning the interpretation of the data are present, because this approach combines the limitations of the previous studies and those of its own. The primary restraint is that the cost estimates are based on the assumption that the changes in the costs of diabetes will be similar to the changes in inflation, utilization, prevalence and mortality rates; this may or may not be true.

Individual-based Estimates from General Population Data

The costs of diabetes have also been estimated from the data of diabetic individuals identified from the general population, diabetes registries, or diabetes clinics, hospitals, practices, etc. Cost estimates derived from this design have been determined from the survey data or reported experience of persons with diabetes. This approach differs from the first design where costs were based upon diagnostic category data. The advantage of surveying individuals is that more precise estimates of the costs of diabetes can be attained, because individual costs and utilization patterns are directly observed, rather than estimated from aggregated categories which mask the influence of subgroups and individuals. In addition, if a representative sample of the population is used, data based upon the reports of diabetic individuals are much more likely to reflect the experience of the diabetes population than are data based upon diagnostic categories. Data based upon diagnostic categories have not been representative of the diabetic population for the reason mentioned earlier, i.e. not all people with diabetes will have diabetes listed as a primary diagnosis. The disadvantage of surveying costs among a representative sample of diabetic individuals is that it is an expensive and lengthy process to complete. Analysis of data grouped by primary diagnosis category is much quicker because of the availability of government statistics and, thus, it is much less expensive to conduct.

Three population sources in the literature have been chiefly used to estimate the costs of diabetes from the data of diabetic individuals. These include:

(1) the estimation of the direct costs in diabetes from surveys of health care use and cost in the general population, such as the National Medical Care Expenditure Survey (NMCES)

and National Medical Care Utilization and Expenditure Survey (NMCUES);

(2) the estimation of selected health care costs in diabetes from the data of diabetes population registries;

(3) the estimation of selected health costs for diabetes from the data of diabetes clinics, practices, etc.

Each has concentrated on estimating the health care costs of diabetes rather than the total costs.

Data on the health care costs of diabetes from the NMCES and NMCUES have recently been reported. In these surveys, the medical costs of a random sample of the general population were recorded in a 1-year period and averaged. Individuals with diabetes were identified in the survey by their responses to questions on medical history. Expenditures for the entire diabetes population were estimated by multiplying the average costs for the individual with diabetes by the prevalence estimate for diabetes. The indirect costs of diabetes have not been studied with this approach, nor (even though the costs of individuals were observed) did the estimates of the NMCES and NMCUES distinguish IDDM from NIDDM.

Individual-based Estimates from Diabetes Registries

Some components of the health care costs of diabetes have also been estimated from the surveys of population-based diabetes registries. In this approach, selected costs of diabetes care, including the costs for daily treatment of diabetes, physician care, and the treatment of diabetic ketoacidosis, were surveyed or determined from diabetic individuals listed in a diabetes registry. These diabetes registries contained individuals who were representative of the diabetes population in a specific geographical region.

The main advantage of surveying costs by this method is that, again, more precise estimates and subgroup analysis of the costs in diabetes care are possible. Costs for IDDM can also be ascertained, as the majority of diabetes registries are composed entirely of insulin dependent cases. The main disadvantage of this methodology is the expense and time required to establish a diabetes registry; furthermore, at present there are few registries for NIDDM. Registries,

on the whole, have been underutilized in the assessment of the costs of diabetes.

Individual-based Estimates from Diabetes Groups

Finally, estimates of the cost for selected components of diabetes care, such as equipment, drug therapy, diagnosis and pregnancy costs, have been generated from diabetes clinics, practices, and organizations. In this approach, the costs associated with diabetic individuals at a particular hospital, physician's office, drug company or organization were surveyed. These cost estimates were not often based on representative samples of the diabetes population. However, this method of cost estimation may be a good source of hypothesis-generating data on the costs of diabetes care, therapies and procedures, and can provide a rough estimate of the overall pattern of costs. Space constraints prevent the detailed discussion of the many diabetes treatment estimates generated in this fashion.

ESTIMATES OF THE COST OF DIABETES MELLITUS

Cost Estimates for the USA

As mentioned before, cost of diabetes studies have been completed largely in the USA. Estimates of the economic costs of diabetes mellitus in the USA are listed in Table 2 and suggest that the costs of this disease are quite substantial. The Statistical Bureau of the Metropolitan Life Insurance Company (SBMLIC) has estimated the costs of diabetes mellitus over a period of years using diagnostic category data on health care utilization, disability and mortality. In their reports, the total economic impact of diabetes rose from US $2.6 billion (thousand million) in 1969 to a projected $13.8 billion in 1984 [14]. The direct costs (or health care costs) of diabetes rose from $1.0 billion in 1969 to a projected $7.4 billion in 1984, and the indirect costs (or the loss of earnings due to diabetes) rose from $1.6 billion to $6.3 billion in the same period.

Several reasons have been cited for this increase in the economic costs of diabetes and the increase seen in the percentage of total costs related to health care: they include the inflation of medical care prices, the increased prevalence of diabetes, the increased utilization of medical

Table 2 Estimates of the economic costs of diabetes mellitus in the USA, by study

Study	Year	Design	Total costs ($ billion)	Direct costs		Indirect costs	
				$ billion	% of total	$ billion	% of total
Statistical Bureau of the Metropolitan Life Insurance Company (SBMLIC) [14]	1969	Costs estimated from diagnostic category data of general population	2.6	1.0	38	1.6	62
SBMLIC	1973	Diagnostic category data	4.0	1.65	41	2.37	59
SBMLIC	1975	Diagnostic category data	5.3	2.5	47	2.8	53
SBMLIC	1977	Diagnostic category data	6.8	3.4	50	3.4	50
NMCES [14]	1977	Costs estimated from diabetic individuals in the general population	–	6.9	–	–	–
Policy Analysis, Inc. [15]	1977	Lifetime costs estimated from diagnostic category data	10.8	3.7	34	7.1	66
Platt, Sudovar [16]	1979	Projections from the 1975 SBMLIC data	15.7 4.8 IDDM	5.6 1.8 IDDM	36	10.0 3.0 IDDM	64
Miller [17]	1979	Costs estimated from diagnostic category data and other cost studies	12.4	7.4	60	5.0	40
SBMLIC	1980	Diagnostic category data	9.7	4.8	49	4.9	51
Smeeding, Booton [18]	1980	Diagnostic category data and other cost studies	18.9	5.7	30	10.0	53
Carter Center [19]	1980	Diagnostic category data and other cost studies	–	7.9	–	–	–
SBMLIC	1984	Projections from 1980 SBMLIC data	13.8	7.4	54	6.3	46
Fox, Jacobs [20]	1987	Diagnostic category data	20.4	9.6	47	10.8	53

services among diabetic patients and the development of new treatment technologies for diabetes. From 1969 to 1980, the estimated health care costs of diabetes rose 380%, while the medical care component of the consumer price index rose 134% [21, 22].

Other studies used design and calculation procedures that differed from that of the SBMLIC to arrive at their estimates for the cost of diabetes. Platt and Sudovar, using cost projections from the 1975 SBMLIC data, estimated the total expense of diabetes in 1979 to be $15.7 billion [16]. Of this figure, the total costs for IDDM were projected to be $4.8 billion. Estimates of the IDDM costs were determined by multiplying the direct (except for nursing-home care) and indirect expenditures for diabetes by 30%—Platt and Sudovar's estimate of the per-

centage of IDDM patients among the total diabetic population. This approach to measuring IDDM costs is inappropriate because of the flawed method of estimating IDDM prevalence from the number of diabetics using insulin and the known increased risk of premature morbidity and mortality for IDDM cases compared with NIDDM cases.

In another study, Miller [17] estimated the total costs of diabetes to be near $12.4 billion in 1979. Smeeding and Booton [18] estimated an $18.9 billion price tag for diabetes in 1980. Both studies relied upon diagnostic category statistics and data from previous cost studies to derive their cost estimates. Although the estimates of these three studies are 1.3–2.0 times higher than the costs estimated by the SBMLIC for 1980, the differences between these estimates and that of the SBMLIC are not large, given the use of different methodologies. This may be a consequence, however, of each of the three studies using data from the SBMLIC to arrive at their estimates.

More recently, Fox and Jacobs [20] estimated the cost of diabetes to be $20.4 billion in 1987. However, their methods differed from the previous studies, which all attributed costs based upon primary diagnosis data. Fox and Jacobs used primary diagnosis data, but went one step further and also estimated the hospitalization and mortality costs in instances where diabetes was listed as a secondary or tertiary diagnosis or cause of death. Roesler and colleagues [35] used this same data to project that the costs of diabetes for the state of Minnesota were $301 million in 1988.

Huse et al [36] estimated the costs of NIDDM based upon yet another technique to consider costs where diabetes was not a primary reason for health care use, disability, or death. Using a 'top down' approach and estimates on the proportion of circulatory, visual, and kidney disease related to NIDDM, they reported that the total costs of NIDDM were $19.8 billion in 1986.

Policy Analysis, Inc. (PAI) [15] has calculated the only estimate to consider the costs of diabetes over the entire lifetime of a diabetic cohort. The other studies estimated the costs of diabetes in a given year for the prevalent diabetes population. Using diagnostic category data, PAI estimated the lifetime costs for all persons diagnosed in 1977 to total $10.8 billion. To interpret this, roughly $11 billion in present and future costs would be saved if all incident cases of diabetes in 1977 were prevented. The methods to compute lifetime costs are discussed elsewhere [23].

The National Medical Care Expenditure Survey has provided the only economic cost figures for diabetes estimated from the experiences of the individual diabetic patient. In 1977, the NMCES estimated that the direct costs of diabetes were $6.9 billion [14]. This figure contrasts sharply with the $3.4 billion estimate reported by the SBMLIC for 1977. The primary reason for this difference lies in the methodological procedures utilized in both studies and suggests that the SBMLIC, which exclusively used primary diagnosis data in its calculations, considerably underestimated the health care costs of diabetes.

As mentioned before, the direct costs of diabetes include the cost of hospital care, physician services, nursing-home care, and drugs and medications, among other medical care needs. Estimates of the costs of these services are listed in Table 3. Although these estimates are not directly comparable between studies, and differ because of the different methodologies used in each study, they do provide a general idea of the expenses related to diabetes in the USA. The majority of the direct costs related to diabetes care were from hospital care: roughly 50% of all health care costs. Costs for nursing-home care (about 25% in 1984), physician services (16–20%) and drugs (about 8%) also accounted for large percentages of the medical care costs in diabetes.

As the methodology of the National Medical Care Expenditure Survey examined the costs of diabetes on the level of the diabetic individual, per-capita costs and their distribution in the diabetes population could be determined. Table 4 presents the per-capita expenses for health care (excluding nursing-home care) in the diabetic and non-diabetic populations with expenditures for health care. On average, persons with diabetes paid roughly three times more for health care than did persons without diabetes ($1514 versus $548) in 1977 [14, 26]. Per-capita expenditures for hospital care were 1.6 times higher in the diabetic population than in the non-diabetic population. Similarly, per-capita expenses for ambulatory care were 1.9 times higher and average expenses for prescribed medicines were 3.2 times higher in the diabetic population. The cost differential between the diabetic and non-diabetic groups was greatest in females and among individuals under 45 years old (which includes most IDDM patients).

Health care utilization is directly related to the cost figures presented and the cost of health care in general. Those individuals who use health services and facilities more frequently are likely to spend more for medical care than those who use the services less frequently. Data from the NMCES and NMCUES have shown that individuals with diabetes use health care services and facilities much more frequently than persons without diabetes [14, 26]. In 1977, 28% of the diabetes population had a hospital stay compared with 11% of subjects without diabetes. About 95% of the diabetic patients had an am-

Table 3 Estimates of direct costs for health care services in diabetes in the USA, by study

Study	Year	Hospital care		Physician visits		Nursing-home care		Drugs, medications	
		($ million)	(%)	($ million)	(%)	($ million)	(%)	($ million)	(%)
Statistical Bureau of the Metropolitan Life Insurance Company (SBMLIC) [24]	1973	800	48	400	24	185	11	225	14
SBMLIC [25]	1975	1050	42	590	23	520	21	300	12
NMCES	1977	4826	–	980	–	–	–	577	–
Miller	1979	4400	59	1395	19	1530	21	661	9
Platt, Sudovar [16]	1979	1119	20	1584	28	830	15	–	–
IDDM		335		475		110		–	
SBMLIC [14]	1980	2200	46	840	18	1240	26	380	8
National Hospital Discharge Survey [19]	1980	6157	–	–	–	–	–	–	–
Sinnock (National Hospital Discharge Survey) [12]	1980	6500	–	–	–	–	–	–	–
National Ambulatory Medical Care Survey [19]	1980	–	–	652	–	–	–	–	–
Van Nostrand (National Nursing Home Survey Data) [19]	1980	–	–	–	–	663	–	–	–
SBMLIC [14]	1984	3540	48	1180	16	1950	26	580	8
Fox, Jacobs [20]	1987	6930	–	724	–	942	–	–	–

bulatory physician visit compared with 76% of the non-diabetic population.

The indirect costs of diabetes include the costs related to premature mortality and morbidity. These costs result from the loss of earnings or wages in those disabled or limited by diabetes, and from the loss of lifetime earnings in those who have died. Estimates of the indirect expenses of morbidity and mortality are presented in Table 5. The SBMLIC has consistently reported that the expenses related to disability (morbidity) make up the majority of indirect costs in diabetes

Table 4 Average expense for persons with expenditures for medical care, excluding nursing-home care, by type of expense and diabetic status, USA, 1977

	Diabetic $	Non-diabetic $	Ratio
Total expenses	1514	548	2.8
Hospital care	3784	2417	1.6
Hospital stay	2831	1783	1.6
Physician care	940	634	1.5
Other	222	214	1.0
Ambulatory care	277	148	1.9
Physician contacts	225	132	1.7
Non-physician contacts	167	88	1.9
Prescribed medicines	132	41	3.2
Vision	82	72	1.1
Dental	115	147	0.8
Other medical expenses	125	62	2.0

From National Medical Care Expenditure Survey, 1977 [14, 26].

—about 70% [14, 24, 25]. Fox and Jacobs, however, found that the costs of premature mortality were much higher than the costs of disability [20]. This difference between studies was probably related to the different methodologies of the studies. Fox and Jacobs considered deaths where diabetes was a contributing cause, as well as an underlying cause of death, but did not account for disability costs related to diabetes as a secondary or tertiary cause of disability. The SBMLIC estimated costs from underlying cause of death and primary cause of disability data.

It seems surprising that the indirect costs associated with mortality were not nearly as large as those for morbidity in the earlier studies. When calculating costs, mortality costs include the value of lost productivity in future years, whereas morbidity costs do not. Indeed, Fox and Jacobs' estimate suggests that mortality costs are severely underestimated when contributing causes of death are not considered in addition to underlying causes of death. The costs of disability will also be underestimated if secondary and tertiary diagnoses are not considered. Given the methodological limitations of the previous studies, the distribution of mortality costs to disability costs remains unknown, but the cost estimates suggest that indirect costs related to diabetes (both mortality and morbidity costs) are sizeable.

Table 5 Estimates of the indirect costs due to morbidity and mortality from diabetes mellitus by year

	1969	1973	1975	1977	1979	1980	1984	1987
Source	SBMLIC	SBMLIC	SBMLIC	SBMLIC	Platt, Sudovar	SBMLIC	SBMLIC	Jacobs, Fox
Indirect costs due to morbidity								
$ million	464	980	1680	2340	7355	3440	4440	3280
% of indirect costs	29	41	61	69	–	70	70	31
Indirect costs due to mortality								
$ million	1129	1385	1070	1040	1529	1460	1880	7500
% of indirect costs	71	59	39	31	–	30	30	69

Cost Estimates for Diabetes Around the World

There are limited data on the cost of diabetes from countries other than the USA. In many nations, defining the costs associated with diabetes could potentially lead to more health care resources being directed to diabetes care. Governments, health care organizations and legislators might be more knowledgeable about the impact of diabetes and more willing to allocate limited resources to diabetes services if they were able to see how diabetes affects the population.

The most thorough study on the cost of diabetes has been conducted by Jonsson in Sweden [27]. On the basis of diagnostic category data, Jonsson estimated the total cost of diabetes to be 1317 million Swedish kronor in 1978. Health care costs accounted for 43% of the total cost, the remainder being attributable to indirect costs due to premature morbidity and mortality.

In Great Britain, Laing [28] used diagnostic category data to estimate the direct costs of diabetes at £83.4 million in 1979; disability costs were approximately £60.9 million. In a subsequent report, Laing and Williams [37] estimated that the direct costs of diabetes in 1986–87 for England and Wales were £484 million. With a similar design, Gerard and colleagues [38] estimated that the total costs of diabetes in England and Wales were at least £259 million.

Cost studies have been completed with other designs as well. In France, Triomphe et al [29] estimated that the average cost of diabetes was 7711 French francs for each IDDM patient and 5892 French francs for each NIDDM patient in 1984. These estimates were based on the charges and utilization data of 109 patients with diabetes in the Paris area. These patients, however, do not appear to constitute a representative sample of French diabetic cases. Figures on the cost of diabetes in Australia and Canada have been projected from the results of cost studies completed in the USA. In Australia, the cost of diabetes was estimated at $1.2 billion Australian for 1986 [30], while costs in Canada approached $1.8 billion Canadian for 1985 [31]. At present, cost comparisons between countries are speculative because there is no standardized methodology for measuring costs across the world.

COST–BENEFIT AND COST-EFFECTIVENESS ANALYSIS IN DIABETES

The second major concept in the economic analysis of diabetes is the use of cost–benefit or cost-effectiveness studies to evaluate treatments, therapies, procedures and programs. In an era of increasing pressure to limit increases in health care costs, these analyses offer an understanding of the costs and benefits involved in different treatments, procedures, etc. and can provide a mechanism for effective allocation of limited resources. Because of the substantial costs involved in diabetes mellitus, intervention strategies may become an important way of reducing the direct and indirect costs related to diabetes. Cost–benefit or cost-effectiveness analysis would, then, be needed to evaluate the appropriateness of the intervention strategies.

Cost–benefit analysis is one form of economic evaluation of alternative programs and procedures. In this evaluation process, all the costs and consequences of a program, procedure or therapy are expressed in monetary terms in an attempt to determine its cost worthiness [32]. The cost–benefit process strives to evaluate all benefits or weaknesses, including health benefits or weaknesses, of the program, or treatment in terms of dollars. However, one limitation of the analysis is that researchers often measure only those outcomes that are easy to measure in monetary terms. Furthermore, the thought that human life and health can have a monetary value could be a sensitive issue for some evaluators.

Cost-effectiveness analysis is another form of economic evaluation for health programs, procedures, treatments, etc. In this method of evaluation, the costs of the program are expressed in monetary terms, but the consequences are expressed in physical units [32]. Results of this analysis are presented as cost per unit of health outcome (e.g. cost per life saved, cost per case prevented, etc.). Often, cost-effectiveness analysis is used to evaluate two different programs that have the same objective [32]. Cost-effectiveness analysis does not attempt to place a monetary value on a health benefit or loss, but rather presents in monetary terms only those costs and consequences that are easily measured in financial form. Health effects are generally presented in physical units that summarize their outcome.

Cost–benefit and cost-effectiveness analyses are similar in concept in that they evaluate one alternative against another. Cost–benefit and cost-effectiveness studies also both consider the costs of starting and managing the program, treatment, etc. Philosophically, though, cost–benefit analysis often seeks to determine if an objective is worthwhole, while cost-effectiveness analysis already assumes that it is [39]. The analyses also differ in the manner in which they assess the outcomes of the program or therapy: cost–benefit analysis places a monetary value on the health outcome of the program, whereas cost-effectiveness analysis does not. If one can accept the notion that health effects can be assigned a monetary value, then comparison of the alternative programs is much easier with the cost–benefit approach.

Use of cost–benefit or cost-effectiveness analysis in the diabetes sector is very limited and often flawed. There is, however, considerable potential for using these procedures. The majority of the cost–benefit procedures completed in diabetes have involved the evaluation of diabetes education and nutrition programs. Kaplan and Davis [33] have critically discussed a large portion of the diabetes education literature. They point out that many of the program analyses have not addressed the main issues in cost–benefit analysis. For example, many studies have neglected to account for the costs of starting and operating the education program, focusing

instead on the benefits of the program. The majority of studies also have not included alternative or control groups for comparative purposes in their evaluation of education programs. Kaplan and Davis also point out the danger of evaluating programs simply on the basis of a reduction of medical costs, because health care costs can be influenced by simple changes in the reimbursement mechanism affecting them.

Two recent reports have modelled the cost-effectiveness of screening for and treating diabetic retinopathy [40, 41]. Javitt et al [40] estimated a cost of $966 per person-year of vision saved for the detection and treatment of proliferative retinopathy in IDDM patients. Dasbach and colleagues [41] went one step further in their model and found that the cost of screening for retinopathy was recovered (in terms of vision-years saved) for persons using insulin, both young and old. The costs of screening, though, were larger than the benefits obtained for those persons diagnosed with diabetes at a later age and not on insulin.

The potential exists for cost–benefit or cost-effectiveness studies in other segments of diabetes care as well. Screening programs, insulin treatment programs (multiple injections compared with single injections and insulin pump therapy), complications treatment programs and home blood glucose monitoring programs are areas that also could be evaluated with cost-benefit analysis. However, further medical evidence on the effectiveness of treatment regimens may need to be accumulated in some of these areas before appropriate economic analyses can be completed.

Economic analysis has utility in scientific evaluations as well as programmatic evaluations. Cost analysis can be easily incorporated into randomized clinical trials, such as the DCCT, where there are multiple end-points, both positive and negative, of concern. The human capital methodology can be easily applied to evaluate both the positive outcomes (e.g. improvements in health) and negative side-effects of the trial. This approach offers an innovative way to analyze the overall effectiveness of the clinical trial.

CONCLUSION

To summarize, it is clear that the economic costs of diabetes are extensive. The total costs of diabetes have risen markedly in the last 18 years. The health care costs of diabetes treatment have risen more rapidly than the medical care component of the consumer price index. Health care costs and utilization are higher in the diabetes population than in the general population and mortality costs in the USA approach $7.5 billion per year.

What, then, are the future needs of economic research into the costs of diabetes? There is a pressing need for more evaluation of the costs of diabetes throughout the world. Economic cost data are important for setting priorities for the use of health care resources, attracting research funds and evaluating health care practices, policies and treatment programs. However, cost studies in much of the world have been non-existent, and more effort needs to be directed towards investigating the cost of diabetes in these areas. In countries that lack appropriate population-based health and demographic statistics, surveys of individuals identified from diabetes registries may be an important source of diabetes-specific data.

A standardized methodology for estimating the impact of diabetes also needs to be developed and applied so that cost data from one country can be compared with data from another country. Currently, cost comparisons between countries are speculative because there is no standardized approach to measuring and evaluating the costs of diabetes. Comparison of the distribution of costs between nations could provide clues about the possible advantages and disadvantages of different health care delivery systems and practices.

There is also a strong need to dissect out costs, to examine costs from the perspective of the individual and family. Governments, health care organizations and legislators might be more understanding, knowledgeable and interested in diabetes care issues if they were able to see how diabetes directly affects the individual. The costs of IDDM and NIDDM need to be estimated, as well as the costs of diabetic complications.

There also is a need to recognize the role of cost–benefit or cost-effectiveness analysis in diabetes research. Use of cost–benefit or cost-effectiveness analysis in the diabetes sector is currently very limited. These types of analyses, however, offer an understanding of the costs and benefits involved in different diabetes programs, treatments and procedures, and can promote the effective allocation of limited health care funds. Economic analyses of randomized trials also offer an innovative way to evaluate the positive and negative health outcomes of the trial and should be considered as a method of evaluation in all trials.

Certainly, estimating the costs of diabetes does not have to be an educated guess; there are many possibilities in this sector that can, and should, be developed.

REFERENCES

1. Simanis JG. Health care expenditures: international comparisons, 1970–80. Soc Sec Bull 1987; 50: 19–24.
2. Simanis JG, Coleman JR. Health care expenditures in nine industrialized countries, 1960–76. Soc Sec Bull 1980; 43: 3–8.
3. Rice DP. Estimating the cost of illness. Health Economic Series no. 6, PHS publ. no. 947-6. Washington, DC: US Govt Printing Office, 1966.
4. Cooper BS, Rice DP. The economic cost of illness revisited. Soc Sec Bull 1976; 39: 21–36.
5. Rice DP, Hodgson TA, Kopstein AN. The economic costs of illness: a replication and update. Health Care Fin Rev 1985; 7: 61–80.
6. Hodgson TA, Meiners MR. Cost-of-illness methodology: a guide to current practices and procedures. Milbank Mem Fund Quar 1982; 60: 429–62.
7. Scitovsky AA. Estimating the direct costs of illness. Milbank Mem Fund Quar 1982; 60: 463–91.
8. Schelling TC. The life you save may be your own. In Chase (ed.) Problems in public expenditure analysis. Washington, DC: Brookings Institute, 1968.
9. Mishan EJ. Evaluation of life and limb: a theoretical approach. J Polit Econ 1971; 79: 687–705.
10. Tolpin HG, Bentkover JD. Economic cost of illness: decision-making applications and practical considerations. In Scheffler, Rossiter (eds) Advances in Health Economics and Health Services Research, vol. 4. Greenwich, CT: JAI Press, 1983.
11. Harris MI, Entmacher PS. Mortality from diabetes. In Diabetes in America: diabetes data compiled 1984. National Diabetes Data Group, NIH publ. no. 85-1468. Washington, DC: US Govt Printing Office, 1985, XXIX, pp 1–48.
12. Sinnock P. Hospital utilization for diabetes. In Diabetes in America: diabetes data compiled 1984. National Diabetes Data Group, NIH publ. no. 85-1468. Washington, DC: US Govt Printing Office, 1985, XXVI, pp 1–11.
13. Palumbo PJ, Elveback LR, Chu-Pin C. Diabetes mellitus: incidence, prevalence, survivorship and

causes of death in Rochester, Minnesota, 1945–1970. Diabetes 1976; 25: 566–73.

14. Entmacher PS, Sinnock P, Bostic E, Harris MI. The economic impact of diabetes. In Diabetes in America: diabetes data compiled 1984. National Diabetes Data Group, NIH publ. no. 85-1468. Washington, DC: US Govt Printing Office, 1985, XXXII, pp 1–13.

15. Policy Analysis, Inc. Evaluation of cost of illness ascertainment methodology, part II: applications of methodology to ascertain lifetime economic costs of illness in an incidence cohort. Final Report to the National Center for Health Statistics. DHHS contract no. 233-79-2048, December 1981.

16. Platt WG, Sudovar SG. The social and economic costs of diabetes: an estimate for 1979. Elkhart, Ind: Home Health Care Group, Ames Division, Miles Laboratories Inc., 1983.

17. Miller LV. Socioeconomic impact of diabetes mellitus. In Brodoff, Bleicher (eds) Diabetes mellitus and obesity. Baltimore: Williams & Wilkins, 1982.

18. Smeeding TM, Booton LA. Measuring and valuing the economic benefits of diabetes control. 19th National Meeting, Public Health Conference on Records and Statistics, August 23–24, 1983; pp 80–5.

19. Carter Center of Emory University. Closing the gap: the problem of diabetes mellitus in the United States. Diabetes Care 1985; 8: 391–406.

20. Fox NA, Jacobs J. Direct and indirect costs of diabetes in the United States in 1987. Alexandria, Va: American Diabetes Association, 1988.

21. Medical care component of the consumer price index, 1940–77. Soc Sec Bull 1978; 41: 67.

22. Medical care component of the consumer price index for all urban consumers, 1977–84. Soc Sec Bull 1984; 47: 62.

23. Hartunian NS, Smart CN, Thompson MS. The incidence and economic costs of major health impairments: a comparative analysis of cancer, motor vehicle injuries, coronary heart disease, and stroke. Lexington, Mass: Lexington Books, 1981.

24. Entmacher PS. The economic impact of diabetes. In Fajans SS (ed.) Diabetes mellitus. International Series on Preventive Medicine. New York: Fogarty, 1976, pp 33–40.

25. Entmacher PS. Report of economic impact of diabetes. In Report of the National Commission of Diabetes: scope and impact of diabetes. NIH publ. no. 76-1022, vol. 3, part 2. Washington, DC: US Govt Printing Office, 1976.

26. Taylor AK. Medical expenditures and insurance coverage for people with diabetes: estimates from the National Medical Care Expenditure Survey. Diabetes Care 1987; 10: 87–94.

27. Jonsson B. Diabetes—the cost of illness and the cost of control. An estimate for Sweden 1978. Acta Med Scand 1983; 671 (suppl.): 19–27.

28. Laing W. The cost of diet-related disease. In Turner M (ed.) Preventive nutrition and society. London: Academic Press, 1981.

29. Triomphe A, Flori YA, Costagliola D, Eschwège E. The cost of diabetes in France. Health Policy 1988; 9: 39–48.

30. Diabetes in Australia 1986. Canberra: Australian Diabetes Foundation, 1986.

31. Bain M, Ross SA. Socio-economic impact of diabetes mellitus. In Chiasson, Hunt, Hepworth, Ross, Tan, Zinman (eds) Status of diabetes in Canada. Report of symposium held at Le Chateau, Montebello, Quebec, 21–23 May 1985. Association du Diabète du Québec, Canadian Diabetes Association and Juvenile Diabetes Foundation Canada, 1987.

32. Drummond MF, Stoddart GL. Principles of economic evaluation of health programs. World Health Stat Quar 1985; 38: 355–76.

33. Kaplan RM, Davis WK. Evaluating the costs and benefits of outpatient diabetes education and nutrition counseling. Diabetes Care 1986; 9: 81–6.

34. Lubeck DP, Yelin EH. A question of value: measuring the impact of chronic disease. Milbank Quarterly 1988; 66: 445–64.

35. Roesler J, Bishop D, Walseth J. Economic cost of diabetes mellitus—Minnesota, 1988. MMWR 1991; 40: 229–31.

36. Huse DM, Oster G, Killen AR, Lacey MJ, Colditz GA. The economic costs of non-insulin-dependent diabetes mellitus. JAMA 1989; 262: 2708–2713.

37. Laing W, Williams R. Diabetes, a model for health care management. Office of Health Economics, paper no. 92, London, October 1989.

38. Gerard K, Donaldson C, Maynard AK. The cost of diabetes. Diabet Med 1989; 6: 164–70.

39. Mills A, Drummond MF. Economic evaluation of health programmes: glossary of terms. World Health Stat Q 1985; 38: 432–4.

40. Javitt JC, Canner JK, Sommer A. Cost-effectiveness of current approaches to the control of retinopathy in type I diabetics. Ophthalmology 1989; 96: 255–64.

41. Dasbach EJ, Fryback DG, Newcomb PA, Klein R, Klein BEK. Cost-effectiveness of strategies for detecting diabetic retinopathy. Med Care 1991; 29: 20–39.

74

Primary Prevention of Diabetes Mellitus

Jaakko Tuomilehto*, Eva Tuomilehto-Wolf*, Paul Zimmet‡,
K.G.M.M. Alberti§ and H. Keen¶

*National Public Health Institute, Helsinki, Finland, ‡ International Diabetes Institute, Caulfield, Victoria, Australia, § The Medical School, Newcastle upon Tyne, UK, and ¶ Guy's Hospital Medical School, London, UK

Recent advances in research into the etiology and natural history of diabetes mellitus have increased our knowledge about different types of diabetes to such an extent that primary prevention of diabetes mellitus is becoming a reality. Until now, only a few studies had attempted to test measures for primary prevention of diabetes; the data supporting the possibility of successful primary prevention are therefore, to a great extent, indirect and need to be tested in preventive trials or in community-based prevention programs. We believe, however, that the time is ripe to take action in those populations where the prevalence of diabetes is known to have increased over recent years, for instance Pima Indians, Nauruans, Maltese, Asian Indians in Fiji and Mauritius, etc.

Primary prevention and secondary prevention are part of the established terminology of preventive medicine [1]. Primary prevention has been defined as all measures designed to reduce the incidence of a certain disease in a population, by reducing the risk of its onset. In other words, this means that the attributable risk related to certain risk factors is modified by influencing the levels of such factors. Using a univariate approach, the relative importance of different risk factors can be determined by calculating from incidence of the exposed (I_e) and non-exposed (I_0) populations the 'attributable risk' $I_e - I_0$, i.e. the rate of disease in exposed individuals that can be attributed to the risk factor exposure. If the incidence in the total population (I_p) can be estimated, it is possible to calculate the 'population attributable risk': $(I_p - I_0)/I_p$. This provides an indicator of the proportion of the disease that could be eliminated by removing the risk factor. However, both insulin dependent diabetes mellitus (IDDM) and non-insulin dependent diabetes mellitus (NIDDM) are multifactorial diseases. Therefore, preventive measures for these diseases, to be effective, must be based on interventions on several potential risk factors simultaneously. This means that univariate estimates of attributable risks must be interpreted with great caution.

Secondary prevention includes all measures designed to reduce the prevalence of a disease in a population, by shortening its course and

International Textbook of Diabetes Mellitus. Edited by K.G.M.M. Alberti, R.A. DeFronzo, H. Keen and P. Zimmet

duration. Both types of prevention are necessary to achieve effective control of chronic non-communicable diseases, as for instance diabetes mellitus. The level of knowledge about the natural history of the disease, the effective intervention methods, the occurrence of the disease and the quality of the existing health care system will dictate which of the possible preventive measures will be selected and used.

Primary prevention can be implemented (a) through a population strategy, i.e. changing the life-style and the environmental determinants that are known to be risk factors for diabetes mellitus, and (b) through a high-risk strategy, i.e. targeting preventive measures only at those specific individuals or groups that are at high risk for the future development of diabetes.

Secondary prevention of diabetes mellitus means (a) very early intervention to avert the progression of the disease and to prolong the partial recovery period commonly known as the 'honeymoon period' in IDDM, and (b) implementation of intervention methods to prevent the development of major complications and disabilities related to diabetes such as cardio-vascular disease, retinopathy, neuropathy and nephropathy.

Prevention of a disease in a whole population requires action from many sectors of the community, in addition to the health care sector. Health personnel have an important role in increasing public awareness through their leadership, their influence on national policy-making and their patient contacts. Some activities that may lead to the prevention of diabetes have been initiated in various countries but, basically, the primary prevention of diabetes mellitus requires new, carefully designed and well-evaluated techniques and programs. Although a full consensus on the relation between certain health habits and diseases is lacking, preventive programs must be based on the best currently available knowledge about the etiology and natural history of different types of diabetes. The increasing incidence of diabetes, the severity of its complications and the increasing socioeconomic costs favor immediate preventive action. To await 'final proof' of the causes of different forms of diabetes mellitus cannot help the ever-increasing number of diabetic subjects. Fortunately, in spite of the gaps in our current knowledge, we probably understand the natural history of diabetes well enough to justify preventive actions.

It is quite surprising that, in spite of dramatic developments in the treatment of diabetes mellitus, there are hardly any serious research projects to explore the possibilities for primary prevention of diabetes. The history of public health is, however, replete with examples of successful preventive actions that were not based on complete knowledge of the etiology and pathophysiology of the disease concerned. Carefully planned and implemented prevention programs have proved to be important in forming a link between basic laboratory and clinical research, and public health, adding to the knowledge of the disease etiology.

INSULIN DEPENDENT DIABETES MELLITUS

Insulin dependent diabetes mellitus (IDDM or type 1 diabetes) is not a genetic disease but a disease with a genetic background. The susceptibility to develop the disease is inherited, but IDDM is only phenotypically expressed through the influence of environmental factors [2]; therefore, primary prevention of IDDM, i.e. reducing the incidence of IDDM in the population through reducing the risk of onset, is theoretically feasible.

Primary prevention of IDDM can be implemented by either a high-risk or a population approach. The high-risk approach would entail identification of susceptible subjects, e.g. first-degree and second-degree relatives of IDDM patients, and then the prevention of the onset of the disease by modifying the underlying genetic susceptibility or the precipitating environmental factors. The population approach would be more difficult and would aim either at altering lifestyle or at eliminating environmental determinants that are known to be risk factors for IDDM [3].

Secondary prevention of IDDM, which is not further discussed in this chapter, is directed at intervening in the progression of the disease once it is manifest. This can be done either by early intervention in newly diagnosed IDDM patients to prolong the 'honeymoon period', or by implementing measures to prevent the major macrovascular and microvascular complications of IDDM [4]. Several trials have already been carried out using immunosuppressive therapy such as cyclosporin A [5, 6], glucocorticoids [7], antilymphocyte serum [8], azathioprine [9] and other antimetabolites in newly diagnosed IDDM patients; interferon [10, 11], plasmapheresis [12] and levamisole [13] have also been tried. Such early intervention trials fall into the category of secondary prevention, although the term 'postprimary prevention' has been used [14]. Early, aggressive antihypertensive treatment trials aimed at reducing the decline in kidney function in diabetic nephropathy also fall into this category [15].

Although the susceptibility to IDDM is inherited, the main problem in prevention of IDDM using the high-risk approach is that only 12–15% of IDDM occurs in families and only in these 'multiplex' families have the predictive markers for IDDM been studied in detail. The majority of IDDM—according to Bennett [16] about 85°—occurs in a sporadic fashion and is therefore unaccounted for in most studies aimed at estimating risk and predictive value of certain markers.

The IDDM disease genotype has a low penetrance, i.e. not all HLA-identical siblings of an IDDM proband will develop the disease. The risk for an HLA-identical sibling (who by definition shares both parental haplotypes with the diabetic proband) for developing diabetes is not more than 10–20%. The risk for an HLA haploidentical sibling who has one parental haplotype in common with the proband is about 5%, and the risk for an HLA non-identical sibling who has no parental haplotype in common with the proband is less than 1% [17].

Genetic Background of IDDM

The HLA System

The susceptibility and resistance to developing IDDM is conferred by genes in the HLA region which is located on the short arm of chromosome 6 in the distal portion of the 6p21.3 band. The HLA region represents about one-thousandth of the total human genome and is about 3.5 million base pairs long (3.5 centimorgans) and contains more than 100 genes, including the gene or genes that confer susceptibility or resistance to IDDM.

Several loci are known to exist in this highly polymorphic region. The loci HLA-A, B and D code for class I antigens, the loci HLA-DR, DP and DQ for class II antigens and the region coding for class III antigens comprises the genes for the complement factors C2, C4A, C4B and Bf [18]. Many more genes are known in the HLA region which do not appear to be relevant for IDDM, such as the genes for 21-hydroxylase deficiency, idiopathic hemochromatosis, tumor necrosis factor and the genes coded by the loci HLA-DZ, DO, E, X, Y and Z.

The HLA genetic characteristics of IDDM are the same for sporadic and familial cases. A very high proportion of IDDM patients (about 95%) possess either HLA-DR3 or DR4, whereas the frequencies of DR2, DR7 and DR5 are decreased in IDDM patients [2, 19, 20]. There is no increase in the recombination frequency in families with IDDM, nor is there an increase in DR3 or DR4 homozygosity. A very important feature is the epistatic effect of B8 and Bw62, and especially of DR3 and DR4: this could indicate that both parents contribute genetically to their offspring's susceptibility to IDDM. The excess of DR3/DR4 heterozygotes in IDDM is well documented, and the coexistence of DR3 and DR4 also seems to influence the concordance rate in identical twins [21].

Most HLA studies in IDDM have compared the HLA frequencies found in unrelated IDDM patients with those found in healthy control subjects. Studies in unrelated patients can only reveal associations between HLA antigens and IDDM. In contrast, family studies are a much more powerful tool to establish linkage between the HLA system and IDDM. Family studies are rarer because they are more difficult to carry out; not enough attention is therefore given to the fact that only particular HLA haplotypes are increased in IDDM [22, 23]. For instance, the well-documented increase in DR4 is due to a selective increase of specific haplotypes. These extended haplotypes are more precise markers for IDDM than the antigens of any single locus, whether it be the B, the DR or the DQ locus. Calculating the relative risk for an HLA antigen of a single locus, for instance for DR4, might lead to the conclusion that the majority of DR4-positive people in the population never develop diabetes; such a conclusion is misleading. A more meaningful approach would be to see how often particular DR4-positive haplotypes, which are made up of certain antigens coded for by the HLA-A to the DQ locus which are in linkage disequilibrium, occur in the general population and then to calculate how often people with specific DR4 haplotypes (for instance the A2, Cw3, Bw62, C2*1, BF*S, C4A*QO, C4B*3, DR4, DRw53, Dw4, DQw8 haplotype or the A2, Cw1, Bw56, DR4, DRw53, DQw8 haplotype [177]) never develop IDDM. It is possible that a number of different genetic interactions between the various HLA loci might confer susceptibility. Unfortunately, there are no methods available that can make use of multiple polymorphic markers coded for at different but closely linked loci which might interact in increasing the liability to develop IDDM. Close linkage of the various HLA markers and linkage disequilibrium between some of them make calculations very difficult, but such analyses might be useful for more precise identification of genetically susceptible individuals.

In recent years, the science of molecular genetics has made it possible to reach the HLA genes themselves, and a new and exciting era has begun [24–26]. It is now quite clear that there are no mutant genes involved in IDDM and that no unique disease alleles exist in IDDM. Thus far, only sequence variations outside the functional genes have been found, so that most hypervariable sites are not in the coding regions but in the flanking sequences and are correlated only because of linkage disequilibrium [27].

Recently, the amino acid sequences of the HLA-DQ β chain derived from healthy people and from IDDM patients have been determined [28]. All haplotypes that were negatively associated or not associated with IDDM had the amino acid aspartic acid in position 57 of the $\alpha2$ helix of the DQ β chain. Whereas the DR $\beta1$ chains from healthy persons and IDDM patients were not very different, the positions 45 to 65 on the DQ β chain and the positions 52 to 56 of the DQw3 α chain seem to mediate susceptibility to IDDM. This discovery will very probably lead to new therapeutic and preventive approaches.

However, neither sequence determination, sequence-specific oligonucleotide hybridization nor restriction fragment length mapping are superior to HLA serology for defining the risk of developing IDDM. All differences detected by DNA typing so far are just more markers for the extended HLA haplotypes that are increased or decreased in IDDM. No different patterns, either of restriction fragment length or of DQ $\beta3$ subgroups, have been found between healthy and diabetic HLA-identical siblings. It seems that studying the HLA system at the DNA level does not advance our knowledge about which susceptible relative of an IDDM patient will develop the disease, and does not give additional clues about sporadic cases in the population.

Even though the determination of the HLA genes themselves is a major breakthrough for our understanding of IDDM, this may not directly contribute a great deal to the prevention of IDDM. It seems unlikely that gene manipulation and gene therapy in humans will be possible for IDDM in the near future.

The attributable risk of genetic factors for susceptibility to IDDM seems to be less than 50% as only about one-third of monozygotic twins become concordant for the disease [29] (see also Chapters 3 and 5). Furthermore, not all inbred non-obese diabetic (NOD) mice and only 60% of Bio-Breeding (BB) rats develop IDDM. It has been argued that the twin data do not have to be taken any more as evidence that environmental factors have a role, and an alternative hypothesis was put forward by Eisenbarth [30]. This postulates that new genes are created in genetically identical twins by a random combination process: 'thus identical twins are not genetically identical for key immunologic genes'; this is even harder to believe.

Non-HLA Genetic Markers

In the NOD mouse, which spontaneously develops IDDM characterized by autoimmune insulitis and lymphocytic infiltration in and around the islet, three recessive genes are necessary for the development of overt diabetes [31]: one gene is closely linked to the $H-2^k$ locus on chromosome 17 (the H-2 region in the mouse is the analog to the human HLA region), another gene is on chromosome 9 near the Thy-1 cluster and one gene is not linked. These results suggest that a polygenic basis for susceptibility to IDDM might exist also in humans, that the search for genes not linked to the major histocompatibility locus should be intensified and, perhaps, that genes on the long arm of chromosome 11 where the human Thy-1 locus is located should be studied.

So far, all attempts to identify additional genetic markers for IDDM outside the HLA region have failed [32–34]. Neither GLO on chromosome 6, nor the Kidd blood group or the Km locus on chromosome 2, nor the Gm locus on chromosome 14, nor the insulin gene locus on chromosome 11 [33], nor the insulin receptor gene locus on chromosome 19 [34], nor the Lewis blood group nor the fast acetylator phenotype, all of which have been implicated in IDDM in a variety of studies, can contribute to a clearer definition of susceptibility to IDDM.

Autoantibodies in IDDM

The clinical onset of IDDM is associated with a number of immune abnormalities [35]. About 50–80% of newly diagnosed IDDM patients have circulating autoantibodies to islet cell components. These antibodies have been divided into cytoplasmic islet cell antibodies (ICA) and islet cell surface antibodies (ICSA). Even though the final proof is still missing, IDDM is most probably an autoimmune disease with a long prodromal period during which autoantibodies to insulin and cytoplasmic ICA can be detected, sometimes up to several years before the first clinical symptoms [36].

Insulin autoantibodies and cytoplasmic ICA fluctuate and become transiently negative like all autoantibodies [29, 37]: cross-sectional studies in populations, therefore, may not reflect the true situation. Thus it remains to be seen how useful large-scale screening for ICA and for insulin autoantibodies will be. A study carried out on 1445 schoolchildren in Pasco County, Florida, found a prevalence of ICA of 0.8% in healthy children; 3 of the 12 positive children had a family history of IDDM and were therefore potentially genetically susceptible, and 4 others had parents with autoimmune diseases [38].

It is now clear that complement fixing islet cell antibodies, which were believed to be better predictive markers in families than conventional ICA [39], represent high-titer cytoplasmic ICA measured in a less sensitive assay.

The target antigens of cytoplasmic and islet cell surface antibodies are not known. It is interesting that cytoplasmic ICA react with all the cells in the islets of Langerhans, even though only B cells are selectively destroyed during the prediabetic phase. In the future, it might just be possible for peptides that mimic sequences of islet cell peptides to be used to prevent IDDM by virtue of their cross-tolerance; they might also prevent other endocrine cells from sustaining the autoimmune reaction.

Insulin autoantibodies occurring spontaneously in people who have never received insulin were first described in Japan in patients with reactive hypoglycemia [40]; they are found with a prevalence of about 40%. Recently, it has been shown that insulin autoantibodies appear after acute infections with common viruses such as mumps, rubella and measles, and especially frequently after chickenpox [41].

Abnormal Immune Reactions in IDDM

Many immunologic abnormalities have been described, not only in animal models for IDDM but also in humans. Increased levels of activated, Ia antigen-positive T lymphocytes and of killer cells, decreased numbers of T lymphocytes, and decreased levels of suppressor cells, have been found in newly diagnosed IDDM patients and in some healthy first-degree relatives [35].

However, these immunologic factors are not specific markers for IDDM and it is of interest that in monozygotic discordant twins, the increase in activated T lymphocytes can remit without leading to diabetes [29].

The specific aim in primary prevention of IDDM is to find a way to prevent the selective destruction of the pancreatic B cells or to increase the generation of new islet cells from pancreatic duct cells [42]. One way to achieve this could be through specific manipulation of the immune system, because in an abnormal immune response the binding of the processed foreign or altered self-antigen might be imperfect and therefore might inhibit the specific proliferation of the T-helper lymphocytes.

Clinical Predictors

Impaired Glucose Tolerance

In a long-term study of siblings of IDDM patients, the 2-hour oral glucose tolerance test identified a group of siblings who had an increased risk for developing IDDM. The predictive power of the positive oral glucose tolerance test was 13.6% [43]. More studies are needed, as little information is available about the relationship of impaired glucose tolerance (IGT) in children and the later development of IDDM, and about the use of the oral glucose tolerance test as a predictor of future disease in first-degree relatives.

First-phase Insulin Response

A slowly progressive loss of the insulin response to intravenous glucose takes place during the long prodromal period in all IDDM patients [44]. Whereas the fasting blood glucose levels are normal, the first-phase insulin response to intravenous glucose is low or virtually absent during the symptomless prediabetic phase. In a prospective study at the Joslin Clinic, 3 out of 5 initially discordant monozygotic twins who developed IDDM had an impaired first-phase insulin response before onset of the disease [45]. Larger studies are needed to assess the value of the progressive impairment of the first-phase insulin response as a predictor for future IDDM.

Viruses

Although a large number of common viruses, e.g. mumps, rubella and the coxsackie B group, have been implicated as having a role in the development of IDDM, this disease is not a common consequence of viral infection. Even though it was suggested in the last century that there might be a connection between mumps and IDDM [46], the part that viruses play in IDDM is still not clear. Many reports have shown a temporal relationship between certain viral infections and IDDM, but whether viruses are directly responsible for damage to the pancreatic B cell in humans or whether they can cause diabetes by triggering an autoimmune response is unknown [47]. In vitro, mumps virus, coxsackie B3 and B4 virus, and reovirus type 3 can infect human pancreatic B cells and destroy them. In mice the encephalomyocarditis virus, the meningovirus and the coxsackie B4 virus are able to destroy pancreatic B cells when inoculated, and in cattle a form of diabetes developed after an outbreak of foot-and-mouth disease [48].

An increased prevalence of IDDM has been found in patients with congenital rubella [49–51] and it has been shown that rubella virus can multiply in the pancreas and cause lesions.

The number of well-documented case reports involving coxsackie B viruses is small. However, they show that virus infections can trigger or be the final insult in the development of IDDM at least in some cases [52]. Viruses are unlikely to be the major precipitating factors in IDDM, otherwise the incidence of IDDM should have changed with a fall during the first decade of immunization against measles, rubella, mumps and poliomyelitis in the USA [53]. In Finland, the country with the highest incidence of IDDM in the world, an immunization scheme against mumps and rubella was started in 1982. Even though it may be too soon to see results, it is interesting to note that the incidence of IDDM is still increasing in Finland [54].

It must be borne in mind that many virus variants are grouped together under one name: for instance, the term 'coxsackie virus B4' signifies at least 13 variants. It may be that only a rare variant of the coxsackie virus B group is diabetogenic and that vaccination against this variant might be possible in the future.

The costs and benefits of a theoretical vaccine for diabetes have been estimated [55]. It was calculated that vaccinating the whole population rather than high-risk individuals would be the preferred policy and this would reduce the annual incidence of IDDM by 29% and the annual costs of the disease by 18%.

It has been reported that diabetic patients had reduced titers of antibodies to reoviruses and reduced titers of IgG and IgM antibodies to mumps, compared with healthy controls, whereas mumps-specific IgA antibodies were found more frequently [56]. These results suggest that the immunologic response to certain viruses is different in IDDM patients compared with healthy people and may indicate that IDDM patients have selective defects in their humoral response to certain viral antigens. This is clearly an area for further research with respect to prevention of IDDM.

Dietary Factors: Toxins

Some nutritional factors have been implicated in the etiology of IDDM but no firm data linking diet to incidence of the disease exist in humans. There has not yet been any prospective study to obtain accurate dietary information on a representative sample of genetically susceptible first-degree relatives of IDDM patients with follow-up to determine IDDM incidence.

Borch-Johnsen et al [57] proposed an inverse correlation between the frequency and duration of breastfeeding and the frequency of IDDM in the three areas of Norway, Sweden and Denmark. They postulated that breast milk provides protection against environmental factors that lead to the selective destruction of pancreatic B cells in genetically susceptible children. It could also be that commercially available milk substitutes or baby foods contain chemicals toxic to the pancreatic B cells or that cow's milk contains certain proteins that could be harmful to islet B cells. If it could also be shown in other countries that the duration of breastfeeding is relevant to the incidence of diabetes, then education campaigns for prolonged breastfeeding could be started. This might also have other beneficial health aspects besides IDDM prevention.

In the BB rat it was possible to reduce the incidence of diabetes by feeding the weanling rats a semisynthetic diet in which the proteins were replaced by L-amino acids [58]. In this study, the presence of intact protein in the diet was necessary for the development of diabetes, and even small amounts of dietary protein increased the incidence in the BB rat. It was suggested that people with a low protein diet might also have a low incidence of IDDM. A more recent study showed that diet has a dramatic effect on the immune system in the BB rat [59]: thymus weight and total white cell count were increased through a more pure diet, insulitis decreased, and the ratio of T helper to T suppressor cells was doubled.

Other studies have also shown that dietary factors could precipitate the expression of diabetes. In Iceland the traditional high intake of smoked and cured mutton during Christmas and New Year was correlated with an excess of boys under the age of 15 years born in October, who developed IDDM [60]; N-nitroso compounds were found in the smoked and cured mutton, and it was postulated that nitrosamines (which are known to cause cancer) are also capable of damaging the pancreatic B cells before or shortly after conception. This hypothesis was tested in pregnant Swiss mice, with suggestive results [61]. Nitrosamines are toxic substances that are related to the rodenticide Vacor, which has also been shown to cause diabetes in humans after ingestion [62]. Nitrosamines are also related to streptozotocin, an agent used to induce experimental diabetes in mice. It would be of extreme interest to study the content of nitrosamines in the diet of countries with a high or a low incidence of IDDM, as this may also have important implications for prevention of IDDM.

Conclusion

At present, the only practical advantage of determining HLA genotypes and other predictive markers for IDDM in relatives of IDDM patients is that those with a high risk of developing the disease can be observed for hyperglycemic symptoms so that ketoacidosis at the onset of overt diabetes can perhaps be avoided. According to a survey in Japan, 1 in 200 children die in ketoacidosis [63].

It is to be hoped that the high-risk approach will be of more use in the future when a better understanding of the pathophysiologic mechanism of the disease has been achieved and the environmental factors have been clarified. As not all siblings or offspring defined to be at high risk by HLA genotyping and with the existing immunologic and clinical markers develop diabetes, it is unethical to attempt immunotherapy in these still healthy children [64, 65].

Even though it is possible to define HLA antigens on fetal cells obtained through amniocentesis to ascertain the HLA status prenatally, this does not help in IDDM as yet.

An even more difficult approach is to try to prevent IDDM in the entire population. The environmental factors that precipitate IDDM are not well understood and more research in this area is definitely needed. Even though a rapid method of screening for HLA antigens within 5 minutes, using immunomagnetic beads and monoclonal antibodies, has been described recently [66], which would allow faster screening for susceptible individuals in the population, the costs of such screening would outweigh the potential benefit. HLA screening programmes will be useful only when the environmental determinants of IDDM are better understood.

NON-INSULIN DEPENDENT DIABETES MELLITUS

Genetic Susceptibility

NIDDM has a strong familial basis and it has been estimated that almost 40% of the siblings of NIDDM patients can expect to develop diabetes, assuming a maximum life expectancy of 80 years [67]. The risk of first-degree relatives developing NIDDM before the age of 65 years is of the order of 5–10%. The empiric recurrence risk to first-degree relatives for IGT is as high as 15–25%, but each year only about 2% of these will develop clinical diabetes [68, 69]. Firm evidence of the importance of genetic factors has been obtained from twin studies which have shown that there is about 90% concordance in NIDDM [70]; it can be argued, therefore, that environmental factors unmask this susceptibility in genetically predisposed individuals [71]. Unfortunately, specific genetic markers or determinants still remain to be identified. Several markers, independent of blood glucose concentration, that have been proposed so far have failed to clarify this problem [72–74].

While the search for specific genetic markers for NIDDM still continues, recent studies relating foreign genetic admixture to the prevalence of NIDDM have confirmed the important role of genetic factors. In Nauru, among people aged 60 years or more, the prevalence of NIDDM was 83% in full-blooded Naurans, compared with only 17% in part-Nauruans, suggesting that ancestral foreign genes have a protective effect against the disease [75]. In a study of Mexican-Americans, a positive relationship was demonstrated between the prevalence of NIDDM and estimates of the proportion of native American genes [76, 77]. An ecological correlation study with population-based data from six semitraditional Pacific communities showed a gradient of increasing mean 2-hour plasma glucose concentration after controlling for age and obesity [78]. However, as little can be done at present to change genetic susceptibility, one of the major challenges in diabetes prevention remains the modification of the environmental factors identified as being associated with the risk of NIDDM in particular populations.

Hyperinsulinemia and Obesity

During a lengthy period, at a given level of plasma glucose, basal insulin levels (and especially the insulin levels in response to glucose and to tolbutamide) are higher in obese patients compared with those of normal weight; this is accepted as a sign of insulin resistance in the former. Obese individuals exhibit hyperinsulinemia after glucose, suggesting that such individuals produce excessive quantities of insulin after glucose challenge, but insulin is, in fact, ineffective, as glucose tolerance is relatively impaired even in the face of massive hyperinsulinemia [79]. Data from Pima Indians [80], Micronesians [81] and Mexican-Americans [82]

have suggested that these populations, who are at high risk for NIDDM, have a greater degree of hyperinsulinemia than can be accounted for by their adiposity alone.

In normal-weight individuals, abnormal glucose tolerance implies either impaired insulin secretion or insulin resistance. In the obese with abnormal glucose tolerance, however, insulin resistance is consistently present whereas impaired secretion is rarely found [83]. At the stage of overt diabetes in normal-weight subjects, insulin secretion in response to intravenous glucose is markedly decreased when fasting glycemia exceeds 5.5 mmol/l, whereas this same phenomenon is observed in obese diabetic patients only when the fasting glucose level is more than 11.0 mmol/l. Responsiveness to tolbutamide, although greater than that to glucose in any diabetic, displays the same difference between normal weight and obese patients [83, 84].

At a given blood glucose level, hyperinsulinism and thus insulin resistance are the corollary to obesity, of which the initial causative mechanism remains to be established. The existence of a 'vicious circle' involving hyperinsulinism, diminished number of receptors by downward regulation and increased insulin resistance is established [85]. The subsequent hyperglycemia results in islet cell exhaustion as shown by reduced insulin secretion—a situation described as glucotoxicity. It has not yet been shown, however, that either insulin resistance or diminished insulin secretion are causal determinants of NIDDM.

A Japanese study has suggested that diminished insulin response following oral glucose is an independent predictor of the development of diabetes over the following 5–12 years, regardless of the initial postchallenge blood glucose [86]. In the Bedford study the adjustment for glucose concentration removed the association between insulin concentration and deterioration of IGT to overt diabetes [87]. In Pima Indians, insulin concentrations decreased with increasing fasting blood glucose values starting from 7.8 mmol/l and 2-hour post-challenge plasma glucose starting from 11.1 mmol/l, suggesting that inadequate insulin secretion contributed to the transition from IGT to NIDDM [80].

Obesity is often mentioned in connection with NIDDM, as the association between obesity and NIDDM is consistent, strong and graded. It has been shown that as many as 80% of NIDDM patients are obese at the time of onset of the disease [88, 89]. The incidence of NIDDM increases exponentially with an increasing degree of obesity. The obese children of diabetic parents have a much higher risk of developing NIDDM than obese children of non-diabetic parents [88-91]. Thus, genetic susceptibility and obesity seem to act synergistically [90, 91]. Many cross-sectional and longitudinal studies support the theory of a causal relationship between obesity and NIDDM [66-68, 92-94] but some (especially cross-sectional) studies do not [93-95]. It is clear that there is heterogeneity in the occurrence of obesity and in the impact of obesity on diabetes between populations.

Vague proposed in 1956 that complications of obesity were more prevalent in android obesity (excess fat in the upper part of the body) than in gynoid obesity (excess fat in the gluteal and femoral parts of the body) [96] (see also Chapter 21). This theory has been replicated many times recently [97-103]. The findings from several studies have suggested that this association is more pronounced in women than men. There is some evidence that subjects with predominantly upper body fat distribution are more insulin resistant then equally heavy subjects with predominantly lower body fat [104, 105]. Little is known about changes in the pattern of body fat distribution in obese subjects during weight loss. A modest weight loss, of course, does not seem to have much influence on this pattern [106].

NIDDM in the Elderly

The prevalence of NIDDM increases greatly with age, so that the majority of patients are over 60 years old. In populations with a high frequency of NIDDM the disease can be prevalent even in younger age groups [107-110]. Circulating plasma insulin levels do not decline with age, but tend to rise [111, 112]; increasing glucose intolerance with age cannot, therefore, be accounted for by a fall in insulin secretory capacity. Although obesity measured by body mass index often decreases with aging, more subtle changes in body fat distribution and a marked relative decrease in muscle mass may be important determinants of insulin insensitivity and glucose intolerance in the elderly [113, 114]. It has been suggested that a significant proportion of the insulin resistance that occurs in

older subjects might be avoidable if these people could remain physically active and if excess body weight gain during adulthood could be avoided. Unfortunately, there are no data from intervention studies among older subjects to support this argument, simply because such studies have not been carried out.

Impaired Glucose Tolerance

It is well documented that the condition of people with IGT may deteriorate to overt diabetes [67, 68, 80, 86, 87, 115]. IGT may be a critical stage in the development of NIDDM, because it is detectable and treatment may prevent or delay its progression. IGT is the first recognizable stage in the process from genetic susceptibility to NIDDM, and therefore it is potentially important with regard to the prevention of NIDDM. IGT is, however, a heterogeneous category which contains not only individuals who, indeed, are either in transition to NIDDM or are already at an early stage of disease, but also people whose casual 2-hour blood glucose values are high by random testing only [116]. Recent results from the Finnish study show that in a repeated glucose tolerance test two-thirds of the subjects with IGT at the first measurement will no longer fulfil the criteria for IGT [117].

IGT is a major problem in terms of number of people affected. The prevalence of IGT increases with age until about 65 years, when it exceeds 20% in several populations [95, 109, 110, 118, 119]. The duration of the IGT phase varies markedly, and some people may develop overt diabetes without this intermediate stage being diagnosed at all. The present criteria for IGT are arbitrary and the association between the 'baseline' blood glucose level and the subsequent risk of NIDDM is probably linear or exponential, without any clear threshold.

The rate of progression from IGT to diabetes is about 2-3% per year in studies carried out in the UK and USA. In populations in which the occurrence of diabetes is not very high, about half of those with IGT seem to return to normal within a 10-year follow-up period [67, 68, 86, 120]. In populations that have a higher prevalence of diabetes, it is likely that a greater proportion of persons with IGT will develop diabetes, as shown in Pima Indians [110].

Nauruans [121] and recently also in the Maltese population (J. Tuomilehto, unpublished).

In the Whitehall study, the initial blood glucose values, i.e. the degree of impairment of glucose tolerance, appeared to be the best predictor of worsening from IGT to diabetes in a 5-year study [67]. The second-best predictor was the presence of diabetes in the parents [67, 90, 91]. The importance of these factors has also been shown in other studies.

Hypertension

Hypertension is strongly associated with diabetes: in fact it is so frequently associated with NIDDM and obesity that common underlying mechanisms have been suggested [122, 123]. Recent data from Israel and Taiwan have shown that insulin resistance or hyperinsulinemia are present in the majority of hypertensives and could possibly explain the association between obesity, hypertension and glucose intolerance [124]. It can be argued that the hypertension and IGT are related, partially through genetic factors and partially through dietary factors [122–128]. Obesity per se is an important factor but is not sufficient to explain this association. Other important environmental factors are a high dietary fat intake [129, 130] and low dietary fibre intake [131, 132]. Whatever mechanisms of action may be involved in this association, hypertensive subjects are at higher risk of developing diabetes than normotensive ones. Moreover, commonly used antihypertensive agents may unmask glucose intolerance [128].

Fat Intake

A recent analysis of data from a Seventh-Day Adventist population living in California showed that, in this particular population, the risk of diabetes as an underlying cause of death during 21 years of follow-up was approximately half of that for all US whites [133]. Within the male Adventist population, vegetarians had a substantially lower risk of diabetes as an underlying or contributing cause of death than non-vegetarians. Furthermore, the prevalence of self-reported diabetes was lower in vegetarians than in non-vegetarians. The authors proposed the hypothesis that the reduced rates of diabetes could be due to lower meat or saturated fat intake in vegetarians. It has been shown that

saturated fat consumption may increase insulin secretion and possibly lead to insulin insensitivity [134]. Other pathophysiological mechanisms, such as an increased synthesis of estrogens [129] and an increased intake of *N*-nitroso compounds [57], have also been suggested.

Physical Inactivity

Experimental studies have demonstrated that regular physical activity improves glucose tolerance in patients with NIDDM through increasing insulin sensitivity [135], even if the effect of a single exercise bout has only a short duration [136]. The evaluation of a community-based exercise intervention among the Zuni Indians of New Mexico, USA, suggested that active participation in the program produced a significant weight loss of about 4 kg, and improvement in glycemic control among 30 participants with NIDDM [137]. Participants were also significantly more likely than non-participants to have stopped their hypoglycemic medication (relative risk 4.2) and to have decreased their medication dosage (relative risk 2.2). In non-diabetic people, physical training seems to have only a small, though positive effect on glucose tolerance [138, 139]. It has also been suggested that a high level of physical activity could partially prevent the deterioration of glucose tolerance with aging [139, 140]. At present, epidemiological data on the role of physical activity in the etiology of NIDDM or in the worsening of glucose tolerance are still sparse, but promising. A recent report described the lower prevalence of diabetes in female former college athletes as compared with non-athletes using a questionnaire method with a relative risk of 2.24 for the non-athletes [141]. Results from cross-sectional studies suggest that physical inactivity is an independent risk factor for NIDDM [142, 143].

In a recent study in Malta, which is known for the high occurrence of NIDDM, the influence of physical inactivity on the risk of NIDDM was assessed during a 2-year follow-up (J. Tuomilehto, unpublished data). The age-standardized 2-year risk of glucose intolerance, i.e. IGT or diabetes, was consistently and inversely related to the level of physical activity. Among subjects with normal glucose tolerance at baseline, those with low physical activity had a 2.7 times higher risk of glucose intolerance during follow-up than those with high physical activity and even a 3.7-fold risk of glucose intolerance when both normal and IGT subjects at baseline were considered together. Similar trends were observed for the risk of diabetes.

High physical activity may be more helpful in maintaining normal glucose tolerance, than in stabilizing or improving glucose tolerance in subjects in whom a deterioration of glucose tolerance has already occurred. Exercise is actually regarded as a useful adjunct to the therapy of NIDDM [144]. However, a recent review came to the conclusion that exercise appears to be effective in normalizing glucose tolerance only in patients who still have an adequate capacity to secrete insulin, and in whom insulin resistance is the major cause of abnormal glucose tolerance [140].

It has been shown that the response of pancreatic B cells to oral glucose improves at decreased glucose levels, and the pancreas seems to have an important role in improvement in glucose tolerance after long-term physical exercise [139, 145, 146]. A recent experimental study, which assessed the relative contributions of impaired insulin secretion and insulin sensitivity to glucose intolerance, suggested that an impaired B-cell response was the major determinant of glucose intolerance [147]; prospective population studies from Japan [86] and Nauru [121] are in agreement with these findings. It has been proposed that the training enhances insulin sensitivity in peripheral tissues [148, 149]. It has also been suggested that decreased physical fitness is related to peripheral insulin insensitivity in addition to the decreased insulin secretion of individuals with familial aggregation of NIDDM [150].

Pregnancy

Glucose intolerance may occur or be detected during pregnancy as gestational diabetes [151, 152]. There is uncertainty about the prognostic significance of testing glucose tolerance in pregnant women [153]. However, the incidence of subsequent overt diabetes mellitus in women with gestational diabetes is quite high, about 3–5% per year, which cumulatively means 35–40% of individuals in a 15-year follow-up [154, 155]. Gestational diabetes in the mother may mean an increased risk of the offspring for developing diabetes: in the Pima Indians an extraordinarily high incidence of diabetes before

the age of 20 years was seen in offspring of women with gestational diabetes [156].

Intervention Measures to Prevent NIDDM

High-risk Approach

The potential for primary prevention of NIDDM exists in families in which a positive family history for NIDDM has been confirmed. People aged 40–65 years (in some populations up to 75 years) should be the main target group. All women with gestational diabetes should be considered to be at high risk. Hypertensive patients form another high-risk group. Obese and physically inactive people should be considered as additional risk groups, especially if the family history for diabetes is positive.

The best predictor of the development of diabetes in high-risk groups (apart from the genetic predisposition) is the degree of glucose intolerance, and such groups should be screened for IGT. The screening should probably be repeated at regular intervals of about 2–5 years, depending on the presence of other risk factors for progression to diabetes. Subjects with IGT should be given individual health education, counselling and treatment, to improve the metabolic state.

Unfortunately, too little is known and too few controlled, long-term intervention studies have been performed with the aim of preventing the worsening to diabetes in people with IGT, to establish which are the most efficient preventive measures to be employed. On the other hand, the recommendations concerning dietary and health behavior changes listed below are not harmful and also have beneficial effects on general health, in addition to the potential improvement in glucose metabolism. The following actions are recommended for people at high risk for NIDDM.

Weight control in the obese. This should be especially intensive in obese patients with high glucose levels and high blood pressure. In hypertensive patients treated with antihypertensive drugs, the need for drug treatment will become less through weight reduction [157] and the impairment of glucose tolerance due to these drugs may be thus avoided [128, 158].

Increase in physical activity. This should be especially considered in people with IGT and in those who are obese. Physical activity seems to protect also against coronary heart disease [159], which is a very common macrovascular complication in diabetic patients. The increasing occurrence of diabetes with age in the elderly, together with the decreasing level of physical activity, calls for special attention to this issue.

Dietary regulation avoiding excessive energy intake. Rapidly absorbed carbohydrates should be replaced by complex carbohydrates and dietary fiber. It has been suggested that food rich in fiber is a protective factor against NIDDM [131]. Certainly, NIDDM is rare in populations living on a traditional diet which is rich in complex carbohydrates and fiber. A high-fiber dietary regimen in diabetic patients produces a significant decrease in postprandial blood glucose [132, 160–162], and it seems to reduce the need for oral hypoglycemic agents and insulin [158]. Dietary fiber (especially guar gum) seems to lower serum cholesterol levels [132, 163] and elevated blood pressure [132, 164], which means a significant decrease in the overall risk of atherosclerosis, especially in hyperlipidemic and hypertensive people.

The long-term effects of high-fiber diets in diabetic patients are not well known, and the addition of therapeutic doses of active fiber such as guar may result in problems with compliance. However, the preventive approach in promoting the use of high-fiber diets in population groups at high risk of diabetes is feasible and well demonstrated, for instance in traditional cultures and vegetarian groups. Controlled studies comparing low-carbohydrate, high-fat diets with high-carbohydrate, low-fat diets, with low and high fiber contents respectively, have shown that it is not the enhancement in the percentage of carbohydrates itself but the addition of crude fibers that is responsible for the beneficial effects of a high-carbohydrate diet on glucose control and lipoprotein profile [165]. Thus, natural foods rich in polysaccharides and fibers, such as wholemeal bread, fruits and vegetables, should be preferred. There are many data suggesting that such a high-fiber diet in vegetarians is associated with a lower risk of diabetes [133], cardiovascular disease [133, 134] and cancer [166].

Blood glucose lowering with oral antidiabetic agents. Although there is disagreement about

prevention of NIDDM in people with IGT using oral hypoglycemic drugs [66], tolbutamide treatment combined with diet regulation may prevent or postpone progression from IGT to manifest diabetes [115]. Such a pharmacological preventive measure can carry some additional risks [167] and should be used only for selected patient groups.

Reduction of saturated fat intake. It is suggested that a diet high in fat reduces glucose tolerance, and hastens the onset and increases the incidence of diabetes mellitus [129, 130, 134]. High serum cholesterol is a good marker for a high intake of saturated fats. People with a positive family history of NIDDM who have high serum cholesterol values should be especially advised to avoid saturated fat intake [168]. Such dietary recommendations for the control of diabetes are also suitable with regard to the primary prevention of NIDDM. With improved facilities for the control of blood glucose and a better understanding of the different effects of various carbohydrates, fibers and fats on the glucose–insulin axis and cardiovascular risk respectively, a new diet strategy for diabetes has been proposed [169]. These high-carbohydrate, low-fat diets offer 50–60% of the energy in the form of carbohydrates and limit the fat consumption to below 30% of energy intake.

Non-pharmacological treatment of hypertensive patients with a positive family history of NIDDM. Many antihypertensive drugs have a diabetogenic effect [128, 158] and, therefore, their use in patients with a positive history of NIDDM should be avoided. The merits of non-pharmacological therapy (weight control, restricted intake of sodium, saturated fats, calcium and alcohol, increased intake of potassium, magnesium and dietary fiber) to lower blood pressure are clear [170]. Simultaneously, these measures not only control blood pressure but are also beneficial for glucose metabolism.

Screening for genetically predisposed individuals. Whether or not early detection of NIDDM is useful has been debated frequently [167]. Now seems to be the time to take an active role in facilitation of the early detection of diabetes [171–173].

A more complicated issue is whether genetic screening for NIDDM is needed or feasible. As there is no biological genetic marker for NIDDM, the only way of assessing genetic predisposition is to take a complete and detailed family history with regard to NIDDM. The number of first-degree and second-degree relatives affected by the disease, and the age of onset, could be useful in evaluating the degree of genetic predisposition. There are some problems in establishing precise family histories because a number of people will transmit the genetic disposition without having manifest diabetes. It is agreed that genetic counselling as a way of primary prevention of NIDDM is not possible at present. However, people with a positive family history should be a specific target group for health education in order to reduce the environmental risk factors. In most communities it is neither feasible nor cost-effective to start specific screening programs among family members of NIDDM patients, but this should be considered in high-risk populations.

General Population

The basis of primary prevention using a population approach is to shift the average blood glucose level of the population in the direction of lower ('normal') glucose values. Although the risk for NIDDM is usually reflected only in the upper range of the glucose distribution, there are populations where the entire distribution of blood glucose is positioned at higher levels [106–109]. Such a displacement reflects environmental influences; it should be therefore possible to improve the situation through a community-based environmental intervention. It is possible that these populations, which have undergone recent and rapid environmental changes, evolved a metabolic ('thrifty') genotype that is conservative and non-wasteful [131, 174]. Natural selection has favoured a metabolic state with a high storage capacity of energy. As the environment has changed, these people now have an excessive energy intake and the evolved metabolic genotype may be disadvantageous (see Chapter 22). If this is true, the population approach for prevention of NIDDM is the only appropriate way, supported by the high-risk strategy.

The feasibility and effectiveness of reducing coronary disease risk factors (smoking, blood pressure and serum cholesterol) have been demonstrated [175]. Therefore, it is reasonable to assume that a healthier life-style would also reduce the levels of the known risk factors of NIDDM. In fact, there is not much difference between the preventive measures for NIDDM and coronary heart disease at the community level. Because coronary heart disease is the major complication associated with NIDDM, any large-scale prevention program for NIDDM must be integrated with coronary heart disease prevention activities.

Even though it could be argued that uncertainty still exists as to whether large-scale prevention can be justified on the basis of existing data for NIDDM, very little will be learned about prevention of NIDDM without trying it.

In 1921, Dr E. P. Joslin in his article 'The prevention of diabetes mellitus' [176] expressed his opinion in the following way: '. . . it is proper at the present time to devote time not alone to treatment, but still more, as in the campaign against typhoid fever, to prevention. The results may not be quite so striking or as immediate, but they are sure to come and to be important.' Looking back over nearly 70 years, there is no cause to be proud about the achievements in relation to Dr Joslin's recommendations. The list of serious attempts at primary prevention of diabetes is not very long. Dr Joslin was suggesting intervention against overweight, especially. Should we not be a little ashamed that not even the hypothesis of weight control in the prevention of NIDDM has been scientifically tested in proper population-based studies by 1992?

REFERENCES

1. Hogarth J. Glossary of health care. Public health in Europe 5. Copenhagen: WHO/EURO, 1975: p 302.
2. Wolf E, Spencer KM, Cudworth AG. The genetic susceptibility to Type 1 (insulin-dependent) diabetes: analysis of the HLA-DR association. Diabetologia 1983; 24: 224–30.
3. Tuomilehto J, Wolf E. Primary prevention of diabetes mellitus. Diabetes Care 1987; 10: 238–48.
4. Hawthorne VM, Cowie CC. Some thoughts on early detection and intervention in diabetes mellitus. J Chron Dis 1984; 37: 667–9.
5. Stiller CR, Laupacis A, Dupre J et al. Cyclosporin for treatment of early Type 1 diabetes: preliminary results. New Engl J Med 1983; 308: 1226–7.
6. Assan R, Feutren G, Debray-Sachs M et al. Metabolic and immunological effects of cyclo-

sporin in recently diagnosed Type I diabetes mellitus. Lancet 1985; i: 67–71.

7. Elliot RB, Grossley JR, Berryman CC, James AG. Partial preservations of pancreatic B-cell function in children with diabetes. Lancet 1981; ii: 631–2.

8. Leslie RDG, Pyke DA. Immunosuppression of acute insulin dependent diabetics. In Irwine WJ (ed.) Immunology of diabetes. Edinburgh: Teviot, 1980: 101–7.

9. Spencer KM, Dean BM, Bottazzo GF, Medbak S, Cudworth AG. Preliminary evidence for a possible therapeutic intervention in early Type 1 (insulin-dependent) diabetes. Diabetologia 1982; 23: 474(A).

10. Rand KH, Rosenbloom AL, Maclaren NK et al. Human leukocyte interferon treatment of two children with insulin dependent diabetes. Diabetologia 1981; 21: 116–19.

11. Koivisto VA, Aro A, Cantell K et al. Remissions in newly diagnosed Type 1 (insulin-dependent) diabetes: influence of interferon as an adjunct to insulin therapy. Diabetologia 1984; 27: 193–7.

12. Ludvigsson J, Heding L, Lieden G, Marner B, Lernmark Å. Plasmapheresis in the initial treatment of insulin-dependent diabetes mellitus in children. Br Med J 1983; 286: 176–8.

13. Cobb WE, Jackson IMD, Reichlin S. Failure of levamisole, a putative immunosuppressive agent, to modify the course of early insulin-dependent diabetes mellitus. New Engl J Med 1980; 303: 1065–6.

14. WHO Study Group on Diabetes Mellitus. Technical Report Series 727. Geneva: WHO, 1985.

15. Parving HH, Andersen AR, Smidt U, Svendsen PA. Early, aggressive antihypertensive treatment reduces rate of decline in kidney function in diabetic nephropathy. Lancet 1983; i: 1175–9.

16. Bennett PH. Changing concepts of the epidemiology of insulin-dependent diabetes. Diabetes Care 1985; 8 (suppl. 1): 29–33.

17. Tuomilehto-Wolf E, Tuomilehto J. HLA antigens in insulin dependent diabetes mellitus. Ann Med 1991 (in press).

18. Crumpton MJ. HLA in medicine. Br Med Bull 1987; 43: 1–240.

19. Christy M, Green A, Cristau B et al. Studies of the HLA system and insulin-dependent diabetes mellitus. Diabetes Care 1979; 2: 209–14.

20. Deschamps I, Lestradet H, Bonaiti C et al. HLA genotype studies in juvenile insulin-dependent diabetes. Diabetologia 1980; 19: 189–93.

21. Johnston C, Pyke DA, Cudworth AG, Wolf E. HLA-DR typing in identical twins with insulin-dependent diabetes: difference between concordant and discordant pairs. Br Med J 1983; 286: 253–5.

22. De Jongh BM, Bruning GJ, Schreuder GNT et al. HLA and Gm in insulin-dependent diabetes in the Netherlands: report on a combined multiplex family and population study. Hum Immunol 1984; 10: 5–21.

23. Bertrams J, Hintzen U, Schlicht S, Schoeps S, Gries FA, Louton TK, Baur MP. Gene and haplotype frequencies of the fourth component of complement (C4) in type 1 diabetics and normal controls. Immunobiology 1984; 166: 335–44.

24. Owerbach D, Lernmark I, Platz P et al. HLA-DR-chain DNA endonuclease fragments differ between healthy and insulin-dependent individuals. Nature 1983; 303: 815–17.

25. Cohen D, Cohen O, Marcadet A et al. HLA class IIB DC DNA restriction fragments differentiate among HLA-DR2 individuals in insulin-dependent diabetes and multiple sclerosis. Proc Natl Acad Sci USA 1984; 81: 1774–8.

26. Owerbach D, Hugglik B, Lernmark I, Holmgren G. Susceptibility to insulin-dependent diabetes defined by restriction enzyme polymorphism of HLA-D region genomic DNA. Diabetes 1984; 33: 958–65.

27. Niven MJ, Hitman GA. The molecular genetics of diabetes mellitus. Biosci Rep 1986; 6: 501–12.

28. Todd JA, Bell JI, McDevitt HO. HLA-DQ beta gene contributes to susceptibility and resistance to insulin-dependent diabetes mellitus. Nature 1987; 329: 599–604.

29. Millward BA, Alviggi L, Hoskins PJ et al. Immune changes associated with insulin dependent diabetes may remit without causing the disease: a study in identical twins. Br Med J 1986; 292: 793–6.

30. Eisenbarth GS. Genes, generator of diversity, glycoconjugates, and autoimmune beta-cell insufficiency in type 1 diabetes. Diabetes 1987; 36: 355–64.

31. Prochazka M, Leiter EH, Serreze DV, Coleman DL. Three recessive loci required for insulin-dependent diabetes in nonobese diabetic mice. Science 1987; 237: 286–9.

32. Cudworth AG, Wolf E. Genetic basis of Type 1 (insulin-dependent) diabetes. In Gupta S (ed.) Immunology of clinical and experimental diabetes. New York: Plenum, 1984: pp 271–94.

33. Neumer C, Brandt R, Zahlke H. The human insulin gene and diabetes mellitus. Exp Clin Endocrinol 1986; 87: 89–103.

34. Ullrich A, Bell JR, Chen EY et al. Human insulin receptor and its relationship to the tyrosine kinase family of oncogenes. Nature 1985; 313: 756–61.

35. Drell DW, Notkins AL. Multiple immunological abnormalities in patients with Type 1

(insulin-dependent) diabetes mellitus. Diabetologia 1987; 30: 132–43.

36. Gorsuch AN, Spencer KM, Lister J, McNally JM, Dean BM, Bottazzo GF, Cudworth AG. Evidence for a long prediabetic period in Type 1 (insulin-dependent) diabetes mellitus. Lancet 1981; ii: 1363–5.

37. Spencer KM, Tam A, Dean BM, Lister J, Bottazzo GF. Fluctuating islet-cell autoimmunity in unaffected relatives of patients with insulin-dependent diabetes. Lancet 1984; i: 764–6.

38. Maclaren NK, Horne G, Spillar RP, Barbour H, Harrison D, Duncan J. Islet cell autoantibodies (ICA) in US school children. Diabetes 1985; 34 (suppl. 1): 84.

39. Gorsuch AN, Spencer KM, Wolf E, Cudworth AG. HLA and family studies. In Kibberling J, Tattersall R (eds) The genetics of diabetes mellitus. London: Academic Press, 1982: pp 43–53.

40. Hirata Y, Ishizu H, Ouchi N et al. Insulin autoimmunity in a case of spontaneous hypoglycaemia. Japan Diab Soc 1970; 13: 312–20.

41. Bodansky HJ, Grant PJ, Dean BM, McNally J, Bottazzo GF, Hambling MH, Wales JK. Islet-cell antibodies and insulin autoantibodies in association with common viral infections. Lancet 1986; ii: 1351–3.

42. Gepts W, Lecompte PM. The pancreatic islets in diabetes. Am J Med 1981; 70: 105.

43. Rosenbloom AL, Hunt SS, Rosenbloom EK, Maclaren N. Ten year prognosis of impaired glucose tolerance in siblings of patients with insulin-dependent diabetes. Diabetes 1982; 31: 385–7.

44. Srikanta S, Ganda OP, Gleason RE, Jackson RA, Soeldner JS, Eisenbarth GS. Pre-type I diabetes: linear loss of beta cell response to intravenous glucose. Diabetes 1984; 33: 717–20.

45. Srikanta S, Ganda OP, Jackson RA et al. Type I diabetes mellitus in monozygotic twins: chronic progressive beta cell dysfunction. Ann Intern Med 1983; 99: 320–6.

46. Harris HF. A case of diabetes mellitus quickly following mumps. Boston Med Surg J 1899; 140: 465–9.

47. Yoon JW, Ray UR. Perspectives on the role of viruses in insulin-dependent diabetes. Diabetes Care 1985; 8 (suppl. 1): 39–44.

48. Barboni E, Manocchio J. Alterazionia pancreatiche in bovini con diabete mellito post-aftoso. Arch Veter Ital 1962; 13: 477–89.

49. Hay DR. The relation of maternal rubella to congenital deafness and other abnormalities in New Zealand. NZ Med J 1949; 48: 604–8.

50. Ginsberg-Fellner F, Witt ME, Yagihashi S et al. Congenital rubella syndrome as a model for Type 1 (insulin-dependent) diabetes mellitus: increased prevalence of islet cell surface antibodies. Diabetologia 1984; 27: 87–9.

51. Menser MA, Forrest JM, Honeyman MC, Burgess JA. Diabetes, HLA-antigens and congenital rubella. Lancet 1974; ii: 1508–9.

52. Barrett-Connor E. Is insulin-dependent diabetes mellitus caused by coxsackievirus B infection? A review of the epidemiologic evidence. Rev Infect Dis 1985; 7: 207–15.

53. Fleegler FM, Rogers KD, Drash A, Rosenbloom AL, Travis LB, Court JM. Age, sex, and season of onset of juvenile diabetes in different geographic areas. Pediatrics 1979; 63: 374–9.

54. Tuomilehto J, Rewers M, Reunanen A et al. Increasing trend in type 1 (insulin-dependent) diabetes mellitus in childhood in Finland. Analysis of age, calendar time and birth cohort effects during 1965 to 1984. Diabetologia 1991; 34: 282–7.

55. England WL, Roberts SD. Immunization to prevent insulin-dependent diabetes mellitus? The economics of genetic screening and vaccination for diabetes. Ann Intern Med 1981; 94: 395–400.

56. Toniolo A, Conaldi PG, Garzelli C et al. Role of antecedent mumps and reovirus infections on the development of type 1 (insulin-dependent) diabetes. Eur J Epidemiol 1985; 1: 172–9.

57. Borch-Johnsen K, Joner G, Mandrup-Poulsen T et al. Relation between breast-feeding and incidence rates of insulin-dependent diabetes mellitus. Lancet 1984; ii: 1083–6.

58. Elliot RB, Martin JM. Dietary protein: a trigger of insulin-dependent diabetes in the BB rat? Diabetologia 1984; 26: 297–9.

59. Scott FW, Mongeau R, Kardish M, Hatina G, Trick KD, Wojcinsky Z. Diet can prevent diabetes in the BB rat. Diabetes 1985; 34: 1059–62.

60. Helgason T, Jonasson MR. Evidence for a food additive as a cause of ketosis-prone diabetes. Lancet 1981; ii: 716–20.

61. Helgason T, Ewen SW, Ross IS, Stowers JM. Diabetes produced in mice by smoked/cured mutton. Lancet 1982; ii: 1017–22.

62. Prosser PR, Karam JH. Diabetes mellitus following rodenticide ingestion in man. JAMA 1978; 239: 1148–51.

63. Japan and Pittsburgh Childhood Diabetes Research Groups. Coma at onset of young insulin-dependent diabetes in Japan: the result of a nationwide survey. Diabetes 1985; 34: 1241–6.

64. Rossini AA. Immunotherapy for insulin-dependent diabetics? New Engl J Med 1983; 308: 333–5.

65. Cyclosporin for diabetes? (editorial). Lancet 1986; ii: 140–1.

66. Gaudernack G, Lundin KE, Thorsby E. Immunomagnetic HLA typing in a single step (abstr.). 10th International Histocompatibility Conference, New York, November 18–21, 1987; A28.

67. Köbberling J, Tillil H. Empirical risk figures for first-degree relatives of non-insulin-dependent diabetics. In Köbberling J, Tattersall R (eds) The genetics of diabetes mellitus. London: Academic Press, 1982: pp 201–10.

68. Jarrett RJ, Keen H, Fuller JH, McCartney P. Worsening to diabetes in men with impaired glucose tolerance ('borderline diabetes'). Diabetologia 1979; 16: 25–30.

69. Keen H, Jarrett RJ, McCartney P. Ten year follow-up of the Bedford survey (1962–1972): glucose tolerance and diabetes. Diabetologia 1982; 22: 73–8.

70. Barnett AH, Eff C, Leslie RDG, Pyke DA. Diabetes in identical twins—a study of 200 pairs. Diabetologia 1981; 20: 87–93.

71. Simpson NE. Heritabilities of liability to diabetes when sex and age at onset are considered. Ann Hum Genet 1969; 32: 283.

72. Keen H, Track NS. Age of onset and inheritance of diabetes: importance of examining relatives. Diabetologia 1968; 4: 317–24.

73. Pyke DA. Diabetes: the genetic connections. Diabetologia 1979; 17: 333–43.

74. Rotwein PS, Chirgwin J, Province M et al. Polymorphism in the 5'-flanking region of the human insulin gene: a genetic marker for non-insulin dependent diabetes. New Engl J Med 1983; 308: 65–71.

75. Serjeantson SW, Owerbach D, Zimmet P, Nerup J, Thoma K. Genetics of diabetes in Nauru: effects of foreign admixture, HLA antigens and the insulin-gene-linked polymorphism. Diabetologia 1983; 25: 13–17.

76. Gardner LI, Stern MP, Haffner SM et al. Prevalence of diabetes in Mexican Americans: relationship to percent of gene pool derived from native American sources. Diabetes 1984; 33: 86–92.

77. Brosseau JD, Eelkema RC, Crawford AC, Abe TA. Diabetes among the three affiliated tribes: correlation with degree of Indian inheritance. Am J Publ Health 1979; 69: 1277–8.

78. King H, Zimmet P, Bennett P, Taylor R, Raper LR. Glucose tolerance and ancestral genetic admixture in six semitraditional Pacific populations. Genet Epidemiol 1984; 1: 315–28.

79. Efendic S, Luft R, Wajngot A. Aspects of the pathogenesis of type 2 diabetes. Endocr Rev 1984; 5: 395–409.

80. Bennett PH, Knowler WC, Pettitt DJ, Carraher MJ, Vasquez B. Longitudinal studies of the development of diabetes in the Pima Indians. In Eschwège E (ed.) Advances in diabetes epidemiology. Amsterdam: Elsevier, 1982: pp 65–74.

81. King H, Zimmet P, Pargeter K, Raper LR, Collins V. Ethnic differences in susceptibility to noninsulin-dependent diabetes: a comparative study of two urbanized Micronesian populations. Diabetes 1984; 33: 409–15.

82. Haffner SM, Stern MP, Hazuda HP, Pugh JA, Patterson JK. Hyperinsulinemia in a population at high risk for non-insulin-dependent diabetes mellitus. New Engl J Med 1986; 315: 220–4.

83. Vague PH, Ramahandridona G, Vialettes B, Lassmann V, Altomare E. Insulin secretion at the different stages of diabetes. In Vague J, Vague PH (eds) Diabetes and obesity. Amsterdam: Excerpta Medica, 1979: pp 203–13.

84. Reaven GM. Insulin resistance in the first stages of diabetes. In Vague J, Vague PH (eds) Diabetes and obesity. Amsterdam: Excepta Medica, 1979: pp 188–98.

85. Vague PH, Ramahandridona G, Gerolami A. Insulin response to glucose and tolbutamide in 'essential' versus 'pancreatic' mild glucose intolerance. Diabetes 1974; 23: 896.

86. Kadowaki T, Miyake Y, Hagura R et al. Risk factors for worsening to diabetes in subjects with impaired glucose tolerance. Diabetologia 1984; 26: 44–9.

87. O'Sullivan JB, Mahan CM. Blood sugar levels, glycosuria and body weight related to development of diabetes mellitus. JAMA 1965; 194: 117–22.

88. Köbberling J. The respective place of obesity and heredity in the development of diabetes. In Vague J, Vague PH (eds) Diabetes and obesity. Amsterdam: Excerpta Medica, 1979: pp 83–90.

89. Keen H, Jarrett RJ, Thomas BJ, Fuller JH. Diabetes, obesity and nutrition: epidemiological aspects. In Vague J, Value PH (eds) Diabetes and obesity. Amsterdam: Excerpta Medica, 1979: pp 91–103.

90. Knowler WC, Pettitt DJ, Savage PJ, Bennett PH. Diabetes in Pima Indians: contributions of obesity and parental diabetes. Am J Epidemiol 1981; 113: 114–56.

91. Ostrander LD, Butler WJ. Diabetes and blood glucose: the Tecumseh study. In Eschwège E (ed.) Advances in diabetes epidemiology, INSERM Symp. no. 22. Amsterdam: Elsevier, 1982: pp 57–64.

92. Medalie JH, Papier CM, Goldbourt U, Herman JB. Major factors in the development of diabetes mellitus in 10 000 men. Arch Int Med 1975; 135: 811–17.

93. Zimmet P. Type 2 (non-insulin-dependent)

diabetes—an epidemiological overview. Diabetologia 1982; 22: 399–411.

94. Lee ET, Anderson PS Jr, Bryan J et al. Diabetes, parental diabetes, and obesity in Oklahoma Indians. Diabetes Care 1985; 8: 107–13.

95. Tuomilehto J, Nissinen A, Kivelä S-L et al. Prevalence of diabetes mellitus in elderly men aged 65 to 84 years in eastern and western Finland. Diabetologia 1986; 29: 611–15.

96. Vague J. The degree of masculine differentiation of obesities: a factor determining predisposition to diabetes, arteriosclerosis, gout and uric calculus disease. Am J Clin Nutr 1956; 4: 20–34.

97. Stern MP, Haffner SM. Body fat distribution and hyperinsulinemia as risk factors for diabetes and cardiovascular disease. Arteriosclerosis 1986; 6: 123–30.

98. Feldman R, Sender AJ, Siegelaub AB. Difference in diabetic and nondiabetic fat distribution patterns by skinfold measurements. Diabetes 1969; 18: 478–86.

99. Sims EAH. Definitions, criteria, and prevalence of obesity. In Bray GA (ed.) Obesity in America. US Dept of Health, Education and Welfare, NIH publication no. 79–359. Washington DC: US Government Printing Office, 1979.

100. Kissebah AH, Vydelingum N, Murray R et al. Relation of body fat distribution to metabolic complications of obesity. J Clin Endocrinol Metab 1982; 54: 254–60.

101. Hartz AJ, Rupley DC, Kalkhoff RD, Rimm AA. Relationship of obesity to diabetes: influence of obesity level and body fat distribution. Prev Med 1983; 12: 351–7.

102. Larsson B, Svärdsudd K, Welin L et al. Abdominal adipose tissue distribution, obesity, and risk of cardiovascular disease and death: 13-year follow-up of participants in the study of men born in 1913. Br Med J 1984; 288: 1401–4.

103. Joos SK, Mueller WH, Hanis CL, Schull WJ. Diabetes Alert Study: weight history and upper body obesity in diabetic and nondiabetic Mexican American adults. Ann Hum Biol 1984; 11: 167–71.

104. Kissebah AH, Vydelingum N, Murray R et al. Relationship of body fat distribution to metabolic complications of obesity. J Clin Endocrinol Metab 1982; 54: 254–60.

105. Krotkiewski M, Björntorp P, Sjöström L, Smith U. Impact of obesity on metabolism in men and women: importance of regional adipose tissue distribution. J Clin Invest 1983; 72: 1150–62.

106. Kissebah AH, Evans DJ, Peiris A, Wilson CR. Endocrine characteristics in regional obesities: role of sex steroids. Proceedings of the International Symposium on the Metabolic Complications of Human Obesities, Marseille, May 30–June 1 1985 (ICS no. 682). Amsterdam: Elsevier, 1986.

107. West KM. Epidemiology of diabetes and its vascular lesions. New York: Elsevier/North Holland, 1978.

108. Jarret RJ. The epidemiology of diabetes mellitus. In Boström H, Ljungstedt N (eds) Recent trends in diabetes research. Stockholm: Almqvist & Wiksell, 1982: 24–36.

109. Zimmet P, Taft P, Guinea A, Guthrie W, Thoma K. The high prevalence of diabetes mellitus on a Central Pacific Island. Diabetologia 1977; 13: 111–15.

110. Knowler WC, Bennett BH, Hamman RF, Miller M. Diabetes incidence and prevalence in Pima Indians: a 19-fold greater incidence than in Rochester, Minnesota. Am J Epidemiol 1978; 108: 497–504.

111. Reaven GM, Reaven EP. Effects of age on various aspects of glucose and insulin metabolism. Mol Cell Biochem 1980; 31: 37.

112. Reaven GM, Reaven EP. Insulin and glucose metabolism during aging. In Adelman RC, Roth GS (eds) Endocrine and neuroendocrine mechanisms of aging. Boca Raton, Fla: CRC Press, 1983: p 1.

113. Yki-Järvinen H, Koivisto VA. Effects of body composition on insulin sensitivity. Diabetes 1983; 32: 965.

114. Rosenthal M, Haskell WL, Solomon R et al. Demonstration of a relationship between level of physical training and insulin-stimulated glucose utilization in normal humans. Diabetes 1983; 32: 408.

115. Sartor G, Schersten B, Carlstrom S, Melander A, Norden A, Persson G. Ten-year follow-up of subjects with impaired glucose tolerance prevention of diabetes by tolbutamide and diet regulation. Diabetes 1980; 29: 41–9.

116. Stern MP, Rosenthal M, Haffner SM. A new concept of impaired glucose tolerance: relation to cardiovascular risk. Arteriosclerosis 1985; 5: 311–14.

117. Tuomilehto J, Salomaa V, Korhonen H, Kartovaara L. The repeatability of classification and factors related to it in two consecutive oral glucose tests. Helsinki: National Public Health Institute (abstr.).

118. Harris MI, Hadden WC, Knowler WC, Bennett PH. Prevalence of diabetes and impaired glucose tolerance and plasma glucose levels in US population aged 20–74 yr. Diabetes 1987; 36: 523–34.

119. Zimmet P, Taylor R, Ram P et al. Prevalence of diabetes and impaired glucose tolerance in the biracial (Melanesian and Indian) population of Fiji: a rural–urban comparison. Am J Epidemiol 1983; 118: 673–88.

120. Crombie DL, Pike LA, Malins JM, FitzGerald

MG, Goodwin RP, Thompson J. Ten-year follow-up report on Birmingham Diabetes Survey of 1961. Br Med J 1976; 2: 35–7.

121. Sicree R, Zimmett P, King H, Coventry J. Plasma insulin response among Nauruans: prediction of deterioration in glucose tolerance over 6 years. Diabetes 1987; 36: 179–86.

122. Cederholm J, Wibell L. Glucose intolerance in middle-aged subjects—a cause of hypertension? Acta Med Scand 1985; 217: 363–71.

123. Fuh MM-T, Shieh S-M, Wu D-A, Chen Y-DI, Reaven GM. Abnormalities of carbohydrate and lipid metabolism in patients with hypertension. Arch Int Med 1987; 147: 1035–8.

124. Modan M, Halkin H, Almog S et al. Hyperinsulinemia. A link between hypertension, obesity and glucose intolerance. J Clin Invest 1985; 75: 809–17.

125. Jarrett RJ, Keen H, McCartney M, Fuller JH, Hamilton PJS, Reid DD, Rose G. Glucose tolerance and blood pressure in two population samples: their relation to diabetes mellitus and hypertension. Int J Epidemiol 1978; 7: 15–24.

126. Christlieb AR, Warram JH, Krolewski AS et al. Hypertension—the major risk factor in insulin-dependent diabetics with juvenile onsets. Diabetes 1981; 30 (suppl. 2): 90.

127. Florey C, du Uppal VS, Clowy C. Relation between blood pressure, weight, and plasma sugar and serum insulin levels in school children aged 9–12 years in Westland, Holland. Br Med J 1976; 1: 1368–71.

128. Murphy MB, Kohner E, Lewis PJ, Schumer B, Dollery CT. Glucose intolerance in hypertensive patients treated with diuretics: a fourteen-year follow-up. Lancet 1982; ii: 1293–5.

129. Addanki S. Roles of nutrition, obesity, and estrogens in diabetes mellitus: human leads to an experimental approach to prevention. Prev Med 1981; 10: 577–89.

130. Himsworth HP. Diet and incidence of diabetes mellitus. Clin Sci 1935; 2: 117–48.

131. Trowell H. Diabetes mellitus and dietary fiber of starchy foods. Am J Clin Nutr 1978; 31: 553–7.

132. Uusitupa M, Tuomilehto J, Karttunen P, Wolf E. Long term effects of guar gum on metabolic control, serum cholesterol and blood pressure in Type 2 (non-insulin dependent) diabetic patients with high blood pressure. Ann Clin Res 1984; 16 (suppl. 43): 126–31.

133. Phillips RL, Lemon FR, Beeson WL, Kuzuma JW. Coronary heart disease mortality among Seventh-day Adventists with differing dietary habits: a preliminary report. Am J Clin Nutr 1978; 31: S191–8.

134. Snowdon DA, Phillips RL, Fraser GE. Meat consumption and fatal ischemic heart disease. Prev Med 1984; 13: 490–500.

135. Kemmer FW, Berger M. Exercise and diabetes mellitus: physical activity as a part of daily life and its role in the treatment of diabetic patients. Int J Sports Med 1983; 4: 77–88.

136. Lampman RM, Santinga JT, Savage PJ et al. Effect of exercise training on glucose tolerance, in vivo insulin sensitivity, lipid and lipoprotein concentrations in middle-aged men with mild hypertriglyceridemia. Metabolism 1985; 34: 205–11.

137. Heath GW, Leonard BE, Wilson RH, Kendrick JS, Powell KE. Community-based exercise intervention: Zuni Diabetes Project. Diabetes Care 1987; 10: 579–83.

138. Schneider SH, Amorosa LF, Khachadurian AK, Ruderman NB. Studies on the mechanism of improved glucose control during regular exercise in Type 2 (non-insulin-dependent) diabetes. Diabetologia 1984; 26: 355–60.

139. Björntorp P. Physical activity, plasma insulin and glucose tolerance in relation to coronary heart disease. Finn Sports Exer Med 1983; 2: 87–92.

140. Holloszy IO, Schultz I, Kusnierkiewicz I, Hagberg IM, Ehsani AA. Effects of exercise on glucose tolerance and insulin resistance. Acta Med Scand 1986; suppl. 711: 55–65.

141. Seals DR, Hagberg JM, Allen WK et al. Glucose tolerance in young and older athletes and sedentary men. J Appl Physiol 1984; 56: 1521–5.

142. Taylor R, Ram P, Zimmet P, Raper LR, Ringrose H. Physical activity and prevalence of diabetes in Melanesian and Indian men in Fiji. Diabetologia 1984; 27: 578–82.

143. Cederholm J, Wibell L. Glucose tolerance and physical activity in a health survey of middle-aged subjects. Acta Med Scand 1985; 217: 373–8.

144. Cooppan R. Determining the most appropriate treatment for patients with non-insulin-dependent diabetes mellitus. Metabolism 1987; 36 (suppl. 1): 17–21.

145. Rönnemaa T, Mattila K, Lehtonen A, Kallio V. A controlled randomized study on the effect of long-term physical exercise on the metabolic control in type 2 diabetic patients. Acta Med Scand 1986; 220: 219–24.

146. Bogardus C, Ravussin E, Robbins DC, Wolfe RR, Horton ES, Sims EAH. Effects of physical training and diet therapy on carbohydrate metabolism in patients with glucose intolerance and non-insulin-dependent diabetes mellitus. Diabetes 1984; 33: 311–18.

147. O'Rahilly SP, Nugent Z, Rudenski AS et al. Beta-cell dysfunction, rather than insulin insensitivity, is the primary defect in familial type 2 diabetes. Lancet 1986; ii: 360–4.

148. Sato Y, Hayamizu S, Yamamoto C et al.

Improved insulin sensitivity in carbohydrate and lipid metabolism after physical training. Int J Sports Med 1986; 7: 307–10.

149. Saltin B, Lindgärde F, Houston M, Hurlin R, Nygaard E, Gad P. Physical training and glucose tolerance in middle-aged men with chemical diabetes. Diabetes 1979; 28 (suppl. 1): 30.

150. Berntorp K, Lindgärde F. Impaired physical fitness and insulin secretion in normoglycaemic subjects with familial aggregation of type 2 diabetes mellitus. Diabetes Res 1985; 2: 151–6.

151. National Diabetes Data Group. Classification and diagnosis of diabetes mellitus and other categories of glucose intolerance. Diabetes 1979; 28: 1039–57.

152. WHO Expert Committee on Diabetes Mellitus. Second report. Technical Report Series 646. Geneva: WHO, 1980.

153. Jarret RJ. Reflections on gestational diabetes mellitus. Lancet 1981; ii: 1220–2.

154. O'Sullivan JB, Mahan CM. Prospective study of 352 young patients with chemical diabetes. New Engl J Med 1968; 278: 1038–41.

155. Pettitt DJ, Knowler WC, Baird HR, Bennett PH. Gestational diabetes: infant and maternal complications of pregnancy in relation to third trimester glucose tolerance in Pima Indians. Diabetes Care 1980; 3: 458–64.

156. Pettitt DJ, Baird HR, Aleck KA, Knowler WC. Diabetes mellitus in children following maternal diabetes during gestation. Diabetes 1982; 31 (suppl. 2): 66A.

157. Langford GH, Blaufox A, Oberman CM et al. Dietary therapy slows the return of hypertension after stopping prolonged medication. JAMA 1985; 253: 657–69.

158. Christlieb AR, Maki PC. The effect of beta-blocker therapy on glucose and lipid metabolism. Prim Cardiol 1980; 1: 47.

159. Powell KE, Thompson PD, Caspersen CJ, Kendrick JS. Physical activity and the incidence of coronary heart disease. Am Rev Publ Health 1987; 8: 253–87.

160. Jenkins DJA, Wolever TMS, Taylor RH, Barker HM, Fieldman H. Exceptionally low blood glucose response to dried beans: comparison with other carbohydrate foods. Br Med J 1980; 281: 578–80.

161. Jenkins DJA, Wolever TMS, Hockaday TDR et al. Treatment of diabetes with guar gum. Reduction in urinary glucose loss in diabetics. Lancet 1977; ii: 779–80.

162. Kiehm TG, Anderson JW, Ward K. Beneficial effects of high carbohydrate. High fiber diet on hyperglycaemic diabetic men. Am J Clin Nutr 1976; 29: 895–9.

163. Jenkins DJA, Leeds AR, Slavin B, Mann J, Jepson EM. Dietary fiber and blood lipids: reduction of serum cholesterol in type II hyperlipidemia by guar gum. Am J Clin Nutr 1979; 32: 16–18.

164. Tuomilehto J, Karttunen P, Vinni S, Uusitupa M. A double-blind evaluation of guar gum in patients with dyslipidaemia. Hum Nutr Clin Nutr 1983; 373: 109–16.

165. Riccardi G, Rivellese A, Pacioni D, Genovese S, Mastranzo P, Mancini M. Separate influence of dietary carbohydrate and fibre on the metabolic control in diabetes. Am J Clin Nutr 1984; 26: 116–21.

166. Phillips RL, Snowdon DA. Brin BN. Cancer in vegetarians. In Wynder EL, Leveille GA, Weisburger JH, Livingston GE (eds) Environmental aspects of cancer—the role of macro and micro components of foods. Westport, Conn: Food & Nutrition Press, 1983.

167. Screening for carbohydrate intolerance (editorial). Lancet 1980; i: 1174–5.

168. Savage PJ, Bennion LJ, Flock EV et al. Diet-induced improvement of abnormalities and glucagon secretion and in insulin receptor binding in diabetes mellitus. J Clin Endocrinol Metab 1979; 48: 999–1007.

169. American Diabetes Association. Principles of nutrition and dietary recommendations for individuals with diabetes. Diabetes Care 1979; 2: 520–3.

170. Rose IL, Beilin LJ. Vegetarian diet and blood pressure. J Hypertens 1984; 2: 231–40.

171. International Collaborative Group. Joint discussion on asymptomatic hyperglycemia and coronary heart disease. J Chron Dis 1979; 32: 829–37.

172. Bennett PH, Knowler WC. Early detection and intervention in diabetes mellitus—is it effective? J Chron Dis 1984; 37: 653–66.

173. Hawthorne VM, Cowie CC. Some thoughts on early detection and intervention in diabetes mellitus. J Chron Dis 1984; 37: 667–9.

174. Neel JV. Diabetes mellitus: a thrifty genotype rendered detrimental by 'progress'? Am J Hum Genet 1962; 14: 353–62.

175. Puska P, Tuomilehto J, Salonen J et al. The North Karelia Project. Evaluation of a comprehensive community programme for control of cardiovascular disease in North Karelia, Finland 1972–1977. Copenhagen: WHO/EURO, 1981.

176. Joslin EP. The prevention of diabetes mellitus. JAMA 1921; 76: 79–84.

177. Tuomilehto-Wolf E, Tuomilehto J, Cepaitis Z, Lounamaa R, DIME Study Group. A new susceptibility haplotype in type 1 diabetes. Lancet 1989; 2: 299–302.

Index

Page numbers in **bold** indicate main discussions

The following abbreviations have been used in subheadings: AGE, advanced glycation end-products; GFR, glomerular filtration rate; HDL, high-density lipoprotein; IDDM, insulin dependent diabetes mellitus; IGT, impaired glucose tolerance; IVGTT, intravenous glucose tolerance test; LDL, low-density lipoprotein; MODY, maturity onset diabetes of young; NIDDM, non-insulin dependent diabetes mellitus; OGTT, oral glucose tolerance test; VLDL, very low-density lipoprotein

The alphabetical arrangement is letter-by-letter

Abdominal pain
  chronic pancreatitis, management
    187–8
  diabetic ketoacidosis 1031,
    1034–5, 1154, 1158
  fibrocalculous pancreatic diabetes
    183, 184
Abdominal wall, insulin absorption
  844
Abducens (sixth) nerve palsies
  1367–8
Abortions, spontaneous 76, 1087
  diabetic nephropathy and 1301
Abscesses
  insulin injection site 885–6
  perinephric 1302
Acanthosis nigricans syndromes
  248, **539**
  type A 38, 40, **369–72**, 539
  type B 38, 539
  type C 539
Acarbose 809, 826
Accidents, motor vehicle 1633,
  1634
Accu-Chek 973
A cells
  gastrointestinal tract 204, 334
  isolated preparations 262
  pancreatic 223, **225**, 226, 334
    chronic pancreatitis 246
    development 224
    distribution in islets 227
    fibrocalculous pancreatic
      diabetes 186
    paracrine interactions 420
    type 1 diabetes 231, 236,
      237
Acesulphame K 696

Acetoacetate 287, 1153
  extrahepatic utilization 463
  insulin deficiency and 465
  synthesis 462
Acetohexamide 746, **757**
  elderly patients 1120, 1121
Acetone 462, 1153
Acetylcholine, insulin secretory
  response 274
Acetyl-CoA
  insulin resistance in NIDDM and
    607, 608
  metabolism 462, 463
  regulation of synthesis 390
Acetyl-CoA carboxylase **391–2**,
  398, 399, 400
Acetyl-CoA carboxylase kinase
  399, 400
N-Acetyl-β-D-glucosaminidase
  (NGA) 1289
Acetylsalicylate, GFR reduction
  1286
Achondroplasia 39
Acid–base balance, diabetic
  ketoacidosis 1153
Acidosis, hyperkalaemic
  hyperchloraemic 1303
Acromegaly 247, **295**
  insulin resistance 295, 365, 534
ACTH (adrenocorticotrophic
  hormone) 394
Actin, islet cells 264
Actomyosin, diabetic nephropathy
  1292
Acute-phase proteins 1448
Addison's disease 47
Adenosine deaminase gene, MODY
  and 72

Adenosine diphosphate, see ADP
Adenosine triphosphate, see ATP
Adenylate cyclase
  drug actions 798
  glucagon actions 276–7, 808
  insulin-induced inhibition 401
  nutrient-mediated activation 272
  see also Cyclic AMP
Adhesive capsulitis, shoulder
  1420–1
Adipocytes
  glucagon actions 335
  glucose transport 387–8, 603–4
  insulin receptors 358, 365
    IDDM 369
    NIDDM 367
    obesity 366, 367
  lipid metabolism 391–3, 394
  visceral fat depots 554
Adipose tissue
  distribution, steroid hormone
    effects **560–4**
  glucose uptake 555, 586
  insulin actions on specific
    mRNAs 396
  ketone body metabolism **460**,
    461, 463
  lipid metabolism 391
  protein degradation 477
  pyruvate dehydrogenase activity
    390
  visceral accumulation
    and metabolic aberrations,
      syndrome of 561–4
    metabolic effects 554–5
    steroid hormone-induced
      560–1
  see also Obesity, abdominal

Adolescents **1025–53**
  blood glucose self-monitoring
    1041–2, 1043
  brittle diabetes 1064–5
  diabetes education 936, **941**,
    1039, **1044–7**
  IDDM epidemiology 1025–6
  insulin resistance 541
  long-term IDDM management
    1037–53
  see also Children
ADP
  insulin secretion and 271
  platelet aggregation and 1452,
    1453
Adrenal autoantibodies 47, 123
Adrenaline (epinephrine)
  adrenergic symptoms of
    hypoglycaemia 1135
  as counterregulatory hormone
    1137, 1137–8, 1139–40
  exercise and 727, 728, 729
  glycogen synthase activity and
    389
  hyperglycaemia after myocardial
    infarction and 1199–201
  IDDM, deficient responses
    1140–1
  insulin-mediated glucose disposal
    and 433
  insulin secretion and 275–6,
    288, 289
  insulin suppression test 425,
    520, 578, 1074
  ketogenic effects 464
  lipid metabolism and 394
  outcome of myocardial infarction
    and 1193
  pancreatectomized patients 212
  platelet aggregation and 1452
Adrenal insufficiency
    (hypoadrenalism) 366, 1063
Adrenal sex steroids, obesity 556,
    557
Adrenergic agonists
    (sympathomimetics)
  insulin secretion and 289
  neuropathic foot oedema
    1541
α-Adrenergic agonists, B cell
    function and 420
β-Adrenergic agonists
  B cell function and 420
  insulin receptor activity and
    363, 365
  lipid metabolism and 391,
    392
  premature labour 1094
α-Adrenergic blockers
  brittle diabetes 1065
  hypertension 1529, 1530
  insulin secretion and 290
β-Adrenergic blockers (beta-
    blockers)

after myocardial infarction
    1196–7
  brittle diabetes 1065
  hypertension **1529–30**, 1531
  insulin secretion and 289
  pregnancy 1093, 1094
Adrenergic receptors, islet B cells
    275
α-Adrenergic receptors, insulin
    secretion and 288
α₂-Adrenergic receptors, insulin
    secretion and 274, 275
β-Adrenergic receptors
  insulin secretion and 274,
    288
  visceral fat 560
β₂-Adrenergic receptors, adrenaline-
    induced hyperglycaemia and
    1137
Adrenergic system
  diet-induced thermogenesis and
    431
  glucagon release and 336
  insulin secretion and **274–6**
Adrenocorticotrophic hormone
    (ACTH) 394
Advanced glycation end-products,
    see Glycation end-products,
    advanced
Affinity chromatography
  glycated haemoglobin 993–4
  glycated serum proteins 995
Africa
  diabetes prevalence 1614–15
  dietary management of diabetes
    711–17
  dietary patterns and food
    consumption 711–13
  energy needs 713
  fibrocalculous pancreatic diabetes
    182
  see also Tanzania
Africans
  complications in NIDDM 180
  HLA and IDDM associations
    139–42
  IDDM frequency **137–9**
  NIDDM frequency 179
Agar gel electrophoresis, glycated
    haemoglobin measurement
    993, 994–5
Age
  hypoglycaemia and 1137
  NIDDM frequency and 154–5,
    1103–4
  prevalence of diabetes and IGT
    and 1103–5, 1106
AGE, *see* Glycation end-products,
    advanced
Age at onset **34**
  diabetes subtypes 42
  IDDM subtypes 48, 49
  limited joint mobility and
    1422–3

NIDDM 34, 62
  tropical countries 179
  pancreatic diabetes 210
  risk of diabetic nephropathy and
    1268
Aging **1103–24**
  counterregulatory hormones and
    1111
  diet and 1109–10
  exercise and 1110–11
  free fatty acids and 1111
  glucose absorption and 1109
  glucose transport and 1109, 1110
  hepatic glucose production and
    1109
  insulin binding and 1108–9
  insulin resistance and 288–9,
    541, **1106–7**, 1108
  insulin secretion and 1107–8
  lean body mass and 1109
  mechanisms for glucose
    intolerance of 1105–11
  non-insulin-mediated glucose
    uptake and 1109
  rhesus monkeys, NIDDM
    development 598, 599
  see also Elderly
AIR, *see* Insulin response, acute
Airline cabin attendants 1639–40
Airline pilots 1638–9
Air traffic controllers 1640
AL1567 809
Alanine
  biguanide actions 780
  interorgan exchange 496–7,
    498–9
  pancreatectomized patients 208,
    209, 210
  pancreatic diabetes 210
Alaninuria 38
Albumin
  basement membrane binding
    672, 1252–3
    diabetic nephropathy 1277,
    1292
  glycated **995**, 996
    assay 995
    flux across glomerular
    membrane 1278
    pregnancy 1002
  synthesis 1448
    insulin actions 396, 492
  urinary excretion rates (UAER)
    1272–3, 1287–8
    antihypertensive therapy and
    1524–5, 1526
    blood pressure and 1289,
    1466, 1524, 1525
    glycaemic control and
    1218–19, 1235, 1298,
    1299
    renal morphology and 1294
  see also Microalbuminuria;
    Proteinuria

Albumin/creatinine ratio 1272, 1274
Alcohol (ethanol)
  biguanide interactions 788
  chronic pancreatitis and 199
  insulin secretion and 289
  sulphonylurea interactions 766
Alcohol consumption
  Africa 714–15
  hypoglycaemia awareness and 1136
  hypoglycaemia induction 1146
  NIDDM development and 157
  pancreatic diabetes and 212, 215, 216
  recommendations 697
Alcoholic ketoacidosis 1158
Alcoholic pancreatitis 182, 190
Aldimines (Schiff base adducts) 670–1, 986, 987
Aldose reductase 1233, 1255
  kidney 1278
  neutrophil function and 1167, 1168
  role in humans **1389–90**
Aldose reductase inhibitors (ARI) **809**, 1550
  autonomic neuropathy 1558
  basement membrane changes and 1256
  diabetic neuropathy 809, 1387–8, **1390**, 1400, 1555
  diabetic retinopathy 1335, 1552
  early diabetic nephropathy 1278–9, 1299
Aleuts, IDDM frequency 134, 135
Alkaline phosphatase 402, 1417
1-Alkyl-2-formyl-3,4-diglycosyl pyrroles (AFGP) 671
Allergy
  insulin 884–5, **887–8**
    injection site 836, 887–8
    systemic 836, 887
    treatment 888
  retarding agents in insulin preparations 889–90
Alloxan
  B-cell destruction 249
  diabetogenic effects 61, 289–90
Alloxan-induced animal diabetes
  retinopathy 1231
  somatostatin production 345, 346
Alpha-1-antitrypsin deficiency 38
α-Fetoprotein 1093
  maternal serum (MSAFP) 76–7
Alpha-glucosidase inhibitors **808–9**
  sulphonylureas combined with 765
  triglyceride reduction 826
Alstrom's syndrome 38, 1028

Amadori glycation products 670, 671, 986, 987
Ambulatory diabetes care programme
  advantages 959
  caveats 961–2
  economics 962–3
  initiation of therapy 958–9
  intercurrent illness and other crises 960
  ongoing management 959–60
  screening for complications 960–1
Ambulatory glucose profile (AGP) 1016, 1017
American blacks, *see* Black Americans
American Diabetes Association (ADA)
  dietary recommendations 685, 708, 1040
  employment policy 1634–5, 1639, 1640
  screening for NIDDM 1574, 1580
Americans
  non-Caucasoid, IDDM epidemiology 129–36
  see also specific population groups
Amino acids
  branched chain (BCAA), interorgan exchange 496, 497–8, 499
  glucagon and 336
  glucose and fatty acid interactions 431, 433
  hepatic glucose production and 418
  insulin secretion and
    in vitro 277–8
    in vivo 288
  interorgan exchange **496–9**
    postabsorptive state in IDDM 498–9
    protein feeding in IDDM 499
    protein feeding in normal humans 497–8
  islet cells 268
  metabolism in pancreatic diabetes 209–10, 211
  plasma appearance rate 480
  protein metabolism and 474–5
    animal studies 478
    human studies 483
    IDDM 485, 487
  see also specific amino acids
Amino acid tracer techniques 479–80
Amino acid transport **489–90**
  system A 489, 490
  system ASC 489–90
  system L 489–90

2-Aminobicyclo[2,2,1]-heptane-2-carboxylic acid (BCH) 266, 267, 269, 271
Aminoguanidine 677–8, 1277, 1401
Amphetamines 289
Amputations 1535, **1544**, 1545
  minor, arterial reconstruction and 1515
  rates in NIDDM 1465
  ray 1539, 1544
  renal replacement therapy and 1307
Amylase 491, 492
Amylin, *see* Islet amyloid polypeptide
Amyloidosis, islet, *see* Islet amyloidosis
Amyotrophy, diabetic 1114
Amyotrophy of Garland 1398
Anabolic hormones 1173
Anaemia
  blood glucose self-monitoring and 975
  glycated haemoglobin levels and 999
  pernicious 47, 75
  pregnancy in diabetic nephropathy and 1301
Anaphylactic reactions, protamine-induced 889–90
Anaphylactic shock, insulin-induced 887
Androgen receptors 560
Androgens
  abdominal obesity 557–9
  actions in visceral adipose tissue 554
  adipose tissue distribution and 560
  insulin resistance and **539–40**, 556–7, 558, 559
  stress-induced hypothalamic arousal and 562
  see also Testosterone
Angina pectoris 1498
  hypoglycaemia and 1143
  postinfarction 1500
Angiography
  fluorescein, *see* Fluorescein angiography
  peripheral vascular disease **1512–15**, 1543
Angiopathy, *see* Vascular disease
Angioplasty, limb ischaemia 1544
Angiotensin-converting enzyme (ACE) inhibitors 1296–7, 1529, **1530**, 1531, 1550–1
  early diabetic nephropathy 1296–7, 1530, 1554
  pregnancy 1094
Animal models of diabetes, *see* Experimental diabetes

Anion gap, diabetic ketoacidosis
    1154
Ankle–arm blood pressure ratio
    1465
Ankle jerks 1545, 1556, 1557
Ankle pressure index (API) 1400,
    1536, 1542, 1545
Anorexia, elderly 1118–19
Anorexia nervosa 1065
Anosmia–hypogonadism syndrome
    39
Antiandrogen compounds 546
Antibiotic therapy, foot infections
    1539, 1543
Anticoagulants
    natural 1450
    prophylactic therapy 1157,
        1160, 1196
Antidiabetic drugs, new, *see* New
    antidiabetic drugs
Antidiuretic hormone (ADH,
    vasopressin), sulphonylurea-
    induced secretion 752, 1121
Antihypertensive therapy 1528,
    1529–31, 1550–1, 1666
    autonomic neuropathy and 1276
    choice of drug 1530–1
    diabetic nephropathy 1219,
        1296–7, 1524–5, 1526,
        1554
    elderly 1114
    threshold for initiation 1527–8
Antilymphocytic globulins (ALG)
    917
Antimicrosomal antibodies 123
Antinuclear factor 123
Antiplatelet agents 1454–5
    after myocardial infarction
        1196–7
    diabetic retinopathy 1357–9
    stroke prevention 1204
Antithrombin III 1450, 1473
Anxiety, screening for diabetic
    complications 1559
Aorta
    increased stiffness 1439
    metabolic changes 1441
    morphological changes 1436,
        1437–8, 1439
Aorto-iliac arteries, occlusive
    disease 1510, 1543
Apolipoprotein(s) 439, 440, **443–5**
    chylomicrons 440, 441
    molecular biology 447–8
Apolipoprotein A (apo-A) 1495
Apolipoprotein AI (apo-AI) 441,
    444, 447, 448
    biguanide therapy and 781, 782
    IDDM 818
    insulin actions 450
    NIDDM 454–5
Apolipoprotein AI/CIII/AIV gene
    complex, NIDDM and 70
Apolipoprotein AI gene 448

polymorphisms, NIDDM
    associations 150
Apolipoprotein AI (apo-AI)
    receptors 447
Apolipoprotein AII (apo-AII) 441,
    444, 447, 448
    IDDM 818
    insulin actions 450
Apolipoprotein B (apo-B)
    biguanide therapy and 781,
        782–3
    glycation 454, 1473
    IDDM 818
    insulin actions 449
    molecular biology 447–8
    NIDDM 448, 452–3, 818
    obesity 451–2
Apolipoprotein B gene 70, 448
Apolipoprotein B receptors 441
Apolipoprotein B48 (apo-B48)
    440, 441, 444
Apolipoprotein B100 (apo-B100)
    441, 444, 445, 553, 554
Apolipoprotein C (apo-C)
    HDL 443
    VLDL 441, 442
Apolipoprotein CI (apo-CI) 441,
    444, 448
Apolipoprotein CII (apo-CII) 441,
    444, 448
Apolipoprotein CIII (apo-CIII)
    441, 444, 446, 448
Apolipoprotein CIII gene 448
Apolipoprotein E (apo-E) 441,
    444, 448
    HDL 443
    NIDDM 454
    VLDL 441, 442
Apolipoprotein E (apo-E) receptors
    441, 446
Apolipoprotein genes 448
    NIDDM and 67, 70, 448
Appendicitis, diabetic ketoacidosis
    and 1034–5
Aprotinin (Trasylol) 546, 1062,
    1067–8
Arachidonate metabolism, platelets
    1453
Aredlyd syndrome 38
Arginine-induced insulin responses
    chronic hyperglycaemia and
        637, 638, 641
    chronic pancreatitis 200, 201
    in vitro 277–8
    NIDDM rat model 577
    normal humans 287
    pancreas transplantation and
        918
Argon laser photocoagulation
    1349, 1353, 1354
Armanni–Ebstein lesion, diabetic
    nephropathy 1292
Arm, upper, insulin absorption
    844

Arterial blood sampling, glucose
    levels 522
Arterial calcification, medial
    (Mönckeberg's sclerosis)
    1438–9, 1471, 1511, 1536
    diabetic nephropathy 1276,
        1544
Arterial cannulation, forearm blood
    flow measurement 525
Arterial reconstruction 1510, 1511,
    1514, **1515**, **1543–4**
Arterial wall
    biology, hyperglycaemia and
        1472
    cellular components 674–7
    changes in composition 1437–9
    changes in experimental diabetes
        1440
    increased stiffness 1439, 1536
    protein components 671–4
    thickening 1436, 1437
    tunica media thinning 1436,
        1437
Arteriography
    digital subtraction (DSA) 1513
    peripheral vascular disease
        1512–15, 1543
Arteriolar lesions, diabetic
    nephropathy 1292, 1293
Arthus reaction, insulin allergy
    888
Artificial endocrine pancreas
    871–9, 979
    alternative open-loop systems
        873–4
    closed-loop system 872–3
    optimized conventional therapy
        874–9
Asia
    HLA and IDDM associations
        122–3, 142–3
    IDDM aetiopathogenesis **122–5**
    IDDM epidemiology **117–22**
    South East, dietary management
        of diabetes **701–6**
    see also China; India; Japan;
        Malaysia
Asian Americans, IDDM frequency
    136
Asian Indians
    complications in NIDDM 180
    genetic factors in NIDDM 179
    HLA and IDDM associations
        142–3
    IDDM frequency 120, **121–2**,
        139
    insulin resistance in NIDDM
        179–80
    MODY 10, 35, 71, 179, 1602
    NIDDM frequency 151–2,
        178–9
    prevalence of diabetes 1602
L-Asparaginase therapy 1029
Aspartame 696

Aspartate transaminase 1191,
1199, 1200
Aspirin 1454
after myocardial infarction
1196, 1197
diabetic nephropathy progression
and 1286, 1299
diabetic retinopathy 1357–9,
1551–2
stroke prevention 1204
sulphonylurea interactions 766
Ataxia telangiectasia 38, 248,
540
Atenolol 1196
Atherosclerosis 1185, 1487
diabetic macroangiopathy vs.
1436
elderly 1115
epidemiology **1459–65**
experimental diabetes 1440
hyperglycaemia and **1472–81**,
1495–6
diabetics 1476–8
intervention studies 1478–9
mechanisms 672, 1472–4
non-diabetics 1474–6
role of metabolic control in
prevention 1479–81
hyperinsulinaemia and 450,
1472, **1496–7**
mortality and morbidity in IDDM
1461–2
mortality and morbidity in
NIDDM 1463–5
outcome of myocardial infarction
and 1191–2
pathogenesis, role of diabetes
1495–9
pathology 1489–90
peripheral arteries 1509–15,
1541
progression in diabetes 1490
see also Cerebrovascular
disease; Coronary artery
disease; Peripheral vascular
disease
Atherosclerotic plaque 1490
Atherosclerotic vascular disease
(ASVD), *see* Atherosclerosis
ATP
costs of futile cycles 423
glucose phosphorylation in islet
B cells 267
insulin secretion and 269,
270–1, 272
ATP/ADP ratio, insulin secretion
and 271
ATP-citrate lyase **392–3**, 392, 398,
400
ATP-dependent proteolysis 475–6,
496
Atrial natriuretic peptide (ANP),
glomerular hyperfiltration and
1286

Audiovisual aids 932–4
Audit 1592
Australia
economic cost of diabetes
1651
health care provision 956
NIDDM prevalence 150
Autoantibodies
autoimmune polyendocrine
syndromes 109–10
IDDM 47, 123, 133, 1659
NIDDM 123
see also specific autoantibodies
Autoimmune B cell destruction
56–8, 1027–8
hypothetical mechanisms 232–9
transplanted islets 904–5
Autoimmune diseases
IDDM associations 42, **47**, 48,
123, 232
multiple endocrine organs
109–10
screening and prevention 75
Autoimmune polyendocrine
syndromes (APS) **109–10**
islet changes 239
type 1 109, 110
type 2 109, 110
Automatisms, subacute
neuroglycopenia 1134–5
Autonomic function tests 1393,
1401–3, 1545, 1558
Autonomic neuropathy **1401–5**
adrenaline responses to
hypoglycaemia 1140–1
antihypertensive therapy and
1276
bladder function 1276, **1300–1**,
1405
clinical features and treatment
1403–5
exercise and 731
histopathological features
1386–7
hypoglycaemia awareness and
1136
neuropathic foot 1400, 1536
outcome of myocardial infarction
and 1193
painless myocardial infarction
1190, 1498
pancreatic diabetes 215
pancreatic polypeptide responses
and 349
peripheral neuropathy and 1403
prevention 1557–8
pupillary effects 1371, 1402
screening 1558
Autophagocytic protein degradation
474, 475
Autoregulation of blood flow,
impaired 1526–7
Aviation industry 1638–40
Axoglial dysjunction 1386, 1388

Axonal atrophy 1386
Axonal degeneration 1386
Axonal transport **1388**
Azathioprine, pancreas
transplantation 917, 918

Bangladesh, IDDM frequency 138
Bantus, pancreatic iron infiltration
204
Bardet–Biedl (Lawrence–Moon–
Biedl–Bardet) syndrome 39,
248, 1028
Bargaining stage 926
Basement membranes **1245–61**
changes in diabetes 672, 673–4,
1250–3
aminoguanidine therapy and
677
pathogenesis 1255–8
pathophysiological
consequences 1253–4
role in microvascular
complications
1258–60
composition 1246, 1249
function 1246–50
glycation 674, 1251, 1254,
1256–7
normal morphology 1246, 1247
serum factors promoting
accumulation 1443
thickening 673, 1250–1
adverse effects 1254
pathogenesis 1229–31, 1237,
1238, 1255–8
B cells, pancreatic 223, **225–6**
aberrant MHC class II expression
109, 233–5, 236
autoimmune destruction 56–8,
1027–8
hypothetical mechanisms
232–9
transplanted islets 904–5
bioelectrical activity 265
blood supply 227–30
cellular interaction, heterogeneity
and recruitment 264–5
chronic pancreatitis 200, 201–2,
246
congenital absence 245
cystic fibrosis 207
degranulation and hydropic
transformation 240, 252
desensitization to sulphonylureas
657–8
development 224
distribution in islets 227
excessive iron deposition 247
"exhaustion" in NIDDM 166,
655–6
fibrocalculous pancreatic diabetes
186
functional organization **262–5**
see also Insulin secretion

B cells, pancreatic (*cont.*)
  glucose toxicity 166, 244,
    636–44
  glucose transport 265, 266, 603,
    642
  hyperplasia and hypertrophy
    250, 251, 252
  hypertrophy of nuclei 252
  IDDM, pathological changes
    231–2, 234
  isolated preparations 262
  mechanism of insulin release
    262–4
  NIDDM
    function during development
      165–6
    pathological changes 240,
      241–2, 243–4, 292, 575
  paracrine interactions 264, 420
  proinsulin biosynthesis and
    conversion 262
  regeneration 252
  secretory output 303
  sulphonylureas, effects of
    746–50
  virus infections 60, 61
BCH (2-aminobicyclo[2,2,1]-
    heptane-2-carboxylic acid)
    266, 267, 269, 271
Bed rest, foot ulceration 1539
Beef insulin, *see* Bovine insulin
Beta-blockers, *see* β-Adrenergic
    blockers
Bethanechol chloride 1300
Bezafibrate 825, 826, 827
Biases, evaluation of screening
    programmes 1571–2
Bicarbonate
  plasma levels, diabetic
    ketoacidosis 1031
  therapy, ketoacidosis 1034,
    1036, **1156**
Biguanides **773–91**
  adverse effects 789–91
    lactic acidosis 773, 789–91
    symptomatic side-effects
      789
    vitamin B$_{12}$ malabsorption
      789
  chemistry 774
  mechanism of action 774–85
    gastrointestinal function
      784–5
    glucose levels 775
    haemorheology and
      haemostasis 784
    hepatic glucose production
      779–80
    insulin action and peripheral
      glucose utilization 368,
      776–9
    insulin levels 775
    insulin secretion 775–6
    lactate metabolism 780–1

  lipid metabolism 781–4
  pharmacodynamics 774–85
  pharmacokinetics 785–6
    absorption 785
    distribution 785–6
    dose–response relationship
      786
    elimination 786
    metabolism 786
  sulphonylureas combined with
    765, 787
  sulphonylureas vs. 763, 787
  therapeutic use 786–9
    alcohol interactions 788
    clinical trials 786–8
    contraindications and
      precautions 788
    dosage 789
    drug interactions 788
    indications and treatment
      schedules 788
    pregnancy 788–9
  see also Metformin
Bile acid-sequestering resins 824,
    825, 826, 827
Binge eating 1065
Bio-Breeding (BB) rat 117, 1658
  autoantibodies 111
  dietary influences 1661
  genetic susceptibility 40, 45,
    46, 54, 108
  immune-related B-cell
    destruction 56, 232, 238
  islet transplantation 904
  neuropathy 1386, 1388, 1391
  prevention of diabetes
    development 115
Bioelectrical activity, pancreatic B
    cells 265
Biothesiometer 1394, 1545, 1556
Birth order effect, IDDM 57
Black Americans
  IDDM **129–33**
    a different type? 131
    genetic and immunological
      markers 132–3, 142
    incidence 131
    prevalence 129–31
    rising frequency 131–2
  IDDM progressing to NIDDM
    10, 33, 72, 131
Bladder dysfunction 1276,
    1300–1, 1405
Blindness 1112
  causes 1378–9
  incidence 1377–8, 1379
  prevalence 1373–7
  see also Visual impairment
Blood flow
  biguanide therapy and 784
  endoneurial 1391
  glucose uptake and 411–12
  impaired autoregulation 1526–7
  islets of Langerhans 227–30

  measurement through forearm
    muscle bed 525
  neuropathic foot 1399–400,
    1536
  retinal 1525–7
  subcutaneous, insulin absorption
    and 1062
  uteroplacental, reduced 1088,
    1093
  see also Haemodynamic
    changes
Blood pressure, arterial **1465–7**
  ankle–arm ratio 1465
  biguanide therapy and 784
  blood glucose levels and 1473–4
  diabetic retinopathy and 1348,
    1525–7
  ephedrine therapy and 1541
  IDDM 1465–6, 1474
  lower extremity 1511, 1542
  measurement 1527
  NIDDM 1466–7, 1474
  postural change 1558
  proteinuria and 1274
    IDDM 1462, 1463
    NIDDM 1467
  urinary albumin excretion and
    1289, 1466, 1524, 1525
  see also Hypertension
Blood–retinal barrier 1250
Blood transfusions
  glycated haemoglobin levels and
    999
  multiple chronic 203
  pancreas transplantation and
    916
Body mass, lean, aging and 1109,
    1110
Body mass index (BMI) 10
  Africans 713, 714
  desirable 686
  health and 563
  insulin secretion and 552
  NIDDM frequency and 155, 156
  protein deficient diabetes mellitus
    181
Bone mineral loss 1415–18
  IDDM 1416–17
  NIDDM 1417–18
Bone scanning, isotopic,
    neuropathic foot 1536, 1540
Bovine insulin 884, 1039–40
  extended-acting 848
  short-acting 847
Brain
  energy requirements 1133
  glucose transport 410–11, 603
    chronic hyperglycaemia and
      649
    NIDDM 593–4
  glucose uptake 1133–4
    basal state 421, 422, 581–2
    NIDDM 586, 593–4
  insulin receptors 358–9

Brain damage, hypoglycaemia-
    induced 1134, 1143, 1144
Breast, fibrous disease 1424–5
Breastfeeding
    diabetic mothers 1095
    IDDM frequency and 1660–1
British Diabetic Association (BDA),
    audiovisual aids 932–4
Brittle diabetes **1059–69**
    clinical features of "idiopathic"
        1065–6
    investigation 1066
    measurement of brittleness
        1059–60
    natural history 1068
    pancreatic disease 210–12, 215
    possible causes 1060–5
        accelerated insulin clearance
            1062–3
        counterregulatory hormone
            defects 1063
        eating disorders 1065
        endogenous insulin production
            and 1061–2
        factitious disease and
            malingering 1063–4
        impaired subcutaneous insulin
            absorption 1062
        intercurrent illness 1063
        overinsulinization and
            Somogyi effect 1061
        psychosocial factors 1064–5
    treatment 972, 1066–8
        augmented subcutaneous
            insulin absorption
            1067–8
        extracorporeal infusion
            systems 866, 1066–7
        implantable pumps 1067
        psychotherapy 1068
        somatostatin 347–8
Brunzell syndrome 38
Buformin 773, 774, 789
Bulbocavernous reflex latency
    1405
Bulimia 1065

C1q, serum levels 1169
C3, serum levels 1169
C4, serum levels 1169
C57BL/6J mouse strain 63
C57BL/KsJ (BL/Ks) mouse strain
    63
Cabin attendants, airline
    1639–40
Cachexia, diabetic neuropathic
    1114, 1397–8
Caesarian section 1094, 1096,
    1180–1
Calbindin, islet cells 280
Calcitonin gene-related peptide
    (CGRP)
    insulin resistance in NIDDM and
        611–12

insulin secretion and 288, 576
Calcium (Ca^{2+})
    cytosolic
        actions of sulphonylureas
            747, 749
        cholinergic effects in islet cells
            274
        insulin actions 395
        insulin secretion and 263,
            272, 274, 277
    dietary intake, Japan 708
    urinary excretion 1417
Calcium (Ca^{2+}) channels,
    pancreatic B cells 264
Calcium-dependent proteolysis
    475, 496
Calcium entry blockers 1529,
    1530, 1531
    pregnancy 1093–4
Callosities (skin callus)
    foot 1538
    management 1539, 1545
Callus, fracture, neuropathic foot
    1537
Calmodulin 1453
    insulin secretion and 264, 272
Calorimetry, indirect 422, 480
Calpins I and II 475
cAMP, *see* Cyclic AMP
Camps, children and adolescents
    936, 941
Canada
    economic cost of diabetes
        1651
    IDDM frequency 101, 140
Cancer, insulin resistance and
    541
Candida albicans, phagocyte killing
    in diabetes 1167
Candidate genes
    IDDM 46–7
    NIDDM **67–70**, 150
Capillaries
    barrier function in diabetes
        1253–4
    islets of Langerhans 227–8
    subcutaneous, insulin absorption
        and 841, 843, 844
    see also Basement membranes
Capillary blood flow, neuropathic
    foot 1536
Capillary density, muscle
    abdominal obesity 556
    NIDDM 610–11
    physical training and 736
Capillary permeability, *see* Vascular
    permeability
Capsular drop lesion, diabetic
    nephropathy 1291, 1293
Captopril 1530
Carbamylcholine, insulin secretion
    and 273, 274
Carbohydrate metabolism, insulin
    actions **385–91**

Carbohydrates, dietary (CHO)
    423, **687–91**
    African diets 711, 712, 716
    aging and 1109–10
    Chinese diet 719–20
    drugs inhibiting absorption
        808–9
    hypoglycaemic episodes 1145
    Indian and South East Asian
        diets 702–3
    insulin resistance and 545
    Japanese diet 708
    NIDDM prevention 1666
    prevention of exercise-induced
        hypoglycaemia 732–3,
        1041
Carbon dioxide production 422
γ-Carboxyglutamic acid 1450
Carbutamide 746
Carcinoid syndrome 247
Cardiac dysrhythmias
    frequency in diabetes 1499
    postmyocardial infarction 1188,
        1189, 1190
Cardiac failure, congestive, *see*
    Heart failure, congestive
Cardiac function
    autonomic neuropathy 1403–4
    limited joint mobility and 1424
Cardiac surgery
    anaphylactic reactions to
        protamine 889–90
    open heart, management 1180
Cardiogenic shock, postinfarction
    1188, 1189, 1499
Cardiomyopathy, diabetic 1471–2,
    1490
    congestive heart failure and
        1193, 1471–2, 1498
Cardiovascular disease 1185
    diabetic nephropathy and, *see*
        Nephropathy, diabetic,
        cardiovascular disease and
    epidemiology in diabetes 1215,
        1459–67, 1488
    fibrinogen plasma levels and
        1449
    see also Atherosclerosis;
        Macrovascular disease
Cardiovascular risk factors 451,
    1471, **1491–5**
    diabetic nephropathy and
        1218
    elderly 1115
    IDDM 1492, 1493, 1495
    lipid and lipoprotein-mediated
        686, 817, 821–2
    NIDDM 1492, 1493, 1494,
        1495
        generation 554–5
        physical training and 737
Care, diabetes, *see* Diabetes care
Carnitine acyltransferase (CAT)
    inhibitor 805

Carnitine palmitoyl transferase I
  (CPT-I)   392, 393, 461–2,
  463
Carnitine palmitoyl transferase II
  392, 461, 462
Carnitine shuttle   461–2
Carotid arteries, frequency of
  stenoses   1461
Carpal tunnel syndrome   1398,
  1419, 1424
Case-finding   1566
Casein kinase II   392, 399, 472,
  494
Cassava hypothesis, fibrocalculous
  pancreatic diabetes   188–9
Catabolic hormones   1173–4
  see also Counterregulatory
    hormones
Cataracts   **1370–1**
  secondary (cataracta complicata)
    1370–1
  senile   1112, 1370
  snowflake (metabolic)   1370
  surgery   1112–13, 1370
Catecholamines
  brittle diabetes and   1063
  as counterregulatory hormones
    1140
  exercise and   726, 727, 728,
    729, 730
  hepatic glucose production and
    419, 420
  hyperglycaemia after myocardial
    infarction and   1199–201
  insulin resistance and   **534**
  insulin secretion and   275–6
  ketone body metabolism and
    460, 464
  lipolysis and   554
  outcome of myocardial infarction
    and   1193
  plasma levels
    autonomic neuropathy
      1402
    hypertension in diabetes
      1522
  surgical trauma and   1174
  see also Adrenaline;
    Noradrenaline
Catheterization, urinary   1300
Caucasians, HLA and IDDM
  associations   142
Caudal regression syndrome   1087
Causalgia (shoulder–hand
  syndrome)   1420–1, 1424
Cellulitis, foot   1537, 1538, 1539
Centrally acting antihypertensive
  drugs   1529, 1530
Central nervous system,
  hypoglycaemia and
  1133–7
Central venous pressure monitoring
  1157
Cereals   694

Cerebral hypoxia, cerebral oedema
  of diabetic ketoacidosis and
  1036
Cerebral oedema of diabetic
  ketoacidosis   **1035–7, 1157–8**
  assessment   1037
  pathogenesis   1035–7, 1157–8
  treatment   1037
Cerebrovascular disease   1185,
  1490
  elderly   1115
  frequency in diabetes   1461
  hyperglycaemia and   1203,
    1475, 1476–7, 1478
  mortality and morbidity in IDDM
    1462
  mortality and morbidity in
    NIDDM   1464–5
  see also Stroke
Cervical spine, limited mobility
  1421
Charcot (neuropathic) joint   1537,
  1540–1
Checklists, diabetic clinics   1592
Cheiroarthropathy, juvenile diabetic
  1422
  see also Joint mobility, limited
Chemical agents
  diabetes/IGT caused by   12
  islet changes   **248–9**
  IDDM induction   61, 1027
Chemical injuries, foot   1538
Chemstrip bG   974, 975
Children   **1025–53**
  aetiology of diabetes   1026–9
  blood glucose self-monitoring
    972, 1039, 1041–2, 1043
  brittle diabetes   1064–5
  criteria for metabolic control
    1042–4
  diabetes education   936, **941,**
    1039, **1044–7**
  diabetic ketoacidosis   1030–7
  diagnosis of IDDM   1029–30
  epidemiology of IDDM   32–3,
    1025–6
    Asia   117–22
  exercise   1041
  hypoglycaemia   **1047–8**, 1142,
    1144
  insulin therapy   851–2, **1037–40**
    overinsulinization   1061
  less common causes of diabetes
    1028–9
  long-term complications   1051–3,
    1559
  management of IDDM
    1037–47
  meal planning   1040–1
  monitoring   1041–2
  nerve function   1396
  OGTT   20, 26, 1029–30
  psychosocial support   1044–7
  sick day rules   1031, 1048–51

China
  dietary management   **719–23**
  HLA associations with IDDM
    102–3, 123
  IDDM frequency   104, **119–20,**
    140, 141
Chinese hamster, diabetic,
  somatostatin in   345, 346
Chinese populations
  HLA and IDDM associations
    123, 142
  IDDM frequency   120, 121
  NIDDM frequency   152–3
Chiropodists   1596
Chiropody   1539, 1543, 1545
4-(2-(5-Chloro-2-
  methoxybenzamido)-ethyl)-
  benzoic acid (HB699)   798
2-Chloropropionate   803–4
Chloroquine phosphate   1068
Chlorpropamide   **757**
  clinical efficacy   753
  contraindications   760–1
  dosage intervals   763
  elderly patients   1120, 1121
  extrapancreatic effects   752
  glibenclamide vs.   757
  hypoglycaemic reactions   757,
    765
  potency and intrinsic activity
    754
  rate of onset and duration of
    action   755
  structure   746
Chlorpropamide alcohol-induced
  flushing, MODY   72
Cholangiopancreatography,
  endoscopic retrograde (ERCP),
  fibrocalculous pancreatic
  diabetes   185, 186
Cholecystitis, emphysematous
  1166
Cholecystokinin (CCK), insulin
  secretion and   230, 287, 288,
  800
Cholecystokinin-pancreozymin
  (CCK-PZ)
  chronic pancreatitis   201
  glucagon release and   336
Cholera toxin   276–7, 401
Cholesterol (CH)   446
  dietary intake   693, 720
  HDL
    biguanide therapy and   781
    cardiovascular disease risk and
      1495
    dietary fat intake and   692,
      693
    endogenous
      hypertriglyceridaemia
      451
    NIDDM   454, 455
    obesity   452
    target levels in diabetes   821

Cholesterol (CH) (*cont.*)
 LDL
  biguanide therapy and   781
  cardiovascular disease risk and
   1493–4
  dietary fat intake and   691–2,
   693
  NIDDM   454
 metabolism, diabetes   820
 serum levels
  benefits of reduction   821–2
  biguanide therapy and   781,
   782–3
  cardiovascular disease risk and
   1493–4
  children with IDDM   1044
  IDDM   450
  large vessel abnormalities and
   1440
  NIDDM   452
  NIDDM prevention and
   1666
  pancreatic diabetes   209
  sex differences   1491
  target levels in diabetes   821,
   1481
  see also Hypercholesterolaemia
 synthesis, insulin actions   391,
  394–5
Cholesterol esterase   391, 395
Cholesterol esters
 breakdown   391, 395
 synthesis   445
 transfer   447
Cholesterol transfer proteins   447
Cholesterol transport pathway,
 reverse   **443**
Cholesteryl-β-D-glucoside hydrolase
 1441
Cholestyramine   825, 827
Choline acetyltransferase (CHAT),
 axonal transport   1388
Cholinergic neurons, islets of
 Langerhans   230
Cholinergic stimulation, insulin
 secretion and   **273–4**, 288
Chondrocalcinosis, acute
 symptomatic   1415
Christian's syndrome   39
Chromogranin A   225, 226
Chylomicrons   439, **440–1**, 442,
 446
 IDDM   818
 NIDDM   818
Chymotrypsin test, faecal   187
Cimetidine, metformin interactions
 788
Cirrhosis of liver
 and diabetes (Naunyn's diabetes)
  248
 glucose potassium and insulin
  infusion   1178, 1179
 insulin regimens   852–3
 insulin resistance   **541**

proinsulin levels   320, 322
cis-acting DNA elements   468, 490
Cisapride   1404
Citrate, Randle cycle and   607,
 608
Classification of diabetes,
 see Diabetes mellitus,
  classification
Claudication, intermittent   1465,
 1488, 1512
 see also Peripheral vascular
  disease
Clawing of toes   1537
Clinistix   968
Clinitest   968, 969
Clonidine, inhibition of insulin
 release   273, 275
Clot retraction, protein glycation
 and   1451
Clotting disorders   **1447–55**
 cellular changes   1452–3
 clinical implications   1453–4
 collagen changes and   1451–2
 plasma factors and   1447–51
 see also Haemostatic changes
Clotting factors, plasma   **1447–51**,
 1473
Coagulation, blood
 atherogenesis and   1495, **1497**
 effects of diabetes   **1447–55**
Cockayne's syndrome   39
Cognitive function
 elderly diabetics   1114–15
 hypoglycaemia and   1134
Colestipol   825, 827
Collagen
 aminoguanidine therapy and
  677, 1277
 changes in diabetes   672–3,
  1251–2
 Dupuytren disease   1419
 glycated   672–3, 674, 1277,
  1451–2
  atherogenesis and   672, 1472
  skin thickening and   1426
 increased synthesis   1251, 1256,
  1279
 limited joint mobility and   1425,
  1426, 1427–8
 platelet aggregation and   1452
 role in coagulation   1451–2
Collagenase
 pancreatic duct injection   896–7,
  906
 vascular wall changes and   675
Collagen type I
 diabetic nephropathy   1292
 increased crosslinking   673,
  1251, 1257
 serum factors promoting
  synthesis   1442–3
Collagen type IV
 changes in diabetes   674,
  1251–2

 characteristics   1246, 1249,
  1250
 decreased crosslinking   1251–2,
  1254, 1257
 diabetic nephropathy   1292
 glycation   1252, 1254, 1256–7
 increased synthesis   1251, 1256
 vascular wall   1438
Collagen type VI, diabetic
 nephropathy   1292
Colour vision defects   1379
 blood glucose self-monitoring
  and   975
 urine testing and   968
Coma
 diabetic ketoacidosis   1031,
  1154
 hyperosmolar non-ketotic, *see*
  Hyperosmolar non-ketotic
  coma
 hypoglycaemic, *see*
  Hypoglycaemic coma
 pancreatic diabetes   212
Communication problems
 India   1603–4
 insulin resistance and   1080
Community
 costs and benefits of screening
  1570–1, 1572
 diabetes care in, *see* Primary
  care
Community analysis (diagnosis)
 1624–5
Community programmes, diabetes
 control   **1619–28**
 design   1623–4
 evaluation   1625–6
 implementation   1625
 intervention strategies   1621–2
 main components   1624–6
 major constraints   1627–8
 as model for other non-
  communicable diseases
  1626–7
 need for demonstration
  programmes   1622–3
 planning   1624–5
Complement
 abnormalities in diabetes
  1169
 diabetic nephropathy   1292
Compliance
 blood glucose self-monitoring
  977–8
 dietary, India and South East
  Asia   704–6
 factors affecting   925–7
 problems in Tanzania/African
  countries   1617
Complications of diabetes   22
 changing impact   **1213–20**
 children and adolescents
  1051–3
 elderly   **1111–16**

Complications of diabetes (*cont.*)
  exercise and 731
  fibrocalculous pancreatic diabetes
      185–6
  insulin resistance and **542**
  islet transplantation and 900–1
  MODY 72
  NIDDM at diagnosis 957
  pancreas transplantation and
      895–6, **920**
  pancreatic diabetes 213–15
  pathogenesis 669, 670,
      1225–41, 1261
    capillary basement membrane
        changes and 1258–60
    clinical studies 1233–9
    epidemiological studies
        1226–8
    hypotheses 1228–33
    role of hyperglycaemia 635,
        636, 1232–3
  patient education **942–3**, 961
  prevention and screening 762,
      960–1, **1549–59**, 1580
    early treatment 1551
    elderly patients 1123
    glycated haemoglobin
        measures 1000–1,
        1043–4
    methods of prevention
        1550–1
    methods of screening 1551
    one-visit package 1559
    primary vs. secondary
        prevention 1550
    psychological aspects 1559
    renal replacement therapy and
        1305–7
  treatment 961
  tropical/developing countries
      180, 1609
  see also Macrovascular disease;
      Microvascular disease;
      specific complications
Composite insoles 1539
Compound I (2,4-diamino-5-
    cyano-6-bromopyridine)
    799–800
Computer-assisted education (CAI)
    934, **949–53**, 1013
  advantages and disadvantages
      950, 952
  cost–effectiveness 952–3
  educational strategies 951–2
  effectiveness 952
  neural network computers and
      1018–19
  programs available 950–1
  uses 953
Computer-assisted sensory
    examination 1395
Computers
  applications 949, **1009–19**
    future directions 1013–19

historical perspective
    1009–13
  clamping plasma glucose 522,
      1074–5
  hand-held
    clinical decision-making
        1011–12, 1013–15
    and memory-based reflectance
        meters 1015–18
  insulin dosage adjustments
      877–8, 879, 979, 1018
  neural network 1018–19
  patient management systems
    development 1012–13
    integrated 1015–18
  simulation models of diabetes
      1019
Condiments, Indian and Asian diets
    704
Conduction velocity, nerve, *see*
    Nerve conduction velocity
Cone dystrophy, progressive,
    degenerative liver disease,
    endocrine dysfunction and
    hearing defect 39
Congenital malformations 76
  IDDM 1087
  maternal diabetic nephropathy
      and 1301
  NIDDM 1095
  prenatal diagnosis 76–7, 1093
Connective tissue disorders
    1415–28
Conn's syndrome 247
Consanguineous marriages 1602
Constipation 1404
Contact lenses 1368–9
Contrast media, radiological,
    nephrotoxicity 1512–13
Control, locus of 925–6
Convulsions, hypoglycaemia-
    induced 1143, 1144
Corn cures, foot trauma 1538
Cornea, diabetic **1368–9**
Coronary arteries
  changes in composition
      1437–8
  experimental diabetes 1440
  morphological changes 1436–7,
      1438, 1472–3
  spontaneous reperfusion after
      thrombosis 1192
Coronary artery bypass surgery
    1197, **1500–1**
  results 1500–1
Coronary artery disease (CAD,
    CHD) 1459–61, **1487–501**
  assessment before renal dialysis
      or transplantation 1304
  diabetic nephropathy and, *see*
      Nephropathy, diabetic,
      cardiovascular disease and
  dietary fat intake and 691–2
  elderly 1115

hyperglycaemia and
    diabetics 1476–8
  non-diabetics 1474–6,
      1488–9, 1491
  hypoglycaemia and 1143
  IDDM 1190, 1478, 1491
  insulin resistance syndrome
      534–5
  mortality and morbidity in IDDM
      1461–2
  mortality and morbidity in
      NIDDM 1463–4
  obesity and 563, 564, 1493
  pathology 1489–90
  prevention 1667
  progression in diabetes 1490
  risk factors, *see* Cardiovascular
      risk factors
  role of diabetes in pathogenesis
      1495–9
  sex differences 1491
  see also Myocardial infarction
Corticosteroids
  insulin resistance and 559
  insulin secretion and 288
  muscle fibre composition and
      556
  see also Glucocorticoids
Cortisol
  adipose tissue lipolysis and 560
  brittle diabetes and 1063
  as counterregulatory hormone
      1137, 1138, 1139, 1140
  exercise and 726, 729, 730
  hepatic glucose production and
      419, 420
  hyperglycaemia after myocardial
      infarction and 1199–200,
      1202
  IDDM, response to
      hypoglycaemia 1141
  insulin-mediated glucose disposal
      and 433
  ketone body metabolism and
      460, 464
  obesity and 559–60
  peripheral insulin sensitivity and
      556
  stress-induced hypothalamic
      arousal and 561, 562, 563
  surgical trauma and 1174
Cost–benefit analysis **1651–2**
  screening programmes 1570–1,
      1572
Cost–effectiveness analysis
    1651–2
  computer-assisted education
      952–3
Costs, economic **1644–51**
  blood and urine glucose testing
      974
  direct 1644
  estimates around the world 1651
  estimates in USA 1647–50

Costs, economic (*cont.*)
  indirect 1644, 1650, 1651
  methodology in estimation
    1644–7
    general methods 1644
    study designs 1644–7
    psychosocial 1644
  urine and blood test strips 968
Cotton-wool spots (soft exudates)
  1333–4, 1335
Coumarin anticoagulants 1450
Counselling
  antismoking 1558
  brittle diabetes 1068
  diabetic complications **942–3**
  nutritional, India and South East
    Asia 705–6
  prepregnancy 942, 1087
Counterregulatory hormones
  abnormalities in IDDM 1140–1,
    1145
  aging and 1111
  brittle diabetes and 1063
  diabetic ketoacidosis and
    1152–3
  glycaemic thresholds for release
    1135, 1136
  hepatic glucose production and
    419–20
  hypoglycaemia in normal humans
    and 1137–40
  identification of abnormalites
    1146
  insulin-mediated glucose disposal
    and 433
  insulin receptor function and
    365–6
  insulin resistance and 365,
    533–4, 1080
  new drugs inhibiting 807–8
  normal glucose balance 1137
  Somogyi effect and 1061, 1142
  surgical trauma and 1173, 1174
  see also Adrenaline; Cortisol;
    Glucagon; Growth
    hormone; Noradrenaline
Coxsackie B viruses 59, 1026
  B-cell destruction and 60,
    236–7
  protein deficient diabetes 181
Coxsackie B4 virus 59, 60, 1660
  HLA-DR4-associated IDDM and
    49, 60
Coxsackie B5 virus 59
Coxsackie viruses 245, 1168
C-peptide 225, **305–18**
  biosynthesis 262, 303, 304
  brittle diabetics 1061–2
  chronic pancreatitis 200, 201
  classification and management of
    diabetes 317–18
  cleavage site mutations 71
  clinical applications 313–18
  cystic fibrosis and 207

degradation in plasma 305
equimolar secretion with insulin
  306
fibrocalculous pancreatic diabetes
  186, 187
hepatic extraction 306–7
IDDM 9, 108, 290, 307,
  313–17
  subtypes 48, 49
  vs. NIDDM classification
    10–11
kinetics and metabolic clearance
  rate 307–10
as marker of insulin secretion
  303–5, **306–10**
as measure of hepatic insulin
  extraction 310–11
MODY and 72
obesity 553
pancreas transplantation and
  918
pancreatic carcinoma 204
physiological plasma profiles
  845–7
radioimmunoassay 305–6
renal extraction 307, 311
two-compartment model of
  kinetics 308–10
urinary, as measure of insulin
  secretion 311–13
C-peptide/insulin molar ratio 310
Cranial nerve palsies 1367–8,
  1398
Creatinine, serum
  caveats 1274–5
  diabetic ketoacidosis 1158
  measurement 1554
Creatinine clearance
  aging and 1113
  caveats 1274–5
  measurement 1554
  pregnancy 1091, 1301
m-Cresol, insulin preparations
  837–8
Cuba, IDDM frequency 139, 140,
  141
Cushing's disease 247
  insulin resistance 533
  muscle fibre composition 556
Cushing's syndrome 247, 295
Cyanide ingestion, fibrocalculous
  pancreatic diabetes and
  188–9
Cyclamates 696
Cyclic AMP
  drug actions 798
  fatty acid metabolism and 460
  glucagon-induced generation
    276–7, 335
  insulin secretion and 272, 275
  mode of action in pancreatic B
    cells 277
  role in insulin actions 387, 394,
    398, 401

Cyclic AMP analogues, insulin
  receptor function 365, 399
Cyclic AMP phosphodiesterase
  401, 798
Cyclic GMP, role in insulin actions
  401–2
Cyclic nucleotides, role in insulin
  action 401–2
Cyclosporin
  islet transplantation 903, 906
  newly diagnosed IDDM 317
  pancreas transplantation 917,
    918
Cyproheptadine 249
Cystic fibrosis 38, **207–8**, 210,
  1029
  diabetic complications 213
  frequency of diabetes 198, 207
  hormone secretion 207–8
  pancreatic pathology 207, 247,
    248
  therapy of diabetes 215
Cytochalasin B 387
Cytokine production, vascular wall
  674–6
Cytomegalovirus (CMV) 59, 60

"Dawn phenomenon" 347, 546,
  1142
  children 1040
  measurement 1060
DBA/2J mouse strain 63
db/db mouse 63, 345, 346
D cells 223–4, 225, **226**, 343
  animal models of diabetes
    345–6
  development 224
  distribution in islets 227
  type 1 diabetes 231
Death
  causes
    cardiac disease 1460
    diabetics in Tanzania 1613
    IDDM 1214, 1215
    postmyocardial infarction
      1188–9
    proteinuria and 1216
    sudden cardiac 1188–9, 1404
    sudden hypoglycaemia-associated
      1143–4
Death, sudden, patients on
  haemodialysis 1305
Decision-making
  computer-based 1011–12,
    1013–15
  evaluation 944
Deconvolution method of
  estimating insulin secretion
  308–10
Defence mechanisms 926
Dehydration
  diabetic ketoacidosis 1031
  hyperosmolar non-ketotic coma
    1159, 1160

Demyelination, segmental   1386
Dendritic cells, islets of Langerhans
    230
Denial stage   926
Denmark
    IDDM frequency   101, 140
    life-insurance   1632
Dentures, poorly fitting   1119
3-Deoxyglucosone   670, 671
Depression
    elderly   1115
    hopeful   926–7
Developing countries
    chronic pancreatitis   190
    community-based diabetes care
        1594
    IDDM frequency   **136–9**, 143,
        177–8, 1603
    organization of care and
        problems   **1601–17**
    see also Tropical countries;
        specific countries
Dexamethasone
    induction of insulin resistance
        289, 294, 533
    insulin receptor function and
        365
Dextrans, urinary clearance   1288,
    1296
Diabetes care   **955–63**
    availability   955–6
    community-based   1594, 1597
    computers in   **1009–19**
    cost–benefit or cost–effectiveness
        analysis   1651–2
    diagnosis and assessment
        957–8
    economics   962–3, **1643–53**
    India   **1601–5**
    initiation of therapy and
        stabilization   958–9
    integrated, and diabetes care
        centre   1597
    intercurrent illness/other crises
        960
    Malaysia   **1607–10**
    monitoring control and ongoing
        management   959–60
    organization   **1589–628**
        developing countries
            1601–17
        diabetes care centre   1593–7
        diabetes community
            programmes   1619–28
        diabetic clinic   1589–92
        surgical diabetic patients
            1179
    related issues   961–2
    screening for complications
        960–1
    Tanzania   **1611–17**
    treating complications   961
Diabetes care centre   **1593–7**
    design   1595–6

health service organization and
    1597
integrated care and   1597
role   1595
structure   1595
team   1596–7
Diabetes community control
    programmes, *see* Community
    programmes, diabetes
    control
Diabetes Control and Complications
    Trial (DCCT)   1238–9, 1240,
    1241, 1479
Diabetes insipidus–diabetes
    mellitus–optic atrophy–
    deafness (Wolfram's or
    DIDMOAD) syndrome   39,
    109, 248, 1028
Diabetes Key-Facts   950
Diabetes mellitus (DM)
    adult onset, *see* Non-insulin
        dependent diabetes mellitus
    age at onset, *see* Age at onset
    age-related prevalence   1103–5,
        1106
    atypical, in American blacks
        10, 33, 72, 131
    classification   **3–16**, 32, 1085
        C-peptide measurement in
            317–18
        islet morphology and   231
        tropical countries   177,
            178
    conditions and syndromes
        associated with   11, 12–13
    congenital (permanent neonatal),
        islet changes   245
    diagnosis   **19–27**, 32, 957–8
        glucose tolerance test   22–7
        glycaemic criteria   19–20,
            24–6
        glycation products in   27,
            1003
        recognition of diabetic state
            20–2
    duration
        atherosclerotic vascular
            disease and   1476,
            1477–8
        diabetic nephropathy and
            1267–8
        hypoglycaemia awareness and
            1136
        limited joint mobility and
            1422–3
        macroangiopathy and   1437,
            1439
        microalbuminuria and   1289
        mortality and   1214, 1215
        retinopathy and   1217, 1226,
            1227, 1340–2
    epidemiology   **32–6**
        demographic characteristics
            34–6

disease frequency   32–4
    methodological problems
        32
genetic susceptibility, *see*
    Genetic susceptibility
gestational, *see* Gestational
    diabetes mellitus
juvenile onset, *see* Insulin
    dependent diabetes mellitus
latent, *see* Glucose tolerance,
    impaired; Glucose
    tolerance, previous
    abnormality
malnutrition related, *see*
    Malnutrition related
    diabetes mellitus
maturity onset, of young, *see*
    Maturity onset diabetes of
    young
neonatal   245, 1028
and other non-communicable
    diseases   1619–21
other types   5, **11**, 12–13
potential, *see* Glucose tolerance,
    potential abnormality
primary prevention   **1655–67**
screening   **1565–83**
    elderly   1116–17, 1118
secondary   5, 197
    see also Pancreatic disease,
        diabetes secondary to
subclasses, difficulties in
    assigning patients to
    13–14, 32
tropical   4, 11
type 1, *see* Insulin dependent
    diabetes mellitus
type 1.5   10, 33
type 2, *see* Non-insulin
    dependent diabetes mellitus
undiagnosed
    hyperglycaemia after
        myocardial infarction
        and   1197–8
    stroke and   1203
Diabetic clinics   **1589–92**, 1593–4
    developing countries   1604
    organization   1591
    patient–staff encounter   1590–1
    regular staff meetings   1592
    role of knowledge   1589–90
    self-help groups   1592
    service management concept
        1590
    support routines   1591–2
Diabetic clinic staff   1590, 1591
Diabetic complications, *see*
    Complications of diabetes
Diabetic foot clinic   1544–5,
    1557
Diabetic hand syndrome   1419,
    1424
Diabur-Test 5000   968
Diacare Monitor   1018

Diacylglycerol (DAG) 274, 395, 643, 644
Diacylglycerol acyltransferase 394
2,4-Diamino-5-cyano-6-bromopyridine (compound I) 799–800
2,4-Diamino-5-cyano-6-halopyridines 799–800
Diarrhoea
  biguanide-associated 789
  diabetic 1404
Diascan 973
Diastix 968
Diazoxide 249, 250, 278, 289, 643
Dibutyryl cyclic AMP 275
Dichloroacetate and analogues 803–4
DIDMOAD (diabetes insipidus–diabetes mellitus–optic atrophy–deafness, Wolfram's) syndrome 39, 109, 248, 1028
Diet(s)
  African 711–13
  aging and 1109–10
  American Diabetes Association 685, 708, 1040
  atherogenic, large vessel changes and 1439–40
  Chinese 719–20
    therapeutic use 720–3
  fibrocalculous pancreatic diabetes and 188–9
  healthy 1627
  IDDM aetiology and 1660–1
  Indian 701–2
    therapeutic use 702–4
  insulin receptor function and 364
  Japanese 707–8
    therapeutic use 708–9
  low-protein 693–6, 1114, 1297–8, 1553–4
  myo-inositol-supplemented 1279
  NIDDM development and 153, 156–8
  NIDDM prevention 1666
  Pacific Islanders 153
  very low-calorie (VLCD), NIDDM 686–7
Dietary management
  Africa **711–17**
    dietary education 715–17
    dietary patterns 711–13
    energy needs and 713
    factors affecting 713–15
  atherosclerosis prevention and 1481
  carbohydrate and fibre intake 687–91
  children and adolescents 1040–1
  China **719–25**

diabetic nephropathy 1114, **1297–8**
early diabetic nephropathy (microalbuminuria) 693–6, 1298, 1553–4
elderly 1118–19
energy intake 685–7
Europe and North America **685–98**
exercise and 716, 732–3, 854, 1041
fat intake 691–3
hypertension 1528
hypoglycaemia 1145
IDDM 685, 687
  carbohydrate and fibre intake 689–90
  China 720–2
  exercise and 732–3
  fat intake 691
IGT 1581
implementation 697–8
India and South East Asia **701–6**
  compliance with dietary advice 704–6
  historical perspective 701
  meal planning 706
  special foods 706
  therapeutic use of traditional diets 702–4
  traditional diets 701–2
insulin resistance 545
insulin therapy and 854, 876
Japan **707–9**
NIDDM 685, 697, 1118–19
  carbohydrate and fibre intake 689–90
  China 722–5
  fat intake 691
  insulin receptor function 368
  normal-weight patients 687
  overweight patients 685–7
pancreatic diabetes 216
patient education 705–6, 715–17, **940**
pregnancy 1092
protein intake 693–6
Dietitians 717, 1596
Digital subtraction arteriography (DSA) 1513
1,25-Dihydroxyvitamin D$_3$ 1417, 1418
Diphenylhydantoin (phenytoin) 249, 289
2,3-Diphosphoglycerate (2,3-DPG)
  atherosclerosis and 1496
  diabetic ketoacidosis 1036, 1154, 1156
Diplopia 1367, 1368
Dipyramidole 1299, 1357–8
Direct 30/30 Glucose Sensor 973
Disability
  diabetes self-management and 972, 1117–18

economic costs 1650
  employment and 1637–8
Diuretics **1529**, 1531
  insulin secretion and 289
  potassium-sparing 1529
DNA 468, 469
  AGE-induced damage **676–7**
Doctors (physicians)
  care of diabetic patients **955–63**
  computer-based patient management systems and 1015, 1017–18
  developing countries 1603, 1616
  diabetes care centre 1596
  hospital-based, role in diabetes care 956, 958
  insulin dosage adjustments 876
Domperidone 1404
Doppler ultrasound
  ankle pressure index (API) 1400
  diabetic impotence 1405
  peripheral vascular disease 1512, 1536, 1542
Down's syndrome (trisomy 21) 39, 108–9, 110, 1028
Driving **1633–6**
  heavy goods (commercial) vehicles 1634–6, 1638
  occupational licences 1634
Drug interactions
  biguanides 788
  sulphonylureas 766, 1121, 1122
Drugs
  diabetes/IGT caused by 12, 248–9
  insulin secretion and **289–90**
  new antidiabetic, *see* New antidiabetic drugs
Duchenne muscular dystrophy, insulin resistance 540
Dulcitol 1167
Dupuytren disease (DD) **1419**, 1423, 1424
Duration of diabetes, *see* Diabetes mellitus, duration
Dwarfism
  hereditary panhypopituitary 38
  Laron 38
Dyslipoproteinaemia
  diabetes 817–18
  diagnosis in diabetes 820–1
  treatment in diabetes 821–7
  see also Hyperlipidaemia

Eating disorders, brittle diabetes and 1065
Economic factors, dietary compliance and 705
Economics of diabetes care 962–3, **1643–53**
Edema, *see* Oedema

Education, diabetes **923–45**
  blood glucose self-monitoring
    939, 976
  children and adolescents 936,
    941, 1039, **1044–7**
  community programmes 1626
  computer-assisted 934, **949–53**,
    1013
  developing countries, problems in
    715, 1603
  diabetic clinics 1591
  diabetic complications 942–3,
    961
  dietary 705–6, 940
    Africa 715–17
  factors affecting ability to learn
    925–7
  families of children with
    IDDM 1044–7
  foot care 940–1, 1545, 1557
  glucagon injection 1047–8
  hypoglycaemia 937–9, 1146
  initiation of insulin therapy 937
  insulin dosage adjustments 877,
    878
  neural network computers and
    1018–19
  oral agents 941–2
  pregnancy 942
  prevention of diabetic
    ketoacidosis 1031, 1158–9
  "sick day" rules 941
Education, further 1637
Educational programmes **923–45**,
  953
  audiovisual aids 932–4
  benefits 923–4
  children and adolescents 1044–7
  controlled studies 925
  cost–benefit analysis 1652
  evaluation 943–5
    developing methods 943
    outcome measures 943–4
    process 943, 945–6
  group learning 934–6
  one-to-one learning 936–7
  planning 927–32
    context of learning 927
    curriculum 929–32
    instructional objectives
      927–9, 930
  shortcomings 924–5
  specific problems 937–43
Educators, diabetes 962, 1603
Edward's syndrome 38
Eicosapentaenoic acid (EPA)
  692–3, 707
eIF-2, *see* Initiation factor-2 (eIF-2)
eIF-2α kinase 472
Elderly 1103
  blood glucose self-monitoring
    972
  complications of diabetes
    1111–16

exercise 737–8, 1119
glucose potassium and insulin
  infusion 1178
hyperosmolar non-ketotic coma
  1115–16, 1159
hypoglycaemia 1137
insulin resistance 288–9, 541,
  1106–7, 1108
NIDDM prevention 1663
screening for diabetes 1116–17,
  1118
treatment of diabetes **1117–23**
  dietary guidelines 1118–19
  evaluation 1117–18
  goals 1123
  insulin therapy 850, 851,
    1123
  metformin 791, 1122–3
  sulphonylureas 765, 1120–2
  symptomatic patients 1123
  see also Aging
Electrocardiography
  autonomic function tests
    1401–2, 1404
  diabetic ketoacidosis 1158
Electroencephalography (EEG)
  elderly diabetics 1114
  hypoglycaemia and 1134
Electrolyte balance, diabetic
  ketoacidosis 1033–4, 1153–4
Electrophysiological measurements
  1393–4, 1556
Elongation factor-1 (EF-1, eEF-1)
  472, 473
Elongation factor-2 (eEF-2) 473
Embryopathy, diabetic **1087**
  pancreatic pathology **249–50**,
    251
Emergency surgery **1181**
Emphysematous pyelitis 1302
Emphysematous pyelonephritis
  1166, 1302
Employment **1636–40**
  aviation industry 1638–40
  commercial vehicle drivers
    1634–6, 1638
  disabled status and 1637–8
Enalapril 1297, 1530
Encephalomyocarditis (EMC) virus
  60, 237, 238, 1660
Endocrine adenomatosis/neoplasia
  syndrome, multiple 38, 40
Endocrine disorders
  brittle diabetes 1063
  diabetes/IGT secondary to 11,
    12, 38
  fibrocalculous pancreatic diabetes
    184
  hypertension and 1521, 1522
  insulin therapy 852
  islet-cell changes 247
Endoneurial basement membranes,
  plasma protein deposition
    672

Endoneurial blood flow 1391
Endoneurial oxygen tension 1391
Endoscopic retrograde
  cholangiopancreatography
    (ERCP), fibrocalculous
    pancreatic diabetes 185, 186
Endothelial cells 1453
  AGE-modified protein receptors
    674, 675, 676
  barrier function 1249–50
  decreased adhesion to basement
    membranes 1254
  glucose toxicity 676–7,
    1279–80, 1472
  islet capillaries 227
  muscle capillaries, NIDDM
    610–11
  responses to vascular injury
    1248
Endothelium, insulin uptake 1063
Energy intake, total **685–7**
  Africa 712, 713, 716
  children and adolescents
    1040–1
  China 719
  India and South East Asia
    701–2
  Japan 707
  normal-weight NIDDM and
    IDDM 687
  overweight NIDDM patients
    685–7
  pregnant women 1092
Energy supply, exercise and 726
England, IDDM frequency 101,
  140
Enkephalins, insulin secretion and
  288
Entactin 1246, 1249, 1250
Enteroglucagon 204
Enuresis 1030
Environmental factors
  IDDM 43, **58–61**, 104, 110,
    236–9
  NIDDM 62, **153–7**
Epalrestat 809
Ephedrine
  insulin secretion and 289
  neuropathic foot oedema
    1541
Epidermal growth factor (EGF)
  receptors 403
Epinephrine, *see* Adrenaline
Epiphyseal dysplasia and infantile
  onset diabetes mellitus 39
Erythrocytes
  aggregation 1454–5
  blood coagulation and 1453
  deformability 1451
  glucose transport 409–10, 603
  insulin receptors 368, 369
Erythropoiesis, extramedullary,
  infants of diabetic mothers
    1090

Erythropoietin, infants of diabetic
    mothers 1090
Eskimos
    abnormal glucose tolerance
        63–4
    IDDM frequency **133–4**
Estrogens, *see* Oestrogens
Ethanol, *see* Alcohol
Ethiopia
    health care provision 956
    IDDM frequency 122, 137–8
    protein deficient diabetes mellitus
        181
Ethnic differences
    diabetes incidence/prevalence
        35, 40–1, 1602
    diabetic nephropathy in NIDDM
        1270, 1271
    glucose tolerance 64
    IDDM frequency 35, 1026
    models of IDDM inheritance and
        53
    NIDDM frequency 149, 150
    osteopenia 1416–17
Etofibrate 825, 826, 827
Eukaryotic initiation factors, *see*
    Initiation factors, eukaryotic
Europe
    dietary management of diabetes
        685–98
    driving regulations 1633–4
    employment problems 1636
    life-insurance 1632–3
European Association for the Study
    of Diabetes (EASD)
    Diabetes and Nutrition Study
        Group 685
    NIDDM Policy Group 745
Evoked potentials, somatosensory
    1393
ExacTech 973, 975
Exchange lists, *see* Food exchange
    lists
Exercise (physical activity)
    725–38
    aging and 1110–11
    cardiovascular responses,
        impaired 1404
    children and adolescents 1041
    dietary advice 716, 732–3, 854,
        1041
    elderly 737–8, 1119
    fuel sources 726
    glucagon levels 337, 726, 728,
        729, 730
    hypertension and 731, 1528
    hypoglycaemia induced by 730,
        732–3, 738, 1146
    insulin receptor function and
        364, 727, 735–6
    insulin resistance and 156, 545,
        734–6, 1664–5
    insulin-treated diabetics
        729–33, 876

clinical implications 730–3,
    738
pathophysiology 729–30
NIDDM **733–8**
    acute effects 733–4
    effects on glucose tolerance
        652, 653
    insulin sensitivity/glucose
        tolerance and 734–6
    pathogenic significance 153,
        156, **1664–5**
    prevention 1665–6
    therapeutic use 736–8
normal humans 726–9
regulation of fuel fluxes 726–9
urinary albumin excretion and
    1273, 1289
Exocrine pancreatic function,
    pancreatic diabetes 187,
    212
Exocytosis, compound 263
Exons 469
Experimental diabetes
    diabetogenic viruses 60, 61
    genetic heterogeneity 40
    IDDM 45, 46, 117
        inheritance of susceptibility
            54
    large vessel abnormalities
        1439–40
    large vessel metabolism 1440–1
    late complications 1231–2,
        1276–7
    NIDDM 63
    peripheral nerve changes 1386
    protein metabolism 476–7
    somatostatin in 345–6
    see also specific animal models
Extracellular fluid volume,
    hypertension in diabetes
    1522, 1523
Extracellular matrix
    glomerular, changes in diabetes
        1279
    glycated
        accumulation in blood vessels
            672–3
        functional abnormalities
            673–4
        plasma protein binding 672
    see also Basement membranes;
        Collagen
Extramedullary erythropoiesis,
    infants of diabetic mothers
    1090
Exudative lesions, diabetic
    nephropathy 1291–2, 1293
Eye care
    elderly patients 1112
    recommendations 1382
Eye disease
    diabetic non-retinal **1367–71**
    elderly diabetic patients
        1112–13

see also Retinopathy, diabetic
Eye pain 1367, 1398

Facial (VII) nerve palsy 1398
Factitious disease
    brittle diabetes 1063–4
    insulin resistance 1080
    investigation 1066
Factor V 1473
Factor VII 1449, 1473
Factor VIII 1449, 1473, 1497
Factor Xa 676
Factor XIII 1451
Faecal chymotrypsin test 187
Faecal incontinence 1404
Family
    children with brittle diabetes
        1064–5
    diabetes education and
        psychosocial support
        1044–7
    dietary advice 704
Family studies
    diabetes 36
    diabetic nephropathy 1219,
        1281–3
    fibrocalculous pancreatic diabetes
        189
    IDDM 123–4, 1657
    limited joint mobility 1427
    NIDDM 64, 148–9
        glycogen synthesis 606, 617
        insulin secretion vs. insulin
            sensitivity 598–9, 600
        physiological studies 65–7
    see also Insulin dependent
        diabetes mellitus, high-risk
        individuals; Non-insulin
        dependent diabetes mellitus,
        high-risk individuals
Fanconi's syndrome–
    hypophosphataemia 38
Fasciculation, muscle 1398
Fasting
    hepatic glucose production 415,
        420
    insulin receptor function and
        364
    insulin-stimulated protein
        synthesis and 477
    ketogenesis and 461
    pregnancy 1087
    protein degradation 474, 477
    religious, dietary advice 704,
        716–17
    see also Starvation
Fasting ascending glycaemic
    excursions (FAGE) 1060
Fat, dietary **691–3**, 1481
    African diets 711, 716
    children and adolescents 1040
    Chinese diet 719, 720
    fibrocalculous pancreatic diabetes
        and 189

Fat, dietary (*cont.*)
  Indian and South East Asian
      diets 702, 703–4
  insulin resistance and 545
  Japanese diet 707
  NIDDM development and 1664
  NIDDM prevention 1666
Fat cells, *see* Adipocytes
Fathers, IDDM, risks to offspring
      73, 74, 1028, 1098
Fat tissue, *see* Adipose tissue
Fatty acid(s)
  monounsaturated (MUFA) 692
  omega-3 (long-chain)
      polyunsaturated 692–3,
      703, 707
  polyunsaturated (PUFA) 692
  saturated 691–2, 693
Fatty acid(s), free (FFA, NEFA)
  aging and 1111
  atherogenesis and 1473
  biguanide therapy and 781–4
  diabetic ketoacidosis and 538,
      1153
  glucagon and 335, 336
  glucose and amino acid
      interactions 431, 433
  hepatic insulin clearance in
      obesity and 553–4
  hormonal regulation of
      metabolism 460, 461–2
  hyperosmolar non-ketotic coma
      and 1159
  plasma levels
      after myocardial infarction
          1193
      aging and 1111
      biguanide actions 779
      hepatic glucose production and
          168, 555
      insulin actions 428, 430,
          448, 449
      insulin resistance in NIDDM
          and 607–10
      NIDDM 514, 516, 536
      pancreatic diabetes 209
  re-esterification
      hormonal regulation 460,
          461
      quantitation of insulin actions
          428–31
  regulation during exercise 728
  regulation of glucose production
      418–19
  use by exercising muscles 726
Fatty acid oxidation
  biguanide actions 779, 784
  gluconeogenesis and 553–4,
      804–5
  hepatic glucose production and
      610
  insulin actions 391, **393**,
      461–2
      quantitation 428–31

insulin resistance in NIDDM and
    607–10, 611
pathways 392, 461, 462, 806
Fatty acid synthase 392
Fatty acid synthesis 445
  insulin actions **391–3**, 463
Fatty acyl-CoA 461
Fatty acyl-CoA synthetase 392,
    393, 394
Federal Aviation Administration
    (FAA) 1638–9, 1640
Federal Highway Administration
    (FHA) 1634–5
Federal Rehabilitation Act (1973)
    1637
Femoral artery
  medial calcification 1439
  morphological abnormalities
      1437
Femoral artery angioplasty
    1544
Femoral pulses 1510
Fenofibrate 825, 826, 827
Fetal growth retardation 1088,
    1089, 1093
Fetal hypoxia 1090, 1094
Fetal macrosomia 76, 1087–8
  NIDDM and 1096
  pathogenesis 1089–90
  perinatal problems 1090
  screening 1093
Fetal monitoring 1094
Fetal pancreas transplantation
    905–6
Fetopathy, diabetes **1087–8**
Fibre, dietary **687–91**
  artificial supplements 808
  Chinese diet 720
  Indian and South East Asian
      diets 702–3
  insoluble 688
  Japanese diet 708
  NIDDM prevention 1666
  as part of mixed diet 689–90
  purified soluble 688–9
  soluble 688
Fibric acid derivatives 825–6,
    827
Fibrin cap lesion, diabetic
    nephropathy 1291, 1293
Fibrin cleavage products 1256,
    1292, 1448–9
Fibrinogen 1256, **1447–9**
  control of synthesis 1448
  glycation 1450, 1473
  molecular properties 1448
  plasma levels 1447–8, 1454,
      1473
      agents reducing 1454–5
      biguanide therapy and 784
      cardiovascular disease and
          1449
  role in blood coagulation
      1448–9

turnover 1447–8, 1473
Fibrinolysis 1450–1, 1473
  biguanide therapy and 784
  spontaneous, after myocardial
      infarction 1192
  sulphonylurea therapy and 752
Fibrinopeptide A 1448–9
Fibroblasts
  binding of glycated LDL 1441
  dermal, collagen synthesis
      1427–8
Fibrocalculous pancreatic diabetes
    (FCPD) 4, 11, 177, **182–90**,
    199–200
  clinical features 183–4
  diabetic complications 185–6
  diagnostic criteria 190
  exocrine pancreatic function
      187
  historical perspective 182
  ketosis resistance 186
  lipid studies 185
  management of chronic
      pancreatitis 187–8
  nature of diabetes 184
  pancreatic pathology 186–7
  pathogenesis 188–9
  prevalence and incidence 182
  radiological features 184, 185
  ultrasonography and ERCP
      184–5, 186
Fibronectin 1246, 1249, 1250
  changes in diabetes 1252
  diabetic nephropathy 1292
  glycation 1277
  serum factors promoting
      synthesis 1442–3
  vascular wall 1438, 1439
Fibrous breast disease 1424–5
Fiji
  IDDM frequency 121, 138
  NIDDM prevalence 150
Filter paper method, blood glucose
    measurement 974
Financial resources
  India 1604–5
  Malaysia 1608
  Tanzania 1613–14
  see also Economics
Finger-joint limitation, *see* Joint
    mobility, limited
Fingers, gangrene, diabetic
    nephropathy and 1544
Finland
  IDDM frequency 103, 104, 140
  risk of IDDM development
      100, 101
Firbush scheme 936
Fish 693, 694, 702, 707
Flexor tenosynovitis (FTS)
    1419–20, 1423, 1424
Fludrocortisone 1113, 1404
Fluid overload, therapy of diabetic
    ketoacidosis 1157

Fluid replacement therapy
 diabetic ketoacidosis   1032,
  1155
  cerebral oedema and   1036–7,
   1157
  hyperosmolar non-ketotic coma
   1160
  intercurrent illness   1049
Fluid retention
 end-stage renal failure   1275–6
 hypertension in diabetes   1522,
  1523
Fluorescein angiography
 retinal oedema   1331
 screening for retinopathy   1553
Foam cells   446, 1495
Food exchange lists   697–8, 1041
 China   720
 Japan   708–9
Food ingestion, surreptitious   1080
Food intake regulation
 pancreatic polypeptide and   348
 somatostatin and   344
Foods
 availability in Africa   714–15
 glycaemic index, *see* Glycaemic
  index
 guidelines on choice   694–5
 special diabetic   697, 706
 staple   702, 711–12, 713, 719
Foot   **1535–48**
 diabetic nephropathy and   1276,
  1544
 ischaemic   **1541–4**
  investigations   1542
  pathophysiology   1541–2
  ulceration and gangrene
   1542–4, 1545
  see also Peripheral vascular
   disease
 neuropathic   1398, **1535–41**
  assessment   1403
  complications   1538–41
  examination   1511
  pain   1399–400
  pathophysiology   1535–6
  peripheral vascular disease and
   1510, 1542
  pressure and deformity   1537
  sweating   1537
  treatment   1512
  ulceration, *see* Foot ulceration,
   neuropathic
Foot-and-mouth disease   1660
Foot care
 clinic organization   1544–5,
  1557
 early treatment   1551
 patient education   **940–1**, 1545,
  1557
 preventive   960–1, 1545, 1555–7
 professionals' views on
  preventive measures   928,
   929

screening of high-risk patients
  1556–7
Foot deformities   1545, 1557
 Charcot osteoarthropathy   1537,
  1540
 footwear   1539–40
 medial convexity   1540
 neuropathy and   1537
 rocker-bottom   1540
Foot drop   1398
Foot oedema
 management   1541
 pathogenesis   1536, 1537–8
Foot pressures, elevated   1537
Foot processes, glomerular
  epithelial, *see* Glomerular
  epithelial foot processes
Foot ulceration   1535
 chronic sensory neuropathy
  1397
 high-risk patients   1556–7
 ischaemic   1542–4, 1545
  medical treatment   1543
  pathogenesis   1542–3
  surgical treatment   1543–4
 neuropathic   **1538–40**, 1545
  management   1538–40
  pathogenesis   1538
Footwear, special   1539–40, 1543,
  1545
Forearm perfusion technique
 insulin-mediated glucose uptake
  430, 432
 method   525
 NIDDM   585–6, 593
 protein metabolism   483
Forskolin   276, 277
C-fos, insulin actions   396, 397,
  491
Fourth (trochlear) nerve palsies
  1367–8
Fractures
 callus formation, neuropathic foot
  1537
 Charcot osteoarthropathy   1540
 risk in diabetes   1416
France
 economic cost of diabetes   1651
 IDDM frequency   101, 140
Frey's hairs, sensory testing   1393
Friedreich's ataxia   39, 540, 1028
Frozen shoulder   1420–1
Fructosamine
 assay   995
 blood glucose levels and   998–9
 diagnosis of diabetes   27
 diagnosis of gestational diabetes
  1097
 hyperglycaemia after myocardial
  infarction and   1198
 screening for diabetes   1577
 uraemic patients   1306
Fructose
 diabetic nerve   1389

dietary   696–7, 720
Fructose 1,6-biphosphate   987,
  988
Fructose 1,6-bisphosphatase   386
Fructose 2,6-bisphosphate   1152
Fructose 2,6-bisphosphate kinase
  386, 387
Fruit   694, 716
"Fuel" concept of insulin secretion
  266
Fungal infections, foot   1538
2-Furoyl-4(5)-(2-furanyl)1-*H*-
  imidazole (FFI)   671
Futile metabolic cycles   423
F-wave latencies   1393

Galactose, polyol pathway of
  metabolism   1255–6
Galanin   230, 288, 576
Gamma-linolenic acid   1401
Gangliosides   1400–1
Gangrene
 digital, diabetic nephropathy and
  1544
 ischaemic foot   1542–4
  medical treatment   1543
  pathogenesis   1542–3
  surgical treatment   1543–4
 neuropathic foot   1538, 1539
Gas, subcutaneous, foot sepsis
  1538
Gastric acid secretion, biguanide
  actions   785
Gastric emptying
 biguanide actions   785
 glucose absorption and   433,
  434
 impaired (gastroparesis)
  autonomic neuropathy   1404
  children and adolescents
   1052
  insulin resistance   1080
Gastric inhibitory polypeptide (GIP)
  800–1
 chronic pancreatitis   201
 cystic fibrosis   208
 glucagon release and   336
 insulin secretion and   287, 288
 pancreatectomy and   204
Gastric parietal cell antibodies   47,
  57, 123
Gastrin
 insulin secretion and   287, 288
 pancreatectomy and   204
Gastrin-releasing peptide (GRP)
  288
Gastritis, atrophic, screening   75
Gastrointestinal function, biguanides
  and   784–5
Gastrointestinal hormones
 biguanide actions   785
 incretins   800–1
 insulin secretion and   276, 287,
  288

Gastrointestinal insulin
 administration **867–8**
Gastrointestinal symptoms
 autonomic neuropathy
  1404–5
 biguanide-associated 789
 diabetic ketoacidosis 1158
 metformin-associated 1122
Gastroparesis, *see* Gastric emptying,
 impaired
Gc genotype 67
Gemfibrozil 825–6, 827
Gender differences, *see* Sex
 differences
Gene dosage model, IDDM
 inheritance 51
General practitioners
 care of diabetic patients 955,
  958, 961, 963
 screening for diabetic retinopathy
  1382
Genes 468
 candidate, *see* Candidate genes
Genetic counselling **73–7**
 diagnosis and 73
 female diabetics 76–7
 IDDM 73–5, 76, 1028
 MODY 1029
 NIDDM 74, 75–6
Genetic heterogeneity
 animal models 40
 diabetes 37–41
 IDDM 47–9
  biological models 54–6
 MODY 71–2
Genetic linkage 43–4
Genetic markers
 IDDM 46–7, 132, 1658–9
 MODY 71–2
 NIDDM 67–70, 149–50
 see also HLA
Genetic models, IDDM inheritance
 49–54
Genetic susceptibility **31–77**
 abdominal obesity 561
 development of diabetic
  complications **1225–41**,
  1258
  clinical studies 1233–9
  epidemiological studies
   1226–8
  genetic vs. metabolic
   hypotheses 1228–33
 diabetes
  Asia 123–4, 1602
  epidemiology and ethnic
   differences 32–6
  evidence for genetic
   heterogeneity 37–41
  family and twin studies 36–7
 diabetic nephropathy 1219,
  1230–1, 1281–3
 fibrocalculous pancreatic diabetes
  189

heterogeneity between IDDM
 and NIDDM 41–2
IDDM **43–61**, 108–9, 1657–9
 autoimmune associations 47
 biological models of
  heterogeneity 54–6
 difficulties in genetic analysis
  43–4
 genetic heterogeneity within
  47–9
 HLA region and 44–6
 interaction of genetic and
  environmental factors
  58–61
 models of inheritance 49–54
 non-HLA genes and 46–7
 pathophysiology and natural
  history 56–8
 see also Insulin dependent
  diabetes mellitus, high-
  risk individuals
 insulin resistance 66, 167–8,
  598–9, 600
 limited joint mobility 1427
 MODY 71–2, 151
 NIDDM **61–73**, 148–51,
  1661–2
  approaches to studying 64–5
  candidate genes 67–70, 150
  difficulties in genetic analysis
   62–3
  evidence from animal models
   63
  maternal effects 72–3
  mutant insulins 70–1
  physiological evidence for
   disease heterogeneity
   65
  physiological studies in
   high-risk groups 37,
   65–7
  physiological variability in
   populations 63–4
  screening for 1666–7
  tropical countries 179
  twin and family studies 64,
   148–9
  see also Non-insulin
   dependent diabetes
   mellitus, high-risk
   individuals
Genetic syndromes, IGT/diabetes
 associated with 11, 13,
 37–40, 248
Geographic differences
 diabetes incidence/prevalence
  35
 HLA allele prevalence 102–4
 IDDM incidence/prevalence 35,
  100–2
Germany, driving regulations 1634
Gestational diabetes mellitus
 (GDM) 5, **11–13**, **1096–7**,
 1665

congenital malformations and
 76
definition 1096
diagnostic criteria 20, 21–2,
 1085–6, 1581–2
follow-up 1097
former, insulin secretory capacity
 289, 294–5
long-term prognosis of offspring
 1097–8
medical care 1097
obstetric care 1097
reclassification as previous
 abnormality of glucose
 tolerance 13, 15
risk of NIDDM development
 after 159
screening 1096–7, 1578,
 1581–3
GH, *see* Growth hormone
Ghana, IDDM frequency
 138
GIP, *see* Gastric inhibitory
 polypeptide
Glare, visual problems due to
 1379–80
Glaucoma **1369–70**
 acute angle closure (narrow
  angle) 1369
 neovascular 1349, 1369–70
 open-angle 1112, 1369
Glibenclamide (glyburide) 734,
 758–9, 798
 biguanides vs. 787
 chlorpropamide vs. 757
 clinical efficacy 753
 dosage intervals 763
 elderly patients 1120–1
 extrapancreatic effects 752
 glipizide vs. 758–9
 hypoglycaemic reactions 755,
  758, 765
 mechanisms of action 747–8,
  754
 potency and intrinsic activity
  754
 rate of onset and duration of
  action 755–6
 structure 746
Glibornuride 746, 755, **760**
Glicazide 746, 755, **759**, 763
Glicentin 225, 334
Glipizide **759–60**, 763, 1303
 clinical efficacy 753
 elderly patients 1120, 1121
 glibenclamide vs. 758–9
 plasma membrane binding sites
  748
 potency and intrinsic activity
  754
 rate of onset and duration of
  action 755
 structure 746
Gliquidone 748, 755, **760**, 1303

Glisoxepide 746, 760
Glomerular basement membrane
    (GBM)
    aminoguanidine therapy and
        677
    changes in diabetes 1251–3,
        1277–8, 1279
    glycation 673, 1251, 1277
    normal structure 1246, 1248,
        1250
    plasma protein deposition 672,
        1277
    thickening
        electron microscopy 1292–3
        pathogenesis 1280, 1281
Glomerular capillary hydraulic
    pressure, increased 1280,
    1283–4
Glomerular disease, concurrent non-
    diabetic 1295
Glomerular epithelial foot processes
    (podocytes)
    barrier function 1253–4
    basement membrane adhesion
        1254
    pathological changes 1293
Glomerular filter **1287–8**
    diabetes 1253–4, 1288
Glomerular filtration rate (GFR)
    decline 1274–5, 1303–4
        antihypertensive therapy and
            1219, 1296, 1524–5,
            1526
        low-protein diet and 693,
            1297–8
        pathophysiology **1290**
    determinants 1283–5
    increased, *see* Glomerular
        hyperfiltration
Glomerular hyperfiltration **1271–2**,
    1273
    dietary protein restriction
        693–5, 1553–4
    glomerular injury induced by
        1280
    glycaemic control and 1271,
        1299
    metabolic and hormonal
        mediators **1285–6**
    pathophysiology **1283–5**
Glomerular hypertrophy, diabetic
    nephropathy 1292, 1293
Glomerular lesion, diffuse 1291
Glomerular ultrafiltration coefficient
    1284–5
Glomerulopressin 1286
Glomerulosclerosis, diabetic 985
    extent, in relation to renal
        function 1293–4
    haemodynamic factors 1280–1
    pancreatic diabetes 213–14
    pathology 1291–2
Glucagon 225, **333–8**
    acute pancreatitis 199

biguanide actions 785
brittle diabetes and 1063
chronic pancreatitis 202
control of release 336, 337, 344
as counterregulatory hormone
    336–7, 1137–8, 1139–40
cystic fibrosis and 207–8
deficiency in pancreatic diabetes
    186, 208, 210, 212, 213
diabetes and 337
diabetic ketoacidosis and
    1152–3
in exercise **337**, 726, 728, 729,
    730
glomerular filtration rate and
    1285–6
glycogen synthase activity and
    389
haemochromatosis 203
hepatic glucose production and
    335, 419, 420
hyperosmolar non-ketotic coma
    and 1159
IDDM 337
    residual B-cell function and
        314
    response to hypoglycaemia
        1140, 1141
injection
    hypoglycaemic coma 1145
    patient education 938,
        1047–8
insulin resistance and 533
insulin secretion and 276–7,
    287, 288
ketone body metabolism and
    335, 460, 464–5
ketosis resistance and 186
lipid metabolism and 335, 391,
    392, 394
in neonates 337
new drugs suppressing activity
    807–8
pancreas transplantation and
    918, 919
pancreatectomized patients 204,
    205
pancreatic carcinoma 204
physiological actions 335–6
protein metabolism and 486–7
somatostatin and 344, 347
in starvation 337
in stress 337
structure and biosynthesis
    333–5
sulphonylurea therapy and 750
surgical trauma and 1174
Glucagon analogues (antagonistic)
    807–8
Glucagon-like peptide 1 (GLP-1)
    334–5
Glucagon-like peptide 2 (GLP-2)
    334–5
Glucagon-like peptides (GLPs) 225

Glucagonoma 247, 295, 533, 1080
Glucagon-producing cells, *see* A
    cells
Glucagon test 317–18
Glucochek 973
Glucocorticoid receptors (GR)
    554, 559, 560
Glucocorticoids
    actions in visceral adipose tissue
        554
    insulin receptor gene regulation
        359
    insulin resistance and 365, 533
    insulin secretion and 289
    in NIDDM, insulin secretion and
        289, 294
    therapy, *see* Steroid therapy
Glucokinase
    insulin actions 396, 491, 492
    islet cells 267, 268
    starvation and 279
Glucometer 973
Gluconeogenesis
    basal 415–17
    biguanide actions 780
    fatty acid oxidation and 553–4,
        804–5
    hormones facilitating 335, 420
    insulin actions 387, 498–9
    new drugs inhibiting 804–7
    NIDDM 583, 584, 610
    pancreatic diabetes 208
Gluconeogenic precursors
    basal state 416–17
    biguanide actions 780
Glucoscan 973
Glucose **409–36**
    anomeric specificity of insulin
        response 266
    blood water 410
    distribution and exchange in
        body 409–12
    extraction ratio (fractional
        extraction) 414–15, 420–1
    hepatic production, *see* Glucose
        production, hepatic
    metabolic clearance rate (MCR)
        522–3
        NIDDM 591–2, 593
    metabolic cycles **423**
    net organ (body region) balance
        410
    phosphorylation in islet B cells
        267, 268
    proinsulin biosynthesis and 262
    regulation of insulin secretion
        261, 274, 285, 286–7
    renal threshold, variability 968,
        1576
    renal tubular reabsorption 1289
    urinary, *see* Glycosuria
    urinary loss (U_{gl}) 521
    urine testing, *see* Urine testing,
        glucose

Glucose, blood 410
  ambulatory glucose profile
      (AGP) 1016, 1017
  atherosclerotic vascular disease
      and
    diabetics 1476–8
    non-diabetics 1474–6
  bedside monitoring 1179
  biguanide actions 775, 787
  blood pressure and 1473–4
  diabetic ketoacidosis 1031
  diagnosis of diabetes/IGT 20
  fasting 542
    aging and 1105–6
    diagnosis of diabetes/IGT 20
    screening for diabetes
        1578–9
    standard deviation (SD) 1060
  glucose potassium and insulin
      infusion and 1179
  glycated haemoglobin/protein
      levels and 995–7
  goals
    children 1042
    elderly 1123
    IDDM 875, 876
    IDDM-predisposed individuals
        58, 114
  insulin dosage adjustments
      853
  mean of daily differences
      (MODD) 1060
  measurement 875
    filter paper method 974
    meters, *see* Glucose
        reflectance meters
    reagent strips 973–4
    in vivo sensors 872–3,
        979–80
  measures of brittleness
      1059–60
  normal 20
  physiological profiles 845–7
  postprandial 1578
  pregnancy 1086–7
  random (casual)
    diagnosis of gestational
        diabetes 1096, 1097
    diagnostic criteria 24–6
    screening for diabetes
        1577–8
  screening for diabetes 1577–9
  self-monitoring, *see* Self-
      monitoring of blood glucose
  see also Glycaemic control;
      Hyperglycaemia
Glucose, plasma 409, 410
  after myocardial infarction
      1194, 1197–8, 1199,
      1200
  diagnosis of diabetes 20
  diagnosis of gestational diabetes
      22
  diagnosis of IGT 20

  fasting 513–14, 515
    diagnosis of diabetes 20,
        1029, 1104
    NIDDM 571–2
    screening for diabetes 1117,
        1578–9
    screening test for NIDDM
        1569, 1571, 1572
  glycated haemoglobin levels and
      998
  hypoglycaemic symptom
      awareness and 1135
  level at half maximal response
      (PG_{50})
    NIDDM 293
    normal 287
  postprandial 514–15, 516
  random (casual)
    diagnostic criteria 24–6,
        1029
    screening for diabetes 1578
  steady state (SSPG) 520–1
Glucose absorption 433–4
  aging and 1109
  biguanide actions 784
Glucose administration
  chronic infusion technique,
      insulin secretion and 636,
      638, 642
  glycaemic clamp studies 522,
      1074–5
  hypoglycaemia 1145
  intravenous 423–5
    children undergoing surgery
        1050–1
    diabetic ketoacidosis 1032,
        1155, 1156
    hepatic insulin extraction and
        311
    hypoglycaemic coma 1145
    insulin response in NIDDM
        572, 573–4
    metabolic studies **425–33**
    surgery 1177–8
    see also Intravenous glucose
        tolerance test
  oral
    hepatic insulin extraction and
        311
    insulin response in NIDDM
        572–3
    metabolic studies **433–6**
    see also Oral glucose
        tolerance test
Glucose–alanine cycle 496–7
Glucose appearance rate, total (R_a)
    413, 434, 521, 524–5
Glucose balance, *see* Glucose
    homeostasis
Glucose clamp techniques 425,
    521–4, 542–3
  euglycaemic insulin clamp 425,
      426, **521–2, 1074–5**
    aging and 1107, 1108

  effects of hyperglycaemia
      646
  free fatty acid levels and lipid
      oxidation 607–10
  frequent sampling IVGTT
      (FSIGT) vs. 519
  measures of insulin sensitivity
      522–4, 525
  NIDDM 166, 167, 579–80,
      583–6, 595
  hyperglycaemic 425, 426,
      523–4
    aging and 1106–7
    glucose uptake 646
Glucose clearance (CR) 414–15
  NIDDM 591–2, 593
  specific organs and tissues 421
Glucose disposal (uptake)
  adipose tissue 555, 586
  basal state **420–2**, 569, 570
  brain, *see* Brain, glucose uptake
  glucose toxicity and **644–50**
  hepatic (splanchnic), *see* Liver,
      glucose uptake
  hypoglycaemia and 1139
  insulin-mediated 426–33, 1137
    biguanide actions 776–9
    correction of hyperglycaemia
        and 647–8
    during exercise 726–7
    haemodynamic effects 432–3
    hyperglycaemia and 644–5,
        646
    inter-individual variability
        427
    NIDDM 580, 581, 583–5,
        586, 589–94, 595–6
    NIDDM-predisposed
        individuals 599, 600
    physical training and 735–6
    potentiation by sulphonylureas
        751
    quantitation of components
        428–31
    see also Insulin sensitivity
  muscle (peripheral), *see* Muscle,
      skeletal, glucose uptake
  non-insulin (glucose) mediated
    aging and 1109
    effects of hyperglycaemia
        645–7, 648–50
    NIDDM 537, 588
  non-oxidative (glucose storage)
    lipid oxidation in NIDDM and
        607, 609, 610
    NIDDM 536, 595–6, 604–5
    NIDDM-predisposed
        individuals 599, 600
    obesity 604, 605
    physical training and 736
    quantitation 428–31
  oral glucose load 434–5
    NIDDM **587–9**
  specific tissues 525

Glucose disposal rates (*M* values)
  euglycaemic glucose clamp
    425, 426, 521–2
  hyperglycaemic glucose clamp
    425, 426, 523–4
Glucose disposal rate, total (R_d)
    413, 521, 524
  oral glucose load 434, 435
Glucose–fatty acid cycle 555
Glucose homeostasis 569, 570,
    1137
  exercise and 726, 728–9
    IDDM 730
  hypoglycaemia 1137–40
  role of glucagon 336–7
  steady state 285–6
  see also Counterregulatory
    hormones
Glucose insulin and potassium
  infusion, *see* Glucose
    potassium and insulin (GKI)
    infusion
Glucose/insulin ratio 514, 587
Glucose–insulin tolerance test
  519–20
Glucose intolerance 1103
  of aging **1105–11**
  classification **3–16**
  mortality of myocardial
    infarction and 1187
  screening **1565–83**
  see also Glucose tolerance,
    impaired
Glucose isotopes, *see* Glucose tracers
Glucose metabolism **413–36**
  basal state 415–23, 569, 570
    glucose cycles 422–3
    glucose disposal 420–2
    glucose production 415–20
  diabetic ketoacidosis and
    1152–3
  fed state 423–36
    intravenous glucose 425–33
    methods 423–5
    oral glucose 433–6
  glucose toxicity and 612–16,
    644–50
  insulin actions **385–91**, 1137
  methods of investigation
    413–15
  organ–circulation model 420–1
  pancreatic diabetes 208
  polyol pathway, *see* Polyol
    metabolism
  regulation in islet B cells
    266–9
  vascular, experimental diabetes
    1441
Glucose oxidation
  IDDM 538
  lipid oxidation in NIDDM and
    607, 609, 610
  NIDDM 536, 585, 595–6,
    606–7

quantitation 428–31
Glucose-6-phosphatase (G6Pase)
    412
Glucose-6-phosphate dehydrogenase
    1441
Glucose-6-phosphate (G6P) 418,
    987, 988
  hepatic production, sulphonylurea
    therapy and 296
  islet cells 267, 268
  Randle cycle and 607, 608
Glucose potassium and insulin
  (GKI) infusions **1178–9**,
    1180
  advantages 1181
  after myocardial infarction
    1195
  special surgical situations
    1180–1
Glucose potentiation slope 287
  IDDM 290
Glucose production, hepatic (HGP,
    HGO)
  aging and 1109
  autoregulation 646, 1139
  basal state **415–20**, 569, 570
    NIDDM 581–2
  biguanide actions 779–80
  diabetic ketoacidosis and
    1152–3
  exercise and 726, 728–9
  glucagon actions 335, 419,
    420
  glucose clamp techniques and
    521, 523
  hypoglycaemia 1138–9
    IDDM 538
  insulin actions 425–6, 427, 428,
    429, 525
    hypoglycaemia and 1137
    IDDM 419–20
    NIDDM 582–3
  insulin suppression test and
    520
  measurement 415, 524
  NIDDM 168, 535–6, **581–3**,
    584
    effects of therapy 651–3
    fatty acid oxidation and 610,
      611
    oral glucose load 587–9
    role in hyperglycaemia
      589–93, 594
  oral glucose and 434
  pancreatectomized patients
    206–7
  pancreatic diabetes 208
  regulation 417–20
Glucose profile, ambulatory (AGP)
    1016, 1017
Glucose reflectance meters **973**
  computerization of patient-
    collected data 1010
  development 1010–11

memory-based 973, 977,
    1010–11
  integrated computer-based
    patient management
    systems 979, 1015–18
  new generation 1015
  screening for diabetes 1577
"Glucose resistance" 537, 582,
    646–7
Glucose sensors, in vivo 872–3,
    979–80
Glucose system 413
Glucose tolerance
  exercise and 156, **734–6**
  impaired (IGT) 5, 7, **14–15**
    acromegaly 295
    acute pancreatitis 199
    after myocardial infarction
      1198
    aging and 1103–5
    atherosclerosis and
      1474–6
    chronic pancreatitis 199
    conditions and syndromes
      associated with 11,
      12–13
    Cushing's syndrome 295
    diagnostic criteria 20, 23–6,
      1085, 1086
    fibrocalculous pancreatic
      diabetes and 184
    genetic counselling 74
    genetic factors 36, 65
    genetic heterogeneity in
      animals 40
    genetic syndromes 11, 13,
      37–40
    glucagonoma 295
    glycated haemoglobin and
      1003, 1117
    IDDM-predisposed individuals
      1659
    individual variability 27
    insulin resistance 167
    insulin secretion 164–6, 573,
      574
    insulin therapy and 295–6
    pancreatic tumours 204
    phaeochromocytoma 295
    physical training effects 736
    progression to NIDDM
      158, 1581, 1663–4
      prevention 1666
    proinsulin levels 320, 322
    screening 1574, 1575–6,
      1578–9, **1581**
    stress-associated 15
  maintenance of normal 569,
    570
  pancreas transplantation and
    918
  population studies 63–4
    bimodal frequency
      distributions 64, 161–2

Glucose tolerance (*cont.*)
  population studies (*cont.*)
    diabetes diagnosis and 23,
      24, 25
    potential abnormality (PotAGT)
      6, 7, **15–16**
    previous abnormality (PrevAGT)
      6, 7, 13, **15**
    sulphonylurea treatment and
      296–7
    weight loss and 297
Glucose tolerance tests, *see*
    Intravenous glucose tolerance
    test; Oral glucose tolerance
    test
Glucose toxicity **635–58**
  definition 635
  endothelial cells 676–7,
    1279–80, 1472
  glucose metabolism 644–50
    cellular mechanisms 648–50
    clinical implications 650
    insulin resistance and glucose
      uptake 534, 612–16,
      644–7
    reversibility of effects 647–8
  "honeymoon period" in IDDM
    and 658
  insulin secretion 166, 244, 573,
    576–8, **636–44**
    acute and chronic
      hyperglycaemia
      636–7
    cellular mechanisms 642–4
    non-glucose secretagogues
      637–9
    reversibility of effects
      639–42
  pathogenesis of diabetic
    nephropathy and
    1279–80
  pathogenesis of NIDDM 618,
    654–6
    clinical implications 656–8
    therapeutic approach 650–3
  see also Hyperglycaemia
Glucose tracer methods
  basal hepatic glucose production
    415, 416
  hepatic insulin sensitivity 524
  IVGTT 424–5
  measurement of glucose turnover
    413–14
  metabolic fate of glucose 422
  NIDDM 167, 587
  non-steady state conditions
    583
  regional glucose metabolism
    414–15
Glucose tracers (isotopes) 413
  "isotope effect" 524
  recycling 415, 524
Glucose transport 409–12
  aging and 1109, 1110

brain, *see* Brain, glucose
  transport
  effects of hyperglycaemia
    648–50
  glucose-stimulated 645–7, 649
  insulin actions **387–9**, 601
  islet cells 265, 266, 603, 642
  NIDDM **603–4**, 612
  Randle cycle and 607, 608
Glucose transporters 70, 409–10
  gene polymorphisms in NIDDM
    67, **70**, 150
  insulin actions 386, 387–8, 422
    sulphonylureas and 750–1
  NIDDM 537, 603–4
  physical training effects 736
  see also Glut1; Glut2; Glut3;
    Glut4
Glucose turnover rate (TR) 413
  glucose clearance (CR) and
    414–15
  methods of measurement
    413–14
  non-steady state conditions 414
  steady-state conditions 414
Glucose uptake, *see* Glucose disposal
Glucostix 974
Glut1 70, 388, 409–10, 603
Glut2 70, 412, 603
Glut3 70, 410, 603
Glut4 70, 388, 409, 603
  NIDDM 604
Glutamate dehydrogenase 266,
  267
Glutamic acid decarboxylase (64K
  autoantigen) autoantibodies
  107, 111, 232, 239, 1027
Glutamine
  interorgan exchange 496
  stimulation of protein synthesis
    478
Gluten-sensitive enteropathy 54
Glyburide, *see* Glibenclamide
Glycaemic control
  acceptable limits 1000–1
    children 1042–4
    IDDM 875
  antihypertensive drugs and
    1529, 1530
  blood glucose self-monitoring
    and 977–8
  computer-based patient
    management systems
    1014–15
  continuous ambulatory peritoneal
    dialysis and 1306
  continuous subcutaneous
    insulin infusion 856–7,
    858
  control systems for optimizing
    871–9
  development of complications
    and **1225–41**, 1550
    clinical studies 1233–9

    epidemiological studies
      1226–8
    genetic vs. metabolic
      hypotheses 1228–33
  diabetic embryopathy and 1087
  diabetic nephropathy and, *see*
    Nephropathy, diabetic,
    glycaemic control and
  diabetic neuropathy and
    1395–6, 1555
  diabetic retinopathy and, *see*
    Retinopathy, diabetic,
    glycaemic control
  educational programmes and
    924
  glycated haemoglobin levels and
    988–91
  hypoglycaemia awareness and
    1135, 1136
  IDDM
    basement membrane changes
      and 1229–30
    exercise and 730–2
    insulin sensitivity and
      615–16, 650, 651
    preservation of B-cell function
      316–17
    role of residual B-cell function
      313–14, 315, 316
  infections and 1165
  insulin antibodies and 890–1
  limited joint mobility and
    1426–8
  lipid/lipoprotein abnormalities
    and 817–18, 821, 822–4
  macrovascular disease and
    1471–81, 1490, 1495–6
  myocardial infarction and
    1194–6, 1499
  NIDDM
    biguanide therapy and 787
    high-carbohydrate, high-fibre
      diet and 689–90
    insulin secretion and 578,
      579, 650, 652
    insulin sensitivity and
      615–16, 650, 651
    physical training and 736–7
    sulphonylurea therapy and
      752–3
  pancreas transplantation 918–20
  pregnancy 1002–3, 1091–2
  somatostatin therapy and 347–8
  stroke patients 1203–4
  surgery and 1175
Glycaemic excursions
  fasting ascending (FAGE)
    1060
  mean amplitude (MAGE)
    1060
Glycaemic index **691**, 692, 708
  Chinese foods 720, 722
Glycaemic instability, *see* Brittle
  diabetes

Glycation, non-enzymatic
  basement membranes 674,
    1251, 1254, 1256–7
  diabetic nephropathy and
    1277–8
  diabetic neuropathy and 1389,
    1401
  nomenclature 988
Glycation end-products, advanced
  (AGE) **669–78**, 1277
  cellular receptors 674–5, 1278
  chemical properties 669–71
  diabetic neuropathy 1389
  limited joint mobility and 1426,
    1428
  pharmacological intervention
    677–8
  vessel wall cellular components
    and 674–7
  vessel wall protein components
    and 671–4
Glycation products
  diabetes diagnosis **27**, 1003
  reversible 669, 670–1
  see also Haemoglobin, glycated;
    Proteins, glycated
Glyceraldehyde-3-phosphate
  dehydrogenase 397, 491,
    492
Glycerol 460
  hepatic glucose production and
    418, 419
  insulin preparations 837
Glycerol-3-phosphate 391, 460,
  464
Glycerol phosphate acyltransferase
  393, 394
Glycoaldehyde 671
Glycogen **412**
  pancreatic B cells 277
Glycogen-laden hepatomegaly,
  insulin-induced 891
Glycogenolysis 387, 412
  exercising muscles 726, 727,
    728
  hormones facilitating 335, 420
  rates during fasting 416
Glycogen storage disease, type I
  (von Gierke's disease) 38
Glycogen synthase
  chronic hyperglycaemia and
    649–50
  inhibition by fatty acids 418–19
  insulin actions 386, 387,
    389–90, 398, 402
  NIDDM 536, 606
  Randle cycle and 607, 608
Glycogen synthesis 387, 412
  effects of hyperglycaemia
    649–50
  hepatic 436
  insulin-mediated 428–31
  muscles, after exercise 727
  NIDDM 595–6, **604–6**

NIDDM-predisposed individuals
  599, 606, 617
NMR spectroscopy 605–6
potentiation by sulphonylureas
  751
Randle cycle and 607, 608
Glycolysis
  insulin actions 387
  islets in starved rats 279
Glycosaminoglycans, glomerular
  content 1279
Glycosuria 413
  acceptable limits in IDDM 875,
    876
  acute pancreatitis 199
  decompensation in NIDDM and
    292
  diabetes diagnosis 21
  glucose clearance in NIDDM and
    592
  renal 21
  screening for diabetes and
    1576
Glycosyltransferase activity
  1279
Goniophotocoagulation 1370
Gout 1415
G-proteins, *see* GTP-binding
  regulatory proteins
Grieving responses 926
Group learning 930, **934–6**
  dietary management 940
  hypoglycaemia 938
Group-specific component (Gc),
  NIDDM and 67
Growth
  children with IDDM 484, 1030
  cultured arterial smooth muscle
    cells 1442
  fetal, factors affecting
    1088–90
  limited joint mobility and 1423
  pubertal, insulin requirements
    1038
Growth hormone (GH)
  brittle diabetes and 1063
  as counterregulatory hormone
    1137, 1138, 1139, 1140
  exercise and 729, 730
  glomerular filtration rate and
    1285–6
  hepatic glucose production and
    419
  hereditary deficiency 38
  hyperostosis and 1418
  IDDM, response to
    hypoglycaemia 1141
  increased, insulin resistance
    295, **533–4**
  insulin receptor function and
    365
  insulin secretion and 288
  ketone body metabolism and
    460, 464

pathogenesis of macroangiopathy
  1442, 1443
retinopathy and 347
somatostatin analogues and
  807, 808
somatostatin and 344, 347
surgical trauma and 1174
Growth retardation, fetal 1088,
  1089, 1093
GSK-3 389
G-subunit, glycogen synthase
  dephosphorylation 389
GTP
  hydrolysis in translation 473
  ternary complex formation 471,
    472
GTP-binding regulatory proteins
  (G-proteins)
  cholinergic-stimulated insulin
    release and 273
  Ni, islet cells 275, 276
  Ns, islet cells 276–7
  role in insulin actions 401
Guanidine triphosphate, *see* GTP
Guanine nucleotide exchange factor
  (GEF) 473, 494
Guar gum 688, 785, 808
Gustatory sweating 1405
Gut
  amino acid flux 496, 497
  glucose disposal in basal state
    421

H_2-receptor antagonists 216
Haematemesis, glycated
  haemoglobin levels and
    999
Haematocrit, blood glucose self-
  monitoring and 975
Haematuria, diabetic nephropathy
  1275, 1294–5
Haemochromatosis 190, 198, 211
  diabetic complications 214
  glycated haemoglobin levels and
    999
  pancreatic pathology 247
  primary 38, 114, **203**
    diabetes onset 210
    diabetic complications 213
    hormone secretion 203
    pathology 203
  secondary **203–4**, 247
  therapy of diabetes 215
Haemodialysis **1304–6**
  insulin resistance and 541
  metformin-associated lactic
    acidosis 791
  quality of life 1305–6
Haemodynamic changes
  capillary basement membrane
    thickening and 1257
  diabetic nephropathy and
    1280–1
  hyperglycaemia and 1256

Haemodynamic changes (*cont.*)
  retinopathy and 1260
  see also Blood flow
Haemofiltration 1307
Haemoglobin
  carbamylation 999–1000
  synthesis of adult, infants
    of diabetic mothers
    1090
Haemoglobin, glycated
  985–1003
  assays 991–5
    "charge"-dependent 991–3
    choice 994–5
    ketoamine linkage-based
      993–4
  biochemistry 986–8
  children and adolescents 1042,
    1043–4
  clinical application 999–1002
    confounding medical
      conditions 999–1000
    duration of diabetes and
      1000
    frequency of measurement
      1002
    "quick on–slow off" glycation
      reaction and 1000
    reasonable goals 1000–1
  complications of diabetes and
    1230, 1231
  diabetes diagnosis and 27, 1003
  diabetic neuropathy and 1396
  early studies identifying 985–6
  feasibility of achieving normal
    levels 1239, 1240
  IGT and 1003, 1117
  "labile" 989–91
  myocardial infarction and
    hospital outcome and 1190
    hyperglycaemia after 1198,
      1199, 1200
  NIDDM vs. IDDM 997–9
  nomenclature 988
  pregnancy and 1002–3
  relationship to glycaemic control
    988–91
  screening for diabetes 1117,
    1576–7
  stroke patients 1203
  uniqueness of information
    derived 995–7
  uraemic patients 1306
  see also Haemoglobin A_{1c}
Haemoglobin A_0 (HbA$_0$) 987, 989
Haemoglobin A_1 (HbA$_1$) 986, 989
  blood glucose levels and 996–7
  glycaemic control and 988–9
  measurement 991–4
  NIDDM 997–8
  pregnancy and 1002
  target levels 1001
Haemoglobin A_{1a} (HbA$_{1a}$) 986,
  987

Haemoglobin A_{1a1} (HbA$_{1a1}$) 988,
  989
Haemoglobin A_{1a2} (HbA$_{1a2}$) 988,
  989
Haemoglobin A_{1b} (HbA$_{1b}$) 986,
  988, 989
Haemoglobin A_{1c} (HbA$_{1c}$) 986
  biochemistry **986–7**
  children and adolescents 1043–4
  diabetes diagnosis and 1003,
    1097
  feasibility of achieving normal
    levels 1239, 1240
  glycaemic control and 988, 989
  "labile" 989–91
  measurement 991–4
  myocardial infarction and 1499
  pancreas transplantation and
    919, 920
  physical training in NIDDM and
    736
  pregnancy and 1002, 1087,
    1092
  see also Haemoglobin, glycated
Haemoglobin C (HbC) 992, 993
Haemoglobin F (HbF) 991–2, 993,
  1043
Haemoglobin S (HbS) 992, 993
Haemoglobin variants, glycated
  haemoglobin assay and
  991–2, 993, 999, 1043
Haemolytic anaemia, glycated
  haemoglobin levels and 999
Haemorheological changes
  biguanides and 784
  diabetic nerve 1392
Haemostatic changes
  atherogenesis and 1473
  biguanide therapy 784
  outcome of myocardial infarction
    and 1192
  see also Clotting disorders
Handbooks 932–4
Hands
  diabetic hand syndrome 1419,
    1424
  flexor tenosynovitis 1419–20,
    1423, 1424
  vascular disease (stiff hand
    syndrome) 1419, 1424
Haptoglobin (Hp), NIDDM and
  67–8
Hard exudates, diabetic retinopathy
  1329, 1331–2, 1333
HB699 (4-(2-(5-chloro-2-
  methoxybenzamido)-ethyl)-
  benzoic acid) 798
Health assistants 961
Health beliefs 925
Health education 1626
Health locus of control 925–6
Health personnel
  diabetes care centre 1596
  diabetic clinic 1591, 1592

"intermediate" 961
  Malaysia 1608–9
  Tanzania 1612, 1616
  teams, *see* Teams, health care
  training 962, 1590, 1591, 1626
  views on educational objectives
    928, 929
Health planning, developing
  countries 1609–10
Health services
  community diabetes control
    programmes and
    1626–7
  costs and benefits of screening
    1570, 1572
  India 1604–5
  Malaysia 1607–8
  organization and reorganization
    1597
  Tanzania 1611–12
Heart
  glucose disposal in basal state
    421
  methylpalmoxirate actions
    806–7
  microvascular disease 1490
  protein degradation 477
  protein synthesis 476, 493–4
Heart conduction disorders 1188,
  1189, 1490
Heart failure, congestive 1488,
  1498
  diabetic cardiomyopathy and
    1193, 1471–2, 1498
  glucose potassium and insulin
    infusion 1178
  postmyocardial infarction 1188,
    1189, 1193, 1498–9
  sex differences 1491
Heart muscle disease, diabetic, *see*
  Cardiomyopathy, diabetic
Heart rate
  fixed, autonomic neuropathy
    1404
  response to standing 1402
Heart-rate monitoring, fetal 1094
Heart rate variation (R–R intervals)
  during respiration 1401–2,
    1403, 1558
  Valsalva manoeuvre 1558
Hemiplegic hypoglycaemia 1143
Heparan sulphate proteoglycan
  changes in diabetes 674, 1252,
    1255
  characteristics 1246, 1249,
    1250
  glomerular basement membrane
    1279, 1290
Heparin
  activity in diabetes 1450
  binding to glycated basement
    membranes 674, 677
  subcutaneous therapy 1157,
    1160, 1196

Hepatic glucose production,
  see Glucose production,
  hepatic
Hepatic triglyceride lipase, *see*
  Triglyceride lipase, hepatic
Hepatitis, viral 190
Hepatocytes
  glucagon actions 335
  insulin receptors 358
  NIDDM 367
  obesity 366, 367
Hepatomegaly
  insulin-induced **891**, 1061
  limited joint mobility and 1423
Herrmann syndrome 39
Heterogeneity model, three-allele,
  IDDM inheritance 51–3, 54
Hexokinase 267, 268, 603
Hexose monophosphate shunt
  (HMPS) 1167, 1168
High-density lipoproteins (HDL)
  439, 440
  biguanide therapy and 781,
    782–3
  cardiovascular disease risk and
    1495
  dietary fat intake and 692, 693
  glycaemic control and 823–4
  IDDM 450, 818
  insulin actions 449, 450
  metabolism 442, **443**, 444, 445,
    447
    diabetes **820**
  NIDDM 452, 454–5, 818
  obesity 452
  target levels in diabetes 821
High-performance liquid
  chromatography (HPLC),
  glycated haemoglobin
  measurement 992, 1043
Hispanic/Mexican Americans
  IDDM frequency **135–6**
  insulin receptor region
    polymorphisms 69
  NIDDM 1662
  physiological studies 66
Histamine release test 887
HLA
  autoimmune polyendocrine
    syndrome type 2 and 109
  diabetes secondary to chronic
    pancreatitis and 200
  gene loci 44
  IDDM associations 8, 41–2,
    44–6, 1657–8
    Africans **139–42**
    Asians **122–3**, 142–3
    black Americans 132
    Eskimos 135
    Hispanic Americans 136
    pathogenesis of diabetes and
      108, 1027–8
    tropical countries 178
  insulin allergies and 887

matching, pancreas
    transplantation 916
  microvascular complications and
    1229–31
  NIDDM associations 67, **68**,
    123, 150
  population frequencies vs. IDDM
    incidence 101, 102
  typing
    children at risk of IDDM
      1030
    genetic counselling and 73,
      74–5
    IDDM prevention 1661
  see also MHC
HLA-B8
  Eskimos 135
  IDDM associations 41, 44
HLA-B8-DR3
  complement serum levels and
    1169
  immunoglobulin serum levels
    and 1168
  immunological correlates 48,
    50, 55
HLA-B15
  Eskimos 135
  IDDM associations 41, 44
HLA-B15-DR4, immunological
  correlates 48, 50, 55
HLA-DQ alpha chain variations
  46
HLA-DQ beta chain
  non-Asp 57-allele 45–6, 53–4,
    108, 1027, 1658
    geographical variations in
      prevalence 102–4
    IDDM pathogenesis and 56,
      1028
  variations 45–6
HLA-DQw8 (formerly DQw3.2)
  45, 46, 49, 54
HLA-DR2, IDDM and 45, 108
HLA-DR3
  high- and low-risk haplotypes
    45–6
  IDDM associations 41, 44–6,
    108, 1027, 1657
    black Americans 132
    tropical countries 178
  inheritance 53–4
  risks of IDDM development 54,
    74
  type 1.5 diabetes 10
HLA-DR3-associated IDDM
  characteristics 48–9, 50
  immunogenetic models of
    pathogenesis 54–6
  late-onset, islet changes 239
  models of IDDM inheritance and
    52
HLA-DR3/DR4 compound
  heterozygotes 44–5
  characteristics of IDDM 48, 49

immunogenetic models of IDDM
    pathogenesis 55, 56
  models of IDDM inheritance and
    52, 53
  risks of IDDM 48
HLA-DR4
  high- and low-risk haplotypes
    45–6
  IDDM associations 41, 44–6,
    108, 1027, 1658
    black Americans 132
  inheritance 53–4
  microvascular complications and
    1230, 1231
  risks of IDDM development 54,
    74
  tropical countries 178
  type 1.5 diabetes 10
HLA-DR4-associated IDDM
  characteristics 48, 49, 50
  coxsackie B4 virus and 49, 60
  immunogenetics models of
    pathogenesis 54–6
  models of IDDM inheritance and
    52
HLA-DR5, IDDM and 45
HMG-CoA reductase, *see*
  Hydroxymethylglutaryl-CoA
  reductase
Home
  initiation of insulin therapy at
    937, 941
  see also Ambulatory diabetes
    care programme
Homeostatic model assessment
  (HOMA) model 514
Homoarginine 278
"Honeymoon period", IDDM, *see*
  Insulin dependent diabetes
  mellitus, "honeymoon period"
Hong Kong, IDDM frequency 138
Hopeful depression 926–7
Hormone response element (HSE)
  490
Hormones
  capillary basement membrane
    changes and 1258
  counterregulatory, *see*
    Counterregulatory hormones
  insulin secretion and **276–7**,
    287, 288
  see also Endocrine disorders;
    specific hormones
Hormone-sensitive lipase (HSL,
  triacylglycerol lipase) 391,
  394, 460
Hospital admission
  diabetic ketoacidosis 1031–2
  economics 962–3
  educational programmes and
    923–4
  indications 959–60
  initiation of therapy and
    stabilization 937, 959

Hospital admission (*cont.*)
  pregnancy 1093
Human capital approach, estimating
  costs of illness 1644
Human insulin 884–5, 1039–40
  extended-acting 848–9
  hypoglycaemia unawareness and
    1040, 1136
  immunogenicity 835, 885
  short-acting 847
  sudden unexplained deaths
    1144
Human leukocyte antigens, *see*
  HLA
Huntington's disease 39
Hybrid populations, NIDDM
  frequency 149
Hydralazine 1093–4, 1530
Hydrazonopropionic acids 804
Hydroxyacyl-CoA dehydrogenase
  1441
3-Hydroxybutyrate 1153
  extrahepatic utilization 463
  insulin deficiency and 465
  pancreas transplantation and
    919
  synthesis 462
5-Hydroxymethyl furfural (5-HMF)
  986, 987, 993
Hydroxymethylglutaryl-CoA (HMG-
  CoA) reductase 446, 448,
  1494
  regulation by insulin 391, 395,
    398
Hydroxymethyl glutaryl CoA (HMG
  CoA) reductase inhibitors
  824, 825, 826–7
25-Hydroxyvitamin D_3 1417,
  1418
Hyperandrogenaemia
  hyperinsulinaemia and 558
  insulin resistance and **539–40**,
    558
  risk of NIDDM development and
    558–9
Hypercholesterolaemia
  familial 448
  NIDDM prevention 1666
  treatment in diabetes **824–5**
Hyperglycaemia 413
  acute pancreatitis 199
  after myocardial infarction,
    see Myocardial infarction,
    hyperglycaemia after
  after pancreas transplantation
    917
  AGE and 669–78
  atherosclerosis and **1472–81**,
    1495–6
  basement membrane changes and
    1255–7
  biguanide actions 775, 787
  complications of diabetes and
    635, 636, 669, 670, 1232–3

coronary artery disease and
  1474–8, 1488–9, 1491
cystic fibrosis 208
diabetic nephropathy and 1228,
  1276–8
diabetic neuropathy and 1387
diagnosis of diabetes 19–20,
  21, 24–6
exercise and 1041
fetal macrosomia and 1087–8
glomerular filtration rate and
  1285, 1290
glucagon release and 336
glucose uptake and 645–7,
  648–50
hepatic glucose production and
  417, 418
historical recognition 20–1
hyperosmolality 1035
hyperosmolar non-ketotic coma
  1159
immunological effects 1166–7
insulin secretion and, *see*
  Glucose toxicity, insulin
  secretion
ketoacidosis without 1158
NIDDM
  effects of exercise 733–4
  effects on glucose uptake
    537, 588
  hepatic glucose production and
    582–3
  insulin resistance and 612–16
  pathogenesis 291–2, **589–94**
  role in disease pathogenesis
    618, **654–6**
  sulphonylureas and 749–50,
    752, 755
pancreatic diabetes 211
postoperative 1175
proinsulin secretion 322
rebound posthypoglycaemic, *see*
  Somogyi effect
recurrent, blood glucose self-
  monitoring 972
refractive errors and 1371
stress-induced 15
stroke patients 1203
thiazide-induced 1529
see also Glucose toxicity;
  Glycaemic control
Hyperinsulinaemia
atherogenic effects 450, 1472,
  1496–7
biguanide actions 775
cirrhosis of liver 541
fetal macrosomia and 1087,
  1088–90
glucagon release and 336
hepatic glucose production and
  417
hyperandrogenaemia and 558
hypertension and 554, 1523
hypoglycaemia and 1145

insulin receptor downregulation
  363–4
insulin resistance and 288, 289,
  531, 534
lipoprotein metabolism 450–5
neonatal complications and
  1090–1
NIDDM 592–3
  Asian Indians 179–80
  preceding disease onset 158,
    159, 573, 578
  role in pathogenesis 617–18,
    1662–3
obesity 288, 309, 535, 1662
  abdominal type 551–2, 554
  mechanisms 560
vascular wall changes and 1440
see also Insulin resistance
Hyperkalaemia
diabetic ketoacidosis 1154
end-stage renal failure 1276
hyporeninaemic
  hypoaldosteronism 1113
patients on haemodialysis 1305
Hyperkalaemic hyperchloraemic
  acidosis 1303
Hyperlipidaemia
abdominal obesity 554
cardiovascular disease risk and
  1493–5
diabetes 817–18
diagnosis in diabetes 820–1
familial, association with diabetes
  38, 448, 1495
progression of diabetic
  nephropathy and 1290–1
treatment in diabetes 821–7
  alpha-glucosidase inhibitors
    826
  drug dosages and side-effects
    826–7
  hypercholesterolaemia 824–5
  hypertriglyceridaemia 825–6
  indications 822
  optimization of glycaemic
    control 822–4
Hyperlipoproteinaemia
biguanide therapy and 781
type III 445
Hypernatraemia, hyperosmolar non-
  ketotic coma 1160
Hyperosmolality
cerebral oedema and 1035
hyperosmolar non-ketotic coma
  1159
intravenous fluid therapy 1032
Hyperosmolar non-ketotic coma
  (HONK) **1159–60**
diagnosis 1160
elderly patients 1115–16, 1159
epidemiology 1159
pathophysiology 1159–60
precipitating factors 1159
treatment 1160

Hyperostosis **1418**
Hyperostosis frontalis interna 1418
Hyperostotic spondylosis (HS) 1418
Hyperproinsulinaemia 320, 322, **532**
  C-peptide cleavage site mutations 71
  insulin gene polymorphisms and 68
Hypersensitivity reactions, insulin-induced 887, 888
Hypertension 451, **1465–7, 1521–31**
  biguanide therapy and 784
  blood glucose levels and 1473–4
  borderline 1527
  capillary basement membrane thickening and 1257
  cardiovascular disease risk and 1492–3
  classification 1521, 1522
  definition 1527–8
  diabetic microangiopathy and 1230, 1524–7
  diabetic nephropathy and 1270, 1275, 1280, **1524–5**
    genetic factors 1219, 1230–1, 1282
    pathogenesis 1522–3
    progression during antihypertensive therapy 1219, 1296–7, 1524–5, 1530
  diabetic retinopathy and 1348, 1525–7
  elderly 1115
  essential 1522
  exercise and 731, 1528
  gestational (pre-eclampsia) 1093, 1301
  hyperinsulinaemia and 554, 1523
  IDDM, *see* Insulin dependent diabetes mellitus, hypertension
  investigation in diabetes 1527
  NIDDM, *see* Non-insulin dependent diabetes mellitus, hypertension
  obesity and 561, 563, 564, 1493, 1523
  pathogenesis in diabetes 1522–4
  pregnancy **1093–4**
  treatment **1528–31**, 1554
    non-pharmacological 697, 1528, 1666
    pharmacological, *see* Antihypertensive therapy
Hyperthyroidism, *see* Thyrotoxicosis

Hypertriglyceridaemia
  cardiovascular disease risk and 1494–5
  endogenous, lipoprotein metabolism **451**
  familial 448
  IDDM 818, 823
  NIDDM 818, 819, 823
  treatment 823, 825–6
Hyperventilation, diabetic ketoacidosis 1031, 1154
Hypoadrenalism (adrenal insufficiency) 366, 1063
Hypoglycaemia 413, **1131–47**
  blood glucose self-monitoring and 976
  causes in IDDM 1145
  central nervous system and 1133–7
  central (neuroglycopenic) symptoms 1132, 1134–5
  children and adolescents **1047–8**, 1142, 1144
  chronic renal failure 1303
  classification 1132
  complications 1141–4
  continuous subcutaneous insulin infusion and 858, 874, 1067
  definitions 1131–2
  driving and 1634, 1635
  exercise-induced 730, 732–3, 738, 1146
  factitious 323, 1064
  factors modifying symptoms 1135–7
  frequency 1132–3
  glucagon release and 336, 337
  glucose counterregulation 1137–41
  hemiplegic 1143
  hepatic glucose production and 417
  insulin absorption and 843
  insulinoma 323
  insulin tolerance test 519
  intensive insulin therapy and 1001, 1133, 1239
  loss of warning 1132, 1136
  mortality in IDDM 1215
  neurological defects 1134
  nocturnal
    children 1040, 1048
    fasting glucose levels and 1142
    frequency 1132–3
    prevention 1146–7
  pancreatic diabetes 210–11, 216
  patient education **937–9**, 1146
  peripheral (adrenergic) symptoms 1132, 1135
  physiology 1133–4
  prediction 1146–7
  pregnancy and 1092

  prevention 1146–7
  prognosis 1143–4
  recurrent
    management 851, 854, 972, 1067
    see also Brittle diabetes
  sulphonylurea-induced 755, 757, 758, **765**, 1121–2, 1144
  symptom complexes 1134–5
  symptom generation 1135
  terminology 1132
  treatment 1145–6
  unawareness 1132
    beta-blocker therapy and 1529–30
    human insulin and 1040, 1136
Hypoglycaemic coma
  frequency 1133
  patient education 938
  treatment **1145–6**
Hypoglycaemic neuropathy 1399
Hypoglycaemic reaction, controlled 937
Hypogonadism in men, insulin resistance 559, 562
Hypokalaemia
  diabetic ketoacidosis 1154, 1156
  hypoglycaemia 1143
Hypolipidaemic agents **817–27**
  after myocardial infarction 1197
  dosages and side-effects 826–7
  guidelines in diabetes 821–2
  hypercholesterolaemia 824–5
  hypertriglyceridaemia 825–6
  indications 822
Hypomagnesaemia, diabetic ketoacidosis 1153
Hyponatraemia
  diabetic ketoacidosis 1157
  glucose potassium and insulin infusion and 1178–9
  sulphonylurea-associated 1121
Hypophosphataemia, diabetic ketoacidosis 1034, 1036, 1154, **1156**
Hypophysectomy
  brittle diabetes 1063
  diabetic retinopathy 1348–9
Hyporeninaemic hypoaldosteronism 1113
Hypotension, postural 1403–4, 1528
Hypothalamic arousal syndromes 561–4
Hypothalamus
  insulin secretion and 288
  somatostatin-containing neurons 343
  somatostatin functions 344

Hypothalamus (*cont.*)
    somatostatin levels in diabetes
        346
Hypothermia, hypoglycaemia 1143
Hypoxia
    atherosclerosis and 1496
    diabetic nerve 1391
    fetal 1090, 1094

IAPP, *see* Islet amyloid polypeptide
IgA deficiency
    diabetes 48, 1168
    malabsorption and diabetes,
        hereditary 38
IgE, anti-insulin 836, 887
IgG
    anti-insulin 836
    basement membrane binding in
        diabetes 672, 1252–3,
        1277
    renal deposition in diabetic
        nephropathy 1292
    serum levels in diabetes 1168
    urinary clearance 1287–8
IgM, deposition in basement
        membranes 672
IGT, *see* Glucose tolerance,
        impaired
Iliac artery
    angioplasty 1544
    occlusive disease 1543
Illness, intercurrent
    ambulatory care programme
        960
    brittle diabetes and 1063
    diabetic ketoacidosis and 1152
    dietary advice 716
    sick day management rules 941,
        1031, **1048–51**
Imipramine, painful neuropathy
        1400
Immunity **1165–9**
    hyperglycaemia and ketosis and
        1166–7
    primary abnormalities 1167–9,
        1659
Immunogenetic immune response
        model, IDDM pathogenesis
        55, 56
Immunogenetic models, IDDM
        pathogenesis 54–6
Immunoglobulin heavy chain
        allotypes (Gm) 46
Immunoglobulins
    abnormalities in diabetes 1168
    antiviral, IDDM 1660
Immunosuppressive therapy
    islet transplantation 904–5
    newly diagnosed IDDM 75,
        115, 317, 1656–7
    pancreas transplantation 917,
        918
Immunotherapy, IDDM prevention
        114–15

Impaired glucose tolerance, *see*
    Glucose tolerance, impaired
Implanted insulin pumps 866, **867**,
    1067
Implants, subcutaneous insulin 868
Impotence **1405–6**
    antihypertensive drugs and
        1528, 1529
Incontinence, faecal 1404
Incretins 800–1
India
    autoantibodies in IDDM 123
    communication and transport
        problems 1603–4
    dietary management of diabetes
        701–6
    fibrocalculous pancreatic diabetes
        182, 183
    HLA and IDDM associations
        142
    IDDM frequency 121–2, 138,
        178
    limited financial resources
        1604–5
    literacy 1603
    maldistribution of physicians
        1603
    organization of care and
        problems **1601–5**
    prevalence of diabetes 1601–3
    religious beliefs and taboos
        1604
    see also Asian Indians
Indomethacin, glomerular
        hyperfiltration and 1286
Indonesia
    fibrocalculous pancreatic diabetes
        182
    IDDM frequency **121**, 136–7,
        138
Infants of diabetic mothers
    long-term prognosis 1097–8
    neonatal care 1095
    pancreatic pathology **249–50**,
        251
    pathogenesis of complications
        1088–91
    perinatal morbidity 1095, 1096
    proinsulin levels 322
    see also Congenital
        malformations; Parents,
        diabetic
Infections **1165–9**
    brittle diabetes and 1063
    diabetic ketoacidosis and
        1030–1, 1152
    foot ulcers 1538
    glucose potassium and insulin
        infusion 1178, 1179
    hyperosmolar non-ketotic coma
        and 1159
    immunological abnormalities and
        1166–9
    insulin injection site 885–6

insulin resistance and 541
ischaemic foot 1543
mortality in IDDM 1215
mortality in Tanzania 1613
postoperative 1175
predisposition to 1165–6
sick day rules 1048–50
Infectious agents, IDDM aetiology
        59–61, 110, 198
Inflammatory responses, neuropathic
        foot 1537
Information systems, community
        diabetes control programmes
        1627
Inhibitor 1 389, 398
Initiation (start) codon 471
Initiation complex, 80S 472, 473
Initiation factor-2 (eIF-2) 397
    effects of insulin 494
    function 471, 472, 473
Initiation factors, eukaryotic (eIF)
        471–3
Injection site
    infections 885–6
    lipoatrophy 836, 886, **888–9**
    lipohypertrophy 844, **886–7**
    local complications 885–7
    reactions 836, 887–8
Inositol phosphates 395, 643, 644
Insoles, moulded 1539–40
Insulin 225
    accelerated clearance 1062–3
    assays, specificity 514
    atherogenic effects 1472,
        1496–7
    biosynthesis **262**, 303, 304, 470
        chronic hyperglycaemia and
        642–3
    chemical synthesis 833–4
    chemistry and its clinical
        consequences 832
    Chicago 71
    evolutionary origin 224
    feedback inhibition of its own
        secretion 265
    glomerular filtration rate and
        1285–6
    glucose disposal and, *see*
        Glucose disposal, insulin-
        mediated
    glucose production and, *see*
        Glucose production,
        hepatic, insulin actions
    growth promoting effects in
        arteries 1442
    hepatic extraction 303
        C-peptide as measure
        310–11
    obesity subgroups 552,
        553–5
    sulphonylureas and 752
insulin receptor binding, *see*
    Insulin receptors, insulin
    binding to

Insulin (*cont.*)
  insulin receptor regulation 361,
    363–4, 365
  intracellular actions **385–404**
    carbohydrate metabolism
      385–91
    lipid metabolism 391–5
    NIDDM **600–7**
    possible mechanisms
      397–403, 600–1
    protein metabolism 395–7,
      488–96
  islet cells of type 1 diabetes
    231–2, 235
  Los Angeles 71
  metabolic clearance rate (MCR),
    aging and 1108
  mutant 42, **70–1**, 532, 576
  overnight basal requirements,
    measurement 1080–1
  pharmacological preparations, *see*
    Insulin preparations
  plasma levels
    basal (fasting) 513–14, 515,
      542, **571–2**
    biguanide actions 775
    physiological profiles 845–7
    postprandial 514–15, 516
    prereceptor antagonists 532–4
    purification from animal pancreas
      832–3
  renal tubular function and 1289
  thoracic duct levels 611
  Wakayama 71
Insulin absorption
  intramuscular 840, 844
  subcutaneous **840–4**
    absorption process 841–3
    augmentation in brittle
      diabetes 1067–8
    factors affecting 836, 843–4,
      1062
    impaired, brittle diabetes and
      1062
Insulin actions in vivo
  assessment **513–26**
  glucose metabolism **413–36**,
    1137
  ketone body metabolism
    459–66
  lipoprotein metabolism **448–55**
  protein metabolism **467–99**
  see also Insulin resistance;
    Insulin sensitivity
Insulin allergy, *see* Allergy, insulin
Insulin analogues **839**, 847, 1039
  absorption 842
Insulin antibodies 834–6
  clinical significance 836, **890–1**
  human insulin 835
  IDDM subtypes 48, 49, 50
  insulin absorption and 836, 844
  insulin resistance 533, 546,
    836, 891, 1081

measurement 836
purity of insulin preparations and
  834
transfer to fetus 1090
Insulinase, sulphonylureas and 752
Insulin autoantibodies (IAA, CIAA)
  111, **112–13**, 232, 835–6,
  1659
  assays 112–13
  IDDM pathogenesis and 1027
  IDDM subtypes 48
  insulin resistance and **533**
  newly diagnosed IDDM 8, 112
  as predictor of IDDM
    development 58, 107
Insulin clamp studies, *see* Glucose
  clamp techniques, euglycaemic
  insulin clamp
Insulin deficiency
  diabetic ketoacidosis and
    464–5, 1152, 1153
  exercise and 729–30
  IDDM 8
  NIDDM 596–8
    aetiology **575–8**, 618
  outcome of myocardial infarction
    and 1193
  protein degradation 474–5, 477,
    483–8, 495–6
  protein synthesis 476, 483–8
  see also Insulin secretion
Insulin degradation
  increased 532–3, 1062
  inhibition 546, 1067–8
  sulphonylureas and 752
Insulin delivery systems **871–9**
  closed-loop (artificial pancreas)
    872–3, 979
  open-loop 873–4
  optimized conventional therapy
    874–9
Insulin dependent diabetes mellitus
  (IDDM, type 1 diabetes)
  aetiopathogenesis 8–9, 1026–8
    Asia **122–5**
    autoimmune polyendocrine
      syndromes 109–10
    genetic factors 108–9
    prodromal metabolic
      abnormalities 113–14
    stages in development 56–8,
      107–8
    target antigens 110–13
    triggering events 110
    Western Society **107–15**
  amino acid metabolism 498–9
  atherosclerotic vascular disease
    1185
    intervention studies 1479
    mortality and morbidity
      1461–2
    prevention 1480–1
  autoimmune associations 42,
    47, 48, 123, 232

biguanide therapy 788
blood glucose self-monitoring
  972
cardiovascular risk factors
  1492, 1493, 1495
children and adolescents
  1025–53
classification 4, **8–9**, 317–18
  difficulties 14, 32, 41–2
  heterogeneity in clinical
    course and 10–11
coronary artery bypass surgery
  1500
coronary artery disease 1190,
  1478, 1491
C-peptide, *see* C-peptide,
  IDDM
developing/tropical countries
  136–9, 143, 177–8, 1603
diabetic nephropathy 1227–8
  clinical course and natural
    history 1271–6
  epidemiology 1267–9
  other manifestations of renal
    disease 1299–302
  pathogenesis 1230–1, 1235,
    1236, 1276–83
  pathology 1291–5
  pathophysiology 1283–91
  treatment 1296–9
diagnosis 1029–30
dietary management, *see* Dietary
  management, IDDM
driving regulations 1634, 1638
economic costs 1646, 1647,
  1648
educational programmes 928–9,
  930, 932, 933, 935, 1044–7
elderly 1117
employment problems 1636–7,
  1638, 1639
epidemiology **99–105**, 1025–6
  age at onset 34
  Asia **117–22**
  environmental factors 104
  ethnic differences 35
  future 104–5
  geographic (world-wide)
    patterns 35, 100–2
  HLA antigen prevalence and
    102–4
  incidence and prevalence
    32–3
  non-Caucasoid populations
    129–43
  north–south gradient 124
  seasonal influences 8–9,
    35–6
  sex ratio 34
  socioeconomic status and
    35
  time trends in incidence 33,
    124–5
exercise **729–33**, 738, 876

Insulin dependent diabetes mellitus
(IDDM, type 1 diabetes)
(*cont.*)
  genetic counselling **73–5**, 1028
    congenital malformations and
      76
    empiric risks 73, 74
    screening for other
      autoimmune diseases
      75
    screening and prevention
      73–5
  genetic susceptibility **43–61**,
    108–9, 1657–9
  glucagon levels 337
  glucose counterregulation
    1140–1, 1145
  glycated haemoglobin/protein
    levels 997–9, 1000, 1001,
    1002
  high-risk individuals 15–16,
    1656
    capillary basement membrane
      thickening 1229
    first-phase insulin secretion
      113–14, 1660
    identification 73–5, 114,
      1579
    IGT 1659
    monitoring 1030
    progression to IDDM 58,
      114
  HLA associations, *see* HLA,
    IDDM associations
  "honeymoon period" 290–1,
    296, 658, 1026–7, 1042
    C-peptide secretion 313, 314
    insulin therapy 850, 1038
  hypertension 1465–6, 1474
    diabetic microangiopathy and
      1524–5, 1526, 1527
    pathogenesis 1522–3
  hypoglycaemia, causes 1144–5
  immunogenetic models 54–6
  immunological abnormalities
    1167–9, 1659
  immunosuppressive therapy in
    newly diagnosed 75, 115,
    317, 1656–7
  insulin receptor function 368–9
  insulin resistance, *see* Insulin
    resistance, IDDM
  insulin secretion, *see* Insulin
    secretion, IDDM
  insulin therapy, *see* Insulin
    therapy
  islet morphology **231–9**
  ketoacidosis, *see* Ketoacidosis,
    diabetic
  late-onset, islet morphology
    239
  life-insurance 1219–20, 1632
  limited joint mobility 1421,
    1422, 1424–8

lipid/lipoprotein abnormalities
  817–18, 1472–3
  management 822–3
lipoprotein metabolism 450,
  819, 820
long-term management
  1037–53
osteopenia 1416–17
pancreatic polypeptide levels
  349
pregnancy **1087–95**
prevention
  primary 73–5, 114–15, 1579,
    1656–61
  secondary 316–17, 1656–7
prognosis **1213–20**
  declining mortality 1213–14,
    1215
  life insurance risks and
    1219–20
  methods of improving
    1218–19
  proteinuria and cause of death
    1216
  proteinuria and mortality
    1214–16
  renal–retinal syndrome
    1216–17
  type of angiopathy and
    1217–18
progressing to NIDDM ("black"
  diabetes) 10, 33, 72, 131
progressive (PIDDM) 10
proinsulin levels 320, 322
protein metabolism **483–8**, 488
retinopathy 1112, 1226–7,
  1228, 1340–2
  pathogenesis 1230, 1235–9
  screening 1553
screening 73–5, **1579**
somatostatin secretion 346–7
somatostatin therapy 347–8
surgery 1174, 1176, **1177–9**,
  1180
urinary C-peptide excretion
  311, 312, 313
urine testing 967, 968, 969
visual impairment 1112,
  1373–8, 1379
Insulin dosage adjustment
  algorithms
  children and adolescents 1038
  computer-implemented 877–8,
    879, 979, 1012, 1014–15,
    1018
  educating patients to use 877,
    878
  meal-related 1014–15
Insulin dosage adjustments 853,
  876
  children and adolescents
    1038–9, 1042–3
  evaluation of educational
    programmes 944

exercise and 732
sick day management 1048
"sliding scale" 1039
Insulin dose
  indicating insulin resistance
    531–2
  residual B-cell function and
    314, 315, 316
  see also Insulin therapy, injection
    regimens
Insulin dose adaptation system
  (IDAP) 1014
Insulin dose–response curves
  1075–8
  slope of linear interval 1077–8
Insulin gene
  DNA polymorphisms, in NIDDM
    67, **68**, 150
  DNA variable region near,
    IDDM 42, 46–7, 108
  genes activating transcription
    576
  mutations (mutant insulins) 42,
    70–1, 532, 576
  structure 470
Insulin/glucose ratio 587
Insulin infusion
  continuous intramuscular, brittle
    diabetes 1067
  continuous subcutaneous, *see*
    Subcutaneous insulin
    infusion, continuous
  intravenous, *see* Intravenous
    insulin infusion
Insulin-like growth factor 1 (IGF-1)
  AGE-induced production 674,
    675, 676
  protein metabolism and 486–7
  receptors 320, 368
Insulin-like growth factor 2 (IGF-2)
  receptors 388
Insulin neuritis 1399
Insulin oedema 891
Insulinoma
  diagnosis 323
  proinsulin levels 320, 322, 323
  Somogyi effect 1061
Insulin preparations **836–40**, 875
  absorption characteristics
    841–3
  animal, purification methods
    832–3
  choice 847–9
  extended-acting 838–9
    absorption 842–3
    choice 848–9
    not in general use 838
  historical development 883–5
  hypoglycaemia awareness and
    1136
  immunogenicity 834–6, 884–5,
    889–90
  insulin analogues 839
  premixed formulations 839

Insulin preparations (*cont.*)
  purity 834, 884, 888
  short-acting 836–8
    absorption 841–2
    choice 847–8
  standardization 840
  storage and stability 839–40
  synthetic 833–4
  unmodified (regular) insulin, *see*
    Unmodified insulin
  see also specific preparations
Insulin pumps
  continuous subcutaneous infusion
    855
  implanted 866, **867**, 1067
  intraperitoneal insulin delivery
    866
Insulin receptor gene **359**, 360,
  448
  mutations 39–40, 66, 69,
    369–74, 602–3
    acanthosis nigricans type A
      syndrome 40, 369–72,
      539
    polymorphisms, NIDDM and
      67, **69–70**, 150
    regulation 359
Insulin receptors **357–74**
  antibodies 533, 544, 546,
    1081–2
  assessment of defects causing
    insulin resistance 1075–7
  autophosphorylation 362, 398–9
    effects of insulin 364
  biguanide actions 776–9
  biosynthesis and processing
    359–60
  genetic disorders 12, 369–74
  IDDM 368–9
  insulin binding to **361–2**
    aging and 1108–9
    assessment 1077
    exercise and 364, 727,
      735–6
    new drugs promoting 802
    NIDDM **366–8**, 536, **601**,
      1078–9
    obesity 366, 367, 535, 1078
    physical training and 364,
      735–6
    proinsulin affinity 320
  recycling and down regulation
    (internalization) 358,
    360–1, 388–9, 403–4, 489
  regulation **363–9**
    counterregulatory hormones
      365–6
    diet 364
    exercise 364, 727, 735–6
    insulin 361, 363–4, 365
  serine/threonine phosphorylation
    362, 363, 365, 398, 399
  signal transduction 362,
    397–403, 488–9, 600–1

NIDDM **601–3**
  structure 357–8, 488
    NIDDM 601–2
  tissue distribution 358–9
  tyrosine kinase activity 357,
    358, **362**, 363
    dietary effects 364
    glucocorticoids and 365
    IDDM 369
    NIDDM 367–8, 602
    obesity 366, 535
    role in insulin actions **398–9**,
      488–9
    type A severe insulin
      resistance 370–2
Insulin resistance 363, **531–46**
  acanthosis nigricans syndromes
    248, **369–72**, 539
  acromegaly 295, 375, 534
  aging and 288–9, 541, **1106–7**,
    1108
  androgens and **539–40**, 556–7,
    558, 559
  biguanide therapy and 775
  brittle diabetes 1062–3, 1068
  cellular 532, **534–41**, 1081
    assessment 1075–7
    NIDDM 366–7, 536–7,
      600–7, 1078–9
    treatment 1082
  clinical **1073–82**
  clinical approach 1079–82
  counterregulatory hormones
    inducing 365, **533–4**,
    1080
  definition 531–2, 1079
  diabetic complications and 542
  diabetic nephropathy and 540,
    1282, 1283
  diagnosis and investigation
    542–4, 1079–81
  exercise and 156, 545, 734–6,
    1664–5
  experimental methods of
    assessment 525–6, **1073–8**
  genetic syndromes associated
    with 38, 39–40, 248,
    369–74, 540
  glucose toxicity and **644–50**
    cellular mechanisms 648–50
    clinical implications 650
    correction of hyperglycaemia
      and 647–8
  haemochromatosis 203
  hepatic, *see* Liver, insulin
    sensitivity
  hyperglycaemic 542–3
  IDDM 368–9, **537–9**,
    1079–81
    acute untreated (without
      ketoacidosis) 538
    diabetic ketoacidosis 537–8
    glycaemic control and
      615–16, 650, 651

longstanding diabetes 538–9
  treatment 296, 546, 1081–2
insulin antibodies inducing 533,
  546, 836, 891, 1081
insulin secretion and 165,
  288–9
lipoatrophic diabetes syndromes
  373–4, 540
location of cause 1081
long-term follow-up and
  reassessment 1082
new drugs acting on 801–4
NIDDM 525–6, **535–7**, 569–70,
  578–90
  Asian Indians 179–80
  cellular mechanisms 366–7,
    536–7, **600–7**, 1078–9
  genetic susceptibility 66,
    167–8, 598–9, 600
  interactions with insulin
    secretion 292, 293–4,
    594–9
  lipid disturbances and 819,
    820
  non-cellular mechanisms
    607–16
  OGTT and 587–9
  risk factor for disease
    development 158–9,
    1662–3
  role in pathogenesis **166–8**,
    617–18
  site 581–6
  treatment 295–6, 546, 650,
    651, 1082
NIDDM-predisposed individuals
  66, 167, 599, 600
non-diabetics 63, 64
normoglycaemic/hyperinsulinaemic
  542
obesity 164, 167, 288, 1078
  abdominal type 542, 552,
    555–7
  cellular mechanism 366, **535**
  hyperandrogenaemia and
    539, 556–7
  NIDDM and 159
  treatment 1082
pancreas transplantation and
  919–20
pancreatectomized patients
  206
pathophysiological states
  532–41, 1078–9
  abnormal B cell secretory
    products 532
  diagnosis 542–4
  prereceptor antagonists of
    insulin action 532–4
  target cell defects, *see* Insulin
    resistance, cellular
physiological states inducing
  541
pregnancy 541, 1086, 1092

Insulin resistance (*cont.*)
 receptor/postreceptor mechanisms
   mediating, *see* Insulin
   resistance, cellular
 steroid-induced 289, 294, 365,
   533, 556–7
 stress-induced hypothalamic
   arousal and 562
 subcutaneous 1062, 1067–8,
   1081
 surgical trauma 1174
 treatment 544–6, 1081–2
 type A severe, *see* Acanthosis
   nigricans syndromes, type
   A
Insulin resistance syndrome
 (syndrome X) **534–5**
Insulin response, acute (AIR) 286
 to arginine 287
 to IV glucose (AIR$_{glucose}$),
   IDDM 290
 maximum potentiation (AIR$_{max}$)
   287
   NIDDM 293, 294
   NIDDM-predisposed
     individuals 295
 NIDDM 292–3, 294
 see also Insulin secretion, first-
   phase
Insulin secretagogues
 new pharmacological agents
   797–800
 non-glucose, chronic
   hyperglycaemia and
   637–9
 non-nutrient **273–8**
 nutrient
   identification 266
   metabolism in islet cells
     268–9
   proinsulin biosynthesis and
     262
   stimulation of insulin secretion
     266–73
Insulin secretion **285–97**
 acromegaly 295
 acute pancreatitis 199
 adrenergic pathway 274–6
 aging and **1107–8**
 amino acid-induced
   in vitro studies 277–8
   normal humans 287
 biguanide actions 775–6
 biphasic pattern 286
 cholinergic pathway 273–4, 288
 chronic pancreatitis 200–2
 C-peptide measurements as
   marker 303–5, **306–10**
 Cushing's syndrome 295
 cystic fibrosis 207
 deconvolution method of
   estimation 308–10
 diazoxide and 278
 drugs affecting **289–90**

exercise and 726, 728, 734
fat-mediated 287
first-phase
 abnormalities preceding IDDM
   onset 113–14, 290,
   1660
 actions of sulphonylureas
   746–9, 750
 NIDDM 166, 292, 571,
   573–4, 639
 pancreas grafts 917
 see also Insulin response,
   acute
"fuel" concept 266
glucagonoma 295
glucose (carbohydrate)-mediated
 286–7
glucose toxicity and, *see* Glucose
   toxicity, insulin secretion
haemochromatosis 203
IDDM 41, 42, 107–8, **290–1**,
 292, 1038
 C-peptide as measure **313–17**
 metabolic stability and
   1061–2
 urinary C-peptide as measure
   311, 313
IGT 164–6, 573, 574
insulin-mediated feedback
 inhibition 265
insulin resistance and 165,
 288–9
in vitro studies **261–80**
mechanism **262–4**
 dynamic aspects 264
 effector system 262–3
 role of protein kinases 263–4
minimal model method of
 estimation 310
MODY 72
neural regulation 288
NIDDM 41, 42, **291–5**, 639
 basal 291–2, 571–2
 C-peptide as measure 309,
   311
 effects of therapy 639, 650,
   651–3, 657
 genetic factors 66
 glucose toxicity and 654–6
 interactions with insulin
   sensitivity 292,
   293–4, 594–9
 natural history 164–6
 postprandial regulation
   292–3, 572–3
 pulsatile **574–5**
 role in pathogenesis 569,
   570–8, 618–19
 variability 65
NIDDM-predisposed individuals
 66–7, 294–5
non-nutrient pathways **273–8**
normal human
 basal 285–6

meal-related 286–8
variability 64
nutrient pathway **266–73**, 749
 coupling of metabolic to distal
   events 269–73
 identification of nutrient
   secretagogues 266
 regulation of glucose
   metabolism 266–9
obesity 279, 553
 subgroups 551–3
pancreas transplantation and
 918–19
pancreatectomized patients
 206
pancreatic carcinoma 204
peptidergic pathway 276–7
phaeochromocytoma 295
in populations, variability 64
pregnancy 1086
regulation 261
 basal state 285–6
 hypoglycaemia 1138
 insulin resistance and 288–9
 long-term 278–80
 meal-related 286–8
 somatostatin and 276, 287, 288,
   344
 sulphonylurea-mediated 278,
   290
 acute effects **746–9**
 chronic effects **749–50**
surgical trauma 1174
treatment implications 295–7
urinary C-peptide as measure
 311–13
Insulin sensitivity
 assessment **513–26**, **1073–8**,
   1106–7
   direct methods 425, 514,
     519–22, 1074–8
   indirect methods 513–19
   specific tissues 524–5
 biguanide actions 776–9
 chronic pancreatitis 202
 exercise and 727–8, **734–6**
 extrahepatic 525
 glucose clamp-based measures
   522–4, 1074–5
 hepatic 167, 524–5, 555,
   581–3
 insulin therapy and 295–6, 546,
   614–16
 minimal model approach 424,
   517–19, 1077, 1107
 new drugs promoting 801–4
 NIDDM, *see* Insulin resistance,
   NIDDM
 pancreatectomized patients
   204–6
 pancreatic diabetes 208
 sulphonylurea actions 545,
   614–15, **750–2**
 see also Insulin resistance

Insulin sensitivity index (S_{IP}) 523, 1077
Insulin suppression test 425, **520–1**, 578–9, 1073–4
Insulin therapy **831–59**
  after myocardial infarction 1194–6, 1197, 1499–500
  artificial endocrine pancreas **871–9**, 979
  brittle diabetes **1066–8**
  chemistry and manufacture of insulin 832–4
  children and adolescents 851–2, **1037–40**, 1061
  complications **883–91**
    allergy to retarding agents 889–90
    glycogen-laden hepatomegaly 891
    injection site problems 885–7
    insulin allergy 836, 884–5, 887–8
    insulin antibodies, *see* Insulin antibodies
    insulin oedema 891
    lipoatrophy 836, 886, 888–9
    refractive changes 891
  continuous subcutaneous infusion, *see* Subcutaneous insulin infusion, continuous
  control systems, *see* Insulin delivery systems
  diabetic ketoacidosis 1032–3, **1155–6**
  diabetic neuropathic cachexia 1397
  dietary management and 854, 876
  dosage adjustments, *see* Insulin dosage adjustments
  dose, *see* Insulin dose
  elderly patients 850, 851, 1123
  exercise and **729–33**, 876
    clinical implications 730–3, 738
    pathophysiology 729–30
  gestational diabetes 1097
  "honeymoon period" in IDDM 290, 296, 313, 314, 850, 1038
  hyperosmolar non-ketotic coma 1160
  immunogenicity 834–6
  initiation 958–9
    children and adolescents 1037–8
    patient education **937**, 941
  injection regimens 844–54
    basal/bolus (multiple daily injections) 851, 1040
    children and adolescents 851–2, 1037–8

    choice of insulin preparation 847–9
    once-daily 849–50
    physiological plasma insulin profiles and 845–7
    special groups of patients 851–3
    surgery 1050–1, 1177
    twice-daily 850–1
  insulin sensitivity and 295–6, 546, 614–16
  intensive 851, 1040
    albumin excretion rates and 1298
    blood glucose self-monitoring 972
    cardiovascular complications and 1478–9
    children and adolescents 1040
    diabetic retinopathy progression and 1344–8
    disadvantages 1133, 1239, 1241
    hypoglycaemia awareness and 1135, 1136
    lipid/lipoprotein profiles and 450, 823
    microvascular disease progression and 1234–9
    NIDDM 653
    pregnancy 1092
    preservation of B-cell function in IDDM 115, 316–17
    see also Glycaemic control; Subcutaneous insulin infusion, continuous
  intraperitoneal 866, 1306
  labour and delivery 1094–5
  NIDDM
    injection regimens 850
    insulin sensitivity and 295–6, 546, 614–16
    lipid/lipoprotein profiles and 454, 823–4
    obese patients 852
  optimizing **874–9**
    acceptable limits for glucose control 875
    computer-implemented dose adjustments 877–8
    human component 875–7
    insulins and glucose-measuring instruments 875
  oral hypoglycaemic agents combined with 297, 764–5, 1123
  pancreatic diabetes 215–16
  pharmacological preparations, *see* Insulin preparations
  pregnancy 852, **1092**, 1096
  proinsulin levels and 306
  protein deficient diabetes mellitus 181

  psychological aspects 854
  routes of administration 840, **865–8**
  subcutaneous injection, *see* Subcutaneous insulin injection
  sulphonylureas combined with 297, 764–5, 1123
  sulphonylureas vs. 763
  surgery 1174, 1176
  visually impaired diabetics 1383
Insulin tolerance test (ITT) **519**, 542–3, 1080–1
Insulin-zinc suspensions **838–9**
  absorption 842–3
  crystalline (ultralente) 837, 838, 848
  mixed (lente) 837, 838, 848
Insulitis
  experimental 232, 238
  IDDM 60, 231, 234
  transplanted islets/pancreas 239, 904
Insurance **1631–3**
Integrins 674
Intellectual ability
  children of diabetic mothers 1098
  hypoglycaemia and 1144
  patient education and 927
Intercostal nerve palsy 1398
α-Interferon, B-cell destruction and 236
Interleukin-1 (IL-1)
  AGE-induced production 674, 675, 676
  glucose toxicity and 1280
Intermediate-density lipoproteins (IDL) 439
Interview skills, training 1590, 1591
Intestinal function, biguanide actions 784–5
Intralipid infusion 607, 608, 609
Intramuscular insulin infusion, continuous 1067
Intramuscular insulin injection 865
  absorption 840, 844
  diabetic ketoacidosis 1032–3, 1155–6
  unintentional 885
Intranasal insulin administration **867**, 1038–9
Intraperitoneal (IP) insulin delivery **866**, 867, 1067
Intraretinal microvascular abnormalities (IRMA) 1333–4, 1335
Intravenous fluids
  diabetic ketoacidosis 1032, 1155
  high rates 1036–7, 1157

Intravenous fluids (*cont.*)
  glucose-containing 1177
  hyperosmolar non-ketotic coma
    1160
  intercurrent illness 1049
Intravenous glucose administration,
  see Glucose administration,
  intravenous
Intravenous glucose tolerance test
  (IVGTT) 22, 423–5
  advantages 287
  assessment of insulin sensitivity
    517–19
  disadvantages 424
  frequent sampling (FSIGT) 424,
    517–19, 1107
  NIDDM 571
  prediction of IDDM development
    113–14
  prediction of NIDDM
    development 166
Intravenous insulin infusions
  866–7
  after myocardial infarction
    1499–500
    diabetics 1194–6, 1197
    non-diabetics 1202
  continuous (CIVII) 866–7,
    1067
  diabetic ketoacidosis 1032–3,
    1155–6
  glucose potassium and insulin
    (GKI) **1178–9**, 1180–1,
    1195
  surgery 1177–8, 1180
Introns 469
Inuit, *see* Eskimos
Ion-exchange chromatography,
  glycated haemoglobin
  measurement 991–2, 1043
Iontophoresis of insulin 868
Iron deficiency anaemia, glycated
  haemoglobin levels and 999
Iron deposition, excessive 203–4,
  247
Ischaemia
  diabetic nerve 1391
  resistance of diabetic nerve to
    1392
Ischaemic foot, *see* Foot, ischaemic
Ischaemic heart disease, *see*
  Coronary artery disease
Islet amyloidosis
  B-cell function and 576
  NIDDM 239, 240, 241, 242,
    244–5
  type 1 diabetes 232
Islet amyloid polypeptide (IAPP,
  amylin) 225–6, 240, 242,
  244
  insulin resistance in NIDDM and
    611–12
  insulin secretion in NIDDM and
    576

Islet cell antibodies (ICA) 16,
  110–11, 112, 1659
  before onset of IDDM 9, 57–8,
    107
  diagnosis of IDDM 8, 41, 42,
    317, 1030
  IDDM in Asia 123
  IDDM subtypes 48
  IDDM in tropical countries 178
  monitoring, children at risk of
    IDDM 1030
  North American Indians 133
  pathogenesis of IDDM and 232,
    239, 1027
  predictive value 57–8, 74, 75,
    111, 1579
  protein deficient diabetes mellitus
    181
  standardized assay 111
Islet cell surface antibodies (ICSA)
  123, 232, 1659
Islets of Langerhans **223–30**
  anatomy 226–7
  blood flow 227–30
  chronic pancreatitis 200, 245–7
  congenital absence 38, 245
  cystic fibrosis 207, 247, 248
  diabetes-related morphological
    changes **231–50**
  embryology and fetal
    development 224
  endocrine cell types 225–6
  evolutionary origin 224–5
  fibrocalculous pancreatic diabetes
    186
  IDDM **231–9**
    aetiology and pathogenesis of
      changes 232–9
    macroscopic changes 231
    microscopic changes 231–2
    pancreas transplantation and
      57, 232, **239**
  innervation 230
  isolated 261–2
  NIDDM **239–45**
    aetiology and pathogenesis of
      changes 242–5
    microscopic changes 239–42
  non-diabetes-related
    morphological changes
    251–2
  non-endocrine cells 230
  obesity and 241, 244
  regeneration 252
Islet transplantation **895–908**
  clinical trials 906–7
  effect on diabetic complications
    900–1
  fetal and neonatal 905–6
  future prospects 907–8
  islet isolation and transplantation
    techniques 896–7, 907
  metabolic function 897–900
    canine studies 898–9

    rat studies 898
    simian studies 899–900
  recurrent autoimmune disease
    904–5
  rejection 901–3, 907–8
    mechanisms 901–2
    prevention 902–3
3-Isobutyl-1-methylxanthine
  (IBMX) 638
Isoelectric focusing, glycated
  haemoglobin assay 992–3
Isophane (NPH) 837, **838**
  absorption 842
  childhood diabetes 1037–8
  clinical applications 848–9
  immunogenicity 889, 890
Isoprenaline (isoproterenol) 274,
  287, 365, 638
"Isotope effect", glucose tracer
  studies 524
Israel
  IDDM frequency 101, 140,
    141
  NIDDM frequency 152, 179
IVGTT, *see* Intravenous glucose
  tolerance test

Japan
  autoantibodies in IDDM 123
  dietary management of diabetes
    707–9
  genetic factors in IDDM 124
  HLA and IDDM associations
    122, 142
  IDDM frequency **117–19**, 122,
    140, 141
  north–south gradient in
    IDDM/multiple sclerosis
    prevalence 124
  risk of IDDM development
    100, 101
Japanese Americans
  IDDM frequency 136
  NIDDM frequency 152
  physiological studies 65–6
Japanese Diabetes Society (JDS)
  dietary recommendations 708
  food exchange lists 708–9
Japanese Hawaiians
  NIDDM frequency 152
  NIDDM risk factors 157
Japanese sumo wrestlers 157
Joint, neuropathic (Charcot joint)
  1537, **1540–1**
Joint disease **1418**
Joint mobility, limited (LJM)
  1420, **1421–8**
  association with microvascular
    disease 1425–6
  biochemical studies 1426
  cardiac function and 1424
  constitutional vs. metabolic
    causes 1426–8
  differential diagnosis 1423–4

Joint mobility, limited (LJM) (*cont.*)
    examination and classification
        1421–2
    fibrous breast disease and
        1424–5
    growth effects 1423
    natural history 1422–3
    neuropathy and 1424
    pulmonary changes and 1424
    skin changes 1425
J-type diabetes, *see* Protein deficient
    diabetes mellitus

Kearns–Sayre mitochondrial
    myopathy 39
Kemptide kinase 399, 400
Kenya, IDDM frequency 138
Ketoacidosis, alcoholic 1158
Ketoacidosis, diabetic (DKA)
    1151–9
    children **1030–7**
    complications of treatment
        1157–8
        adult respiratory distress
            syndrome 1158
        cerebral oedema 1035–7,
            1157–8
        fluid overload 1157
    diagnosis and assessment
        1031–2, 1154
    elderly patients 1115–16
    epidemiology 1151–2
    factitious 1064
    fibrocalculous pancreatic diabetes
        184, 186
    IDDM subtypes 48
    insulin receptor function and
        369
    insulin resistance in 537–8
    mortality 1151–2, 1215, 1613
    myocardial infarction and 1189,
        1194, 1499
    pancreatic diabetes 208–9,
        212–13
    pathophysiology 464–5, **1152–4**
    precipitating factors 858, 1041,
        1152
    prevention 1031, 1158–9
    problems in diagnosis and
        management 143, 1158
    recurrent 1152
        causes 1031
        treatment 1066–7
        see also Brittle diabetes
    residual B-cell function and
        314
    treatment **1155–7**
        bicarbonate 1034, 1036,
            1156
        children 1032–7
        electrolytes 1033–4, 1156
        fluid replacement 1032,
            1155
        insulin 1032–3, 1155–6

    monitoring 1034–5, 1156–7
    without hyperglycaemia 1158
Keto-Diabur-Test 5000 967
KetoDiastix 967, 968
Ketogenesis
    extrahepatic tissues 463
    glucagon-induced 335
    hepatic 461–2
    insulin actions 463–4
    regulation 459, 461–2
α-Ketoisocaproate (KIC) 480
Ketonaemia
    diabetic ketoacidosis 1031
    pregnant women during fasting
        1087
Ketone bodies (ketones)
    antilipolytic effects 460
    glomerular filtration rate and
        1285
    glucose urine testing and 969
    insulin secretion and 288
    methylpalmoxirate actions
        805–6
    pancreatic diabetes 209, 210
    peripheral utilization 463, 464
    physiological plasma profiles
        846, 847
    smell on breath 1154
    urine testing, *see* Urine testing,
        ketones
Ketone body metabolism **459–66**
    diabetic ketoacidosis and 1153
    regulation 459–63
        adipose tissue 460, 461, 463
        extrahepatic tissues 463, 464
        liver 461–2, 463–4
    role of insulin 463–4
Ketonuria 1042
    diabetic ketoacidosis 1031
    exercise and 1041
    pregnancy 1092
Ketosis
    immunological effects 1166–7
    NIDDM 9
    protein deficient diabetes mellitus
        181
Ketosis-resistant diabetes of the
    young, *see* Malnutrition
    related diabetes mellitus
Ketostix 967
Kidd blood group 46
Kidney capsule
    fetal pancreas transplantation
        905
    islet implantation 897, 898
Kidney enlargement, *see* Renal
    hypertrophy
Kidneys
    amino acid flux 496, 497
    C-peptide extraction 307, 311
    glucose disposal in basal state
        421
    glucose transport 412
    proinsulin clearance 319

    protein synthesis 476
Klinefelter's syndrome 39, 1028
Knowledge
    propositional 1589
    tacit 1589, 1590
Kobberling–Dunnegan syndrome
    (familial partial lipodystrophy)
        38
Korea, IDDM prevalence and
    incidence **119**
Kuwait, IDDM frequency 101,
    122, 139, 140

Labetalol, pregnancy 1093,
    1094
Laboratory facilities, India 1604
Labour
    management 1094–5
    premature 1094
Lactate
    antilipolytic effects 460
    hepatic glucose production and
        418
    incorporation into glucose
        416–17
    metabolism, biguanide actions
        780–1
    production 422, 435–6, 585
Lactation 1095
    insulin release 279
Lactic acidosis
    biguanide-associated 773,
        789–91
    diabetic ketoacidosis 1153
    metformin-associated (MALA)
        789–91, 1122
Lamina densa 1246
Lamina rara 1246
Laminin
    changes in diabetes 674, 1252,
        1255
    characteristics 1246, 1249,
        1250
    diabetic nephropathy 1292
    glycation 1254
    vascular wall 1438
Language problems, India 1603
Laron dwarfism 38
Laser photocoagulation therapy, *see*
    Photocoagulation therapy
Lawrence–Moon–Biedl–Bardet
    (Bardet–Biedl) syndrome 39,
        248, 1028
Lead-time bias, evaluation of
    screening programmes 1571
Leaflets, educational 934
Lean body mass, aging and 1109,
    1110
Learned hopelessness, blood
    glucose self-monitoring 939
Lecithin cholesterol acyltransferase
    (LCAT) 443, 445
Ledderhose disease 1419
Legal issues 961–2, 1635–6

Leg perfusion technique
  glucose disposal in NIDDM
    585, 586, 593
  protein metabolism 483, 484
Length bias, evaluation of screening
    programmes 1571
Lens implant surgery 1112–13,
    1370
Lente insulin 837, 838
  clinical applications 848
Leprechaunism 38, 40, 248
  insulin receptor defects 371,
    372–3
  insulin resistance 372–3, 540
Leucine
  stimulation of protein synthesis
    478
  tracers, measurement of protein
    metabolism 480, 481, 482,
    483
Life-insurance 1219–20, **1631–3**
Life problems **1631–40**
Life-style
  promotion of healthier 1667
  Westernized, NIDDM
    development and 34, 153,
    160–1
Lignocaine derivatives 1401
Limited joint mobility, *see* Joint
    mobility, limited
Linkage, genetic 43–4
Linkage disequilibrium 44
  IDDM markers 48, 53, 132
Linogliride 798–9, 802–3
γ-Linolenic acid 1401
Lipid(s)
  diabetic nerve 1388–9
  insulin secretion and 287
  serum
    atherogenesis and 1472–3
    biguanide therapy and 781,
      782–3
    children with IDDM 1044
    diabetes 817–18
    monitoring 821
    pancreatic diabetes 209
    screening 820–1
    sulphonylurea therapy and
      752
    target values in diabetes 821
  see also Cholesterol; Fatty
      acid(s), free; Triglycerides
Lipid-lowering agents, *see*
    Hypolipidaemic agents
Lipid metabolism
  biguanide actions 781–4
  insulin actions 385, **391–5**,
    422–3
  pancreatic diabetes 208–9
  see also Fatty acid oxidation;
      Fatty acid synthesis
Lipid transfer protein (LTP) 447
Lipoatrophic diabetes syndromes
    37, 38, 248

insulin receptor defects **373–4**
insulin resistance 373–4, 540
Lipoatrophy, injection site 836,
    886, **888–9**
Lipodystrophy
  congenital generalized, insulin
    resistance 540
  familial partial (Kobberling–
    Dunnegan syndrome) 38
  partial, with Rieger's syndrome
    38
Lipohypertrophy
  brittle diabetes and 1062, 1066
  injection sites 844, **886–7**
Lipolysis (triacylglycerol breakdown)
  basal state 422–3
  biguanide therapy and 781–4
  hormonal regulation 335, 460,
    461
  insulin actions 391, **394**, 463
  visceral fat depots 554
Lipomatosis, symmetric 39
Lipoprotein(s) **439–55**
  composition 440–3
  serum profiles
    advancing renal disease
      1290–1
    atherogenesis and 1472–3
    biguanide therapy and 781,
      782–3
    diabetes 817–18
    fibrocalculous pancreatic
      diabetes 185
    glycaemic control and 822–4
    microalbuminuria and 1289
    pancreatic diabetes 209
    sex differences 1491
    sodium–lithium
      countertransporter
      activity and 1282
  structure and classification
    439–40
  see also High-density
      lipoproteins; Low-density
      lipoproteins; Very low-
      density lipoproteins
Lipoprotein lipase (LPL) 1450
  hypertriglyceridaemia and
    1494–5
  IDDM 819
  insulin actions 402, 449, 450
  metabolic function 440, 441,
    442, 445
  molecular biology 448
  NIDDM 455, 819
  steroid hormones and 560
Lipoprotein metabolism 440–3
  apolipoproteins and 443–5
  cholesterol transfer proteins 447
  diabetes 818–20
  endogenous
    hypertriglyceridaemia 451
  endogenous pathway 441–3
  enzymes 445

exogenous pathway 440–1
hyperinsulinaemic states 450–5
IDDM 450
insulin actions **448–55**
molecular biology and 447–8
NIDDM 452–5
obesity 451–2
receptors 445–7
reverse cholesterol transport
    pathway 443
Literacy, developing countries
    715, **1603**
Liver
  amino acid flux 496, 497
  C-peptide extraction 306–7
  glucagon actions 335
  glucose production, *see* Glucose
      production, hepatic
  glucose transport 412, 603
  glucose uptake
    basal state 421
    NIDDM **583–5**, 586, 587
    oral glucose load 434–5
  glycogen 412
  glycogen synthesis 436
  insulin effects on mRNA levels
    396
  insulin extraction, *see* Insulin,
      hepatic extraction
  insulin sensitivity
    abdominal obesity 555
    assessment 524–5
    NIDDM 167, 581–93
  islet grafts 898–9
  ketogenesis
    insulin actions 463–4
    regulation 461–2
  lipid metabolism 391, 393,
    394–5
  proinsulin extraction 319
  protein degradation 474, 477,
    478, 483
  protein synthesis 483
  ribosomal protein synthesis
    495
Liver disease, glucose potassium
    and insulin infusion 1178,
    1179
Liver transplantation, islet
    transplantation and 907
Locus of control 925–6
Lovastatin 825, 827
Low-density lipoprotein (LDL)
    receptors 443, 445–6, 448,
    1494
Low-density lipoproteins (LDL)
    439, 440
  accumulation in blood vessel
    walls 672
  benefits of reduction 821–2
  biguanide therapy and 781,
    782–3
  cardiovascular disease risk and
    1493–4

Low-density lipoproteins (LDL)
(*cont.*)
dietary fat intake and 691–2,
693
glycaemic control and 823
glycation 454, 819–20, 1441,
1494, 1496
hepatic synthesis 553, 554
IDDM 450, 818
insulin actions 449, 450
metabolism **441–3**, 445, 446
diabetes **819–20**, 1473
NIDDM 452, 453–4, 818
obesity 451
receptor-mediated uptake and
processing 445–6
small dense 1494
subfractions 439–40, 441
Lower extremity
examination 1510–12
ischaemic 1541–4
see also Foot
Low-molecular weight mediators,
insulin actions 389, 390–1,
402–3
Lp(a) antigen 67, 70, 445
Lumbar sympathectomy, foot
ischaemia 1544
Lundh meal test, tropical calcific
pancreatitis 187
Lymphocytes
function in diabetes 1166,
1167–8
insulin receptors 365
Lysosomes, protein degradation
474–5, 496
Lysyl hydroxylase activity
1279

Machado disease (ataxia) 39
Macrophages
AGE-modified protein receptors
674–5, 1278
atherogenesis and 1495
binding of glycated LDL 1441
Macrosomia, fetal, *see* Fetal
macrosomia
Macrovascular disease
(macroangiopathy)
acute events **1185–204**
concept of specific diabetic
1435–6, 1444
elderly **1115–16**
epidemiology **1459–65**
experimental diabetes 1439–40
fibrocalculous pancreatic diabetes
186
in vitro tissue culture studies
1441–3
metabolic changes in
experimental diabetes
1440–1
metabolic control and **1471–81**,
1490, 1495–6

morphological abnormalities
1436–9
mortality and morbidity in IDDM
1461–2
mortality and morbidity in
NIDDM 180, 1463–5
pathogenesis **1435–44**
pathology 1489–90
prevention 1558, 1580, 1667
see also Atherosclerosis;
Cerebrovascular disease;
Coronary artery disease;
Peripheral vascular disease
Macular degeneration, senile 1112
Macular oedema 1331–3
diabetes type and duration and
1342
photocoagulation 1349, 1350,
1355–6, 1381, 1552
screening 1552
visual impairment and 1331–3,
1379, 1382
Maillard fluorescent product 1
(MFP-1) 671
Major histocompatibility complex,
see MHC
Malaria 1152
Malaysia **1607–10**
IDDM frequency **120–1**, 138
organization of health care
1607–8
problems of organization of
diabetes care 1608–10
Malic enzyme 492
Malingering 1063–4
Malnutrition
cancer-associated, insulin
resistance and 541
fibrocalculous pancreatic diabetes
and 183, 188
Malnutrition related diabetes
mellitus (MRDM) 4, **11**, 200
age at onset 34
problems of management
1602–3
sex ratio 35
tropical countries 177, **180–90**
Malonyl-CoA 392, 393, 462, 463
Mammary gland
insulin effects on mRNA levels
396
lipid metabolism 391
pyruvate dehydrogenase activity
390
Manipulative behaviour 1063–4,
1080
Mannitol, intravenous 1037
Mannoheptulose 249
Mannose, anomeric specificity of
insulin response 266
MAP-2 kinase 399, 400
Marriages, consanguinous 1602
Massage, insulin absorption and
843

Maturity onset diabetes of young
(MODY) 42, **71–2**, 190,
1029
Asian Indians 10, 35, 71, 179,
1602
black Americans 10, 133
clinical variability 72
epidemiology
age at onset 34
ethnic and geographic
differences 35
incidence and prevalence 33
sex ratio 35
genetic counselling 75, 1029
genetics 71–2, 151
Mauriac syndrome 248
Mauritius, NIDDM prevalence
150
Meal patterns, Africa 712–13, 716
Meal planning 696
children and adolescents 1040–1
India and South East Asia 706
insulin therapy and 848, 850,
854, 1038
sulphonylurea therapy and 755
see also Dietary management
Mean amplitude of glycaemic
excursions (MAGE) 1060
Mean of daily differences (MODD)
in blood glucose 1060
Medial arterial calcification, *see*
Arterial calcification, medial
Medial plantar sensory action
potential (MPSAP) 1394
Medicolegal issues 961–2, 1635–6
Mediterranean islands 102
Megaloblastic anaemia
biguanide-induced 784–5
thiamine responsive (with
deafness) 38
Melaena, glycated haemoglobin and
999
Membranous nephropathy,
concurrent 1295
Meningovirus 1660
Menstrual disorders, brittle diabetes
1066
Mental retardation, children of
diabetic mothers 1098
Mental status, diabetic ketoacidosis
1031, 1154
Mesangial hypertrophy
adverse effects 1254
pathogenesis 1280, 1281
pathological appearance 1293,
1294
proteinuria and 1259
Mesangial matrix, changes in
diabetes 1252–3, 1279
Messenger RNA (mRNA)
non-transcriptional regulation by
insulin 492–3
posttranscriptional processing
469–70

Messenger RNA (mRNA) (*cont.*)
   synthesis   468–70
      insulin actions   396–7, 490–2
      translation   470–3
         regulation by insulin   493–4
Metabolic acidosis, diabetic
   ketoacidosis   1153
Metabolic control, *see* Glycaemic
   control
Metabolism, inborn errors   38
Metageria   39
Metformin   773–4, 1303
   adverse effects   789–91
   elderly patients   1120, 1121,
      1122–3
   insulin resistance and   545
   pharmacodynamics   774–85
   pharmacokinetics   785–6
   sulphonylureas vs.   763
   surgery and   1176
   therapeutic use   786–9
   see also Biguanides
Metformin-associated lactic acidosis
   (MALA)   789–91, 1122
Methionine, protein synthesis and
   478
Methionine-tRNA (Met-tRNA)
   471, 472, 473
Methyl-2-tetradecylglycidate
   (methylpalmoxirate)   805–7
Methyl 4-hydroxybenzoate   837–8,
   839
2-(3-Methyl-cinnamylhydrazone)-
   propionate   804
Methyldopa, pregnancy   1093–4
Metoclopramide   1404
Mexican Americans, *see*
   Hispanic/Mexican Americans
Mexiletine   1401
MHC
   class I antigens, hyperexpression
      on islet cells   235–6
   class II antigens, aberrant
      expression on pancreatic
      B cells   109, 233–5, 236
   compatibility, islet allograft
      rejection and   901, 904
   see also HLA
Microalbuminuria   **1272–4**
   antihypertensive therapy   1219,
      1296–7
   children and adolescents
      1052
   concomitants   1288–9
   detection   1554–5
   dietary protein restriction
      693–5, 1298, 1553–4
   glycaemic control and
      progression   1218–19,
      1235, 1236, 1273–4,
      1298–9, 1554
   hypertension and   1466, 1522–3,
      1524–5, 1554
   pathophysiology   **1287–9**

Microaneurysms, retinal capillary
   1329–31, 1332, 1358
Microencapsulation, grafted islets
   902
β_2-Microglobulin, urinary excretion
   1287, 1290
Microneurography   1394
Micronutrients   690, 696
   fibrocalculous pancreatic diabetes
      and   189
Microtubular–microfilamentous
   system, pancreatic B cells
   263
Microvascular disease
   children and adolescents   1051–2
   diabetic nerve   **1390–2**
   effect of pregnancy on   1091
   foot   1541–2
   heart   1490
   hypertension and   1230, 1524–7
   limited joint mobility and
      1425–6
   pancreatic diabetes   213–15
   pathogenesis   **1225–41**, 1261
      capillary basement membrane
         changes and   1258–60
      clinical studies   1233–9
      epidemiological studies
         1226–8
      hypotheses   1228–33
   pregnancy complications and
      1088
   prevention in NIDDM   1580
   tropical countries   180
   see also Nephropathy, diabetic;
      Neuropathy, diabetic;
      Retinopathy, diabetic
Middle East, IDDM frequency
   139
Migrant populations   35
   IDDM   102, 103
   NIDDM frequency   **151–3**
Military services   1637
Mineral intake   690, 696
Minimal model approach
   insulin secretion rates   310
   insulin sensitivity   424, 517–19,
      1077, 1107
Mitochondrial myopathy, Kearns–
   Sayre   39
Mitochondrial oxidative events, islet
   cells   268
MK-678 (somatostatin analogue)
   342
Mönckeberg's sclerosis, *see* Arterial
   calcification, medial
Monoacylglycerol lipase   394, 460
Monoamine oxidase inhibitors
   804
Monocytes
   atherogenesis and   1472, 1495
   insulin receptors   364, 369
   islets of Langerhans   230
Mononeuropathies   1367–8, 1398

Mortality
   diabetic ketoacidosis   1151–2,
      1215, 1613
   economic costs   1650, 1651
   IDDM   1213–14
   myocardial infarction in diabetics
      1186–8
Mothers, diabetic
   risks of diabetes in offspring
      72–3, 74, 1028, 1097
   see also Infants of diabetic
      mothers; Pregnancy
Motilin   204
Motor neuropathy
   diffuse symmetrical   1398
   proximal   1398
Motor vehicle accidents   1633,
   1634
mRNA, *see* Messenger RNA
Mucormycosis, rhinoculocerebral
   1166
Multiple endocrine
   adenomatosis/neoplasia
   syndrome   38, 40
Multiple sclerosis, epidemiology in
   prevalence   124
Mumps virus   49, 59, 1026, 1660
Muscarinic receptors, islet cells
   273
Muscle, skeletal
   amino acid flux   496–7, 498,
      499
   calcitonin gene-related peptide
      levels   612
   capillary basement membrane
      thickening   1229–30, 1231,
      1237, 1238, 1258–9
      distance below heart level and
         1251, 1257
      sex hormones and   1258
   capillary density
      abdominal obesity   556
      NIDDM   610–11
      physical training and   736
   endothelial insulin transport,
      NIDDM   610–11
   exercising
      fatty acid uptake   728
      fuel sources   726
      glucose uptake   **726–8**, 735–6
   fibre type composition
      abdominal obesity   555–6
      NIDDM   610–11
      steroid hormones and   556–7
   glucose transport   603–4
   glucose uptake
      basal state   421, 422
      biguanide actions   779
      capillary density and   610
      exercise and   726–8, 735–6
      hyperglycaemia and   648,
         649–50
      insulin-mediated   426–7, 428
      NIDDM   **585–6**, 587–8, 593

Muscle, skeletal (*cont.*)
glycogen 412
glycogen synthesis in NIDDM
605–6
insulin receptors
NIDDM 367–8
obesity 366, 367
insulin sensitivity
abdominal obesity 555–6
measurement 525
protein degradation 474–5, 477,
478, 483
protein synthesis 476, 477, 478,
483, 493–4
pyruvate dehydrogenase 390
ribosomal protein synthesis 495
Muscle fasciculation 1398
Muscle strength, testing 1393
Muscle wasting 1397, 1398
Muscle weakness 1397
Muscular dystrophies 39, 540
Muslim women 1604
M value (index of blood sugar
control) 1060
M values, *see* Glucose disposal
rates
Mycobacterium cheloni, injection
site infections 886
Myelin
destruction 1386
glycation 1389
Myelin basic protein kinase 399
Myocardial infarction **1185–97**,
1215, 1498–500
causes of poor prognosis
1191–4
complications 1498–9
diabetic ketoacidosis and 1189,
1194, 1499
elderly 1115
hospital mortality 1186–8
hospital outcome vs. patient
characteristics 1190
hyperglycaemia after 15,
1197–202
determinants and importance
1198–201
diabetic patients 1190, 1194
management in non-diabetics
1201–2
undiagnosed diabetes and
1197–8
intervention studies 1194
long-term prognosis 1194, 1500
management 1194–7, 1499–500
mode of death 1188–9
referral patterns 1193–4
silent 1190–1, 1497–8
site 1191, 1461, 1499
size 1191, 1199
spontaneous coronary artery
reperfusion 1192
Myocardial ischaemia, silent
1497–8

Myofibrillar proteins, degradation
474–5, 477, 478
Myo-inositol
diabetic neuropathy and
1387–8, 1389
dietary supplementation 1279
reduced intracellular 1255, 1278
Myopathy, late-onset proximal (with
cataracts) 39
Myopic shifts 891, 1371
Myotonic dystrophy 38, 540

Na^+, K^+-ATPase 269–70, 1255,
1387, 1392
$NADH/NAD^+$ ratio
pancreatic B cells 269–70
Randle cycle and 607, 608
$NADPH/NADP^+$ ratio, pancreatic B
cells 269–70
Nasal insulin administration **867**,
1038–9
National Diabetes Data Group
(NDDG) 3, 23
IDDM subclass 132
National Diabetes Data Group
(NDDG)/World Health
Organization (WHO)
classification system 3, 4–6,
7–8
diagnostic glycaemic criteria
20, 23–4, 1104
standard oral glucose tolerance
test 26, 1578
National Health and Nutrition
Examination Survey
(NHANES II, 1976–80) 32,
1104–5
National Health Interview Surveys
32, 130, 155
National Medical Care Expenditure
Survey (NMCES) 1646–7,
1649–50
National Medical Care Utilization
and Expenditure Survey
(NMCUES) 1647, 1649–50
Naunyn's diabetes (cirrhosis and
diabetes) 248
Nauruans
genetic susceptibility to NIDDM
65, 1662
IGT 158
insulin secretion 164–5
NIDDM frequency 34, 62
screening for NIDDM 1575
Neonatal diabetes 245, 1028
Neonatal pancreas transplantation
905–6
Neonates **1095**
glucagon levels 337
morbidity 1095
proinsulin levels 320, 322
routine care 1095
Neoprene, pancreatic duct injection
915, 916, 918

Nephropathy, diabetic **1267–308**,
1553–5
aminoguanidine therapy and
677
cardiovascular disease and 1276
IDDM 1216, 1217, 1218,
1269, 1462, 1478
NIDDM 1271
cause of death 1216
children and adolescents 1052
clinical (late phase) **1274–5**
see also Proteinuria
clinical course and natural
history 1271–6
early phase **1271–4**
elderly **1113–14**
end-stage renal failure, *see* Renal
failure, end-stage
epidemiology 1267–71
foot problems 1276, 1544
genetic susceptibility 1219,
1230–1, 1281–3
glycaemic control and 1233,
1298–9, 1553
epidemiological studies
1227–8
glomerular hyperfiltration
1271, 1299
progression of
microalbuminuria and
1218–19, 1235, 1236,
1273–4, 1298–9, 1554
renal hypertrophy 1272, 1299
transplantation studies
1231–2
hypertension and, *see*
Hypertension, diabetic
nephropathy and
incipient, *see* Microalbuminuria
insulin resistance and 540,
1282, 1283
islet transplantation and 900–1
mortality and 1214–16
non-renal complications 1275
other glomerular diseases in
diabetics 1295
other manifestations of diabetic
renal disease 1299–302
pancreas transplantation and
895–6, 1232
pancreatic diabetes 213–14
pathogenesis 1261, **1276–83**
basement membrane changes
1258–9, 1279
familial and genetic pathways
1281–3
glucotoxicity 1279–80
haemodynamic and
hypertrophic pathways
1280–1
hyperglycaemia and non-
enzymatic glycation
1276–8
polyol pathway 1278–9

Nephropathy, diabetic (*cont.*)
  pathogenesis of hypertension
      1522–3
  pathology   1291–5
    electron microscopy   1292–3
    immunopathology   1292
    light microscopy   1291–2
    structure in relation to
        function   1293–4
  pathophysiology   1283–91
  pregnancy and   1086, 1091,
      1301
  prevention   1271, 1553–4
  renal biopsy, indications for
      1294–5
  retinopathy and (renal–retinal
      syndrome)   1216–17, 1275,
      1294
  risk factors   1228
  screening   960, 1554–5
  treatment   **1296–9**
    blood pressure control, *see*
        Antihypertensive therapy,
        diabetic nephropathy
    dietary   693, 1297–8
    early (secondary prevention)
        1218–19, 1235, 1236,
        1298–9, 1554
    glycaemic control   1298–9
Nephrotic syndrome, glycated
    protein levels and   1000
Nephrotoxicity, radiological contrast
    media   1512–13
Nerve conduction velocity (CV)
  aldose reductase inhibitors and
      1390
  biochemical mechanisms of
      changes   1387–8
  glycaemic control and   1396
  impotence   1405
  ischaemia and   1392
  measurement   1393–4, 1395,
      1556
Nerve growth factor (NGF)   1389
Nesidioblastosis   252
Netherlands, IDDM frequency
    101, 140
Neural network computers
    1018–19
Neuroglycopenia   1132
  acute   1134
  chronic   1135
  subacute   1134–5
Neurological assessment   **1392–3**,
    1556
  lower extremity   1511
Neurological disability score (NDS)
    1393
Neurological disorders
  elderly diabetics   **1114–15**
  offspring of diabetic mothers
      1098
Neurological symptom score (NSS)
    1392–3

Neuropathic cachexia, diabetic
    1114, 1397–8
Neuropathic foot, *see* Foot,
    neuropathic
Neuropathic (Charcot) joint   1537,
    1540–1
Neuropathy, diabetic   **1385–406**,
    1419, **1555–7**
  aldose reductase inhibitors   809,
      1387–8, **1390**, 1400, 1555
  assessment   1392–5, 1545
  biochemical mechanisms
      1387–90
  children and adolescents   1052
  elderly   1114
  glycaemic control and   1395–6,
      1555
  histopathological changes
      1386–7
  hypoglycaemic   1399
  impotence   1405–6
  limited joint mobility and   1424
  microvascular disease in   1390–2
  newly-diagnosed diabetes   1399
  pain in   1399–400
  pancreas transplantation and
      895, 920
  pancreatic diabetes   215
  peripheral vascular disease and
      1510, 1542
  pregnancy and   1091
  prevalence   1395
  prevention   1555–6
  screening   1556–7
  staging/grading system   1393
  treatment   1390, 1400–1
  treatment-induced (insulin
      neuritis)   1399
  see also Autonomic neuropathy;
      Peripheral neuropathy
Neuropeptides, insulin secretion and
    288
Neuropeptide Y (NPY)   288
Neurophysiological tests   **1393–4**,
    1556
Neuropsychological function,
    hypoglycaemia and   1134
Neurotensin   204
Neutral protamine Hagedorn (NPH)
    insulin, *see* Isophane
Neutrophils
  diabetic ketoacidosis   1154
  function in diabetes   1166, 1167
New antidiabetic drugs   **797–810**
  future developments   809–10
  gluconeogenesis inhibitors   804–7
  incretins   800–1
  inhibitors of counterregulatory
      hormones   807–8
  insulin secretagogues   797–800
  promoting insulin sensitivity
      801–4
  retarding carbohydrate absorption
      808–9

New Caledonia, driving regulations
    1634
New Zealand, IDDM frequency
    101, 140
Nicotinamide therapy, IDDM   317
Nicotinic
  acid, hypercholesterolaemia
      824
Nifedipine   1094
Nigeria, IDDM frequency   137,
    138
Nitrogen balance technique,
    shortcomings   478–9
Nitrosamines   1661
NMR imaging spectroscopy, muscle
    glycogen synthesis   605–6
Nocturia   1030
Nocturnal hypoglycaemia, *see*
    Hypoglycaemia, nocturnal
Nocturnal penile tumescence (NPT)
    1405
Nodular lesions, diabetic
    nephropathy   1291
Non-communicable diseases (NCD)
  community control programmes
      1623–6
  diabetes and   1619–21
  prevention and control   1621–2
Non-insulin dependent diabetes
    mellitus (NIDDM, type 2
    diabetes)
  atherosclerotic vascular disease
      1185
    hyperglycaemia and   1477
    intervention studies   1478–9
    mortality and morbidity
        1463–5
    pathogenesis   1496
    prevention   1480–1
  autoantibodies   123
  biguanide therapy   786–9
  blood pressure and hypertension
      1466–7, 1474
  cardiovascular risk factors, *see*
      Cardiovascular risk factors,
      NIDDM
  classification   4, **9–10**, 317–18
    difficulties   14, 32
  coronary artery bypass surgery
      1500
  decompensated   292
  diabetic nephropathy   1113
    early phase   1271–2, 1273–4
    epidemiology   1269–71
    genetic factors   1281–2
    indications for renal biopsy
        1294, 1295
    non-renal complications
        1275
    pathology   1291
  dietary management, *see* Dietary
      management, NIDDM
  diet-induced thermogenesis
      431

Non-insulin dependent diabetes
mellitus (NIDDM, type 2
diabetes) (*cont.*)
driving regulations 1634
early onset 72
economic costs 1646, 1647,
1649
educational programmes 928,
932, 933, 935, 942
elderly 1117–23, 1663
environmental factors 62,
151–7
epidemiology **147–69**
age at onset 34, 179
age-specific
incidence/prevalence
154–5, 1103–4
ethnic and geographic
differences 35, 149,
150, 151–3
incidence and prevalence 33
non-Caucasoid Americans
133, 134, 135
secular changes in prevalence
33–4, 154
sex ratio 34–5, 154, 179
socioeconomic status and 35
tropical countries 178–9
exercise, *see* Exercise, NIDDM
genetic counselling **75–6**
empiric risks 74, 75
female diabetics 76
screening and prevention
75–6
genetic susceptibility, *see*
Genetic susceptibility,
NIDDM
glucagon levels 337
glycated haemoglobin levels
997–9, 1001, 1002
glycated protein levels 997–9
heterogeneity **10–11**, 41–2, 65,
148, 163
high-risk individuals 15
glycogen synthesis 599, 606,
617
insulin resistance 66, 167,
599, 600
insulin secretion 66–7, 294–5
insulin secretion vs. insulin
sensitivity 598–9, 600
intervention measures 1665–7
physiological studies 65–7
screening for 1666–7
HLA associations 67, **68**, 123,
150
hypertension 1466–7, 1474,
1664
pathogenesis 1523–4
retinopathy and 1525
treatment 1528, 1529,
1530–1
IGT progressing to 158, 1581,
1663–4

insulin receptor function **366–8**,
536, **601**, 1078–9
insulin resistance, *see* Insulin
resistance, NIDDM
insulin secretion, *see* Insulin
secretion, NIDDM
insulin therapy, *see* Insulin
therapy, NIDDM
islet morphology **239–45**
life-insurance 1632
limited joint mobility 1421,
1422
lipid/lipoprotein abnormalities
817–18, 1473
management 823–4
lipoprotein metabolism **452–5**,
819–20
myocardial infarction 1190,
1500
natural history **161–8**
hepatic glucose production and
168
insulin resistance and 166–8
insulin secretion and 164–6
non-obese form 163
obesity and 163–4
non-obese 163
obesity and, *see* Obesity,
NIDDM and
oral hypoglycaemic agents, *see*
Oral hypoglycaemic agents
pancreatic polypeptide levels
349
pathogenesis **569–619**
cellular mechanisms of insulin
resistance 600–7
fasting hyperglycaemia and
589–94
glucose toxicity and 618,
654–8
insulin action/insulin secretion
interaction 594–9
insulin resistance and 578–89
insulin secretion and 570–8
non-cellular mechanisms of
insulin resistance
607–16
primary cellular defect
617–18
primary insulin secretory
defect 618–19
summary 616–19
pathophysiological subtypes
65
peripheral vascular disease
1465
pregnancy
management 852, **1095–6**
risk factors for diabetes in
159, 1665
prevention (primary) 75–6,
1481, 1621, **1661–7**
high-risk approach 1665–7
population approach 1667

risk factors, *see* Non-insulin
dependent diabetes
mellitus, risk factors and
determinants
proinsulin levels 320, 322, **575**
protein metabolism **488**
retinopathy 1112, 1340–2, 1553
risk factors and determinants
62, **148–61**, 558–9, 563,
564, **1661–5**
"thrifty gene" hypothesis 67,
160
"Westernization" hypothesis
160–1
screening 75–6, 1574, 1575–6,
1580
fasting plasma glucose for
1569, 1571, 1572
methods 1577
screening for complications of
diabetes 957, 1553, 1555
skeletal changes 1416, 1417–18
somatostatin synthesis 347
somatostatin therapy 347, 348
sulphonylurea therapy 296–7,
745, 761–3
surgery and 1174, **1176–7**,
1180
therapeutic approach to glucose
toxicity 650–3
tropical countries 177, **178–80**
undiagnosed 32
urinary C-peptide excretion
312, 313
urine testing 967, 968, 969
visual impairment 1373–8,
1379
weight reduction, *see* Weight
loss, NIDDM
of young (NIDDY), *see*
Maturity onset diabetes of
young
Non-obese diabetic (NOD) mouse
117
autoantibodies 111, 113
genetics 40, 45, 46, 54, 108,
1658
immune-related B-cell
destruction 56, 232
islet transplantation 904
prevention of diabetes
development 115, 125
Non-steroidal anti-inflammatory
agents, insulin secretion and
290
Noradrenaline (norepinephrine)
as counterregulatory hormone
1137, 1138
exercise and 729
insulin secretion and 275, 288,
289
ketone body metabolism and
464
lipid metabolism and 393

Noradrenaline (norepinephrine)
  (*cont.*)
  myocardial infarction and   1193,
    1199–200, 1201
  pancreatectomized patients   212
  plasma levels, autonomic
    neuropathy   1402
Norepinephrine, *see* Noradrenaline
North America, dietary management
  of diabetes   **685–98**
North American Indians, IDDM
  frequency   **133–4**
North–south gradient, IDDM and
  multiple sclerosis prevalence
  124
Norway, IDDM frequency   101,
  140
NPH insulin, *see* Isophane
Nurse educators   936
Nurse specialists   941
  care of diabetic patients   **955–63**
  diabetes care centre   1596–7
  medicolegal issues   961–2

Obese Zucker rats, physical training
  736, 737
Obesity   **551–64**
  abdominal (android)   551
    hepatic insulin clearance
      553–5
    insulin resistance   542, 555–7
    insulin secretion, metabolism
      and efficacy   551–2
    lipoprotein metabolism   452
    and metabolic aberrations,
      syndrome with   561–4
    role of steroid hormones in
      560
    steroid hormone secretion
      557–60
  Africans   713
  black Americans   132
  cardiovascular disease risk and
    451, 1493
  China   722
  definition   10
  diagnosis of diabetes and   21
  diet-induced thermogenesis   431
  duration, NIDDM frequency and
    156
  fat distribution   1663
    insulin secretion, metabolism
      and efficacy   551–3
    NIDDM frequency and   155–6
    steroid hormones and   560–4
    see also Waist-to-hip ratio
  glucose disposal, non-oxidative
    604, 605
  glucose potassium and insulin
    infusion   1178, 1179
  glycogen synthesis   606
  health and   564
  hyperinsulinaemia, *see*
    Hyperinsulinaemia, obesity

hyperostosis and   1418
hypertension and   561, 563, 564,
  1493, 1523
insulin absorption and   844
insulin receptor function   366,
  367, 535, 1078
insulin resistance, *see* Insulin
  resistance, obesity
insulin secretion   279, 553
islet changes   241, 244
lipid oxidation and insulin
  resistance   610
lipoprotein metabolism   **451–2**
NIDDM and   10, **163–4**, 551
  epidemiological studies   153,
    155–6
  insulin receptor defects   602
  insulin sensitivity/insulin
    secretion interactions
    594–8
  insulin therapy   852
  role in aetiology   554–5,
    1662–3
NIDDM prevention   1665
offspring of diabetic mothers
  1098
peripheral (gynoid)   551
  cortisol secretion   559–60
  insulin resistance   542
  insulin secretion, metabolism
    and efficacy   552
  lipoprotein metabolism   452
pregnancy and   1096
proinsulin levels   320, 322
steroid hormone secretion
  557–60
weight loss, *see* Weight loss
ob/ob mouse   63, 345, 346, 349
Obstetric care
  gestational diabetes   1097
  IDDM   **1092–5**
    fetal monitoring   1094
    hypertensive disorders
      1093–4
    lactation   1095
    premature labour   1094
    timing and mode of delivery
      1094–5
  NIDDM   1096
Octreotide (SMS 201-995)   342,
  348, 807, 808
Ocular hypertension, steroid-
  induced   39
Oculomotor (third) nerve palsies
  1367–8, 1398
Oedema
  end-stage renal failure
    1275–6
  foot   1536, 1541, 1543
  insulin   891
Oesophageal immotility   1404
Oestrogens
  adipose tissue distribution and
    560

muscle fibre composition and
  556
obesity   557
OGTT, *see* Oral glucose tolerance
  test
OK-432 streptococcal preparation
  125
Okadaic acid   388
Oncotic pressure, systemic
  1285
One-to-one learning   936–7
Ophthalmoplegia   **1367–8**, 1398
Ophthalmoscopic examination
  adolescents   1051–2
  elderly patients   1112
  microaneurysm detection   1331
  screening for retinopathy   961,
    1382, 1552–3
Optic disc oedema   1335–7
Optic fundus examination, *see*
  Ophthalmoscopic examination
Oral drug therapy, patient education
  941–2
Oral glucose tolerance test (OGTT)
  7, **22–7**
  aging and   1105–6
  assessment of insulin sensitivity
    515–17
    NIDDM   **587–9**
  children   20, 26, 1029–30
  diagnosis
    diabetes   20, 23–6, 1085,
      1086
    gestational diabetes   1085–6,
      1096, 1097
    IGT   20, 23–6, 1085, 1086
  individual variability in response
    26–7, 286–7
  insulin secretory response,
    NIDDM   570–1, 596–7
  obesity   596–7
  pancreas transplantation and
    918, 919
  screening
    abbreviated test   26
    diabetes/IGT   1116, 1575–6,
      1577–9
    gestational diabetes   1582–3
    WHO/NDDG standard method
      26, 1578
Oral hydration
  diabetic ketoacidosis   1032
  intercurrent illness   1049
Oral hypoglycaemic agents
  cardiovascular complications and
    1478–9
  combined with insulin   297,
    764–5, 1123
  complications of diabetes and
    1580
  elderly   1120–3
  hypoglycaemia and   1144
  IGT, NIDDM prevention   1581,
    1666

Oral hypoglycaemic agents (*cont.*)
insulin receptor function and 368
myocardial infarction and 1189, 1190, 1500
osteopenia and 1417, 1418
pancreatic diabetes 215
see also Biguanides; Sulphonylureas; *specific agents*
Oral insulin administration 867
Organ–circulation model, glucose metabolism 420–1
Organ donors, living related 920
Organophosphorus poisoning 1158
Ornithine 277–8
Osmolality, serum, diabetic ketoacidosis 1035
Osmoles, idiogenic 1035, 1157
Osteitis condensans ilii 1418
Osteoarthritis 1418
Osteoarthropathy, Charcot 1537, **1540–1**
Osteolysis 1418, 1540
Osteopenia **1415–18**
IDDM 1416–17
neuropathic foot 1536–7
NIDDM 1417–18
Otitis, malignant external 1166
Outpatient care programme, *see* Ambulatory diabetes care programme
Overinsulinization 1061
Overweight
diabetes prevalence and 40
diagnosis of diabetes and 21
see also Obesity
Oviduct, chick, insulin effects on mRNA levels 396
Oxidant stress, fibrocalculous pancreatic diabetes and 189
3-Oxoacid CoA transferase 463
Oxygen-derived free radicals, myocardial infarction and 1193
Oxygen supply, exercise and 726
Oxygen tension
endoneurial 1391
transcutaneous (TcPo$_2$), peripheral vascular disease 1512, 1542
Oxyntomodulin 334, 335

PACBERG computer program 522, 1075
Pacific Islanders
genetic susceptibility to NIDDM 65, 67, 1662
NIDDM frequency 34, 62, 147, **153**
screening for NIDDM 1572
Pain, diabetic neuropathy **1399–400**

Painful neuropathy
acute 1386, **1397–8**
treatment 1400
Pain sensation, neuropathic foot 1535
Pancreas
artificial endocrine **871–9**, 979
congenital absence 38, 245, 1089
embryology and fetal development 224
exocrine function, pancreatic diabetes 187, 212
fibrosis, chronic pancreatitis 245–6
insulin effects on mRNA levels 396
isolated perfused 261
normal morphology **223–30**
pathology
chronic pancreatitis 200, 245–7
cystic fibrosis 207, 247, 248
diabetes-related **231–50**
fibrocalculous pancreatic diabetes 186–7
haemochromatosis 203
pancreatic carcinoma 204, 247
unrelated to diabetes 251–2
see also Islets of Langerhans
Pancreas transplantation
fetal and neonatal 905–6
allografts 905–6
clinical studies 906–7
isografts 905
islet lesions 57, 232, **239**
progression of nephropathy after 895–6, 1232
progression of retinopathy and 895, 920, 1237–8
whole organ and segmental **915–21**
clinical results 917–18
diabetic complications and 895–6, 920
diagnosis of rejection 917
immunological aspects 916–17
living related donor 920
metabolic results 918–20
renal transplantation and 916, 917–18, 920, 1307
surgical techniques 915–16
see also Islet transplantation
Pancreatectomized animals
insulin secretion
effects of hyperglycaemia 636–7, 638
phlorhizin therapy and 576–7, 640–2
insulin sensitivity, phlorhizin therapy and 612, 614, 647–8, 649

islet transplantation 897, 898
Pancreatectomy **204–7**
clinical features of diabetes 211, 212, 1063
diabetes development 198
diabetic complications 213
hormone secretion 205–7
metabolic profile 208, 209–10, 211
subtotal 198, 205–6
therapy of diabetes 215–16, 850
total 198, 205
Pancreatic acinar cells, atrophy in type 1 diabetes 231, 232, 233
Pancreatic atrophy, type 1 diabetes 231, 233
Pancreatic calculi, fibrocalculous pancreatic diabetes 184, 185, 186–7
Pancreatic carcinoma 198, 204
diabetes onset 210
hormone secretion 204, 205
pancreatic pathology 204, 247
Pancreatic disease, diabetes secondary to (pancreatic diabetes) 11, 12, 182, **197–217**
aetiology 198–205 208
clinical manifestations 210–13
diabetic complications 213–15
islet pathology 245–7
metabolic profile 208–10
therapy 215–17, 852
thickened capillary basement membranes 1229, 1230, 1258
see also Malnutrition related diabetes mellitus
Pancreatic ducts
collagenase injection 896–7, 906
fibrocalculous pancreatic diabetes 185, 186
polymer injection 915–16, 918
Pancreatic enzyme therapy 216
Pancreatic hypoplasia, congenital 38
Pancreaticoduodenal transplantation 916
Pancreaticoduodenectomy (Whipple's resection) 205
Pancreatic polypeptide (PP) 225, 226, **348–9**
actions 348
acute pancreatitis 199
cells secreting, *see* PP cells
chronic pancreatitis 202–3, 348
circulating levels 348
diabetes and 349
gut endocrine tumours secreting 348
pancreatectomized patients 204

Pancreatic (insulin) suppression test
    425, **520–1**, 578–9, 1073–4
Pancreatic tissue, pieces   261
Pancreatic tumours   **204**
Pancreatitis
    acute   **198–9**, 245
        hormone secretion   199
        management   215
    alcoholic   182, 190
    chronic   182, **199–203**, 206
        aetiology in developing
            countries   190
        clinical features of diabetes
            211
        diabetic complications   213,
            214
        diagnostic criteria   190
        heterogeneity in tropics   188,
            189–90
        hormone secretion   200–3
        management   187–8, 215–16
        metabolic profile   208, 210
        pancreatic pathology   200,
            245–7
        pancreatic polypeptide
            202–3, 348
        subtotal pancreatectomy   205
    hereditary relapsing   38, 200
    tropical calcific (TCP)   182
        exocrine pancreatic function
            187
        spectrum of glucose tolerance
            184
Panhypopituitarism, brittle diabetes
    852
Panhypopituitary dwarfism,
    hereditary   38
Papaverine, intracavernous injection
    1406
Papillopathy, diabetic   1335–7
Papua New Guinea, NIDDM
    prevalence   150
Parasympathetic fibres, islets of
    Langerhans   230
Parasympathetic nervous system,
    tests of function   1401
Parasympathetic stimulation
    hepatic glucose production and
        417
    insulin secretion and   288
Parents, diabetic
    NIDDM in offspring   163
    risks of IDDM in offspring   73,
        74, 1028, 1097–8
Parity, risk of NIDDM development
    and   159
Parotid glands, fibrocalculous
    pancreatic diabetes   187
PAS-positive material, vascular
    wall   672, 1437–8, 1439,
    1443
Patient management systems
    development   1012–13
    integrated   1015–18

Patients
    acceptability of continuous
        subcutaneous insulin
        infusion   859
    accuracy of blood glucose self-
        monitoring   974–5
    education, *see* Education,
        diabetes
    evaluation of attitudes   944
    locus of control   925–6
    non-acceptance of disease
        926–7
    perceptions of diabetes and its
        treatment   925–7
    reliability in reporting blood
        glucose values   939, 977,
        1010–11
    self-help groups   1592
"Peak L1"   671
Pectin   688
Pedal artery, arterial reconstruction
    surgery   1515
Penile prostheses   1406
Penile tumescence, nocturnal (NPT)
    1405
Pen-injectors, insulin   851, 852, 858
Pentosidine   671
Pepsinogen I/pepsinogen II ratio
    75
Peptide hormones, insulin secretion
    and   **276–7**
Peptidergic neurons, islets of
    Langerhans   230
Percentage desirable weight (PDW)
    10
Periarticular tissue disorders
    1418–28
Perinatal morbidity   1095
    diabetic nephropathy and   1301
    IGT in pregnancy and   1582
    pathophysiology   1088–91
Perinatal mortality   1086
Perinephric abscesses   1302
Peripheral blood flow, neuropathic
    foot   1536
Peripheral nerves
    aminoguanidine therapy and
        678
    measurement of function
        1392–5
    microvascular disease   1390–2
Peripheral neuropathy   **1396–9**
    autonomic neuropathy and   1403
    children and adolescents   1052
    classification   1396–7
    elderly   1114
    end-stage renal failure   1276
    exercise and   731
    focal and multifocal neuropathies
        1397
    histopathological features   1386
    mononeuropathies   1367–8, 1398
    symmetrical polyneuropathies
        1396–7

    treatment   809, 1400–1
Peripheral tissues
    fate of ingested glucose   435–6
    glucose uptake   434
        NIDDM   **585–6**, 587–8, 593
    ketone body utilization   463
    see also Adipose tissue; Muscle,
        skeletal
Peripheral vascular disease   1490,
    1509–15
    angiography   1512–15, 1543
    arterial reconstruction   1515,
        1543–4
    clinical presentation and
        evaluation   1510–12, 1542
    diabetic nephropathy   1276,
        1544
    frequency in diabetes   1461
    hyperglycaemia and   1475,
        1477, 1478
    mortality and morbidity in
        NIDDM   1465
    neuropathic foot problems and
        1510, 1542
    prevention   1558
    see also Foot, ischaemic
Peritoneal cavity, fetal and
    neonatal pancreas
    transplantation   905
Peritoneal dialysis, continuous
    ambulatory (CAPD)
    1306–7
    insulin resistance and   541
    intraperitoneal insulin delivery
        866, 1306
    visual impairment and   1380
Peritonitis   1306 Pernicious
    anaemia   47, 75
Peroneal artery, occlusive disease
    1509, 1515
Pertussis toxin   275
Peyronie disease   1419
PH
    arterial, diabetic ketoacidosis
        1031, 1154
    intracellular, pancreatic B cells
        269–70
Phaeochromocytoma   38, 247, 295,
    1080
Phagocytes, function in diabetes
    1166–7
Pharyngitis, streptococcal, brittle
    diabetes and   960
Phenformin   773, 774, 789
    cardiovascular complications and
        1478–9
    lactate metabolism and   780, 781
    pharmacokinetics   785, 786
Phenol, insulin preparations
    837–8, 839
Phenprocoumon, metformin
    interactions   788
Phentolamine, intracavernous
    injection   1406

Phenylalanine hydroxylase 398

Phenylalanine tracers, measurement of protein metabolism 480, 483

Phenylpropanolamine, insulin secretion and 289

Phenylpyruvate 269

Phenytoin (diphenylhydantoin) 249, 289

Philippines, IDDM frequency **120**, 138

Phlorhizin therapy
insulin secretion and 576–7, 640–2, 647–9
insulin sensitivity and 612, 614, 647–8, 649

Phorbol esters
glucose transport and 388
insulin-like effects on transcription 396
insulin receptor function and 362, 363, 365, 399

Phosphate
administration in diabetic ketoacidosis 1034, 1036
renal tubular reabsorption 1289
serum levels, diabetic ketoacidosis 1034, 1156
urinary excretion 1417

Phosphatidate phosphohydrolase 393, 394

Phosphatidyl inositol 3-kinase 403

Phosphoenol-pyruvate 269

Phospho-enol-pyruvate carboxykinase (PEPCK) 396, 491–2

Phosphoenol pyruvate carboxylase 397

Phosphofructokinase (PFK) 386
islet cells 268
Randle cycle and 607, 608
starvation and 279

Phosphoinositide hydrolysis
cholinergic activation 273
insulin actions **395**
insulin secretion and 272, 643, 644

Phosphoinositol glycans, role in insulin actions **402–3**

Phospholipase A₂, islet cells 273

Phospholipase C
cholinergic activation 273
insulin-activated 402, 403
insulin secretion and 272

Phospholipase C-gamma 403

Phospholipids, biguanide actions 775, 776

Phosphorylase 386, 387, 398

Phosphorylase kinase 386, 387, 398

Photocoagulation therapy **1349–56**
macular oedema 1349, 1350, 1355–6, 1381, 1552
mechanisms of action 1349–50
neovascular glaucoma 1369–70

panretinal (scatter) 1349
proliferative diabetic retinopathy 1349, 1350–5, 1381, 1552
visual problems due to 1380

Photon absorptiometry 1416–17

Phrenic nerve palsy 1398

Physical activity, *see* Exercise

Physical training (fitness)
insulin sensitivity and glucose tolerance and 167, 734–6
therapy of NIDDM 736–8

Physician assistants 961

Physicians, *see* Doctors

Pilots, airline 1638–9

Pima Indians 147
development of NIDDM 598
diabetic nephropathy 1269
glucose tolerance 64, 158, 161, 162
glycogen synthase activity 606
half-blooded, NIDDM frequency 149
IDDM prevalence and incidence 133, 134
insulin receptor function 367
insulin receptor region polymorphisms 69
insulin resistance 66, 167, 536, 603
insulin secretion 164–5, 166
NIDDM frequency 154, 155
NIDDM risk factors 155, 157, 158, 159, 163

Pirogliride 798–9, 802–3

Pituitary ablation, diabetic retinopathy **1348–9**

Pituitary adenoma, insulin resistance 1080

Pituitary autoantibodies 123

Placenta
diabetic pregnancy 1088, 1089
glucose transport 410
insulin receptors 359

Plasma proteins, *see* Proteins, serum

Plasma volume, hypertension in diabetes 1522, 1523

Plasmin 1450–1

Plasminogen activator
biguanide therapy and 784
production in diabetes 1280, 1450–1, 1473, 1497
sulphonylurea actions 752
therapy of myocardial infarction 1196

Plasminogen activator inhibitor (PAI-I) 1192, 1451

Plastozote insoles 1539

Platelet adhesion 1452, 1497

Platelet aggregation 1452, 1453, 1473, 1497
biguanide therapy and 784
spontaneous 1452

Platelet α-granule proteins 1192, 1200–1

Platelet-derived growth factor (PDGF) 674, 676

Platelet-derived growth factor receptors 403

Platelet factor 4 1473

Platelets
arachidonate metabolism 1453
atherogenesis and 1497
effects of diabetes 1452
size changes 1453

Plethysmography 1511–12, 1542

Pneumonia 1165

Podocytes, *see* Glomerular epithelial foot processes

POEMS syndrome 110

Poland, IDDM frequency 140

"Polar antigen" autoantibodies 107, 111, **113**

Polycystic ovary syndrome
abdominal obesity in women and 557, 558
insulin resistance 539, 546
metabolic abnormalities 557–8

Polycythaemia
blood glucose self-monitoring and 975
infants of diabetic mothers 1090

Polydipsia 1030, 1154

Polyendocrine deficiency disease (Schmidt's syndrome) 38

Polyneuropathies, symmetrical 1396–7

Polyol metabolism 1167, 1168, 1232–3
basement membrane changes and **1255–6**, 1260–1
diabetic nephropathy and **1278–9**
diabetic neuropathy and 1389–90
diabetic retinopathy and 1334–5
sex steroids and 1258
see also Sorbitol

Polysomes 471

Polyuria 21, 1154

Popliteal artery
angioplasty 1544
occlusive disease 1510, 1543–4

Population attributable risk 1655

Populations
glucose tolerance, *see* Glucose tolerance, population studies
high-prevalence, screening for diabetes 1569, 1571, 1572, 1580
primary prevention of NIDDM 1667

Pork insulin 884–5, 1039–40
extended-acting 848–9
short-acting 847

Porphyria, acute intermittent 38

Portal vein
    fetal and neonatal pancreas
        transplantation 905
    insulin delivery into 867
    islet transplantation 897, 898–9,
        906
Postural hypotension 1403–4,
    1528
Potassium (K$^+$)
    administration
        diabetic ketoacidosis 1033–4,
            1156
        hyperosmolar non-ketotic
            coma 1160
        see also Glucose potassium
            and insulin infusion
    pancreatic B cells 269
    serum levels
        after myocardial infarction
            1195
        diabetic ketoacidosis 1031,
            1033, 1153–4
        hyporeninaemic
            hypoaldosteronism
            1113
        insulin secretion and 289
Potassium acetate, diabetic
    ketoacidosis 1034
Potassium (K$^+$) channels
    actions of sulphonylureas 747,
        748–9
    pancreatic B cells 265, 269,
        270–1, 278, 643
Potassium chloride, diabetic
    ketoacidosis 1034
Potassium phosphate, diabetic
    ketoacidosis 1034
PP, *see* Pancreatic polypeptide
PP cells 223–4, 225, **226**, 348
    chronic pancreatitis 246
    distribution in islets 227
    type 1 diabetes 231
Prader–Willi (Prader–Labhart–Willi)
    syndrome 39, 248, 1028
Prausnitz–Küstner reaction 887
Prediabetes 16
    see also Insulin dependent
        diabetes mellitus, high-risk
        individuals; Non-insulin
        dependent diabetes mellitus,
        high-risk individuals
Predictive value (PV), screening
    tests 1568–9, 1570, 1571
Pre-eclampsia 1093, 1301
Pregnancy 76–7, **1085–98**
    biguanides in 788–9
    blood glucose self-monitoring
        972
    diabetic nephropathy and 1086,
        1091, **1301**
    glycation products in **1002–3**
    hormonal and metabolic changes
        276, 1086–7
    IDDM 1087–95

diabetes fetopathy 1087–8
    embryopathy 1087
    fetal supply line 1088
    medical care 852, 1091–2
    microvascular disease and
        1091
    newborn infant 1095
    obstetric care 1092–5
    pathophysiology of perinatal
        problems 1088–91
insulin resistance 541, 1086,
    1092
NIDDM
    management 852, 1095–6
    risk to offspring 159
patient education **942**
perinatal mortality 1086
risk factors for NIDDM
    development after 159,
    1665
White's classification 1086
see also Gestational diabetes;
    Infants of diabetic mothers
Preinitiation complex
    43S 471, 472
    48S 472–3
Premature labour 1094
Prenatal diagnosis, congenital
    malformations 76–7, 1093
Preoperative assessment
    1175–6
Prepregnancy
    counselling 942, 1087
    insulin regimens 852
Preproglucagon 334
Preproinsulin 303
Preprosomatostatin 341, 342
Pressure neuropathies 1398
Prevention
    autoimmune diseases 75
    autonomic neuropathy 1557–8
    complications of diabetes, *see*
        Complications of diabetes,
        prevention and screening
    diabetes **1655–67**
    diabetic nephropathy 1271,
        1553–4
    diabetic neuropathy 1555–6
    diabetic retinopathy 1551–2
    experimental IDDM 115, 125
    foot problems 960–1, 1545,
        1555–7
    IDDM, *see* Insulin dependent
        diabetes mellitus,
        prevention
    macrovascular disease 1558,
        1580, 1667
    NIDDM, *see* Non-insulin
        dependent diabetes mellitus,
        prevention
    non-communicable diseases
        1621–2
    primary 1566
    secondary 1566, 1655–6

Primary care
    diabetes care 1594, 1597
    diabetes control programmes
        1619–28
    Malaysia 1607–8
    Tanzania 1612, 1615–16
Primary-care physicians, *see*
    General practitioners
Probucol 824–5
Procoagulant factors 1449
Progeroid syndromes 39
Progesterone
    adipose tissue distribution and
        560
    obesity 557
    stress-induced hypothalamic
        arousal and 562
Proglucagon 225, 334
Progressive cone dystrophy,
    degenerative liver disease,
    endocrine dysfunction and
    hearing defect 39
Proinsulin 225, 305, **318–23**
    biosynthesis **262**, 303
    chronic hyperglycaemia and
        643
    clinical applications 323
    contaminating insulin
        preparations 884
    conversion process 262, 303,
        304
    hepatic extraction 319
    insulin receptor affinity 320
    interference with C-peptide
        measurement 305–6
    kinetics and metabolism 319–21
    measurement 318–19
    NIDDM 320, 322, **575**
    renal clearance 319
    secretion in humans 320,
        321–3
    sulphonylurea-mediated
        inhibition 750
    therapeutic use 323
Proinsulin immunoreactive material
    (PIM) 303, 319
    conditions with elevated 320,
        321–3
Proinsulin immunoreactive material
    (PIM)/insulin (I) ratio 320
Proislets 906
Prolactin 534
Promoter sites 468, 469
Properdin factor B (BF) alleles 49,
    142–3, 178
Propranolol
    insulin suppression test 425,
        520, 578, 1074
    recovery from hypoglycaemia in
        IDDM and 1140
Prosomatostatin 341, 342
Prostacyclin 1472, 1497
Prostaglandin E, insulin secretion
    and 288

Prostaglandin E$_2$ (PGE$_2$), insulin
  secretion and   643–4
Prostaglandins
  atherogenesis and   1473
  glomerular filtration rate and
    1286
Protamine   838
  immunogenicity   889–90
Protamine-zinc insulin   837, **838**
  absorption   843
  clinical applications   848
Proteases
  AGE-modified protein-induced
    secretion   675
  calcium-dependent   475, 496
Protein, dietary   **693–6**
  African diets   711
  Chinese diet   719, 720
  IDDM frequency and   1661
  Indian and South East Asian
    diets   702
  restriction   693–6, 1114,
    1297–8, 1553–4
Protein C   1450
Protein deficient (pancreatic)
  diabetes mellitus (PDDM)
    177, **180–1**
  classification   4, 11
  a separate entity?   181, 190
Protein degradation (proteolysis)
  amino acids and   478, 481–3
  ATP-dependent   475–6, 496
  calcium-dependent   475, 496
  IDDM   483–8
  insulin actions   468
    animal and in vitro studies   477
    intracellular mechanisms
      495–6
    in vivo human studies   481–3
  lysosomal pathway   474–5, 496
  measurement in humans   478–80
  NIDDM   488
  normal regulation   **473–6**
Protein–energy malnutrition   188
Protein feeding
  IDDM   499
  normal humans   497–8
Protein kinase A (cAMP-dependent
  protein kinase)
  insulin actions   389
  insulin secretion and   264
  lipid metabolism and   394, 395
Protein kinase C (PKC)
  diabetic neuropathy   1388
  insulin secretion and   264, 273–4
Protein kinases
  glycogen synthase
    phosphorylation   389–90
  insulin-mediated activation   398,
    399–401
  role in insulin secretion   263–4
Protein metabolism   **467–99**
  amino acid interorgan exchange
    and   496–9

animal and in vitro studies   478
  amino acids and   478
  insulin and diabetes and
    476–7
  human   478–88
    IDDM   483–8
    insulin and amino acids and
      481–3
    methodology   478–80
    NIDDM   488
  mechanisms of insulin actions
    488–96
    amino acid transport   489–90
    insulin receptor signal
      transduction   488–9
    regulation of protein synthesis
      490–5
    regulation of proteolysis
      495–6
  normal regulation   468–76
Protein phosphatase 1   389
Protein phosphatase 2A   389
Proteins
  AGE-modified   671, 1277, 1278
  axonal transport   1388
  glycated   988, 1232
    atherogenesis and   1472,
      1496
    clot retraction and   1451
    diabetic nephropathy and
      1277–8
    glomerular filtration   1288
    screening for diabetes
      1576–7
  insulin-stimulated
    phosphorylation   397–401
  vascular wall, AGE-induced
    alterations   671–4
Proteins, serum
  accumulation in vessel walls
    671–2
  basement membrane binding
    1252–3, 1277
  glycated   **995**
    assay   995
    blood glucose levels and
      997, 998–9
    clinical application   999
    confounding medical
      conditions   1000
    diabetes diagnosis and   1003
    pregnancy and   1002–3
    see also Fructosamine
  see also Albumin
Protein synthesis
  amino acid levels and   478,
    481–3
  IDDM   483–8, 488
  insulin actions   467–8
    animal and in vitro studies
      476–7
    intracellular mechanisms
      395–7, **488–96**
    in vivo human studies   481–3

measurement in humans   478–80
  NIDDM   488
  normal regulation   **468–73**
Proteinuria
  antihypertensive therapy and
    1296
  blood pressure and
    IDDM   1462, 1463
    NIDDM   1467
  cause of death and   1216
  detection using test strips   1554,
    1555
  early vs. late onset   1295
  experimentally-induced   1250,
    1253–4
  life-insurance and   1632
  mesangial hypertrophy and
    1259
  mortality and   1214–16
  NIDDM   1113
  pancreatic diabetes   214
  persistent/clinical   1272, 1274–5
    see also Nephropathy, diabetic
  in pregnancy   1091, 1301
  progression   1290
Proteoglycan, heparan sulphate,
  see Heparan sulphate
  proteoglycan
Proteolysis, *see* Protein degradation
Proteosomes   476
Protons (H$^+$)
  cerebral oedema of diabetic
    ketoacidosis and   1035–6
  pancreatic B cells   269–70
Pseudodisease   1572
Pseudogout   1415
Pseudo-Refsum's syndrome   39
Psychological problems
  brittle diabetes and   1064
  diabetic impotence and   1405–6
  insulin injection therapy   854
  screening for diabetic
    complications   1559
Psychosocial problems
  brittle diabetes and   1064–5
  elderly   1118
Psychosocial support, children and
  adolescents   1044–7
Psychotherapy, brittle diabetes
  1068
Pulmonary changes, limited joint
  mobility   1424
Pulmonary maturation, infants of
  diabetic mothers   1090–1
Pulmonary oedema
  end-stage renal failure   1276
  postmyocardial infarction   1188,
    1189
Pulses, peripheral   1510, 1536,
  1545, 1558
Pulse volume recording   1511–12,
  1542
Pupillary function, autonomic
  neuropathy   1371, 1402

Pupils, dilatation in fundus
    examination 1552
Pyelitis, emphysematous 1302
Pyelonephritis, emphysematous
    1166, 1302
Pyridine compounds 799–800
N-3-Pyridylmethyl-*N'*-*p*-
    nitrophenylurea (PNU, RH-
    787, Vacor) 61, 249, 1661
Pyruvate dehydrogenase (PDH)
    386
    IDDM 538
    insulin actions 387, **390–1**, 398,
        402
    NIDDM 536, 606–7
    Randle cycle and 607, 608
Pyruvate dehydrogenase
    phosphatase 390
Pyruvate kinase 386, 387, 398,
    492

Quadruple infusion technique, *see*
    Insulin suppression test
Quality control, blood glucose self-
    monitoring 975
Questionnaires, evaluation of
    educational programmes
    944

Rabson–Mendenhall syndrome 38
Racial differences, *see* Ethnic
    differences
Radiogrammetry 1416
raf-1 kinase 399
Randle cycle 607, 608
    activity in NIDDM 607–10
Rat poison (*N*-3-pyridylmethyl-
    N'-*p*-nitrophenylurea, PNU,
    Vacor) 61, 249, 1661
Reagent strips
    blood glucose 973–4
    proteinuria detection 1554,
        1555
    urinary glucose 968
    urinary ketones 967
Records, patient 1591–2
Rectal insulin administration 867–8
Red blood cells, *see* Erythrocytes
Red cell casts, urinary 1275, 1294–5
Reflectance meters, blood glucose,
    see Glucose reflectance meters
Reflex sympathetic dystrophy
    (shoulder–hand syndrome)
    1420–1, 1424
Refractive errors 891, **1371**
Refsum's syndrome 1028
Registers, diabetes 1591, 1592,
    1595, 1613
    estimates of care costs from
        1647
Regular insulin, *see* Unmodified
    insulin
Rehabilitation, visually impaired
    patients 1382–3

Reliability, screening tests 1567–8
Religious beliefs
    dietary management and 704,
        716–17
    India 1604
Renal biopsy, indications 1294–5
Renal dialysis **1304–8**
    initiation 1304
    renal transplantation vs. 1307–8
    visual impairment and 1305–6
    see also Haemodialysis;
        Peritoneal dialysis,
        continuous ambulatory
Renal disease
    hyperosmolar non-ketotic coma
        and 1159–60
    urinary clearance of C-peptide
        307, 312
Renal failure
    acute, radiocontrast-induced
        1512–13
    end-stage (ESRF) 1113, 1267,
        1275–6, **1302–8**
        IDDM 1269
        NIDDM 1270, 1271
        visual impairment and 1380
    glycated haemoglobin assay and
        999–1000
    insulin resistance **540–1**
    insulin therapy 851
    intraperitoneal insulin delivery
        866
    pancreas and renal
        transplantation 916,
        917–18
    proinsulin levels 319, 320, 322
Renal function
    angiography and 1513
    dietary protein restriction and
        693–5
    metformin therapy and 786,
        788, 790, 1122
    pathological changes in diabetic
        nephropathy and 1293–4
    sulphonylurea therapy and 760–1
Renal–hepatic–pancreatic dysplasia
    38
Renal hypertrophy 1272
    pathogenesis of diabetic
        nephropathy and 1281
    pathophysiology **1286–7**
    reversibility 1272, 1287, 1299
Renal interstitium, pathological
    changes 1292
Renal papillary necrosis (RPN)
    1299–300
Renal plasma flow (RPF), increased
    1271–2, 1280, 1283
Renal replacement therapy **1302–8**
    initiation 1303–4
    size of problem 1302–3
    treatment options 1304–7
Renal–retinal syndrome 1216–17,
    1275, 1294

Renal threshold for glucose,
    variability 968, 1576
Renal transplantation 1304, **1307**
    dialysis vs. 1307–8
    genesis of diabetic nephropathy
        and 1231–2
    islet transplantation and 902–3,
        906, 907
    pancreas transplantation and
        916, 917–18, 920, 1307
Renal tubular basement membrane,
    changes in diabetes 1252–3
Renal tubular function,
    pathophysiology of changes
    1289
Renal tubules, pathological changes
    1292
Renin, glomerular hyperfiltration
    and 1286
Renin–angiotensin–aldosterone
    system (RAAS)
    hypertension with nephropathy
        1522–3
    hypertension without
        nephropathy 1523–4
Reovirus 3 virus 1660
Repeatability, screening tests
    1567–8
Resins, bile acid-sequestering 824,
    825, 826, 827
Respiratory distress syndrome
    adult, complicating diabetic
        ketoacidosis 1158
    infants of diabetic mothers
        1091, 1095
Respiratory quotient (RQ) 422
Restriction fragment length
    polymorphisms (RFLPs)
    150
    glucose transporter regions 70
    insulin gene region 68
    insulin receptor gene region
        69–70
Retina, featureless 1334, 1336
Retinal blood flow 1525–7
Retinal capillaries
    basement membrane changes
        1251, 1258–60, 1330
    blood–retinal barrier 1250
    microaneurysms **1329–31**,
        1332, 1358
Retinal colour photography 1553
Retinal detachment, tractional
    1338, 1340
Retinal haemorrhages 1333–4
Retinal oedema (thickening) 1329,
    1331–3
Retinal vascular occlusion, diabetic
    retinopathy 1329, **1333–5**
Retinal vein dilation (venous
    beading) 1260, 1334, 1335
Retinopathy, diabetic **1329–59**,
    1551–3
    aminoguanidine therapy 677

Retinopathy, diabetic (*cont.*)
  blood glucose self-monitoring
    and 975
  blood pressure and 1348, 1525–7
  children and adolescents 1051–2
  classification of severity 1343
  diabetic nephropathy and (renal–
    retinal syndrome)
    1216–17, 1275, 1294
  elderly 1112
  exercise and 731
  fibrocalculous pancreatic diabetes
    185
  glycaemic control and **1342–8**,
    1551
    clinical studies 1233–9
    epidemiological studies
      1226–7, 1228
    experimental and
      transplantation studies
      1231
    transient worsening
      phenomenon 1235,
      1236, 1237, 1346–7
  glycated haemoglobin levels and
    1043–4
  growth hormone and 347
  limited joint mobility and
    1425–6
  natural course 1329–40
    contraction of vitreous
      and fibrovascular
      proliferations
      1338–40
    excessive vascular
      permeability 1331–3
    microaneurysms 1329–31
    proliferation of new vessels
      and fibrous tissue
      1335–8
    vaso-obliteration 1333–5
  non-proliferative (NPDR)
    1329–35
    risk of progression to PDR
      1342
    severe (preproliferative)
      1334
  pancreas transplantation and
    895, 920, 1237–8
  pancreatic diabetes 213, 214
  pathogenesis 1261
  pregnancy and 1091
  prevention 1551–2
  proliferative (PDR) 1329,
    1335–8
    contraction of vitreous
      and fibrovascular
      proliferations 1338–40
    new vessels on disc (NVD)
      1335–7
    new vessels elsewhere (NVE)
      1335, 1337
    photocoagulation 1349,
      1350–5, 1381, 1552

  type and duration of diabetes
    and 1340–2
  renal replacement therapy and
    1305–7
  risk factors 1228, 1348
  screening 957, 960, 1552–3
    cost-effectiveness analysis
      1652
  specificity 1435–6
  treatment 1348–59, 1551, 1552
    antiplatelet agents 1357–9
    photocoagulation 1349–56
    pituitary ablation 1348–9
    vitrectomy 1356–7
  type and duration of diabetes and
    1340–2
  visual impairment and 1378–9,
    1381
RF termination factor 473
Rhesus monkeys, NIDDM
  development 598, 599
Rheumatoid arthritis 1423
Ribosomal protein S6, *see* S6
  ribosomal protein
Ribosomal proteins
  degradation 495
  synthesis 495
Ribosomal RNA (rRNA) 470, 471
  effects of insulin 495
Ribosomes 471
  regulation by insulin 493, **495**
Rice-based diets 701, 702, 708
Rieger's syndrome, partial
  lipodystrophy with 38
RINm5F tumoral islet cell line,
  insulin secretion 271
Risk, population attributable 1655
Ristocetin cofactor, *see* von
  Willebrand factor
RNA
  synthesis 468–70
  see also Messenger RNA;
    Ribosomal RNA; Transfer
    RNA
RNA polymerase I 495
RNA polymerase II 468–9, 470,
  490
  inhibition by insulin 491
Rocker-bottom foot deformity 1540
Rodenticide 1661
Roussy–Lévy syndrome 39
Rubella virus
  congenital, IDDM in 61, 110,
    1026, 1660
  IDDM and 59, 60, 61
Rubeosis iridis 1369–70
Rural areas
  Africa
    food availability 714
    nutritional status 713, 714
  distribution of resources and
    expertise 1603, 1609,
    1616
  NIDDM frequency 159–60

S6 kinase(s) 397, 399
S6 kinase (70 K) 399, 400
S6 kinase II (90 K) 389–90, 399,
  400
S6 ribosomal protein 397, 398,
  400, 489
Saccharin 696
St Vincent Declaration (Italy 1989)
  1597, 1598–9
Salicylates
  glucose urine testing and 969
  insulin secretion and 290
Salivary glands, glucagon secretion
  204
Saphenous vein grafts 1543–4
Scandinavia, IDDM frequency 140
Schiff base adducts 670–1, 986,
  987
Schmidt's syndrome (polyendocrine
  deficiency disease) 38
Scleroderma diabeticorum
  1418–19
Scotland, IDDM frequency 101,
  140
Screening
  autoimmune diseases 75
  autonomic neuropathy 1558
  complications of diabetes, *see*
    Complications of diabetes,
    prevention and screening
  cost–effectiveness analysis 1652
  definition and rationale 1566
  diabetes and glucose intolerance
    1565–83
    blood glucose and OGTT
      1577–9
    elderly 1116–17, 1118
    glycated proteins 1576–7
    history 1573–4
    limitations 1574–6
    methods 1576–9
    recommendations 1579–83
    urine glucose testing 1576
  diabetic nephropathy 960,
    1554–5
  diabetic neuropathy 1556–7
  diabetic retinopathy 957, 960,
    1552–3
  foot problems 1556–7
  gestational diabetes 1096–7,
    1581–3
  IDDM 73–5, 1579
  IDDM-predisposed individuals
    73–5, 114, 1579
  multiphasic 1567
  NIDDM, *see* Non-insulin
    dependent diabetes mellitus,
    screening
  NIDDM-predisposed individuals
    1666–7
  scope 1566–7
  see also Prevention
Screening programmes
  desirable characteristics 1567–9

Screening programmes (*cont.*)
  evaluation 1569–73
    costs and benefits 1570–1, 1572
    measures and pitfalls 1571–2
    methods 1572–3
Screening tests 1567–9, 1570
  high-prevalence populations 1569, 1571, 1572
  predictive value (PV) 1568–9, 1570, 1571
  repeatability/reliability 1567–8
  sensitivity 1568, 1569, 1570, 1571
  specificity 1568, 1569, 1570
Seasonality of onset, IDDM 8–9, 35–6, 119
Secretin 287, 800
Secretin–pancreozymin test 187
Seip–Berardinelli syndrome 38
Self-help groups, patient 1592
Self-monitoring of blood glucose (SMBG) 967, 968, **971–80**
  accuracy 974–7
    clinical significance 976–7
    quality control 975–6
    sources of error 975
  children and adolescents 972, 1039, 1041–2, 1043
  computer-based diabetes management 979, 1011–12
  effect on glycaemic control 977–8
  evaluation of performance 944
  future developments 979–80
  inappropriate use of data 978–9
  indications 972
  intercurrent illness 1048
  methods 972–4
  objectives and advantages 971
  patient education **939**, 976
  pregnancy 1091, 1092
  reliability of patient-collected data 939, 977, 1010–11
Semilente insulin 838, 849
Seminole Indians 64, 65
Senegal, IDDM frequency 138
Sensitivity, screening tests 1568, 1569, 1570, 1571
Sensorimotor neuropathy
  chronic 1386
  hypoglycaemia-induced 1399
Sensory action potential, medial plantar (MPSAP) 1394
Sensory examination, computer-assisted 1395
Sensory function, testing 1393–5, 1556
Sensory impairment
  ischaemic foot 1542
  neuropathic foot 1535–6
  risk of foot problems and 1557

Sensory neuropathy
  chronic insidious **1397**
  painful 1399
Serine phosphorylation
  glycogen synthase 389
  insulin receptors 362, 363, 365, 399
  insulin-stimulated 397–8, 399–401
Serum proteins, *see* Proteins, serum
Seventh (facial) nerve palsy 1398
Sex (gender) differences
  cardiovascular disease in diabetes 1491
  diabetic nephropathy 1268, 1289
  myocardial infarction 1189, 1190, 1194
  osteopenia 1416–17
Sex hormone binding globulin (SHBG) 557, 558–9
Sex hormones
  adipose tissue distribution and 560–1
  capillary basement membrane changes and 1258, 1260–1
  diabetic nephropathy and 1268
  insulin resistance and 534, 556
  stress-induced hypothalamic arousal and 561, 562
Sex ratio
  diabetes frequency **34–5**
  NIDDM frequency 34–5, 154, 179
"Shared care" approach 958, 962
Shock
  anaphylactic, insulin-induced 887
  cardiogenic, postmyocardial infarction 1188, 1189, 1499
  islet lesions 251–2
Shoulder
  adhesive capsulitis **1420–1**
  frozen 1420–1
Shoulder–hand syndrome **1420–1**, 1424
SHR/N-cp rat strain 63
Sialoproteins
  basement membrane 1246, 1250
  glomerular, changes in diabetes 1254, 1279
Siblings
  IDDM patients, proinsulin levels 320, 322–3
  IDDM risks 74–5, 1028
Sick day management rules 941, 1031, **1048–51**
Simulation models of diabetes, computers 1019
Simvastatin 825, 827
Singapore
  HLA associations with IDDM 123

IDDM prevalence and incidence **121**
NIDDM prevalence 150
Sixth (abducens) nerve palsies 1367–8
Skeletal changes **1415–18**, 1540
Skin
  connective tissue disorders **1418–28**
  high-risk foot 1557
  limited joint mobility and 1425
Skin biopsies, insulin allergies 887–8
Skin infections 1165
  continuous subcutaneous insulin infusion 858, 886
  insulin injection site 885–6
Skin problems, continuous subcutaneous insulin infusion 858
Skin testing, insulin allergies 887
Skin thickening 1425
Small-molecular weight mediators, insulin actions 389, 390–1, **402–3**
Smoking, cigarette
  cardiovascular disease risk and 1492
  cessation advice 1197, 1558
  fibrinogen levels and 1449
Smooth muscle cells, arterial
  atherosclerosis and 1472
  growth and proliferation 1442
SMS 201-995 (octreotide) 342, 348, 807, 808
Sociocultural factors, dietary management and 704, 713–14
Socioeconomic status (SES) 35
Sodium (Na$^+$)
  cerebral oedema of diabetic ketoacidosis and 1035–6
  diabetic ketoacidosis 1153
  pancreatic B cells 269
  renal tubular reabsorption 1289
  retention in hypertension 1522, 1523
  serum levels, diabetic ketoacidosis 1034, 1154
Sodium chloride (salt)
  dietary intake **697**, 708, 1528
  insulin preparations 837
Sodium (Na$^+$)/hydrogen (H$^+$)
  plasma membrane transporter
  cerebral oedema of diabetic ketoacidosis and 1035–6, 1157–8
  diabetic nephropathy and 1282–3
Sodium–lithium countertransport, red cell 1219, 1230–1, 1282, 1289

Soft exudates (cotton-wool spots) 1333–4, 1335
Solomon Islands, NIDDM prevalence 150
Somatomedins, fetal growth and 1089–90
Somatosensory evoked potentials (SEP) 1393
Somatostatin (SRIF) 225, 226, **341–8**
  actions 344, 345, 807
  carbohydrate absorption and 808
  chronic pancreatitis 203
  conditions with raised levels 344
  diabetes and 344–7
    animal studies 345–6
    humans 346–7
  distribution 343
  hyperglycaemic glucose clamp 523
  inhibition of insulin secretion 276, 287, 288, 344
  insulin suppression test 425, 520, 578, 1074
  pancreatectomized patients 204
  protamine zinc 807
  release 343–4
  sulphonylurea therapy and 750
  synthesis and structure 341, 342
  treatment of diabetes 347–8
Somatostatin-14 341, 342
Somatostatin-28 341, 342
Somatostatin analogues 341, 342
  antidiabetic actions 807, 808
  carbohydrate absorption and 808
  therapy in NIDDM 348
Somatostatin-containing neurons 343
Somatostatinomas 344
Somatotropin release inhibiting factor (SRIF), *see* Somatostatin
Somogyi effect 347, **1141–2**
  brittle diabetes and 1061
  children 1040
Sorbinil 809, 1278, 1335
Sorbitol 696, 1255
  atherosclerotic vascular disease and 1472
  cataracts and 1370
  diabetic nephropathy and 1278
  diabetic neuropathy and 809, 1387–8, 1389
  diabetic retinopathy and 1334–5
  phagocyte function and 1167
  red cell 1389–90
Sorbitol pathway of metabolism, *see* Polyol metabolism
South Africa
  HLA and IDDM associations 140–2

IDDM frequency 138, 139
  NIDDM frequency 179
South African Cape Coloured subjects 35, 140–2
South East Asia, dietary management of diabetes **701–6**
Specificity, screening tests 1568, 1569, 1570
Spectrin, glycation 1451
Spermine 389, 390
Spices, Indian and Asian diets 704
Spine
  cervical, limited mobility 1421
  hyperostosis 1418
Spleen, islet grafts 897, 898, 899
Splicing, mRNA 469–70
SRIF, *see* Somatostatin
Staff, health care, *see* Health personnel
Standard deviation (SD) of fasting blood glucose 1060
Staphylococcus aureus skin infections, insulin injection site 885–6
Starling's curve of the pancreas 571–2, 597
Start codon 471
Starvation
  accelerated, pregnancy 1087
  glucagon levels 337
  protein degradation 478, 496
  regulation of insulin release 279
  see also Fasting
Statil (ICI-128,436) 809, 1278–9
Statistical Bureau of the Metropolitan Life Insurance Company (SBMLIC) 1647–9, 1650, 1651
Steatorrhoea
  fibrocalculous pancreatic diabetes 183, 184
  management 187, 216
Steroid hormones
  actions in visceral adipose tissue 554
  adipose tissue distribution and **560–4**
  obesity **557–60**
  peripheral insulin sensitivity and 556–7
  see also Androgens; Cortisol; Glucocorticoids; Oestrogens
Steroid-induced ocular hypertension 39
Steroid therapy
  diabetes induced by 852
  glucose potassium and insulin infusion 1178, 1179
  insulin antibody-mediated insulin resistance 546, 1081
  pancreas transplantation 917, 918

Stiff hand syndrome **1419**, 1424
Stiff man syndrome 39
Streptococcal preparation, OK-432 125
Streptococcus milleri infections 886
Streptokinase 1196
Streptozotocin 61, 249, 289–90, 1027
Streptozotocin-induced experimental diabetes
  chronic hyperglycaemia 636, 638
  fetal pancreas transplantation 905
  insulin resistance 612, 613
  islet transplantation 897, 898, 900
  lipoprotein metabolism 449
  pancreatic polypeptide levels 349
  somatostatin in 345, 346
Stress
  brittle diabetes and 1065
  glucagon levels 337
  hyperglycaemia and IGT 15
  hypothalamic arousal 561–4
  insulin resistance and 534, 541, 1080
  insulin secretion and 288
Stress hormones, *see* Counterregulatory hormones
Stroke 1185, **1202–4**, 1488
  acute hyperglycaemia after 1203
    outcome and 1203
  diabetic patients 1115, 1202–4
  metabolic control and 1475, 1476–7, 1478
  mortality and morbidity in NIDDM 1464–5
  obesity and 563, 564
  tight glycaemic control after 1203–4
Subcutaneous insulin implants 868
Subcutaneous insulin infusion, continuous (CSII) **854–9**
  acceptability 859
  blood glucose self-monitoring 972
  children and adolescents 1040
  clinical application 856–9
  complications and problems 858–9, 874, 886
  concept and implementation 855
  diabetic ketoacidosis and 1152
  exercise and 733
  indications 857, 1066–7
  insulin dose distribution 857–8
  metabolic control achieved 856–7
  multiple daily injections vs. 874

Subcutaneous insulin infusion,
  continuous (CSII) (*cont.*)
  optimizing glycaemic control
    873–4
  pharmacokinetics 855–6
  pregnancy 1092
  progression of microvascular
    complications and
    1218–19, 1234–7, 1344–8
  see also Insulin therapy,
    intensive
Subcutaneous (SC) insulin injection
  after myocardial infarction 1195
  alternatives **865–8**
  diabetic ketoacidosis 1032–3
  disadvantages 865, 874
  injection site complications
    885–7
  insulin absorption, *see* Insulin
    absorption, subcutaneous
  local insulin degradation 533,
    546
  surgical management in IDDM
    1177
  technique 854
Substance P, insulin secretion and
  288
Sucrose 690, 691
Sudeck atrophy (shoulder–hand
  syndrome) 1420–1, 1424
Sugars, simple 690
Suicide deaths, IDDM 1214, 1215
Sulindac 1278
Sulphonamides, sulphonylurea
  interactions 1122
Sulphonylureas **745–67**, 1303
  adverse effects 765–7, 1121–2
    hypoglycaemia 755, 757,
      758, **765**, 1121–2, 1144
    interactions 766, 1121, 1122
    toxicity 766–7
  biguanides combined with 765,
    787
  biguanides vs. 763, 787
  chemistry and structure 745–6
  choice of agents 760–1
  clinical effects 752–3
  clinical use 761–3
    contraindications 767
    discontinuous exposure
      761–2
    dose and dosage 762–3
    early intervention 761
    indications 761
    therapeutic goals 762
  combination therapy 764–5
  elderly 1120–2, 1123
  exercise and 734, 738
  failures 764
    primary 764
    secondary 657–8, 753, 764
    and insulin therapy in
      NIDDM 297, 764–5,
      1123

insulin therapy vs. 763
lipoprotein metabolism and 454
mechanisms of action 296–7,
  650–1, 653, 654, **746–52**,
  802
  extrapancreatic effects 368,
    545, 614–15, 750–2
  pancreatic effects 278, 290,
    746–50
new 798
pancreatic diabetes 215
pharmacodynamics and
    pharmacokinetics 753–60
  kinetic–dynamic relations
    756
  potency and intrinsic
    molecular activity 754
  rate of onset and duration of
    action 754–6
  specific agents 756–60
pharmacology and clinical
    pharmacology 745–61
plasma membrane binding sites
  747–8, 751
surgery and 1176
tachyphylaxis 750
Sumo wrestlers, Japanese 157
Superficial femoral artery,
  occlusive disease 1510,
  1511, 1543–4
Suppositories, insulin 867–8
Surgery **1173–82**
  aims of treatment 1175
  Caesarian section 1180–1
  children with diabetes 1050–1
  emergency 1181
  management in IDDM 1177–9,
    1180
    glucose potassium and insulin
      infusion 1178–9
    historical aspects 1177–8
  management in NIDDM
    1176–7, 1180
  metabolic responses 1173–4
  open heart 1180
  organization of care 1179
  preoperative assessment of
    diabetes 1175–6
  principles of management of
    diabetes 1174, 1175
  protocol for diabetic care 1180
  risks associated with diabetes
    1174–5
Surinam, NIDDM prevalence 150
Sweating
  gustatory 1405
  neuropathic foot 1537, 1557
Sweden
  community-based diabetes care
    1594
  economic cost of diabetes
    1651
  genetics of NIDDM 66
  IDDM frequency 101, 140

Sweeteners **696–7**, 720
Sympathectomy, limb ischaemia
  1544
Sympathetic denervation,
  neuropathic foot 1536
Sympathetic dystrophy, reflex
  (shoulder–hand syndrome)
  1420–1, 1424
Sympathetic fibres, islets of
  Langerhans 230
Sympathetic nervous system
  activation during exercise 729
  tests of function 1401
Sympathetic stimulation, hepatic
  glucose production and
  417
Sympathomimetic agents, *see*
  Adrenergic agonists
Syndrome X (insulin resistance
  syndrome) **534–5**

Taboos 1604
Taiwan, IDDM prevalence and
  incidence **120**
Tanzania **1611–17**
  complications in NIDDM 180
  diagnosis of diabetic ketoacidosis
    143
  IDDM frequency 138–9
  medical services 1611–12
  NIDDM frequency 179
  prevalence of diabetes 1614–15
  problems in organization of
    diabetes care 1613–17
  prognosis for diabetic patients
    1612–13
Tanzania Diabetes Association
  1614
T-cell receptor, beta chain 46–7,
  108
T cells
  function in diabetes 1166,
    1167–8, 1659
  IDDM pathogenesis and 57
Teams, health care 955, 957–8,
  1046–7
  diabetes care centre 1596–7
  diabetic clinic 1591
  surgical patients 1179
Telephone advice 959, 960
  brittle diabetes 1066
  sick day management 1031
Tenosynovitis, flexor (FTS)
  1419–20, 1423, 1424
Ternary complex 471, 472
  effects of insulin 494
Tes-tape 968
Testosterone
  actions in visceral adipose tissue
    554
  adipose tissue distribution and
    560
  insulin resistance and 539–40,
    556–7

Testosterone (*cont.*)
  obesity 557
  plasma levels, diabetic impotence 1405
  stress-induced hypothalamic arousal and 562
Test strips, *see* Reagent strips
12-*O*-Tetradecanoylphorbol-13-acetate (TPA) 274, 275–6
Thailand
  fibrocalculous pancreatic diabetes 182
  HLA and IDDM associations 123, 142
  IDDM prevalence and incidence **121**
Thalassaemia 38, 247
Thalassaemia major 203–4
Thermal discrimination threshold **1394–5**, 1556
Thermal injuries, foot 1538
Thermal sensation, neuropathic foot 1535
Thermogenesis, diet-induced (DIT) 431–2
  facultative 431
  obligatory 431
Thiamine responsive megaloblastic anaemia (with deafness) 38
Thiazide diuretics 1529
Thigh, insulin absorption 844
Thiobarbituric acid (TBA) 986, 993
Thiolase 463
Third (oculomotor) nerve palsies 1367–8, 1398
Thirst 21, 1154
Three-allele heterogeneity model, IDDM inheritance 51–3, 54
Threonine phosphorylation
  insulin receptors 362, 363, 365, 399
  insulin-stimulated 397–8, 399–401
"Thrifty gene" hypothesis 67, **160**
Thrombin 1448
  control of generation 1450
  generation 1449
Thromboembolism
  diabetic ketoacidosis 1154
  hyperosmolar non-ketotic coma 1160
  postmyocardial infarction 1188, 1189
β-Thromboglobulin 1192, 1453, 1473
Thrombolytic therapy 1196
Thrombomodulin production 676
Thromboxane 1453, 1473
Thromboxane A$_2$ 1497
Thrombus formation, pathogenesis 676
Thyrogastric autoimmunity 46
Thyroglobulin antibodies 123

Thyroid autoantibodies 57, 123
Thyroid disease, autoimmune
  IDDM 47, 48, 136
  screening and prevention 75
Thyroid function testing 75
Thyroid hormones
  diet-induced thermogenesis and 431
  hepatic glucose production and 420
  insulin-mediated glucose disposal and 433
  insulin resistance induction 534
Thyroid microsomal antibodies (TMA) 47, 123, 136
Thyrotoxicosis (hyperthyroidism) 247
  brittle diabetes 1063
  insulin resistance 534
  proinsulin levels 320, 322
Thyroxine, ketone body metabolism and 460
Tibial artery, occlusive disease 1509, 1514, 1515
Ticlopidine 1358, 1454
Timolol 1196
Tissue cultures, vascular cells 1441–3
Tissue factor, glucose toxicity and 1280
Tissues, insulin sensitivity of specific **524–5**
Toes
  blood pressure 1511, 1542
  clawing 1537
  gangrene, diabetic nephropathy and 1544
Tolazamide 746, 755, **757–8**
  elderly patients 1120–1
Tolbutamide **756–7**
  cardiovascular complications and 1478–9
  clinical efficacy 753
  elderly patients 1120, 1121
  extrapancreatic effects 752
  frequent sampling IVGTT 517, 518
  insulin response after pancreas transplantation 918
  mechanisms of action 747
  potency and intrinsic activity 754
  rate of onset and duration of action 755
  structure 746
Tolrestat 809
Topical insulin 868
Toxins, IDDM aetiology and 1660–1
TPA (12-*O*-tetradecanoylphorbol-13-acetate) 274, 275–6
Traditional medicine
  India 1604

Tanzania 1616
Training
  diabetes specialist nurses 962, 1596
  health personnel 962, 1590, 1591, 1626
trans-acting factors 468, 469, 490
Transcomplementation model, IDDM pathogenesis 55
Transcription 467
  insulin actions **396–7, 490–2**
  normal regulation **468–70**
Transcutaneous oxygen tension (TcPo$_2$), peripheral vascular disease 1512, 1542
Transdermal insulin absorption 868
Transferrin receptors, insulin actions 388
Transfer RNA (tRNA) 470
  function 470–1
Transglutaminase, insulin secretion and 264
Translation 467
  initiation 471–3, 493–4
  insulin actions **397, 493–4**
  normal regulation **470–3**
  peptide chain elongation 473, 494–5
  peptide chain termination 473, 494–5
Transport problems, India 1603–4
Trauma
  foot ulceration and 1538
  ischaemic limb 1543
Triacylglycerol
  breakdown, *see* Lipolysis
  phospholipid metabolism and 395
  synthesis (esterification), insulin actions 391, **393**, 394
Triacylglycerol (TG-) lipase (hormone-sensitive lipase, HSL) 391, 394, 460
Tricyclic antidepressants, painful neuropathy 1400
Trigger finger (flexor tenosynovitis) **1419–20**, 1423, 1424
Triglyceride lipase 398
  hepatic (HTGL) 441, 445, 448
  insulin actions 449, 450
  NIDDM 455, 819
Triglycerides (TG)
  HDL, NIDDM 455
  hepatic glucose production and 419
  insulin actions 449
  insulin secretion and 287
  metabolism 447
  obesity 451
  serum levels
    biguanide therapy and 781, 782–3
    cardiovascular disease risk and **1494–5**

Triglycerides (TG) (*cont.*)
    IDDM 450, 818, 1044
    NIDDM 452, 685–6, 818
    pancreatic diabetes 209
    target values in diabetes
        821
    see also Hypertriglyceridaemia
Triiodothyronine (T$_3$), hepatic
    glucose production and 419
(1-N^α-Trinitrophenylhistidine,12-
    homoarginine)-glucagon
    (THG) 807–8
Trisomy 21 (Down's syndrome)
    39, 108–9, 110, 1028
Trochlear (fourth) nerve palsies
    1367–8
Tropical countries 41, **177–90**
    classification of diabetes 177,
        178
    fibrocalculous pancreatic diabetes
        182–90
    future research issues 190
    IDDM in 177–8
    malnutrition related diabetes
        mellitus 180–90
    NIDDM in 177, 178–80
        complications 180
        genetic factors 179
        hyperinsulinaemia and insulin
            resistance 179–80
        prevalence 178–9
        sex ratio reversal 179
        younger age at onset 179
    protein deficient diabetes mellitus
        180–1
Tropical diabetes 4, 11
    see also Malnutrition related
        diabetes mellitus
Trypsin, serum levels 187
Tuberculosis 1152, 1165
Tubulin 492
Tumour necrosis factor (TNF),
    AGE-induced production
    674, 675, 676
Turner's syndrome 39, 110,
    1028
Twins
    discordant for IDDM,
        proinsulin levels 320,
        322–3
    risks of IDDM 74, 1658
Twin studies **36–7**
    IDDM 41, 42, 43
    islet cell antibodies (ICAs)
        58
    NIDDM 37, 41, 42, 64, 149
Two-compartment model of C-
    peptide kinetics 308–10
Tyrosine aminotransferase 396
Tyrosine kinase, insulin receptor,
    see Insulin receptors, tyrosine
    kinase activity
Tyrosine phosphorylation, insulin
    receptor-mediated 362

Ubiquitin 475–6
Ubiquitin-conjugate degrading
    enzyme 475, 476
Ubiquitin proteolytic pathway 475
Ultralente insulin 837, 838
    absorption 843
    clinical applications 848
Ultrasonography
    fetal monitoring 1093
    fibrocalculous pancreatic diabetes
        184–5
    kidneys 1294
United Kingdom (UK)
    economic cost of diabetes 1651
    IDDM frequency 140
United States of America (USA)
    dietary management of diabetes
        685–98
    driving regulations 1633
    economic cost of diabetes
        1647–50, 1651
    employment legislation 1637–8
    IDDM frequency 101, 140
    interstate truck driving 1634–6
    NIDDM frequency 150, 155
    non-Caucasoid populations,
        IDDM epidemiology and
        aetiopathogenesis 129–36
    see also specific population
        groups
Unmodified (regular) insulin **836–8**
    absorption 841, 842
    childhood diabetes 1037–8
    clinical applications 847–8, 849
    intravenous infusion, diabetic
        ketoacidosis 1032–3
Uraemia
    glycated protein assays and
        999–1000
    insulin resistance 540–1
    mortality in IDDM from 1214,
        1215, 1216
Urban areas
    Africa
        food availability 714
        nutritional status 713, 714
    distribution of resources and
        expertise 1603, 1609,
        1616
    NIDDM frequency 159–60
Urea
    blood glucose self-monitoring
        and 975
    serum levels, glycated
        haemoglobin and
        999–1000
Urinary diversion, pancreas
    transplantation and 916
Urinary tract infections 1300,
    1301–2
Urine testing **967–9**
    glucose 875, 967, 972
        advantages and disadvantages
            967–8, 1060–1

    children and adolescents
        1041–2, 1043
    diagnosis of diabetes 21
    false readings 969
    Japan 118
    methods **968**
    screening for diabetes 1576
    use in diabetes 969
    ketones **967**, 1042, 1060–1
        intercurrent illness 1048
        pregnancy 1092
Uteroplacental blood flow, reduced
    1088, 1093

Vaccination, diabetogenic viruses
    61, 1660
Vacor (N-3-pyridylmethyl-N'-p-
    nitrophenylurea, PNU) 61,
    249, 1661
Vagus nerve
    glucagon release and 336
    insulin secretion and 273, 288
Valsalva manoeuvre 1402, 1403,
    1558
Vanadate 649
Vascular access, haemodialysis
    1305
Vascular disease (angiopathy)
    1435–6
    aminoguanidine therapy and
        677
    Chinese diabetics 723
    diabetic impotence 1405
    elderly 1115, 1116
    end-stage renal failure 1276
    hands (stiff hand syndrome)
        1419, 1424
    malignant and benign types in
        IDDM 1217–18
    pathogenesis **671–7**
    peripheral, see Peripheral
        vascular disease
    see also Macrovascular disease;
        Microvascular disease
Vascular events, acute **1185–204**
Vascular neuropathies, focal
    1398
Vascular permeability
    changes in diabetes 1253–4
    diabetic retinopathy **1331–3**
    hyperglycaemia and 1256
    sex steroids and 1258
Vascular surgery, see Arterial
    reconstruction
Vascular wall, see Arterial wall
Vasoactive intestinal peptide (VIP)
    230, 288, 785
Vasoconstriction
    impaired, neuropathic foot 1536
    insulin absorption and 843
    insulin-mediated glucose disposal
        and 432–3
Vasodilation
    hyperglycaemia-induced 1285

Vasodilation (*cont.*)
  insulin absorption and 843
  insulin-mediated glucose disposal
    and 432–3
Vasodilators, arterial 1529
Vasopressin (antidiuretic hormone,
    ADH), sulphonylurea-induced
    release 752, 1121
Vegetables 694, 716
Vegetarian diet, renal function and
    1298
Vegetarians 690, 702, 1664, 1666
Vein grafts, arterial reconstruction
    1515, 1543–4
Venous blood sampling 522
Venous pressure, central, monitoring
    1157
Ventilatory reflexes, testing
    1402–3
Ventricular fibrillation 1189, 1190
Very low-calorie diets (VLCD),
    NIDDM 686–7
Very low-density lipoproteins
    (VLDL) 439, 440
  biguanide therapy and 781
  cardiovascular disease risk and
    1494
  endogenous
    hypertriglyceridaemia 451
  hepatic synthesis 553, 554
  IDDM 450, 818
  insulin actions 448–9, 450
  metabolism **441–3**, 446–7
    diabetes **819**
    NIDDM 452–3, 685–6, 818
    obesity 451–2
  shunt pathway 447
Vibrameter 1394
Vibration perception threshold
    (VPT) **1394**, 1395, 1556
  glycaemic control and 1396
  ischaemia and 1392
  neuropathic foot 1535–6, 1545
Videotapes 932–4
Viruses
  B-cell destruction 236–9
  fibrocalculous pancreatic diabetes
    and 189
  IDDM aetiology **59–61**, 110,
    1026, 1168, **1660**
  insulin autoantibodies and 1659
  pancreas destruction 198
  pancreatic inflammatory
    responses 245
Visidex II 974
Visual acuity, regular assessment
    957, 1552
Visual impairment 1117,
    1373–83
  causes 1378–9
  epidemiology 1373–8
  foot care and 1557

incidence 1377–8, 1379
  macular oedema and 1331–3,
    1379, 1382
  prevalence 1112, 1373–7
  prevention 1352–5, 1356,
    1380–2
  prognosis 1380
  rehabilitation 1382–3
  renal dialysis and 1305–6,
    1380
  types 1379–80
Vitamin B$_{12}$ deficiency
  biguanide-induced 784–5, 789,
    1122–3
  testing for 75
Vitamin C, glucose urine testing
    and 969
Vitamin D deficiency, insulin
    secretion and 279–80
Vitamin intake 690, 696
Vitamin K 1450
Vitrectomy **1356–7**, 1381
Vitreous, posterior detachment
    1338–40
Vitreous haemorrhage 1338–40
  vitrectomy 1356–7
Vomiting
  diabetic ketoacidosis 1031
  intercurrent illness 1049
von Gierke's disease (glycogen
    storage disease type I) 38
von Willebrand factor (vWF)
    1280, 1451, 1472, 1497

Waist-to-hip ratio (WHR)
  cardiovascular disease risk and
    1493
  cortisol secretion and
    559–60
  hepatic insulin clearance and
    552
  lipoprotein metabolism and
    452
  NIDDM frequency and 155,
    156
  stress-induced hypothalamic
    arousal and 561–2
  stroke risk and 563, 564
Weak-acid hydrolysis
  glycated haemoglobin **993**, 994,
    995
  glycated serum proteins 995
Weight, percentage desirable (PDW)
    10
Weight loss
  African diabetics 716
  diabetes onset 21
  diabetic ketoacidosis 1030,
    1154
  diabetic neuropathic cachexia
    1114, 1397
  hypertension 1528

NIDDM 297, 685–7
  biguanide therapy 787–8
  Chinese diet 722
  effects on insulin secretion
    651–3, 654, 657
  glucose tolerance and 297
  insulin receptor function and
    368, 602
  insulin resistance and
    614–15
NIDDM prevention 1665
pancreatic diabetes 212
patient education 940
Werner's syndrome 39, 248, 1028
West Africa, HLA and IDDM
    associations 140
Westernized life-style, NIDDM
    development and 34, 153,
    160–1
Whipple's resection
    (pancreaticoduodenectomy)
    205
White's classification of diabetes
    1086
"Willingness to pay" approach,
    estimating costs of illness
    1644
Wolfram's (diabetes mellitus–optic
    atrophy–diabetes insipidus–
    deafness, or DIDMOAD)
    syndrome 39, 109, 248,
    1028
Woodhouse–Sakati syndrome 39
Work routine, dietary patterns in
    Africa and 713–14
World Health Organization (WHO)
  Collaborating Centre for diabetes
    registries 101
  dietary recommendations 703
  Expert Committee on Diabetes
    3, 23, 147–8
  Multinational Project on
    Childhood Diabetes 100,
    105
  see also National Diabetes Data
    Group (NDDG)/World
    Health Organization (WHO)
Wound healing, postoperative
    1175

Xenon arc photocoagulation 1349,
    1353, 1354
Xylitol 720

Yoghurt 703–4

Zimbabwe, IDDM frequency 138
Zinc (Zn^{2+})
  immunogenicity 889
  insulin–zinc suspensions 838
  unmodified insulin preparations
    837

Index compiled by Liza Weinkove